	Hydroxyzine	Meperidine	Metoclopramide	Midazolam	Morphine	Nalbuphine	Pentazocine	Pentobarbital	Perphenazine	Prochlorperazine	Promazine	Promethazine	Ranitidine	Scopolamine Hbr	Secobarbital	Thiethylperazine
	C	C	C	C	C	C	C	C	C	C	C	C	C	C	I	
	C	C	C	C	C		C	I	C	C		C		C	I	C
	C	C	C	C	C		C	I	C	C	C	C	C	C	I	
								I							I	
	I	I	I		I	I	I	I	I	I	I	I		I	I	I
	I	C	C	I	C		C	I	C	I	I	I	C	C	I	
	C	C	C	C	C		C	I	C	C	C	C	C	C	I	
	C	C	C		C	C	C	I	C	C	C	C		C	I	
	C	C	C		C		C	I	C	C	C	C	C	C	I	
	C	C			C		I	I		C	C	C	C	C	I	
		I			I		I					I				
		C	C		C	C	C	I		C	C	C	I	C	I	
	C		C		I		C	I	C	C	C	C	C	C	I	
	C	C			C		C		C	C	C	C	C	C	I	
	C		C		C	C		I	I	I	C	C	I	C		C
	C	I	C				C	I	C	C	C	C	C	C	I	
	C							I		C		C	C	C	I	C
	C	C	C		C			I	C	C	C	C	C	C	I	
	I	I			I	I	I		I	I	I	I		C	I	
		C	C		C		C	I		C		C	C	C	I	I
	C	C	C		C	C	C	I	C		C	C	C	C	I	
	C	C	C		C		C	I		C		C		C	I	
	C	C	C		C	C	C	I	C	C	C		C	C	I	
		C	C	I	C	C	C		C	C		C		C		C
	C	C	C		C	C	C	C	C	C	C	C	C		I	
	I	I	I		I	I	I	I	I	I	I	I		I		I
						C			I				C		I	

Parenteral compatibility occurs when two or more drugs are successfully mixed without liquefaction, deliquescence, or precipitation.

Mosby's Drug Guide for Nurses

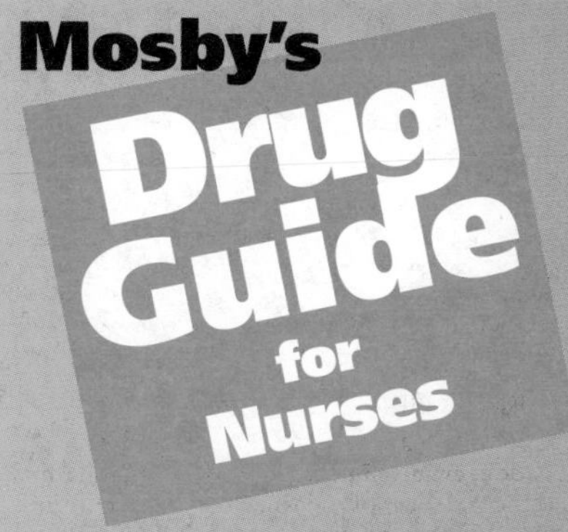

Linda Skidmore-Roth, R.N., M.S.N., N.P.
Formerly, Nursing Faculty,
New Mexico State University,
Las Cruces, New Mexico;
El Paso Community College,
El Paso, Texas

with 44 *illustrations and* 1 *color insert*

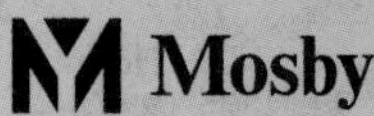

St. Louis Baltimore Boston
Carlsbad Chicago Naples New York Philadelphia Portland
London Madrid Mexico City Singapore Sydney Tokyo Toronto Wiesbaden

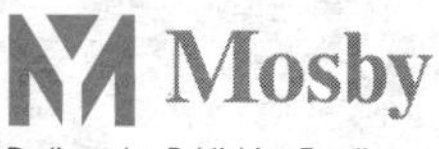

Dedicated to Publishing Excellence

A Times Mirror Company

Publisher: Nancy Coon
Editor: Robin Carter
Developmental editor: Gina Gay Wright
Project manager: Carol Sullivan Weis
Production editor: Christine Carroll
Designer: Sheilah Barrett
Cover illustrator: Ken Joudrey
Manufacturing supervisor: Betty Richmond

A NOTE TO THE READER

The author and publisher have made every attempt to check dosages and nursing content for accuracy. Because the science of pharmacology is continually advancing, our knowledge base continues to expand. Therefore we recommend that the reader always check product information for changes in dosage or administration before administering any medication. This is particularly important with new or rarely used drugs.

Printed in the United States of America
Composition by Graphic World, Inc.
Printing/binding by Rand McNally

Mosby–Year Book, Inc.
11830 Westline Industrial Drive
St. Louis, Missouri 63146

Library of Congress Cataloging-in-Publication Data

Mosby's drug guide for nurses / Linda Skidmore-Roth.
p. cm.
Includes bibliographical references and indexes.
ISBN 0-8151-7808-5
1. Drugs—Handbooks, manuals, etc. 2. Nursing—Handbooks, manuals, etc. I. Skidmore-Roth, Linda.
[DNLM: 1. Drugs—nurses' instruction—handbooks. 2. Drug Therapy—nurses' instruction—handbooks. QV 39 M895 1995]
RM301.12.M66 1996
615'.1—dc20
DNLM/DLC 95-11282
for Library of Congress CIP

95 96 97 98 99 / 9 8 7 6 5 4 3 2 1

Consultants

Barbara A. Brunow, R.N., M.S.N.
Instructor, Providence Hospital,
School of Nursing,
Sandusky, Ohio

Connie L. Bush, R.N., M.S.
Associate Professor, Nursing,
Niagara County Community College,
Sanborn, New York

Shari L. Clarke, R.N.C.
Nursing Unit Coordinator,
Emory at Crawford Long Hospital,
Fayetteville, Georgia

Judy E. Davison, R.N., M.S., C.C.R.N.
Clinical Nurse Specialist,
University of California San Diego Medical Center,
San Diego, California

Jane Doyle, R.N., B.S.N., M.S., M.B.A.
Nursing Faculty,
Mount Wachusett Community College,
Gardner, Massachusetts

Laurel A. Eisenhauer, R.N., Ph.D.
Professor of Nursing,
Boston College School of Nursing,
Chestnut Hill, Massachusetts

Tim Engelhardt, B.Sc., Pharm.D.
Manager, Pharmacy Services,
Calgary District Hospital Group,
Calgary, Alberta

Linda A. Howe, R.N., M.S., M.A.E.
Director,
Roper Hospital School of Nursing,
Charleston, South Carolina

Theresa M. Hulub, R.N., M.S.Ed., M.S.N.
Professor of Nursing Education,
Niagara County Community College,
Sanborn, New York

Kimberly A. Hunter, Pharm.D.
Assistant Professor of Pharmacy Practice,
Washington State University College of Pharmacy;
Geriatric Clinical Pharmacist,
Sacred Heart Medical Center,
Spokane, Washington

Jon E. Lewis, B.A., Ph.D.
Senior Research Scientist and Director,
Respiratory Diseases,
Marion Merrell Dow Research Institute,
Cincinnati, Ohio

Edwina A. McConnell, R.N., Ph.D.
Independent Nurse Consultant,
Madison, Wisconsin

Janet R. Paul, B.S.N., M.S.N., R.N.
Assistant Professor of Nursing,
Hahnemann University,
Philadelphia, Pennsylvania

Rosemary A. Pine, R.N., M.S.N.
Assistant Professor of Nursing,
Department Chair, ADN Program,
Houston Baptist University,
Houston, Texas

Carolyn Smith Powell, A.D.N., B.S.N., M.S.N.
Assistant Professor of Nursing,
Abraham Baldwin College,
Tifton, Georgia

Mary Quintas, R.N.
Miles Community College,
Department of Nursing,
Miles City, Montana

Roberta Roynayne, R.N., B.Sc.N., M.Sc.
Assistant Professor,
University of Ottawa,
School of Nursing,
Ottawa, Ontario

Carol Ruscin, R.N., B.S.
Level I Faculty,
Baptist Medical System,
School of Nursing,
Little Rock, Arkansas

Lori Schoonover, Pharm.D.
Assistant Professor, Pharmacy,
Washington State University,
Spokane, Washington

Roberta J. Secrest, Ph.D., Pharm.D., R.Ph.
Associate Scientist,
Marion Merrell Dow Research Institute,
Cincinnati, Ohio

Denice Sheehan, R.N., M.S.N., O.C.N.
Nursing Supervisor,
Hospice of the Western Reserve,
Mentor, Ohio

John R. White, Jr., Pharm.D.
Assistant Professor,
Washington State University,
College of Pharmacy,
Spokane, Washington

Preface

Mosby's Drug Guide for Nurses presents more than 7500 generic and trade name drugs—those most commonly administered by students—including 16 new drugs recently approved by the FDA. A **software disk** for drug therapy care planning is included inside the back cover. Brief introductory chapters on principles of drug action, drug calculation, and drug therapy across the lifespan, as well as a **four-color photo atlas** of drug administration, provide invaluable reviews for practitioners and students. **Key drugs** are highlighted with a special icon, ⚷, at the individual monograph and within the drug classifications section to call attention to important drugs. More than 60 drug classifications are provided. IV content includes detailed coverage of both drug compatibilities and incompatibilities and site-specific information. The five-step nursing process format includes rationales. To aid application of the nursing process, therapeutic outcomes are prominently stated at the beginning of each monograph, and positive **therapeutic outcomes** are highlighted under the evaluation heading. Treatment of overdose is included after evaluation when appropriate.

Drug monographs are arranged in alphabetical order by generic name, and trade names are given for all medications commonly used in the United States and Canada. Drugs available only in Canada are identified by a maple leaf, ✤. The following information is provided whenever possible for safe and effective administration of each drug:

Pronunciations: Pronunciations are provided to help the nursing student master the more complex generic names.

Functional and chemical classifications: All known broad functional and chemical classifications are given. These classifications allow the nurse to see similarities and dissimilarities among drugs that are in the same functional class and different chemical classes.

Pregnancy category: FDA pregnancy categories A, B, C, D, or X are noted at the beginning of the monograph and under precautions. Appendix F provides a detailed explanation of each category.

Controlled substance schedule: Schedules are included for the United States (I, II, III, IV, V) and Canada (F, G, H). Appendix E provides a chart correlating the two systems with examples.

Action: Pharmacologic properties are described in detail. Action is discussed to the cellular level when known.

Therapeutic outcome: All possible results of medication use are detailed.

Uses: Provides drug application.

Investigational uses: Provides drug application for those uses a student may encounter in practice, although they are not FDA approved.

Dosage and route: May be given if known for uses not FDA approved but encountered in practice.

Available forms: All available forms — including tablets, capsules, extended-release, injectables (IV, IM, SC, ID, IC), solutions, creams, ointments, lotions, gels, shampoos, elixirs, suspensions, suppositories, sprays, aerosols, and lozenges — are provided.

Side effects/adverse reactions: Grouped by body system, common side effects are in *italic type,* and life-threatening reactions are in ***bold italic type,*** allowing the nurse to quickly identify common and life-threatening reactions. Separate headings for Following IV and Following IM include route-specific or unusual side effects. All side effects/adverse reactions are reported for an incidence of 1% or greater.

Contraindications: Contraindications are instances in which a medication absolutely should not be given. When the FDA has assigned pregnancy safety category D or X, it appears here.

Precautions: Special precautionary steps are given here, including FDA pregnancy safety categories A, B, and C.

Pharmacodynamics: When known, absorption, distribution, elimination, and half-life are reported here in an easily accessible chart format.

Pharmacokinetics: Also presented in a handy chart format are onset, peak, and duration, if known.

Interactions/incompatibilities: This section includes confirmed drug, food, and smoking interactions. The drugs are listed in alphabetical order first, followed by the reaction(s) caused by that drug.

Lab test interferences: When known, lab test interferences are provided. Lab interference includes false negative and false positive results and increase or decrease interferences.

Nursing considerations: Highlighted nursing considerations are organized to foster use of the nursing process: Assessment, Associated nursing diagnoses, Implementation, Patient/family education, and Evaluation with positive therapeutic outcomes.

Treatment of overdose: Drugs and treatment for overdoses are provided for appropriate drugs.

Appendixes: The following appendixes are included to further enhance the usability of this reference: Infusion Rate Tables, Drugs Not to Crush, Routine Pediatric and Adult Immunizations, Combination Products, Controlled Substance Chart, FDA Pregnancy Categories, Nomogram for Body Surface Area Calculation, Commonly Used Abbreviations, Bibliography, and IV/Drug Solution Compatibility Chart.

Disorders index: This book includes both a general index and a disorders index, an innovative feature. For easy application with integrated medical-surgical nursing courses, the disorders index lists major disorders and major drugs used in their management, followed by the page number for each drug listed.

Inside the cover: A syringe compatibility chart is printed inside the front cover for quick access, and a software disk for drug therapy care planning is inside the back cover.

Design: This book features a functional, user-friendly, two-color design that includes alphabetical tabs; icons for key drugs, therapeutic outcome →, and lifespan content G P; colored monograph headings; and screened pages for the category drugs and index to facilitate information retrieval. The type and format of the book is spacious to enhance visual appeal and user-friendliness.

I am indebted to the nursing and pharmacology consultants who reviewed the manuscript, and I thank them for their thoughtful comments and encouragement. I would also like to thank Robin Carter and Gina Wright, my editors, whose active encouragement and enthusiasm have made this book better than it might otherwise have been. I am likewise grateful to Carol Sullivan Weis, Christine Carroll, Betty Richmond, Pat Stinecipher, and Graphic World, Inc. for the careful coordination of the production process, and the book's designer, Sheilah Barrett, for her creativity and cooperative spirit. In addition, I want to extend a special note of gratitude to Don Ladig, who has supported and encouraged my efforts since I began my relationship as an author with Mosby.

Linda Skidmore-Roth

Contents

Mosby's Drug Guide for Nurses

SECTION I

PHARMACOLOGY PRINCIPLES

Chapter 1

Principles of Drug Action

DRUG ATTACHMENT

Drugs participate in chemical reactions that change the physiologic activity of the body. They do this most commonly when the medication bonds chemically at a specific site in the body called a **receptor site** (see the box on p. 4.) The chemical reactions are possible only when the receptor site and the chemical can fit together like pieces of a jigsaw puzzle or like a key fitting into a lock. If the chemical fits the receptor site well, the chemical response is generally good. We call these drugs **agonists.** Some drugs compete with other chemicals that are already bonded to a receptor site and replace them, producing a different action.

Some drugs attach at the receptor site, but then produce no new chemical reaction. These drugs are called **antagonists.** Other drugs attach, but produce only a small chemical response and may even prevent other reactions from occurring. These drugs are called **partial agonists.**

BASIC DRUG PROCESSES

All drugs go through four basic processes in the body. Each drug has different characteristics of absorption, distribution, metabolism, and excretion. To understand how a drug works, the nurse must understand each of these processes for the drug being administered.

Medication absorption

Absorption describes how a drug enters the body and passes into the body fluids and tissues. Absorption takes place through processes of diffusion, filtration, or osmosis. The rate of absorption depends on: solubility of the drug, route of administration, and degree of blood flow through the tissue where the medication is found.

All medication must be dissolved in body fluid before it can enter body tissues. The ability of the medication to dissolve is called **solubility.** Sometimes the medication must be dissolved quickly; sometimes it should be dissolved slowly. Solubility of the drug is often controlled by the form of the medication: solutions are more soluble

Drug Receptor Sites

Agonist: Chemical fits receptor site well; chemical response is usually good.
Antagonist: Drug attaches at drug receptor site, but then remains chemically inactive; no chemical drug response is produced.
Partial agonist: Drug attaches at drug receptor site, but only a slight chemical action is produced.

than capsules. Enteric-coated capsules are covered with a substance that slows absorption. An injection with an oil base may be given to delay absorption from the tissue. When the patient takes water with a tablet, it helps dissolve the medication and increase its solubility, as well as eases swallowing.

The route of administration also influences absorption. Medication routes are **enteral** (directly into the gastrointestinal tract through oral, nasogastric tube, or rectal administration); **parenteral** (directly into dermal, subcutaneous, or intramuscular tissue, or into the blood stream through intravenous injections); or **percutaneously** (through topical [skin]; sublingual [under the tongue]; or inhalation [breathing]) administration.

In areas where the blood flow through tissues is very high, medication will be rapidly absorbed. Medications injected intravenously into the bloodstream have the fastest action. Oral or rectal medications usually take much longer because they must dissolve and diffuse across the gastric mucosa and then be transported to the body tissues.

Medication distribution

Once the medication is absorbed, it must travel throughout the body. The term **distribution** refers to the ways in which drugs move from circulating body fluids to the sites of action in the body. The drug is usually carried by the bloodstream and lymphatic system throughout the whole body. The organs that have the greatest blood supply receive the medication quickly, and areas of skin and fat receive the medication more slowly. Some drugs cannot pass through some cell barriers, such as the placenta or into the brain. Thus the distribution is selective for some types of drugs.

The chemical properties of the drug also influence how the drug is distributed. Some chemicals bind with proteins, such as albumin (found in the blood plasma), which serves as a carrier for drugs that are not easily dissolved. Thus a drug may be a complex, with part of its chemicals locked to the protein and part of its chemicals free to diffuse into the tissues. The ratio of bound chemical to free chemical remains the same in the blood. As more of the free chemical diffuses into the tissues, more of the bound chemical becomes unlocked and thus available to diffuse.

Medication metabolism

Once the medication is absorbed and distributed, the body's enzymes use it in chemical reactions through the process of metabolism. The medication is gradually broken down, primarily in the liver, through complex chemical reactions until it becomes chemically inactive. This process is called **biotransformation.** A great deal of medication is actually inactivated by the liver before it can be distributed to other portions of the body.

Medication excretion

All inactive chemicals, chemical by-products, and waste (often referred to as metabolites) are eventually discarded from the body through the process of **excretion.** Fibrous or insoluble waste is usually excreted through the gastrointestinal tract as feces. Chemicals that are more easily dissolved may be filtered out as they pass through the kidneys and are then excreted in the urine. Some chemicals are exhaled from the lungs or lost through evaporation from the skin. Very small amounts of medication may also escape in tears, saliva, or milk of breast-feeding mothers.

Half-life. Some chemicals are quickly excreted from the body. Other drugs remain for a long time. A standard method of expressing how long it takes to metabolize and excrete a drug is the **half-life,** or the time it takes to eliminate 50% of the drug from the body. Because these rates are usually the same for most individuals, the half-life helps determine the dosage and frequency needed for the administration of different drugs. If a drug has a long half-life, it may need to be administered only once a day. If a person takes too much medication with a long half-life, it may cause a serious situation because the action lasts for such a long time. If the half-life of a drug is short, such as for many antibiotics, the person must take frequent doses to maintain an effective level in the blood. If an individual's liver or kidneys do not function correctly, medications may not be properly metabolized or excreted, thus causing higher dosages of medication to circulate for a longer time and producing symptoms of overdosage. Therefore it is important to monitor kidney and liver function through renal and hepatic tests and to alert the physician if there are any problems.

BASICS OF DRUG ACTION

When a drug is given to a patient, a predictable chemical reaction is anticipated. However, because each patient is different, many unpredictable chemical reactions also occur. With each patient, giving a medication is somewhat of a therapeutic experiment, and the patient must be monitored closely to determine the effects of the medication. For a summary of common responses to medications, see the box on p. 7.

The expected response of the medication is called the **desired action.** When the desired action occurs, the medication produces the action the physician intended and the therapeutic goal is achieved.

Because the medication also has the potential to influence many body systems at the same time, the action of the medication is often inspecific. Other reactions may be produced, which are called side effects or adverse reactions. **Side effects** are usually regarded as mild but annoying responses to the medication. **Adverse reactions,** or adverse effects, usually imply more severe symptoms or problems that develop because of the drug. Because substantial testing is required for each drug before it can be placed on the market, most side effects and adverse reactions are predictable. Some side effects, such as drowsiness, may go away after the patient takes the medication for a while. Some side effects, such as nausea, may be eliminated if the dosage is reduced. Some side effects are such a problem that the medication must be changed or discontinued. An example of this might be hyperactivity or inability to sleep. Certainly if adverse effects such as bleeding or liver damage develop, the medication must be stopped.

Occasionally a patient may experience a reaction to a drug that is not anticipated. Strange, unique, or unpredicted responses are called **idiosyncratic responses.** These reactions usually are caused by underlying enzyme deficiencies from genetic or hormonal variation. They often produce either an unanticipated result, such as pain or bleeding, or an overresponse to the drug. These types of reactions are rare.

A second type of unanticipated reaction is that produced by hypersensitivity or allergy. Some medications and some individuals are more likely to be associated with allergic reactions than others. Allergic

Common Responses to Medications

Desired effect
When the desired effect takes place, the therapeutic goal is achieved. The drug does what it is supposed to do. An example would be temperature reduction after taking aspirin.

Side effects
Side effects are mild but annoying responses to medication. An example would be gastric burning caused by aspirin.

Adverse effects
Adverse effects are more severe symptoms or problems that arise because of the medication. An example would be that the patient might develop severe gastric bleeding from an ulcer caused by the aspirin.

Idiosyncratic response
Idiosyncratic responses are strange, unique, or unpredicted reactions. An example would be blood in the urine caused by the aspirin. This is rare.

Allergic response
An allergic response is an antigen-antibody reaction. The body develops hives, rashes, itching, or swelling of the skin. A rash or shortness of breath may occur in patients allergic to aspirin. These responses are occasionally seen.

Anaphylactic response
An anaphylactic response is a severe form of allergic reaction that is life threatening. The patient develops severe shortness of breath, may stop breathing, or have cardiac collapse.

reactions usually occur when an individual has been exposed to a drug and his or her body has developed antibodies to it. When the body is reexposed to the drug, the antigen-antibody reaction produces hives, rash, itching, or swelling of the skin. These mild allergic reactions are extremely common, and the nurse should always question patients about them. Patients with an allergy to one medication may be more likely to develop an allergy to another medication, and individuals commonly develop a reaction to medications that they have taken previously without problem.

Occasionally the allergic reaction is so severe that the patient has difficulty breathing and may even have cardiovascular collapse. This life-threatening allergic response is called an **anaphylactic reaction.** If a patient has had a mild reaction to a medication, he or she is much more likely to develop the more severe anaphylactic reaction if the medication is given again. These individuals should always be warned about their allergy so they will not take the drug again, and they should wear a Medic-Alert badge or carry identification regarding their allergy.

Patients commonly report allergy to medication that does not represent a true allergy, but only a common side effect. It is important to clarify the nature of the response to the drug if a patient claims to be allergic to a particular medication.

Common Drug Interactions

Additive
An additive effect takes place when two drugs are given together and double the effect is produced.

Antagonistic
An antagonistic effect takes place when one drug interferes with the action of another drug.

Displacement
A displacement effect takes place when one drug replaces another at the drug receptor site, increasing the effect of the first drug.

Incompatibility
Incompatibility occurs when two drugs mixed together in a syringe produce a chemical reaction so they cannot be given.

Interference
Interference occurs when one drug promotes the rapid excretion of another, thus reducing the activity of the first.

Synergistic
A synergistic effect takes place when the effect of two drugs taken at the same time is greater than the sum of each drug given alone.

DRUG INTERACTIONS

When one drug alters the action of another drug, a **drug interaction** is present (see the box on p. 8). Some medications are given together because the drug interactions are helpful. For example, probenecid is given with penicillin to increase the absorption of penicillin in treating venereal disease. Other drug interactions produce adverse effects. For example, some antibiotics make birth control pills less effective, thus placing a woman at risk for pregnancy.

Several types of effects are seen with drug interactions. If two drugs given together double the effect produced, an **additive effect** is seen. If one drug interferes with the action of another drug, it is described as an **antagonistic effect.** At times, one drug may replace another drug at a receptor site, increasing the effect of the first drug. This is called **displacement.** Sometimes drugs are chemically **incompatible.** Attempts to mix them together in a syringe produce a chemical reaction so the drugs cannot be given. **Interference** is sometimes seen when one drug promotes the rapid excretion of another drug, thus reducing its activity. Finally, if the effect of two drugs taken at the same time is greater than the sum of each drug given alone, the drugs have a **synergistic effect.**

PATIENT VARIABLES THAT MAY AFFECT DRUG ACTION

Extensive research is conducted on all drugs before they are marketed. A great deal of information is known about every medication, and certain parameters have been established. These drug parameters include the therapeutic response, side effects, adverse effects, and probable interactions with other drugs. This information is listed by the manufacturer on a slip of paper inserted into the product container. All pharmaceutical companies publish this same information each year for all drugs on the market in the *Physician's Desk Reference* (PDR).

Just as medications vary, variations among individuals influence the absorption, distribution, metabolism, and excretion of the medications also. General variables that influence drug activity often help the nurse anticipate individual response to medication. Some of these patient variables are summarized in the box on p. 10.

Patient Variables Influencing Drug Action

Body weight

An *overweight* individual requires a larger dosage. An *underweight* individual requires a smaller dosage.

Age

Infants and *children* require smaller dosages because they have lower fat and total water content, immature enzyme systems, reduced kidney function, and variation in circulating blood proteins.
Elderly individuals may require smaller dosages because of changes in cellular composition and functioning throughout the body, (especially in the liver and kidneys), the presence of several disease processes, and the necessity for many medications.

Illness

The type of pathologic process influences body processes. *Nephrotic syndrome, dehydration, malabsorption, or malnutrition* may cause changes in blood volume and protein composition. *Kidney* disease produces changes in blood and electrolyte concentration. *Liver* disease leads to decreased metabolism of drugs. *Hyperthyroidism* may produce higher metabolic rate, which increases drug metabolism. A patient in *shock* may have reduced circulation with delays in drug distribution in tissues.

Cumulative drug effects

A drug may reach a higher level than needed because it is administered too often, the dosage is too high, or other drugs or chemicals (such as alcohol) that increase the effect of the drug are taken at the same time. The drug may accumulate in a high concentration and produce side effects.

Psychologic overlay

The patient's attitude about drug acceptability and effectiveness is important. *Placebos,* inert or ineffective substances, given to some individuals may be as effective as the real medication. Other patients develop *tolerance,* or a need for an increased dosage over time to produce the same effects.

Dependence

An individual may develop both a physical and a psychologic need for a drug, usually a controlled substance. This may also be termed *addiction* or *habituation.*

Chapter 2

Drug Calculations Review

CALCULATION METHODS

Calculating dosages involves the following three steps:

1. Determine whether the drug dosage desired (what is written in the prescriber's order) is in the same measurement system as the drug dosage available. If they are not in the same measurement system, convert between the two systems.
2. Simplify by reducing to the lowest terms whenever possible.
3. Calculate the dosage quantity to be administered. This may be done by using fractions, ratios, or proportions.

Fraction method

When using fractions to compute drug dosages, write an equation consisting of two fractions. First set up a fraction showing the number of units to be given over x, the unknown number of tablets or milliliters. For example, if the physician's order states "ibuprofen 600 mg," you would put $\frac{600\text{ mg}}{x}$. On the other side of the equation, write a fraction showing the drug dosage as listed on the medication bottle over the number of tablets or milliliters. The ibuprofen bottle label states "200 mg per tablet," so the second fraction would be $\frac{200\text{ mg}}{1}$. The fractions then read:

$$\frac{600\text{ mg}}{x\text{ tab}} = \frac{200\text{ mg}}{1\text{ tab}}$$

You will note that the same units of measure are in both numerators and the same measures are in both denominators. Now, solve for x:

$$\frac{600\text{ mg}}{x\text{ tab}} = \frac{200\text{ mg}}{1\text{ tab}}$$

$$\frac{600}{x} = \frac{200}{1}$$

$$200\,x = 600$$

$$x = 3\text{ tablets}$$

Ratio method

In using the ratio method, first write the amount of the drug to be given and the quantity of the dosage (*x*) as a ratio. Using the example above this would be 600 mg : *x* tab. Next, complete the equation by forming a second ratio consisting of the number of units of the drug in the dosage form and the quantity of that dosage form, as taken from the bottle. Again, using the example above, the second ratio would be 200 mg : 1 tablet. Solving for *x* determines the dosage.

$$200 \text{ mg} : 1 \text{ tab} :: 600 \text{ mg} : x \text{ tab}$$

Multiply the means (inside); divide by the extremes (outside).

$$600 \times 1 = 600$$

$$200x\overline{)600} = 3$$

$$600$$

This, again, gives us three tablets.

Desired over available method

A third method for drug dosage calculation combines the conversion of ordered units into available units and the computation of drug dosage into one step. The equation for doing this is:

$$\begin{matrix}\text{DESIRED} \\ \text{Units}\end{matrix} \times \begin{matrix}\text{Conversion} \\ \text{Factor}\end{matrix} \times \frac{\begin{matrix}\text{Quantity} \\ \text{(Caps, tabs, etc)}\end{matrix}}{\begin{matrix}\text{Dosage} \\ \text{AVAILABLE}\end{matrix}} = \begin{matrix}x\text{(Quantity} \\ \text{to give)}\end{matrix}$$

If a physician orders 10 grains of a drug and the drug is available only in 300 mg tablets, the dose may be easily calculated with this formula.

Substitute 10 gr (DESIRED) for the first element of the equation. Then use the conversion fraction $^{60\text{ mg}}/_{1\text{ gr}}$ as the second portion of the formula. The third element of the equation shows the quantity of dosage form (capsule or tablet) for the dosage AVAILABLE. One tablet contains 300 mg. The completed equation then is:

$$10 \text{ gr} \times \frac{60 \text{ mg}}{1\text{gr}} \times \frac{1 \text{ tab}}{300 \text{ mg}} = x = 10 \times \frac{60}{1} \times \frac{1}{300} = \frac{600}{300} = 2 \text{ tablets}$$

Solving for x, you find that the patient should receive two 300 mg tablets.

As you can see, all three methods of drug calculation (fractions, ratios, or proportions) use the same information and much of the same format in solving the problems. With minor variations, they do the same thing. Some methods will seem to make more sense to you or be easier for you to follow. Throughout the calculation sections, use the method of drug calculation that makes the most sense to you. Return here for review if you have difficulty.

CALCULATING DOSAGES

Oral medications

Although there are many forms of oral products, oral medications usually come in capsules, tablets, or liquids. Medications dispensed via the unit-dose system are packaged by the pharmacist according to the dosage ordered.

When medication is ordered individually or through an open-stock system, the nurse usually calculates the proper drug dosage. These drug calculations are required when

1. The drug available is in a smaller dose than that ordered.
2. The drug available is in a larger dose than that ordered.
3. The drug available is in a different unit of measure than that ordered.

Capsules and tablets

Capsules cannot be broken or divided. This makes calculating the drug dosage more difficult. More than one capsule may be given to provide an accurate dosage; a part of one capsule cannot be given. Manufacturers of drugs provide capsules in different dosages to help in arriving at the proper dosage. If your calculations specify that you should give a fraction of a capsule, give an additional capsule if the fraction is ½ or more; do not give an additional capsule if the fraction is less than ½. (For example, if you find the calculations work out to 2¾, give three capsules; if it is 2¼, give two.)

Some tablets may be easily divided if they are "scored." Examples of unscored tablets include coated tablets and layered tablets. If a tablet is not scored, it should *not* be broken or cut apart.

The medication order usually states the dosage of grams, grains, or milligrams to give. Therefore the nurse understands the dosage DESIRED. The order also specifies how often the medication is to be given, such as twice a day (bid) or four times a day (qid). It may or may not specify for how many days the medication is to be given. If the order does not indicate a specific length of time (such as give for 5 days), the drug is given on a continuous basis, unless the institution has a specific policy limiting the length of time a drug may be given without reordering. Therefore the nurse may also need to calculate how much medication to order, depending on the length of time the patient will receive the medication. The nurse needs to know how much medication is NEEDED.

For example, the order reads: diazepam (Valium) 10 mg PO stat and 2 mg bid × 10 days. The medication DESIRED is diazepam 10 mg and diazepam 2 mg. The nurse must know the dosage AVAILABLE of the medication. A check with the pharmacy reveals that diazepam comes in 2 mg, 5 mg, and 10 mg tablets.

The nurse NEEDS one 10 mg diazepam tablet and enough 2 mg tablets for 10 days, or enough 2 mg tablets to fill the whole order (bid means twice a day). Thus the nurse needs to order:

One 10 mg tablet plus
One 2 mg tablet × 2 times a day × 10 days =
$1 \times 2 \times 10 = 20$ 2 mg tablets plus 1 10 mg tablet

or because five 2 mg tablets are the same as one 10 mg tablet, the nurse may order:

Five 2 mg tablets plus one 2 mg tablet ×
2 times a day × 10 days =
$5 + (1 \times 2 \times 10) = 25$ tablets

The formula to calculate the number of capsules or tablets to order is a basic proportion problem

$$\frac{\text{Dose}}{\text{DESIRED}} : \frac{\text{Dose}}{\text{AVAILABLE}} :: \begin{array}{c}\text{Tablets or}\\ \text{capsules}\\ \text{per dose}\end{array} : \frac{\text{Drug form}}{\text{(tablets or capsules)}} = \begin{array}{c}\text{Numbers of tablets}\\ \text{or capsules per dose}\end{array}$$

For example, the order reads: sulfadiazine 1.0 gm q6h × 3 days. Sulfadiazine comes in 300 or 500 mg tablets.

DESIRED: 1.0 gm

AVAILABLE: 500 mg = 0.5 gm (converted from mg to gm)

$$\frac{1.0\text{ gm}}{0.5\text{ gm}} = 2\text{ tablets}$$

Therefore give two 500 mg tablets every 6 hours for 3 days. Two tablets given four times a day for 3 days equals 24 tablets total. In simple terms this means:

$$\frac{\text{(Dose DESIRED)}}{\text{(Dose AVAILABLE)}} \times \frac{\text{Tablet}}{\text{or capsule}} = \frac{\text{Number of tablets}}{\text{or capsules per dose}}$$

To illustrate, let's try a few examples. Order: ASA gr *x* stat and prn for temperature elevation. ASA is labeled as 0.3 gm/tab.

$$\frac{\text{(Dose DESIRED)}}{\text{(Dose AVAILABLE)}}\ \frac{\text{gr } x}{0.3\text{ gm}}$$

$$\left(\text{gr } 16 = 1\text{ gm, so } \frac{\text{gr } x}{16} = 0.6\text{ gm}\right)$$

$$\frac{D}{A} = \frac{0.6\text{ mg}}{0.3\text{ mg}} \times 1 = 2\text{ tablets}$$

Order: methocarbamol 1.5 gm qd. The medication comes in 750 mg tablets.

$$\frac{\text{(Dose DESIRED)}}{\text{(Dose AVAILABLE)}}\ \frac{1.5\text{ gm}}{750\text{ mg}} \times 1 = ?$$

$$(1.5\text{ gm} = 1500\text{ mg})$$

$$\frac{D}{A} = \frac{1500\text{ mg}}{750\text{ mg}} \times 1 = 2\text{ tablets}$$

Liquids

The process and formulas used to calculate dosages of liquids are the same as those used to compute dosages of capsules or tablets. Only the unit of measure is different.

To review:

$$\frac{\text{(Dose DESIRED)}}{\text{(Dose AVAILABLE)}} \times \frac{\text{Drug form}}{\text{(minims, ml, drams)}} = \frac{\text{Amount of liquid}}{\text{per dose}}$$

Order: phenobarbital elixir 0.2 gm hs. The drug is available in 20 mg/5 ml.

$$\frac{\text{(Dose DESIRED)}}{\text{(Dose AVAILABLE)}} \; \frac{0.2\text{ gm}}{20\text{ mg/5 ml}} = \frac{200\text{ mg}}{20\text{ mg/5 ml}}$$

$$20\text{ mg} : 5\text{ ml} :: 200\text{ mg} : x\text{ ml} = 50\text{ ml/dose}$$

Parenteral medications

When medication is to be injected, it comes in the following three different forms:

1. A prefilled syringe labeled with a certain dosage in a certain volume (for example, meperidine [Demerol] 100 mg in 1 ml).
2. A single- or multiple-dose ampule labeled with a certain dosage in a certain volume (for example, epinephrine [Adrenalin] 1:1000 in 0.1 ml).
3. A vial with a powder or crystals that must be mixed or reconstituted with sterile water or normal saline solution. The drug may be measured in grains, grams, milligrams, or units. The amount of solution to be added varies and must be calculated according to the instructions with the vial. Medications given intradermally or subcutaneously generally involve very small amounts of solution, whereas IV preparations may involve 50 ml or more of solution.

Again, proportion is the standard method for calculating this dosage.

$$\text{Drug AVAILABLE} : \text{Dilution} :: \text{Drug DESIRED} : x$$

To illustrate, let's try a few examples.

Order: digoxin 0.2 mg IM. Drug is available as 0.5 mg/ml.

$$\frac{\text{(Dose DESIRED)}}{\text{(Dose AVAILABLE)}} \; \frac{0.2\text{mg}}{0.5\text{ mg}} \times 1\text{ ml} = \frac{2}{5} \times 1\text{ ml} = 0.4\text{ ml or 6 minims}$$

Order: KCl 24 mEq stat PO. Solution labeled potassium chloride contains 20 mEq/10 ml.

$$\frac{\text{(Dose DESIRED)}}{\text{(Dose AVAILABLE)}} \; \frac{24\text{ mEq}}{20\text{ mEq}} \times 10\text{ ml} = \frac{6}{5} = 12\text{ ml}$$

Order: Cedilanid-D 0.6 mg IM qd. Drug is available in 0.8 mg/4 ml ampules.

$$\frac{\text{(Dose DESIRED)}}{\text{(Dose AVAILABLE)}}\ \frac{0.6\text{ mg}}{0.8\text{ mg}} \times 4\text{ ml} = \frac{3}{4} \times 4\text{ ml} = 3\text{ ml (0.6 mg)}$$

Some medications come as powders or crystals, making them more stable. When the medication is ordered, liquid must be added to the drug to dissolve the medication in the solution (reconstitute the drug). The medication must then be given within a few hours or it will decay.

Some chemicals come in a single-dose vial. When the medication is ordered, usually 1 to 2 ml of liquid is added, the solution is gently shaken to dissolve it, and the whole amount is drawn into a syringe and injected.

At other times, an ampule will contain several doses of the powdered medication. The instructions for adding the liquid (diluent) must be followed carefully. Some multiple-dose vials for steroids contain the diluent in the top part of the bottle, separated from the powder in the bottom part of the container. Pushing on the top part forces the liquid down into the bottom part, dissolving the medication. The instructions are usually found on the package, on the ampule label, or on the package insert in the box, and they must be followed exactly. If instructions are not included, it is common to dissolve the drug in enough diluent so that the dose ordered may be given in no more than 0.5 to 1 ml.

Once powders have been dissolved in liquid or reconstituted, the bottle must be carefully labeled so that further doses may be accurately given from it. It is especially important to note the date and time the powder was dissolved, as well as the concentration of the reconstituted medication.

If instructions are not given for diluting the medication, the following modification of the familiar proportion formula may be used:

Dose desired : 1 ml :: Total drug available : *x*

The dose desired to the known amount of liquid is compared to the total amount of the drug to an unknown amount of liquid.

Multiply the means, divide by the extremes. (NOTE: In this formula, the dose AVAILABLE is on the top of the formula, the dose DESIRED is on the bottom. Think clearly as you establish your problems. Keep the logic of the proportions clear. DESIRED doesn't always go over AVAILABLE!)

For example, order: cephalothin (Keflin) 500 mg q6h IM. It comes in a multiple-dose vial containing 3 gm of powder. Prepare it so that 500 mg equals 1 ml. Convert 3 gm to 3000 mg.

$$500 \text{ mg} : 1 \text{ ml} :: 3000 \text{ mg} : x = 6 \text{ ml diluent to add to obtain } 1 \text{ ml} = 500 \text{ mg/ml}$$

or

$$\frac{\text{(Dose AVAILABLE)}}{\text{(Dose DESIRED)}} \frac{3000 \text{ mg}}{500 \text{ mg}} \times 1 \text{ ml} = 6 \text{ ml to add}$$

Order: give 500,000 U penicillin IM. Dilute 1,000,000 U penicillin so that 500,000 U equals 1 ml.

$$1{,}000{,}000 \text{ U} : x :: 500{,}000 \text{ U} : 1 \text{ ml} = 2 \text{ ml diluent}$$

or

$$\frac{\text{(Dose AVAILABLE)}}{\text{(Dose DESIRED)}} \frac{1{,}000{,}000 \text{ U}}{500{,}000 \text{ U}} \times 1 \text{ ml} = 2 \text{ ml diluent added}$$

Order: Give cephalosporin 200 mg in 1 ml IM. The drug comes in 1 gm units of powder. What is the amount of diluent to add?

$$\frac{\text{(Dose AVAILABLE)}}{\text{(Dose DESIRED)}} \frac{1 \text{ gm}}{200 \text{ mg}} = \frac{1000 \text{ mg}}{200 \text{ mg}} \times 1 \text{ ml} = 5 \text{ ml diluent}$$

Hypodermic tablets

Some narcotics come as sterile tablets. A tablet is put into a syringe, 1 to 2 ml of diluent is drawn into the syringe, and the medication is dissolved by gently turning the syringe. Rather than breaking the tablet, the proper amount is calculated and any extra solution is discarded before the medication is injected. The usual dilution is 1 ml. The following standard formula is used:

$$\text{Amount available} : 1 \text{ ml} :: \text{Amount desired} : x \text{ ml}$$

For example, the order reads: give morphine gr $\frac{1}{6}$. The available tablets are gr $\frac{1}{4}$.

$$\frac{\text{(Dose DESIRED)}}{\text{(Dose AVAILABLE)}}\ \frac{\text{gr } 1/6}{\text{gr } 1/4} \times 1\text{ ml} = \frac{1}{6} \times \frac{4}{1} \times 1\text{ ml}$$

$$= \frac{2}{3}\text{ ml or 11 minims}$$

Insulin

Great accuracy is important in preparing and administering insulin because the quantity given is very small and even minor variations in dosage may produce adverse symptoms in the patient.

Calculating and preparing insulin dosage is unique in the following three ways:

1. There are many kinds of insulin, but they all come in a standardized measure called a *unit*. Insulin is available in 10 ml vials and in two strengths (concentrations): U-100 (100 units per 1 ml solution) and U-500 (500 units per 1 ml solution). U-500 is five times stronger (more concentrated) than U-100. This preparation is rarely used.
2. Insulin should be drawn up in a special insulin syringe that is calibrated in units. If an insulin syringe is not available, a tuberculin syringe that is calibrated in minims may be used.
3. The insulin order, the insulin bottle, and the insulin as drawn up should always be rechecked by another nurse for maximum accuracy. Small errors can cause big problems.

Let's try some examples.

Order: 48 U Lente insulin U-100 (insulin zinc suspension) 1 hour before breakfast.

$$\frac{\text{(Dose DESIRED)}}{\text{(Dose AVAILABLE)}}\ \frac{48\text{ U}}{100\text{ U}} \times 1 = 48\text{ U}$$

It is easy to see then, that if the insulin and the syringe are both U-100, all you have to do is draw up the number of units ordered.

When the order calls for two different types of insulin, both may be given at the same time in the same syringe. One will be short-acting (regular) insulin and the other will be an intermediate or longer-acting type (NPH or zinc suspension). Draw up the regular insulin first, then the longer acting. Give both in the same syringe.

For example, order: 20 U regular (Iletin) insulin U-100 and 30 U NPH (isophane insulin suspension) U-100 before breakfast. Using a U-100 syringe, draw up 20 U regular insulin; then draw up 30 U NPH insulin to equal 50 U in the syringe.

Sometimes U-100 syringes are not available and a tuberculin (TB) syringe must be used. The number of minims that will equal the units ordered must be calculated. The formula for determining insulin dosage when a TB syringe is used is as follows:

$$\frac{\text{(Insulin DESIRED)}}{\text{(Insulin AVAILABLE)}} \times 16 \text{ minims} = \begin{matrix}\text{Number of minims} \\ \text{to administer}\end{matrix}$$

Order: 80 U of regular (Iletin) U-100 insulin, to be given in a TB syringe.

$$\frac{\text{(Dose DESIRED)}}{\text{(Dose AVAILABLE)}} \frac{80 \text{ U}}{100 \text{ U}} \times 16 = \frac{64}{5} = 12.8 \text{ minims}$$

Intravenous infusions

Flow rates: Regulating the intravenous infusion rate is a common nursing task. The completeness of prescribers' orders for intravenous infusions varies widely. Some prescribers are more specific in their instructions than others. A complete order specifies the type of solution and the volume to be infused (usually 500 or 1000 ml), as well as the length of time that the medication should be given. More commonly, the nurse is left to calculate the flow rate, or how fast the infusion will be completed.

There are three mathematical procedures that the nurse must be familiar with regarding intravenous infusions

1. Calculating the flow rate for IV fluid administration.
2. Making modifications in flow rates for infants.
3. Calculating total administration time for IV fluid.

To *calculate the flow rate for IV fluid administration,* two concepts must be understood—the flow rate and the drop factor. The rate at which IV fluids are given is the flow rate, and this is measured in drops per minute. The drop factor is the number of drops per milliliter of liquid and is determined by the size of the drops. The drop factor is different for different manufacturers of IV infusion equipment, and it must be checked by reading it on the infusion set itself. Regular infusion sets generally range between 10 and 15 drops per milliliter. Infusion sets have different drop factors for use with blood infusion sets (usually 10 to 12 drops per milliliter) because the drops are larger, whereas pediatric setups use very small drops called microdrops (often with 50 or 60 microdrops per milliliter).

Once the nurse has learned the drop factor for the equipment being used, the flow rate may be calculated by using the following formula:

Drop factor × Milliliters per minute = Flow rate (drops/minute)

Order: IV infusion to run at a slow rate to keep vein open. The rate is to be at 2 ml/minute. The IV infusion set delivers 10 drops/ml. The goal is to determine the flow rate in drops/minute.

10 (drop factor) × 2 ml/min = 20 drops/minute

Order: 1000 ml NS to be administered in 5 hours.
The drop factor is 15.
Use:

$$\frac{\text{Total of fluid to give}}{\text{Total time (minutes)}} \times \text{Drop factor} = \text{Flow rate (drops/minute)}$$

$$\frac{1000 \text{ ml}}{300 \text{ min}} \times 15 = \frac{15{,}000 \text{ ml}}{300 \text{ min}} = 50 \text{ drops/minute}$$

Flow rates for infants and children: Infants and small children are very sensitive to extra amounts or volumes of fluids. Smaller total amounts of IV fluids are often given, and the infusions are given in very small drops to avoid quickly overloading the infant's circulation. This is a built-in safety mechanism to prevent fluid overload resulting from accidental delivery of too much fluid.

The drop factor must be determined from the infusion setup. Usually 60 microdrops per ml is the drop factor for infants. For calculating the flow rates in infants, the same formula is used, but the microdrop drop factor must be substituted into the formula for the adult drop factor.

$$\frac{\text{Total of fluid to give}}{\text{Total time (minutes)}} \times \text{Drop factor} = \text{Flow rate (drops/minute)}$$

For example, give 50 ml of D_6W IV in 4 hours. The drop factor is 60 microdrops/ml.

$$\frac{50 \text{ ml}}{240 \text{ min}} \times 60 = \frac{300}{24} = 12.5 \text{ microdrops/minute}$$

Total infusion time

Sometimes prescribers order how fast they want infusions to run. To plan nursing care of the patient and to anticipate when new IV bottles may be needed, the nurse needs to calculate the total time the infusion will run.

Calculating the total administration time for IV fluid depends on calculating the total number of drops to be infused. Using this information, plus the drop factor, the total infusion time can be easily determined by using the following formula:

$$\frac{\text{Total drops to be infused}}{\text{Flow rate (drops/min)} \times 60} = \begin{array}{l}\text{Total infusion time}\\ \text{(hours or minutes)}\end{array}$$

For example, if the prescriber orders 1000 ml 5% dextrose in water (D_5W) to be given at 50 drops per minute with a drop factor of 10 drops/ml:

1. *Determine the total number of drops ordered.* The total number of drops to be infused comes from the prescriber's order for the amount of fluid (such as 1000 ml) × the drop factor (read from the infusion setup).
2. *Determine the number of minutes that the IV is to flow.* The number of drops per minute (50) is multiplied by 60 to give the number of drops infused in 1 hour (3000). This figure is then divided into the total number of drops. This will give the number of minutes for the total infusion. For example:

$$1000 \text{ ml} \times 10 \text{ drops/ml} = 10{,}000 \text{ drops}$$

$$\frac{10{,}000 \text{ drops}}{3{,}000 \text{ drops/hr}} = 3.33 \text{ hr or 3 hours, 20 minutes}$$

Other factors influencing flow rates: There are many other factors that influence the flow rate of an infusion. The nurse has no control over many of them, such as the age, size, and condition of the patient, the size of the vein, the type of fluid, and the need for the fluid. Other factors, such as the size of the needle, the needle's position in the vein, the height of the IV pole, the condition of the filter, the air in the air vent, and movement of the patient, may be altered to assist in infusion of IV fluids. If the fluid does not infuse at the calculated rate, the IV should be carefully checked from the IV bottle to the site of the needle's insertion.

Chapter 3

Drug Therapy Across the Life Span

CHILD-BEARING CLIENTS

Any substance ingested or absorbed by a pregnant or nursing woman is likely to reach the fetus by way of maternal circulation or to be transferred to the breast-fed neonate by way of breast milk if the substance is in sufficient concentration and is well distributed. These drugs taken by the mother potentially can cause serious harm to the fetus or neonate. No drug is known to be *absolutely* safe for the developing embryo, but some oral medications that are inactivated in the mother's stomach or not absorbed by the maternal gastrointestinal tract are assumed to be relatively safe. However, many drugs and other substances have yet to be identified as harmful to the fetus.

Considerations for drug therapy in the child-bearing client center on the effects of drugs administered to the mother on the developing fetus or nursing infant. The child-bearing client takes, on average, four or more drugs (other than vitamins) during pregnancy, and the fetal effects of these drugs are unknown. Based on animal experiments, there are more than 600 substances with some degree of "teratogenicity," or ability to cause developmental abnormalities of offspring when taken by a parent. Only about 25 substances are known to cause human malformations.

Parents now ask health professionals more questions than in the past. Nurses are called on to supply accurate information, provide rationales, discuss the options available, and support parents' decisions. Prescribers and parents may have to make difficult choices between the benefits to the mother and the risks to the fetus or neonate. A judgment may need to be made between the risks to both if the mother's illness is not treated by a certain drug and the risks to the fetus if the drug is administered.

Drug transfer to the fetus

Pregnancy does not seem to have much effect on drug absorption from the gastrointestinal tract, but protein binding is decreased, freeing more drug for placental transfer. Biotransformation of drugs in the liver is probably delayed in pregnancy, but renal excretion may be more rapid

Drugs That Cross the Placenta Rapidly*	
ampicillin	meperidine
barbiturates	penicillin G
cephalothin	phenytoin
diazepam	propranolol
ethanol	salicylates
kanamycin	streptomycin
lidocaine and other local anesthetics	sulfonamides
	tetracycline

*Especially if administered intravenously.

because renal blood flow increases dramatically as a result of increased cardiac output and glomerular filtration rate.

At the placental interface, transfer of drugs and other substances is affected primarily by simple diffusion and partly by active transport. Transfer across the placenta depends on the chemical properties of the drug: its molecular weight, spatial configuration, protein-binding capabilities, pK_a (the point when half the amount of drug in the body is ionized and half is nonionized), and lipid solubility, as well as its distribution and concentration gradient. The potential for transfer is proportional to the period of time the drug remains in the maternal bloodstream. Transfer is greater during late gestation because of enhanced uteroplacental blood flow, increased placental surface at the interface, thinner membranes separating maternal blood flow and placental capillaries, and an increased proportion of free drug available to the circulation. Pathologic processes in the placenta, such as inflammation, degeneration, or partial separation, can increase blood flow and thus drug transfer. Not much is known about drug metabolism in the placenta itself, but it is thought to be a less active process. Certain drugs can alter placental enzyme activity necessary for degradation of substances and for energy-dependent transport mechanisms.

Many drugs are carried across the placenta within minutes, especially if administered intravenously (see box above). Thus the historical concept of the placenta as a completely protective barrier to circulating substances must be discarded. Most drugs that cross the placenta stabilize in the fetus at a level between 50% and 100% of the maternal level. Some (such as diazepam and local anesthetics) stabilize at levels even higher than the mother's blood levels. However, continued exposure of the fetus to a drug is more important than the rate of placental transport.

Within the fetus, drug effects may be more significant and prolonged than in the mother because of (1) probable lower enzyme concentrations and enzymatic reaction rates of drug metabolism and (2) slower excretion rates. Fetal excretion of drugs takes place via maternal resorption and by excretion by the fetal kidneys into amniotic fluid, which, under ordinary circumstances, the fetus often swallows.

On occasion, various fetal complications such as anemia and syphilis exposure have been actively treated by drugs in utero. The drug delivery routes chosen have been either the passive, transplacental approach or direct instillations into the amniotic fluid. These modes are still controversial.

It is, however, well documented that many unintended fetal drug doses via maternal circulation produce harmful fetal effects. The embryo or fetus runs the risk of developing the usual side or toxic effects, just as the mother does. Also, doses can be lethal or **teratogenic** (causing fetal organ defects), **mutagenic** (causing genetic mutation), or **carcinogenic** (causing or accelerating the development of cancer, sometimes much later).

Every embryo undergoes a series of precisely programmed steps from cell proliferation, differentiation, and migration to organogenesis. The critical periods for drug effects on the fetus are the first 2 weeks of rapid cell proliferation, when drug exposures can be lethal to the embryo, and the third through the tenth weeks of pregnancy, when the axial skeleton, muscles, limbs, and organs are developing most rapidly. Beyond the tenth week of pregnancy, the results are more likely to be physiologic or behavioral alterations and delays in growth.

Abuse of cocaine by pregnant women has resulted in reports of frequent miscarriages, fetal hypoxia, and low-birth-weight infants in the United States. In utero, cocaine exposure has induced fetal tremors, strokes, and an increase in stillbirth rates. Exposed infants are also at high risk for developing congenital heart disease, skull defects, and other congenital malformations. The newborn often has symptoms of increased irritability, increased respiratory and heart rates, diarrhea, irregular sleeping patterns, and poor appetite. It has been reported that behavioral patterns of infants born from cocaine-abusing mothers may also be affected—that is, they may have poor attention spans and a decrease in organizational skills.

Advice that all drugs be avoided during pregnancy and breastfeeding cannot always be followed. Some maternal conditions (such as hypertension, epilepsy, diabetes, and infection) place both mother and fetus in serious jeopardy if left untreated. Although authoritative

Drugs Contraindicated in Pregnant Women*	
aminopterin	oral contraceptives
sodium iodide (^{125}I, ^{131}I)	clomiphene
	measles vaccine
iodinated glycerol	mumps vaccine
diethylstilbestrol (DES)	rubella vaccine
chlorotrianisene	smallpox vaccine
dienestrol	vitamin A, high doses (25,000 units or more daily)
estradiol	
estrogens, conjugated	isotretinoin
estrone	menadione
ethinyl-estradiol	menadiol
mestranol	phencyclidine

*These are listed in category X on the FDA pregnancy scale.

literature and drug package inserts routinely warn that drugs have not been tested for use in pregnancy, during breast-feeding, or for infants, much empiric data and some research data are accumulating. The FDA now rates drugs as to their safety for use during pregnancy. (See Appendix F)

Certain categories of drugs are expressly contraindicated during pregnancy or are used only when the risk-benefit situation has been carefully considered and thoroughly discussed with the client. These are listed in the box above. Some drugs are considered relatively safe during pregnancy, depending on the situation. However, their use should be severely curtailed, being limited to only those pregnant women whose life or that of the fetus would be in jeopardy without drug treatment. One variable to be considered is the dose that reaches the embryo or fetus. This depends on the maternal dosage, the maternal volume of distribution, and the metabolic clearance rate of the mother. The fetal gestational age at time of exposure, duration of therapy planned, fetal and maternal genotypes, and any other drugs administered concurrently are also factors in prescribing decisions. Dosages, dosing intervals, and duration of treatment may be manipulated carefully to avoid harmful effects. Ethyl alcohol, especially at or near time of conception, is associated with the **fetal alcohol syndrome,** which produces both growth and mental retardation. Other very common substances such as aspirin, vitamin supplements, caffeine, and nicotine are suspected to cause adverse reactions in the fetus.

One difficulty with these and other substances is that effects on the embryo may occur before the woman is aware that she is pregnant. Women of child-bearing age who are not using contraceptives and who are sexually active should be prescribed for carefully and should be instructed to use over-the-counter medications cautiously. Education and prevention are considered the best therapy.

Medication administration in childbearing clients

Most nursing goals related to these topics should be aimed at ensuring that parents know that any foreign substance absorbed by the mother may have lifelong effects on the child. A balance must be maintained between protecting the child and dealing constructively with the family; creating unnecessary family concern is not appropriate. Essential to these aims is cooperating with the prescribing clinician, providing an environment for free exchange of information, and, if possible, forestalling parental feelings of guilt or fear associated with drug administration, whether planned or inadvertent. The following information should be conveyed:

1. Potential harm to the child resulting directly from substances the mother is exposed to and potential danger to both mother and child if treatment is not begun must both be weighed. These decisions must be made with the prescriber whenever exposure to an unfamiliar substance or drug is contemplated. Not everything is known at this time about effects on the child; and as more information becomes available, accepted guidelines may change.
2. Over-the-counter medications and other common substances such as aspirin, high-dose or multiple vitamin supplements, alcohol, caffeine, and nicotine may also have detrimental effects on the fetus.
3. Any prescription written by a professional who is not a specialist in the care of pregnancies or nursing mothers should be evaluated by an obstetrician or pediatrician. The prescription may need to be changed by the specialist to a safer drug or dosage.
4. If a questionable substance is absorbed by the mother, close health care supervision is essential. If real potential for fetal or infant injury results, the parents need ongoing support as they endure the sometimes long wait for effects to be manifested. If birth defects or toxic effects are present or if invasive diagnostic tests or a therapeutic abortion is to be performed, objective psychologic intervention may help the parents endure this critical period.

PEDIATRIC CLIENTS

Neonates

Because newborns are small and immature, lacking many of the protective mechanisms that allow older children and adults to be relatively resistant to stressors of all kinds, they require special considerations. Their skin is thin and permeable, their stomachs lack acid, and their lungs lack much of the mucous barrier. Neonates regulate body temperature poorly and become dehydrated easily. Their liver and kidneys are immature and cannot manage foreign substances as well as those of older children and adults.

Breast-fed infants

Almost *all* forms of drugs in maternal circulation can be readily transferred to the colostrum and breast milk. Because drugs or their biotransformed products are handled by different pathways in the infant and the fetus, the impact of maternal medications on the infant probably differs (is probably less) from that on the fetus. This difference can serve as a guide in prescribing for the breast-feeding mother. Typical nontherapeutic outcomes in the breast-fed infant are signs of the drug's usual side or toxic effects. Adverse effects may occur, such as gray-brown stains of the later-erupting teeth as a result of tetracycline therapy more than 10 days in length or allergic sensitization to penicillin. Most drug products that reach the neonate via breast milk have undergone maternal biotransformation and are probably less than the original dose. However, immaturity of the neonate's liver and kidney systems limits its capacity for further metabolism and excretion.

Data about infants' capabilities for drug absorption, digestion, distribution, metabolism, and excretion are scant and conflicting. In general, the proved benefits of continuing breast-feeding must be weighed on an individual basis against the risks of maternal medication to the infant. Although the mammary glands are a relatively insignificant route for maternal drug excretion and the drug level in breast milk is usually less than the actual maternal dose, the infant's actual dose depends largely on the volume of milk consumed. Thus a single measurement of a drug in human milk will not accurately reflect the total dose the infant receives.

The concentration of the drug in maternal circulation depends on the relationship among several factors: dosing and route of administration, the drug's distribution, its protein binding, and maternal metabolism and excretion. The mammary alveolar epithelium presents to any potentially transferable substance a lipid barrier with water-filled pores. It is more permeable to drugs during the colostrum stage of milk production—during the first week of life. Drug factors that enhance drug excretion into milk are nonionization, low molecular weight, solubility in fat, and plasma binding versus milk-protein binding. Transfer of an active or passive form of a drug's metabolites into maternal plasma and then to milk depends mainly on passive diffusion. The absorptive processes of the infant's gastrointestinal tract and drug distribution are estimated to be similar to those in the adult, which means that lipid-soluble substances are well absorbed. The infant's age (thus the amount of drug-containing milk consumed) and the relative immaturity of the infant's important organs bear greatly on the outcome. If the drug is fat soluble, it may be more highly concentrated in breast milk at the end of feedings and at midday. Because the infant's total serum protein is lower in comparison to the adult's, more free drug is available to the circulation. Metabolic reactions in the infant's liver are slower than in the older child's; consequently, drug biotransformation may likewise be delayed. Other factors in the neonatal period may present risks: inadequate body temperature control, hypoxemia, or inadequate nutrition, for example. Drug excretion is delayed in the neonate because it is largely via the kidneys, where immature glomerular filtration rates and tubular functioning are maintained for several months. The extreme variability among drug effects and infants' capabilities makes it difficult to decide whether the mother should take a drug and whether or not she should breast-feed.

Human milk contains small, fixed amounts of many substances absorbed by the mother. Considerable evidence shows that certain other substances are incontrovertibly contraindicated unless necessary for survival and unless their effects are closely monitored. The usual recommendation is that breast-feeding be temporarily interrupted (usually for 24 to 72 hours) and the breasts pumped to remove drug-containing milk. Less often, it is advisable to cease breast-feeding altogether. Dosages and routes may also be changed. It is recommended that certain drugs be avoided while breast-feeding; see the box on p. 31.

Drug effects may be minimized by substituting formula for the midday breast-feeding, since that is the feeding highest in fat content and thus more likely to contain higher amounts of fat-soluble drug products. In addition, breast-feeding mothers who must be treated with medications can time their doses to be taken right *after* breast-

Drugs Contraindicated During Breast-Feeding	
The American Academy of Pediatrics committee on drugs has suggested that the following drugs be avoided in the woman who is breast-feeding:	
bromocriptine	gold salts
cimetidine	methimazole
clemastine	methotrexate
cyclophosphamide	phenindione
ergotamine	thiouracil

feeding so as much time as possible elapses and the drug can reach a relatively low concentration before the next feeding.

With radioactive substances, therapy is of short duration; or if merely a diagnostic radioisotope test is to be done, breast-feeding must be interrupted until all radiation is absent from milk samples. Breast-feeding will probably be terminated when the drug is so potent that minute amounts may profoundly affect the infant, when the drug has high allergenic potential, when the mother exhibits evidence of decreased renal function (which augments drug excretion into breast milk), or when serious pathologic conditions require prolonged drug administration of high dosages.

Changes in the activity levels of the fetus or nursing infant signal dangerous effects resulting from drug administration; parents should be taught how to assess and report unusual fetal inactivity or infant apathy.

Alternatives to drug therapy. Both health professionals and clients place high value on pharmaceutical solutions to health concerns. However, many illnesses are self-limited or cause only minor discomforts that end or decrease without medication or with non-drug alternatives, such as relaxation techniques rather than tranquilizers. The effect of any medication should be weighed against the mother and child's physical and psychologic stress of abrupt weaning.

Other considerations might be to delay the mother's pharmacologic therapy until the infant is weaned on his or her own or to select another drug to meet the therapeutic goal without interfering with breast-feeding. The age and maturity of the child must be considered also; as the infant develops physiologically the drug's ability to cause harmful effects will diminish. The frequency of feedings should also be considered. An infant dependent on breast milk for total nutrition will receive higher doses of drugs than an infant breast-feeding only once or twice a day and taking other forms of nourishment.

Other pediatric clients

Drug administration to pediatric clients requires special knowledge and approaches. Physicians may prescribe the dosage of medication, but it is the nurse's responsibility to know the safe dosage range of any medication administered to children. A standard dosage of medication is nonexistent in pediatrics; medications are usually ordered according to the weight or body surface area of the child. Some pharmaceutical companies continue to supply medications in a standard adult dosage strength, and the nurse must be able to evaluate the correct dosage before administering the medication.

Weight as a basis. Following is a formula for calculating estimated safe dosages based on weight alone (Clark's rule). Because this is based on weight alone, it is a somewhat imprecise calculation for children.

$$\frac{\begin{matrix}\text{Average}\\ \text{adult dose}\end{matrix} \times \begin{matrix}\text{Weight of}\\ \text{child in pounds}\end{matrix}}{150} = \text{Estimated safe dose}$$

A nurse preparing calculated dosages of digitalis, insulin, barbiturates, and narcotics should have the calculations as well as the prepared medication dosage checked by another nurse or pharmacist before the drug is administered. Pediatric dosages are often minute, and a slight mistake in calculating the amount of medication to be administered results in greater proportional error.

Pediatric dose calculation based on weight alone implies that the pediatric client is a small adult, which is not true. Physiologic differences in the infant when compared to an adult may definitely affect the amount of drug needed to produce a therapeutic effect. For example, infants have a body composition that is approximately 75% water (adults have 50% to 60%) and less fat content than the adult. Therefore, water-soluble drugs are generally administered in larger doses to infants and children per body weight than to an adult.

Rules based on weight, such as Clark's rule, are generally taught and used by students in clinical areas to assess pediatric dosages. While useful as a guide, their accuracy for a number of drugs is questionable.

Body surface area as a basis. More than 100 years ago, Hufeland suggested that drug doses should be calculated on size or proportional amount of body surface area (BSA) to weight. Many physicians continue to use weight as the basis for calculating drug doses and body surface area for calculating fluid requirements. Most clinicians advocate using body surface area for determining drug dosage for adults as well as children. Physicians usually carry a simple slide rule or nomogram, such as the West nomogram (see Appendix G) to make rapid BSA conversions from weight and height. It is believed that the larger amount of total body water (TBW) in children, as well as the percentage of water in body weight and the part of that percentage formed by extracellular water, accounts for the fact that children tolerate or require larger doses of some drugs on a mg/m^2 basis.

For the 75% of drugs that have no established pediatric dosage, calculating the child's dosage as a fraction of the average adult dose using Clark's rule is really too imprecise for most applications, yet it may be used (mg per kg) where the dosage according to body surface area has not been established. The surface area rule is the most accurate. As a relationship between height and weight, it can provide a more precise guide to the maturity of the child's organs and metabolic rate of functioning for effective pharmacokinetics. The dosage should be tailored to the individual child according to the amount of medication per square meter of body surface area. The BSA rule for children's dosages follows:

$$\text{Child's approximate dose} = \frac{\dfrac{\text{Child's BSA in square}}{\text{meters (from nomogram)}} \times \text{Adult dose}}{1.73}$$

Medication administration in pediatric clients

Although these rules have been devised for relating adult doses to infants and children, it must be emphasized that *no rules or charts are adequate to guarantee safety of dosage at any age,* particularly in the neonate. No method takes into account all variables, particularly individual tolerance differences. Astute, accurate nursing observations of how individual children react to drugs can assist in choosing drugs and dosages.

The administration of medications to infants and children is both challenging and frustrating. Giving injections skillfully will enhance security and help gain a child's cooperation. A sound knowledge of growth and development also provides the nurse with information about how a child might be approached, whether reasoning will help or hinder the process, and whether assistance will be needed. The

Pediatric Drug Administration

1. Parents are frequently good sources of information about successful methods or vehicles of giving medications to their children.
2. Try to avoid using essential foods such as milk, cereal, or orange juice, because the child may refuse to accept that food in the future.
3. Never underestimate children's reactions. They may not require that the taste of medication be disguised.
4. A sip of cold fruit juice, ice chips, a frozen fruit-bar, or a mint-flavored substance before and after the administration of an unpalatable medicine may effectively dull its taste.
5. Sugarless vehicles such as those sweetened by saccharin should be used to disguise the taste of medications given to diabetic children or those on a ketogenic diet.
6. Honey and syrup are ideal for suspending drugs that do not dissolve easily in water.
7. Since fruit syrups are usually acid, they should not be used for medicines that react in an acid medium (such as sodium bicarbonate, soluble barbiturates, and penicillin).
8. Elixirs have an alcohol base that, when undiluted, may cause the child either to refuse them or to cough and choke; they may also cause a drug-drug interaction. Small amounts of water added to elixirs of phenobarbital or chloral hydrate occasionally help.
9. Nursing time can be saved by recording the most successful method of administering medications and pertinent nursing orders on the child's care plan. This notation also saves the child frustration, fear, and anxiety.

principles of safe administration of medication apply to all age groups, but children differ from adults, and the nurse has added responsibilities. (See box above.)

Ideally, a child will cooperate more readily with a nurse who has established a positive relationship. The child may also find it easier to accept the discomforts accompanying injections and some oral medications from the nurse who is associated with daily hygiene, feeding, holding, play, and happy times. In addition, the nurse will feel less guilty when the child associates the nurse with pleasure and comfort most of the time, and discomfort only when necessary to get well.

When a child is afraid or anxious, the natural response is to strike out at the frustration or avoid it. By accepting this behavior as a natural response, the nurse will be able to deal with it and be honest when a medication or procedure will be unpleasant or painful.

Truthful explanations to children are essential. Children have a right to some explanation of any procedure that concerns them. The timing and type of explanation should be geared to the child's ability to perceive and understand. For the child 2 years of age or younger very simple explanations such as "I have some medicine for you to drink" or "I have an injection to give you, and it will hurt a little" are sufficient. Long explanations to children through 5 years of age do little more than prolong the anticipation and increase anxiety or fear. Telling 4-year-olds to stop kicking, hitting, or other avoidance behavior only conveys to them that they are not understood and they will receive little or no help with their feelings of frustration about being medicated. Providing the preschool-age child opportunities at play (for example, to give a doll an "injection" [empty syringe without a needle] or "drops") affords an important outlet and allows the child to work through the trauma of the experience.

Many children are courageous, or like to be considered so, and appealing to their courage is sometimes effective. Children 4 years old or over may choose to hold their own medicine cup, or drink unassisted, and to take pills from the container without any assistance from the nurse. Children of this age are motivated by social reinforcers, such as being praised for their cooperation, or "your job is to stay very still," which enhance their self-esteem and feelings of competence. Because of the sense of achievement that follows, they may want to save the medicine cups to show their parents.

Oral medications. Success in administering oral medications usually requires a kind yet firm approach with a positive attitude. No doubt that the child will take the medicine should be reflected in choice of words or tone of voice. The nurse might say, "Jimmy, it's time to take your yellow medicine" or "Do you want to take your pill now or with your Jell-O?" This indicates that Jimmy is expected to cooperate and to do it willingly. It also allows the child some control over the situation. An unwise approach that reveals doubt on the nurse's part might be: "I have your yellow pill, Jimmy. Will you take it for me, please?"

Nurses should try to be aware of how a medicine tastes so that they can answer such questions as, "Does it taste bad? Will it burn my mouth?" A helpful reply would be, "It tastes like cherry to me. Tell me what it tastes like to you." Often the child will accept the suggestion to taste and find out. However, if the medication is bad tasting, attempting deceit or lying to the child is as futile and destructive as it is to an adult.

Disagreeable-tasting medications should be disguised if at all possible. Small amounts of honey, syrup, jam, fruit, and some fruit juices are suitable sweet vehicles for less palatable drugs. Some pills can be crushed and suspended in small amounts of these substances as long as the two are compatible. Infants and children swallow many liquid medications more readily if mixed with a sweet substance or diluted with a small amount of water. (If large amounts of water or other substances are used and the child refuses to take all of the mixture, estimating the amount of medication the child received is difficult.) Fortunately, many drugs are available in palatable syrups or suspension form well suited for administration to infants and children. Suspensions, however, should be thoroughly agitated to ensure that doses are not offered in unequal concentrations.

Caution must be exercised to prevent aspiration when giving oral medications to children. Medications must be given to infants slowly and in small amounts to avoid choking. Liquid medications may be administered by nipple, plastic medicine cup, plastic dropper, or a plastic syringe without the needle. Water should be swished through the inside of these *first* to prevent medication from sticking, thereby undermedicating. Glass cups, droppers, or syringes should be avoided because of the obvious danger of breakage in the child's mouth. A dropper or syringe is best suited for placing a liquid medication along one side of the infant's tongue. Older infants and toddlers seem to prefer to take their medications from a plastic medicine cup. If children are held or placed in a sitting position, they are less likely to aspirate the medication than if lying on their backs. When administering a medication with a dropper or syringe, the nurse may purse the infant's lips with one hand to keep the medicine from running out of the mouth. Droppers and syringes used for medication should be kept clean, they should be reserved for only one client's use, and they should be rinsed or washed before being returned to the medication bottle.

If the child refuses to cooperate even after explanations and encouragement, the nurse may have to ask whether the child will take the medication alone or will need the nurse to give it. Physical coercion is seldom necessary, but if used, it should be mild and used with dispatch and firmness, since aspiration is a danger. The nurse must not combine force with anger or resort to force when one nurse has been unable to administer the medication. Careful consideration should be given to such factors as: Why does the child resist? Does the child disapprove only of one nurse? Have past experiences with medications given at home or in the hospital frightened the child? Will forcing a medication cause a struggle that will negate the effects of a drug given for sedation? If mild restraint is necessary, the nurse should explain to the child that this form of treatment is necessary. The child will not cooperate if force is seen as a punishment for inability to cooperate; often the child loses confidence in all personnel.

Topical medications. Children have a large skin surface area in proportion to total body weight. Their skin, especially neonates', is particularly thin, permeable, and without much protective oil. Although adults absorb much more medication through intact skin than was previously believed, the child is at increased risk for systemic medication administration. The discovery that hexachlorophene can cause encephalopathy in newborns and that topically applied boric acid can cause systemic poisoning testifies to the hazard of applying drugs to children's skin, especially for prolonged contact or over broken skin areas. Plain soap and water may be preferred for abrasions or open lesions, replacing medicated dressings.

Subcutaneous injections. There are wide swings in the amounts of subcutaneous fat during the childhood years. Neonates have proportionately smaller amounts; these increase slightly to 23% by 1 year of age. From 1 to 5 years of age they drop to between 8% and 12%. Then the amounts of bodily fat climb to about 20% when the child reaches age 10. Lipid-soluble drugs have an affinity for fat tissue; less subcutaneous fat means that lower dosages of drugs such as diazepam and barbiturates are necessary to maintain blood levels. In addition, less subcutaneous tissue for injections may be available. An alternate route may need to be selected—oral, intramuscular, or intravenous.

Intramuscular injections. The principles and techniques of the administration of injections are similar to those for adults.

Most authorities believe that the risk of sciatic nerve injury is too great to warrant the use of the gluteal site of administration. The sciatic nerve is the largest nerve in the body; its normal pathway is the hollow midway between the ischial tuberosity and the greater trochanter, covered by the gluteus maximus muscle. This pathway, however, varies a great deal from individual to individual. In addition, the small size of the gluteal mass in the infant or neonate and the potential neurotoxicity of many drugs enhance the possibility of iatrogenic trauma secondary to IM injections. Trauma of this kind is the leading cause of sciatic neuropathy in infancy. A lesion at this height of the sciatic nerve is usually tragically associated with marked permanent disability.

The younger the child, the less muscle tissue may be available for IM injections anywhere on the body. If repeated injections are necessary, the available sites may become overused, inflamed, or dystrophic, requiring concerted efforts by the nurse to develop systematic plans for rotating sites and communicating them to the rest of the staff. The vastus lateralis muscle is the site of choice for IM injections in children under 3 (see Figure 11, color plates). The ventrogluteal site is preferred for the child over 3 years old who has been walking for a year or two (see Figure 10, color plates). The dorsogluteal muscles should not be used for injections in the child under 6 years old if other IM sites are available. These muscles should not be used for injections at all until the younger child has been walking for at least 1 year.

For injection into the left gluteals, the thumb is placed on the trochanter and the middle finger on the iliac crest. The index finger placed midway between the thumb and middle finger will indicate a safe injection area. Infants should receive no more than 0.5 ml in each injection site. Small children can tolerate a volume of up to 1 ml at each site. The deltoid muscle is likewise not used for children under 5 years of age because of its underdevelopment. Rather than the skin being held taut, as for adults, the muscle mass may instead be pinched up. The needle will thus avoid striking deeper-lying structures such as nerves, bones, or blood vessels. The IM injection is still made at a 90-degree angle to the top of the massed flesh. Preferred needle sizes for pediatric IM injections are 25- to 27-gauge and ½ to 1 inch in length. A 21- or 22-gauge needle may be preferred if a viscous medication such as procaine penicillin is to be given. In the interest of safety, the child should usually be restrained for an injection, and the injection should be given rapidly. Two or more persons should be available for children over 4 years of age despite promises that they will "hold still." An extra sterile needle may be carried in a pocket in case a needle becomes contaminated when a child moves unexpectedly. A child's attention may be distracted from the injection by asking the youngster to wiggle the toes. Because children enjoy trying out each other's beds, the identifying armband must be checked before giving each medication.

Rectal administration. When oral administration is difficult or contraindicated, the rectal route is often advised. Many children perceive use of the rectal route as an extreme invasion of their bodies or anticipate pain as a result. It may help to let them insert the suppository. Several drugs, such as sedatives, aspirin, and antiemetics, are available in suppository form. Suppositories made with a cocoa butter base will melt rapidly at normal body temperature, releasing the drug for absorption. After a suppository is inserted in an infant, the buttocks should be held or taped together for 5 to 10 minutes to relieve pressure on the anal sphincter and thereby help to ensure retention and absorption of the medication. Infants and children with diarrhea, however, may easily expel suppositories with explosive stools. Likewise, a suppository inserted into a child with a constipation problem or a rectum full of stool will be surrounded with stool and will have little chance for absorption of its contents.

Pharmacists and nurses often divide suppository doses by cutting them to obtain correct doses. This is a dangerous practice because all the medication might be contained in one area of the suppository. If divided doses must be administered, the pharmacist should be contacted for alternate product advice and guidance.

Nose drops, eardrops, and eyedrops. Aqueous preparations of nose drops are the only safe preparations to use, if it is deemed necessary to use them at all, because of the danger of aspiration. Many nose drop preparations contain vasoconstrictors, and prolonged or excessive use may be harmful. Infants are nose breathers, and nasal congestion will inhibit their sucking. For this reason, nose drops, if necessary, should be instilled 20 to 30 minutes before feedings.

To instill *nose drops* (see Figure 20, color plates):

1. Hold the infant in your arm, allowing the head to fall back over the edge of your arm, or place a small pillow under the shoulders and allow the head to fall back over the edge of the pillow.
2. Place your free arm so that the forearm is around the far side of the child's head, stabilizing the head between your forearm and your body. Use your hand to stabilize the arms and hands.
3. With your free hand you can then instill the prescribed drops with minimum struggle and maximum accuracy.

The instillation of *eardrops* requires a knowledge of anatomic structure because the shape of the auditory canal of a young child is different from that of an adult. Gentle massage of the area immediately anterior to the ear will facilitate the entry of the drops into the ear canal (see Figure 19, color plates). Before the initial administration of a course of therapy with eardrops, the nurse should assess whether the child has excessive cerumen. If so, it may be necessary to consult with the physician about its removal with cerumen softeners and/or irrigation before instilling the eardrops.

Eyedrop instillation is done in the same way with children as with adults except that the head may be stabilized by an assistant. Many eyedrops cause a burning sensation for a few seconds, so if both eyes are to be medicated it is wise to do the second instillation quickly before the client begins to blink and tear as a reaction to the burning sensation occurring in the first eye medicated. Mild pressure for 30 seconds over the inner canthus next to the nose will prevent premature drainage of the medication away from the eye. (See Figure 18, color plates.)

Aqueous preparations of nose, ear, and eye drops may support the growth of bacteria and fungi. For this reason small volumes of such medications are ordered and should be used for only *one* individual (not shared by family members). The dropper (especially eye droppers) should not be permitted to become contaminated by touching anything but medication or rinsing water from the tap at any time. It should never be inverted so that medication or water runs into the rubber bulb to form a medium for microbiologic growth or to flavor the medication with a rubber taste. A dropper from one medication should usually not be used to measure and administer another type of medication because droppers are not standardized—all droppers are not manufactured to deliver drops of the same volume. Viscosity of drugs also varies, affecting the drop size.

Eyedrops and eardrops are more comfortably tolerated if they are warmed (if not contraindicated) before instillation. Warming can be achieved by running warm water over the side of the bottle without the label or immersing the bottle in some warm water in a medicine cup. Even carrying the bottle in a pocket for half an hour or so will take the chill off the drops.

Intravenous medications. The use of IV drug therapy is widespread on most pediatric services for several reasons. In children with vomiting and diarrhea, medications given by mouth may be vomited, losing precious time in drug management. These same children may have poor absorption of drugs and fluids as a result of dehydration or peripheral vascular collapse, so that drugs administered via the IM route may be equally ineffective. For premature or physiologically distressed neonates, it may be preferable to give certain high-osmolality drugs by IV rather than give the syrup or elixir forms by the oral route. These infants are prone to necrotizing enterocolitis (NEC) and death when administered feedings or oral drugs that have an osmolality

Pediatric IV Drug Administration

1. IV drug therapy should be used only if other channels of drug administration are impracticable. Pediatric nurses skilled in giving medications to children via other routes may be able to influence prescribers' decisions regarding successful routes of drug administration.
2. For small infants a scalp vein or a superficial vein of the wrist, hand, foot, or arm may be most convenient and most easily stabilized. Scalp veins have no valves, and thus infusions may be in either direction. They are the most frequent sites for infant infusions. Older children may receive infusions through any accessible vein.
3. A too-rapid IV infusion or injection may cause "speed shock": rapid fall in blood pressure, respiratory irregularity, blood incoagulability, and even death. Preventive measures include use of the minidropper (note that the milliliter per hour in the order translates to the drops per minute with this tubing), calibrated volume control chambers, and infusion pumps.
4. Total parenteral nutrition (TPN) solutions are usually infused into the vena cava or innominate or subclavian veins approached via the external or internal jugular veins. Occasionally the inferior vena cava is entered via the femoral vein.
5. Once a drug is injected intravenously, the drug's action is relatively irreversible.
6. Drugs must be properly diluted. Too much emphasis cannot be placed on the caution: GIVE THE SMALLEST POSSIBLE DOSE AT THE SLOWEST POSSIBLE RATE.

greater than that of body fluids. Although elixirs of theophylline, phenobarbital, calcium, digoxin, and dexamethasone all have osmolalities 10 times greater than body fluids and have been implicated in causing NEC, analysis shows that the contained additives actually raise the medication's osmolality. Related studies continue.

The pediatric nurse responsible for the administration of IV drugs may find the suggesstions in the box above helpful. Most older children may be given fluids or drugs intravenously following the same principles and techniques used for adults. The younger and smaller the child, the greater the margin for error.

Neonates, infants, and children must be adequately restrained so as not to dislodge or pull out an infusion needle or catheter once it is in place. Some of the following may be helpful hints to the nurse caring for a client receiving IV therapy:

1. The needle or catheter should be fixed with plastic tape.
2. When a loop of tubing directly above the needle is secured to the tape, tension is relieved from the needle should it be pulled by sudden movement.
3. Because most children move about or are restless, it is necessary to support the limb with a padded arm board and immobilize the site of IV therapy. Support should extend to the joints above and below the site (with arm boards or IV boards).
4. If the infusion bottle is too high, the pressure in the vein will increase, causing fluid seepage into the surrounding tissues.

Other factors influencing drug dosages. Again, the dosage of most agents is related to the child's age, weight, and height. A child's bodily systems grow and develop at varying rates. This makes for unpredictable primary and secondary effects in pediatric medication administration. One example of secondary effects specific to children is discoloration of teeth and depression of enamel growth in the child under 8 years of age with administration of tetracycline liquid medications. (This adverse reaction is well-documented, but many prescriptions for this drug are still being written for this age group, according to the FDA.) Skeletal growth of children receiving long-term adrenocortical steroids is similarly impaired.

Individual variations are noted in children's response to digitalis, insulin, opiates, and oral enzyme products; dosages require careful titration. Paradoxical responses are noted with a few drugs; responses may be directly opposite that which could be expected in the adult. Excessive reactivity to atropine by infants may be related to immaturity of the central nervous system. In addition, many drugs that are safe and effective for adults have not been tested for use with children, nor have dosages been established, because of the complex medicolegal issues involved in experimentation on children.

GERIATRIC CLIENTS

Although individuals age 65 and over represent 12% of the total population in the United States today, they use approximately 35% of all health care goods and services, 25% to 30% of all prescribed drugs, and considerable quantities of OTC, self-treatment medications. Today the elderly comprise 1 of every 9 Americans, but within 50 years (by the year 2040) it has been projected that 1 of every 5 Americans will be 65 years or older (Lamy, 1988; Sloan, 1986).

At the turn of the century, only 1 person in 25 was over 65 years old. People died from parasitic and infectious diseases (pestilence and famine) then, while today the primary causes of death result from degenerative, chronic diseases. Three out of every four elderly deaths today are caused by heart disease, cancer, or stroke.

The elderly are usually affected by age-related, altered pharmacokinetics and pharmacodynamics and an increased incidence of chronic diseases, which generally result in an increase in physician's prescriptions or self-treatment with various medications and home remedies. The age of specialization has in some ways added to this problem in that multiple physicians usually prescribe a variety of medications often without discontinuing any previous drugs the client is taking. This practice, often referred to as *polypharmacy,* too often has a disastrous outcome.

The practice of polypharmacy has resulted in an increased risk of inducing drug interactions, adverse reactions, and the need for, or prolonging of, hospitalization. Pray (1989) has reported that persons receiving two medications have a 5.6% potential for having a drug interaction, while clients that receive five or eight different medications have a 50% and 100% drug interaction risk, respectively. Dr. Robert Kane (1989) reported that "adverse drug reactions in the elderly in 1985 were responsible for 243,000 hospitalizations; 32,000 hip fractures; 160,000 mental impairments, and 2,000,000 addictions." While the magnitude of problems with polypharmacy is enormous, it is frequently overlooked as the causative factor. It is important that health care providers realize that the vast majority of undesirable drug effects resulting from polypharmacy are preventable.

Physiologic changes

As people age they undergo a variety of physiologic changes that increase their sensitivity to drugs and drug-induced disease. General loss in body weight of many elderly clients may require reevaluation of dosages used for them; the criterion for dosage should be shifted from age to weight. Some older clients weigh no more than the average large child, and some weigh a lot less; yet they are prescribed the larger "adult" doses. In another case, stimulants are generally less effective in elderly individuals, and large doses are often necessary. However, CNS depressants produce intensified effects in the elderly. Sedatives and hypnotics can produce paradoxical side effects of irritability, incontinence, confusion, and disorientation.

Pharmacokinetics are altered in the aging client because of reduced gastric acid and slowed gastric motility, resulting in unpredictable rates of dissolution and absorption of drugs. Changes in absorption may occur when acid production decreases, altering the absorption of weakly acidic drugs such as barbiturates. However, few studies of drug absorption have shown clinically significant changes occurring with advanced age.

Changes in body composition, such as increased proportion of body fat and decreased total body water, plasma volume, and extracellular fluid, have been noted in the elderly. The increased proportion of body fat increases the body's ability to store fat-soluble compounds such as phenothiazines and barbiturates, and thus increase the accumulation of those drugs. The reduced lean body mass affects drug distribution by decreasing the volume in which the drug circulates, thereby causing higher peak levels. The risk of toxicity with water-soluble drugs increases as total body water decreases. Decreased serum albumin for binding drugs leads to increased amounts of free drug in the circulation. Disorders common to the aging person such as congestive heart failure (CHF), which may impair liver function, influence biotransformation by decreasing the metabolism of drugs and increasing the risk of drug accumulation and toxicity. Renal function may be impaired because of loss of nephrons, decreased blood flow, and glomerular filtration rate. A reduction in renal function is also secondary to CHF. Decreased renal clearance may cause increased plasma drug concentrations and longer half-lives of drugs and active metabolites that the kidney usually excretes. Special precautions include careful monitoring of the elderly client for a safe drug regime.

Problem medications in the elderly

The potent medications available to treat the diseases or illnesses of the elderly often have a narrow index between drug effectiveness and toxicity.

Responsibility of health care providers. The primary responsibility of a health care provider is to reduce or eliminate the potentially adverse risk factors associated with various drug regimens. This can be accomplished by the following:

1. Identify the client at special risk, such as the elderly person with potential altered pharmacokinetics, multiple illnesses, or

liver or kidney impairment. Other factors that may affect selected medications include a history of alcoholism, smoking, or specific dietary habits.

2. Take a complete medication history, preferably in the client's home. Note all medications on hand, ordering physician(s), expiration dates, and their storage. A thorough history should include prescribed drugs, OTC medications, and home remedies (such as herbal or health food store purchases), if used.
3. If unfamiliar with a drug, look it up for its primary and secondary effects. Also check recommended dosage, side and adverse effects, and contraindications.
4. Check all medications for possible drug interactions by using a current reference guide or by consulting a pharmacist.
5. Discuss drug regimen with the primary physician (or encourage the client to do so) if problem areas are identified (for example, duplicate medications have been prescribed, possible drug interactions are present, or the client has had side effects that may be attributable to one or more of the medications).
6. Educate clients on their medications, safe storage, and proper method of disposing of discontinued medications.
7. Monitor therapy closely so that therapeutic response and development of side effects or adverse effects can be detected early in treatment.

Ideally the prescriber will individualize and simplify drug therapy for the client. Keeping medications to a minimum with the least frequent dosage administration necessary will help reduce the potential for drug interactions and also improve client compliance with the drug regimen.

Nursing management of medication administration for geriatric clients

In view of the effects just outlined and the multiplicity of drugs prescribed for elderly clients, their occasionally unreliable memories and senses, inadequate financial status, and propensity for adverse secondary effects, nurses must make every attempt to simplify the geriatric drug therapy plan. Suspect medications as the cause whenever you note a change in an elderly client's behavior, particularly restlessness, irritability, and confusion. These alterations of thought processes may be the earliest signs of drug toxicity. Encourage nursing assistants to report to a nurse any changes they notice in the client's behavior. Often what passes for senility is drug-induced lethargy or confusion.

In the administration of medications, the geriatric client may have special needs. The elderly frequently have dry mucous membranes, which impede swallowing, so offer water before and after oral medications if the client's condition permits. Position the elderly client so that gravity will assist the drug through the esophagus and minimize the possibility of aspiration. Because of diminished sensation, the client may be unaware that the tablet is stuck between the lip and gum, so examine the client's mouth to ensure that the medication has been swallowed. Geriatric clients may have slowed reflexes and reduced understanding of treatment. It helps to organize the dispensing of medication so that enough time is allowed for clients who require a great deal of attention, possibly by medicating them last, and yet so that all clients will receive their medication on time. A nurse has roughly an hour's range in which to distribute all the medications during one administration period.

Diminished taste sensation usually keeps unpalatable drugs from being much of a problem, but many older individuals may have difficulty swallowing, especially if they have sustained a cerebrovascular accident (stroke).

Selection of sites for injectable medications in elderly clients may present the nurse with a challenge. Because muscle mass declines with age, suitable sites for intramuscular injection may be fewer than in younger individuals and will require more skill and effort in palpating to detect muscles of adequate body and size. On the other hand, decreased sensory perception, including perception of pain, may make injections less painful.

Physical problems often interfere with the ability of the older client to comply with prescribed drug regimens. Some older clients may be unable to read labels or locate drugs because of failing eyesight; others, such as arthritic clients, may have difficulty opening bottles (particularly child-proof containers) or handling small pills, while the hard-of-hearing client may not hear all of the instructions. The logistics of obtaining drugs and the economic cost may be a deterrent to complying with therapy. Multiple drug therapy may simply be too complex for the client to manage without assistance. The nurse can simplify drug administration and scheduling as much as possible. Dosage schedules and calendars often help the forgetful client. Drug packaging that is easy to use and clearly labeled, as well as printed directions and drug information, help ensure compliance in the older client.

The elderly client's functional capabilities must be assessed to determine the educational requirements for safe and accurate self-administration of medications in the home. The nurse's creativity and skill are essential in devising teaching plans to enhance client compliance with the home medication regimen. Discuss OTC medications with clients and their family and friends and have them describe in detail how and when they take all medications.

Probably the most important part of the nursing process for aging clients is the nurse's ability to communicate patience, warmth, and understanding and to treat the elderly as persons with dignity and with the ability to reason, to feel, and to contribute.

SECTION II

INDIVIDUAL DRUG MONOGRAPHS

acebutolol
(ase-bute'oh-lole)
Monitan ✤, Sectral
Func. class.: Antihypertensive
Chem. class.: Selective β-blocker; group II antidysrhythmic
Pregnancy category B

Action: Competitively blocks stimulation of β-adrenergic receptor within vascular smooth muscle; produces chronotropic, inotropic activity (decreases rate of SA node discharge, increases recovery time), slows conduction of AV node, decreases heart rate, which decreases O^2 consumption in myocardium; also decreases renin-aldosterone-angiotensin system at high doses, inhibits β_2-receptors in bronchial system (high doses)

➡ **Therapeutic Outcome:** Decreased B/P, heart rate, AV conduction, control of dysrhythmias

Uses: Mild to moderate hypertension, sinus tachycardia, persistent atrial extrasystoles, tachydysrhythmias, prophylaxis of angina pectoris

Investigational uses: Prophylaxis of MI, treatment of angina pectoris, tremor, mitral valve prolapse, thyrotoxicosis, idiopathic hypertrophic subaortic stenosis

Dosage and routes

Hypertension

Adult: PO 400 mg qd or in 2 divided doses; may be increased to desired response

Ventricular dysrhythmia

Adult: PO 200 mg bid, may increase gradually; usual range 600-1200 mg daily

Available forms: Caps 200, 400 mg, tabs 200, 400 mg (Canada only)

Side effects/adverse reactions

CNS: Insomnia, fatigue, dizziness, mental changes, memory loss, hallucinations, depression, lethargy, drowsiness, strange dreams, catatonia
CV: ***Profound hypotension, bradycardia, CHF, cold extremities, postural hypotension, 2nd or 3rd degree heart block***
EENT: Sore throat, dry burning eyes
ENDO: Increased hypoglycemic response to insulin
GI: Nausea, diarrhea, vomiting, ***mesenteric arterial thrombosis, ischemic colitis***
GU: Impotence
HEMA: ***Agranulocytosis, thrombocytopenia, purpura***
INTEG: Rash, fever, alopecia
RESP: ***Bronchospasm,*** dyspnea, wheezing

Contraindications: Hypersensitivity to β-blockers, cardiogenic shock, heart block (2nd or 3rd degree), sinus bradycardia, CHF, cardiac failure

Precautions: Major surgery, pregnancy: **B**, lactation, diabetes mellitus, renal disease, thyroid disease, COPD, asthma, well-compensated heart failure, aortic or mitral valve disease

Pharmacokinetics

Absorption	Well (PO)
Distribution	Crosses placenta, minimal CNS
Metabolism	Liver to diacetolol
Excretion	Kidneys, unchanged
Half-life	8-13 hr diacetolol, 3-4 hr acebutolol

Pharmacodynamics

	PO (ANTIHYPERTENSIVE)	PO (ANTIDYSRHYTHMIAS)
Onset	1-1½ hr	1 hr
Peak	2-4 hr	4-6 hr
Duration	12-24 hr	8-10 hr

Interactions

Drug/drug:

Individual drugs

Alcohol: ↑ hypotension (large amounts)
Epinephrine: Bradycardia stimulation
Hydralazine: ↑ hypotension, bradycardia
Indomethacin: ↓ antihypertensive effect
Insulin: ↑ hypoglycemia
Phenytoin (IV): ↑ myocardial depression
Prazosin: ↑ hypotension, bradycardia
Thyroid: ↓ effectiveness
Verapamil: ↑ myocardial depression

Drug classifications

Antihypertensives: ↑ hypertension
Cardiac glycosides: ↑ bradycardia
Nitrates: ↑ hypotension
Theophyllines: ↓ bronchodilatation

Lab test interferences

Interference: Glucose/insulin tolerance tests
Increase: Uric acid, potassium, triglyceride, lipoproteins

NURSING CONSIDERATIONS

Assessment

- Monitor B/P during beginning treatment, periodically thereafter; pulse q4h; note rate, rhythm, quality; apical/radial pulse before administration; notify prescriber of any significant changes (pulse <50 bpm)
- Check for baselines in renal, liver function tests before therapy begins
- Assess for edema in feet, legs daily, monitor I & O, daily weight; check for jugular vein distention, rales bilaterally, dyspnea (CHF)
- Monitor skin turgor, dryness of mucous membranes for hydration status, especially elderly [G]

Associated nursing diagnoses

- ✓ Cardiac output, decreased (side effects)
- ✓ Injury, risk for physical (side effects)
- ✓ Knowledge deficit (teaching)
- ✓ Noncompliance (teaching)

Implementation

PO route

- Given ac, hs; tablet may be crushed or swallowed whole; give with food to prevent GI upset; reduced dosage in renal dysfunction; check pulse before giving, hold dose and notify prescriber if pulse is <50 bpm
- Store protected from light, moisture; place in cool environment

Patient/family education

- Teach patient not to discontinue drug abruptly, taper over 2 wk; may cause precipitate angina if stopped abruptly
- Teach patient not to use OTC products containing α-adrenergic stimulants (such as nasal decongestants, cold preparations); to avoid alcohol, smoking; and to limit sodium intake as prescribed
- Teach patient how to take pulse and B/P at home, advise when to notify prescriber
- Instruct patient to comply with weight control, dietary adjustments, modified exercise program
- Tell patient to carry/wear Medic Alert ID to identify drug(s) that patient is taking, allergies; tell patient that drug controls symptoms but does not cure
- Caution patient to avoid hazardous activities if dizziness or drowsiness is present
- Teach patient to report symptoms of CHF: difficult breathing, especially on exertion or when lying down, night cough, swelling of extremities or bradycardia, dizziness, confusion, depression, fever
- Teach patient to take drug as prescribed, not to double or skip doses; take any missed doses as soon as remembered if several hours until next dose

Evaluation

Positive therapeutic outcome

- Decreased B/P in hypertension (after 1-2 wk)
- Absence of dysrhythmias

Treatment of overdose:

Lavage, **IV** atropine for bradycardia, **IV** theophylline for bronchospasm, digitalis, O_2, diuretic for cardiac failure, hemodialysis, **IV** glucose for hyperglycemia, **IV** diazepam (or phenytoin) for seizures

acetaminophen

(a-seat-a-mee'noe-fen)

Acetaminophen Uniserts, Anacin-3 Infant's Drops, Anacin-3 Maximum Strength, Apacet, Aspirin Free Pain Relief, Atasol ♣, Banesin, Campain ♣, Children's Feverall, Dapa Extra Strength, Datril Extra-Strength, Dolane, Dorcol Children's Fever and Pain Reducer, Genapap Extra Strength, Genapap Infant's Drops, Genebs Extra Strength, Halenol Children's, Junior Strength Feverall, Liquiprin Elixir, Liquiprin Infant Drops, Meda Cap, Myapap Drops, Oraphen PD, Panadol, Panadol Infant's Drops, Panex-500, Parten, Pedric, Phenaphen Caplets, Redutemp, Robigesic ♣, Rounax ♣, St. Joseph Aspirin-free Infant Drops, Tapanol Extra Strength, Tempra, Tempra Drops, Tylenol, Tylenol Caplets, Tylenol Extra Strength, Tylenol Infant's Drops

Func. class.: Nonnarcotic analgesic

Chem. class.: Nonsalicylate, paraaminophenol derivative

Pregnancy category **B**

Action: May block pain impulses peripherally that occur in response to inhibition of prostaglandin synthesis; does not possess antiinflammatory properties; antipyretic action results from inhibition of prostaglandins in the CNS (hypothalamic heat-regulating center)

➔ **Therapeutic Outcome:** Decreased pain, fever

Uses: Mild to moderate pain or fever

Dosage and routes

P ***Adult and child >10 yr:*** PO 325-650 mg q4h prn, not to exceed 4 g/day; REC 325-650 mg q4h prn, not to exceed 4 g/day

P ***Child 0-3 mo:*** 40 mg/dose

P ***Child 4-11 mo:*** 80 mg/dose

P ***Child <1 yr:*** PO/REC 15-60 mg/dose q4-6h, not to exceed 65 mg/kg/day

P ***Child 1-2 yr:*** PO/REC 60 mg/dose

P ***Child 2-3 yr:*** PO/REC 120 mg/dose

P ***Child 3-4 yr:*** PO/REC 180 mg/dose

P ***Child 4-5 yr:*** PO/REC 240 mg/dose

P ***Child 5-10 yr:*** PO/REC 325 mg/dose

Available forms: Rec supp 120, 125, 325, 600, 650 mg; chewable tabs 80, 160 mg; caps 500 mg; elix 120, 160, 325 mg/5 ml; liq 120, 160 mg/5 ml, 500 mg/15 ml; sol 100 mg/1 ml, 120 mg/2.5 ml; tabs 160, 325, 500, 650 mg; granules 80 mg/pkg or cup

A

Side effects/adverse reactions

CNS: Stimulation, drowsiness
GI: Nausea, vomiting, abdominal pain, ***hepatotoxicity***
HEMA: ***Leukopenia, neutropenia, hemolytic anemia (long-term use), thrombocytopenia, pancytopenia***
INTEG: Rash, urticaria, ***angioedema***
SYST: ***Anaphylaxis***
TOXICITY: ***Cyanosis, anemia, neutropenia, jaundice, pancytopenia, CNS stimulation, delirium followed by vascular collapse, convulsions, coma, death***

Contraindications: Hypersensitivity; intolerance to tartrazine (yellow dye no. 5), alcohol, table sugar, saccharin

Precautions: Anemia, hepatic disease, renal disease, chronic alcoholism, pregnancy **B**, G elderly, lactation

Pharmacokinetics

Absorption	Well absorbed (PO), variable (rec)
Distribution	Widely distributed; crosses placenta
Metabolism	Liver 85%-95%; metabolites are toxic at high levels
Excretion	Kidneys—metabolites, breast milk
Half-life	3-4 hr

Pharmacodynamics

	PO	REC
Onset	½-1 hr	½-1 hr
Peak	1-3 hr	1-3 hr
Duration	3-4 hr	3-4 hr

Interactions

Drug/drug:

Individual drugs
Alcohol: ↑ hepatotoxicity
Caffeine: ↑ effects of acetaminophen
Cholestyramine: ↓ effects of acetaminophen
Colestipol: ↓ effects of acetaminophen

NURSING CONSIDERATIONS

Assessment

- Monitor liver function studies: AST (SGOT), ALT (SGPT) bilirubin, creatinine before therapy if long-term therapy is anticipated
- Monitor renal function studies: BUN, urine creatinine, occult blood; albumin indicates nephritis
- Monitor blood studies: CBC, pro-time if patient is on long-term therapy
- Check I&O ratio; decreasing output may indicate renal failure (long-term therapy)
- Assess for fever and pain: type of pain, location, intensity, duration, temperature, diaphoresis
- Assess mucosa, fingernail beds for cyanosis; inquire about dyspnea, vertigo, headache, weakness; symptoms indicate methemoglobinemia; notify prescriber immediately
- Assess for chronic poisoning: rapid, weak pulse, dyspnea, cold, clammy extremities; report immediately to prescriber
- Assess hepatotoxicity: dark urine, clay-colored stools, yellowing of skin and sclera; itching, abdominal pain, fever, diarrhea if patient is on long-term therapy

• Assess allergic reactions: rash, urticaria; if these occur, drug may have to be discontinued

Associated nursing diagnoses

✓ Pain (uses)
✓ Mobility, impaired physical mobility (uses)
✓ Injury, risk for (side effects)
✓ Knowledge deficit (teaching)

Implementation

PO route

• Administer to patient crushed or whole; chewable tabs may be chewed
• Give with food or milk to decrease gastric symptoms; give 30 min before or 2 hr after meals; absorption may be slowed

Patient/family education

• Teach patient not to exceed recommended dosage; acute poisoning with liver damage may result; acute toxicity includes symptoms of nausea, vomiting, and abdominal pain; prescriber should be notified immediately
• Tell patient to read label on other OTC drugs; many contain acetaminophen and may cause toxicity if taken concurrently
• Teach patient to recognize signs of chronic overdose: bleeding, bruising, malaise, fever, sore throat
• Inform patient that urine may become dark brown as a result of phenacetin (metabolite of acetaminophen)
• Tell patient to notify prescriber for pain or fever lasting over 3 days

Evaluation

Positive therapeutic outcome

• Decreased pain
• Decreased fever

Treatment of overdose: Drug level q4h, gastric lavage, activated charcoal; administer oral acetylcysteine to prevent hepatic damage (see acetylcysteine monograph, p. 63)

acetazolamide

(a-set-a-zolé-a-mide)

Acetazolam ✤, Generic acetazolamide, AK-ZOL, Diamox, Diamox sequels, Hydrazol, Diamox Parenteral

Func. class.: Diuretic carbonic anhydrase inhibitor

Chem. class.: Sulfonamide derivative

Pregnancy category **C**

Action: Decreases the aqueous humor in the eye, which lowers intraocular pressure by the inhibition of carbonic anhydrase; also inhibits carbonic anhydrase activity in proximal renal tubules to decrease reabsorption of water, sodium, potassium, bicarbonate; decreases carbonic anhydrase in CNS, increasing seizure threshold; prevents uric acid or cystine buildup in the renal system by the decrease in pH causing alkaline urine

➔ **Therapeutic Outcome:** Decreased intraocular pressure;

control of seizures; prevention and treatment of acute mountain sickness; prevention of uric acid/cystine renal stones; decreased edema in lung tissue and peripherally; decreased B/P

Uses: Open angle glaucoma, narrow angle glaucoma (preoperatively if surgery delayed), epilepsy (petit mal, grand mal, mixed), edema in CHF, drug-induced edema, acute mountain sickness

Investigational uses: Prevention of uric acid/cystine renal stones

Dosage and routes

Closed angle glaucoma

Adult: PO/IM/**IV** 250 mg q4h or 250 mg bid, to be used for short-term therapy or 500 mg ES bid

Open angle glaucoma

Adult: PO/IM/**IV** 250 mg-1g/day in divided doses for amounts over 250 mg

Edema

Adult: IM/**IV** 250-375 mg/day in AM

P *Child:* IM/**IV** 5 mg/kg/day in AM

Seizures

Adult: PO/IM/**IV** 8-30 mg/kg/day, usual range 375-1000 mg/day in divided doses tid or qid, or 300-900 mg/m^2/day, not to exceed 1.5 g/day

Mountain sickness

Adult: PO 250 mg q8-12h

Renal stones

Adult: PO 250 mg hs

Available forms: Tabs 125, 250 mg; caps ext rel 500 mg; inj IM/**IV** 500 mg

Side effects/adverse reactions

CNS: Drowsiness, paresthesia, anxiety, depression, headache, dizziness, confusion, stimulation, fatigue, ***convulsions,*** sedation, nervousness
EENT: Myopia, tinnitus
ENDO: Hyperglycemia, hypokalemia, hypocalcemia, hypomagnesemia, hyponatremia, hyperchloremia
GI: Nausea, vomiting, anorexia, constipation, diarrhea, melena, weight loss, ***hepatic insufficiency,*** taste alterations
GU: Frequency, hypokalemia, polyuria, ***uremia,*** glucosuria, hematuria, dysuria, crystalluria, renal calculi
HEMA: **Aplastic anemia, hemolytic anemia, leukopenia, agranulocytosis, thrombocytopenia, purpura, pancytopenia**
INTEG: Rash, pruritus, urticaria, fever, ***Stevens-Johnson syndrome,*** photosensitivity

Contraindications: Hypersensitivity to sulfonamides, severe renal disease, severe hepatic disease, electrolyte imbalances, (hyponatremia, hypokalemia), hyperchloremic acidosis, Addison's disease, long-term use in narrow angle glaucoma

Precautions: Hypercalcemia, pregnancy **C**

Pharmacokinetics

Absorption	GI tract–65% if fasting (75%) with food); IV—complete
Distribution	Crosses placenta; widely distributed
Metabolism	None
Excretion	Kidneys, unchanged (80% within 24 hr), breast milk
Half-life	2½-5½ hr

Pharmacodynamics

	PO	PO–EXT REL	IV
Onset	1½ hr	2 hr	2 min
Peak	2-4 hr	8-12 hr	15 min
Duration	6-12 hr	18-24 hr	4-5 hr

Interactions

Drug/drug:

Individual drugs

Amphotericin B: ↑ hypokalemia
Aspirin: ↑ excretion of aspirin
Ephedrine: ↑ action, toxicity
Flecainide: ↑ action, toxicity
Lithium: ↑ excretion of lithium
Procainamide: ↑ action, toxicity
Pseudoephedrine: ↑ action

Drug classifications

Amphetamines: ↑ action
Barbiturates: ↑ excretion
Diuretics: ↑ hypokalemia
Salicylates: ↑ toxicity
Tricyclics, antidepressants: ↑ action, toxicity

Lab test interferences

False positive: Urinary protein, 17-hydroxysteroids

NURSING CONSIDERATIONS

Assessment

- Assess patient for tinnitus, hearing loss, ear pain; periodic testing of hearing is needed when high doses of this drug are given by **IV** route
- Monitor manifestations of hypokalemia: *RENAL:* acidic urine, reduced urine osmolality, nocturia, polyuria, polydipsia; *CARDIAC:* hypotension, broad T wave, U wave, ectopy, tachycardia, weak pulse; *NEURO:* muscle weakness, altered LOC, drowsiness, apathy, lethargy, confusion, depression; *GI:* anorexia, nausea, cramps, constipation, distention, paralytic ileus; *RESP:* hypoventilation, respiratory muscle weakness
- Monitor for CNS, GI, cardiovascular, integumentary, neurologic manifestations of hypocalcemia: *CNS:* personality changes, anxiety, disturbances, depression, psychosis, nausea, vomiting; *GI:* constipation, abdominal pain from muscle spasm; *CV:* decreased contractility, decreased cardiac output, hypotension, lengthened ST segment, prolonged QT interval; *INTEG:* scaling eczema, alopecia, hyperpigmentation; *NEURO:* tetany, muscle twitching, cramping, grimacing, seizure, altered deep tendon reflexes, spasm
- Monitor for manifestations of hypomagnesemia: *CNS:* agitation; *NEURO:* muscle twitching, paresthesias, hyperactive reflexes, positive Babinski's reflex, dysphagia, nystagmus seizures, tetany; *GI:* nausea, vomiting, diarrhea, anorexia, abdominal distention;

CARDIAC: ectopy, tachycardia, broad, flat or inverted T waves, depressed ST segment, prolonged QT, decreased cardiac output, hypotension

- Monitor for manifestations of hyponatremia: *CV:* increased B/P, cold, clammy skin, hypovolemia, or hypervolemia, vomiting, diarrhea, abdominal cramps; *NEURO:* lethagy, increased intracranial pressure, confusion, headache, seizures, coma, fatigue, tremors, hyperreflexia
- Monitor for manifestations of hyperchloremia: *NEURO:* weakness, lethargy, coma; *RESP:* deep, rapid breathing
- Assess fluid volume status: I&O ratio and record, count or weigh diapers as appropriate, distended neck veins, crackles in lung, color, quality and sp gr of urine, skin turgor, adequacy of pulses, moist mucous membranes, bilateral lung sounds, peripheral pitting edema; dehydration symptoms of decreasing output, thirst, hypotension, dry mouth, and mucous membranes should be reported
- Monitor electrolytes: potassium, sodium, calcium, magnesium; also include BUN, blood pH, ABGs, uric acid, CBC, blood sugar
- Assess B/P before and during therapy with patient lying, standing, and sitting as appropriate; orthostatic hypotension can occur rapidly
- Monitor blood, urine glucose in diabetic patients; glucose levels may be increased
- Assess for eye pain, change in vision when using drug for intraocular pressure
- Assess neurologic status when using drug for seizures
- Assess for decreased symptoms of acute mountain sickness: headache, nausea, vomiting, dizziness, fatigue, drowsiness, shortness of breath, insomnia

Associated nursing diagnoses

- ✓ Sensory-perceptual alterations: visual (uses)
- ✓ Fluid volume deficit (side effects)
- ✓ Fluid volume excess (uses)
- ✓ Knowledge deficit (teaching)

Implementation

- Give in AM to avoid interference with sleep
- Administer fluids 2-3 L/day to prevent renal calculi, unless contraindicated
- Potassium replacement if potassium level is <3.0 whole

PO route

- Give with food, if nausea occurs, crush tabs and mix with sweet substance to counteract bitter taste; ES caps may be opened and sprinkled on food; do not crush or chew caps

IV **IV route**

- Do not use solution that is yellow or has a precipitate or crystals

IV: Dilute 500 mg of drug/5 ml or more sterile water for inj: use within 24 hr

***Direct* IV:** Give over 1 min or more

Intermittent infusion: May be added to NS, D_5W, $D_{10}W$, 0.45% NaCl; give over 4-8 hr

Additive compatibility:

Cimetidine

Additive incompatibilities: Multivitamins

Patient/family education

- Teach patient to take the medication early in the day to prevent nocturia
- Instruct patient to take with food or milk if GI symptoms of nausea and anorexia occur
- Teach patient to maintain a record of weight on a weekly basis and notify prescriber of weight loss of >5 lb
- Caution patient that this drug causes a loss of potassium so food rich in potassium should be added to the diet; refer to a dietician for assistance in planning
- Advise patient to wear protective clothing and sunscreen in the sun to prevent photosensitivity
- Teach patient not to use alcohol or any OTC medications without prescriber's approval; serious drug reactions may occur
- Emphasize the need to contact prescriber immediately if muscle cramps, weakness, nausea, dizziness, or numbness occurs
- Teach patient to take own B/P and pulse and record
- Teach patient to continue taking medication even if feeling better; this drug controls symptoms but does not cure the condition
- Teach patient to see ophthalmologist periodically; glaucoma is a slow process

Evaluation

Positive therapeutic outcome

- Decreased intraocular pressure
- Decreased edema
- Decreased seizures
- Prevention of mountain sickness
- Prevention of uric acid/cystine stones

Treatment of overdose: Lavage if taken orally, monitor electrolytes, administer dextrose in saline, monitor hydration, CV, renal status

acetohexamide

(a-set-oh-hex'a-mide)

acetohexamide, Dimelor ✤, Dymelor

Func. class.: Antidiabetic, oral

Chem. class.: Sulfonylurea (1st generation)

Pregnancy category C

Action: Causes functioning β-cells in pancreas to release insulin, leading to drop in blood glucose levels; may improve binding between insulin and insulin receptors or increase number of insulin receptors with prolonged administration; may also reduce basal hepatic glucose secretion; not effective if patient lacks functioning β-cells

➔ **Therapeutic Outcome:** Decreased blood glucose levels in diabetes mellitus

Uses: Stable adult-onset diabetes mellitus (type II), NIDDM

Dosage and routes

Adult: PO 250 mg-1.5 g/day; usually given before breakfast, unless large dose is required; then dose is divided in two

Available forms: Tabs 250, 500 mg scored

Side effects/adverse reactions

CNS: Headache, weakness, tinnitus, fatigue, dizziness, vertigo
ENDO: Hypoglycemia, hyponatremia
GI: Nausea, vomiting, diarrhea, ***hepatotoxicity, jaundice,*** heartburn
HEMA: Leukopenia, thrombocytopenia, agranulocytosis, aplastic anemia, hemolytic anemia, increased AST (SGOT), ALT (SGPT), alkaline phosphatase
INTEG: Rash, allergic reactions, pruritus, urticaria, eczema, photosensitivity, erythema

Contraindications: Hypersensitivity to sulfonylureas, juvenile or brittle diabetes, renal failure

Precautions: Pregnancy **C**, G elderly, cardiac disease, renal disease, hepatic disease, thyroid disease, severe hypoglycemic reactions

Pharmacokinetics

Absorption	Well absorbed (PO)
Distribution	Bile
Metabolism	Liver to metabolites
Excretion	Kidneys
Half-life	Parent drug 1.3 hr, metabolites 6 hr

Pharmacodynamics

	PO
Onset	10-30 min
Peak	½-2 hr
Duration	3-4 hr

Interactions

Drug/drug:

Individual drugs

Cimetidine: ↑ hypoglycemia
Chloramphenicol: ↑ hypoglycemia
Diazoxide: ↓ effect of both drugs
Guanethidine: ↑ hypoglycemia
Insulin: ↑ hypoglycemia
Methyldopa: ↑ hypoglycemia
Phenytoin: ↓ action of acetohexamide
Rifampin: ↓ action of acetohexamide

Drug classifications

Anticoagulants, oral: ↑ hypoglycemia
Corticosteroids: ↓ action of acetohexamide
Diuretics, thiazide: ↓ action of acetohexamide
Estrogens: ↓ action of acetohexamide
MAOI: ↑ hypoglycemia
NSAIDs: ↑ hypoglycemia
Oral contraceptives: ↓ action of acetohexamide
Phenothiazines: ↓ action of acetohexamide
Salicylates: ↑ hypoglycemia
Sulfonamides: ↑ hypoglycemia

NURSING CONSIDERATIONS

Assessment

• Assess for hypoglycemic/hyperglycemic reactions that can occur soon after meals; hypoglycemic reactions: sweating, weakness, dizziness, anxiety, tremors, hunger

- Monitor CBC (baseline, q3mo) during treatment; check liver function tests (AST [SGOT], LDH) periodically and renal studies (BUN, creatinine) during treatment

Associated nursing diagnoses

- ✓ Nutrition, altered: More than body requirements (uses)
- ✓ Nutrition altered: Less than body requirements (adverse reactions)
- ✓ Injury, risk for physical (adverse reactions)
- ✓ Knowledge deficit (teaching)
- ✓ Noncompliance (teaching)

Implementation

- Conversion from other oral hypoglycemic agents or insulin dosage of <40 U/day, change may be made without gradual dosage change; patients taking insulin of >40 U/day convert gradually by receiving oral hypoglycemic and 50% of previous insulin dosage for 3-5 days; monitor serum or urine glucose and ketones 3 times/day during conversion

PO route

- Give drug 30 min before breakfast; if large dose is required, may be divided into two; give with meals to decrease GI upset and provide best absorption
- Give tabs crushed and mixed with meal or fluids for patients with difficulty swallowing
- Store in tight container in cool environment

Patient/family education

- Teach patient to check for symptoms of cholestatic jaundice: dark urine, pruritus, yellow sclera; if these occur, notify prescriber
- Teach patient to use capillary blood glucose test or Chemstrip 3 times a day
- Teach patient symptoms of hypoglycemia and hyperglycemia and what to do about each
- Tell patient that drug use must be continued daily; explain consequence of discontinuing drug use abruptly
- Teach patient to take drug in AM to prevent hypoglycemic reactions at night
- Tell patient to avoid OTC medications unless prescribed
- Teach patient that diabetes is lifelong illness; that this drug is not a cure
- Tell patient that all food included in diet plan must be eaten to prevent hypoglycemia
- Tell patient to carry Medic Alert ID for emergency purposes and to carry a glucagon emergency kit

Evaluation

Positive therapeutic outcome

- Decrease in polyuria, polydipsia, polyphagia; clear sensorium, absence of dizziness, stable gait, blood glucose, WNL

Treatment of overdose:

Glucose 25 g **IV**, via dextrose 50% sol, 50 ml or 1 mg glucagon

acetylcysteine ⊶

(a-se-til-sis'tay-een)

Airbron ♣, Mucomyst, Mucosil

Func. class.: Mucolytic; antidote—acetaminophen

Chem. class.: Amino acid L-cysteine

Pregnancy category **B**

Action: Decreases viscosity of secretions in respiratory tract by breaking disulfide links of mucoproteins; increases hepatic glutathione, which is necessary to inactivate toxic metabolites in acetaminophen overdose

➔ **Therapeutic Outcome:** Decreased hepatotoxicity from acetaminophen overdose (PO); decreased viscosity of mucus in respiratory disorders (inh)

Uses: Acetaminophen toxicity; bronchitis; pneumonia; cystic fibrosis; emphysema; atelectasis; tuberculosis; complications of thoracic surgery and cardiovascular surgery; diagnosis in bronchial lab tests

Dosage and routes

Mucolytic

P *Adult and child:* Inh 2-20 ml (10% sol) q1-4h prn, or 1-10 ml (20% sol)

Acetaminophen toxicity

P *Adult and child:* PO 140 mg/kg, then 70 mg/kg q4h × 17 doses to total 1330 mg/kg

Available forms: Sol 10%, 20%

Side effects/adverse reactions

CNS: ***Dizziness, drowsiness,*** headache, fever, chills

CV: Hypotension

EENT: *Rhinorrhea,* tooth damage

GI: *Nausea,* stomatitis, constipation, vomiting, anorexia, ***hepatotoxicity***

INTEG: Urticaria, rash, fever, clamminess

RESP: ***Bronchospasm,*** burning, ***hemoptysis,*** chest tightness

Contraindications: Hypersensitivity, increased intracranial pressure, status asthmaticus

Precautions: Hypothyroidism, Addison's disease, CNS depression, brain tumor, asthma, hepatic disease, renal disease, COPD, psychosis, alcoholism, convulsive disorders, lactation, pregnancy **B**

Pharmacokinetics

Absorption	Extensive (PO), locally (INH)
Distribution	Unknown
Metabolism	Liver
Excretion	Kidneys
Half-life	Unknown

Pharmacodynamics

	PO	INH
Onset	Unknown	1 min
Peak	Unknown	Unknown
Duration	up to 4 hr	5-10 min

Interactions

Drug/drug:

Individual drugs

Activated charcoal: ↓ absorption of acetylcysteine

Iron, copper, rubber: Do not use with acetylcysteine

NURSING CONSIDERATIONS

Assessment

Mucolytic use

• Assess cough: type, frequency, character, including sputum

• Assess characteristics, rate, rhythm of respirations, increased dyspnea; discontinue if bronchospasm occurs; ABGs for increased CO_2 retention in asthma patients

• Monitor VS, cardiac status including checking for dysrhythmias, increased rate, palpitations

Antidotal use

• Assess liver function tests, acetaminophen levels; inform prescriber if dose is vomited or vomiting is persistent; provide adequate hydration; decrease dosage in hepatic encephalopathy

Associated nursing diagnoses

✓ Injury, risk for physical (uses) (antidote)

✓ Impaired gas exchange (uses) (mucolytic)

✓ Airway clearance ineffective (uses) (mucolytic)

✓ Poisoning, risk for (uses) (antidote)

✓ Knowledge deficit (teaching)

Implementation

• Give decreased dosage to G elderly patients; their metabolism may be slowed; give gum, hard candy, frequent rinsing of mouth for dryness of oral cavity

• Use only if suction machine is available

PO route: *Antidotal use*

• Lavage, then give within 24 hr; give with cola or soft drink to disguise taste; can be given with H_2O through tubes; use within 1 hr

• **Inh route:** *Mucolytic use*

• Use ac ½-1 hr for better absorption, to decrease nausea; only after patient clears airway by deep breathing, coughing

• Give by syringe 2-3 doses of 1-2 ml of 20% or 2-4 ml of 10% sol; 20% sol diluted with NS or water for injection; may give 10% sol undiluted

• Store in refrigerator: use within 96 hr of opening

• Provide assistance with inhaled dose: bronchodilator if bronchospasm occurs; wash face and rinse mouth after use to remove sticky feeling

• Use mechanical suction if cough insufficient to remove excess bronchial secretions

Patient/family education

Mucolytic use

• Tell patient to avoid driving or other hazardous activities until patient is stabilized on this medication; avoid alcohol, other CNS depressants; will enhance sedating properties of this drug

• Teach patient that unpleasant odor will decrease after repeated use; that discoloration of solution after bottle is opened does not impair its effectiveness; avoid smoking, smoke-filled rooms, perfume, dust, environmental pollutants, cleaners

Evaluation

Positive therapeutic outcome
- Absence of purulent secretions when coughing (mucolytic use)
- Clear lung sounds bilaterally (mucolytic use)
- Absence of hepatic damage (acetaminophen toxicity)
- Decreasing blood toxicology (acetaminophen toxicity)

acrivastine/ pseudoephedrine

Semprex-D
Func. class.: Antihistamine
Chem. class.: H_1-histamine antagonist
Pregnancy category **B**

Action: Acts on blood vessels, GI, respiratory system by competing with histamine for H_1-receptor site; decreases allergic response by blocking pharmacologic effects of histamine; less sedation rate than with other histamines; causes increased heart rate, vasodilation, increased secretions

Therapeutic Outcome: Absence of allergy symptoms and rhinitis

Uses: Rhinitis, allergy symptoms, chronic idiopathic urticaria

Dosage and routes

P *Adult and child > 12 yr:* PO 8 mg q4-6 hrs

Available forms: Caps 8 mg/60 mg

Side effects/adverse reactions

CNS: ***Headache,*** dizziness, nervousness, insomnia
GI: ***Nausea,*** dry mouth
GU: Dysmenorrhea
RESP: Cough, pharyngitis

Contraindications: Hypersensitivity to this drug or triprolidine, severe hypertension, cardiac disease

Precautions: Pregnancy **B,** G elderly, P children, respiratory disease, hypertension, diabetes mellitus, ignemic heart disease, increased intraocular pressure, prostate hypertrophy

Pharmacokinetics

Absorption	Well absorbed (PO), rapidly
Distribution	Not known
Metabolism	Liver
Excretion	Kidneys, feces
Half-life	1½ hr

Pharmacodynamics

	PO
Onset	Unknown
Peak	1-1½ hr
Duration	12 hr

Interactions

Drug/drug:

Individual drugs
Alcohol: ↑ CNS depression

Drug classifications

Beta agonists: Hypertensive crisis

MAOI: Hypertensive crisis

Narcotics: ↑ CNS depression

Sedative/hypnotics: ↑ CNS depression

Lab test interferences

False negative: Skin allergy tests (discontinue antihistamine 3 days before testing)

NURSING CONSIDERATIONS

Assessment

- Assess respiratory status: rate, rhythm, increase in bronchial secretions, wheezing, chest tightness; provide fluids to 2L/day to decrease secretions thickness

Associated nursing diagnoses

✓ Airway clearance, ineffective (uses)

✓ Knowledge deficit (teaching)

Implementation

PO route

- Give with food or fluid for GI symptoms
- Store in tight, light-resistant container

Patient/family education

- Teach all aspects of drug usage; to avoid driving or other hazardous activity if drowsiness occurs; to avoid alcohol or other CNS depressants that may potentiate effect
- Caution patient not to exceed recommended dose
- Advise patient hard candy, gum, frequent rinsing of mouth may be used for dryness

Evaluation

Positive therapeutic response

- Absence of running or congested nose, rashes

Treatment of overdose:

Administer ipecac syrup or lavage, diazepam, vasopressors, barbiturates (short-acting)

activated charcoal

Acta-char, Acta-Char Liquid-A, Actidose-Aqua, Aqueous Charcodote ✤, Charac-50 ✤, Charcoaide, Charcocaps, Charcodote, Charcotabs, Digestalin, Insta-Char, Insta-Char Aqueous Suspension, Liqu-Char, Super-Char, Super-Char Aqueous

Func. class.: Antiflatulent/antidote

Pregnancy category **C**

Action: Binds poisons, toxins, irritants; increases adsorption in GI tract; inactivates toxins and binds until excreted

➔ **Therapeutic Outcome:** Prevention of toxicity and death resulting from absorption of drugs

Uses: Flatulence, poisoning, dyspepsia, distention, deodorant in wounds, diarrhea

Dosage and routes

Poisoning

P ***Adult and child:*** PO 5-10 × weight of substance ingested; minimum dosage 30 g/250 ml of water; may give 20-40g q6h for 1-2 days in severe poisoning

Flatulence/dyspepsia

Adult: PO 520-975 mg pc up to 4.16 g/day

Available forms: Powder 15, 30, 40, 120, 125, 240 g/container; oral susp 12.5 g/60 ml, 15 g/72 ml, 15 g/120 ml, 25 g/120 ml, 30 g/120 ml, 50 g/240 ml; Canada 15 g/120 ml, 25 g/125 ml, 50 g/225 ml, 50 g/250 ml

Side effects/adverse reactions

GI: Nausea, black stools, vomiting, constipation, diarrhea

Contraindications: Hypersensitivity to this drug, unconsciousness, semiconsciousness, poisoning of cyanide, mineral acids, alkalies

Precautions: Pregnancy **C**

Pharmacokinetics	
Absorption	None
Distribution	None
Metabolism	None
Excretion	Feces (unchanged)
Half-life	Unknown

Pharmacodynamics	PO
Onset	1 min
Peak	Unknown
Duration	4-12 hr

Interactions

Drug/drug:

Individual drugs

Ipecac: ↓ effectiveness of both drugs

Drug classifications

Laxatives: ↓ effectiveness of both drugs

Drug/food:

Dairy products: ↓ effect of activated charcoal

NURSING CONSIDERATIONS

Assessment

- Assess neurologic status including LOC, pupil reactivity, cough reflex, gag reflex, and swallowing ability before administration; do not give if neurologic status is impaired; aspiration may occur unless a protected airway is present
- Assess toxin, poison ingested, time of ingestion, and amount
- Monitor respiration, pulse, B/P to determine charcoal effectiveness if taken for barbiturate/narcotic poisoning

Associated nursing diagnoses

- ✓ Injury, risk for (uses)
- ✓ Poisoning, risk for (uses)
- ✓ Knowledge deficit (teaching)

Implementation

PO route

- Give after inducing vomiting unless vomiting contraindicated (i.e., cyanide or alkalies); mix with 8 oz water or fruit juice to form thick syrup; do not use dairy products to mix charcoal; repeat dose if vomiting occurs soon after dose

• Space at least 2 hr before or after other drugs, or absorption will be decreased; use a laxative to promote elimination; constipation occurs often
• Give alone; do not administer with ipecac; give through a nasogastric tube, if patient unable to swallow, dilute to a less thick sol; keep container tightly closed to prevent absorption of gases

Patient/family education

• Tell patient stools will be black
• Teach patient about overdose/poison prevention and about keeping poison control chart available

Evaluation

Positive therapeutic outcome
• Alert, PERL (poisoning)
• Absence of distention
• Absence of odor in wounds

acyclovir

(ay-sye′kloe-ver)
Zovirax
Func. class.: Antiviral
Chem. class.: Acylic purine nucleoside analog
Pregnancy category **C**

Action: Interferes with DNA synthesis by conversion to acyclovir triphosphate, causing decreased viral replication, time of lesional healing

Therapeutic Outcome: Decreased amount and time of healing of lesions

Uses: Mucocutaneous herpes simplex virus, herpes genitalis (HSV-1, HSV-2), herpes zoster; simple mucocutaneous herpes simplex, in immunocompromised clients with initial herpes genitalis; herpes simplex encephalitis

Dosage and routes

Herpes simplex

P *Adult and child >12 yr:* **IV** inf 5 mg/kg over 1 hr q8h × 5 days

P *Child <12 yr:* **IV** inf 250 mg/m^2 over 1 hr q8h × 5 days

Genital herpes

Adult: PO 200 mg q4h 5 times a day while awake × 5 days to 6 mo depending on whether initial, recurrent, or chronic

P *Adult and child:* top apply to all lesions q3h while awake, 6 times a days × 1 wk

Herpes simplex encephalitis

P *Child >6 mo:* **IV** 500 mg/m^2 q8h × 10 days

Herpes zoster

Adult: PO 800 mg q4h while awake × 7-10 days; **IV** 5 mg/kg q8h

Children with immunosuppression

P *Child >2 yr:* 20 mg/kg qid × 5 days

Available forms: Caps 200 mg; inj **IV** 500 mg; top ointment 5% (50 mg/g); tabs, susp

Side effects/adverse reactions

CNS: Tremors, confusion, lethargy, hallucinations, ***convulsions, dizziness, headache,*** encephalopathic changes
EENT: Gingival hyperplasia
GI: Nausea, vomiting, diarrhea, increased ALT (SGPT), AST (SGOT), abdominal pain, glossitis, colitis
GU: ***Oliguria, proteinuria, hematuria,*** vaginitis, moniliasis, ***glomerulonephritis, acute renal failure,*** changes in menses, polydipsia
INTEG: Rash, urticaria, pruritus, pain or phlebitis at **IV** site, unusual sweating, alopecia, stinging, burning, vulvitis
MS: Joint pain, leg pain, muscle cramps

Contraindications: Hypersensitivity

Precautions: Lactation, hepatic disease, renal disease, electrolyte imbalance, dehydration, pregnancy **C**

Pharmacokinetics

Absorption	Minimal (PO)
Distribution	Widely distributed, crosses placenta, CSF concentration 50% plasma
Metabolism	Liver, minimal
Excretion	Kidneys, 95% unchanged
Half-life	2.0-3.5 hr, increased in renal disease

Pharmacodynamics

	PO	IV	TOP
Onset	Unknown	Rapid	Unknown
Peak	1½-2½	Infusion's end	Unknown

Interactions

Drug/drug:

Individual drugs

Amphotericin B: ↑ neurotoxicity, nephrotoxicity
Interferon: ↑ neurotoxicity, nephrotoxicity
Methotrexate: ↑ neurotoxicity
Probenecid: ↑ neurotoxicity, nephrotoxicity

Drug classification

Aminoglycosides: ↑ neurotoxicity, nephrotoxicity

NURSING CONSIDERATIONS

Assessment

- Monitor for signs of infection, type of lesions, area of body covered, purulent drainage
- Check I&O ratio; report hematuria, oliguria, fatigue, weakness; may indicate nephrotoxicity; check for protein in urine during treatment
- Monitor any patient with compromised renal system, since drug is excreted slowly in poor renal system function; toxicity may occur rapidly
- Monitor liver studies: AST (SGOT), ALT (SGPT)
- Monitor blood studies: WBC, RBC, Hct, Hgb, bleeding time; blood dyscrasias may occur; drug should be discontinued
- Monitor renal studies: urinalysis, protein, BUN, creatinine, CrCl; increased BUN, creatinine indicates renal failure
- Obtain C&S before drug therapy; drug may be taken as soon as culture is taken; repeat C&S after treatment; determine the presence of other sexually transmitted diseases

- Monitor bowel pattern before, during treatment; if severe abdominal pain with bleeding occurs, drug should be discontinued
- Assess allergies before treatment, reaction of each medication; place allergies on chart in bright red letters; allergic reaction: burning, stinging, swelling, redness, rash, vulvitis, pruritus

Associated nursing diagnoses

✓ Infection, risk for (uses)
✓ Knowledge deficit (teaching)

Implementation

PO route

- Give with food to lessen GI symptoms
- Store at room temperature in dry place

Topical route

- Use finger cot or rubber glove to prevent further infection
- Enough medication to cover lesions completely
- After cleansing with soap and water before each application, dry well

IV **IV route**

- Provide increased fluids to 3 L/day to decrease crystalluria when given **IV**
- Give by int inf after reconstituting with 10 ml sterile water for injection/500 mg of drug (50 mg/ml); shake; dilute in 0.9% NaCl, LR, D_5W, D_5/0.25% NaCl, D_5/0.45% NaCl, D_5/0.9% NaCl (7 mg/ml); give over at least 1 hr (constant rate) by infusion pump to prevent nephrotoxicity; do not reconstitute with sol containing benzyl alcohol or parabens; check infusion site for redness, pain, induration; rotate sites
- Lower dosage in acute or chronic renal failure
- Store at room temperature for up to 12 hr after reconstitution; if refrigerated, sol may show a precipitate that clears at room temperature

Y-*site compatibilities:*

Amikacin, ampicillin, cefamandole, cefazolin, cefonicid, cefoperazone, ceforanide, cefotaxime, cefoxitin, ceftazidime, ceftizoxime, ceftriaxone, cefuroxime, cephapirin, chloramphenicol, cimetidine, clindamycin, co-trimoxazole, dexamethasone sodium phosphate, dimenhydrinate, diphenhydramine, erythromycin lactobionate, gentamicin, heparin, hydrocortisone sodium succinate, hydromorphone, imipenem/cilastatin, lorazepam, magnesium sulfate, meperidine, methylprednisolone sodium succinate, metoclopramide, metronidazole, morphine, multivitamin infusion, nafcillin, oxacillin, penicillin G potassium, pentobarbital, perphenazine, piperacillin, potassium chloride, ranitidine, sodium bicarbonate, tetracycline, theophylline, ticarcillin, tobramycin, vancomycin, zidovudine

Y-*site incompatibilities:*

Dobutamine, dopamine, ondansetron, verapamil

Additive incompatibilities:

Blood products, protein-containing solutions, dobutamine, dopamine

Patient/family education

Topical route

• Tell patient not to use in eyes; for use when there is no evidence of infection; apply with glove to prevent further infection

• Instruct patient to avoid use of OTC creams, ointments, lotions unless directed by prescriber; may cause reinfection, delayed healing

• Teach patient to use asepsis (hand washing) before, after each application and avoid contact with eyes; to adhere strictly to prescribed regimen to maximize successful treatment outcome

PO route

• Teach patient that drug may be taken orally before infection occurs; that drug should be taken when itching or pain occurs, usually before eruptions; that partners need to be told that patient has herpes; they can become infected, so condoms must be worn to prevent reinfections; that drug does not cure infection, just controls symptoms and does not prevent infection to others

• Tell patient to report sore throat, fever, fatigue; may indicate superinfection; that drug must be taken in equal intervals around the clock to maintain blood levels for duration of therapy

• Tell patient to notify prescriber of side effects: bruising, bleeding, fatigue, malaise; may indicate blood dyscrasias

• Tell patient to seek dental care during treatment to prevent gingival hyperplasia

• Teach female patients with genital herpes to have regular Pap smears to prevent undetected cervical cancer

Evaluation

Positive therapeutic outcome

• Absence of itching, painful lesions

• Crusting and healed lesions

Treatment of overdose:
Discontinue drug, hemodialysis, resuscitate if needed

adenosine

(ah-den'oh-seen)

Adenocard

Func. class.: Antidysrhythmic misc.

Chem. class.: Endogenous nucleoside

Pregnancy category **C**

Action: Slows conduction through AV node, can interrupt reentry pathways through AV node, and can restore normal sinus rhythm in patients with paroxysmal supraventricular tachycardia (PSVT)

➡ Therapeutic Outcome: Normal sinus rhythm in patients diagnosed with PSVT

Uses: PSVT

Dosage and routes

Adult: **IV** bol 6 mg; if conversion to normal sinus rhythm does not occur within 1-2 min, give 12 mg by rapid **IV** bol; may repeat 12 mg dose again in 1-2 min

Available forms: Inj 3 mg/ml

Side effects/adverse reactions

CNS: Lightheadedness, dizziness, arm tingling, numbness, apprehension, blurred vision, headache
CV: Chest pain, ***atrial tachydysrhythmias***, sweating, palpitations, hypotension, *facial flushing*
GI: *Nausea,* metallic taste, throat tightness, groin pressure
RESP: *Dyspnea, chest pressure,* hyperventilation

Contraindications: Hypersensitivity, 2nd or 3rd degree heart block, AV block, sick sinus syndrome, atrial flutter, atrial fibrillation, ventricular tachycardia

Precautions: Pregnancy **C**, P lactation, children, asthma, G elderly

Pharmacokinetics

Absorption	Complete bioavailability (IV)
Distribution	Erythrocytes, cardiovascular endothelium
Metabolism	Liver, converted to inosine and adenosine monophosphate
Excretion	Kidneys
Half-life	10 sec

Pharmacodynamics

	IV
Onset	Rapid
Peak	Unknown
Duration	1-2 min

Interactions

Drug/drug:

Individual drugs

Caffeine: ↓ effects of adenosine
Carbamazepine: ↑ heart block
Dipyridamole: ↑ effects of adenosine
Theophylline: ↓ effects of adenosine

Drugs/smoking: ↑ tachycardia

Lab test interferences

Increase: Liver function tests

NURSING CONSIDERATIONS

Assessment

- Monitor I&O ratio, electrolytes (potassium, sodium, chloride)
- Assess cardiac status: pulse, respiration, ECG intervals (PR, QRS, QT); check for transient dysrhythmias (PVCs, PACs, sinus tachycardia, AV block); B/P continuously for fluctuations
- Assess respiratory status: rate, rhythm, lung fields for rales, watch for respiratory depression; lung fields, bilateral rales may occur in CHF patient; if increased respiration, increased pulse occurs, drug should be discontinued
- Assess CNS effects: dizziness, confusion, paresthesias; drug should be discontinued

Associated nursing diagnoses

✓ Cardiac output, decreased (uses)
✓ Impaired gas exchange (adverse reactions)
✓ Knowledge deficit (teaching)

Implementation

IV route

- Give **IV** bol undiluted; give 6 mg or less over 1 min; if using an **IV** line, use port near insertion site, flush with NS (50 ml); warm to room temperature before giving
- Store at room temperature; sol should be clear

Patient/family education

- Tell patient to report facial flushing, dizziness, sweating, palpitations, chest pain
- Instruct patient to rise from sitting or standing slowly to prevent orthostatic hypotension

Evaluation

Positive therapeutic outcome

- Decreased B/P, dysrhythmias

albumin, human

(al-byoo'min)

Albuminar 5%, Albutein 5%, Buminate 5%, Plasbumin 5%, Albuminar 25%, Albutein 25%, Buminate 25%, Plasbumin-25%

Func. class.: Blood derivative—volume expander

Chem. class.: Placental human plasma

Pregnancy category **C**

Action: Exerts colloidal oncotic pressure, which expands volume of circulating blood by pulling fluid from extravascular to intravascular spaces, and maintains cardiac output

Therapeutic Outcome: Restoration of plasma volume by extravascular to intravascular fluid shift

Uses: Restores plasma volume in burns, hyperbilirubinemia, shock, hypoproteinemia, prevention of cerebral edema, cardiopulmonary bypass procedures, ARDS, hemorrhage; also replacement in nephrotic syndrome, hepatic failure

Dosage and routes

Burns

Adult: **IV** dose to maintain plasma albumin at 30-50 g/L, use 5% sol initially, then 25% sol after 24 hr

Shock

Adult: **IV** 500 ml of 5% sol q30 min, as needed

Child: ¼-½ adult dose in nonemergencies

Hypoproteinemia

Adult: **IV** 1000-2000 ml of 5% sol qd, not to exceed 5-10 ml/min or 25-100 g of 25% sol qd, not to exceed 3 ml/min, titrated to patient response

Hyperbilirubinemia/erythroblastosis fetalis

Infant: **IV** 1 g of 25% sol/kg before transfusion

Available forms: Inj IV 50, 250 mg/ml; (5%, 25%)

Side effects/adverse reactions

CNS: Fever, chills, flushing, headache

CV: Fluid overload, hypotension, erratic pulse, tachycardia
GI: Nausea, vomiting, increased salivation
INTEG: Rash, urticaria
RESP: Altered respirations, ***pulmonary edema***

Contraindications: Hypersensitivity, CHF, severe anemia, renal insufficiency

Precautions: Decreased salt intake, decreased cardiac reserve, lack of albumin deficiency, hepatic disease, renal disease, pregnancy **C**

Pharmacokinetics

Absorption	Complete bioavailability (IV)
Distribution	Intravascular spaces
Metabolism	Liver
Excretion	Unknown
Half-life	Unknown

Pharmacodynamics

	IV
Onset	15-30 min
Peak	Unknown
Duration	Unknown

Interactions: None

Lab test interferences

False increase: Alkaline phosphatase

NURSING CONSIDERATIONS

Assessment

• Monitor blood studies: Hct, Hgb; if serum protein declines, dyspnea, hypoxemia can result; check for decreasing B/P, erratic pulse, respiration

• Monitor CVP; pulmonary wedge pressure will increase if overload occurs; I&O ratio: urinary output may decrease; CVP reading: distended neck veins indicate circulatory overload; shortness of breath, anxiety, insomnia, expiratory rales, frothy blood-tinged sputum, cough, cyanosis indicate pulmonary overload

• Assess for allergy: fever, rash, itching, chills, flushing, urticaria, nausea, vomiting, hypotension; requires discontinuation of infusion, use of new lot if therapy reinstituted

Associated nursing diagnoses

✓ Fluid volume deficit (uses)
✓ Injury, risk for physical (uses)
✓ Fluid volume excess (adverse reactions)
✓ Knowledge deficit (teaching)

Implementation

IV **IV route**

• Check type of albumin; some are stored at room temperature, some need to be refrigerated; use only amber-colored sol without precipitate; solution should be clear

• Give **IV** slowly to prevent fluid overload; 5% may be given undiluted; 25% may be given diluted (D_5W, 0.9% NaCl) or undiluted; give over 4 hr, use infusion pump

• Provide adequate hydration before, during administration; whole blood may need to be given to prevent anemia; monitor hydration during treatment

Solution compatibilities:

0.9% NaCl, D_5W, D_5/0.9% NaCl, D_5/0.45%, D_5/LR, LR

Patient/family education

• Explain use, reason for albumin; provide information on what to report to prescriber (hypersensitivity, fluid overload)

Evaluation

Positive therapeutic outcome
• Increased B/P, decreased edema (shock, burns)
• Increased serum albumin levels
• Increased plasma protein (hypoproteinemia)

albuterol

(al-byoo'ter-ole)
albuterol,
Novosalmol ✱, Proventil,
Proventil Repetabs,
Salbutamol ✱, Ventolin,
Ventolin Rotacaps,
Volmax

Func. class.: Bronchodilator
Chem. class.: Adrenergic β_2- agonist
Pregnancy category **C**

Action: Causes bronchodilatation by action on β_2 (pulmonary) receptors by increasing levels of cyclic adenosine monophosphate (cAMP), which relaxes smooth muscle; produces bronchodilatation; CNS, cardiac stimulation, increased diuresis, and increased gastric acid secretion; longer acting than isoproterenol

➔ Therapeutic Outcome:

Increased ability to breathe because of bronchodilatation

Uses: Prevention of exercise-induced asthma, bronchospasm

Dosage and routes

To prevent exercise-induced asthma

Adult: Inh 2 puffs 15 min before exercising, NEB/IPPB 5 mg tid-qid

Bronchospasm

Adult: Inh 1-2 puffs q4-6h, PO 2-4 mg tid-qid, not to exceed 8 mg

Available forms: Aerosol 90, 100 μg/actuation; tabs 2, 4 mg; oral sol 2 mg/5 ml, ✱ cont rel 4, 8 mg; inh sol 0.83, 1, ✱ 5 mg/ml; inh caps (Rotacaps) 200 mg

Side effects/adverse reactions

CNS: *Tremors, anxiety,* insomnia, headache, dizziness, stimulation, *restlessness,* hallucinations, flushing, irritability
CV: Palpitations, tachycardia, hypertension, angina, hypotension, dysrhythmias
EENT: Dry nose, irritation of nose and throat
GI: Heartburn, nausea, vomiting
MS: Muscle cramps

Contraindications: Hypersensitivity to sympathomimetics, tachydysrhythmias, severe cardiac disease

Precautions: Lactation, pregnancy **C**, cardiac disorders, hyperthyroidism, diabetes mellitus, hypertension, prostatic hypertrophy, narrow angle glaucoma, seizures, exercise-induced bronchospasm (aerosol) in children <12 years

Pharmacokinetics

Absorption	Well absorbed (PO)
Distribution	Unknown
Metabolism	Liver extensively, tissues
Excretion	Unknown, breast milk
Half-life	3-4 hr

Pharmacodynamics

	PO	PO–EXT REL	INH
Onset	½ hr	½ hr	5-15 min
Peak	2½ hr	2-3 hr	1-1½ hr
Duration	4-6 hr	12 hr	4-6 hr

Interactions

Drug/drug:

Drug classifications

β-Adrenergic blockers: Block therapeutic effect
Bronchodilators, aerosol: ↑ action of bronchodilator
MAOI: ↑ chance of hypertensive crisis
Sympathomimetics: ↑ adrenergic side effects

NURSING CONSIDERATIONS

Assessment

• Assess respiratory function: vital capacity, forced expiratory volume, ABGs, lung sounds, heart rate, rhythm (baseline and during therapy)
• Determine that patient has not received theophylline therapy before giving dose, to prevent additive effect; client's ability to self-medicate
• Monitor for evidence of allergic reactions; paradoxic bronchospasm; withhold dose; notify prescriber

Associated nursing diagnoses

✓ Airway clearance, ineffective (uses)
✓ Impaired gas exchange (uses)
✓ Knowledge deficit (teaching)

Implementation

PO route
• Give PO with meals to decrease gastric irritation; oral sol for children (no alcohol, sugar)
Aerosol route
• Give after shaking; have patient exhale and place mouthpiece in mouth, inhale slowly, hold breath, remove inhaler, exhale slowly; allow at least 1 min between inhalations
• Store in light-resistant container; do not expose to temperatures over 86° F (30° C)

Patient/family education

• Tell patient not to use OTC medications before consulting prescriber; extra stimulation may occur; instruct patient to use this medication before other medications and allow at least 5 min between each to prevent overstimulation; to limit caffeine products such as chocolate, coffee, tea, and cola
• Teach patient to use inhaler; review package insert with patient; to avoid getting aerosol in eyes or blurring may result; to wash inhaler in warm water and dry qd; to rinse mouth after using; to avoid smoking, smoke-filled rooms, persons with respiratory infections

• Teach patient that if paradoxic bronchospasm occurs to stop drug immediately and notify prescriber if so
• Instruct patient on administration of dose, not to use more than prescribed; serious side effects may occur; if taking PO regularly and dose is missed, take when remembered; space other doses on new time schedule; do not double doses

Evaluation

Positive therapeutic outcome
• Absence of dyspnea and wheezing after 1 hr
• Improved airway exchange
• Improved ABGs

Treatment of overdose: Administer a β_2-adrenergic blocker

aldesleukin (interleukin-2, IL-2)

(al-dess-loo'kin)
Proleukin
Func. class.: Miscellaneous antineoplastics
Chem. class.: Interleukin-2, human recombinant
Pregnancy category **C**

Action: Enhancement of lymphocyte mitogenesis and stimulation of IL-2–dependent cell lines; enhancement of lymphocyte cytotoxicity; induction of killer cell activity; induction of interferon-γ-production; results in activation of cellular immunity & cytokines and inhibition of tumor growth

➔ Therapeutic Outcome: Prevention of rapid growth of malignant cells

Uses: Metastatic renal cell carcinoma in adults

Dosage and routes

Adult: **IV** inf 600,000 IU/kg (0.037 mg/kg) q8h over 15 min × 14 doses; off 9 days; repeat schedule for another 14 doses, for a maximum of 28 doses/course

Available forms: Powder for inj, lyophilized

Side effects/adverse reactions

CNS: Mental status changes, dizziness, sensory dysfunction, syncope, motor dysfunction, fever, chills, headache
CV: Hypotension, sinus tachycardia, dysrhythmias, bradycardia, PVCs, PACs, myocardial ischemia, ***myocardial infarction, cardiac arrest***
GI: Nausea, vomiting, diarrhea, stomatitis, anorexia, GI bleeding, dyspepsia, constipation, ***intestinal perforation/*** ileus, jaundice, ascites
GU: ***Oliguria/anuria, proteinuria, hematuria,*** dysuria, ***renal failure***
HEMA: Anemia, ***thrombocytopenia, leukopenia, coagulation disorders, leukocytosis, eosinophilia***
INTEG: Pruritus, erythema, rash, dry skin, ***exfoliative dermatitis,*** purpura, petechiae, urticaria

MS: Arthralgia, myalgia
RESP: Pulmonary congestion, dyspnea, ***pulmonary edema, respiratory failure,*** tachypnea, pleural effusion, wheezing
SYST: Infection

Contraindications: Hypersensitivity, abnormal thallium stress test or pulmonary function tests, organ allografts

Precautions: CNS metastases, bacterial infections, renal/hepatic disease, pregnancy **C**, P lactation, children, anemia, thrombocytopenia

Pharmacokinetics

Absorption	Complete bioavailability (IV)
Distribution	Rapid extracellular, intravascular
Metabolism	Kidneys (convoluted tubules)
Excretion	Kidneys
Half-life	85 min

Pharmacodynamics

	IV
Onset	Unknown
Peak	Unknown
Duration	Unknown

Interactions
Drug/drug:
Individual drugs
Indomethicin: ↑ toxicity
Radiation: ↑ toxicity, bone marrow suppression
Drug classifications
Aminoglycosides: ↑ toxicity
Antihypertensives: ↑ hypotension
Antineoplastics: ↑ toxicity, bone marrow suppression
Corticosteroids: ↓ tumor effectiveness

Lab test interferences
Increase: Bilirubin, BUN, serum creatinine, transaminase, alkaline phosphatase, hypomagnesemia, acidosis hypocalcemia, hypophosphatemia, hypokalemia, hyperuricemia, hypoalbuminemia, hypoproteinemia, hyponatremia, hyperkalemia, alkalosis

NURSING CONSIDERATIONS
Assessment
- Monitor CBC, differential, platelet count weekly; withhold drug if WBC is <4000/mm³ or platelet count is <75,000/mm³; notify prescriber of these results; transfusion of RBCs, platelets may be required
- Identify capillary leak syndrome (CLS), including a drop in mean arterial pressure (2-12 hr after initiating therapy); hypotension and hypoperfusion will occur; monitor ECG, CVP in cardiac patients
- Monitor renal function studies: BUN, serum uric acid, urine CrCl, electrolytes before, during therapy; I&O ratio; report fall in urine output to <30 ml/hr
- Monitor temperature q4h; fever may indicate beginning infection
- Check liver function tests before, during therapy: bilirubin, AST (SGOT), ALT (SGPT), alkaline phosphatase as needed or monthly
- Monitor ECG; watch for ST-T wave changes, low QRS and T, possible dysrhythmias (sinus tachycardia, PVCs)

• Monitor baselines in pulmonary function; document FEV >2 L or ≥75% before therapy
• Obtain stress thallium study before therapy; document normal ejection fraction, unimpaired wall motion
• Assess for bleeding: hematuria, guaiac, bruising or petechiae, mucosa, or orifices q8h
• Assess for GI symptoms: frequency of stools, cramping
• Assess for acidosis, signs of dehydration: rapid respirations, poor skin turgor, decreased urine output, dry skin, restlessness, weakness
• Assess for cardiac status: B/P, pulse, character, rhythm, rate, ABGs, ECG
• Assess for infection: sore throat; antibiotics may be prescribed prophylactically

Associated nursing diagnoses

✓ Injury, risk for (adverse reactions)
✓ Body image disturbance (adverse reactions)
✓ Infection, risk for (adverse reactions)
✓ Knowledge deficit (teaching)

Implementation

IV **IV route**
• Give by intermittent **IV** inf after diluting 22 million IU (1.3 mg)/1.2 ml sterile (1.1 mg/ml) H_2O for inj at side of vial and swirl, do not shake; dilute dose with 50 ml D_5W and give over 15 min; use plastic bag; do not use an in-line filter; give through Y-tube or 3-way stopcock
• Give hydrocortisone, dexamethasone, or sodium bicarbonate (1 mEq/1 ml) for extravasation, apply ice compresses
• Store in refrigerator any diluted drug; do not freeze; administer within 48 hr; bring to room temperature before infusing; discard unused portion

Additive incompatibility:

Do not mix with any other drugs

Patient/family education

• Teach patient to avoid use of products containing aspirin or ibuprofen, razors, commercial mouthwash because bleeding may occur; to report symptoms of bleeding hematuria, tarry stools
• Tell patient to report signs of anemia: fatigue, headache, irritability, faintness, shortness of breath
• Tell patient to report any changes in breathing or coughing even several months after treatment
• Advise patient that contraception will be necessary during treatment; teratogenesis may occur
• Teach patient to report signs/symptoms of infection: fever, chills, sore throat; patient should avoid crowds or persons with known infections

Evaluation

Positive therapeutic outcome
• Decreased spread of malignancy

alfentanil
(al-fen'ta-nil)
Alfenta, Rapifen ♣
Func. class.: Narcotic analgesic
Chem. class.: Opiate, synthetic
Pregnancy category C
Controlled substance schedule II

Action: Inhibits ascending pain pathways in limbic system, thalamus, midbrain, hypothalamus by binding to opiate receptor sites; this alters pain perception and response

➡ **Therapeutic Outcome:** Relief of pain (moderate, severe pain), anesthesia

Uses: In combination with other drugs in general anesthesia; as a primary anesthetic in general surgery usually used with barbiturates, oxygen, nitrous oxide

Dosage and routes
Anesthesia <30 min
Combination
Adult: **IV** 8-50 μg/kg, may increase by 3-15 μg/kg

Anesthetic induction
Adult: **IV** 3-5 μg/kg, then 0.5-1.5 μg/kg/min; total dose is 8-40 μg/kg

Anesthesia 30-60 min
Induction
Adult: **IV** 20-50 μg/kg

Maintenance
Adult: **IV** 5-15 μg/kg; may give up to 75 μg/kg total dose

Continuous anesthesia >45 min
Induction
Adult: **IV** 50-75 μg/kg

Maintenance
Adult: **IV** 0.5-3.0 μg/kg/min; rate should be decreased by 30%-50% after 1 hr maintenance inf; may be increased to 4 μg/kg/min or bol doses of 7 μg/kg

Induction of anesthesia >45 min
Adult: **IV** 130-245 μg/kg, then 0.5-1.5 μg/kg/min or general anesthesia

Available forms: Inj 500 μg/ml

Side effects/adverse reactions
*CNS: **Drowsiness, dizziness, confusion, headache, sedation, euphoria,*** delirium, agitation, anxiety
CV: Palpitations, bradycardia, change in B/P, facial flushing, syncope, asystole
EENT: Tinnitus, blurred vision, miosis, diplopia
*GI: **Nausea, vomiting, anorexia, constipation, cramps,*** dry mouth
GU: Urinary retention, dysuria
*INTEG: **Rash,*** urticaria, bruising, flushing, diaphoresis, pruritus
MS: Rigidity
RESP: Respiratory depression, apnea

P **Contraindications:** Child <12 yr, hypersensitivity

Precautions: Pregnancy **C**, lactation, increased intracranial pressure, acute MI, severe heart disease, renal disease, hepatic disease, asthma, respiratory conditions, convulsive disorders, elderly G

Pharmacokinetics

Absorption	Complete (IV)
Distribution	Crosses placenta; 90% bound to plasma proteins
Metabolism	Liver, up to 100%
Excretion	Kidneys
Half-life	1-2 hr

Pharmacodynamics

	IV
Onset	Immediate
Peak	1-1½ min
Duration	30 min

Interactions

Drug/drug:

Individual drugs

Alcohol: ↑ respiratory depression, hypotension, ↑ sedation
Cimetidine: ↑ recovery time
Erythromycin: ↑ recovery time
Nalbuphine: ↓ analgesia
Pentazocine: ↓ analgesia

Drug classifications

Antihistamines: ↑ respiratory depression, hypotension
Benzodiazepines: ↑ hypotension
CNS Depressants: ↑ respiratory depression, hypotension
MAOI: Do not use within 2 wk of alfentanil
Phenothiazines: ↑ respiratory depression, hypotension
Sedative/hypnotics: ↑ respiratory depression, hypotension

Lab test interferences

Increase: Amylase, lipase

NURSING CONSIDERATIONS

Assessment

• Respiratory status: respiratory depression, character, rate, rhythm; notify prescriber if respirations are <12/min; CV status; bradycardia, syncope; monitor ECG continuously

Associated nursing diagnoses

✓ Pain (uses)
✓ Sensory perceptual alteration: visual, auditory (adverse reactions)
✓ Breathing pattern, ineffective (adverse reactions)
✓ Knowledge deficit (teaching) (preoperatively)

Implementation

General

• Administer pain medications for postoperative pain, since alfentanil effect is short; medication for severe pain may be required

• Benzodiazepines are given after surgery to reduce alfentanil dosage and reduce anesthesia recovery time

IV **IV route**

• Give direct **IV** over 1½-3 min; use tuberculin syringe for accurate dosing

• Give cont **IV** by diluting 20 ml of drug in 230 ml of diluent (0.9% NaCl, D_5W, LR) (40 μg/ml); discontinue infusion 15 min before surgery is completed

• Store in light-resistant area at room temperature

Patient/family education

- Tell patients to avoid CNS depressants (alcohol, sedative/hypnotics) for at least 24 hr after use of this drug
- Discuss with patient that dizziness, drowsiness, and confusion are common; to avoid getting up without assistance
- Discuss in detail all aspects of the drug and the purpose of this drug and what to expect after anesthesia
- Tell patient to make position changes to lessen orthostatic hypotension

Evaluation

Positive therapeutic outcome

- Maintenance of anesthesia
- Absence of motor activity during surgery

Treatment of overdose: Narcan 0.2-0.8 **IV**, O_2, **IV** fluids, vasopressors; have resuscitation equipment available

allopurinol

(al-oh-pure'i-nole)

Alloprin ♣, Generic allopurinol, Apo Allopurinol ♣, Novopurol ♣, Lopurin, Purinol ♣, Zyloprim

Func. class.: Antigout drug

Chem. class.: Xanthine enzyme inhibitor

Pregnancy category **C**

Action: Inhibits the enzyme xanthine oxidase, reducing uric acid synthesis

Therapeutic Outcome: Decreasing serum uric acid levels, decreasing joint pain

Uses: Chronic gout, hyperuricemia associated with malignancies, recurrent calcium oxalate calculi

Dosage and routes

Gout/hyperuricemia

Adult: PO 200-600 mg qd depending on severity, not to exceed 800 mg/day

P *Child 6-10 yr:* 300 mg qd

P *Child <6 yr:* 150 mg qd

Impaired renal function

Adult: PO 200 mg qd when CrCl is 20-10 ml/min

Recurrent calculi

Adult: PO 200-300 mg qd

Uric acid nephropathy prevention

Adult: PO 600-800 mg qd × 2-3 days

Available forms: Tabs 100, 300 mg

Side effects/adverse reactions

CNS: *Headache,* drowsiness, neuritis, paresthesia
EENT: Retinopathy, cataracts, epistaxis
GI: *Nausea, vomiting, anorexia, malaise,* metallic taste, cramps, peptic ulcer, diarrhea, stomatitis
HEMA: ***Agranulocytosis, thrombocytopenia, aplastic anemia, pancytopenia, leukopenia, bone marrow depression, eosinophilia***

INTEG: Fever, chills, dermatitis, pruritus, purpura, erythema, ecchymosis, alopecia
MISC: Myopathy, arthralgia, hepatomegaly, ***cholestatic jaundice, renal failure***

Contraindications: Hypersensitivity

Precautions: Pregnancy **C**, lactation, renal disease, hepatic disease, children

Pharmacokinetics

Absorption	80% (PO)
Distribution	Widely distributed
Metabolism	Liver to oxypurinol
Excretion	Kidneys
Half-life	2-3 hr, terminal 18-30 hr

Pharmacodynamics

	PO
Onset	Unknown
Peak	2-4 hr
Duration	Unknown

Interactions

Drug/drug:

Individual drugs

Ampicillin: ↑ risk of rash
Azathioprine: ↑ bone marrow depression
Chlorpropamide: ↑ action of chlorpropamide
Cyclophosphamide: ↑ action of allopurinol
Mercaptopurine: ↑ bone marrow depression
Theophylline: ↑ action of chlorpropamide

Drug classifications

ACE inhibitors: ↑ action of ACE inhibitors
Aluminum salts: ↓ effects of allopurinol
Anticoagulants, oral: ↑ action of oral anticoagulants
Diuretics, thiazide: ↑ hypersensitivity

Lab test interferences

Increase: AST (SGOT), ALT (SGPT), alkaline phosphatase
Decrease: Hct/Hgb, leukocytes, serum glucose

NURSING CONSIDERATIONS

Assessment

- Assess for pain including location, characteristics, onset/duration, frequency, quality, intensity or severity of pain, precipitating factors
- Monitor uric acid levels q2 wk; normal uric acid levels are 6 mg/dl; check I&O ratio; increase fluids to 2-3 L/day to prevent stone formation, toxicity
- Monitor CBC, AST (SGOT), BUN, creatinine before starting treatment, monthly; check blood glucose in diabetic patients receiving oral antidiabetic agents
- Nutritional status: discourage organ meat, sardines, salmon, legumes, gravies (high-purine foods)

Associated nursing diagnoses

- ✓ Nutrition, more than body requirements (uses)
- ✓ Knowledge deficit (teaching)

Implementation

PO route

- Give with meals to prevent GI symptoms; crush and mix with food or fluids for patients with swallowing difficulties
- Give a few days before antineoplastic therapy if using for hyperuricemia associated with malignancy

Patient/family education

- Tell patient to increase fluid intake to 3-4 L/day; to avoid taking large doses of vitamin C; kidney stone formation may occur; to maintain a diet enhancing urine alkalinity (e.g., milk, other dairy products)
- Tell patient to report skin rash, stomatitis, malaise, fever, aching; drug should be discontinued
- Advise patient to avoid hazardous activities if drowsiness or dizziness occurs; response may take several days to determine
- Tell patient to avoid alcohol, caffeine; these substances increase uric acid levels and decrease allopurinol levels
- Teach patient to report side effects and adverse reactions to prescriber, including rash, itching, nausea, vomiting

Evaluation

Positive therapeutic outcome

- Decreased pain in joints
- Decreased stone formation in kidney
- Decreased uric acid level to 6 mg/dl

alprazolam

(al-pray'zoe-lam)

Apo-Alpraz ✦, Novo-Alprazol ✦, Nu-Alpraz ✦, Xanax

Func. class.: Antianxiety/sedative/hypnotic

Chem. class.: Benzodiazepine

Pregnancy category **D**

Controlled substance schedule **IV**

Action: Depresses subcortical levels of CNS, including limbic system, reticular formation; potentiates GABA (γ-aminobutyric acid)

Therapeutic Outcome: Decreased anxiety

Uses: Anxiety, panic disorders, anxiety with depressive symptoms

Dosage and routes

Adult: PO 0.25-0.5 mg tid, not to exceed 4 mg/day in divided doses

G *Elderly:* PO 0.25 mg bid-tid

Available forms: Tab 0.25, 0.5, 1, 2 mg

Side effects/adverse reactions

CNS: Dizziness, drowsiness, confusion, headache, anxiety, tremors, stimulation, fatigue, depression, insomnia, hallucinations

CV: Orthostatic hypotension, ***ECG changes, tachycardia,*** hypotension

EENT: *Blurred vision,* tinnitus, mydriasis
GI: Constipation, dry mouth, nausea, vomiting, anorexia, diarrhea
INTEG: Rash, dermatitis, itching

Contraindications: Hypersensitivity to benzodiazepines, narrow angle glaucoma, psychosis, pregnancy **D**, child <18 yr

Precautions: Elderly, debilitated, hepatic disease, renal disease

Pharmacokinetics

Absorption	Slow, complete (PO)
Distribution	Widely distributed; crosses placenta; crosses blood-brain barrier
Metabolism	Liver, to active metabolites
Excretion	Kidneys, breast milk
Half-life	12-15 hr

Pharmacodynamics

	PO
Onset	1 hr
Peak	1-2 hr
Duration	4-6 hr, therapeutic response 2-3 days

Interactions
Drug/drug:
Individual drugs
Alcohol: ↑ CNS depression
Cimetidine: ↑ action of alprazolam
Disulfiram: ↑ action of alprazolam
Levodopa: ↑ action of alprazolam

Drug classifications
Anticonvulsants: ↑ CNS depression
Antidepressants: ↑ CNS depression
Antihistamines: ↑ CNS depression
Oral contraceptives: ↑ action of alprazolam
Sedative/hypnotics: ↑ CNS depression

Lab test interferences
Increase: AST (SGOT)/ALT (SGPT), serum bilirubin
False increase: 17-Hydroxycorticosteroids
Decrease: RAIU

NURSING CONSIDERATIONS
Assessment
- Assess mental status: mood, sensorium, anxiety, affect, sleeping pattern, drowsiness, dizziness, especially elderly; physical dependency, withdrawal symptoms: anxiety, panic attacks, agitation, convulsions, headache, nausea, vomiting, muscle pain, weakness; suicidal tendencies; indications of increasing tolerance and abuse
- Monitor B/P (with patient lying, standing), pulse; if systolic B/P drops 20 mm Hg, hold drug, notify prescriber
- Monitor blood studies: CBC during long-term therapy; blood dycrasias have occurred rarely; decreased hematocrit, neutropenia may occur
- Monitor hepatic studies: AST (SGOT), ALT (SGPT), bilirubin, creatinine LDH, alkaline phosphatase
- Monitor I&O; indicate renal dysfunction

Associated nursing diagnoses

- ✓ Anxiety (uses)
- ✓ Depression (uses)
- ✓ Injury, risk for (adverse reactions)
- ✓ Knowledge deficit (teaching)

Implementation

PO route

- Give with food or milk for GI symptoms; tab may be crushed, if patient is unable to swallow medication whole, and mixed with foods or fluids
- Give sugarless gum, hard candy, frequent sips of water for dry mouth

Patient/family education

- Tell patient that drug may be taken with food or fluids, and tab may be crushed or swallowed whole
- Tell patient not to use for everyday stress or longer than 3 mo unless directed by prescriber; not to take more than prescribed amount; may be habit forming; not to double doses or skip doses
- Tell patient to avoid OTC preparations unless approved by prescriber; alcohol and CNS depressants will increase CNS depression
- Tell patient to avoid driving, activities that require alertness, since drowsiness may occur; to avoid alcohol ingestion or other psychotropic medications; to rise slowly or fainting G may occur, especially elderly; that drowsiness may worsen at beginning of treatment
- Tell patient not to discontinue medication abruptly after long-term use; withdrawal symptoms include vomiting, cramping, tremors, seizures

Evaluation

Positive therapeutic outcome

- Decreased anxiety, restlessness, sleeplessness (short-term treatment only)

Treatment of overdose: Lavage, VS, supportive care

alprostadil

(al-pros'ta-dil)

prostaglandin E_1, Prostin VR Pediatric, Prostin VR ♣

Func. class.: Hormone

Chem. class.: Prostaglandin E_1

Pregnancy category **C**

Action: Relaxes smooth muscles of ductus arteriosus; results in increased O_2 content perfusion throughout body

➔ Therapeutic Outcome: Maintenance of patent ductus arteriosus with increased O_2 in neonates with congenital heart defects

Uses: To maintain patent ductus arteriosus (temporary treatment)

Dosage and routes

P *Infants:* **IV**/Intra-arterial inf 0.1 μg/kg/min, until desired response, then reduce to lowest effective amount; 0.4 μg/kg/min not likely to produce greater beneficial effects

Available forms: Inj **IV** 500 μg/ml

Side effects/adverse reactions

CNS: Fever, ***convulsions,*** lethargy, hypothermia, stiffness, hyperirritability, ***cerebral bleeding***
CV: ***Bradycardia, tachycardia, hypotension, CHF, ventricular fibrillation, shock,*** flushing, **cardiac arrest,** edema
GI: Diarrhea, regurgitation, hyperbilirubinemia
GU: Oliguria, hematuria, ***anuria***
HEMA: ***DIC, thrombocytopenia,*** anemia, ***bleeding***
MISC: ***Sepsis,*** hypokalemia, ***peritonitis,*** hypoglycemia, hyperkalemia
RESP: ***Apnea, bradypnea, wheezing, respiratory depression***

Contraindications: **Hypersensitivity,** respiratory distress syndrome (RDS)

Precautions: Bleeding disorders, pregnancy **C**

Pharmacokinetics

Absorption	Complete bioavailability (IV)
Distribution	Unknown
Metabolism	80% lungs, rapidly
Excretion	Kidneys to metabolites
Half-life	Up to 10 min

Pharmacodynamics

Onset	1½-3 hr
Peak	Up to 11 hr
Duration	Infusion's end

Interactions: None

NURSING CONSIDERATIONS

Assessment

- Monitor ABGs, arterial pH, arterial pressure, continuous ECG; if arterial pressure decreases, reduce or stop drug; check for increased pH, B/P, urinary output, decreased ratio of PA to AP (restricted systemic blood flow)
- Assess neurologic status: level of consciousness, reflexes, muscle tone, response to stimuli during administration; if convulsions, stiffness, or hyperirritability occurs, drug should be discontinued; have [P] ventilator available; neonates <2 kg or infusion >48 hr means increased risk for CNS adverse reactions
- Assess respiratory and cardiac status: rate, rhythm, depth, and effort of respirations; check for bradypnea, tachypnea, apnea, wheezing, respiratory depression; monitor arterial B/P by use of umbilical artery catheter, auscultation, Doppler transducer; check for bradycardia, hypotension
- [P] Assess neonate with bleeding tendencies for DIS
- [P] Check neonate for flushing, which indicates a need to reposition the intraarterial catheter

Associated nursing diagnoses

- ✓ Tissue perfusion, altered (cardiopulmonary, cerebral) (uses)
- ✓ Injury, risk for physical (uses, adverse reactions)
- ✓ Impaired gas exchange (uses)
- ✓ Knowledge deficit (teaching)

Implementation

IV **IV route**

- Give only with emergency equipment available by trained clinicians
- Administer by cont inf, after diluting with 0.9% NaCl or D_5W inj to a concentration of 500 μg/ml; dilute further with 0.9% NaCl, D_5W; 500 μg of drug/250 ml = 2 μg/ml; 0.1 μg/kg/min; run at 0.05 ml/kg/min, (2 μg/ml); at 0.02 ml/kg/min (5 μg/ml) use inf pump and arterial pressure measurement during inf; do not use sol with benzyl alcohol; stable for 24 hr at room temperature
- Refrigerate drug; discard all mixed unused portion
- Do not mix with other drugs or sol

Patient/family education

- Teach family about diagnosis, prognosis, treatment; in- P form parents of neonate's condition

Evaluation

Positive therapeutic outcome

- Increased urine output (noncyanotic heart disease)
- Increased PO_2 (cyanotic heart disease)
- Absence of metabolic acidosis

Treatment of overdose: Discontinue drug, provide supportive measures

alteplase

(al'te-plase)

Activase, Activase rt-PA ✱, tissue plasminogin activator, t-PA

Func. class.: Thrombolytic

Chem. class.: Tissue plasminogen activator (TPA)

Pregnancy category C

Action: Produces fibrin conversion of plasminogen to plasmin; able to bind to fibrin, convert plasminogen in thrombus to plasmin, which leads to local fibrinolysis, limited systemic proteolysis

➔ **Therapeutic Outcome:** Lysis of thrombi in MI, pulmonary emboli (life threatening)

Uses: Lysis of obstructing thrombi associated with acute MI; although not currently approved, alteplase will be used for other conditions requiring thrombolysis, (e.g., PE, DUT, unclotting arteriovenous shunts)

Dosage and routes

Adult: **IV** a total of 100 mg; 6-10 mg given **IV** bol over 1-2 min, 60 mg given over 1st hr, 20 mg given over 2nd hr, 20 mg given over 3rd hr; or 1.25 mg/kg given over 3 hr for smaller patients

Available forms: Powder for inj 20 mg (11.6 million IU)/vial, 50 mg (29 million IU)/vial

Side effects/adverse reactions

CV: Sinus bradycardia, ventricular tachycardia, accelerated idioventricular rhythm
INTEG: Urticaria, rash
SYST: GI, GU, intracranial, retroperitoneal bleeding, surface bleeding

Contraindications: Hypersensitivity, active internal bleeding, recent CVA, severe uncontrolled hypertension, intracranial/intraspinal surgery/trauma, aneurysm

Precautions: Pregnancy **C**, P lactation, children

Pharmacokinetics

Absorption	Complete
Distribution	Unknown
Metabolism	>80% liver
Excretion	Kidneys
Half-life	30 min

Pharmacodynamics

	IV
Onset	Unknown
Peak	½-2 hr
Duration	Unknown

Interaction

Drug/drug:

Individual drugs
Aspirin: ↑ bleeding
Dipyridamole: ↑ bleeding
Heparin: ↑ bleeding
Plicamycin: ↑ bleeding
Valproic acid: ↑ bleeding
Drug classifications
Cephalosporins: ↑ bleeding
Anticoagulants, oral: ↑ bleeding
NSAIDs: ↑ bleeding

Lab test interferences

Increase: PT, APTT, TT

NURSING CONSIDERATIONS

Assessment

- Monitor VS q15 min, B/P, pulse, respirations (including peripheral), neurologic signs, temp at least q4h; temp >104° F (40° C) indicates internal bleeding; monitor rhythm closely; ventricular dysrhythmias may occur with hyperfusion; monitor heart, breath sounds, neurologic status, and peripheral pulses
- Assess for bleeding during first hr of treatment: hematuria, hematemesis, bleeding from mucous membranes, epistaxis, ecchymosis, puncture sites; guaiac all body fluids and stools; obtain blood studies (Hct, platelets, PTT, PT, TT, APTT) before starting therapy; PT or APTT must be less than 2 times control before starting therapy; TT or PT q3-4h during treatment; draw CPK—MB drawn to identify drug effectiveness
- Assess allergy: fever, rash, itching, chills; mild reaction may be treated with antihistamines; report to prescriber
- Monitor ECG; on monitor, watch for segment changes, changes in rhythm: sinus bradycardia, ventricular tachycardia, accelerated idioventricular rhythm may occur due to reperfusion

Associated nursing diagnoses

- ✓ Pain (uses)
- ✓ Tissue perfusion, altered (uses)
- ✓ Injury, risk for (adverse reactions)

Implementation

IV route

- Give after reconstituting with provided diluent; add appropriate amount of sterile water for injection (no preservatives); 20-mg vial/20 ml or 50-mg vial/50 ml (1 mg/ml); mix by slow inversion or dilute with NaCl, D_5W to a concentration of 0.5 mg/ml further dilution; 1.5 to <0.5 mg/ml may result in precipitation of drug; use 18-gauge needle; flush line with NaCl after administration; use reconstituted **IV** sol within 8 hr, within 6 hr of coronary occlusion for best results
- Give heparin therapy after thrombolytic therapy is discontinued and when TT, ACT, and APTT less than 2 times control (about 3-4 hr)
- Avoid invasive procedures, inj, rec temp; apply pressure for 30 sec to minor bleeding sites; 30 min to sites of atrial puncture, followed by pressure dressing; inform prescriber if this does not attain hemostasis; apply pressure dressing
- Store powder at room temperature or refrigerate; protect from excessive light

Y-site incompatibilities:
Dobutamine, dopamine, heparin, nitroglycerin

Y-site compatibility:
Lidocaine

Patient/family education

- Teach patient reason for alteplase, signs and symptoms of bleeding, allergic reactions, when to notify prescriber

Evaluation

Positive therapeutic outcome

- Lysis of pulmonary thrombi
- Adequate hemodynamic state
- Absence of congestive heart failure

altretamine

(al-tret'a-meen)

Hexalen, hexamethylmelamine, Hexastat ✦

Func. class.: Misc. antineoplastic

Chem. class.: *S*-Triazine derivative (formerly known as hexamethylmelamine)

Pregnancy category **D**

Action: Products of metabolism form covalent bonds with tissue macromolecules including DNA, which may be responsible for cytotoxicity; activity is not cell cycle phase specific

Therapeutic Outcome: Prevention of rapid growth of malignant cells

Uses: Palliative treatment of recurrent, persistent ovarian cancer following first-line treatment with cisplatin or alkylating agent–based combination

Dosage and routes

Adult: PO 260 mg/m^2 day for 14 or 21 days in a 28-day cycle; give in 4 divided doses pc and hs

A

Available forms: Caps 50, 100 ✦ mg

Side effects/adverse reactions

CNS: Peripheral sensory neuropathy, fatigue, ***seizures,*** mood disorders, disorders of consciousness, ataxia, dizziness, vertigo
GI: Nausea, anorexia, vomiting, increased alkaline phosphatase, ***hepatic toxicity***
GU: Increased BUN, serum creatinine
HEMA: Leukopenia, thrombocytopenia, anemia
INTEG: Rash, pruritus, alopecia

Contraindications: Hypersensitivity, severe bone marrow depression, severe neurologic toxicity

Precautions: Pregnancy **D,** P lactation, children

Pharmacokinetics

Absorption	Well (PO)
Distribution	Concentrated in liver, kidneys, small intestine
Metabolism	Liver (99%)
Excretion	Kidneys
Half-life	4½-10½ hrs

Pharmacodynamics

	PO
Onset	Unknown
Peak	½-3 hr
Duration	Unknown

Interactions

Drug/drug:

Individual drugs
Cimetidine: ↑ toxicity
Radiation: ↑ toxicity

Drug classifications
Antineoplastics: ↑ bone marrow depression
MAOI: ↑ orthostatic hypotension

NURSING CONSIDERATIONS

Assessment

- Monitor CBC, differential, platelet count weekly; withhold drug if WBC is <4000 or platelet count is <75,000; granulocytes <1000 mm^3 notify prescriber of results; nadir (leukopenia/thrombocytopenia) occurs in 1 mo; resolves in 6 wk
- Monitor renal function studies: BUN, serum uric acid, urine CrCl before, during therapy; I&O ratio; report fall in urine output of 30 ml/hr; monitor for decreased hyperuricemia
- Monitor for cold, fever, sore throat (may indicate beginning infection)
- Assess for bleeding: hematuria, guaiac, bruising or petechiae, mucosa or orifices q8h, no rec temp; identify inflammation of mucosa, breaks in skin; use viscous lidocaine (Xylocaine) for oral pain
- Identify food preferences; list likes, dislikes
- Identify edema in feet, joint or stomach pain, shaking
- Assess neurologic status: paresthesia, numbness, tingling; pyridoxine may minimize neurologic reaction

Associated nursing diagnosis

- ✓ Injury, risk for (adverse reactions)
- ✓ Infection, risk for (adverse reactions)
- ✓ Knowledge deficit (teaching)

Implementation

PO route

- Give 1 hr before or 2 hr after meals to lessen nausea and vomiting or antacid before oral agent; give drug after evening meal, before bedtime; antiemetic 30-60 min before giving drug to prevent vomiting
- Antibiotics for prophylaxis of infection may be prescribed, since infection potential is high
- Store in tight container

Patient/family education

- Tell patient that contraceptive measures are recommended during therapy; teratogenic effects occure
- Teach patient to avoid use of products containing alcohol, aspirin, or ibuprofen, razors, hard bristle toothbrush, and commercial mouthwash because bleeding may occur; to report symptoms of bleeding (hematuria, tarry stools)
- Tell patient to report signs of anemia, (fatigue, headache, irritability, faintness, shortness of breath)
- Tell patient to report any changes n breathing or coughing even several months after treatment
- Tell patient that hair may be lost during treatment; a wig or hairpiece may make patient feel better; new hair may be different in color, texture
- Advise patient to avoid vaccinations during treatment; serious reactions may occur
- Teach patient to report signs/symptoms of infection: fever, chills, sore throat; patient should avoid crowds and persons with known infections

Evaluation

Positive therapeutic outcome

- Decreased size and spread of malignancy

aluminum acetate

Bluboro Powder, Boropak Powder, Burow's Solution, Domeboro, Modified Burow's Solution, Pedi-Boro Soak Paks

Func. class.: Astringent (topical)

Chem. class.: Aluminum product

Pregnancy category **C**

Action: Maintains skin acidity, which is protective to skin surface; an astringent

Therapeutic Outcome: Soothing of skin irritation, decreased skin inflammation

Uses: Skin irritation, inflammation, athlete's foot, insect bites, poison ivy, eczema, acne, rash, bruises, pruritus (anal)

Dosage and routes

P *Adult and child:* Top apply for 15-30 min, q4-8h (1 : 10-40 sol); gargle use 1 : 10 sol prn

Available forms: Sol packets (1 : 40 sol); tabs for dissolving (1 : 20, 1 : 40 sol), cream (Canada only)

A

Side effects/adverse reactions

INTEG: Irritation, increasing inflammation

Contraindications: Tight, occlusive dressing

Precautions: Pregnancy **C**

Pharmacokinetics	
Absorption	Not usually absorbed
Distribution	Unknown
Metabolism	Unknown
Excretion	Unknown
Half-life	Unknown

Pharmacodynamics	TOP
Onset	Immediately
Peak	Unknown
Duration	Unknown

Interactions

Drug/drug:

Individual drugs

Collagenase: Blocks action of collagenase

Soap: ↓ action of aluminum acetate

NURSING CONSIDERATIONS

Assessment

• Check area of body to receive top application for irritation, rash breaks, dryness, lesions, excoriation, drainage

Associated nursing diagnoses

✓ Skin integrity, impaired (uses)
✓ Pain (uses)
✓ Knowledge deficit (teaching)

Implementation

Top route

• Mix 1 packet in 1 pt water (1 : 10-40 warm water); apply wet dressings loosely; do not use precipitate or occlusive dressings; sol is stable for 1 wk at room temperature

• Apply sol and dressings to ⅓ of body at a time; provide bath blanket to prevent chilling to the rest of the body

Patient/family education

• Instruct patient to discontinue use if irritation occurs or becomes worse

• Instruct patient to avoid using near eye area, mucous membranes

• Teach patient or family members on use of sol

Evaluation

Positive therapeutic outcome

• Decreased skin irritation, pain, inflammation

aluminum hydroxide

Alterna GEL, Alu-Cap, Alugel ✤, Aluminett, Aluminum Hydroxide, Aluminum Hydroxide Gel, Alu-Tab, Amphojel, concentrated aluminum hydroxide, Dialume, Nephrox

Func. class.: Antacid-hypophosphatemic

Chem. class.: Aluminum product

Pregnancy category **C**

Action: Neutralizes gastric acidity, binds phosphates in GI tract; these phosphates are excreted

Uses: Peptic, gastric, duodenal ulcers; hyperphosphatemia in chronic renal failure; reflux esophagitis, hyperacidity

Therapeutic Outcome: Decreased acidity, healing of ulcers; decreased phosphate levels in chronic renal failure

Dosage and routes

Adult: Susp 5-10 ml 1 hr pc, hs; PO 600 mg 1 hr pc, hs, chewed with milk or water

Hyperphosphatemia in renal failure

Adult: Susp 500 mg-2 g bid-qid

Available forms

Caps 475, 500 mg; tabs 300, 500 mg; chewable tabs 600 mg; susp (4%) 600 mg/5 ml; liq 320 mg/5 ml, 600 mg/5 ml

Side effects/adverse reactions

GI: *Constipation,* anorexia, ***obstruction,*** fecal impaction
META: *Hypophosphatemia,* hypercalciuria

Contraindications: Hypersensitivity to this drug or aluminum products, abdominal pain of unknown origin

Precautions: Elderly, fluid restriction, decreased GI motility, GI obstruction, dehydration, renal disease, sodium-restricted diets, pregnancy **C**

Pharmacokinetics

Absorption	Not usually absorbed
Distribution	Widely distributed if absorbed; crosses placenta
Metabolism	Unknown
Excretion	Feces, kidneys (small amounts), breast milk
Half-life	Unknown

Pharmacodynamics

	PO
Onset	20-40 min
Peak	½ hr
Duration	½-3 hr

Interactions

Drug/drug:

Individual drugs

Amphetamine: ↑ levels
Chlorpromazine: ↓ absorption
Isoniazid: ↓ absorption
Mexiletine: ↑ levels
Quinidine: ↑ levels
Salicylate: ↓ levels
Tetracycline: ↓ absorption

NURSING CONSIDERATIONS

Assessment

- Assess pain symptoms: location, duration, intensity, alleviating precipitating factors
- Monitor phosphate levels, since drug is bound in GI system; urinary pH, calcium, electrolytes; hypophosphatemia: anorexia, weakness, fatigue, bone pain, hyperreflexia
- Monitor constipation; increase bulk in diet if needed

Associated nursing diagnoses

✓ Pain, chronic (uses)
✓ Constipation (adverse reactions)
✓ Knowledge deficit (teaching)

A

Implementation

PO route

- Give laxatives or stool softeners if constipation occurs, G especially elderly
- Give after shaking liq; follow with water to facilitate passage
- Tab may be chewed if patient is unable to swallow; drink 8 oz of water after chewing; or by nasogastric tube if patient unable to swallow
- Give 1 hr before or after other medications to prevent poor absorption
- Give 15 ml 30 min pc and hs (esophagitis)
- May be given as prescribed q1-2 hr and given by gastric tube after diluting with water (peptic ulcer)

Patient/family education

- Instruct patient to increase fluids to 2000 ml/day unless contraindicated
- Instruct patient to avoid phosphate foods (most dairy products, eggs, fruits, carbonated beverages) during drug therapy; to add cheese, corn, pasta, plums, prunes, lentils after drug (hypophosphatemia)
- Instruct patient not to use for prolonged periods if serum phosphate is low or if on a low-sodium diet; CHF patients should check for sodium content and use sodium-reduced products
- Instruct patient that stools may appear white or speckled; constipation may result; to report black tarry stools, which indicate gastric bleeding
- Instruct patient to check with prescriber after 2 wk of self-prescribed antacid use; may be used for 4-6 wk after symptoms subside or as prescribed

Evaluation

Positive therapeutic outcome

- Absence of pain, decreased acidity
- Increased pH of gastric secretions
- Decreased phosphate levels

amantadine

(a-man'ta-deen)

amantadine HCl, Symadine, Symmetrel

Func. class.: Antiviral, antiparkinsonian agent

Chem. class.: Tricyclic amine

Pregnancy category **C**

Action: Prevents uncoating of nucleic acid in viral cell, preventing penetration of virus to host; causes release of dopamine from neurons

➡ **Therapeutic Outcome:** Decreased Parkinson's symptoms, decreased symptoms of influenza type A or prevention

Uses: Prophylaxis or treatment of influenza type A, extrapyramidal reactions, parkinsonism, respiratory tract infections

Investigational uses: Neuroleptic malignant syndrome, cocaine dependency, enuresis

Dosage and routes

Influenza type A

P ***Adult and child >12 yr:*** PO 200 mg/day in single dose or divided bid

P ***Child 9-12 yr:*** PO 100 mg bid

P ***Child 1-9 yr:*** PO 4.4-8.8 mg/kg/day divided bid-tid, not to exceed 200 mg/day

Extrapyramidal reaction/ parkinsonism

Adult: PO 100 mg bid, up to 400 mg/day in EPS; give for 1 wk then 100 mg as needed up to 400 mg in parkinsonism

Available forms: Caps 100 mg; syr 50 mg/5 ml

Side effects/adverse reactions

CNS: Headache, dizziness, drowsiness, fatigue, anxiety, psychosis, depression, hallucinations, tremors, ***convulsions***
CV: Orthostatic hypotension, ***CHF***
EENT: Blurred vision
GI: *Nausea, vomiting,* constipation, dry mouth
GU: *Frequency, retention*
HEMA: ***Leukopenia***
INTEG: Photosensitivity, dermatitis

Contraindications: Hypersensitivity, lactation, P child <1 yr, eczematic rash

Precautions: Epilepsy, CHF, orthostatic hypotension, psychiatric disorders, hepatic disease, renal disease, peripheral edema, pregnancy **C**

Pharmacokinetics

Absorption	Well absorbed
Distribution	Crosses blood-brain barrier
Metabolism	Not metabolized
Excretion	Kidneys (90%) unchanged, breast milk
Half-life	24 hr

Pharmacodynamics

	PO
Onset	48 hr
Peak	2 wk
Duration	Unknown

Interactions

Drug/drug:

Individual drugs

Atropine: ↑ anticholinergic effects
Disopyramide: ↑ anticholinergic effects
Quinidine: ↑ anticholinergic effects

Drug classifications

Antidepressants, tricylic: ↑ anticholinergic effects
Antihistamines: ↑ anticholinergic effects
Phenothiazines: ↑ anticholinergic effects

NURSING CONSIDERATIONS

Assessment

- Assess for Parkinson's symptoms: tremors, akinesia, rigidity, impaired motor movements; as drug therapy continues, these symptoms should lessen
- Assess for drug toxicity: tremors, convulsions, lability, dysrhythmias; drug should be discontinued and physostigmine given

• Assess for symptoms of influenza A: increased temperature, malaise, aches and pains
• Monitor I&O ratio; report frequency, hesitancy, bowel pattern before, during treatment
• Check for mottling of skin (livedo reticularis), which disappears after several weeks of treatment
• Assess for skin eruptions, photosensitivity after administration of drug
• Monitor respiratory status: rate, character, wheezing, tightness in chest
• Assess for allergies before initiation of treatment, reaction of each medication; place allergies on chart in bright red letters

Associated nursing diagnoses

✓ Infection, risk for (uses)
✓ Knowledge deficit (teaching)

Implementation

• Give before exposure to influenza; continue for 10 days after contact
• Give at least 4 hr before hs to prevent insomnia
• Administer after meals for better absorption, to decrease GI symptoms; caps may be opened and mixed with food for easy swallowing
• Give in divided doses to prevent CNS disturbances: headache, dizziness, fatigue, drowsiness
• Store in tight, dry container

Patient/family education

• Teach patient to change body position slowly to prevent orthostatic hypotension
• Teach patient about aspects of drug therapy: the need to report dyspnea, weight gain, dizziness, poor concentration, dysuria, behavioral changes
• Teach patient to avoid hazardous activities if dizziness, blurred vision occur
• Teach patient to take drug exactly as prescribed; parkinsonian crisis may occur if drug is discontinued abruptly; drug should be tapered slowly
• Tell patient to avoid alcohol, OTC medications until discussed with prescriber, serious side effects can occur

Evaluation

Positive therapeutic outcome
• Absence of fever, malaise, cough, dyspnea in influenza A
• Decreased tremors, shuffling gait in Parkinson's disease, extrapyramidal symptoms

Treatment of overdose: Withdraw drug, maintain airway, administer epinephrine, aminophylline, O_2 IV corticosteroids, physostigmine

amcinonide

(am-sin'oh-nide)
Cyclocort
Func. class.: Topical corticosteroid
Chem. class.: Synthetic fluorinated agent, group II potency
Pregnancy category **C**

Action: Antipruritic, anti-inflammatory; suppresses inflammatory response

Therapeutic Outcome: Decreased itching, inflammation

Uses: Psoriasis, eczema, contact dermatitis, pruritus

Dosage and routes

Adult and child: Apply to affected area bid-tid; rub completely into skin

Available forms: Cream 0.1%; oint 0.1%

Side effects/adverse reactions

INTEG: Burning, dryness, itching, irritation, acne, folliculitis, hypertrichosis, perioral dermatitis, hypopigmentation, atrophy, striae, miliaria, allergic contact dermatitis, secondary infection

Contraindications: Hypersensitivity to corticosteroids, fungal infections

Precautions: Pregnancy **C**, lactation, viral infections, bacterial infections

Pharmacokinetics

Absorption	Minimal; systemic absorption on large areas
Distribution	Site only
Metabolism	Not metabolized
Excretion	Not excreted
Half-life	Unknown

Pharmacodynamics

	TOP
Onset	Up to 1 hr
Peak	Up to several days
Duration	Up to several days

Interactions: None

NURSING CONSIDERATIONS

Assessment

- Assess skin for decreasing inflammation, itching, pruritus, flaking, before and during treatment
- Monitor temperature, worsening of rash; if fever develops, drug should be discontinued
- Monitor for systemic absorption: increased temperature, inflammation, irritation

Associated nursing diagnoses

✓ Skin integrity, impairment (uses)
✓ Infection, risk for (adverse reactions)
✓ Knowledge deficit (teaching)

Implementation

Top route

- Cleanse area before application of drug; use drug for a few days after area has cleared
- Apply only to affected areas (do not get ointment or cream in the eyes); then cover with occlusive dressing (only if prescribed), seal to normal skin, change q12h; systemic absorption may occur; apply only to dermatoses; do not use on weeping, denuded, or infected areas; use gloves to apply
- May be applied to the scalp by parting the hair and rubbing a small amount into area; wait until medication drys before putting anything in the hair
- Store at room temperature

Patient/family education

- Instruct patient to avoid sunlight on affected area; burns may occur

• Instruct patient to discontinue drug, notify prescriber if local irritation or fever develops
• Teach patient all aspects of drug administration including method of application and when to notify prescriber; if dose is missed, the dose should be administered when remembered
• Tell patient that, if area treated is on the face, cosmetics should not be used; if in the hair, hair dressing, hair spray, or styling gel should not be used

Evaluation

Positive therapeutic outcome
• Absence of severe itching, patches on skin, flaking

amikacin

(am-i-kay'sin)
amikacin sulfate, Amikin
Func. class.: Antibiotic
Chem. class.: Aminoglycoside
Pregnancy category **D**

Action: Interferes with protein synthesis in bacterial cell by binding to ribosomal subunit, which causes misreading of genetic code; inaccurate peptide sequence forms in protein chain, causing bacterial death

Therapeutic Outcome: Bactericidal effects for the following organisms: *Pseudomonas aeruginosa, Escherichia coli, Enterobacter, Acinetobacter, Providencia, Citrobacter, Staphylococcus, Serratia, Proteus*

Uses: Severe systemic infections of CNS, respiratory, GI, urinary tract, bone, skin, soft tissues

Dosage and routes

Severe systemic infections

P *Adult and child:* **IV** inf 15 mg/kg/day in 2-3 divided doses q8-12h in 100-200 ml D_5W over 30-60 min, not to exceed 1.5 g; decreased dosages are needed in poor renal function as determined by blood levels, renal function studies; IM 15 mg/kg/day in divided doses q8-12h

P *Neonates:* **IV** inf 10 mg/kg initially, then 7.5 mg/kg q12h in D_5W over 1-2 hr

Severe urinary tract infections

Adults: IM 250 mg bid

Adults with poor renal function: 7.5 mg/kg initially, then increased as determined by blood levels, renal function studies

Available forms: Inj IM, **IV** 50, 250 mg/ml

Side effects/adverse reactions

CNS: Confusion, depression, numbness, tremors, ***convulsions,*** muscle twitching, ***neurotoxicity,*** dizziness, vertigo, tinnitus
CV: Hypotension or hypertension, palpitations
EENT: ***Ototoxicity,*** deafness, visual disturbances
GI: Nausea, vomiting, anorexia, increased ALT (SGPT), AST (SGOT), bili-

rubin, hepatomegaly, ***hepatic necrosis,*** splenomegaly
GU: Oliguria, hematuria, renal damage, azotemia, failure, nephrotoxicity
HEMA: Agranulocytosis, thrombocytopenia, leukopenia, eosinophilia, anemia
INTEG: Rash, burning, urticaria, dermatitis, alopecia

Contraindications: Mild to moderate infections, hypersensitivity to aminoglycosides

Precautions: Neonates, mild renal disease, pregnancy **D**, myasthenia gravis, lactation, hearing deficits, Parkinson's G disease, elderly

Pharmacokinetics

Absorption	Well absorbed (IM), complete absorbed (IV)
Distribution	Widely distributed in extracellular fluids, poor in CSF; crosses placenta
Metabolism	Minimal; liver
Excretion	Mostly unchanged (79%) in kidneys
Half-life	2-3 hr; increased in renal disease

Pharmacodynamics

	IM	IV
Onset	Rapid	Rapid
Peak	1-2 hr	1-2 hr

Interactions

Drug/drug:

Individual drugs
Amphotericin B: ↑ ototoxicity, neurotoxicity, nephrotoxicity
Cisplatin: ↑ ototoxicity, neurotoxicity, nephrotoxicity
Ethacrynic acid: ↑ ototoxicity, neurotoxicity, nephrotoxicity
Furosemide: ↑ ototoxicity, neurotoxicity, nephrotoxicity
Mannitol: ↑ ototoxicity, neurotoxicity, nephrotoxicity
Methoxyflurane: ↑ ototoxicity, neurotoxicity, nephrotoxicity
Polymyxin: ↑ ototoxicity, neurotoxicity, nephrotoxicity
Succinylcholine: ↑ neuromuscular blockade, respiratory depression
Vancomycin: ↑ ototoxicity, neurotoxicity, nephrotoxicity

Drug classifications
Anesthetics: ↑ neuromuscular blockade, respiratory depression
Aminoglycosides: ↑ ototoxicity, neurotoxicity, nephrotoxicity
Nondepolarizing neuromuscular blockers: ↑ neuromuscular blockade, respiratory depression

NURSING CONSIDERATIONS

Assessment

- Assess patient for previous sensitivity reaction
- Assess patient for signs and symptoms of infection, including characteristics of wounds, sputum, urine, stool, WBC >10,000, earache, temp; obtain baseline information and during treatment
- Obtain culture and sensitivity tests before beginning drug therapy to identify if correct treatment has been initiated
- Assess for allergic reactions: rash, urticaria, pruritus
- Identify urine output; if decreasing, notify prescriber (may indicate nephrotoxicity); also notify prescriber of increased BUN and creatinine, urine CrCl <80 ml/min; lower

dosage should be given in renal impairment; urinalysis daily for protein, cells, casts
• Monitor blood studies: AST, ALT, CBC, Hct, bilirubin, LDH, alkaline phosphatase; Coombs' test monthly if patient is on long-term therapy
• Monitor electrolytes: potassium, sodium, chloride monthly if patient is on long-term therapy
• Assess bowel pattern qd; if severe diarrhea occurs, drug should be discontinued
• Monitor for bleeding: ecchymosis, bleeding gums, hematuria, stool guaiac daily if on long-term therapy
• Assess for overgrowth of infection: perineal itching, fever, malaise, redness, pain, swelling, drainage, rash, diarrhea, change in cough, sputum
• Obtain weight before treatment; calculation of dosage is usually based on ideal body weight, but may be calculated on actual body weight
• Monitor VS during infusion, watch for hypotension, change in pulse
• Assess **IV** site for thrombophlebitis including pain, redness, swelling q30 min; change site if needed; apply warm compresses to discontinued site
• Obtain serum peak, drawn 30-60 min after IV infusion or 60 min after IM injection; trough level drawn just before next dose; blood level should be 2-4 times bacteriostatic level
• Urine pH if drug is used for UTI; urine should be kept alkaline
• Deafness by audiometric testing, ringing, roaring in ears, vertigo; assess hearing before, during, after treatment
• Dehydration: high sp gr, decrease in skin turgor, dry mucous membranes, dark urine
• Vestibular dysfunction: nausea, vomiting, dizziness, headache; drug should be discontinued if severe

Associated nursing diagnoses

✓ Infection, risk for (uses)
✓ Diarrhea (side effects)
✓ Knowledge deficit (teaching)
✓ Injury, risk for (side effects)

Implementation

IM route
• Give deeply in large muscle mass

IV **IV route**
• Dilute 500 mg of drug in 100-200 ml of **IV** D_5W, D_5NaCl or 0.9% NaCl and give over ½-1 hr; flush after administration with D_5W or 0.9% NaCl

Patient/family education

• Teach patient to report sore throat, bruising, bleeding, joint pain; may indicate blood dyscrasias (rare)
• Advise patient to contact prescriber if vaginal itching, loose foul-smelling stools, furry tongue occur; may indicate superinfection

Evaluation

Positive therapeutic outcome
• Absence of signs/symptoms of infection: WBC <10,000, temp WNL; absence of red draining wounds; absence of earache
• Reported improvement in symptoms of infection

Treatment of overdose: Withdraw drug; administer epinephrine, aminophylline, O_2, hemodialysis, exchange P transfusion in the newborn; monitor serum levels of drug; may give ticarcillin or carbenicillin

amiloride

(a-mill'oh-ride)

Amiloride HCl, Midamor

Func. class.: Potassium-sparing diuretic

Chem. class.: Pyrazine

Pregnancy category **B**

Action: Acts primarily on distal tubule, secondarily by inhibiting reabsorption of sodium and water and increasing potassium retention and conserving hydrogen ions

➔ **Therapeutic Outcome:** Diuretic and antihypertensive effect while retaining potassium

Uses: Diuretic-induced hypokalemia; used with other agents to treat edema, hypertension

Dosage and routes

Adult: PO 5 mg qd; may be increased to 10-20 mg qd if needed

Available forms: Tabs 5 mg

Side effects/adverse reactions

CNS: Headache, dizziness, fatigue, weakness, paresthesias, tremor, depression, anxiety

CV: Orthostatic hypotension, dysrhythmias, angina

EENT: Loss of hearing, tinnitus, blurred vision, nasal congestion, increased intraocular pressure

ELECT: Acidosis, hyponatremia, ***hyperkalemia,*** hypochloremia

GI: Nausea, diarrhea, dry mouth, *vomiting, anorexia,* cramps, constipation, abdominal pain, jaundice, bleeding

GU: Polyuria, dysuria, frequency, impotence

HEMA: ***Agranulocytopenia, leukopenia, megaloblastic anemia, thrombocytopenia (rare)***

INTEG: Rash, pruritus, alopecia, urticaria

Contraindications: Anuria, hypersensitivity, hyperkalemia, impaired renal function

Precautions: Dehydration, pregnancy **B,** diabetes, acidosis, lactation, hepatic disease

Pharmacokinetics

	PO
Absorption	Variable (10%-15%)
Distribution	Unknown
Metabolism	Unchanged in urine (50%) in feces (40%)
Excretion	Renal; breast milk
Half-life	6-9 hr

Pharmacodynamics

	PO
Onset	2 hr
Peak	6-10 hr
Duration	24 hr

Interactions

Drug/drug:

Individual drugs

Lithium: ↑ action, toxicity

Drug classifications

ACE Inhibitors: ↑ hyperkalemia
Antihypertensives: ↑ action
Diuretics, potassium-sparing: ↑ hyperkalemia
NSAIDs: ↓ effectiveness of amiloride
Potassium products: ↑ hyperkalemia
Salt substitutes: ↑ hyperkalemia

Drug/food:

Potassium foods: ↑ hyperkalemia

Lab test interferences

Interfere: GTT

NURSING CONSIDERATIONS

Assessment

- Monitor manifestations of hyperkalemia: *MS:* fatigue, muscle weakness; *CARDIAC:* dysrhythmias, hypotension; *NEURO:* paresthesias, confusion; *RESP:* dyspnea
- Monitor for manifestations of hyponatremia: *CV:* increased B/P, cold, clammy skin, hypovolemia or hypervolemia; *GI:* anorexia, nausea, vomiting, diarrhea, abdominal cramps; *NEURO:* lethargy, increased ICP, confusion, headache, seizures, coma, fatigue, tremors, hyperreflexia
- Monitor for manifestations of hyperchloremia: *NEURO:* weakness, lethargy, coma; *RESP:* deep rapid breathing
- Assess fluid volume status: I&O ratios and record, weight, distended red veins, crackles in lung, color, quality and sp gr of urine, skin turgor, adequacy of pulses, moist mucous membranes, bilateral lung sounds, peripheral pitting edema; dehydration symptoms of decreasing output, thirst, hypotension, dry mouth and mucous membranes should be reported
- Monitor electrolytes: potassium, sodium, calcium, magnesium; also include BUN, ABGs, uric acid, CBC, blood sugar
- Assess B/P before and during therapy with patient lying, standing, and sitting as appropriate; orthostatic hypotension can occur rapidly

Associated nursing diagnoses

- ✓ Fluid volume deficit (side effects)
- ✓ Fluid volume excess (uses)
- ✓ Knowledge deficit (teaching)

Implementation

- Give in AM to avoid interference with sleep

PO route

- With food, if nausea occurs, absorption may be increased

Patient/family education

General

- Teach patient to take medication early in the day to prevent nocturia
- Instruct patient to take with food or milk if GI symptoms of nausea and anorexia occur
- Teach patient to maintain a weekly record of weight and notify prescriber of weight loss >5 lb
- Caution patient that this drg causes an increase in potassium levels, so foods high in potas-

sium should be avoided; refer to dietician for assistance planning

- Caution patient not to exercise in hot weather or stand for prolonged periods since orthostatic hypotension will be enhanced
- Teach patient not to use alcohol or any OTC medications without prescriber's approval; serious drug reactions may occur
- Emphasize the need to contact prescriber immediately if muscle cramps, weakness, nausea, dizziness, or numbness occurs
- Teach patient to take own B/P and pulse and record
- Advise patient that dizziness and confusion may occur; avoid driving or other hazadous activities if alertness is decreased
- Teach patient to continue taking medication even if feeling better; this drug controls symptoms but does not cure the condition
- Advise patient with hypertension to continue other medical treatment (exercise, weight loss, relaxation techniques, cessation of smoking)

Evaluation

Positive therapeutic outcome

- Prevention of hypokalemia (diuretic use)
- Decreased edema
- Decreased B/P
- Increased diuresis

Treatment of overdose: Lavage if taken orally; monitor electrolytes; administer **IV** fluids; monitor hydration, CV, renal status

amino acid

(a-mee'noe)

Injection:
Aminess, Aminosyn, BranchAmin, NephrAmine, FreAmine HBC, HepatAmine

Solution:
Aminosyn, Aminosyn II, Aminosyn-PF, FreAmine III, Novamine, ProcalAmine, RenAmin, Travasol, Trophamine

Func. class.: Caloric agent

Chem. class.: Nitrogen product

Pregnancy category C

Action: Needed for anabolism to maintain structure; decreases catabolism, promotes healing

Therapeutic Outcome: Positive nitrogen balance, decreased catabolism

Uses: Hepatic encephalopathy, cirrhosis, hepatitis, nutritional support in cancer trauma, intestinal obstruction, short bowel syndrome, severe malabsorption

Dosage and routes

Amino acid inj

Adult: **IV** 80-120 g/day; 500 ml of amino acids/500 ml D_{50} given over 24 hr

Amino acid solution

Adult: **IV** 1-1.5 g/kg/day titrated to patient's needs

P ***Child:*** **IV** 2-3 g/kg/day titrated to patient's needs

Available forms: Inj **IV** 2.75%, 3.5%, 4.25%, 5%, 5.5%, 6%, 8.5%, 10%, 11.4%, 15% amino acids

Side effects/adverse reactions

CNS: Dizziness, headache, confusion, ***loss of consciousness***
CV: Hypertension, ***CHF, pulmonary edema***
ENDO: Hyperglycemia, rebound hypoglycemia, electrolyte imbalances, hyperosmolar syndrome, hyperosmolar hyperglycemic nonketotic syndrome, alkalosis, acidosis, hypophosphatemia, hyperammonemia, dehydration, hypocalcemia
GI: Nausea, vomiting, liver fat deposits, abdominal pain
GU: Glycosuria, osmotic diuresis
INTEG: Chills, flushing, warm feeling, rash, urticaria, extravasation necrosis, phlebitis at injection site

Contraindications: Hypersensitivity, severe electrolyte imbalances, anuria, severe liver damage, maple syrup urine disease, PKU

Precautions: Renal disease, P pregnancy **C**, children, diabetes mellitus, CHF

Pharmacokinetics

Absorption	Complete bioavailability (IV)
Distribution	Widely distributed
Metabolism	Anabolism
Excretion	Kidney to urea nitrogen
Half-life	Unknown

Pharmacodynamics

	IV
Onset	Unknown
Peak	Unknown
Duration	Unknown

Interactions

Drug/drug:

Drug classifications
Diuretics: ↑ negative nitrogen balance
Glucocorticoids: ↑ negative nitrogen balance
Tetracyclines: ↑ negative nitrogen balance

NURSING CONSIDERATIONS

Assessment

- Monitor electrolytes (potassium, sodium, calcium, chloride, magnesium), blood glucose, ammonia, phosphate, ketones; renal, liver function studies: BUN, creatinine, ALT (SGPT), AST (SGOT), bilirubin; urine glucose q6h using Chemstrips, which are not affected by infusion substances; if BUN increases over 15%, therapy may need to be discontinued
- Check injection site for extravasation: redness along vein, edema at site, necrosis, pain; for a hard, tender area
- Monitor respiratory function q4h: auscultate lung fields bilaterally for crackles; monitor respirations for quality, rate, rhythm that indicates fluid overload
- Monitor temperature q4h for increased fever, indicating infection; if infection is suspected, infusion is discontinued and tubing bottle, catheter tip cultured; blood catheter may be obtained

- Monitor for impending hepatic coma: asterixis, confusion, fetor, lethargy
- Hyperammonemia: nausea, vomiting, malaise, tremors, anorexia, convulsions; increased ammonia, ketone levels may occur

Associated nursing diagnoses

✓ Nutrition, less than body requirements (uses)
✓ Injury, risk for physical (uses, adverse reactions)
✓ Infection, risk for (adverse reactions)
✓ Knowledge deficit (teaching)

Implementation

IV **IV route**

- Give up to 40% protein and dextrose (up to 12.5%) via peripheral vein; stronger solutions require central **IV** administration; TPN only mixed with dextrose to promote protein synthesis
- Use immediately after mixing in pharmacy under strict aseptic technique using laminar flowhood; use infusion pump, in-line filter (0.22 μm) unless mixed with fat emulsion and dextrose (3 in 1)
- Use careful monitoring technique; do not speed up infusion; pulmonary edema, glucose overload will result
- Storage depends on type of solution; consult manufacturer
- Change dressing and IV tubing to prevent infection q24-48h or q5-7 days if transparent dressing is used

Y-site incompatibility:

Cephradine

Y-site compatibilities:

Cefamandole, cefazolin, cefoperazone, cefotaxime, cefoxitin, cephalothin, cephapirin, chloramphenicol, clindamycin, digoxin, dobutamine, dopamine, doxycycline, erythromycin lactobionate, fat emulsion, foscarnet, furosemide, gentamicin, isoproterenol, kanamycin, lidocaine, meperidine, methicillin, mezlocillin, miconazole, morphine, nafcillin, netilmicin, norepinephrine, oxacillin, penicillin G potassium, piperacillin, sargramostim, ticarcillin, tobramycin, urokinase, vancomycin

Patient/family education

- Teach reason for use of amino acids as part of nutrition (TPN)
- Instruct patient to report at once to prescriber if chills, sweating are experienced

Evaluation

Positive therapeutic outcome

- Weight gain
- Decrease jaundice in liver disorders
- Increased LOC

aminocaproic acid

(a-mee-noe-ka-proe'ik)
Amicar, aminocaproic acid
Func. class.: Hemostatic
Chem. class.: Synthetic monoaminocarboxylic acid
Pregnancy category **C**

Action: Inhibits fibrinolysis by inhibiting plasminogen activator substances

Therapeutic Outcome: Decreased fibrinolysis, decreased bleeding, increased clot formation

Uses: Hemorrhage from hyperfibrinolysis, adjunctive therapy in hemophilia

Investigational uses: Prevention of recurrent subarachnoid hemorrhage

Dosage and routes

Adult: PO/**IV** 5-g loading dose, then 1-1.25 g q1h if needed, not to exceed 30 g/day

Available forms: **IV** inj 250 mg/ml; tabs 500 mg; syr 250 mg/ml

Side effects/adverse reactions

CNS: Headache, dizziness, malaise, fatigue, hallucinations, delirium, psychosis, ***convulsions,*** weakness
CV: ***Dysrhythmias,*** orthostatic hypotension, bradycardia
EENT: Tinnitus, nasal congestion, conjunctival suffusion
GI: Nausea, vomiting, abdominal cramps, diarrhea
GU: Dysuria, frequency, oliguria, ***renal failure,*** ejaculatory failure, menstrual irregularities
HEMA: ***Thrombosis***
INTEG: Rash

Contraindications: Hypersensitivity, abnormal bleeding, postpartum bleeding, DIC, upper urinary tract bleeding, new burns

Precautions: Neonates/infants, mild or moderate renal disease, hepatic disease, thrombosis, cardiac disease, pregnancy **C**

Pharmacokinetics

Absorption	Well absorbed (PO)
Distribution	Widely distributed
Metabolism	Unknown
Excretion	Kidneys, unchanged
Half-life	Unknown

Pharmacodynamics

	PO/IV
Onset	Unknown
Peak	2 hr
Duration	Unknown

Interactions: None

Lab test interferences

Increased: potassium, CPK, AST (SGOT), aldolase

NURSING CONSIDERATIONS

Assessment

- Monitor I&O ratios if urinary output decreases; notify prescriber and stop drug
- Monitor blood studies: coagulation factors, platelets, protamine coagulation factors, platelets, protamine coagulation test for extravascular clotting, thrombophlebitis; creatinine phosphokinase; check for thromboembolic symptoms (leg pain, redness, positive Homans' sign) edema, dyspnea, chest pain
- Monitor B/P, pulse, respiratory status; watch for increasing B/P and pulse
- Monitor drug level: 0.13 mg/ml is required to decrease fibrinolysis

- Assess for allergy: fever, rash, itching, jaundice
- Monitor myopathy: if weakness, fever, myoglobinemia, or oliguria, discontinue drug; watch for increased CPK, AST (SGOT), aldolase
- Assess for bleeding q15 min: mucous membranes, epistaxis, ecchymosis, petechiae, hematuria, hematemesis
- Monitor neurologic status (LOC, pupils, motor status) in subarachnoid hemorrhage

Associated nursing diagnoses

✓ Tissue perfusion, altered (uses)
✓ Injury, risk for (uses, adverse reactions)
✓ Cardiac output (adverse reaction)
✓ Knowledge deficit (teaching)

Implementation

IV **IV route**

- Give **IV** after dilution with 4-5 g/250 ml NS, D_5W, LR; give over 1 hr; may give by cont inf after loading dose(s); use inf pump; do not give by direct IV; stabilize catheter to prevent thrombophlebitis

Cont IV

- May be diluted in 50 ml of diluent and run at 1 g/hr by inf pump
- Store in tight container in cool environment; do not freeze; do not mix with other drugs

Additive incompatibilities:

Do not mix with other drugs in sol or syringe

Patient/family education

- Instruct patient to report any signs of bleeding (gums, under skin, urine, stools, emesis) or myopathy
- Instruct patient to change position slowly to decrease orthostatic hypotension
- Teach patient proper administration for 8-10 days following dental procedure in hemophilia
- Instruct patient to inform physicians and dentists that drug is being taken

Evaluation

Positive therapeutic outcome

- Decreased bleeding
- Absence of rebleeding (subarachnoid hemorrhage)

aminoglutethimide

(a-meen-oh-gloo-teth'i-mide)

Cytadren

Func. class.: Antineoplastic, adrenal steroid inhibitor

Chem. class.: Hormone

Pregnancy category **D**

Action: Acts by inhibiting DNA, RNA, protein synthesis; is derived from *Streptomyces verticillus;* replication is decreased by binding to DNA, which causes strand splitting; phase specific in G_2 and M phases; blocks biosynthesis of all steroid hormones (cortisol, androgens, progestins)

Therapeutic Outcome: Decreased spread of malignancy; decreased adrenal hormone in Cushing's syndrome

Uses: Suppression of adrenal function in Cushing's syndrome, metastatic breast cancer, adrenal cancer

Investigational uses: Advanced prostate cancer, metastatic postmenopausal breast cancer

Dosage and routes

Adult: PO 250 mg qid at 6-hr intervals; may increase by 250 mg/day q1-2 wk, not to exceed 2 g/day

Available forms: Tabs 250 mg

Side effects/adverse reactions

CNS: Drowsiness , dizziness, headache, lethargy
CV: Hypotension, tachycardia
GI: Nausea, vomiting, anorexia, ***hepatotoxicity***
INTEG: Rash, pruritus, hirsutism, *morbilliform skin rash*

Contraindications: Hypersensitivity, hypothyroidism, pregnancy **D**

Precautions: Renal disease, hepatic disease, respiratory disease

Pharmacokinetics

Absorption	Well absorbed (PO)
Distribution	Unknown
Metabolism	Liver (50%)
Excretion	Kidneys, unchanged (50%)
Half-life	13 hr initially

Pharmacodynamics

	PO
Onset	Unknown
Peak	Unknown
Duration	Unknown

Interactions

Drug/drug:

Individual drugs

Alcohol: ↑ effects of aminoglutethimide
Dexamethasone: ↑ metabolism, ↓ effect of dexamethasone
Digitoxin: ↓ effects of digitoxin
Medroxyprogesterone: ↓ effects of medroxyprogesterone
Theophylline: ↓ effects of theophylline
Warfarin: ↓ effects of warfarin

NURSING CONSIDERATIONS

Assessment

- Monitor renal function studies: BUN, serum uric acid, urine CrCl, electrolytes before, during therapy; I&O ratio; report fall in urine output of 30 ml/hr
- Monitor temperature q4h; may indicate beginning infection
- Monitor liver function tests before, during therapy (bilirubin, AST, ALT, LDH) as needed or monthly; RBC, Hct, Hgb, since these may be decreased
- Monitor inflammation of mucosa, breaks in skin, yellowing of skin and sclera, dark urine, clay-colored stools, itchy skin, abdominal pain, fever, diarrhea

• Assess symptoms indicating severe allergic reaction: rash, pruritus, urticaria, purpuric skin lesions, itching, flushing; if rash develops, drug may need to be discontinued
• Assess for Cushing's syndrome: buffalo hump, moon face, personality changes, hypertension, weakness, hirsutism

Associated nursing diagnoses

✓ Injury, risk for (adverse reactions)
✓ Body image disturbance (adverse reactions)
✓ Infection, risk for (adverse reactions)
✓ Knowledge deficit (teaching)

Implementation

PO route
• Give with food or fluids for GI upset
• Give in equal intervals q6h

Patient/family education

• Instruct patient to report side effects
• Advise patient to avoid use of alcohol, which potentiates this drug

Evaluation

Positive therapeutic outcome
• Prevention of rapid division of malignant cells, postmenopausal cancer, prostate cancer
• Suppression of adrenal function (Cushing's syndrome)

Treatment of overdose: Induce vomiting, provide supportive care

aminophylline

(am-in-off'i-lin)
Corophyllin ✦, Palaron ✦, Phyllocontin, Truphylline
Func. class.: Bronchodilator
Chem. class.: Xanthine, ethylenediamine
Pregnancy category **C**

Action: Relaxes smooth muscle of respiratory system by blocking phosphodiesterase, which increases cyclic AMP; increased cyclic AMP alters intracellular calcium ion movements; produces bronchodilatation, increased pulmonary blood flow, relaxation of respiratory tract

➔ **Therapeutic Outcome:** Increased ability to breathe

Uses: Bronchial asthma, bronchospasm, Cheyne-Stokes respirations

Investigational uses: Apnea P in infancy for respiratory/myocardial stimulation

Dosage and routes

Adult: PO 500 mg, then 250-500 mg q6-8h; cont **IV** 0.3-0.9 mg/kg/hr (maintenance); rect 500 mg q6-8h

P ***Child:*** PO 7.5 mg/kg, then 3-6 mg/kg q6-8h; **IV** 7.5 mg/kg, then 3-6 mg/kg q6-8h injected over 5 min; do not exceed 25 mg/min; may give loading dose of 5.6 mg/kg over ½ hr; cont **IV** 1 mg/kg/hr (maintenance);

P for children/infants use drug without preservative of alcohol

P *Neonates:* **IV**/PO 1 mg/kg initially for plasma increases of each 2 μg/ml, then 1 mg/kg q6h

Available forms: Inj **IV**, IM, rec supp 250, 500 mg; oral liq 105 mg/5 ml; tabs 100, 200 mg; con-rel tabs 225 mg

Side effects/adverse reactions

CNS: Anxiety, restlessness, insomnia, ***dizziness, convulsions,*** headache, lightheadedness, muscle twitching
CV: ***Palpitations, sinus tachycardia,*** hypotension, flushing, dysrhythmias, increased respiratory rate
GI: ***Nausea, vomiting,*** anorexia, diarrhea, bitter taste, dyspepsia, anal irritation (suppositories), epigastric pain
GU: Urinary frequency
INTEG: Flushing, urticaria, *rec supp (irritation)*
RESP: Increased rate

Contraindications: Hypersensitivity to xanthines, tachydysrhythmias

G **Precautions:** Elderly, CHF, cor pulmonale, hepatic disease, active peptic ulcer disease, diabetes mellitus, hyperthyroidism, hypertension,
P children, pregnancy **C**, glaucoma, prostatic hypertrophy

Pharmacokinetics

Absorption	Well absorbed (PO), slow (PO–ext rel), erratic (rec)
Distribution	Widely distributed; crosses placenta
Metabolism	Liver to caffeine
Excretion	Kidneys
Half-life	3-12 hr, increased in renal disease, CHF

Pharmacodynamics

	PO	PO–EXT REL	IV
Onset	15-60 min	Unknown	Immediate
Peak	1-2 hr	4-7 hr	Infusion's end
Duration	6-8 hr	8-12 hr	6-8 hr

Interactions

Drug/drug:

Individual drugs

Allopurinol: ↓ metabolism, ↑ toxicity of aminophylline
Carbamazepine: ↑ or ↓ aminophylline levels
Cimetidine: ↓ metabolism, ↑ toxicity of aminophylline
Disulfiram: ↓ metabolism, ↑ toxicity of aminophylline
Erythromycin: ↓ metabolism, ↑ toxicity of aminophylline
Halothane: ↑ risk of dysrhythmias
Interferon: ↓ metabolism, ↑ toxicity of aminophylline
Isoniazid: ↑ or ↓ aminophylline level
Ketoconazole: ↑ metabolism, ↓ effect of aminophylline
Lithium: ↓ effect of lithium
Mexiletine: ↓ metabolism, ↑ toxicity
Phenytoin: ↑ metabolism, ↓ effect of aminophylline
Rifampin: ↑ metabolism, ↓ effect of aminophylline

Thiabendazole: ↓ metabolism, ↑ toxicity

Drug classifications

Barbiturates: ↓ effect of aminophylline
β-Adrenergic blockers: ↓ metabolism, ↑ toxicity
Diuretics, loop: ↑ or ↓ aminophylline levels
Fluoroquinolones: ↓ metabolism, ↑ toxicity
Glucocorticoids: ↓ metabolism, ↑ toxicity
Sympathomimetics: ↑ CNS, CV adverse reactions

Drug/smoking:

↑ metabolism, ↓ effect

Drug/food:

Caffeinated foods (cola, coffee, tea, chocolate): ↑ CNS, CV, adverse reactions
Charcoal-smoked foods: ↓ effect

Lab test interferences

Increase: Plasma free fatty acids

NURSING CONSIDERATIONS

Assessment

- Monitor theophylline blood levels (therapeutic level is 10-20 μg/ml); toxicity may occur with small increase above 20 μg/ml, especially elderly (G); determine whether theophylline was given recently (24 hr); check for toxicity: nausea, vomiting, anxiety, restlessness, insomnia, tachycardia, dysrhythmias, convulsions; notify prescriber immediately
- Monitor I&O; diuresis will occur; dehydration may result in elderly (G) or children (P) in whom diuresis is great
- Monitor respiratory rate, rhythm, depth; auscultate lung fields bilaterally; notify prescriber of abnormalities; check ECG for tachycardia, PVCs, PACs in patients with cardiac problems
- Monitor allergic reactions: rash, urticaria; if these occur, drug should be discontinued, prescriber notified

Associated nursing diagnoses

- ✓ Airway clearance, ineffective (uses)
- ✓ Activity intolerance (uses)
- ✓ Injury, risk for (uses, adverse reactions)
- ✓ Knowledge deficit (teaching)

Implementation

General

- Give around the clock to maintain blood (theophylline) levels
- If switching from **IV** to PO, give controlled-release dose at time of **IV** infusion discontinuation; if giving tab (immediate release), discontinue **IV** and wait >4 hr

PO route

- Give PO after meals or water to decrease GI symptoms; absorption may be affected with a full glass of water or food; do not crush or chew enteric-coated or controlled-release tabs

IV route

- Give **IV** after diluting in 5% dextrose to decrease burning sensation at inj site; only clear solutions; may be diluted for IV inf in 100-200 ml in D_5W, $D_{10}W$, $D_{20}W$, 0.9% NaCl, 0.45% NaCl, LR

Syringe compatibilities:

Heparin, metoclopramide, pentobarbital, thiopental

Y-site compatibilities:

Amrinone, atracurium, cimetidine, enalaprilat, foscarnet, heparin sodium with hydrocortisone sodium succinate, morphine, netilmicin, pancuronium, potassium chloride, ranitidine, tolazoline, vecuronium

Y-site incompatibilities:

Dobutamine, hydralazine, ondansetron

Additive compatibilities:

Amobarbital, bretylium, calcium gluconate, chloramphenicol, dexamethasone, diphenhydramine, dopamine, erythromycin lactobionate, esmolol, heparin, hydrocortisone, lidocaine, methyldopate, metronidazole, pentobarbital, potassium chloride, ranitidine, secobarbital, sodium bicarbonate, sodium iodide, terbutaline, verapamil

Additive incompatibilities:

Ascorbic acid, bleomycin, cephalothin, cefotaxime, chlorpromazine, cimetidine, clindamycin, codeine, dimenhydrinate, dobutamine, doxorubicin, doxycycline, epinephrine, erythromycin gluceptate, hydralazine, hydroxyzine, insulin, isoproterenol, meperidine, methicillin, morphine, nafcillin, nitroprusside, norepinephrine, oxytetracycline, papaverine, penicillin G, pentazocine, phenobarbital, phenytoin, prochlorperazine, promazine, promethazine, sulfisoxazole, tetracycline, vancomycin

- Avoid IM injection; pain and tissue damage may occur
- Only clear sol; flush **IV** line before dose; store diluted sol for 24 hrs if refrigerated

Rectal route

- Rec dose if patient is unable to take PO; retain rec dose for ½ hour

Patient/family education

- Teach patient to take doses as prescribed, not to skip dose; to check OTC medications, current prescription medications for ephedrine which will increase CNS stimulation; advise patient not to drink alcohol or caffeine products (tea, coffee, chocolate, colas), which will increase action
- Teach patient to avoid hazardous activities; dizziness may occur
- Teach patient if GI upset occurs, to take drug with 8 oz water or food; absorption may be decreased
- Teach patient to remain in bed 15-20 min after rec supp is inserted to prevent removal
- Instruct patient that smoking increases metabolism; dosage may need to be increased
- Teach patient to obtain blood levels of drug every few months to prevent toxicity; not to change brands, since effect may not be the same
- Teach patient to increase fluids to 2 L/day to decrease viscosity of secretions

Evaluation

Positive therapeutic outcome

- Decreased dyspnea

- Respiratory stimulation in infancy
- Clear lung fields bilaterally

amiodarone

(am-ee-oh'da-rone)

Cordarone

Func. class.: Antidysrhythmic (Class III)

Chem. class.: Iodinated benzofuran derivative

Pregnancy category C

Action: Prolongs action potential duration and effective refractory period, slows sinus rate with increasing PR and QT intervals, noncompetitive α- and β-adrenergic inhibition

Therapeutic Outcome: Decreased amount and severity of ventricular dysrhythmias

Uses: Severe ventricular tachycardia, supraventricular tachycardia, ventricular fibrillation not controlled by 1st-line agents

Dosage and routes

Adult: PO loading dose 800-1600 mg/day × 1-3 wk; then 600-800 mg/day × 1 mo; maintenance 200-600 mg/day

Available forms: Tabs 200 mg

Side effects/adverse reactions

CNS: Headache, dizziness, involuntary movement, tremors, peripheral neuropathy, malaise, fatigue, ataxia, paresthesias, insomnia

CV: Hypotension, bradycardia, ***sinus arrest, CHF, dysrhythmias, SA node dysfunction***

EENT: Blurred vision, halos, photophobia, ***corneal microdeposits,*** dry eyes

ENDO: Hyperthyroidism or hypothyroidism

GI: Nausea, vomiting, diarrhea, abdominal pain, anorexia, constipation, ***hepatotoxicity***

INTEG: Rash, photosensitivity, blue-gray skin discoloration, alopecia, spontaneous ecchymosis

MISC: Flushing, abnormal taste or smell, edema, abnormal salivation, coagulation abnormalities

MS: Weakness, pain in extremities

RESP: ***Pulmonary fibrosis,*** pulmonary inflammation

Contraindications: Sinus node dysfunction; 2nd, 3rd degree AV block

Precautions: Goiter, Hashimoto's thyroiditis, SN dysfunction, 2nd- or 3rd-degree AV block, electrolyte imbalances, pregnancy **C**, bradycardia, lactation

Pharmacokinetics

Absorption	Slow, variable (PO) up to 65%
Distribution	Body tissues; crosses placenta
Metabolism	Liver
Excretion	Bile, kidney (minimal)
Half-life	15-100 days

Pharmacodynamics

	PO
Onset	1-3 wk
Peak	Unknown
Duration	Up to months

Interactions

Drug/drug:

Individual drugs

Digoxin: ↑ blood levels, ↑ toxicity
Disopyramide: ↑ levels, ↑ toxicity
Flecainide: ↑ levels, ↑ toxicity
Lidocaine: Bradycardia, cardiac arrest
Mexiletine: ↑ levels, ↑ toxicity
Phenytoin: ↑ blood levels
Procainamide: ↑ levels, ↑ toxicity
Quinidine: ↑ levels, ↑ toxicity
Warfarin: ↑ level, ↑ bleeding

Drug classifications

β-Blockers: ↑ dysrhythmias, cardiac arrest
Calcium channel blockers: ↑ dysrhythmias, cardiac arrest

NURSING CONSIDERATIONS

Assessment

- Monitor I&O ratio; monitor electrolytes: potassium, sodium, chloride
- Monitor liver function studies: AST (SGOT), ALT (SGPT), bilirubin, alkaline phosphatase
- Monitor ECG continuously to determine drug effectiveness; measure PR, QRS, QT intervals; check for PVCs, other dysrhythmias; monitor B/P continuously for hypotension, hypertension; check for rebound hypertension after 1-2 hr
- Monitor for dehydration or hypovolemia
- Assess for CNS symptoms: confusion, psychosis, numbness, depression, involuntary movements; if these occur, drug should be discontinued
- Assess for hypothyroidism: lethargy, dizziness, constipation, enlarged thyroid gland, edema of extremities, cool, pale skin
- Monitor hyperthyroidism: restlessness, tachycardia, eyelid puffiness, weight loss, frequent urination, menstrual irregularities, dyspnea, warm, moist skin
- Assess for pulmonary toxicity: dyspnea, fatigue, cough, fever, chest pain; drug should be discontinued if these occur
- Monitor cardiac rate, respiration: rate, rhythm, character, chest pain, ventricular tachycardia, supraventricular tachycardia or fibrillation
- Assess sight and vision before treatment and throughout therapy; microdeposits on the cornea may cause blurred vision, halos, and photophobia

Associated nursing diagnoses

- ✓ Cardiac output, decreased (uses)
- ✓ Gas exchange, impaired (adverse reactions)
- ✓ Knowledge deficit (teaching)

Implementation

PO route

- Give reduced dosage slowly with ECG monitoring only
- Give with meals for GI upset

Patient/family education

- Instruct patient to report side effects immediately to prescriber
- Instruct patient that skin discoloration is usually reversible but skin may turn bluish on neck, face, arms when used for long periods
- Advise patient that dark glasses may be needed for photophobia
- Instruct patient to use sunscreen and protective clothing to prevent burning associated with photosensitivity
- Instruct patient to take medication as prescribed, not to double doses
- Instruct patient to complete follow-up appointment with health care provider including pulmonary function studies, chest x-ray, ophthalmic examinations

Treatment of overdose: Administer O_2, artificial ventilation, ECG, dopamine for circulatory depression, diazepam or thiopental for convulsions, isoproterenol

amitriptyline

(a-mee-trip'ti-leen)

amitriptyline HCl, Apo-Amitriptyline ✦, Elavil, Endep, Enovil, Levate ✦, Meravil ✦, Novotriptyn ✦, Rolavil ✦

Func. class.: Antidepressant—tricyclic

Chem. class.: Tertiary amine

Pregnancy category C

Action: Blocks reuptake of norepinephrine, serotonin into nerve endings that increase action of norepinephrine, serotonin in nerve cells

Uses: Major depression

Investigational uses: Chronic pain management

➔ **Therapeutic Outcome:** Decreased symptoms of depression after 2-3 wk

Dosage and routes

Adult: PO 30-100 mg hs; may increase to 200 mg qd, not to exceed 300 mg/day; IM 20-30 mg qid, or 80-120 mg hs

P G ***Adolescent/ geriatric:*** PO 30 mg/day in divided doses; may be increased to 150 mg/day

Available forms: Tabs 10, 25, 50, 75, 100, 150 mg; inj IM 10 mg/ml; syrup 10 mg/ 5 ml ✦

A

Side effects/adverse reactions

CNS: Dizziness, drowsiness, confusion, headache, anxiety, tremors, stimulation, weakness, insomnia, nightmares, G EPS (elderly), increased psychiatric symptoms
CV: Orthostatic hypotension, ***ECG changes, tachycardia, hypertension,*** palpitations
EENT: Blurred vision, tinnitus, mydriasis, ophthalmoplegia
GI: Diarrhea, dry mouth, nausea, vomiting, ***paralytic ileus,*** increased appetite, cramps, epigastric distress, jaundice, ***hepatitis,*** stomatitis
GU: Retention
HEMA: **Agranulocytosis, thrombocytopenia, eosinophilia, leukopenia**
INTEG: Rash, urticaria, sweating, pruritus, photosensitivity

Contraindications: Hypersensitivity to tricyclic antidepressants, recovery phase of myocardial infarction

Precautions: Suicidal patients, convulsive disorders, prostatic hypertrophy, schizophrenia, psychosis, severe depression, increased intraocular pressure, narrow angle glaucoma, urinary retention, cardiac disease, hepatic/renal disease, hyperthyroidism, electroshock therapy, elective P surgery, child <12 yr, preg-G nancy **C**, elderly

Pharmacokinetics

Absorption	Well absorbed
Distribution	Widely distributed; crosses placenta
Metabolism	Liver, extensively
Excretion	Kidneys, breast milk
Half-life	10-50 hr

Pharmacodynamics

	PO/IM
Onset	45 min
Peak	2-12 hr
Duration	Unknown

Interactions

Drug/drug:

Individual drugs

Alcohol: ↑ CNS depression
Cimetidine: ↑ levels, ↑ toxicity
Clonidine: ↑ hypertension; avoid use
Disulfiram: Organic brain syndrome
Fluoxetine: ↑ levels, ↑ toxicity
Guanethidine: ↓ effects

Drug classifications

Antihypertensives: Blocked response to antihypertensive
MAOI: Hypertensive crisis, convulsions
Barbiturates: ↑ CNS effects
Benzodiazepines: ↑ CNS effects
CNS depressants: ↑ CNS effects
Sympathomimetics, indirect acting: ↓ effects
Oral contraceptives: ↑ effects, toxicity

Drug/smoking:

↑ metabolism, ↓ effects

Lab test interferences

Increase: Serum bilirubin, blood glucose, alkaline phosphatase

Decrease: VMA, 5-HIAA
False increase: Urinary catecholamines

NURSING CONSIDERATIONS

Assessment

- Monitor B/P (with patient lying, standing), pulse q4h; if systolic B/P drops 20 mm Hg, hold drug, notify prescriber; take vital signs q4h in patients with cardiovascular disease
- Monitor blood studies: CBC, leukocytes, differential, cardiac enzymes if patient is receiving long-term therapy
- Monitor hepatic studies: AST (SGOT), ALT (SGPT), bilirubin
- Check weight weekly; appetite may increase with drug
- Assess ECG for flattening of T wave, bundle branch block, AV block, dysrhythmias in cardiac patients
- Assess for EPS primarily in G elderly: rigidity, dystonia, akathisia
- Assess mental status: mood, sensorium, affect, suicidal tendencies; increase in psychiatric symptoms: depression, panic
- Monitor urinary retention, constipation; constipation is P more likely to occur in children G or elderly
- Assess for withdrawal symptoms: headache, nausea, vomiting, muscle pain, weakness; do not usually occur unless drug was discontinued abruptly
- Identify alcohol consumption; if alcohol is consumed, hold dose until morning

Associated nursing diagnoses

- ✓ Coping, ineffective individual (uses)
- ✓ Injury, risk for physical (side effects)
- ✓ Knowledge deficit (teaching)
- ✓ Noncompliance (teaching)

Implementation

PO route

- Give with food or milk for GI symptoms
- Crush if patient is unable to swallow medication whole
- Give dosage hs if oversedation occurs during day; may G take entire dose hs; elderly may not tolerate once/day dosing
- Store at room temp; do not freeze

Patient/family education

- Teach patient that therapeutic effects may take 2-3 wk
- Instruct patient to use caution in driving or other activities requiring alertness because of drowsiness, dizziness, blurred vision; to avoid rising quickly from sitting to G standing, especially elderly
- Advise patient to avoid alcohol ingestion, other CNS depressants
- Teach patient not to discontinue medication quickly after long-term use; may cause nausea, headache, malaise
- Advise patient to wear sunscreen or large hat, since photosensitivity occurs
- Teach patient to increase fluids, bulk in diet if constipation, urinary retention occur, G especially elderly
- Teach patient to take gum, hard sugarless candy, or fre-

quent sips of water for dry mouth

Evaluation

Positive therapeutic outcome
- Decreased depression
- Absence of suicidal thoughts

Treatment of overdose: ECG monitoring, induce emesis, lavage, activated charcoal, administer anticonvulsant

amlodipine
(am-loe'di-peen)
Norvasc
Func. class.: Calcium channel blocker, antianginal, antihypertensive
Chem. class.: Dihydropyridine
Pregnancy category C

Action: Inhibits calcium ion influx across cell membrane during cardiac depolarization; produces relaxation of coronary vascular smooth muscle, peripheral vascular smooth muscle; dilates coronary vascular arteries; increases myocardial oxygen delivery in patients with vasospastic angina

Therapeutic Outcome: Decreased angina pectoris, dysrhythmias, B/P

Uses: Chronic stable angina pectoris, hypertension, vasospastic angina

Dosage and routes

Angina

Adult: PO 5-10 mg qd

Hypertension

Adult: PO 5 mg qd initially; may increase up to 10 mg/day

Available forms: Tabs 2.5, 5, 10 mg

Side effects/adverse reactions

CNS: Headache, fatigue, dizziness, anxiety, depression, insomnia, paresthesia, somnolence, asthenia
CV: Dysrhythmia, edema, bradycardia, hypotension, palpitations, syncope, AV block
GI: Nausea, vomiting, diarrhea, gastric upset, constipation, abdominal cramps, flatulence, anorexia
GU: Nocturia, polyuria, ***acute renal failure***
INTEG: Rash, pruritus, urticaria, hair loss
MISC: Flushing, nasal congestion, sweating, shortness of breath, sexual difficulties, muscle cramps, cough, weight gain, tinnitus, epistaxis

Contraindications: Sick sinus syndrome, 2nd- or 3rd-degree heart block, hypotension less than 90 mm Hg systolic, hypersensitivity

Precautions: CHF, hypotension, hepatic injury, pregnancy P C, lactation, children, renal G disease, elderly

Pharmacokinetics

Absorption	Well absorbed (PO), up to 90%
Distribution	Crosses placenta
Metabolism	Liver, extensively
Excretion	Kidneys to metabolites (90%)
Half-life	30-50 hr

Pharmacodynamics

	PO
Onset	Unknown
Peak	6-12 hr
Duration	24 hr

Interactions

Drug/drug:

Individual drugs

Alcohol: ↑ hypotension
Fentanyl: ↑ hypotension

Drug classifications

Antihypertensives: ↑ hypotension
Nitrates: ↑ hypotension

NURSING CONSIDERATIONS

Assessment

- Assess fluid volume status: I&O ratio and record, weight, distended red veins, crackles in lung, color, quality and specific gravity of urine, skin turgor, adequacy of pulses, moist mucous membranes, bilateral lung sounds, peripheral pitting edema; dehydration symptoms of decreasing output, thirst, hypotension, dry mouth and mucous membranes should be reported
- Monitor B/P and pulse; if B/P drops call prescriber
- Monitor ALT (SGPT), AST (SGOT), bilirubin daily; if these are elevated, hepatotoxicity is suspected
- Monitor if platelets are <150,000/mm^3; drug is usually discontinued and another drug started
- Monitor cardiac status: B/P, pulse, respiration, ECG

Associated nursing diagnoses

✓ Cardiac output, decreased (uses)
✓ Knowledge deficit (teaching)

Implementation

PO route

- Give once a day, with food for GI symptoms

Patient/family education

- Advise patient to avoid hazardous activities until stabilized on drug, dizziness is no longer a problem
- Instruct patient to limit caffeine consumption; to avoid alcohol and OTC drugs unless directed by prescriber
- Advise patient to comply in all areas of medical regimen: diet, exercise, stress reduction, drug therapy; to notify prescriber of irregular heart beat, shortness of breath, swelling of feet and hands, pronounced dizziness, constipation, nausea, hypotension
- Teach patient to use as directed even if feeling better; may be taken with other cardiovascular drugs (nitrates, β-blockers)

Evaluation

Positive therapeutic outcome

- Decreased anginal pain
- Decreased B/P

Treatment of overdose: Defibrillation, β-agonists, **IV** calcium inotropic agents, diuretics, atropine for AV block, vasopressor for hypotension

amobarbital

(am-oh-bar'bi-tal)

amobarbital sodium, Amytal, Amytal Sodium, Amytal Sodium Pulvules

Func. class.: Sedative/hypnotic barbiturate (intermediate acting) anticonvulsant

Chem. class.: Amylobarbitone

Pregnancy category D

Controlled substance schedule II (USA), schedule G (Canada)

Action: Depresses activity in brain cells primarily in reticular activating system in brainstem; also selectively depresses neurons in posterior hypothalamus, limbic structures; able to decrease seizure activity by inhibition of impulses in CNS; decreases motor activity

Uses: Sedation, preanesthetic sedation, insomnia, anticonvulsant, adjunct in psychiatry, hypnotic

➔ **Therapeutic Outcome:** Sedation, anticonvulsant, improved energy

Dosage and routes

Preanesthetic sedation

P ***Adult and child:*** PO/IM 200 mg 1-2 hr preoperatively

Sedation

Adult: PO 30-50 mg bid or tid; may be 15-120 mg bid-qid

P ***Child:*** PO 2 mg/kg/day in 4 divided doses

Anticonvulsant/psychiatry

Adult: **IV** 65-500 mg given over several min, not to exceed 100 mg/min; not to exceed 1 g

P ***Child less than 6 yr:*** **IV**/IM 3-5 mg/kg over several min

Insomnia

Adult: PO/IM 65-200 mg hs, not to exceed 5 ml in one site

P ***Child:*** IM 3-5 mg/kg hs, not to exceed 5 ml in one site

Available forms: Tabs 30, 50, 100 mg; caps 65, 200 mg; powder for inj IM, **IV** 250, 500 mg/vial

Side effects/adverse reactions

CNS: Lethargy, drowsiness, hangover, dizziness, stimulation in the elderly and children, lightheadedness, physical dependence, CNS depression, mental depression, slurred speech

G P

CV: Hypotension, bradycardia

GI: Nausea, vomiting, diarrhea, constipation

HEMA: Agranulocytosis, thrombocytopenia, megaloblastic anemia (long-term treatment)

INTEG: Rash, urticaria, pain, abscesses at injection site, ***angioedema,*** thrombophlebitis, ***Stevens-Johnson syndrome***

RESP: Depression, apnea, laryngospasm, bronchospasm

Contraindications: Hypersensitivity to barbiturates, respiratory depression, addiction to barbiturates, severe liver impairment, porphyria

Precautions: Anemia, pregnancy **D**, lactation, hepatic disease, renal disease, hypertension, G elderly, acute/chronic pain

Pharmacokinetics

Absorption	Well absorbed (PO, IM)
Distribution	Widely distributed; crosses placenta
Metabolism	Liver
Excretion	Kidneys
Half-life	16-40 hr

Pharmacodynamics

	PO	IM	IV
Onset	45-60 min	30-45 min	10 min
Peak	Unknown	Unknown	Unknown
Duration	6-8 hr	6-8 hr	3-6 hr

Interactions

Drug/drug:

Individual drugs

Acebutolol: ↓ effectiveness
Alcohol: ↑ CNS depression
Chloramphenicol: ↓ effectiveness
Doxycycline: ↑ half-life
Griseofulvin: ↓ effectiveness
Metoprolol: ↓ effectiveness
Propranolol: ↓ effectiveness
Quinidine: ↓ effectiveness
Timolol: ↓ effectiveness

Drug classifications

Antidepressants, tricyclics: ↑ CNS depression
Antihistamines: ↑ CNS depression
Estrogens: ↓ effectiveness
Glucocorticoids: ↓ effectiveness
MAOI: ↑ CNS depression
Narcotics: ↑ CNS depression
Oral contraceptives: ↓ effectiveness
Phenothiazines: ↓ CNS depression
Sedatives/hypnotics: ↑ CNS depression
Tricyclics: ↓ effectiveness

Lab test interferences

False increase: Sulfobromophthalein

NURSING CONSIDERATIONS

Assessment

- Mental status: mood, sensorium, affect, memory (long, G short), especially elderly; if using as a hypnotic, assess sleep patterns during therapy; drug suppresses REM sleep with dreaming; withdrawal insomnia may occur after short-term use; do not start using drug again, insomnia will improve in 1-3 nights; may experience increased dreaming
- Monitor for respiratory dysfunction: respiratory depression, character, rate, rhythm (when using **IV**); hold drug if respirations are <10/min or if pupils are dilated; also check VS q30 min after parenteral route for 2 hr
- Assess for barbiturate toxicity: hypotension, pulmonary constriction, cold, clammy skin, cyanosis of lips, CNS depression, nausea, vomiting, hallucinations, delirium, weakness, coma, pupillary constriction; mild symptoms may occur in 8-12 hr without drug
- Assess for blood dyscrasias: fever, sore throat, bruising,

rash, jaundice, epistaxis (long-term treatment only)

- Assess for pain in postoperative patients; pain threshold is lowered when patients are taking this medication

Associated nursing diagnoses

- ✓ Sleep pattern disturbance (uses)
- ✓ Injury, risk for (adverse reactions)
- ✓ Knowledge deficit (teaching)
- ✓ Noncompliance (teaching)

Implementation

- Use after removal of cigarettes, to prevent fires; after trying conservative measures for insomnia

PO route

- Give 30 min before hs for expected sleeplessness; on empty stomach for best absorption

IM route

- Reconstitute with sterile water for inj (100 mg/ml); mix by rotating vial; do not shake
- Give in deep muscle mass (gluteal) to minimize irritation to tissues; split inj of >5 ml into 2 since irritation to tissues may occur; reconstitute with sterile water for inj (100 mg/ml); mix by rotating vial, do not shake

IV **IV route**

- Reconstitute with sterile water for inj (100 mg/ml); mix by rotating vial; do not shake; may be further diluted with D_5W, $D_{10}W$, $D_{20}W$, D_5/0.9% NaCl, D_5LR, 0.9% NaCl, 3% NaCl, LR; use within 30 min; do not use if cloudy or colored after 5 min of reconstitution

IV **Direct IV route**

- Use large vein to prevent extravasation; if extravasation occurs, use moist heat to the area and procaine sol 5% injected into area; give at 100 mg/min or more (adult); 60 P mg/m^2/min (child); give **IV** only with resuscitative equipment available (only by qualified personnel)

Additive compatibilities:

Amikacin, aminophylline, sodium bicarbonate

Additive incompatibilities:

Cefazolin, cephalothin, cimetidine, chlorpromazine, clindamycin, codeine, diphenhydramine, droperidol, hydroxyzine, regular insulin, levorphanol, meperidine, methadone, morphine, norepinephrine, pentazocine, procaine, streptomycin, tetracycline, vancomycin

Patient/family education

- Teach patient that hangover is common
- Instruct patient that drug is indicated only for short-term treatment of insomnia and is probably ineffective after 2 wk
- Inform patient that physical dependency may result when used for extended time (45-90 days depending on dosage)
- Caution patient to avoid driving or other activities requiring alertness
- Caution patient to avoid alcohol ingestion and CNS depressants; serious CNS depression may result

- Instruct patient not to discontinue medication quickly after long-term use; drug should be tapered over 1 wk
- Emphasize the need to tell all prescribers that a barbiturate is being taken
- Inform patient that withdrawal insomnia may occur after short-term use; do not start using drug again; insomnia will improve in 1-3 nights, may experience increased dreaming
- Inform patient that effects may take 2 nights for benefits to be noticed; teach patient alternate measures to improve sleep: reading, exercise several hours before hs, warm bath, warm milk, TV, self-hypnosis, deep breathing
- Teach patient to make position changes slowly; orthostatic hypotension may occur
- Instruct patient to notify prescriber immediately if bruising or bleeding occurs, which may indicate blood dyscrasias

Evaluation

Positive therapeutic outcome

- Improved sleeping patterns
- Decreased seizure activity
- Improved energy

Treatment of overdose: Lavage, activated charcoal, warming blanket, vital signs, hemodialysis, alkalinize urine; give **IV** volume expanders, **IV** fluids

amoxapine

(a-mox'a-peen)

amoxapine, Asendin

Func. class.: Antidepressant—tricyclic

Chem. class.: Dibenzoxazepine derivative, secondary amine

Pregnancy category C

Action: Blocks reuptake of norepinephrine, serotonin into nerve endings, thereby increasing action of norepinephrine, serotonin in nerve cells

Uses: Depression

Therapeutic Outcome: Decreased symptoms of depression after 2-3 wk

Dosage and routes

Adult: PO 50 mg tid; may increase to 100 mg tid on 3rd day of therapy; not to exceed 300 mg/day unless lower doses have been given for at least 2 wk; may be given daily dose hs; not to exceed 600 mg/day in hospitalized patients

G ***Elderly:*** PO 25 mg BID-TID, may increase to 50 mg BID-TID, not to exceed 300 mg/day

Available forms: Tabs 25, 50, 75, 100, 150 mg

Side effects/adverse reactions

CNS: Dizziness, drowsiness, confusion, headache, anxiety, tremors, stimulation, weak-

ness, insomnia, nightmares, G EPS (elderly), increased psychiatric symptoms, paresthesia, impairment of sexual functioning
CV: Orthostatic hypotension, ECG changes, tachycardia, ***hypertension,*** palpitations
EENT: Blurred vision, tinnitus, mydriasis, ophthalmoplegia
GI: Diarrhea, dry mouth, constipation, nausea, vomiting, ***paralytic ileus,*** increased appetite, cramps, epigastric distress, jaundice, ***hepatitis,*** stomatitis
GU: Retention, ***acute renal failure***
HEMA: ***Agranulocytosis, thrombocytopenia, eosinophilia, leukopenia***
INTEG: Rash, urticaria, sweating, pruritus, photosensitivity

Contraindications: Hypersensitivity to tricyclic antidepressants, recovery phase of myocardial infarction, convulsive disorders, prostatic hypertrophy

Precautions: Suicidal patients, severe depression, increased intraocular pressure, narrow-angle glaucoma, urinary retention, cardiac disease, hepatic disease, hyperthyroidism, electroshock therapy, elective G surgery, elderly, pregnancy **C**

Pharmacokinetics

Absorption	Well absorbed
Distribution	Widely distributed; crosses placenta
Metabolism	Liver, extensively
Excretion	Kidneys, breast milk
Half-life	8 hr

Pharmacodynamics

	PO
Onset	Unknown
Peak	Unknown
Duration	Unknown

Interactions

Drug/drug:

Individual drugs
Alcohol: ↑ CNS depression
Cimetidine: ↑ levels, ↑ toxicity of amoxapine
Clonidine: Severe hypotension; avoid use
Disulfiram: Organic brain syndrome
Fluoxetine: ↑ levels, ↑ toxicity of amoxapine
Guanethidine: ↓ effects of amoxapine

Drug classifications
MAOI: Hypertensive crisis, convulsions
Barbiturates: ↑ effects of amoxapine
Benzodiazepines: ↑ effects of amoxapine
CNS depressants: ↑ effects of amoxapine
Sympathomimetics, indirect acting: ↓ effects of amoxapine
Oral contraceptives: ↑ effects, toxicity of amoxapine

Drug/smoking: ↑ metabolism, ↓ effects

Lab test interferences

Increase: Serum bilirubin, blood glucose, alkaline phosphatase
Decrease: VMA, 5-HIAA
False increase: Urinary catecholamines

NURSING CONSIDERATIONS

Assessment

- Monitor B/P (with patient lying, standing), pulse q4h; if systolic B/P drops 20 mm Hg hold drug, notify prescriber; take vital signs q4h in patients with cardiovascular disease
- Monitor blood studies: CBC, leukocytes, differential, cardiac enzymes if patient is receiving long-term therapy
- Monitor hepatic studies: AST (SGOT), ALT (SGPT), bilirubin
- Check weight weekly; appetite may increase with drug
- Assess ECG for flattening of T wave, bundle branch block, AV block, dysrhythmias in cardiac patients
- Assess for EPS primarily in G elderly: rigidity, dystonia, akathisia
- Assess mental status: mood, sensorium, affect, suicidal tendencies; increase in psychiatric symptoms: depression, panic
- Monitor urinary retention, constipation; constipation is P more likely to occur in children G and elderly
- Assess for withdrawal symptoms: headache, nausea, vomiting, muscle pain, weakness; do not usually occur unless drug was discontinued abruptly
- Identify alcohol consumption; if alcohol is consumed, hold dose until morning

Associated nursing diagnoses

- ✓ Coping, ineffective individual (uses)
- ✓ Injury, risk for physical (side effects)
- ✓ Knowledge deficit (teaching)
- ✓ Noncompliance (teaching)

Implementation

PO route

- Give with food or milk for GI symptoms
- Crush if patient is unable to swallow medication whole
- Store at room temp; do not freeze

Patient/family education

- Teach patient that therapeutic effects may take 2-3 wk
- Instruct patient to use caution in driving or other activities requiring alertness because of drowsiness, dizziness, blurred vision; to avoid rising quickly from sitting to standing, G especially elderly
- Teach patient to avoid alcohol ingestion, other CNS depressants
- Teach patient not to discontinue medication quickly after long-term use: may cause nausea, headache, malaise
- Teach patient to wear sunscreen or large hat, since photosensitivity occurs
- Teach patient to increase fluids, bulk in diet if constipation, urinary retention occur, G especially elderly
- Advise patient to take gum, hard sugarless candy, or frequent sips of water for dry mouth

Evaluation

Positive therapeutic outcome

- Decreased depression
- Absence of suicidal thoughts

Treatment of overdose: ECG monitoring, induce emesis, lavage, activated charcoal, administer anticonvulsant

amoxicillin

(a-mox-i-sill'in)

Amoxican ♣, amoxicillin, Amoxil, Amoxil Pediatric Drops, Apo-Amoxi ♣, Biomox, Novamoxin ♣, Polymox, Polymox Drops, Trimox 125, Trimox 250, Trimox 500, Wymox

Func. class.: Broad-spectrum antibiotic

Chem. class.: Aminopenicillin

Pregnancy category B

Action: Interferes with cell wall replication of susceptible organisms by binding to the bacterial cell wall; the cell wall, rendered osmotically unstable, swells and bursts from osmotic pressure

Uses: Infections of respiratory tract, skin, skin structures, genitourinary tract, otitis media, meningitis, septicemia, sinusitis and endocarditis prophylaxis

Investigational uses: Lyme disease

Therapeutic Outcome: Bactericidal effects for the following organisms: effective for gram-positive cocci (*Streptococcus pyogenes, S. faecalis, S. pneumoniae*), gram-negative cocci (*Neisseria gonorrhoeae, N. meningitidis, Escherichia coli*), gram-negative bacilli (*Haemophilus influenzae, Proteus mirabilis, Salmonella*)

Dosage and routes

Systemic infections

Adult: PO 750 mg-1.5 g qd in divided doses q8h

P *Child:* PO 20-40 mg/kg/day in divided doses q8h

Gonorrhea/urinary tract infections

Adult: PO 3 g given with 1 g probenecid as a single dose

Available forms: Caps 250, 500 mg; chewable tabs 125, 250 mg; powder for oral susp 50, 125, 250 mg/5 ml

Side effects/adverse reactions

CNS: Headache, fever

GI: Nausea, vomiting, diarrhea, increased AST (SGOT), ALT (SPGT), abdominal pain, glossitis, colitis, ***pseudomembranous colitis***

HEMA: Anemia, increased bleeding time, ***bone marrow depression, granulocytopenia***

SYST: ***Anaphylaxis, respiratory distress***

Contraindications: Hypersensitivity to penicillins; P neonates

Precautions: Pregnancy **B**, hypersensitivity to cephalosporins

Pharmacokinetics

Absorption	Well absorbed (90%)
Distribution	Readily in body tissues, fluids, CSF; crosses placenta
Metabolism	Liver (30%)
Excretion	Breast milk, kidney, unchanged (70%)
Half-life	1-1.3 hr

Pharmacodynamics

	PO
Onset	½ hr
Peak	2 hr

Interactions

Drug/drug:

Individual drugs

Aspirin: ↑ amoxicillin levels, ↓ renal excretion
Probenecid: ↑ amoxicillin levels, ↓ renal excretion

Drug classifications

Erythromycins: ↓ antimicrobial effectiveness
Oral anticoagulants: ↑ anticoagulant effects
Oral contraceptives: ↓ contraceptive effectiveness
Tetracyclines: ↓ antimicrobial effectiveness

Lab test interferences

False positive: Urine glucose, urine protein

NURSING CONSIDERATIONS

Assessment

- Assess patient for previous sensitivity reaction to penicillins or other cephalosporins; cross-sensitivity between penicillins and cephalosporins is common
- Assess patient for signs and symptoms of infection, including characteristics of wounds, sputum, urine, stool, WBC >10,000, earache, fever; obtain baseline information and monitor symptoms during treatment
- Obtain C & S before beginning drug therapy to identify if correct treatment has been initiated
- Assess for allergic reactions during treatment: rash, urticaria, pruritus, chills, fever, joint pain; angioedema may occur a few days after therapy begins; epinephrine and resuscitation equipment should be available for anaphylactic reactions
- Identify urine output; if decreasing, notify prescriber (may indicate nephrotoxicity); also, increased BUN, creatinine
- Monitor blood studies: AST (SGOT), ALT (SGPT), CBC, Hct, bilirubin, LDH, alkaline phosphatase, Coombs' test monthly if patient is on long-term therapy
- Monitor electrolytes: potassium, sodium, chloride monthly if patient is on long-term therapy
- Assess bowel pattern qd; if severe diarrhea occurs, notify prescriber; drug should be discontinued; may indicate pseudomembranous colitis
- Monitor for bleeding: ecchymosis, bleeding gums, hematuria, stool guaiac daily if on long-term therapy
- Assess for overgrowth of infection: perineal itching, fever, malaise, redness, pain, swelling, drainage, rash, diarrhea, change in cough, sputum

Associated nursing diagnoses

✓ Infection, risk for (uses)
✓ Diarrhea (side effects)

- ✓ Injury, risk for (side effects)
- ✓ Knowledge deficit (teaching)
- ✓ Noncompliance (teaching)

Implementation

PO route

- Give in even doses around the clock; if GI upset occurs, give with food; drug must be given for 10-14 days to ensure organism death and prevent superinfection; store in tight container
- Shake susp; store in refrigerator for 7-10 days

Patient/family education

- Teach patient to report sore throat, bruising, bleeding, joint pain; may indicate blood dyscrasias (rare)
- Advise patient to contact prescriber if vaginal itching, loose, foul-smelling stools, furry tongue occur; which may indicate superinfection
- Instruct patient to take all medication prescribed for the length of time ordered
- Advise patient to notify prescriber of diarrhea with blood or pus, which may indicate pseudomembranous colitis

Evaluation

Positive therapeutic outcome

- Absence of signs/symptoms of infection (WBC <10,000, temp WNL, absence of red draining wounds or earache)
- Reported improvement in symptoms of infection

Treatment of anaphylaxis:

Withdraw drug, maintain airway, administer epinephrine, aminophylline, O_2, **IV** corticosteroids

A

amoxicillin/clavulanate

(a-mox-i-sill′in)

Augmentin, Clavulin ✦

Func. class.: Broad-spectrum antibiotic (extended spectrum)

Chem. class.: Aminopenicillin-β-lactamase inhibitor

Pregnancy category **B**

Action: Interferes with cell wall replication of susceptible organisms; the cell wall, rendered osmotically unstable, swells and bursts from osmotic pressure; combination increases spectrum of activity, β-lactamase resistance

Uses: Infections of respiratory tract, skin, skin structures, genitourinary tract; otitis media, meningitis, septicemia, sinusitis, and endocarditis prophylaxis

➡ Therapeutic Outcome: Bactericidal effects for the following organisms: *Escherichia coli, Proteus mirabilis, Haemophilus influenzae, Streptococcus faecalis, S. pneumoniae;* and β-lactamase–producing organisms: *Neisseria gonorrhoeae, N. meningitis, Shigella, Salmonella, Enterococcus, Streptococcus*

Dosage and routes

Adult: PO 250-500 mg q8h depending on severity of infection

P *Child:* PO 20-40 mg/kg/day in divided doses q8h

Available forms: Tabs 250, 500 mg; chewable tabs 125, 250 mg; powder for oral susp 125, 250 mg/5 ml

Side effects/adverse reactions

CNS: Headache, fever
GI: Nausea, diarrhea, vomiting, increased AST (SGOT), ALT (SGPT), abdominal pain, glossitis, colitis, black tongue, ***pseudomembranous colitis***
GU: **Oliguria, proteinuria, hematuria,** *vaginitis, moniliasis,* ***glomerulonephritis***
HEMA: Anemia, ***bone marrow depression, granulocytopenia, leukopenia, eosinophilia,*** *thrombocytopenic purpura*
META: Hyperkalemia, hypokalemia, alkalosis, hypernatremia
SYST: Anaphylaxis

Contraindications: Hypersensitivity to penicillins; neonates P

Precautions: Pregnancy **B**, hypersensitivity to cephalosporins, lactation

Pharmacokinetics

Absorption	Well absorbed (90%)
Distribution	Readily in body tissues, fluids, CSF; crosses placenta
Metabolism	Liver (30%)
Excretion	Breast milk; kidney, unchanged (70%)
Half-life	1-1.3 hr

Pharmacodynamics

	PO
Onset	½ hr
Peak	2 hr

Interactions

Drug/drug:

Individual drugs
Aspirin: ↑ amoxicillin levels, decreased renal excretion
Probenecid: ↑ amoxicillin levels, decreased renal excretion

Drug classifications
Erythromycins: ↓ antimicrobial effectiveness
Oral anticoagulants: ↑ anticoagulant effects
Oral contraceptives: ↓ contraceptive effectiveness
Tetracyclines: ↓ antimicrobial effectiveness

Lab test interferences

False positive: Urine glucose, urine protein

NURSING CONSIDERATIONS

Assessment

- Assess patient for previous sensitivity reaction to penicillins or other cephalosporins; cross-sensitivity between penicillins and cephalosporins is common
- Assess patient for signs and symptoms of infection, including characteristics of wounds, sputum, urine, stool, WBC >10,000, earache, fever; obtain baseline information and during treatment
- Complete C & S before beginning drug therapy to identify if correct treatment has been initiated
- Assess for allergic reactions: rash, urticaria, pruritus, chills, fever, joint pain; angioedema may occur a few days after therapy begins; epinephrine and resuscitation equipment

should be available for anaphylactic reaction
- Identify urine output; if decreasing, notify prescriber (may indicate nephrotoxicity); also, increased BUN, creatinine
- Monitor blood studies: AST (SGOT), ALT (SGPT), CBC, Hct, bilirubin, LDH, alkaline phosphatase, Coombs' test monthly if patient is on long-term therapy
- Monitor electrolytes: potassium, sodium, chloride monthly if patient is on long-term therapy
- Assess bowel pattern qd; if severe diarrhea occurs, drug should be discontinued; may indicate pseudomembranous colitis
- Monitor for bleeding: ecchymosis, bleeding gums, hematuria, stool guaiac daily if on long-term therapy
- Assess for overgrowth of infection: perineal itching, fever, malaise, redness, pain, swelling, drainage, rash, diarrhea, change in cough, sputum

Associated nursing diagnoses

- ✓ Infection, risk for (uses)
- ✓ Injury, risk for (side effects)
- ✓ Diarrhea (side effects)
- ✓ Knowledge deficit (teaching)
- ✓ Noncompliance (teaching)

Implementation

PO route
- Give in even doses around the clock; if GI upset occurs, give with food; drug must be taken for 10-14 days to ensure organism death and prevent superinfection; store in tight container; cap can be opened and mixed with food or liq; chewable tabs should be chewed
- Shake susp, store in refrigerator for 2 wk or 1 wk at room temp

Patient/family education

- Teach patient to report sore throat, bruising, bleeding, joint pain; may indicate blood dyscrasias (rare)
- Advise patient to contact prescriber if vaginal itching, loose, foul-smelling stools occur; may indicate superinfection
- Instruct patient to take all medication prescribed for the length of time prescribed
- Advise patient to notify prescriber of diarrhea with blood or pus, which may indicate pseudomembranous colitis

Evaluation

Positive therapeutic outcome
- Absence of signs/symptoms of infection (WBC <10,000, temp WNL, absence of red draining wounds, earache)
- Reported improvement in symptoms of infection

Treatment of anaphylaxis:

Withdraw drug, maintain airway, administer epinephrine, aminophylline, O_2, **IV** corticosteroids

amphetamine
(am-fet'a-meen)
amphetamine sulfate
Func. class.: Cerebral stimulant
Chem. class.: Amphetamine
Pregnancy category C
Controlled substance schedule II

Action: Increases release of norepinephrine in nerve endings, dopamine in cerebral cortex to reticular activating system; increases CNS, respiratory stimulation, pupillary dilatation, vasoconstriction

Therapeutic Outcome: Increased alertness, decreased fatigue, ability to stay awake (treatment of narcolepsy), increased attention span, decreased hyperactivity (ADHD)

Uses: Narcolepsy, ADHD

Dosage and routes

Narcolepsy

Adult: PO 5-60 mg qd in divided doses

P ***Child >12 yr:*** PO 10 mg qd increasing by 10 mg/day at weekly intervals

P ***Child 6-12 yr:*** PO 5 mg qd increasing by 5 mg/wk, max 60 mg/day

ADHD

P ***Child >6 yr:*** PO 5 mg qd-bid increasing by 5 mg/day at weekly intervals

P ***Child 3-6 yr:*** PO 2.5 mg qd increasing by 2.5 mg/day at weekly intervals

Available forms: Tabs 5, 10 mg; long-acting cap 5, 10 mg

Side effects/adverse reactions

CNS: ***Hyperactivity, insomnia, restlessness, talkativeness,*** dizziness, headache, chills, stimulation, dysphoria, irritability, aggressiveness, tremor, dependence, addiction
CV: *Palpitations, tachycardia,* hypertension, dysrhythmias, decreased heart rate
GI: Nausea, vomiting, anorexia, dry mouth, diarrhea, constipation, weight loss, metallic taste, cramps
GU: Impotence, change in libido
INTEG: Urticaria

Contraindications: Hypersensitivity to sympathomimetic amines, hyperthyroidism, hypertension, glaucoma, severe arteriosclerosis, drug abuse, cardiovascular disease, anxiety

Precautions: Gilles de la Tourette's syndrome, lactation, P child <6 yr, pregnancy **C**

Pharmacokinetics

Absorption	Well absorbed (PO), within 3 hr
Distribution	Widely distributed; crosses placenta; high concentrations in brain
Metabolism	Liver
Excretion	Kidneys: pH dependent, increased pH leads to increased reabsorption; breast milk
Half-life	10-30 hr; increased when urine is alkaline, decreased when urine is acidic

Pharmacodynamics

	PO
Onset	½ hr
Peak	1-3 hr
Duration	4-20 hr

Interactions

Drug/drug:

Individual drugs

Acetazolamide: ↓ excretion, ↑ effect
Ammonium chloride: ↓ effect
Ascorbic acid: ↓ effect
Meperidine: Hypertensive crisis
Sodium bicarbonate: ↓ excretion, ↑ effect
Thyroid: ↑ effects

Drug classifications

Antidepressants, tricyclics: ↑ dysrhythmias
β-Blockers: ↑ hypertension
Cardiac glycosides: ↑ dysrhythmias
MAOI: Hypertensive crisis
Sympathomimetics: ↑ effect

Drug/food:

Cranberries/juice: ↑ amphetamine effect

NURSING CONSIDERATIONS

Assessment

- Monitor VS, B/P, since this drug may reverse antihypertensives; check patients with cardiac disease more often for increased B/P
- Monitor CBC, urinalysis; in diabetes blood sugar, urine sugar; insulin changes may be required, since eating will decrease
- Monitor height and weight q3 mo, since growth rate in P children may be decreased; appetite is suppressed, weight loss is common during the first few months of treatment
- Monitor mental status: mood, sensorium, affect, stimulation, insomnia; aggressiveness may occur; depression with crying spells may occur after drug has worn off
- Assess for physical dependency; should not be used for extended time except in ADHD; should be discontinued gradually to prevent withdrawal symptoms
- Assess for narcoleptic symptoms before medication and after; ability to stay awake should increase significantly
- P In children or adults with ADHD, monitor for improved organizational skills, attention span, attending to tasks, impulse control, socialization, and ability to get along better with others
- Assess for withdrawal symptoms: headache, nausea, vomiting, muscle pain, weakness; drug tolerance develops after long-term use; dosage should not be increased if tolerance develops; this medication has a high abuse potential

Associated nursing diagnoses

- ✓ Thought processes, altered (uses, adverse reactions)
- ✓ Coping, impaired individual (uses)
- ✓ Knowledge deficit (teaching)
- ✓ Family coping, impaired individual (uses)

Implementation

PO route

- Give at least 6 hr hs to avoid sleeplessness; titrate to patient's response, lowest dosage should be used to control symptoms
- Use gum, hard candy, frequent sips of water for dry mouth at beginning of treatment; these symptoms tend to lessen with time

Patient/family education

- Advise patient to decrease caffeine consumption (coffee, tea, cola, chocolate), which may increase irritability and stimulation; to avoid OTC preparations unless approved by prescriber; to avoid alcohol ingestion; these may cause serious drug interactions
- Instruct patient to taper off drug over several wks, or depression, increased sleeping, lethargy may occur
- Advise patient to avoid hazardous activities until stabilized on medication
- Instruct patient not to double doses if medication is missed; prescriber may suggest drug holidays (ADHD) during the school year to assess progress and determine continued drug necessity
- Instruct patient/family to notify health care provider if significant side effects occur: tremors, insomnia, palpitations, restlessness, drug changes may be needed
- Inform patient that if dry mouth occurs to use frequent sips of water, sugarless gum, hard candy during beginning therapy; dry mouth lessens with continued treatment
- Tell patient to get needed rest; patients feel more tired at end of day; to give last dose at least 6 hr hs to avoid insomnia

Evaluation

Positive therapeutic outcome

- Decreased activity in ADHD
- Absence of sleeping during day in narcolepsy

Treatment of overdose:

Administer fluids, hemodialysis, peritoneal dialysis, antihypertensives for increased B/P; ammonium chloride for increased excretion

amphotericin B 🔑

(am-foe-ter'i-sin)

amphotericin B, Fungizone IV, Fungizone

Func. class.: Antifungal

Chem. class.: Amphoteric polyene

Pregnancy category B

Action: Increases cell membrane permeability in susceptible organisms by binding sterols in fungal cell membrane; decreases potassium, sodium, and nutrients in cell

➡ Therapeutic Outcome: Fungistatic against histoplasmosis, blastomycosis, coccidioidomycosis, cryptococcosis, aspergillosis, phycomycosis, candidiasis, sporotrichosis

Uses: Treatment of severe, possibly fatal fungal infections (**IV**); treatment of topical fungal infections (top)

Dosage and routes

P *Adult and child:* **IV** inf 1 mg/250 ml D_5W (0.1 mg/ml) over 2-4 hr or 0.25 mg/kg/day over 6 hr; may be increased gradually up to 1 mg/kg/day, not to exceed 1.5 mg/kg; intrathecal 25 µg/0.1 ml diluted in 10-20 ml CSF given by barbotage 2-3 times a wk, gradually increased to 0.5 mg q48-72 hr

Candidal infection of GI tract

Adults: 100 mg PO qid × 2 wk

Candidal oral infection: 1 loz qid × 7-14 days; allow loz to dissolve slowly in mouth

P *Adult and child:* Top bid-qid for 7-21 days or longer if needed

Available forms: Powder for inj 50 mg, cream, lotion, oint 3%

Side effects/adverse reactions

CNS: Headache, fever, chills, peripheral nerve pain, paresthesias, peripheral neuropathy, ***convulsions,*** dizziness
EENT: Tinnitus, deafness, diplopia, blurred vision
GI: Nausea, vomiting, anorexia, diarrhea, cramps, ***hemorrhagic gastroenteritis, acute liver failure***
GU: Hypokalemia, axotemia, hyposthenuria, ***renal tubular acidosis,*** nephrocalcinosis, ***permanent renal impairment, anuria, oliguria***
HEMA: Normochromic and normocytic anemia, ***thrombocytopenia, agranulocytosis, leukopenia, eosinophilia,*** hypokalemia, hyponatremia, hypomagnesemia
INTEG: Burning, irritation, pain, necrosis at inj site with extravasation, flushing, dermatitis, skin rash (top route)
MS: ***Arthralgia, myalgia,*** generalized pain, weakness, weight loss

Contraindications: Hypersensitivity, severe bone marrow depression

Precautions: Renal disease, pregnancy **B**

Pharmacokinetics

Absorption	Complete bioavailability (IV), rapidly absorbed (top)
Distribution	Body tissues
Metabolism	Liver
Excretion	Kidneys, detectable for several weeks
Half-life	Initial 24-48 hr, terminal 15 days

Pharmacodynamics

	IV	TOP
Onset	Immediate	Unknown
Peak	1-2 hr	Unknown

Interactions

Drug/drug:

Individual drugs

Mezlocillin: ↑ hypokalemia
Piperacillin: ↑ hypokalemia
Ticarcillin: ↑ hypokalemia

Drug classifications

Diuretics: ↑ nephrotoxicity, hypokalemia
Glucocorticoids: ↑ hypokalemia
Nephrotoxic drugs: ↑ nephrotoxicity

NURSING CONSIDERATIONS

Assessment

IV **IV route**

- Monitor VS q15-30 min during first inf; note changes in pulse, B/P
- Monitor blood studies: Hgb, Hct, potassium, sodium, calcium, magnesium q2 wk; BUN, creatinine weekly; decreased Hgb, Hct and magnesium are common with increased potassium
- Monitor weight weekly; if weight increases over 2 lb/wk, edema is present; renal damage should be considered
- Monitor for renal toxicity: increasing BUN, serum creatinine; if BUN is >40 mg/dl or if serum creatinine >3 mg/dl, drug may be discontinued or dosage reduced; I&O ratio: watch for decreasing urinary output, change in sp gr; discontinue drug to prevent permanent damage to renal tubules; provide hydration of 2-3 L/day
- Monitor for hepatotoxicity: increasing AST (SGOT), ALT (SGPT), alkaline phosphatase, bilirubin
- Monitor for allergic reaction: dermatitis, rash; drug should be discontinued, antihistamines (mild reaction) or epinephrine (severe reaction) administered; check inj site for thrombophlebitis
- Monitor for hypokalemia: anorexia, drowsiness, weakness, decreased reflexes, dizziness, increased urinary output, increased thirst, paresthesias; if these occur, drug should be decreased or discontinued and potassium administered

Top route

- Monitor for allergic reaction: burning, stinging, swelling, redness

Associated nursing diagnoses

✓ Infection, risk for (uses)
✓ Injury, risk for physical (adverse reaction)
✓ Knowledge deficit (teaching)

Implementation

Top route

- Provide enough medication to cover lesions completely; do not cover with occlusive dressing; apply liberally and rub thoroughly into affected area; administer after cleansing with soap, water before each application, dry well (as ordered), wear gloves during application
- Store at room temp in dry place

IV **IV route**

- Give after diluting 50 mg in 10 ml sterile water (no preservatives); shake well, further dilute with 500 ml of D_5W to concentration of 0.1 mg/ml; do not use other diluents or sol; use large needle

(20 G); change needle for each step; wear gloves

- Use test dosage of 1 mg/20 ml D_5W; give over 10-30 min; if no reaction, drug is administered as ordered
- Administer **IV** using in-line filter (mean pore diameter >1 µm) using distal veins; check for extravasation, necrosis q8h; use an inf pump; administer over 6 hr; rapid inf may result in circulation collapse; may also be given through central line
- Give drug only after C&S confirm organism, drug needed to treat condition; make sure drug is used in life-threatening infections
- Provide protection from light during infusion; cover with foil
- Store protected from moisture and light; diluted sol is stable for 24 hr at room temp, 1 wk refrigerated

Syringe compatibility:
Heparin

Y-site compatibility:
Zidovudine

Y-site incompatibilities:
Enalaprilat, fludarabine, foscarnet, ondansetron

Additive compatibilities:
Heparin, hydrocortisone, methylprednisolone, sodium bicarbonate

Patient/family education

Top route

- Teach patient that skin and clothing may become discolored; to use asepsis (hand washing) before, after each application to prevent further infection
- Instruct patient to apply with glove to prevent further infection; not to cover with occlusive dressing; to continue even if condition improves
- Teach patient to avoid use of OTC creams, ointments, lotions, unless directed by prescriber
- Instruct patient to report increased itching, burning, rash, redness; ointment may irritate most hairy areas; to report if condition worsens

IV **IV route**

- Advise patient that long-term therapy may be needed to clear infection (2 wk-3 mo depending on type of infection)
- Teach patient side effects and when to notify prescriber

Evaluation

Positive therapeutic outcome

- Decrease in size, number of lesions (top)
- Decreased fever, malaise, rash
- Negative C&S for infecting organism

ampicillin
(am-pi-sill'in)
Amcil, Ampicin ✤, Apo-Ampi ✤, D-Amp ✤, Nu-Ampi ✤, NovoAmpicillin ✤, Polycillin, Omnipen, Omnipen-N, Polycillin-N, Supen, Totacillin, Totacillin-N
Func. class.: Broad-spectrum antibiotic
Chem. class.: Aminopenicillin
Pregnancy category **B**

Action: Interferes with cell wall replication of susceptible organisms; the cell wall, rendered osmotically unstable, swells, bursts from osmotic pressure

Therapeutic Outcome: Bactericidal effects for the following organisms: effective for gram-positive cocci (*Streptococcus pyogenes, S. faecalis, S. pneumoniae*), gram-negative cocci (*Neisseria gonorrhoeae, N. meningitidis*), gram-negative bacilli (*Haemophilus influenzae, Proteus mirabilis, Salmonella, Shigella, Listeria monocytogenes*), gram-positive bacilli

Uses: Infections of respiratory tract, skin, skin structures, genitourinary tract; otitis media, meningitis, septicemia, sinusitis and endocarditis prophylaxis

Dosage and routes
Systemic infections
Adult: PO 250-500 mg q6h or 1-2 g qd in divided doses q6h; **IV**/IM 250-500 mg q6h, (up to 2 g q4h in severe infections) or 2-8 g qd in divided doses q4-6h
P *Child:* PO 50-100 mg/kg/day in divided doses q6h; **IV**/IM 100- 200 mg/kg/day in divided doses q6h for septicemia or bacterial meningitis

Meningitis
Adult: **IV** 8-14 g/day in divided doses q3-4h × 3 days
P *Child:* **IV** 200-300 mg/kg/day in divided doses q3-4h × 3 days

Gonorrhea
Adult: PO 3.5 g given with 1 g probenecid as a single dose or IM/**IV** 500 mg q 8-12 hr × 2 doses

Available forms: Powder for inj **IV**, IM 125, 250, 500 mg, 1, 2, 10 g; **IV** inf 500 mg, 1, 2 g; caps 250, 500 mg; powder for oral susp 100/1 ml, 125, 250, 500 mg/5 ml

Side effects/adverse reactions
CNS: Lethargy, hallucinations, anxiety, depression, twitching, ***coma, convulsions***
GI: Nausea, vomiting, diarrhea
GU: Oliguria, proteinuria, hematuria, *vaginitis, moniliasis,* ***glomerulonephritis***
HEMA: Anemia, increased bleeding time, ***bone marrow depression, granulocytopenia***
INTEG: Rash, urticaria
SYST: Anaphylaxis

Contraindications: Hypersensitivity to penicillins

Precautions: Pregnancy **B**; hypersensitivity to cephalosporins; neonates P

Pharmacokinetics

Absorption	Moderate, duodenum (35%-50%)
Distribution	Readily in body tissues, fluids, CSF; crosses placenta
Metabolism	Liver (30%)
Excretion	Breast milk; kidney unchanged (70%)
Half-life	50-110 min

Pharmacodynamics

	PO	IM	IV
Onset	Rapid	Rapid	Rapid
Peak	2 hr	1 hr	Infusion's end

Interactions

Drug/drug:

Individual drugs

Aspirin: ↑ ampicillin levels, ↓ renal excretion

Probenecid: ↑ ampicillin levels, ↓ renal excretion

Drug classifications

Erythromycins: ↓ antimicrobial effectiveness

Oral anticoagulants: ↑ anticoagulant effects

Oral contraceptives: ↓ contraceptive effectiveness

Tetracyclines: ↓ antimicrobial effectiveness

Lab test interferences

False positive: Urine glucose, urine protein

NURSING CONSIDERATIONS

Assessment

- Assess patient for previous sensitivity reaction to penicillins or other cephalosporins; cross-sensitivity between penicillins and cephalosporins is common
- Assess patient for signs and symptoms of infection, including characteristics of wounds, sputum, urine, stool, WBC >10,000, earache, fever; obtain baseline information and during treatment
- Obtain C&S before beginning drug therapy to identify if correct treatment has been initiated
- Assess for allergic reactions: rash, urticaria, pruritus, chills, fever, joint pain; angioedema may occur a few days after therapy begins; epinephrine and resuscitation equipment should be on unit for anaphylactic reaction; also, check for ampicillin rash: pruritic, red, raised
- Identify urine output; if decreasing, notify prescriber (may indicate nephrotoxicity); also, check for increased BUN, creatinine
- Monitor blood studies: AST (SGOT), ALT (SGPT), CBC, Hct, bilirubin, LDH, alkaline phosphatase, Coombs' test monthly if patient is on long-term therapy
- Monitor electrolytes: potassium, sodium, chloride monthly if patient is on long-term therapy
- Assess bowel pattern qd; if severe diarrhea occurs, drug should be discontinued; may indicate pseudomembranous colitis
- Monitor for bleeding: ecchymosis, bleeding gums, hematuria, stool guaiac daily if on long-term therapy

• Assess for overgrowth of infection: perineal itching, fever, malaise, redness, pain, swelling, drainage, rash, diarrhea, change in cough, sputum

Associated nursing diagnoses

✓ Infection, risk for (uses)
✓ Injury, risk for (side effects)
✓ Diarrhea (side effects)
✓ Knowledge deficit (teaching)
✓ Noncompliance (teaching)

Implementation

PO route

• Give in even doses around the clock; if GI upset occurs, give with food; drug must be taken for 10-14 days to ensure organism death and prevent superinfection; store cap in tight container
• Tabs may be crushed or caps opened and mixed with water
• Shake suspension; store in refrigerator for 2 wk or 1 wk at room temp

IM route

• Reconstitute with 125 mg/ 0.9-1.2 ml; 250 mg/0.9-1.9 ml; 500 mg/1.2-1.8 ml; 1 g/2.4-7.4 ml; 2 g/6.8 ml
• Give deep in large muscle mass

IV **IV route**

• Reconstitute with 125 mg/ 0.9-1.2 ml; 250 mg/0.9-1.9 ml; 500 mg/1.2-1.8 ml; 1 g/2.4-7.4 ml; 2 g/6.8 ml
• Give by direct **IV** over 3-5 min in lower dosages (125-500 mg) or over 15 min in higher dosages (1-2 g)
• Give by intermittent inf after diluting with 0.9% NaCl, LR, D_5W, D_5/0.45% NaCl; use 50 ml of sol and dilute to concentration of <30 mg/ml

Syringe incompatibilities:

Erythromycin, gentamicin, kanamycin, lincomycin, metoclopramide, oxytetracycline, streptomycin, tetracycline

Syringe compatibilities:

Chloramphenicol, colistimethate, heparin, procaine, lidocaine

Y-*site incompatibilities:*

Calcium gluconate, epinephrine, fluconazole, hetastarch, hydromorphone, hydralazine, ondansetron, sargramostim, verapamil, vinorelbine

Y-*site compatibilities:*

Acyclovir, cyclophosphamide, enalaprilat, esmolol, famotidine, fludarabine, foscarnet, heparin, hydromorphone, regular insulin, labetalol, magnesium sulfate, melphalan, meperidine, morphine, perphenazine, phytonadione, potassium chloride, tolazoline, vitamin B with C

Additive incompatibilities:

Amikacin, azetreonam, chlorpromazine, dopamine, gentamicin, hydralazine, hydrocortisone, prochlorperazine

Additive compatibilities:

Clindamycin, erythromycin, floxacillin, furosemide, verapamil

Patient/family education

• Teach patient to report sore throat, bruising, bleeding, joint pain; may indicate blood dyscrasias (rare)
• Advise patient to contact prescriber if vaginal itching,

loose, foul-smelling stools, furry tongue occur; may indicate superinfection
- Instruct patient to take all medication prescribed for the length of time ordered
- Advise patient to notify prescriber of diarrhea with blood or pus, which may indicate pseudomembranous colitis

Evaluation

Positive therapeutic outcome
- Absence of signs/symptoms of infection (WBC <10,000, temp WNL, absence of red draining wounds, earache)
- Reported improvement in symptoms of infection

Treatment of anaphylaxis: Withdraw drug, maintain airway, administer epinephrine, aminophylline, O_2, **IV** corticosteroids

ampicillin/sulbactam

(am-pi-sill'in/sul-bak'tam)
Unasyn
Func. class.: Broad-spectrum antibiotic
Chem. class.: Aminopenicillin
Pregnancy category **B** (ampicillin)

Action: Interferes with cell wall replication of susceptible organisms; the cell wall, rendered osmotically unstable, swells and bursts from osmotic pressure; this combination extends the spectrum of activity and inhibits β-lactamase that may inactivate ampicillin

➔ Therapeutic Outcome: Bactericidal against *Pneumococcus, Enterococcus, Streptococcus, Escherichia coli, Proteus mirabilis, Neisseria meningitidis, N. gonorrhoeae, Shigella, Salmonella,* and *Haemophilus influenzae organisms*; use only with β-lactamase–producing strain of infection

Uses: Skin and structure infections, intraabdominal infections, gynecologic infections, soft tissue infections, otitis media, sinusitis, meningitis, septicemia

Dosage and routes

Adult: **IV** 1 g ampicillin and 0.5 g sulbactam or 2 g ampicillin, and 1 g sulbactam q6h, not to exceed 4 g/day sulbactam

Available forms: Powder for inj 1.5 g (1 g ampicillin, 0.5 g sulbactam), 3 g (2 g ampicillin, 1 g sulbactam)

Side effects/adverse reactions

CNS: Lethargy, hallucinations, anxiety, depression, twitching, ***coma, convulsions***
GI: *Nausea, vomiting, diarrhea,* increased AST (SGOT), ALT (SGPT), abdominal pain, glossitis, colitis
GU: Oliguria, proteinuria, hematuria, *vaginitis, moniliasis,* ***glomerulonephritis***
HEMA: Anemia, increased bleeding time, ***bone marrow depression, granulocytopenia***
SYST: ***Anaphalaxis***

Contraindications: Hypersensitivity to penicillins

Precautions: Pregnancy **B**, hypersensitivity to cephalosporins, P neonates

Pharmacokinetics

Absorption	Well absorbed (IM)
Distribution	Readily in body tissues, fluids, CSF; crosses placenta
Metabolism	Liver (10%-50%)
Excretion	Breast milk; kidney unchanged (75%)
Half-life	50-110 min (ampicillin)

Pharmacodynamics

	IM	IV
Onset	Rapid	Immediate
Peak	1 hr	Infusion's end

Interactions
Drug/drug:
Individual drugs

Aspirin: ↑ ampicillin levels, ↓ renal excretion

Probenecid: ↑ ampicillin levels, ↓ renal excretion

Drug classifications

Erythromycins: ↓ antimicrobial effectiveness

Oral anticoagulants: ↑ anticoagulant effects

Oral contraceptives: ↓ contraceptive effectiveness

Tetracyclines: ↓ antimicrobial effectiveness

Lab test interferences
False positive: Urine glucose, urine protein

NURSING CONSIDERATIONS
Assessment
- Assess patient for previous sensitivity reaction to penicillins or cephalosporins; cross-sensitivity between penicillins and cephalosporins is common
- Assess patient for signs and symptoms of infection; including characteristics of wounds, sputum, urine, stool, WBC >10,000, earache, fever; obtain baseline information and during treatment
- Complete C&S before beginning drug therapy to identify if correct treatment has been initiated
- Assess for allergic reactions: rash, urticaria, pruritus, chills, fever, joint pain; angioedema may occur a few days after therapy begins; epinephrine and resuscitation equipment should be on unit for anaphylactic reaction
- Identify urine output; if decreasing, notify prescriber (may indicate nephrotoxicity); also, check for increased BUN, creatinine
- Monitor blood studies: AST (SGOT), ALT (SGPT), CBC, Hct, bilirubin, LDH, alkaline phosphatase, Coombs' test monthly if patient is on long-term therapy
- Monitor electrolytes: potassium, sodium, chloride monthly if patient is on long-term therapy
- Assess bowel pattern qd; if severe diarrhea occurs, drug should be discontinued; may indicate pseudomembranous colitis
- Monitor for bleeding: ecchymosis, bleeding gums, hematuria, stool guaiac daily if on long-term therapy
- Assess for superinfection: perineal itching, fever, malaise, redness, pain, swelling, drainage, rash, diarrhea, change in cough, sputum

A

Associated nursing diagnoses

- Infection, risk for (uses)
- Diarrhea (adverse reactions)
- Injury, risk for (adverse reactions)
- Knowledge deficit (teaching)
- Noncompliance (teaching)

Implementation

IM route

• Reconstitute by adding 3.2 ml/1.5 g or 6.4 ml/3 g; use sterile water, 0.5% or 2% lidocaine; give within 1 hr of preparation; give deep in large muscle mass

• Give after C&S completed; on empty stomach

IV **IV route**

• Give **IV** after diluting 1.5 g/4 ml or more sterile H_2O for inj (375 mg/ml); allow to stand until foaming stops; give directly over 15-30 min; dilute further in 50 ml or more of D_5W, $D_5$10.45% NaCl, 10% invert sugar in water, LR, 6% sodium lactate, isotonic NaCl; administer within 1 hr after reconstitution; give as an intermittent inf over 15-30 min

Y-site incompatibilities: Idarubicin, ondansetron, sargramostim

Y-site compatibilities: Enalaprilat, famotidine, fluconazole, regular insulin, meperidine, morphine, paclitaxel

Additive incompatibility: Aminoglycosides

Patient/family education

• Teach patient to report sore throat, bruising, bleeding, joint pain; may indicate blood dyscrasias (rare)

• Advise patient to contact prescriber if vaginal itching, loose, foul-smelling stools, furry tongue occur; may indicate superinfection

• Instruct patient to use another form of contraception other than oral contraceptives

Evaluation

Positive therapeutic outcome

• Absence of signs/symptoms of infection (WBC <10,000, temp WNL, absence of red draining wounds, earache)

• Reported improvement in symptoms of infection

Treatment of overdose: Withdraw drug, maintain airway, administer epinephrine, aminophylline, O_2, **IV** corticosteroids for anaphylaxis

amrinone

(am′ri-none)

Inocor

Func. class.: Cardiac inotropic agent

Chem. class.: Bipyrimidine derivative

Pregnancy category **C**

Action: Positive inotropic agent with vasodilator properties; reduces preload and afterload by direct relaxation of vascular smooth muscle; increases myocardial contractility

➡ **Therapeutic Outcome:** Increased inotropic effect resulting in increased cardiac output

Uses: Short-term management of CHF that has not responded to other medication; can be used with digitalis products

Dosage and routes

Adult: **IV** bol 0.75 mg/kg given over 2-3 min; start inf of 5-10 μg/kg/min; may give another bol 30 min after start of therapy, not to exceed 10 mg/kg total daily dose

P ***Infant:*** **IV** 3-4.5 mg/kg in divided doses, then start inf of 10 μg/kg/min

P ***Neonates:*** **IV** 3-4.5 mg/kg in divided doses, then start inf of 3-5 μg/kg/min

Available forms:
Inj 5 mg/ml

Side effects/adverse reactions

CV: ***Dysrhythmias, hypotension,*** headache, chest pain
ELECT: Hypokalemia
GI: *Nausea, vomiting, anorexia,* abdominal pain, ***hepatotoxicity, ascites,*** jaundice, hiccups
HEMA: ***Thrombocytopenia***
INTEG: Allergic reactions, burning at inj site
RESP: Pleuritis, ***pulmonary densities, hypoxemia,*** dyspnea

Contraindications: Hypersensitivity to this drug or bisulfites, severe aortic disease, severe pulmonic valvular disease, acute MI

Precautions: Lactation, pregnancy **C**, children, renal disease, hepatic disease, atrial flutter/fibrillation, elderly

Pharmacokinetics

Absorption	Complete bioavailability (IV)
Distribution	Unknown
Metabolism	Liver, 50%
Excretion	Kidney, metabolites (60%-90%)
Half-life	4-6 hr, increased in CHF

Pharmacodynamics

	IV
Onset	2-5 min
Peak	10 min
Duration	Variable

Interactions

Drug/drug:

Individual drugs

Disopyramide: ↑ hypotension

Drug classifications

Antihypertensives: ↑ hypotension

Cardiac glycosides: ↑ inotropic effect

NURSING CONSIDERATIONS

Assessment

- Monitor manifestations of hypokalemia: *renal:* acidic urine, reduced urine, osmolality, nocturia; *CV:* hypotension, broad T wave, U wave, ectopy, tachycardia, weak pulse; *neuro:* muscle weakness, altered LOC, drowsiness, apathy, lethargy, confusion, depression; *GI:* anorexia, nausea, cramps, constipation, distention, paralytic ileus; *resp:* hypoventilation, respiratory muscle weakness
- Assess fluid volume status: I&O ratio and record, weight, distended red veins, crackles in lung, color, quality and sp gr of urine, skin turgor, adequacy of

pulses, moist mucous membranes, bilateral lung sounds, peripheral pitting edema; dehydration symptoms of decreasing output, thirst, hypotension, dry mouth, and mucous membranes should be reported
- Monitor electrolytes: potassium, sodium, calcium, magnesium; also include BUN, blood pH, ABGs
- Monitor B/P and pulse, PCWP, CVP, index, often during infusion; if B/P drops 30 mm Hg, stop infusion and call prescriber
- Monitor ALT (SGPT), AST (SGOT), bilirubin daily; if these are elevated, hepatoxicity is suspected
- If platelets are <150,000/mm^3, drug is usually discontinued and another drug started
- Assess for extravasation: change site q48h

Associated nursing diagnoses

- ✓ Cardiac output, decreased (uses)
- ✓ Fluid volume excess (uses)
- ✓ Knowledge deficit (teaching)

Implementation

General
- Patients with low potassium levels (hypokalemia) should receive potassium supplements before amrinone administration
- Administer potassium supplements if ordered for potassium levels <3.0 mg/dl

IV route
- Do not mix directly with glucose sol; chemical reaction occurs over 24 hr; precipitate forms if amrinone and furosemide come in contact

Direct IV
- Administer into running dextrose inf through Y-connector or directly into tubing; may give undiluted over 2-3 min or dilute with NS to concentration of 1-3 mg/ml; run at prescribed rate; another loading dose may be given in 30 min

Cont IV
- Give after diluting with 0.9%, or 0.45% NaCl (1-3 mg/ml); do not dilute with dextrose sol; decomposition of drug will occur; use inf pump; use sol within 24 hr of dilution; titrate to patient response

Y-*site compatibilities:*

Aminophylline, atropine, bretylium, calcium chloride, cimetidine, dobutamine, dopamine, epinephrine, hydrocortisone sodium succinate, isoproterenol, lidocaine, metaraminol bitartrate, methylprednisolone sodium succinate, nitroglycerin, nitroprusside, norepinephrine, phenylephrine, potassium chloride, procainamide, verapamil

Y-*site incompatibilities:*

Furosemide, sodium bicarbonate

Patient/family education

- Teach patient reason for medication and expected results
- Instruct patient to make position changes slowly; orthostatic hypotension may occur
- Teach patient signs and symptoms of hypersensitivity reactions and hypokalemia

Evaluation

Positive therapeutic outcome

- Increased cardiac output
- Decreased PCWP, adequate CVP
- Decreased dyspnea, fatigue, edema, ECG

Treatment of overdose: Discontinue drug, support circulation

amyl nitrite

(am'il nye'trite)

amyl nitrite, Amyl Nitrite Aspirols, Amyl Nitrite Vaporole

Func. class.: Coronary vasodilator (antianginal, antidote for cyanide)

Chem. class.: Nitrite

Pregnancy category **X**

Action: Relaxes vascular smooth muscle; may dilate coronary blood vessels, resulting in reduced venous return, decreased cardiac output; reduces preload, afterload, which decreases left ventricular end diastolic pressure, systemic vascular resistance; converts hemoglobin to methemoglobin, which is able to bind cyanide

➔ **Therapeutic Outcome:** Decreased amount, severity of angina; prevention of death in cyanide poisoning

Uses: Acute angina pectoris

Investigational uses: Cardiac murmur diagnosis

Dosage and routes

Angina

Adult: Inh 0.18-0.3 ml as needed, 1-6 inhalations from 1 cap; may repeat in 3-5 min

Cyanide poisoning

Adult: Inh 0.3-ml ampule 15 sec until preparation of sodium nitrite infusion is ready

Available forms: Inh pearls 0.18, 0.3 ml

Side effects/adverse reactions

CNS: *Headache, dizziness,* weakness, syncope

CV: *Postural hypotension,* ***tachycardia, cardiovascular collapse,*** palpitations

GI: Nausea, vomiting, abdominal pain

INTEG: *Flushing,* pallor, sweating

MISC: Muscle twitching, ***hemolytic anemia, methemoglobinemia***

Contraindications: Hypersensitivity to nitrites, severe anemia, increased intracranial pressure, hypertension, pregnancy **X**

Precautions: Lactation, P children, drug abuse, head injury, cerebral hemorrhage, hypotension

Pharmacokinetics

Absorption	Well absorbed (inh)
Distribution	Widely distributed
Metabolism	Forms methemoglobin
Excretion	Kidneys (33%)
Half-life	1-4 min

Pharmacokinetics

	INH
Onset	30 sec
Peak	Unknown
Duration	3-5 min

Interactions

Drug/drug:

Individual drugs

Acetylcholine: ↓ effects of acetylcholine
Ephedrine: ↓ antianginal effects
Epinephrine: ↑ hypotension
Histamine: ↓ effects of histamine
Norepinephrine: ↓ effects of norepinephrine
Phenylephrine: ↓ antianginal effects

Drug classifications

Antihypertensives: ↑ hypotension
Sympathomimetics: ↓ antianginal effects

NURSING CONSIDERATIONS

Assessment

- Monitor B/P with patient supine and sitting, pulse during treatment until stable
- Monitor for drug tolerance: need for more medication for each attack
- Monitor for postural hypotension, headache during treatment, which are common side effects because of vasodilatation

Associated nursing diagnoses

✓ Cardiac output, decreased (uses)
✓ Poisoning (uses)
✓ Tissue perfusion, decreased (uses)
✓ Knowledge deficit (teaching)

Implementation

Inh route

- Give after wrapping, crushing ampule to avoid cuts; order analgesic if headache develops
- Give to patient who is sitting or lying down during treatment; keep head low, use deep breaths, which will decrease dizziness; have patient rest for 15 min
- Store in light-resistant area in cool environment or refrigerate

Patient/family education

- Instruct patient to keep a record of angina attacks and what aggravates condition; prolonged chest pain may indicate MI: seek emergency treatment
- Advise patient that medication may explode in presence of flame; to keep drug out of reach of children and in secure place, as there is high abuse potential
- Instruct patient to take several deep breaths despite foul odor; to make position changes slowly to prevent orthostatic hypotension

Evaluation

Positive therapeutic outcome

- Relief of chest pain (angina)
- Absence of death (cyanide poisoning)
- Decreased intensity (heart murmur)

anistreplase (APSAC)

(an-is-trep'lase)

Eminase

Func. class.: Thrombolytic enzyme

Chem. class.: Anisolated plasminogen streptokinase activator complex

Pregnancy category **C**

Action: Promotes thrombolysis by promoting conversion of plasminogen to plasmin; complex is a combination of plasminogen and streptokinase

Therapeutic Outcome: Thrombolysis in coronary arteries

Uses: Management of acute MI; although not yet approved, anistreplase will also be used for other conditions requiring thrombolysis: PE, DUT, unclotting arteriovenous shunts

Dosage and routes

Adult: **IV** 30 U over 4-5 min as soon as possible after onset of symptoms

Available forms: Powder, lyophilized 30 U/vial

Side effects/adverse reactions

CNS: Headache, fever, sweating, agitation, dizziness, paresthesia, tremor, vertigo
CV: Hypotension, dysrhythmias, conduction disorders
GI: Nausea, vomiting
HEMA: Decreased Hct, ***GI, GU, intracranial, retroperitoneal***, surface bleeding, ***thrombocytopenia***
INTEG: Rash, urticaria, phlebitis at site, itching, flushing
MS: Low back pain, arthralgia
RESP: Altered respirations, dyspnea, ***bronchospasm, lung edema***
SYST: ***Anaphylaxis***

Contraindications: Hypersensitivity, active internal bleeding, intraspinal or intracranial surgery, neoplasms of CNS, severe hypertension, cerebral embolism, thrombosis, hemorrhage

Precautions: Arterial emboli from left side of heart, pregnancy **C**, ulcerative colitis/enteritis, renal disease, hepatic disease, hypocoagulation, COPD, subacute bacterial endocarditis, rheumatic valvular disease, intraarterial diagnostic procedure or surgery (10 days), recent major surgery

Pharmacokinetics

Absorption	Complete bioavailability (IV)
Distribution	Unknown
Metabolism	Binds to plasmin
Excretion	Kidneys
Half-life	105 min

Pharmacodynamics

	IV
Onset	Unknown
Peak	45 min
Duration	Unknown

Interactions

Drug/drug:

Individual drugs

Aspirin: ↑ bleeding potential

Dipyridamole: ↑ bleeding potential
Heparin: ↑ bleeding potential
Indomethacin: ↑ bleeding potential
Phenylbutazone: ↑ bleeding potential

Drug classifications

Anticoagulants: ↑ bleeding potential
NSAIDs: ↑ bleeding potential

Lab test interferences

Increase: PT, APTT, TT
Decrease: Fibrinogen, plasminogen

NURSING CONSIDERATIONS

Assessment

- Monitor VS, B/P, pulse, respirations, neurologic signs, temp at least q4h, temp >104° F (40° C) or indicators of internal bleeding, cardiac rhythm after intracoronary administration
- Assess for allergy: fever, rash, itching, chills; mild reaction may be treated with antihistamines; hypersensitivity reactions/dyspnea, wheezing, facial swelling should be treated with epinephrine
- Monitor bleeding during 1st hr of treatment (hematuria, hematemesis, bleeding from mucous membranes, epistaxis, ecchymosis); blood studies (Hct, platelets, PTT, PT, TT, APTT) before starting therapy; PT or APTT must be less than 2 × control before starting therapy; TT or PT q3-4h during treatment

Associated nursing diagnoses

- ✓ Tissue perfusion, decreased (uses)
- ✓ Injury, risk for (uses, adverse reactions)
- ✓ Knowledge deficit (teaching)

Implementation

- Give heparin therapy after thrombolytic therapy is discontinued, TT or APTT less than 2 × control (about 3-4 hr)
- Avoid invasive procedures: inj, rec temp; about 10% of patients have high streptococcal antibody titers, requiring increased loading doses
- Treat fever with acetaminophen
- Provide pressure for 30 sec to minor bleeding sites, 30 min to sites of arterial puncture followed by dressing; inform prescriber if hemostasis not attained; apply pressure dressing

IV IV route

- Give after reconstituting single-dose vial/5 ml sterile water for inj (not bacteriostatic water), and roll (not shake) to enhance reconstitution; give over 2-5 min by direct **IV**; give within 6 hr of thrombi identification for best results; cryoprecipitate or fresh frozen plasma if bleeding occurs; store powder in refrigerator; use within 30 min after reconstitution

Incompatibilities:

Do not mix with other drugs in sol or syringe

Patient/family education

- Teach patient action of drug and expected outcome; alert patient to possible hypersensi-

tivity reactions and symptoms to report
- Advise patient bed rest is needed during entire course of treatment; handle patient as little as possible during therapy

Evaluation

Positive therapeutic outcome
- Absence of thrombolysis in MI
- Improved ventricular function

antihemophilic factor (AHF)

(an-tee-hee-moe-fill'ik)

antihemophilic factor, Humate-P, Hemofil M, Koate-HT, Koate-HS, Kogenate, Kryobulin VH ♣, Monoclate, Monoclate P, Profilate OSD, Recombinate

Func. class.: Hemostatic, blood factor

Chem. class.: Factor VIII

Pregnancy category **C**

Action: Necessary for clotting. Activates factor X in conjunction with activated factor IX; transforms prothrombin to thrombin

Therapeutic Outcome: Control of hemorrhage or excessive bleeding in factor VIII deficiency

Uses: Hemophilia A, patients with acquired circulating factor VIII inhibitors, factor VIII deficiency

Dosage and routes

Depends on severity of deficiency and level of antihemophilic factor

Massive hemorrhage

P *Adult /child:* **IV** 40-50 U/kg, then 20-25 U/kg q8-12h

Bleeding (frank, overt)

P *Adult /child:* **IV** 15-25 U/kg, then 8-15 U/kg q8-12h × 4 days

Hemorrhage near vital organs

P *Adult /child:* **IV** 15 U/kg, then 8 U/kg q8h × 2 days, then 4 U/kg q8h × 2 days

Minor hemorrhage

P *Adult /child:* **IV** 8-10 U/kg/ q24 hr × 2-3 days or 8 U/kg q12h × 2 days, then q24h × 2 days

Joint bleeding

P *Adult/ child:* **IV** 5-10 U/kg q8-12h × 1-2 days

Available forms: Inj **IV** 250, 500, 1000, 1500 U/vial (number of units noted on label)

Side effects/adverse reactions

CNS: Headache, *lethargy, chills, fever, flushing*
CV: *Hypotension,* tachycardia
GI: Nausea, vomiting, abdominal cramps, jaundice, ***viral hepatitis***
HEMA: ***Thrombosis, hemolysis, AIDS***
INTEG: Rash, flushing, *urticaria,* stinging at inj site
RESP: ***Bronchospasm***

Contraindications: Hypersensitivity, monoclonal antibody–derived factor VIII

Precautions: Neonates/infants, hepatic disease, blood types A, B, AB, pregnancy **C**, factor VIII inhibitor

Pharmacokinetics

Absorption	Complete availability (IV)
Distribution	Plasma
Metabolism	Not metabolized
Excretion	No excretion
Half-life	Biphasic 4 hr, 15 hr

Pharmacodynamics

	IV
Onset	Immediate
Peak	Unknown
Duration	12 hr

Interactions: None

NURSING CONSIDERATIONS

Assessment

- Monitor blood studies (coagulation factors assay by % normal: 5% prevents spontaneous hemorrhage, 30%-50% for surgery, 80%-100% for severe hemorrhage; blood group of patient, donors (if applicable; most factor VIII not from specific blood group donors)
- Monitor I&O, urine color; notify prescriber if urine becomes orange, red; change in urine color signifying hemolytic reaction; patients other than blood type O are more at risk
- Monitor pulse: discontinue infusion if significant increase
- Obtain test for factor VIII inhibitors before starting treatment, may require concomitant antiinhibitor coagulant complex therapy; Hct, Coombs' test with blood types A, B, AB
- Assess for allergy: fever, rash, itching, jaundice, wheezing, tachycardia, nausea, vomiting; give diphenhydramine (Benadryl); continue therapy if reaction is mild, discontinue if severe; notify prescriber
- Monitor bleeding at ankles, knees, elbows, other joints; check for rebleeding after 15-30 min

Associated nursing diagnoses

- ✓ Tissue perfusion altered (uses)
- ✓ Injury, risk for (uses, adverse reactions)
- ✓ Knowledge deficit (teaching)

Implementation

IV route

- Administer **IV** slowly; use plastic syringe to reconstitute and administer; do not use glass, drug adheres to glass; use another needle as a vent when reconstituting; rotate gently to mix
- Administer after dilution with warm NS, D_5W, LR; give within 3 hr
- Administer by **IV** inf: give at ≤2 ml/min if concentration exceeds 34 U/ml; or over 3 min if concentration is less than 34 U/ml; filter before using
- Store in refrigerator; do not freeze; after reconstitution, do not refrigerate; give within 3 hr

Additive compatibilities:

Do not mix with other drugs in sol or syringe

Patient/family education

- Advise patient to report any signs of bleeding: gums, under skin, urine, stools, emesis; review methods to prevent bleeding; to be checked q2-3 mo for HIV screen
- Instruct patient to avoid salicylates and ibuprofen; increases bleeding tendencies, decreases clotting
- Instruct patient to prepare, administer factor VIII concentrates at first sign of danger
- Instruct patient to advise health professionals of treatment for hemophilia
- Advise patient that immunization for hepatitis B may be given first
- Instruct patient to report hives, urticaria, chest tightness, hypotension; may be monoclonal antibody–derived factor VII; signs of viral hepatitis, AIDS
- Advise patient to carry identification describing disease process, drugs used

Evaluation

Positive therapeutic outcome

- Absence of bleeding
- Prevention of rebleeding

ascorbic acid (vitamin C)

(as-kor'bic)

Ascorbic Acid, Ascorbicap, Ascorbic Acid Caplets, Apo-C ✤, Cecon, Cenolate, Cemill, Cetane, Cevalin, Cevi-Bid, Ce-Vi-Sol, C-Crystals, Cebid Time Celles, Dull-C, Flavorcee, Kamu-Jay ✤, N'ice Vitamin C Drops, Redoxon ✤, Sunkist Vitamin C, Vita-C

Func. class.: Vitamin C, water-soluble vitamin

Pregnancy category A

Action: Needed for wound healing, collagen synthesis, antioxidant, carbohydrate metabolism, protein, lipid synthesis, prevention of infection

➔ Therapeutic Outcome: Replacement and supplementation of vitamin C

Uses: Vitamin C deficiency, scurvy, delayed wound and bone healing, chronic disease, urine acidification, before gastrectomy; increased need: lactation, pregnancy, hyperthyroidism, emotional stress, trauma, burns

Investigational uses: Acidification of urine, common cold prevention

Dosage and routes

Scurvy

Adult: PO/SC/IM/**IV** 100 mg-500 mg qd, then 50 mg or more qd

P *Child:* PO/SC/IM/**IV** 100-300 mg qd, then 35 mg or more qd

Wound healing/chronic disease/fracture

Adult: SC/IM/**IV**/PO 200-500 mg qd

P *Child:* SC/IM/**IV**/PO 100-200 mg added doses

Urine acidification

Adult: 4-12 g qd in divided doses

Available forms: Tabs 25, 50, 100, 250, 500, 1000, 1500 mg; effervescent tabs 1000 mg; chewable tabs 100, 250, 500 mg; timed release tabs 500, 750, 1000, 1500 mg; timed release caps 500 mg; crystals 4 g/tsp; powder 4 g/tsp; liq 35 mg/0.6 ml; sol 100 mg/ml; syr 20 mg/ml, 500 mg/5 ml; inj SC, IM, **IV** 100, 250, 500 mg/ml

Side effects/adverse reactions

CNS: Headache, insomnia, dizziness, fatigue, flushing
GI: Nausea, vomiting, diarrhea, anorexia, heartburn, cramps
GU: Polyuria, urine acidification, oxalate or urate renal stones
HEMA:* *Hemolytic anemia in patients with G6PD

Contraindications: None significant

Precautions: Gout, pregnancy **A**

Pharmacokinetics

Absorption	Actively absorbed (PO)
Distribution	Widely distributed; crosses placenta
Metabolism	Oxidation
Excretion	Kidneys, inactive; breast milk
Half-life	Unknown

Pharmacodynamics

Onset	Unknown
Peak	Unknown
Duration	Unknown

Interaction

Drug/drug:

Individual drugs

Amphetamine: ↑ excretion in acidic urine
Deferoxamine: ↑ iron toxicity
Mexiletine: ↑ excretion in acidic urine
Primadone: ↑ requirements for vitamin C

Drug classifications

Anticoagulants, oral: ↓ action of anticoagulants
Antidepressants, tricyclic: ↑ excretion in acidic urine
Salicylates: ↑ requirements of vitamin C

Drug/smoking:

Smoking decreases vitamin C levels

Lab test interferences

False positive: negatives in glucose tests (Clinitest, Tes-Tape)
False negative: Occult blood (large dose)

Decreased: Bilirubin, urine oxalate, cysteine

NURSING CONSIDERATIONS

Assessment

- Assess nutritional status for inclusion of foods high in vitamin C: citrus fruits, cantaloupe, tomatoes
- Assess for vitamin C deficiency before, during, and after treatment; scurvy (gingivitis, bleeding gums, loose teeth); poor bone development
- Monitor I&O ratio, polyuria; in patients receiving large doses renal stones may occur
- Monitor ascorbic acid levels throughout treatment if continued deficiency is suspected
- Assess inj sites for inflammation, pain, redness

Associated nursing diagnoses

✓ Nutrition, less than body requirements (uses)
✓ Knowledge deficit (teaching)

Implementation

IV **IV route**

- Give undiluted by *direct* **IV** 100 mg over at least 1 min
- Give by intermittent inf after diluting with D_5W, $D_{10}W$, 0.9% NaCl, 0.45% NaCl, LR, Ringer's sol, dextrose/saline, dextrose/Ringer's combinations; temperature will increase pressure in ampules; wrap with gauze before breaking

Syringe incompatibilities:
Cefazolin, doxapram

Syringe compatibility:
Metoclopramide

Additive incompatibilities:
Bleomycin, cephapirin, nafcillin, sodium bicarbonate, warfarin

Additive compatibilities:
Amikacin, calcium chloride, calcium gluceptate, calcium gluconate, cephalothin, chloramphenicol, chlorpromazine, colistimethate, cyanocobalamin, diphenhydramine, heparin, kanamycin, methicillin, methyldopate, penicillin G potassium, polymyxin B, prednisolone, procaine, prochlorperazine, promethazine, tetracycline, verapamil

PO route

- Mix **oral sol** with foods or fluids; **ext rel caps** should be swallowed whole; do not crush, break, or chew

IM route

- Not to be diluted; give deep in large muscle mass

Patient/family education

- Teach patient necessary foods to be included in diet that are rich in vitamin C: citrus fruits, cantaloupe, tomatoes, chili peppers (red)
- Teach patient that, if oral contraceptives are taken, increased levels of vitamin C are needed; oral contraceptives deplete vitamin C
- Teach patient that smoking decreases vitamin C levels; not to exceed prescribed dose; increases will be excreted in urine, except time release
- Teach patient not to exceed RDA recommended dose, urinary stones may occur
- Teach patient using ascorbic

acid for acidification of urine to test urine pH periodically

Evaluation

Positive therapeutic outcome
- Absence of anorexia, irritability, pallor, joint pain, hyperkeratosis, petechiae, poor wound healing
- Reversal of scurvy: bleeding gums, gingivitis, loose teeth

asparaginase (L-asparaginase)

(a-spar'a-gin-ase)

Colaspase, Elspar, Kidrolase ✱

Func. class.: Antineoplastic

Chem. class.: Escherichia coli enzyme

Pregnancy category D

Action: Indirectly inhibits protein synthesis in tumor cells; without amino acids, DNA, RNA synthesis is halted; asparagine, protein synthesis is halted; G_1 phase of cell cycle specific; a nonvesicant

Therapeutic Outcome: Prevention of rapidly growing malignant cells in leukemia

Uses: Acute lymphocytic leukemia in combination with other antineoplastics unresponsive to other agents

Dosage and routes

In combination

Adult: **IV** 1000 IU/kg/day × 10 days given over 30 min; IM 6000 IU/m^2/day

Sole induction

Adult: **IV** 200 IU/kg/day × 28 days

Available forms: Inj 10,000 IU

Side effects/adverse reactions

CNS: Neuritis, dizziness, headache, ***coma,*** depression, fatigue, confusion, hallucinations
CV: Chest pain
ENDO: Hyperglycemia
GI: Nausea, vomiting, anorexia, cramps, stomatitis, ***hepatotoxicity, pancreatitis***
GU: Urinary retention, ***renal failure,*** glycosuria, polyuria, azotemia, uric acid neuropathy
HEMA: Thrombocytopenia, leukopenia, myelosuppression, anemia, decreased clotting factors
INTEG: Rash, urticaria, chills, fever
RESP: Fibrosis, pulmonary infiltrate
SYST: Anaphylaxis, hypersensitivity

Contraindications: Hypersensitivity, infants, pregnancy **D**, lactation, pancreatitis

Precautions: Renal disease, hepatic disease

Pharmacokinetics

Absorption	Complete bioavailability (IV)
Distribution	Intravascular spaces
Metabolism	Unknown
Excretion	Reticuloendothelial system
Half-life	8-30 hr (IV), 39-49 hr (IM)

Pharmacodynamics

	IV	IM
Onset	Immediate	Immediate
Peak	14-24 hr	Unknown
Duration	3-5 wk	3-5 wk

Interactions

Drug/drug:

Individual drugs

Methotrexate: Blocked action of methotrexate

Vincristine: ↑ neurotoxicity

Drug classifications

Hepatotoxic agents: ↑ hepatotoxicity

Glucocorticosteroids: ↑ hyperglycemia

Lab test interferences

Decrease: Thyroid function tests

Increase: BUN

NURSING CONSIDERATIONS

Assessment

- Assess for signs and symptoms of pancreatitis (nausea, vomiting, severe abdominal pain), anaphylaxis (bronchospasm, dyspnea), cyanosis; monitor amylase, glucose
- Assess symptoms indicating severe allergic reaction: rash, pruritus, urticaria, purpuric skin lesions, itching, flushing; joint pain, bronchospasm, hypotension; epinephrine and crash carts should be nearby
- Monitor for frequency of stools, characteristics: cramping, acidosis; signs of dehydration: rapid respirations, poor skin turgor, decreased urine output, dry skin, restlessness, weakness
- Monitor CBC, differential, platelet count weekly; withhold drug if WBC count is <4000/mm^3 or platelet count is <100,000/mm^3, notify prescriber of results; also monitor PT, PTT and TT, which may be increased
- Monitor pulmonary function tests, chest x-ray studies before, during therapy; chest x-ray film should be obtained q2 wk during treatment
- Monitor renal function studies: BUN, serum uric acid, ammonia urine CrCl, electrolytes before, during therapy
- Check I&O ratio; report fall in urine output of 30/ml/hr
- Monitor temperature q4h; may indicate beginning infection
- Obtain liver function tests before, during therapy (bilirubin, AST [SGOT], ALT [SGPT], LDH) as needed or monthly
- Monitor RBC, Hct, Hgb, since these may be decreased; serum, urine glucose levels
- Assess for bleeding: hematuria, guaiac, bruising or petechiae, mucosa or orifices q8h
- Assess for dyspnea, rales, nonproductive cough, chest pain, tachypnea fatigue, increased pulse, pallor, lethargy, or swelling around eyes or lips; anaphylaxis may occur
- Assess for yellowing of skin and sclera, dark urine, clay-colored stools, itchy skin, abdominal pain, fever, diarrhea

Associated nursing diagnoses

- ✓ Injury, risk for (uses, adverse reactions)
- ✓ Body image disturbance (adverse reactions)

Implementation

- Give after intradermal skin testing and desensitization, give 0.1 ml (2 IU) intradermally after reconstituting with 5 ml sterile H_2O or 0.9% NaCl for injection; then add 0.1 ml of reconstituted drug to 9.9 ml diluent (20 IU/ml); observe for 1 hr, check for wheal
- Use allopurinol or sodium bicarbonate to reduce uric acid levels, alkalinization of urine

IV **IV route**

- Give by **IV** infusion using 21-, 23-, 25-gauge needle; administer by slow **IV** infusion via Y-tube or 3-way stop cock of flowing D_5W or NS infusion over 30 min after diluting 10,000 IU/5 ml of sterile H_2O or 0.9% NaCl (no preservatives) (2000 IU/ml); use of filter may be necessary if fibers are present

Patient/family education

- Teach patient to report any complaints or side effects to nurse or physician
- Teach patient to report any changes in breathing or coughing

Evaluation

Positive therapeutic response

- Decreased replication of leukemia cells

Treatment of anaphylaxis:

Administer epinephrine, diphenhydramine, **IV** corticosteroids

aspirin

(as′pir-in)

Ancasal ✤, A.S.A., Aspergum, Aspirin ✤, Bayer, Bayer Children's aspirin, Easprin, Ecotrin, Ecotrin Maximum Strength, 8-Hour Bayer Timed Release, Empirin, Entrophen ✤, Genprin, Maximum Bayer, Norwich Extra-Strength, Novasen ✤, Sal-Adult ✤, Sal-Infant ✤, St. Joseph Children's, Supasa ✤, Therapy Bayer, ZORprin

Func. class.: Nonnarcotic analgesic

Chem. class.: Salicylate

Pregnancy category D

Action: Blocks pain impulses in CNS that occur in response to inhibition of prostaglandin synthesis; antipyretic action results from vasodilatation of peripheral vessels; decreases platelet aggregation

Therapeutic Outcome: Decreased pain, inflammation, fever; absence of MI, transient ischemic attacks, thrombosis

Uses: Mild to moderate pain or fever including rheumatoid arthritis, osteoarthritis, thromboembolic disorders, transient ischemic attacks in men, rheumatic fever, post-MI, prophylaxis of MI

Dosage and routes

Arthritis

Adult: PO 2.6-5.2 g/day in divided doses q4-6h

P *Child:* PO 90-130 mg/kg/day in divided doses q4-6h

Pain/fever

Adult: PO/rec 325-650 mg q4h prn, not to exceed 4 g/day

P *Child:* PO/rec 40-100 mg/kg/day in divided doses q4-6h prn

Thromboembolic disorders

Adult: PO 325-650 mg/day or bid

Transient ischemic attacks

Adult: PO 650 mg qid or 325 mg qid

Available forms: Tabs 65, 81, 325, 500, 650, 975 mg; chewable tabs 81 mg; caps 325, 500 mg; cont rel tabs 800 mg; time-release tabs 650 mg; supp 60, 120, 125, 130, 195, 200, 300, 325, 600, 650 mg, 1.2 g; cream; gum 227.5 mg

Side effects/adverse reactions

CNS: Stimulation, drowsiness, dizziness, confusion, ***convulsion,*** headache, flushing, hallucinations, ***coma***
CV: Rapid pulse, pulmonary edema
EENT: Tinnitus, hearing loss
ENDO: Hypoglycemia, hyponatremia, hypokalemia
GI: Nausea, vomiting, ***GI bleeding,*** diarrhea, heartburn, anorexia, ***hepatitis***
HEMA: ***Thrombocytopenia, agranulocytosis, leukopenia, neutropenia, hemolytic anemia,*** increased pro-time, PTT, bleeding time
INTEG: Rash, urticaria, bruising
RESP: Wheezing, hyperpnea

Contraindications: Hypersensitivity to salicylates, tartrazine (FDC yellow dye #5), GI bleeding, bleeding disorders, P children <12 yr, children with flulike symptoms, pregnancy **D**, lactation, vitamin K deficiency, peptic ulcer

Precautions: Anemia, hepatic disease, renal disease, Hodgkin's disease, pre/postoperatively

Pharmacokinetics

Absorption	Well absorbed, small intestine (PO); erratic (enteric); slow (rec)
Distribution	Rapidly, widely distributed; crosses placenta
Metabolism	Liver, extensively
Excretion	Inactive metabolites, kidney; breast milk
Half-life	2-3 hr (low doses); 30 hr (high doses)

Pharmacodynamics

	PO	REC
Onset	15-30 min	Slow
Peak	1-2 hr	4-5 hr
Duration	4-6 hr	6-7 hr

Interactions

Individual drugs

Alcohol: ↑ bleeding
Cefamandole: ↑ bleeding
Furosemide: ↑ toxic effects
Heparin: ↑ bleeding

Insulin: ↑ effects of insulin
Methotrexate: ↑ effects of methotrexate
PABA: ↑ toxic effects
Phenytoin: ↑ effects of phenytoin
Plicamycin: ↑ bleeding
Probenecid: ↓ effects of probenecid
Spironolactone: ↓ effects
Sulfinpyrazone: ↓ effects
Valproic acid: ↑ bleeding
Vancomycin: ↑ ototoxicity

Drug classifications

Antacids: ↓ effects of aspirin
Anticoagulants: ↑ bleeding
Carbonic anhydrase inhibitors: ↑ toxic effects
NSAIDs: ↑ gastric ulcers
Penicillins: ↑ effects of penicillins
Salicylates: ↓ blood sugar levels
Steroids: ↓ effects of aspirin, ↑ gastric ulcers
Sulfonylamides: ↓ effects of sulfonylamides
Urinary acidifiers: ↑ salicylate levels
Urinary alkalizers: ↓ effects of aspirin

Lab test interferences

Increase: Coagulation studies, liver function studies, serum uric acid, amylase, CO_2, urinary protein
Decrease: Serum potassium, PBI, cholesterol
Interfere: Urine catecholamines, pregnancy test, urine glucose tests (Clinistix, Tes-Tape)

NURSING CONSIDERATIONS

Assessment

- Monitor liver function studies: AST (SGOT), ALT (SGPT), bilirubin, creatinine if patient is on long-term therapy
- Monitor renal function studies: BUN, urine creatinine if patient is on long-term therapy
- Monitor blood studies: CBC, Hct, Hgb, pro-time if patient is on long-term therapy
- Check I&O ratio; decreasing output may indicate renal failure (long-term therapy)
- Assess hepatotoxicity: dark urine, clay-colored stools, yellowing of the skin and sclera, itching, abdominal pain, fever, diarrhea if patient is on long-term therapy
- Assess for allergic reactions: rash, urticaria; if these occur, drug may have to be discontinued
- Assess for ototoxicity: tinnitus, ringing, roaring in ears; audiometric testing needed before, after long-term therapy
- Assess for visual changes: blurring, halos; corneal, retinal damage
- Check edema in feet, ankles, legs
- Identify prior drug history; there are many drug interactions
- Monitor pain: location, duration, type, intensity, before dose and 1 hr after
- Monitor musculoskeletal status: ROM before dose
- Identify fever: length of time and related symptoms

Associated nursing diagnoses

✓ Pain (uses)
✓ Mobility, impaired physical (uses)
✓ Injury, risk for (side effects)
✓ Knowledge deficit (teaching)

Implementation

PO route

- Administer to patient crushed or whole; chewable tab may be chewed (do not crush enteric product)
- Give with food or milk to decrease gastric symptoms; give 30 min before or 2 hr pc; absorption may be slowed
- Give antacids 1-2 hr after enteric products

Patient/family education

- Teach patient to report any symptoms of hepatotoxicity, renal toxicity, visual changes, ototoxicity, allergic reactions, bleeding (long-term therapy)
- Instruct patient to take with 8 oz of water and sit upright for 30 min after dose
- Instruct patient not to exceed recommended dosage; acute poisoning may result
- Advise patient to read label on other OTC drugs; many contain aspirin
- Inform patient that the therapeutic response takes 2 wk (arthritis)
- Teach patient to report tinnitus, confusion, diarrhea, sweating, hyperventilation
- Advise patient to avoid alcohol ingestion; GI bleeding may occur
- Advise patient with allergies that allergic reactions may develop
- Instruct patient to avoid buffered or effervescent products
- Teach patient not to give to children; Reye's syndrome may develop

Evaluation

Positive therapeutic outcome

- Decreased pain
- Decreased inflammation
- Decreased fever
- Absence of MI
- Absence of transient ischemic attacks, thrombosis

Treatment of overdose: Lavage, activated charcoal, monitor electrolytes, VS

astemizole

(a-stem′mi-zole)

Hismanal

Func. class.: Antihistamine

Chem. class.: H_1-histamine antagonist

Pregnancy category **C**

Action: Acts on blood vessels, GI, respiratory system by competing with histamine for H_1-receptor site; decreases allergic response by blocking pharmacologic effects of histamine; less sedation rate than with other antihistamines; causes increased heart rate, vasodilatation, increased secretions

➔ Therapeutic Outcome: Absence of allergy symptoms and rhinitis

Uses: Rhinitis, allergy symptoms, chronic idiopathic urticaria

Dosage and routes

P *Adult and child >12 yr:* PO 10 mg qd; to reduce time to steady state may take 30 mg day 1, 20 mg day 2, followed by 10 mg daily

Available forms: Tabs 10 mg

Side effects/adverse reactions

CNS: Headache, stimulation, drowsiness, sedation, fatigue, confusion, blurred vision, tinnitus, restlessness, tremors, P paradoxical excitation in G children or elderly

CV: Hypotension, palpitations, bradycardia, tachycardia, ***dysrhythmias*** (rare)

GI: Nausea, diarrhea, abdominal pain, vomiting, constipation

GU: Frequency, dysuria, urinary retention, impotence

HEMA: Hemolytic anemia, thrombocytopenia, leukopenia, agranulocytosis, pancytopenia

INTEG: Rash, eczema, photosensitivity, urticaria

RESP: Thickening of bronchial secretions, dry nose, throat

Contraindications: Hypersen- P sitivity, newborn or premature infants, lactation, severe hepatic disease

Precautions: Pregnancy **C**, G elderly, children, respiratory P disease, narrow angle glaucoma, prostatic hypertrophy, bladder neck obstruction, asthma

Pharmacokinetics

Absorption	Well absorbed (PO)
Distribution	Unknown, 97% bound to plasma proteins
Metabolism	Liver, extensively; converted to desmethylastemizole
Excretion	Kidneys
Half-life	Biphasic 3½, 16-23 hr

Pharmacodynamics

	PO
Onset	Unknown
Peak	1-2 hr
Duration	Unknown

Interactions

Drug/drug:

Individual drugs

Alcohol: ↑ CNS depression
Erythromycin: ↑ CV reaction
Itraconazole: ↑ CV reaction
Ketoconazole: ↑ CV reaction

Drug classifications

Anticoagulants, oral: ↓ action
CNS depressants: ↑ CNS depression
MAOI: ↑ anticholinergic effect
Narcotics: ↑ CNS depression
Sedative/hypnotics: ↑ CNS depression

Drug/food: ↓ absorption

Lab test interferences

False negative: Skin allergy tests (discontinue antihistamine 3 days before testing)

NURSING CONSIDERATIONS

Assessment

• Assess respiratory status: rate, rhythm, increase in bronchial secretions, wheezing, chest tightness; provide fluids to 2 L/day to decrease secretion thickness

- Monitor I&O ratio: be alert for urinary retention, frequency, dysuria, especially G elderly; drug should be discontinued if these occur
- Monitor CBC during long-term therapy; blood dyscrasias may occur but are rare

Associated nursing diagnoses

✓ Airway clearance, ineffective (uses)
✓ Injury, risk for (side effects)
✓ Knowledge deficit (teaching)
✓ Noncompliance (teaching, overuse)

Implementation

PO route

- Give on an empty stomach 1 hr before or 2 hr pc to facilitate absorption
- Store in tight, light-resistant container

Patient/family education

- Teach all aspects of drug uses; to notify prescriber if confusion, sedation, hypotension occur; to avoid driving or other hazardous activity if drowsiness occurs; to avoid alcohol or other CNS depressants that may potentiate effect
- Instruct patient to take 1 hr before or 2 hr pc to facilitate absorption
- Instruct patient not to exceed recommended dose; dysrhythmias may occur
- Teach patient hard candy, gum, frequent rinsing of mouth may be used for dryness

Evaluation

Positive therapeutic outcome

- Absence of running or congested nose, rashes

Treatment of overdose:

Administer ipecac syrup or lavage, diazepam, vasopressors, barbiturates (short acting)

atenolol

(a-ten'oh-lole)

Apo-Atenolol ✱, atenolol, Tenormin

Func. class.: Antihypertensive

Chem. class.: β-Blocker, β_1-, β_2-blocker (high doses)

Pregnancy category C

Action: Competitively blocks stimulation of β-adrenergic receptor within vascular smooth muscle; produces negative chronotropic activity, positive inotropic activity (decreases rate of SA node discharge, increases recovery time), slows conduction of AV node, decreases heart rate, decreases O_2 consumption in myocardium; also decreases renin-aldosterone-angiotensin system at high doses, inhibits β_2-receptors in bronchial system at higher doses

➔ Therapeutic Outcome: Decreased B/P, heart rate, prevention of angina pectoris, MI

Uses: Mild to moderate hypertension, prophylaxis of

angina pectoris, suspected or known MI

Investigational uses:

Dysrhythmia, mitral value prolapse, pheochromocytoma, hypertrophic cardiomyopathy, vascular headaches, thyrotoxicosis, tremors

Dosage and routes

Adult: **IV** 5 mg; repeat in 10 min if initial dose is well tolerated, then start PO dose 10 min after last **IV** dose

Adult: PO 50 mg qd, increasing q1-2 wk to 100 mg qd; may increase to 200 mg qd for angina

Available forms: Tabs 25, 50, 100 mg; **IV** 3 mg/10 ml

Side effects/adverse reactions

CNS: Insomnia, fatigue, dizziness, mental changes, memory loss, hallucinations, depression, lethargy, drowsiness, strange dreams, catatonia

CV: ***Profound hypotension, bradycardia, CHF, cold extremities, postural hypotension, 2nd- or 3rd-degree heart block***

EENT: Sore throat, dry burning eyes

ENDO: Increased hypoglycemic response to insulin

GI: Nausea, diarrhea, vomiting, ***mesenteric arterial thrombosis, ischemic colitis***

GU: Impotence

HEMA: ***Agranulocytosis, thrombocytopenia, purpura***

INTEG: Rash, fever, alopecia

RESP: ***Bronchospasm,*** dyspnea, wheezing

Contraindications: Hypersensitivity to β-blockers, cardiogenic shock, 2nd- or 3rd-degree heart block, sinus bradycardia, CHF, cardiac failure

Precautions: Major surgery, pregnancy **C**, lactation, diabetes mellitus, renal disease, thyroid disease, COPD, asthma, well-compensated heart failure

Pharmacokinetics

Absorption	50%-60% (PO)
Distribution	Crosses placenta; protein binding (5%-15%)
Metabolism	Not metabolized
Excretion	Breast milk, kidneys (50%), feces (50%—unabsorbed drug)
Half-life	6-7 hr

Pharmacodynamics

	PO
Onset	1 hr
Peak	2-4 hr
Duration	24 hr

Interactions

Drug/drug:

Individual drugs

Alcohol: ↑ hypotension (large amounts)

Epinephrine: α-Adrenergic stimulation

Hydralazine: ↑ hypotension, bradycardia

Indomethacin: ↓ antihypertensive effect

Insulin: ↑ hypoglycemia

Methyldopa: ↑ hypotension, bradycardia

Phenytoin (IV): ↓ myocardial depression
Prazosin: ↑ hypotension, bradycardia
Reserpine: ↑ hypotension, bradycardia
Thyroid: ↓ effectiveness of atenolol
Verapamil: ↑ myocardial depression

Drug classifications

Antihypertensives: ↑ hypertension
β_2-Agonist: ↓ bronchodilatation
Cardiac glycosides: ↑ bradycardia
Nitrates: ↑ hypotension
Theophyllines: ↓ bronchodilatation

Lab test interferences

Interference: Glucose insulin tolerance tests
Increase: Uric acid, potassium, triglyceride, lipoproteins

NURSING CONSIDERATIONS

Assessment

- Monitor B/P during beginning treatment, periodically thereafter; pulse q4h; note rate, rhythm, quality: apical/radial pulse before administration; notify prescriber of any significant changes (pulse <50 bpm)
- Check for baselines in renal, liver function tests before therapy begins
- Assess for edema in feet, legs daily, monitor I&O, daily weight; check for jugular vein distention, rales bilaterally, dyspnea (CHF)
- Monitor skin turgor, dryness of mucous membranes for hydration status, especially G elderly

Associated nursing diagnoses

- ✓ Cardiac output, decreased (uses)
- ✓ Injury, risk for physical (side effects)
- ✓ Knowledge deficit (teaching)
- ✓ Noncompliance (teaching)

Implementation

PO route

- Given ac, hs, tablet may be crushed or swallowed whole; give with food to prevent GI upset; reduced dosage in renal dysfunction
- Store protected from light, moisture; place in cool environment

IV **IV route**

- Give **IV** direct over 5 min or diluted in 10-50 ml D_5W, 0.9% NaCl, and give at prescribed rate

Y-*site compatibilities:*

Meperidine, morphine

Patient/family education

- Teach patient not to discontinue drug abruptly; taper over 2 wk; may cause precipitate angina if stopped abruptly
- Teach patient not to use OTC products containing α-adrenergic stimulants (such as nasal decongestants, OTC cold preparations); to avoid alcohol, smoking; to limit sodium intake as prescribed
- Teach patient how to take pulse and B/P at home; advise when to notify prescriber
- Instruct patient to comply with weight control, dietary adjustments, modified exercise program
- Advise patient to carry/wear Medic Alert ID for drugs and

allergies; tell patient drug controls symptoms but does not cure

- Caution patient to avoid hazardous activities if dizziness, drowsiness is present
- Teach patient to report symptoms of CHF: difficult breathing, especially on exertion or when lying down, night cough, swelling of extremities or bradycardia, dizziness, confusion, depression, fever
- Teach patient to take drug as prescribed, not to double doses, skip doses; take any missed doses as remembered if at least 6 hr until next dose

Evaluation

Positive therapeutic outcome

- Decreased B/P in hypertension (after 1-2 wk)
- Absence of dysrhythmias
- Absence of MI
- Decreased angina

Treatment of overdose:

Lavage, **IV** atropine for bradycardia, **IV** theophylline for bronchospasm, digitalis, O_2, diuretic for cardiac failure, hemodialysis, **IV** glucose for hyperglycemia, **IV** diazepam (or phenytoin) for seizures

atovaquone

(a-toe'va-kwone)

Mepron

Func. class.: Antiprotozoal

Chem. class.: Aromatic diamide derivative; analog of ubiquinone

Pregnancy category **C**

Action: Interferes with DNA/RNA synthesis in protozoa, specifically ATP and nucleic acid synthesis

Therapeutic Outcome: Antiprotozoal for *Pneumocystis carinii* only

Uses: *Pneumocystis carinii* infections not sensitive to trimethoprim/sulfamethoxazole (co-trimoxazole)

Dosage and routes

Adult: 750 mg with food tid for 21 days

Available forms: Tabs 250 mg

Side effects/adverse reactions

CNS: Dizziness, headache, anxiety
CV: Hypotension
GI: *Nausea, vomiting, diarrhea,* anorexia, increased AST (SGOT) and ALT (SGPT), acute pancreatitis, constipation, abdominal pain
HEMA: Anemia, ***leukopenia***
INTEG: Pruritus, urticaria, *rash,* oral monilia
META: Hyperkalemia, hyperglycemia, hyponatremia

Contraindications: Hypersensitivity or history of developing life-threatening allergic reactions to any component of the formulation

Precautions: Blood dyscrasias, hepatic disease, diabetes
P mellitus, pregnancy **C**, lacta-
G tion, children, elderly

Pharmacokinetics

Absorption	Poor; increased when taken with fatty foods
Distribution	Unknown
Metabolism	Hepatic recycling
Excretion	Feces, unchanged (94%)
Half-life	2-3 days

Pharmacodynamics

	PO
Onset	Unknown
Peak	1-8 hr

Interactions

Drug/drug:

Drug classifications

Use cautiously with highly protein-bound drugs

Drug/food: ↑ absorption of drug, especially fatty foods

NURSING CONSIDERATIONS

Assessment

• Assess for *Pneumocystis carinii*: monitor WBC, bilateral lung sounds, sputum for C&S; these should be checked before, periodically during, and after treatment; after collection of 1st sputum, therapy may begin
• Monitor for symptoms of hyponatremia: *CV:* increased B/P, cold, clammy skin, hypovolemia or hypervolemia; *GI:* anorexia, nausea, vomiting, diarrhea, abdominal cramps; *neuro:* lethargy, increased ICP, confusion, headache, seizures, coma, fatigue, tremors, hyperreflexia
• Monitor for symptoms of hypoglycemia/hyperglycemia in diabetic patients
• Monitor blood studies: blood glucose, CBC, platelets; I&O ratio; ECG for cardiac dysrhythmias, check B/P; liver studies: AST (SGOT), ALT (SGPT)
• Monitor for signs of infection; anemia; monitor bowel pattern before, during treatment
• Monitor respiratory status: rate, character, wheezing, dyspnea
• Assess for dizziness, confusion, hallucination
• Assess for allergies before treatment, reaction of each medication; place allergies on chart; notify all people giving drugs

Associated nursing diagnoses

✓ Infection, risk for (uses)
✓ Diarrhea (adverse reactions)
✓ Knowledge deficit (teaching)

Implementation

PO route

• Give with food (preferably fatty); increased absorption of the drug and higher plasma concentrations will occur; give TID × 3 wks

Patient/family education

• Instruct patient to take with food, preferably fatty foods, to increase plasma concentrations

• Advise patient to take drug exactly as prescribed

Evaluation

Positive therapeutic outcome

• Decreased temperature
• Ability to breathe
• Three negative sputum cultures

atracurium

(a-tra-cure'ee-um)

Tracrium

Func. class.: Neuromuscular blocker (nondepolarizing)

Chem. class.: Biquaternary ammonium ester

Pregnancy category **C**

Action: Inhibits transmission of nerve impulses by binding with cholinergic receptor sites, antagonizing action of acetylcholine

Therapeutic Outcome: Skeletal muscle paralysis after anesthesia

Uses: Facilitation of endotracheal intubation; skeletal muscle relaxation during mechanical ventilation, surgery, or general anesthesia

Dosage and routes

Adult: **IV** bol 0.4-0.5 mg/kg, then 0.08-0.10 mg/kg 20-45 min after 1st dose if needed for prolonged procedures

Available forms: Inj **IV** 10 mg/ml

Side effects/adverse reactions

CV: Bradycardia, tachycardia, increased, decreased B/P
EENT: Increased secretions
INTEG: Rash, flushing, pruritus, urticaria
RESP: ***Prolonged apnea, bronchospasm, cyanosis, respiratory depression***

Contraindications: Hypersensitivity

Precautions: Pregnancy **C**, cardiac disease, lactation, P children <2 yr, electrolyte imbalances, dehydration, neuromuscular disease, respiratory disease

Pharmacokinetics

Absorption	Complete bioavailability (IV)
Distribution	Extracellular space, crosses placenta
Metabolism	Plasma
Excretion	Unknown
Half-life	Biphasic 2 min, 29 min

Pharmacodynamics

	IV
Onset	2 min
Peak	5 min
Duration	20-60 min

Interactions

Drug/drug:

Individual drugs

Clindamycin: ↑ paralysis
Colistin: ↑ paralysis
Lidocaine: ↑ paralysis
Lithium: ↑ paralysis
Magnesium: ↑ paralysis
Polymyxin B: ↑ paralysis
Procainamide: ↑ paralysis
Quinidine: ↑ paralysis
Succinylcholine: ↑ paralysis

Drug classifications

Aminoglycosides: ↑ paralysis
β-Blockers: ↑ paralysis
Diuretics, potassium-losing: ↑ paralysis
General anesthesia: ↑ paralysis

NURSING CONSIDERATIONS

Assessment

- Assess for electrolyte imbalances (potassium, magnesium); may lead to increased action of this drug
- Monitor vital signs (B/P, pulse, respirations, airway) until fully recovered; rate, depth, pattern of respirations, strength of hand grip
- Monitor I&O ratio; check for urinary retention, frequency, hesitancy
- Assess recovery: decreased paralysis of face, diaphragm, leg, arm, rest of body
- Monitor allergic reactions: rash, fever, respiratory distress, pruritus; drug should be discontinued

Associated nursing diagnoses

✓ Breathing pattern, ineffective (uses)
✓ Communication, impaired verbal (adverse reactions)
✓ Fear (adverse reactions)

Implementation

IV **IV route**

- Anesthesiologist should use nerve stimulator to determine neuromuscular blockade
- Give anticholinesterase to reverse neuromuscular blockade
- Give undiluted direct **IV** over 5 min, or diluted in 10-50 ml of D_5W (½ NaCl or NS) and give as an inf at prescribed rate
- Give only by qualified person, usually an anesthesiologist; do not administer IM
- Give only slightly discolored solution
- Store in light-resistant area

Y-site compatibilities:

Aminophylline, cefazolin, cefuroxime, cimetidine, cotrimoxazole, dobutamine, dopamine, epinephrine, esmolol, fentanyl, gentamicin, heparin, hydrocortisone sodium succinate, isoproterenol, lorazepam, midazolam, morphine, nitroglycerine, ranitidine, sodium nitroprusside, vancomycin

Y-site incompatibility:

Diazepam

Additive incompatibilities:

Barbiturates, sodium bicarbonate

Patient/family education

- Provide reassurance if communication is difficult during recovery from neuromuscular blockade
- Provide explanation of all treatments and procedures before beginning

Evaluation

Positive therapeutic outcome

- Paralysis of jaw, eyelid, head, neck, rest of body

Treatment of overdose:

Edrophonium or neostigmine, atropine; monitor VS; may require mechanical ventilation

A

atropine

(a'troe-peen)

Atropine-Care Ophthalmic, Atropine Sulfate Ophthalmic, atropine sulfate S.O.P., Atropisol Ophthalmic, Isopto Atropine

Atropair, Atro-Pen, I-tropine, Minims Atropine

Func. class.: Anticholinergic parasympatholytic, mydriatic

Chem. class.: Belladonna alkaloid

Pregnancy category **C**

Action: Blocks acetylcholine at parasympathetic neuroeffector sites; increases cardiac output, heart rate by blocking vagal stimulation in heart; dries secretions, decreases sweating, salivation in low doses; mydriasis, increased heart rate and cycloplegia occur at moderate doses; motility of GI, GU systems at high dose

Therapeutic Outcome: Drying of secretions, increased heart rate, cycloplegia, mydriasis

Uses: Bradycardia, bradydysrhythmia, anticholinesterase insecticide poisoning, blocking cardiac vagal reflexes, decreasing secretions before surgery, antispasmodic with GU and biliary surgery, bronchodilator; opthalmically for cycloplegia, mydriasis

Dosage and routes

Bradycardia/bradydysrhythmias

Adult: **IV** bol 0.5-1 mg given q3-5 min, not to exceed 2 mg

P *Child:* **IV** bol 0.01-0.03 mg/kg up to 0.4 mg or 0.3 mg/m^2; may repeat q4-6h

Insecticide poisoning

P *Adult and child:* IM/**IV** 2 mg qh until muscarinic symptoms disappear; may need 6 mg qh

Before surgery

Adult: SC/IM/**IV** 0.4-0.6 mg before anesthesia

P *Child:* SC 0.1-0.4 mg 30 min before surgery

Cycloplegic refraction

Adult: Ophth i-ii gtt of 1% sol 1 hr before exam

P *Child:* Ophth i-ii gtt of 0.5% sol bid-tid for up to 3 days before and 1 hr after exam

GI disorders

Adult: PO 0.3-1.2 mg q4-6h

Available forms: Inj 0.05, 0.1, 0.3, 0.4, 0.5, 0.8, 1 mg/ml; tabs 0.4 mg; tabs soluble 0.4, 0.6 mg

Side effects/adverse reactions

CNS: Headache, dizziness, involuntary movement, confusion, psychosis, anxiety, coma, flushing, drowsiness, insomnia, weakness

CV: Hypotension, paradoxic bradycardia, angina, PVCs, hypertension, tachycardia, ectopic ventricular beats

EENT: Blurred vision, photophobia, glaucoma, eye pain, pupil dilatation, nasal congestion
GI: Dry mouth, nausea, vomiting, abdominal pain, anorexia, constipation, paralytic ileus, abdominal distention, altered taste
GU: Retention, hesitancy, impotence, dysuria
INTEG: Rash, urticaria, contact dermatitis, dry skin, flushing
MISC: Suppression of lactation, decreased sweating

Contraindications: Hypersensitivity to belladonna alkaloids, angle closure glaucoma, GI obstructions, myasthenia gravis, thyrotoxicosis, ulcerative colitis, prostatic hypertrophy, tachycardia/tachydysrhythmias, asthma, acute hemorrhage, hepatic disease, myocardial ischemia

Precautions: Pregnancy **C**, renal disease, lactation, CHF, tachydysrhythmias, hyperthyroidism, COPD, hepatic disease, P child <6 yr, hypertension, G elderly, intraabdominal infections, Down's syndrome, spastic paralysis, gastric ulcer

Pharmacokinetics

Absorption	Well absorbed (PO, SC, IM)
Distribution	Crosses blood-brain barrier, placenta
Metabolism	Liver
Excretion	Kidneys, unchanged (70%-90%); breast milk
Half-life	13-40 hr

Pharmacodynamics

	PO	IM/SC	IV	OPHTH
Onset	½ hr	15 min	2-4 min	½ hr
Peak	½-1 hr	30 min	2-4 min	30-60 min
Duration	4-6 hr	4-6 hr	4-6 hr	1-2 wk

Interactions
Drug/drug:
Individual drugs
Amantadine: ↑ anticholinergic effect
Disopyramide: ↑ anticholinergic effect
Potassium chloride, oral: ↑ GI lesions
Quinidine: ↑ anticholinergic effect
Drug classifications
Antacids: ↓ absorption of atropine
Anticholinergics: ↑ anticholinergic effect
Antidepressants, tricyclic: ↑ anticholinergic effect
Antihistamines: ↑ anticholinergic effect

NURSING CONSIDERATIONS
Assessment

- Monitor I&O ratio; check for urinary retention and daily G output in elderly or postoperative patients
- Monitor ECG for ectopic ventricular beats, PVC, tachycardia
- Monitor for bowel sounds; check for constipation; abdominal distention and constipation may occur
- Monitor respiratory status: rate, rhythm, cyanosis, wheezing, dyspnea, engorged neck veins

• Monitor for increased intraocular pressure: eye pain, nausea, vomiting, blurred vision, increased tearing; discontinue use if pain occurs (optic)
• Monitor cardiac rate: rhythm, character, B/P continuously
• Monitor allergic reaction: rash, urticaria

Associated nursing diagnoses

✓ Cardiac output, decreased (uses)
✓ Sensory-perceptual alteration: visual (adverse reactions)
✓ Constipation (adverse reactions)
✓ Knowledge deficit (teaching)

Implementation

IV **IV route**
• Give **IV** undiluted or diluted with 10 ml sterile H_2O; give at a rate of 0.6 mg/min; give through Y-tube or 3-way stopcock; do not add to **IV** sol; may cause paradoxic bradycardia lasting 2 min

Syringe compatibilities:

Benzquinamide, butorphanol, chlorpromazine, cimetidine, dimenhydrinate, diphenhydramine, droperidol, fentanyl, glycopyrrolate, heparin, hydromorphone, hydroxyzine, meperidine, metoclopramide, midazolam, morphine, nalbuphine, pentazocine, prochlorperazine, promazine, promethazine, propiomazine, ranitidine, scopolamine

Y-site compatibilities:

Amrinone, famotidine, heparin, hydrocortisone sodium succinate, nafcillin, potassium chloride

Additive compatibilities:

Dobutamine, netilmicin, sodium bicarbonate, verapamil

PO route
• PO 30 min ac
• Give increased bulk, water in diet if constipation occurs (anticholinergic effect)
IM route
• Expect atropine flush 15-20 min after inj; it may occur in P children and is not harmful

Patient/family education

• Advise patient not to perform strenuous activity in high temperatures; heat stroke may result
• Instruct patient to take as prescribed; not to skip doses
• Instruct patient to report change in vision; blurring or loss of sight; trouble breathing; sweating; flushing, chest pain, allergic reactions
• Caution patient not to operate machinery if drowsiness occurs
• Advise patient not to take OTC products without approval of physician
Ophthalmic route
• Teach patient method of instillation: pressure on lacrimal sac for 1 min; do not touch dropper to eye
• Instruct patient that blurred vision will decrease with repeated use of drug; to omit next instillation if side effects are present
• Instruct patient not to perform hazardous tasks until able to see
• Advise patient to wait 5 min

to use other drops; not to blink more than usual; use sunglasses to protect eyes

Evaluation

Positive therapeutic outcome

- Decreased dysrhythmias
- Increased heart rate
- Decreased secretions, GI, GU spasms
- Bronchodilatation
- Decrease in inflammation (iritis) or cycloplegic refraction (ophthalmic)

Treatment of overdose: O_2, artificial ventilation, ECG; administer dopamine for circulatory depression; administer diazepam or thiopental for convulsion; assess need for antidysrhythmics

attapulgite

(at-a-pull'gite)

Diar Aid, Diasorb, Fowler's Diarrhea Tablets ✤, Hydrated Magnesium Silicate, Kaopectate, Kaopectate Advanced Formula, Kaopectate Maximum Strength, Parepectolin, Rheaban, St. Joseph Antidiarrheal

Func. class.: Antidiarrheal

Chem. class.: Hydrous magnesium aluminum silcate

Pregnancy class C

Action: Decreases gastric motility, water content of stool; adsorbent, demulcent

Therapeutic Outcome: Decreased diarrhea

Uses: Diarrhea (cause undetermined), mild to moderate

Dosage and routes

Adult: PO 60-120 ml (45-90 ml conc) after each loose bowel movement

P *Child >12 yr:* PO 60 ml after each loose bowel movement

P *Child 6-12 yr:* PO 30-60 ml (30 ml conc) after each loose bowel movement

P *Child 3-6 yr:* PO 15-30 ml (15 ml conc) after each loose bowel movement

Available forms: Susp kaolin 0.87 g/5 ml, pectin 43 mg/5 ml; kaolin 0.98 g/5 ml, pectin 21.7 mg/5 ml

Side effects/adverse reactions

GI: Constipation (chronic use)

Precautions: Pregnancy **C**

Pharmacokinetics

Absorption	Not absorbed
Distribution	Unknown
Metabolism	Unknown
Excretion	Unknown
Half-life	Unknown

Pharmacodynamics

	PO
Onset	Unknown
Peak	Unknown
Duration	Unknown

Interactions

All drugs: ↓ action of all other drugs

Associated nursing diagnoses

✓ Diarrhea (uses)
✓ Constipation (adverse reactions)
✓ Knowledge deficit (teaching)

NURSING CONSIDERATIONS

Assessment

- Assess bowel pattern before, during, and after treatment; check for rebound constipation
- Monitor for dehydration in P children

Implementation

PO route

- For 48 hr only after each diarrhea stool

Patient/family education

- Advise patient not to exceed recommended dosage; notify prescriber if symptoms continue
- Instruct patient to shake well before administration

Evaluation

Positive therapeutic outcome

- Decreased diarrhea

auranofin

(au-ran'oh-fin)

Ridaura

Func. class.: Antiinflammatory (gold)

Chem. class.: Active gold compound (29%)

Pregnancy category **C**

Action: Antiinflammatory action unknown; may decrease phagocytosis, lysosomal activity or decrease prostaglandin synthesis; decreases concentration of rheumatoid factor, immunoglobulins

➔ **Therapeutic Outcome:** Relief of pain, inflammation, slowing of rheumatoid arthritis resistant to other treatment

Uses: Rheumatoid arthritis unresponsive to other treatment

Dosage and routes

Adult: PO 6 mg qd or 3 mg bid, may increase to 9 mg/day after 3 mo

Available forms: Caps 3 mg

Side effects/adverse reactions

CNS: Dizziness, confusion, hallucinations, ***seizures,*** EEG abnormalities

GI: Diarrhea, abdominal cramping, stomatitis, nausea, vomiting, enterocolitis, anorexia, flatulence, metallic taste, dyspepsia, jaundice, increased AST (SGOT), ALT (SGPT), glossitis, gingivitis, melena, constipation

GU: ***Proteinuria, hematuria,*** increased BUN, creatinine, vaginitis

HEMA: ***Thrombocytopenia, agranulocytosis, aplastic anemia, leukopenia, eosinophilia, neutropenia***

INTEG: Rash, pruritus, dermatitis, ***exfoliative dermatitis,*** urticaria, alopecia, photosensitivity

MISC: Iritis, corneal ulcers, gold deposits in ocular tissues

RESP: ***Interstitial pneumonitis, fibrosis,*** cough, dyspnea

Contraindications: Hypersensitivity to gold, necrotizing enterocolitis, bone marrow aplasia, child <6 yr, lactation, pulmonary fibrosis, exfoliative dermatitis, blood dyscrasias, recent radiation therapy, renal/hepatic disease, marked hypertension, uncontrolled CHF

Precautions: Elderly , CHF, diabetes mellitus, allergic conditions, ulcerative colitis, renal disease, liver disease, pregnancy **C**

Pharmacokinetics

Absorption	20%-30% (PO)
Distribution	Widely distributed; concentrated in joints
Metabolism	Unknown
Excretion	Kidneys slow (60%-90%); feces (10%-40%); breast milk
Half-life	1 mo (blood); up to 4 mo (tissue)

Pharmacodynamics

	PO
Onset	Unknown
Peak	2 hr
Durations	8-16 wk (steady state)

Interactions

Drug/drug:

Individual drugs

Penicillamine: ↑ toxicity

Radiation: ↑ bone marrow toxicity

Drug classifications

Antineoplastics: ↑ bone marrow toxicity

Lab test interferences

False positive: TB skin test

NURSING CONSIDERATIONS

Assessment

- Assess symptoms of rheumatoid arthritis: pain in joints, stiffness, poor range of motion, inflammation
- Assess respiratory status: dyspnea, wheezing; if respiratory problems occur, drug should be discontinued; pneumonitis, fibrosis may occur
- Monitor urine; hematuria, proteinuria, increased BUN, creatinine may require decrease in dosage or discontinuation of treatment; I&O ratio
- Monitor blood studies: platelets, WBC, eosinophils, granulocytes monthly; drug should be discontinued if platelets <100,000/mm^3, WBC <4000 mm^3, eosinophils >5%, granulocytes <1500 mm^3
- Monitor hepatic test: ALT (SGPT), AST (SGOT), alkaline phosphatase monthly
- Monitor diarrhea stools; if severe, drug should be discontinued
- Assess allergy: rash, dermatitis, pruritus, angioneurotic edema, nitroid reactions; drug should be discontinued if any of these occur
- Assess gold toxicity: decreased Hgb, WBC <4000/mm^3, granulocytes <1500/mm^3, platelets <150,000/mm^3, severe diarrhea, stomatitis, hematuria, rash, itching, proteinuria; drug should be discontinued and dimercaprol (BAL), with glucocorticoids given

Associated nursing diagnoses

✓ Mobility, impaired (uses)

- ✓ Injury, risk for (adverse reactions)
- ✓ Diarrhea (adverse reactions)
- ✓ Knowledge deficit (teaching)

Implementation

PO route

- Give bid or may give as single dose qAM with food or drink to prevent GI symptoms

Patient/family education

- Instruct patient that drug must be taken as prescribed to be useful; to obtain lab work monthly; that therapeutic effect may take 3-4 mo; patient should not double or skip doses
- Teach patient that diarrhea is common, but if blood appears in stools or urine, notify prescriber at once; that patient should check for bruising, hematemesis, hematuria, petechiae, bleeding gums, which indicate thrombocytopenia
- Advise patient to report abnormal skin conditions, stomatitis, fatigue, jaundice; may indicate blood dyscrasias; to notify prescriber of sore throat, fever, malaise; infection, gold toxicity: severe diarrhea, stomatitis, rash, itching; to avoid exposure to sunlight or ultraviolet light; to use sunscreen to prevent burns
- Teach patient to use dilute hydrogen peroxide for mild stomatitis, avoid hot spicy foods and food with high acidic content; use soft toothbrush, rinse more frequently, floss daily
- Teach patient that contraception should be used during treatment

Evaluation

Positive therapeutic outcome

- Ability to move joints with less pain
- Absence of stiffness, inflammation in joints

aurothioglucose/gold sodium thiomalate

(aur-oh-thye-oh-gloo′kose)

Solganal/Myochrysine

Func. class.: Antiinflammatory (gold)

Chem. class.: Active gold compound (50%)

Pregnancy category C

Action: Antiinflammatory action unknown; may decrease phagocytosis, lysosomal activity, prostaglandin synthesis

➔ **Therapeutic Outcome:** Relief of pain, inflammation; slowing of rheumatoid arthritis

Uses: Rheumatoid arthritis resistant to other treatment, psoriatic arthritis

Dosage and routes

Adult: IM 10 mg; then 25 mg weekly × 2-3 wk; then 50 mg/wk until total of 1 g is administered; then 25-50 mg q3-4 wk if there is improvement without toxicity (aurothioglucose); total of 800 mg-1 g

Adult: IM 10 mg, then 25 mg after 1 wk, then 50 mg weekly for total of 14-20 doses; then 50 mg q2 wk × 4; then 50 mg q3 wk × 4; then 50 mg monthly for maintenance (gold sodium thiomalate)

P *Child 6-12 yr:* IM 1 mg/kg/wk × 20 wk, or ¼ of adult dosage (aurothioglucose)

P *Child:* IM 1 mg/kg/wk × 20 wk, then q3-4 wk if improvement without toxicity (gold sodium thiomalate), not to exceed 2.5 mg

Available forms: IM inj 50 mg/ml, 25 mg/ml

Side effects/adverse reactions

CNS: *Dizziness,* EEG abnormalities, ***encephalitis,*** confusion, hallucinations
CV: Bradycardia, rapid pulse
EENT: Iritis, corneal ulcers
GI: Stomatitis, nausea, vomiting, metallic taste, jaundice, ***hepatitis,*** diarrhea, cramping, flatulence
GU: *Proteinuria,* hematuria, ***nephrosis, tubular necrosis***
HEMA: ***Thrombocytopenia, agranulocytosis, aplastic anemia, leukopenia, eosinophilia, neutropenia***
INTEG: *Rash, pruritus, dermatitis,* urticaria, alopecia, photosensitivity, ***exfoliative dermatitis, angioedema***
RESP: Interstitial pneumonitis, pharyngitis, ***pulmonary fibrosis***
SYST: ***Anaphylaxis***

Contraindications: Hypersensitivity to gold, SLE, uncontrolled diabetes mellitus, marked hypertension, recent radiation therapy, CHF, lactation, renal disease, liver disease

Precautions: Decreased tolerance in elderly, children, blood dyscrasias, pregnancy **C**
G P

Pharmacokinetics

Absorption	Slow (IM)
Distribution	Widely distributed; concentration in joints
Metabolism	Unknown
Excretion	Kidneys, slow (60%-90%); feces (10%-40%); breast milk
Half-life	26 days (blood); up to 4 mo (tissue)

Pharmacodynamics

	IM
Onset	Unknown
Peak	4-6 hr
Duration	8-16 wk (steady state)

Interactions

Drug/drug:

Individual drugs

Penicillamine: ↑ toxicity
Radiation: ↑ bone marrow toxicity

Drug classifications

Antineoplastics: ↑ bone marrow toxicity

Lab test interferences

False positive: TB skin test

NURSING CONSIDERATIONS

Assessment

- Assess symptoms of rheumatoid arthritis: pain in joints, stiffness, poor range of motion, inflammation
- Assess respiratory status: dyspnea, wheezing; if respiratory problems occur, drug should be discontinued; pneumonitis, fibrosis may occur
- Monitor urine; hematuria, proteinuria, increased BUN, creatinine may require decrease in dosage or discontinuation of treatment; I&O ratio

- Monitor blood studies: platelets, WBC, eosinophils, granulocytes monthly; drug should be discontinued if platelets <100,000/mm^3, WBC <4000 mm^3, eosinophils >5%, granulocytes <1500 mm^3
- Monitor hepatic test: ALT (SGPT), AST (SGOT), alkaline phosphatase monthly
- Monitor diarrhea stools; if severe, drug should be discontinued
- Assess allergy: rash, dermatitis, pruritus, angioneurotic edema, nitroid reactions; drug should be discontinued if any of these occur
- Assess gold toxicity: decreased Hgb, WBC <4000/mm^3, granulocytes <1500/mm^3, platelets <150,000/mm^3, severe diarrhea, stomatitis, hematuria, rash, itching, proteinuria; drug should be discontinued and dimercaprol (BAL) with glucocorticoids given

Associated nursing diagnoses

- ✓ Mobility, impaired physical (uses)
- ✓ Injury, risk for (adverse reactions)
- ✓ Diarrhea (adverse reactions)
- ✓ Knowledge deficit (teaching)

Implementation

IM route

- Give deep IM, never **IV**; slow administration; keep recumbent for 10 min after inj; monitor for transient reaction
- Shake well before giving

Patient/family education

- Teach patient that drug must be taken as prescribed to be useful; to obtain lab work monthly; that therapeutic effect may take 3-4 mo; patient should not double or skip doses
- Instruct patient that diarrhea is common, but if blood appears in stools or urine, notify prescriber at once; that patient should check for bruising, hematemesis, hematuria, petechiae, bleeding gums, which indicate thrombocytopenia
- Tell patient to report abnormal skin conditions, stomatitis, fatigue, jaundice; may indicate blood dyscrasias; to notify prescriber of sore throat, fever, malaise (infection); severe diarrhea, stomatitis, rash, itching (gold toxicity); to avoid exposure to sunlight or ultraviolet light; to use sunscreen to prevent burns
- Teach patient to use dilute hydrogen peroxide for mild stomatitis, avoid hot spicy foods and food with high acidic content; use soft toothbrush, rinse more frequently, floss daily
- Teach patient that contraception should be used during treatment

Evaluation

Positive therapeutic outcome

- Ability to move joints with less pain
- Absence of stiffness, inflammation of joints

azatadine
(a-za'ta-deen)
Optimine
Func. class.: Antihistamine
Chem. class.: Piperidine H_1-receptor antagonist
Pregnancy category **B**

Action: Acts on blood vessels, GI, respiratory system by competing with histamine for H_1-receptor site; decreases allergic response by blocking histamine; causes increased heart rate, vasodilatation, secretions

➡ **Therapeutic Outcome:** Absence of allergy symptoms and rhinitis

Uses: Allergy symptoms, rhinitis, allergic dermatoses, nasal allergies

Dosage and routes
Adult: PO 1-2 mg bid, not to exceed 4 mg/day

Available forms: Tabs 1 mg

Side effects/adverse reactions
CNS: Dizziness, drowsiness, poor coordination, fatigue, anxiety, euphoria, confusion, paresthesia, neuritis, sweating, chills
CV: Hypotension, palpitations, tachycardia
EENT: Blurred vision, dilated pupils, tinnitus, nasal stuffiness, dry nose, throat, mouth
GI: Constipation, dry mouth, nausea, vomiting, anorexia, diarrhea
GU: Retention, dysuria, frequency, impotence
HEMA: Thrombocytopenia, agranulocytosis, hemolytic anemia
INTEG: Rash, urticaria, photosensitivity
RESP: Increased thick secretions, wheezing, chest tightness

Contraindications: Hypersensitivity to H_1-receptor antagonist, acute asthma attack, lower respiratory tract disease, P child <12 yr

Precautions: Increased intraocular pressure, renal disease, cardiac disease, bronchial asthma, seizure disorder, stenosed peptic ulcers, hyperthyroidism, prostatic hypertrophy, bladder neck obstruction, pregnancy **B**, G elderly

Pharmacokinetics

Absorption	Well absorbed (PO)
Distribution	Crosses placenta
Metabolism	Liver, extensively
Excretion	Kidneys, unchanged (20%)
Half-life	9-12 hr

Pharmacodynamics

	PO
Onset	15-60 min
Peak	4 hr
Duration	12 hr

Interactions
Drug/drug:
Individual drugs
Alcohol: ↑ CNS depression
Drug classifications
CNS depressants: ↑ CNS depression
MAOI: ↑ anticholinergic effect

Narcotics: ↑ CNS depression
Sedative/hypnotics: ↑ CNS depression

Lab test interferences

False negative: Skin allergy tests (discontinue antihistamines 3 days before testing)

NURSING CONSIDERATIONS

Assessment

• Assess respiratory status: rate, rhythm, increase in bronchial secretions, wheezing, chest tightness; provide fluids to 2 L/day to decrease secretion thickness

• Monitor I&O ratio: be alert for urinary retention, frequency, dysuria, especially G elderly; drug should be discontinued if these occur

• Monitor CBC during long-term therapy; blood dyscrasias may occur but are rare

Associated nursing diagnoses

✓ Airway clearance, ineffective (uses)
✓ Injury, risk for (side effects)
✓ Knowledge deficit (teaching)
✓ Noncompliance (teaching-overuse)

Implementation

PO route

• May give with food to prevent GI upset; absorption is not altered by food

• Store in tight, light-resistant container

Patient/family education

• Teach all aspects of drug uses; to notify prescriber if confusion, sedation, hypotension occur; to avoid driving or other hazardous activity if drowsiness occurs; to avoid alcohol or other CNS depressants that may potentiate effect

• Teach patient to take 1 hr ac or 2 hr pc to facilitate absorption

• Caution patient not to exceed recommended dosage; dysrhythmias may occur

• Teach patient hard candy, gum, frequent rinsing of mouth may be used for dryness

Evaluation

Positive therapeutic outcome

• Absence of running or congested nose, rashes

Treatment of overdose:

Administer ipecac syrup or lavage, diazepam, vasopressors, barbiturates (short acting)

azathioprine

(ay-za-thye'oh-preen)
Imuran

Func. class.: Immunosuppressant
Chem. class.: Purine analog

Pregnancy category **D**

Action: Produces immunosuppression by inhibiting purine synthesis, DNA, RNA in cells

➔ **Therapeutic Outcome:** Absence of graft rejection, slowing of rheumatoid arthritis

Uses: Renal transplants to prevent graft rejection, often used with corticosteroids, cytotoxics; refractory rheumatoid arthritis, refractory ITP, glomerulonephritis, nephrotic syndrome, bone marrow transplant

Dosage and routes

Prevention of rejection

P *Adult and child:* PO, **IV** 3-5 mg/kg/day, then maintenance (PO) of at least 1-2 mg/kg/day

Refractory rheumatoid arthritis

Adult: PO 1/mg/kg/day; may increase dosage after 2 mo by 0.5 mg/kg/day; not to exceed 2.5 mg/kg/day

Available forms: Tabs 50 mg; inj **IV** 100 mg

Side effects/adverse reactions

GI: Nausea, vomiting, stomatitis, esophagitis, ***pancreatitis, hepatotoxicity, jaundice***
HEMA: ***Leukopenia, thrombocytopenia, anemia, pancytopenia***
INTEG: Rash
MS: Arthralgia, muscle wasting

Contraindications: Hypersensitivity, pregnancy **D**

Precautions: Severe renal disease, severe hepatic disease

Pharmacokinetics

Absorption	Readily (PO)
Distribution	Crosses placenta
Metabolism	Liver to mercaptopurine
Excretion	Kidney, minimal
Half-life	3 hr

Pharmacodynamics

	PO	IV
Onset	Unknown	Unknown
Peak	4 hr	Unknown
Duration	Unknown	Unknown

Interactions

Drug/drug:

Individual drugs

Allopurinol: ↑ toxicity
Cyclosporine: ↑ myelosuppression

Drug classification

Antineoplastics: ↑ myelosuppression

NURSING CONSIDERATIONS

Assessment

- Assess symptoms of rheumatoid arthritis: pain in joints, stiffness, poor range of motion, inflammation
- Monitor blood studies: Hgb, WBC, platelets during treatment monthly; if leukocytes are <3000/mm^3 or platelets <100,000/mm^3, drug should be discontinued or reduced; decreased Hgb level may indicate bone marrow suppression
- Monitor liver function studies: alkaline phosphatase, AST (SGOT), ALT (SGPT), amylase, bilirubin; and for hepatotoxicity: dark urine, jaundice, itching, light-colored stools; drug should be discontinued

Associated nursing diagnoses

- ✓ Mobility, impaired (uses)
- ✓ Infection, risk for (uses)
- ✓ Knowledge deficit (teaching)

Implementation

PO route

- Give all medications PO if possible, avoiding IM injections, since bleeding may occur
- Give with meals to reduce GI upset; nausea is common
- For several days before transplant surgery, patients should be placed in protective isolation

IV route

- Give after diluting 100 mg/10 ml of sterile water for inj; rotate to dissolve; may further dilute with 50 ml or more saline or glucose in saline given over >30 min (intermittent inf)

Patient/family education

- Teach patient that therapeutic response may take 3-4 mo in rheumatoid arthritis; that drug is needed for life in renal transplant
- Instruct patient to report fever, rash, severe diarrhea, chills, sore throat, fatigue, since serious infections may occur; or clay-colored stools and cramping (hepatotoxicity)
- Advise patient to use contraceptive measures during treatment for 12 wk after ending therapy; drug is teratogenic
- Tell patient to avoid crowds and persons with known infections to reduce risk of infection
- Instruct patient not to use OTC medications without approval of prescriber

Evaluation

Positive therapeutic outcome

- Absence of graft rejection
- Immunosuppression in autoimmune disorders
- Increased joint mobility without pain in rheumatoid arthritis

azithromycin

(aye-zith'row-my-sin)

Zithromax

Func. class.: Antibacterial

Chem. class.: Macrolide (azalide) antibiotic

Pregnancy category **B**

Action: Binds to 50S ribosomal subunits of susceptible bacteria and suppresses protein synthesis; much greater spectrum of activity than erythromycin

Therapeutic Outcome: Bacteriostatic against the following susceptible organisms: *Moraxella catarrhalis, Streptococcus pneumoniae, S. pyogenes, Staphylococcus aureus, Haemophilus influenzae, Clostridium, Legionella pneumophila; Chlamydia trachomatis, Mycoplasma;* no effect on methicillin-resistant *S. aureus*

Uses: Mild to moderate infections of the upper respiratory tract, lower respiratory tract; uncomplicated skin and skin structure infections, nongonococcal urethritis, or cervicitis

Dosage and routes

Adult: PO 500 mg on day 1, then 250 mg qd on days 2-5 for a total dose of 1.5 g; may give a one-time dose of 1 g for chlamydial infections

Available forms: Caps 250 mg

Side effects/adverse reactions

CNS: Dizziness, headache, vertigo, somnolence
CV: Palpitations, chest pain
GI: Nausea, vomiting, diarrhea, ***hepatotoxicity,*** abdominal pain, stomatitis, heartburn, dyspepsia, flatulence, melena, ***cholestatic jaundice***
GU: Vaginitis, moniliasis, nephritis
INTEG: Rash, urticaria, pruritus, photosensitivity

Contraindications: Hypersensitivity to azithromycin or erythromycin

Precautions: Pregnancy **B**, lactation, hepatic/renal/ G cardiac disease, elderly, P children <16 yr

Pharmacokinetics

Absorption	Rapid (PO) up to 50%
Distribution	Widely distributed
Metabolism	Unknown, minimal metabolism
Excretion	Unchanged (bile); kidneys, minimal
Half-life	11-70 hr

Pharmacodynamics

	PO
Onset	Unknown
Peak	Unknown
Duration	24 hr

Interactions

Drug/drug:

Individual drugs
Astemizole: ↑ toxicity
Carbamazepine: ↑ toxicity
Terfenadine: ↑ toxicity
Theophylline: ↑ toxicity

Drug classifications
Aluminum antacids: ↓ peak serum
Anticoagulants, orals: ↑ effect of oral anticoagulants
Magnesium antacids: ↓ levels of azithromycin

Drug/food: ↓ absorption

Lab test interferences

False increase: 17-OHCS/17-KS, AST (SGOT), ALT (SGPT)
Decrease: Folate assay

NURSING CONSIDERATIONS

Assessment

- Assess for signs and symptoms of infection: drainage, fever, increased WBC >10,000 mm^3, urine culture positive, sore throat, sputum culture positive
- Monitor respiratory status: rate, character, wheezing, tightness in chest; discontinue drug if these occur
- Monitor allergies before treatment, reaction of each medication; place allergies on chart, notify all people giving drugs; skin eruptions, itching
- Monitor I&O ratio, renal studies; report hematuria, oliguria in renal disease; check urinalysis, protein, blood
- Monitor liver studies: AST (SGOT), ALT (SGPT), bilirubin, LDH, alkaline phosphatase
- Monitor C&S before drug therapy; drug may be taken as soon as culture is taken; C&S may be repeated after treatment
- Monitor bowel pattern before, during treatment

Associated nursing diagnoses

- ✓ Infection, risk for (uses)
- ✓ Diarrhea (adverse reactions)
- ✓ Knowledge deficit (teaching)

Implementation

- Provide adequate intake of fluids (2 L) during diarrhea episodes

PO route

- Give with a full glass of water; do not give with food; give 1 hr before or 2 hr pc; do not give with fruit juices
- Store at room temperature

Patient/family education

- Instruct patient to report sore throat, black furry tongue, fever, loose foul-smelling stool, vaginal itching, discharge, fatigue; may indicate superinfection
- Caution patient not to take aluminum/magnesium-containing antacids or food simultaneously with this drug; blood levels of azithromycin will be decreased
- Instruct patient to notify prescriber of diarrhea stools, dark urine, pale stools, yellow discoloration of eyes or skin, severe abdominal pain; cholestatic jaundice is a severe adverse reaction
- Teach patient to take at evenly spaced intervals; complete dosage regimen; to notify prescriber if symptoms continue
- Teach patient that if pregnancy is suspected to notify prescriber
- Inform patient that sunburns may occur; wear protective clothing and sunscreen

Evaluation

Positive therapeutic outcome

- C&S negative for infection
- WBC within 5000-10,000 mm^3

A

aztreonam

(az-tree'oh-nam)

azactam

Func. class.: Misc. antibiotic

Chem. class.: Monobactam

Pregnancy category **B**

Action: Inhibits organisms by inhibiting bacterial cell wall synthesis, which causes death of organism (bactericidal)

➔ Therapeutic Outcome: Bactericidal action against susceptible organisms, specifically gram-negative aerobic organisms: *Escherichia coli, Serratia, Klebsiella, Enterobacter, Haemophilus influenzae, Shigella, Providencia, Salmonella, Neisseria gonorrhoeae, Pseudomonas aeruginosa,* including strains resistant to other drugs

Uses: Urinary tract infection; septicemia; skin, muscle, bone infection and other infections caused by gram-negative organisms

Dosage and routes

Urinary tract infections

Adult: **IV**/IM 500 mg-1 g q8-12h

Systemic infections
Adult: **IV**/IM 1-2 g q8-12h

Severe systemic infections
Adult: **IV**/IM 2 g q6-8h; do not exceed 8 g/day
Continue treatment for 48 hr after negative culture or until patient is asymptomatic

Available forms: Powder for inj 500 mg, 1, 2 g

Side effects/adverse reactions
CNS: Lethargy, hallucinations, anxiety, depression, twitching, ***coma, convulsions,*** malaise
EENT: Tinnitus, diplopia, nasal congestion
GI: *Nausea, vomiting, diarrhea,* increased AST (SGOT), ALT (SGPT), abdominal pain, glossitis, colitis
GU: Vaginal candidiasis, vaginitis, breast tenderness
HEMA: Anemia, increased bleeding time, ***bone marrow depression, granulocytopenia***

Contraindications: Hypersensitivity

Precautions: Pregnancy **B**,
P lactation, children, impaired
G renal/hepatic function, elderly

Pharmacokinetics

Absorption	Well absorbed (IM)
Distribution	Widely distributed; crosses placenta
Metabolism	Liver, minimal
Excretion	Kidneys, unchanged (65%-75%); breast milk
Half-life	1.7 hr; increased in renal disease

Pharmacodynamics

	IM	IV
Onset	Rapid	Rapid
Peak	1 hr	Infusion's end

Interactions
Drug/drug:
Drug classifications
Antiinfectives: ↑ antagonist effect
Clindamycin: ↓ action of clindamycin
Furosemide: ↑ levels
Penicillins: ↑ or ↓ action of penicillins
Probenicid: ↑ levels

NURSING CONSIDERATIONS
Assessment
- Assess patient for previous sensitivity reaction to penicillins or cephalosporins; cross-sensitivity between penicillins, cephalosporins and this drug is common
- Assess patient for signs and symptoms of infection including characteristics of wounds, sputum, urine, stool, WBC >10,000, fever; obtain baseline information before and during treatment
- Complete C&S before beginning drug therapy to identify if correct treatment has been initiated
- Identify urine output; if decreasing, notify prescriber (may indicate nephrotoxicity); also check for increased BUN, creatinine; note color, character, pH of urine if drug is administered for urinary tract infection; output should be

800 ml less than intake; if urine is highly acidic, alkalinization may be needed
- Monitor blood studies: AST (SGOT), ALT (SGPT), CBC, Hct, bilirubin, LDH, alkaline phosphatase, Coombs' test monthly if patient is on long-term therapy
- Monitor electrolytes: potassium, sodium, chloride monthly if patient is on long-term therapy
- Assess bowel pattern daily; if severe diarrhea occurs, drug should be discontinued; may indicate pseudomembranous colitis
- Monitor for bleeding: ecchymosis, bleeding gums, hematuria, stool guaiac daily if on long-term therapy
- Assess for overgrowth of infection: perineal itching, fever, malaise, redness, pain, swelling, drainage, rash, diarrhea, change in cough, sputum

Associated nursing diagnoses

- ✓ Infection, risk for (uses)
- ✓ Diarrhea (side effects)
- ✓ Injury, risk for (side effects)
- ✓ Knowledge deficit (teaching)
- ✓ Noncompliance (teaching)

Implementation

IM route
- Reconstitute 1 g/3 ml or more of sterile water for inj 0.9% NaCl; may be diluted with 0.5% or 1% lidocaine to prevent pain; give deep in large muscle mass, massage; sol stable 1 wk refrigerated

IV **IV route**
- Check for irritation, extravasation, phlebitis daily; change **IV** site q72h
- For direct **IV**, dilute 1 g/10 ml or 2 g/20 ml sterile water for injection, shake, let stand until clear; give over 3-5 min into running **IV**
- For intermittent inf, further dilute with 50-100 ml of D_5W, $D_{10}W$, D_5/0.25% NaCl, D_5/0.45% NaCl, D_5/0.9% NaCl, 0.9% NaCl, D_5/LR, D_5/0.02%, sodium bicarbonate, Ringer's or LR; give over 15-60 min into running **IV**

Syringe compatibility:
Clindamycin

Y-*site compatibilities:*
Ciprofloxacin, enalaprilat, foscarnet, melphalan, ondansetron, vinorelbine, zidovudine

Y-*site incompatibility:*
Vancomycin

Additive compatibilities:
Cefazolin, ciprofloxacin, clindamycin, gentamicin, tobramycin

Additive incompatibilities:
Nafcillin, cephradine, metronidazole

Patient/family education

- Teach patient to report sore throat, bruising, bleeding, joint pain; may indicate blood dyscrasias (rare)
- Advise patient to contact prescriber if vaginal itching, loose, foul-smelling stools, furry tongue occur; may indicate superinfection; report itching, rash, pruritus, urticaria

• Instruct patient to take all medication prescribed for the length of time ordered; drug must be taken around the clock to maintain blood levels; do not give medication to others
• Advise patient to notify prescriber of diarrhea with blood or pus

Evaluation

Positive therapeutic outcome
• Absence of signs/symptoms of infection (WBC <10,000, temp WNL, absence of red draining wounds)
• Reported improvement in symptoms of infection

baclofen

(bak'loe-fen)

baclofen, Lioresal, Lioresal DS, Lioresal Intrathecal

Func. class.: Skeletal muscle relaxant, central acting

Chem. class.: GABA chlorophenyl derivative

Pregnancy category C

Action: Inhibits synaptic responses in CNS by decreasing GABA, which decreases neurotransmitter function; decreases frequency, severity of muscle spasms

Therapeutic Outcome: Decreased spasticity of muscles

Uses: Spinal cord injury, spasticity in multiple sclerosis

Dosage and routes

Adult: PO 5 mg tid × 3 days, then 10 mg tid × 3 days, then 15 mg tid × 3 days, then 20 mg tid x 3 days, then titrated to response; not to exceed 80 mg/day

Intrathecal: Use implantable intrathecal inf pump; use screening trial of 3 separate bol doses if needed (50 μg/ml, 75 μg/1.5 ml, 100 μg/2 ml); initially double screening dose that produced result and give over 24 hr; increase by 10%-30% q24h only; maintenance: 12-1500 μg/day

Available forms: Tabs 10, 20 mg, 10 mg/20 ml (500 μg/ml), 10 mg/5 ml (2000 μg/ml)

Side effects/adverse reactions

CNS: *Dizziness, weakness, fatigue, drowsiness,* headache, disorientation, insomnia, paresthesias, tremors
CV: Hypotension, chest pain, palpitations, edema
EENT: Nasal congestion, blurred vision, mydriasis, tinnitus
GI: *Nausea,* constipation, vomiting, increased AST (SGOT), alkaline phosphatase, abdominal pain, dry mouth, anorexia
GU: Urinary frequency
INTEG: Rash, pruritus

Contraindications: Hypersensitivity

B

Precautions: Peptic ulcer disease, renal disease, hepatic disease, stroke, seizure disorder, diabetes mellitus, G pregnancy **C**, elderly

Pharmacokinetics

Absorption	Rapid
Distribution	Widely, crosses placenta
Metabolism	Liver, partially
Excretion	Kidney, unchanged
Half-life	2½-4 hr

Pharmacodynamics

	PO
Onset	Unknown
Peak	2-3 hr
Duration	>8 hr

Interactions

Drug/drug:

Individual drugs

Alcohol: CNS depression

Drug classifications

Antidepressants, tricyclic: ↑ CNS depression

Barbiturates: ↑ CNS depression

Narcotics: ↑ CNS depression

Sedative/hypnotics: ↑ CNS depression

Lab test interferences

Increase: AST (SGOT), alkaline phosphatase, blood glucose

NURSING CONSIDERATIONS

Assessment

- Monitor B/P, weight, blood sugar, and hepatic function periodically
- Check for increased seizure activity in epilepsy patient; this drug decreases seizure threshold, monitor ECG
- Check I&O ratio; check for urinary retention, frequency, hesitancy
- Allergic reactions: rash, fever, respiratory distress; severe weakness, numbness in extremities
- Assess CNS depression: dizziness, drowsiness, psychiatric symptoms
- Check dosage, as individual titration is required

Associated nursing diagnoses

✓ Mobility, impaired uses
✓ Injury, risk for (adverse reactions)
✓ Knowledge deficit (teaching)

Implementation

PO route

- Give with meals for GI symptoms; gum, frequent sips of water for dry mouth
- Store in airtight container at room temperature

IV **IV route**

- Titration is based on response
- Test dose: 50 mg/ml, give over 1 min or more

Patient/family education

- Advise patient not to discontinue medication quickly; hallucinations, spasticity, tachycardia will occur; drug should be tapered off over 1-2 wk
- Advise patient not to take with alcohol, other CNS depressants
- Caution patient to avoid altering activities while taking this drug; to avoid hazardous activities if drowsiness or dizziness occurs

• Advise patient to avoid using OTC medication: cough preparations, antihistamines unless directed by prescriber
• Tell patient to increase fluid intake >2 L/day

Evaluation

Positive therapeutic outcome
• Decreased pain, spasticity

Treatment of overdose: Induce emesis if conscious patient, lavage, dialysis

beclomethasone

(be-kloe-meth'a-sone)

Beclovent, Beconase, Beconase AQ Nasal, Beconase Inhalation, Vancenase AQ Nasal, Vancenase Nasal, Vanceril

Func. class.: Synthetic glucocorticoid (long acting)

Chem. class.: Beclomethasone diester

Pregnancy category **C**

Action: Antiinflammatory; vasoconstrictive properties; also immunosuppressive

➔ Therapeutic Outcome: Decreased inflammation and normal immunity

Uses: Seasonal, perennial allergic rhinitis, nasal polyps, chronic steroid-dependent asthma

Dosage and routes

P ***Adult and child >12 yr:*** Instill 1-2 sprays in each nostril bid-qid; Inh 2-4 puffs tid-qid

P ***Child 6-12 yrs:*** Instill 1 spray in each nostril tid; Inh 1-2 puffs tid-qid

Available forms: Aero 42 µg/spray (nasal); aero for inh; 42 µg/activation; aerosol for nasal inh 0.042%

Side effects/adverse reactions

CNS: Headache, paresthesia
EENT: *Dryness, nasal irritation, burning, sneezing,* secretions with blood, nasal ulcerations, ***perforation of nasal septum, candidal*** infection, earache, hoarseness
ENDO: ***Adrenal suppression***
INTEG: Rash, urticaria, pruritus
RESP: ***Acute status asthmaticus,*** wheezing

Contraindications: Hypersensitivity, systemic corticosteroid therapy

Precautions: Pregnancy **C**, P children <12, nasal ulcers, recurrent epistaxis

Pharmacokinetics

Absorption	Locally only
Distribution	Not distributed
Metabolism	Minimal
Excretion	Feces
Half-life	3-15 hr

Pharmacodynamics

	INH	NASAL
Onset	10 min	10 min
Peak	Unknown	Unknown
Duration	Unknown	Unknown

NURSING CONSIDERATIONS

Assessment

- Assess adrenal suppression: 17-KS, plasma cortisol for decreased levels, adrenal function periodically for HPA axis suppression
- Check nasal passages during long-term treatment for changes in mucus; check for burning, stinging; assess for glucocorticoid withdrawal: dizziness, hypotension, fatigue, muscle/joint pain; notify prescriber immediately
- Assess respiratory status: rest, rhythm, characteristics; auscultate lung bilaterally before and throughout treatment

Associated nursing diagnoses

✓ Airway clearance, ineffective (uses)
✓ Oral mucous membranes, altered (adverse reactions)
✓ Knowledge deficit (teaching)
✓ Noncompliance (teaching)

Implementation

- Use after cleaning aerosol top daily with warm water; dry thoroughly
- Store in cool environment; do not puncture or incinerate container

Patient/family education

- Teach patient to continue using product even if mild nasal bleeding occurs; is usually transient
- Teach patient method of installation after providing written instructions from manufacturer
- Teach patient to clear nasal passages before administration; use decongestant if needed; shake inhaler, invert, tilt head backward, insert nozzle into nostril, away from septum; hold other nostril closed and depress activator, inhale through nose, exhale through mouth

Evaluate

Positive therapeutic outcome

- Decrease in runny nose, improved symptoms of bronchial asthma

benazepril

(ben-a'ze-pril)
Lotensin
Func. class.: Antihypertensive
Chem. class.: ACE inhibitor
Pregnancy category **D**

Action: Selectively suppresses renin-angiotensin-aldosterone system; inhibits ACE; prevents conversion of angiotensin I to angiotensin II; results in dilatation of arterial, venous vessels

➡ **Therapeutic Outcome:** Decreased B/P in hypertension

Uses: Hypertension, alone or in combination with thiazide diuretics

Dosage and routes

Adult: PO 10 mg qd initially, then 20-40 mg/day divided bid or qd; **renal impairment:** 5 mg qd with CrCl<30 ml/min/1.73 m^2; increase as needed to maximum of 40 mg/day

Available forms: Tabs 5, 10, 20, 40 mg

Side effects/adverse reactions

CNS: Anxiety, hypertonia, insomnia, paresthesia, headache, dizziness, fatigue
CV: *Hypotension, postural hypotension,* syncope, palpitations, angina
GI: *Nausea,* constipation, vomiting, gastritis, melena
GU: Increased BUN, creatinine, decreased libido, impotence, urinary tract infection
HEMA: ***Neutropenia, agranulocytosis***
INTEG: ***Angioedema,*** rash, flushing, sweating
META: Hyperkalemia, hyponatremia
MS: Arthralgia, arthritis, myalgia
RESP: Cough, asthma, bronchitis, dyspnea, sinusitis

Contraindications: Hypersensitivity to ACE inhibitors, P pregnancy **D**, lactation, children

Precautions: Impaired renal/liver function, dialysis patients, hypovolemia, blood dyscrasias, G CHF, COPD, asthma, elderly, bilateral renal artery stenosis

Pharmacokinetics

Absorption	<40% (PO)
Distribution	Unknown; crosses placenta
Metabolism	Liver metabolites; serum protein binding 97%
Excretion	Kidney, breast milk (minimal)
Half-life	10-11 hr (metabolite); increased in renal disease

Pharmacodynamics

	PO
Onset	Unknown
Peak	½-1 hr
Duration	Unknown

Interactions

Drug/drug:

Individual drugs

Alcohol: ↑ hypotension (large amounts)
Allopurinol: ↑ hypersensitivity
Digoxin: ↑ serum levels
Hydralazine: ↑ toxicity
Indomethacin: ↓ antihypertensive effect
Lithium: ↑ serum levels
Prazosin: ↑ toxicity

Drug classifications

Adrenergic blockers: ↑ hypotension
Antacids: ↓ absorption
Antihypertensives: ↑ hypotension
Diuretics: ↑ hypotension
Diuretics, potassium-sparing: ↑ toxicity
Ganglionic blockers: ↑ hypotension
Potassium supplements: ↑ toxicity
Sympathomimetics: ↑ toxicity

Lab test interferences

False positive: Urine acetone

NURSING CONSIDERATIONS

Assessment

- Monitor blood studies: neutrophils, decreased platelets
- Monitor B/P, check for orthostatic hypotension, syncope; if changes occur, dosage change may be required
- Monitor renal studies: protein, BUN, creatinine; watch

for increased levels that may indicate nephrotic syndrome and renal failure; monitor renal symptoms: polyuria, oliguria, frequency, dysuria
- Establish baselines in renal, liver function tests before therapy begins
- Check potassium levels throughout treatment, although hyperkalemia rarely occurs
- Check for edema in feet, legs daily
- Assess for allergic reactions: rash, fever, pruritus, urticaria; drug should be discontinued if antihistamines fail to help

Associated nursing diagnoses

✓ Cardiac output, decreased (uses)
✓ Injury, potential for (side effects)
✓ Knowledge deficit (teaching)
✓ Noncompliance (teaching)

Implementation

PO route
- Store in air-tight container at 86° F (30° C) or less
- Severe hypotension may occur after 1st dose of this medication; decreased hypotension may be prevented by reducing or discontinuing diuretic therapy 3 days before beginning benazepril therapy
- Give **IV** infusion of 0.9% NaCl (as ordered) to expand fluid volume if severe hypotension occurs

Patient/family education

- Instruct patient not to discontinue drug abruptly; advise patient to tell all persons associated with care
- Teach patient not to use OTC products (cough, cold, allergy) unless directed by prescriber; serious side effects can occur; xanthines such as coffee, tea, chocolate, cola can prevent action of drug
- Emphasize the importance of complying with dosage schedule, even if feeling better; to continue with medical regimen to decrease B/P: exercise, cessation of smoking, decreasing stress, diet modifications
- Emphasize the need to rise slowly to sitting or standing position to minimize orthostatic hypotension; not to exercise in hot weather because increased hypotension can occur
- Teach patient to notify prescriber of mouth sores, sore throat, fever, swelling of hands or feet, irregular heartbeat, chest pain, coughing, shortness of breath
- Caution patient to report excessive perspiration, dehydration, vomiting, diarrhea; may lead to fall in B/P
- Caution patient that drug may cause dizziness, fainting, light-headedness; may occur during 1st few days of therapy; to avoid activities that may be hazardous
- Teach patient how to take B/P; teach normal readings for age group; ensure patient takes own B/P

Evaluation

Positive therapeutic outcome
- Decreased B/P in hypertension

Treatment of overdose:

0.9% NaCl **IV** inf, hemodialysis

benzocaine
(ben'zoe-kane)
Anbesol Maximum Strength, Baby Anbesol, Children's Chloraseptic, Medamint, Orabase Baby, Oracin, Ora-Jel, Oratect, Spec-T Anesthetic, T-Caine, Tyrobenz
Func. class.: Topical local anesthetic
Chem. class.: Ester
Pregnancy category C

Action: Inhibits conduction of nerve impulses from sensory nerves

Therapeutic Outcome: Absence of pain, irritation

Uses: Oral irritation, sore throat, toothache, cold sore, canker sore, sunburn, minor cuts, insect bites, pain, itching

Dosage and routes
P *Adult and child >12 yr:* Top apply to affected area; loz suck as needed

Available forms: Cream 1%, 5%; lotion 0.5%, 8%; oint 2%, 5%, 20%; sol 2.1%, 2.5%, 6.3%, 20%; loz 3, 5, 6.25, 10 mg; top aerosol 20%; gel 6.3%, 7.5%, 10%, 20%

Side effects/adverse reactions
EENT: Itching, irritation in ear
INTEG: Rash, urticaria

Contraindications: Hypersensitivity

Precautions: Pregnancy **C**

Pharmacokinetics

Absorption	Poorly absorbed
Distribution	Unknown
Metabolism	Plasma, liver cholinesterase
Excretion	Unknown
Half-life	Unknown

Pharmacodynamics

	TOP
Onset	Unknown
Peak	1 min
Duration	½-1 hr

Interactions: None

NURSING CONSIDERATIONS
Assessment
- Assess pain: location, duration, characteristics before and after administration
- Assess for infection: redness, drainage, inflammation; this drug should not be used until infection is treated

Associated nursing diagnoses
✓ Pain (uses)
✓ Knowledge deficit (teaching)

Implementation
- Apply to gums as needed for teething pain
- Use loz for temporary sore throat pain
- Store in tight, light-resistant container; do not freeze, puncture, or incinerate aerosol container

Patient/family education
- Advise patient to avoid contact with eyes
- Caution patient not to use

for prolonged periods: use for <1 wk; if condition remains, prescriber should be contacted

Evaluation

Positive therapeutic outcome
- Decreased redness, swelling, pain on affected area

benzquinamide
(benz-kwin'a-mide)
Emete-Con
Func. class.: Antiemetic
Chem. class.: Benzoquinolizine amide
Pregnancy category C

Action: Acts centrally by blocking chemoreceptor trigger zone, which in turn acts on vomiting center

Therapeutic Outcome: Absence of nausea, vomiting

Uses: To inhibit nausea, vomiting associated with anesthetic

Dosage and routes

Adult: IM 50 mg or 0.5-1 mg/kg; may be repeated in 1 hr, then q3-4h prn; **IV** 25 mg or 0.2-0.4 mg/kg as a one-time dose

Available forms: Inj 50 mg/vial

Side effects/adverse reactions

CNS: *Drowsiness,* fatigue, restlessness, tremor, headache, stimulation, dizziness, insomnia, twitching, excitement, nervousness, extrapyramidal symptoms

CV: ***PACs or PVCs, atrial fibrillation,*** hypertension, hypotension

EENT: Dry mouth, blurred vision, hiccups, salivation

GI: Nausea, anorexia

INTEG: Rash, urticaria, fever, chills, flushing, hives, shivering, sweating, temperature

Contraindications: Hypersensitivity, hypertension

P G Precautions: Children, pregnancy **C**, lactation, elderly

Pharmacokinetics

Absorption	Rapidly (IM) absorbed; completely (IV)
Distribution	Widely distributed
Metabolism	Liver
Excretion	Kidneys, unchanged; feces
Half-life	40 min

Pharmacodynamics

	IM/IV
Onset	15 min
Peak	Unknown
Duration	3-4 hr

Interactions

Drug/drug:

Individual drugs
Alcohol: ↑ CNS depression
Epinephrine: ↑ hypertension

Drug classifications
Analgesics, narcotics: ↑ CNS depression
Antihistamines: ↑ CNS depression
CNS depressants: ↑ CNS depression
Vasopressors: ↑ hypertension

NURSING CONSIDERATIONS

Assessment

- Monitor vital signs, B/P, I&O; check patients with cardiac disease more often; hypotension, hypertension, dysrhythmias may occur
- Observe for drowsiness; instruct patient not to drive, operate machinery if drowsiness occurs

Associated nursing diagnoses

✓ Fluid deficit (uses)
✓ Nutrition: Less than body requirements (uses)
✓ Knowledge deficit (teaching)

Implementation

IV **IV route**

- Give after reconstituting 50 mg of drug with 2.2 ml sterile water for inj to a concentration of 25 mg/ml, do not use NaCl; give direct **IV** 25 mg over 30-60 sec by Y-tube or 3-way stopcock; **IV** route may cause dysrhythmias
- Reduce dosage if patient is receiving pressor drugs
- Store inj before, after reconstitution in light-resistant, single-dose container

Y-site compatibility:
Foscarnet

Syringe compatibilities:
Atropine, droperidol/fentanyl, glycopyrrolate, hydroxyzine, ketamine, meperidine, midazolam, morphine, naloxone, pentazocine, propranolol, scopolamine

Syringe incompatibilities:
Chlordiazepoxide, diazepam, pentobarbital, phenobarbital, secobarbital, thiopental

IM route

- Give deep in large muscle mass, aspirate to prevent **IV** administration; deltoid is not preferred area

Patient/family education

- Instruct patient to rise slowly from sitting or recumbent position to minimize orthostatic hypotension; to ask for assistance when ambulating; drowsiness may occur
- Teach patient to use gum, hard candy, or frequent sips of water for dry mouth

Evaluation

Positive therapeutic outcome

- Absence of nausea, vomiting

Treatment of overdose:
Supportive care; atropine may be helpful

benztropine 🔑

(benz'troe-peen)
benztropine mesylate, Cogentin
Func. class.: Cholinergic blocker
Chem. class.: Tertiary amine
Pregnancy category **C**

Action: Blockade of central acetylcholine receptors in the CNS, neurotransmitters are balanced

B

Therapeutic Outcome: Decreased involuntary movements

Uses: Parkinsonian symptoms, extrapyramidal symptoms associated with neuroleptic drugs, acute dystonia

Dosage and routes

Drug-induced extrapyramidal symptoms

IV *Adult:* IM/**IV** 1-4 mg qd-bid; give PO dose as soon as possible; PO 1-2 mg bid/tid; increase by 0.5 mg q5-6 days

Parkinsonian symptoms

Adult: PO 0.5-1 mg qd; increased 0.5 mg q5-6 days titrated to patient response

Acute dystonic reactions

Adult: IM/**IV** 1-2 mg, may increase to 1-2 mg bid (PO)

Available forms: Tabs 0.5, 1, 2 mg; inj IM, **IV** 1 mg/ml

Side effects/adverse reactions

CNS: Confusion, anxiety, restlessness, irritability, delusions, hallucinations, headache, sedation, depression, incoherence, dizziness, memory loss
CV: Palpitations, tachycardia, hypotension, bradycardia
EENT: Blurred vision, photophobia, dilated pupils, difficulty swallowing, dry eyes, mydriasis, increased intraocular tension, angle closure glaucoma
GI: Dryness of mouth, constipation, nausea, vomiting, abdominal distress, ***paralytic ileus,*** epigastric distress
GU: Hesitancy, retention, dysuria
INTEG: Rash, urticaria, dermatoses
MISC: Increased temperature, flushing, decreased sweating, hyperthermia, heat stroke, numbness of fingers
MS: Muscular weakness, cramping

Contraindications: Hypersensitivity, narrow angle glaucoma, myasthenia gravis, P GI/GU obstruction, child <3 yr, peptic ulcer, megacolon, prostate hypertrophy

Precautions: Pregnancy **C**, G elderly, lactation, tachycardia, liver, kidney disease, drug abuse history, dysrhythmias, hypotension, hypertension, P psychiatric patients, children

Pharmacokinetics

Absorption	Well (PO, IM), completely (IV) absorbed
Distribution	Unknown
Metabolism	Unknown
Excretion	Unknown
Half-life	Unknown

Pharmacodynamics

	IM/IV	PO
Onset	15 min	1 hr
Peak	Unknown	Unknown
Duration	6-10 hr	6-10 hr

Interactions

Drug/drug:

Individual drugs

Amantadine: ↑ anticholinergic effects
Digoxin: ↑ levels of digoxin
Levodopa: ↓ levels of levodopa

Haloperidol: ↑ schizophrenic symptoms

Drug classifications

Antacids: ↓ absorption of benzotropine

Antidepressants, tricyclic: ↑ anticholinergic effects

Antihistamines: ↑ anticholinergic effects

Phenothiazines: ↑ anticholinergic effects

NURSING CONSIDERATIONS

Assessment

- Monitor I&O ratio; retention commonly causes decreased urinary output, distention, frequency, incontinence
- Assess for parkinsonism, extrapyramidal symptoms: shuffling gait, muscle rigidity, involuntary movements, pill rolling, muscle spasms, drooling before and during treatment
- Monitor for urinary hesitancy, retention; palpate bladder if retention occurs
- Monitor for constipation, cramping, pain in abdomen, abdominal distention; increase fluids, bulk, exercise if this occurs
- Assess for tolerance over long-term therapy; dosage may have to be increased or changed
- Assess for mental status: affect, mood, CNS depression, worsening of mental symptoms during early therapy

Associated nursing diagnoses

✓ Mobility, impaired (uses)
✓ Knowledge deficit (teaching)
✓ Noncompliance (teaching)

Implementation

PO route

- Give with or after meals to prevent GI upset; may give with fluids other than water; hard candy, frequent drinks, gum to relieve dry mouth
- Give hs to avoid daytime drowsiness in patient with parkinsonism
- Store at room temperature

IM route

- Give in large muscle mass for dystonic symptoms

IV **IV route**

- Give parenteral dose with patient recumbent to prevent postural hypotension; give undiluted 2 mg or less >1 min or more

Patient/family education

- Teach patient to use caution in hot weather; drug may increase susceptibility to stroke since perspiration is decreased; patient should remain indoors
- Advise patient not to discontinue this drug abruptly; to taper off over 1 wk; to prevent withdrawal symptoms (insomnia, involuntary movements, anxiety, tachycardias)
- Caution patient to avoid driving or other hazardous activities; drowsiness, dizziness may occur
- Teach patient to avoid OTC medication: cough, cold preparations with alcohol, antihistamines unless directed by prescriber; increased CNS depression may occur
- Advise patient to rise from sitting or recumbent position slowly to minimize orthostatic hypotension
- Teach patient to use gum, hard candy, frequent sips of

water to decrease dry mouth; if dry mouth continues, saliva substitutes may be prescribed
- Instruct patient that doses should not be doubled, but missed dose may be taken up to 2 hr before next dose

Evaluation

Positive therapeutic outcome
- Absence of involuntary movements (pill rolling, tremors, muscle spasms)

bepridil

(be'pri-dil)

Vascor

Func. class.: Calcium channel blocker, antianginal, antihypertensive

Chem. class.: Angina

Pregnancy category **C**

Action: Inhibits calcium ion influx across cell membrane during cardiac depolarization; produces relaxation of coronary vascular smooth muscle, peripheral vascular smooth muscle; dilates coronary vascular arteries; increases myocardial oxygen delivery in patients with vasospastic angina

Therapeutic Outcome: Decreased angina pectoris

Uses: Chronic stable angina, used alone or in combination with propranolol

Dosage and routes

Adult: 200-450 mg qd

Available forms: Tabs, film-coated, 200, 300, 400 mg

Side effects/adverse reactions

CNS: Headache, fatigue, drowsiness, dizziness, anxiety, depression, weakness, insomnia, confusion, lightheadedness, nervousness

CV: Dysrhythmia, edema, CHF, bradycardia, hypotension, palpitations, AV block

GI: Nausea, vomiting, diarrhea, gastric upset, constipation, increased levels in liver function studies

GU: Nocturia, polyuria

Contraindications: Sick sinus syndrome, 2nd- or 3rd-degree heart block, Wolff-Parkinson-White syndrome, hypotension less than 90 mm Hg systolic, cardiogenic shock, history of serious ventricular arrhythmias

Precautions: CHF, hypotension, hepatic injury, pregnancy P C, lactation, children, renal disease, IHSS, concomitant β-blocker therapy

Pharmacokinetics	
Absorption	Well absorbed (PO)
Distribution	Plasma protein bound (99%), crosses placenta
Metabolism	Liver
Excretion	Urine, feces
Half-life	42 hr

Pharmacodynamics	
Onset	Unknown
Peak	2-3 hr
Duration	Unknown

Interactions

Drug/drug:

Individual drugs

Fentanyl: ↑ hypotension
Digoxin: ↑ levels of digoxin

Drug classifications

β-Blockers: ↑ adverse reactions

Lab test interferences

Increase: Liver function tests, aminotransferase, CPK, LDH

NURSING CONSIDERATIONS

Assessment

- Assess fluid volume status: I&O ratio and record, weight, distended red veins, crackles in lung, color, quality, and sp gr of urine, skin turgor, adequacy of pulses, moist mucous membranes, bilateral lung sounds, peripheral pitting edema
- Assess cardiac status: B/P, pulse, respiration, ECG intervals (PR, QRS, QT), dysrhythmias
- Obtain digoxin levels if cardiac glycosides are given with bepridil

Associated nursing diagnoses

✓ Cardiac output, decreased (uses)
✓ Knowledge deficit (teaching)

Implementation

PO route

- Give once a day, with food for GI symptoms

Patient/family education

- Instruct patient to avoid hazardous activities until stabilized on drug and dizziness is no longer a problem
- Instruct patient to limit caffeine consumption; to avoid alcohol and OTC drugs unless directed by prescriber
- Advise patient to comply in all areas of medical regimen: diet, exercise, stress reduction, drug therapy; to notify prescriber of irregular heart beat, shortness of breath, swelling of feet and hands, pronounced dizziness, constipation, nausea, hypotension
- Teach patient to use as directed even if feeling better; may be taken with other cardiovascular drugs (nitrates, β-blockers)

Evaluation

Positive therapeutic outcome

- Decreased anginal pain

Treatment of overdose:

Defibrillation, atropine for AV block, vasopressor for hypotension

P beractant

(bear-ac'tant)
Survanta
Func. class.: Natural lung surfactant
Pregnancy category **N/A**

Action: Replenishes surfactant and restores surface activity to P the lungs in premature infants

➔ **Therapeutic Outcome:** Ability of neonate to breathe without assistance

Uses: Prevention and treatment (rescue) of respiratory

distress syndrome in premature infants

P

Dosage and routes

Intratracheal instill: 4 doses can be administered in the 1st 48 hr of life; give doses no more frequently than q6h; each dose is 100 mg of phospholipids/kg birth weight (4 ml/kg)

Available forms:

Susp 25 mg phospholipids/ml in 0.9% NaCl in single-use vials containing 8 ml susp

Side effects/adverse reactions

RESP: Pulmonary air leaks, pulmonary interstitial emphysema, apnea, pulmonary hemorrhage

SYST: Patent ductus arteriosus, intracranial hemorrhage, severe intracranial hemorrhage, necrotizing entercolitis, posttreatment sepsis, posttreatment infection, bradycardia, oxygen desaturation, pallor, vasoconstriction, hypotension, hypertension

Precautions:

Bradycardia, rales, infections

Pharmacokinetics

Absorption	Unknown
Distribution	Lung
Metabolism	Recycled
Excretion	Unknown
Half-life	Unknown

Pharmacodynamics

	INTRATRACHEAL INSTILL
Onset	Few min
Peak	Unknown
Duration	Becomes lung associated within hours of administration

Interactions:

None

NURSING CONSIDERATIONS

Assessment

- Assess respiratory rate, rhythm, character, chest expansion, color, transcutaneous saturation, ABGs; monitor ECG
- Check endotracheal tube placement before dosing; monitor for apnea after endotracheal administration
- Check for reflux of drug into the endotracheal tube during administration; stop drug administration if this occurs, and if needed increase peak inspiratory pressure on the ventilator by 4-5 cm H_2O until tube is cleared
- P Assess infant for repeat dosing using radiographic confirmation of respiratory distress syndrome; repeat doses should be given as noted above; ventilator settings for repeat doses FIO_2 are decreased by 0.2 or amount to prevent cyanosis; ventilator rate of 30/min; inspiratory time <1 sec; if infant's pretreatment rate was >30, leave unchanged during dosing; resume usual ventilator management after dosing

Associated nursing diagnoses

- ✓ Gas exchange, impaired (uses)
- ✓ Knowledge deficit (teaching)

Implementation

- Administer after suctioning; give by endotracheal administration only by persons trained in neonatal intubation and ventilation
- Use a no. 5 Fr end-hole catheter inserted into the endotracheal tube with the tip protruding just beyond the end of the endotracheal tube; shorten the catheter before insertion; do not insert the drug into the mainstem bronchus
- Divide each dose into quarters and administer with infant in different positions
- Determine the dosing by weight of infant; slowly withdraw the contents into the plastic syringe through a 20-G needle; do not filter or shake; attach the premeasured no. 5 Fr catheter to syringe; fill with drug and discard excess through the catheter so only dose to be given remains in syringe
- For **prevention dosing,** stabilize, weigh, and intubate the infant; give drug within 15 min of birth if possible; position infant and inj first quarter dose through catheter over 2-3 sec; remove catheter and manually ventilate with O_2 to prevent cyanosis (60 bpm) and sufficient positive pressure to promote adequate air exchange and chest wall excursion
- For **rescue dosing,** give drug as soon as infant is placed on ventilator after birth; immediately before administering dose, change ventilator settings to 60/min, inspiratory time 0.5 sec, FIO_2 l; position infant and inj first quarter through catheter over 2-3 sec; remove catheter; return to mechanical ventilator
- Ventilate infant for >30 sec or until stable after prevention or rescue strategy; reposition for next dose; same procedure for subsequent dosing; do not suction for at least 1 hr after dosing unless airway obstruction is evident; resume ventilator therapy after dosing
- Reduce peak ventilator inspiratory pressures immediately if chest expansion improves substantially after dose
- Reduce in FIO_2 in small, repeated steps when infant becomes pink and transcutaneous oxygen saturation is in excess of 95%; oxygen saturation should remain between 90% and 95%
- Suction all infants before administration to prevent mucus plugging; if endotracheal tube obstruction is suspected, remove the obstruction and replace tube immediately
- Store in refrigerator; protect from light, warm to room temp for >20 min or warm in hand 8 min before giving; do not use artificial warming methods; enter a vial only once; unopened, unused vials that have been warmed to room temp may be rerefrigerated within 8 hr of warming; do not warm and return to refrigerator more than once

Patient/family education

- Explain disease process and purpose of medication to parents; communicate neonate's progress

Evaluation

Positive therapeutic outcome
- Significant improvement in respiratory status (oxygenation, arterial blood gases WNL)

betamethasone/ betamethasone sodium phosphate/ betamethasone disodium phosphate/ betamethasone acetate/ betamethasone sodium phosphate

(bay-ta-meth'a-sone)

Beclovent, Beconase AQ Nasal, Beconase Inhalaton ✱, Benisone, Betaderm ✱, betamethasone dipropionate, betamethasone valerate, Betatrex, Beta-Val, Betnelan, Celestone/ Alphatrex, Celestone Phosphate, Cel-U-Jec, Diprolene AF/ betamethasone sodium phosphate, Diprosone, Maxivate, Selestoject, Teladar/Diprolene, Uticort, Valisone, Valisone Reduced Strength, Vancenase AQ Nasal, Vancenase Nasal Beta Cort, Vanceril

Func. class.: Corticosteroid, synthetic

Chem. class.: Glucocorticoid, long acting

Pregnancy category **C**

Action: Decreases inflammation by suppression of migration of polymorphonuclear leukocytes, fibroblasts, reversal of increased capillary permeability and lysosomal stabilization

➔ **Therapeutic Outcome:** Decreased inflammation and normal immunity

Uses: Immunosuppression, severe inflammation, prevention of neonatal respiratory distress syndrome (by administration to mother), chronic asthma, rhinitis (inh); psoriasis, eczema, contact dermatitis, pruritus (TOP)

Dosage and routes

Adult: PO 0.6-7.2 mg qd; IM/**IV** 0.6-7.2 mg qd in joint or soft tissue (sodium phosphate)

Pregnant adult: IM 12 mg 36-48 hr, before premature delivery, then same dose in 24 hr (betamethasone acetate)

P *Adult and child:* Apply to affected area qid; (top)

Adult: Inh 2-4 puffs tid-qid; not to exceed 20 inh/day

P *Child: 6-12 yr:* Inh 1-2 puffs tid-qid; not to exceed 10 inh/day

P *Adult and child >12 yr:* Instill 1-2 sprays in each nostril bid-qid

Available forms: Tabs 0.6 mg; syr 0.6 mg/5 ml; inj 3, 4 mg/ml; oint 0.025%, 0.1%; cream 0.025%, 0.01%, 0.1%; lotion 0.025%, 0.1%; gel 0.025%; aero 42 μg/spray

Side effects/adverse reactions

CNS: *Depression, flushing, sweating,* headache, ecchymosis, bruising, mood changes
CV: *Hypertension,* ***circulatory collapse, thrombophlebitis, embolism,*** tachycardia, ***necrotizing angiitis, CHF***
EENT: Fungal infections, increased intraocular pressure, blurred vision
GI: *Diarrhea, nausea, abdominal distention,* ***GI hemorrhage, increased appetite, pancreatitis***
HEMA: ***Thrombocytopenia***
INTEG: *Acne, poor wound healing, ecchymosis, bruising,* petechiae
MS: Fractures, osteoporosis, weakness

Contraindications:
Psychosis, hypersensitivity, idiopathic thrombocytopenia, acute glomerulonephritis, amebiasis, fungal infections, nonasthmatic bronchial disease, P child <2 yr, AIDS, TB

Precautions:
Pregnancy **C**, diabetes mellitus, glaucoma, osteoporosis, seizure disorders, ulcerative colitis, CHF, myasthenia gravis, renal disease, esophagitis, peptic ulcer

Pharmacokinetics

Absorption	Well absorbed (PO); systemic (top)
Distribution	Crosses placenta
Metabolism	Liver, extensively
Excretion	Kidney, breast milk
Half-life	3-5 hr, adrenal suppression 3-4 days

Pharmacodynamics

	PO	IM	IV	TOP
Onset	1-2 hr	Unknown	Rapid	Unknown
Peak	2 hr	4-8 hr	4-8 hr	Unknown
Duration	3 days	1-1½ days	1-1½ days	Unknown

Interactions
Drug/drug:
Individual drugs
Amphotericin B: ↑ hypokalemia
Insulin: ↑ need for insulin
Mezlocillin: ↑ hypokalemia
Phenytoin: ↓ action, ↑ metabolism
Rifampin: ↓ action, ↑ metabolism
Ticarcillin: ↑ hypokalemia
Drug classifications
Barbiturates: ↓ action, ↑ metabolism
Diuretics: ↑ hypokalemia
Hypoglycemic agents: ↑ need for hypoglycemic agents

Lab test interferences
Increase: Cholesterol, sodium, blood glucose, uric acid, calcium, urine glucose
Decrease: Calcium, potassium, T_4, T_3, thyroid ^{131}I uptake test, urine 17-OHCS, 17-KS, PBI
False negative: Skin allergy tests

NURSING CONSIDERATIONS
Assessment
Systemic route
- Monitor potassium, blood sugar, urine glucose while on long-term therapy; hypokalemia and hyperglycemia; check weight daily; notify prescriber of weekly gain >5 lb

• Monitor B/P q4h, pulse; notify prescriber if chest pain occurs
• Monitor I&O ratio; be alert for decreasing urinary output and increasing edema
• Check plasma cortisol levels during long-term therapy (normal level: 138-635 nmol/L [SI units] when drawn at 8 AM); adrenal function periodically for HPA axis suppression
• Assess for symptoms of infection: increase temperature, WBC even after withdrawal of medication; drug masks infection symptoms
• Assess for symptoms of potassium depletion: paresthesias, fatigue, nausea, vomiting, depression, polyuria, dysrhythmias, weakness
• Monitor for edema, hypertension, cardiac symptoms
• Assess for mental status: affect, mood, behavioral changes, aggression

Top route
• Check temperature; if fever develops, drug should be discontinued
• Assess for systemic absorption: increased temperature, inflammation, irritation

Associated nursing diagnoses

✓ Infection, risk for (adverse reactions)
✓ Knowledge deficit (teaching)
✓ Noncompliance (teaching)

Implementation

IV **IV route**
• Give **IV** (only sodium phosphate product); give over >1 min; may be given by **IV** inf in compatible sol after shaking susp (parenteral)
• Give titrated dose; use lowest effective dose

Y-site compatibilities:

Heparin, hydrocortisone sodium succinate, potassium chloride

IM route
• Give IM injection deep in large mass, rotate sites, avoid deltoid, use 21-G needle; in one dose in AM to prevent adrenal suppression; avoid SC administration; may damage tissue

PO route
• Give with food or milk to decrease GI symptoms

Inh route
• Give inh with water to decrease possibility of fungal infections; titrated dose; use lowest effective dose
• Use after cleaning aerosol top daily with warm water; dry thoroughly
• Store in cool environment; do not puncture or incinerate container

Top route
• Apply only to affected areas; do not get in eyes; apply medication, then cover with occlusive dressing (only if prescribed), seal to normal skin, change q12h; syst absorption may occur
• Apply only to dermatoses; do not use on weeping, denuded, or infected area
• Cleanse before applying drug; use treatment for a few days after area has cleared
• Store at room temperature

Patient/family education

Syst route

- Advise patient that long-term therapy may be needed to clear infection (1-2 mo depending on type of infection); that ID as steroid user should be carried; dosage adjustment may be needed
- Instruct patient to notify prescriber if therapeutic response decreases; caution patient not to discontinue abruptly; adrenal crisis can result
- Instruct patient to avoid OTC products: salicylates, alcohol in cough products, cold preparations unless directed by prescriber
- Teach patient all aspects of drug usage including cushingoid symptoms
- Teach patient symptoms of adrenal insufficiency: nausea, anorexia, fatigue, dizziness, dyspnea, weakness, joint pain

Top route

- Caution patient to avoid sunlight on affected area; burns may occur

Evaluation

Positive therapeutic outcome

- Ease of respirations, decreased inflammation (systemic)
- Absence of severe itching, patches on skin, flaking (top)

bethanechol ⚷

(be-than′e-kol)

bethanechol chloride, Duvoid, Myotonachol, Urecholine

Func. class.: Cholinergic stimulant

Chem. class.: Synthetic choline ester

Pregnancy category **C**

Action: Stimulates muscarinic acetylcholine receptors directly; mimics effects of parasympathetic nervous system stimulation; stimulates gastric motility, micturition

➔ **Therapeutic Outcome:** Absence of continued urinary retention

Uses: Urinary retention (postoperative, postpartum), neurogenic atony of bladder with retention

Dosage and routes

Test dose

Adult: SC 2.5 mg repeated 15-30 min intervals × 4 doses to determine effective dose

Adult: PO 10-50 mg bid-qid; SC 2.5-10 mg tid-qid prn

Available forms: Tabs 5, 10, 25, 50 mg; inj SC 5 mg/ml

Side effects/adverse reactions:

CNS: Dizziness

CV: Hypotension, bradycardia, orthostatic hypotension, reflex tachycardia, ***cardiac arrest, circulatory collapse***

EENT: Miosis, increased salivation, lacrimation, blurred vision
GI: Nausea, bloody diarrhea, belching, vomiting, cramps, fecal incontinence
GU: Urgency
INTEG: Rash, urticaria, flushing, increased sweating
RESP:* *Acute asthma, dyspnea

Contraindications: Hypersensitivity, severe bradycardia, asthma, severe hypotension, hyperthyroidism, peptic ulcer, parkinsonism, seizure disorders, CAD, coronary occlusion, mechanical obstruction, peritonitis, recent urinary or GI surgery

Precautions: Hypertension, P pregnancy **C**, lactation, child <8 yr, urinary retention

Pharmacokinetics

Absorption	Poorly absorbed (PO); well absorbed (SC)
Distribution	Does not cross blood-brain barrier
Metabolism	Unknown
Excretion	Kidneys
Half-life	Unknown

Pharmacodynamics

	PO	SC
Onset	30-90 min	5-15 min
Peak	1 hr	15-30 min
Duration	1-6 hr	2 hr

Interactions

Drug/drug:

Individual drugs
Procainamide: ↓ action of bethanechol
Quinidine: ↓ action of bethanechol

Drug classifications
Cholinergics: ↑ action of bethanechol
Ganglionic blockers: ↑ hypotension

Lab test interferences

Increase: AST (SGOT), lipase/amylase, bilirubin

NURSING CONSIDERATIONS

Assessment

- Monitor B/P, pulse, respirations; observe after parenteral dose for 1 hr
- Check I&O ratio; check for urinary retention or incontinence; if bladder emptying does not occur, notify prescriber; catheterization may be needed
- Assess for bradycardia, hypotension, bronchospasm, headache, dizziness, convulsions, sweating, cramping, respiratory depression; drug should be discontinued if toxicity occurs; atropine administration

Associated nursing diagnoses

- ✓ Urinary elimination, altered patterns (uses)
- ✓ Injury, risk for (adverse reactions)
- ✓ Knowledge deficit (teaching)

Implementation

SC route

- Give parenteral dose by SC route; use of IM, **IV** may result in cardiac arrest or cholinergic crisis (diarrhea with blood, cramping, hypotension, circulatory collapse)
- Administer only with atropine sulfate available for cho-

linergic crisis; give only after all other cholinergics have been discontinued
• Do not use sol with a precipitate, or if discolored

PO route
• Give increased doses if tolerance occurs as prescribed
• To avoid nausea and vomiting, take on an empty stomach; 1 hr ac or 2 hr pc
• Store at room temperature

Patient/family education
• Instruct patient to take drug exactly as prescribed; do not double doses; if dose is missed take within 1 hr of scheduled dose
• Caution patient to make position changes slowly; orthostatic hypotension may occur
• Instruct patient to report cramping, diarrhea with blood, flushing to prescriber

Evaluation
Positive therapeutic outcome
• Absence of urinary retention
• Absence of abdominal distention

Treatment of overdose: Administer atropine 0.6-1.2 mg **IV** or IM (adult)

biperiden
(bye-per'i-den)
Akineton
Func. class.: Cholinergic blocker, antiparkinsonian agent
Pregnancy category **C**

Action: Centrally acting competitive anticholinergic; blocks cholinergic responses in the CNS

Therapeutic Outcome: Decreased involuntary movements

Uses: Parkinsonian symptoms, extrapyramidal symptoms secondary to neuroleptic drug therapy

Dosage and routes
Extrapyramidal symptoms
Adult: PO 2 mg qd-tid; IM/**IV** 2 mg q30 min, if needed, not to exceed 8 mg/24 hr

Parkinsonian symptoms
Adult: PO 2 mg tid-qid; max 16 mg/24 hr

Available forms: Tabs 2 mg; inj IM/**IV** 5 mg/ml (lactate)

Side effects/adverse reactions
CNS: Confusion, anxiety, restlessness, irritability, delusions, hallucinations, headache, sedation, depression, incoherence, dizziness, euphoria, tremors, memory loss
CV: Palpitations, tachycardia, postural hypotension, bradycardia
EENT: Blurred vision, photophobia, dilated pupils, difficulty swallowing, mydriasis, increased intraocular tension, angle closure glaucoma
GI: Dryness of mouth, constipation, nausea, vomiting, abdominal distress, ***paralytic ileus***
GU: Hesitancy, retention, dysuria

INTEG: Rash, urticaria, dermatoses
MISC: Increased temperature, flushing, decreased sweating, hyperthermia, heat stroke, numbness of fingers
MS: Weakness, cramping

Contraindications: Hypersensitivity, narrow angle glaucoma, myasthenia gravis, GI/GU obstruction, megacolon, stenosing peptic ulcers, prostatic hypertrophy

Precautions: Pregnancy **C**, G elderly, lactation, tachycardia, dysrhythmias, liver, kidney disease, drug abuse, hypotension, hypertension, psychiatric P patients, children

Pharmacokinetics

Absorption	Well absorbed (PO, IM)
Distribution	Unknown
Metabolism	Unknown
Excretion	Unknown
Half-life	18-24 hr

Pharmacodynamics

	IM/IV	PO
Onset	15 min	1 hr
Peak	Unknown	Unknown
Duration	6-10 hr	6-10 hr

Interactions

Drug/drug:

Individual drugs
Amantadine: ↑ anticholinergic effects
Digoxin: ↑ levels of digoxin
Levodopa: ↓ levels of levodopa
Haloperidol: ↑ schizophrenic symptoms

Drug classifications
Antidepressants, tricyclic: ↑ anticholinergic effects
Antihistamines: ↑ anticholinergic effects
Phenothiazines: ↑ anticholinergic effects

NURSING CONSIDERATIONS

Assessment

- Monitor I&O ratio; retention commonly causes decreased urinary output, distention, frequency, incontinence
- Assess for parkinsonism, extrapyramidal symptoms: shuffling gait, muscle rigidity, involuntary movements, pill rolling, muscle spasms, drooling before and during treatment
- Monitor for urinary hesitancy, retention; palpate bladder if retention occurs
- Monitor for constipation, cramping, pain in abdomen, abdominal distention; increase fluids, bulk, exercise if this occurs
- Assess for tolerance over long-term therapy; dosage may have to be increased or changed
- Assess for mental status: affect, mood, CNS depression, worsening of mental symptoms during early therapy

Associated nursing diagnoses

✓ Mobility, impaired (uses)
✓ Knowledge deficit (teaching)

Implementation

PO route

- Give with food or pc to prevent GI upset; may give

with fluids other than water; hard candy, frequent drinks, gum to relieve dry mouth
- Give hs to avoid daytime drowsiness in patients with parkinsonism
- Store at room temp

IV **IV route**
- Give parenteral dose with patient recumbent to prevent postural hypotension; give undiluted 2 mg or less over 1 min or more

Patient/family education
- Teach patient to use caution in hot weather; drug may increase susceptibility to stroke since perspiration is decreased; patient should remain indoors
- Teach patient not to discontinue this drug abruptly; to taper off over 1 wk to prevent withdrawal symptoms (insomnia, involuntary movements, anxiety, tachycardias)
- Teach patient to avoid driving or other hazardous activities; drowsiness, dizziness may occur
- Teach patient to avoid OTC medication: cough, cold preparations with alcohol, antihistamines unless directed by prescriber; increased CNS depression may occur
- Caution patient to rise from sitting or recumbent position slowly to minimize orthostatic hypotension
- Teach patient to use gum, hard candy, frequent sips of water to decrease dry mouth; if dry mouth continues, saliva substitutes may be prescribed
- Instruct patient that doses should not be doubled, but missed dose may be taken up to 2 hr before next dose

Evaluation
Positive therapeutic outcome
- Absence of involuntary movements (pill rolling, tremors, muscle spasms)

bisacodyl
(bis-a-koe'dill)
Apo-Bisacodyl ✤, bisacodyl, Bisacodyl Uniserts, Bisco-Lax, Dulcagen, Dulcolax, Fleet Bisacodyl
Func. class.: Laxative, stimulant
Chem. class.: Diphenylmethane
Pregnancy category C

Action: Acts directly on intestine by increasing motor activity; thought to irritate colonic intramural plexus; increases water in the colon

➔ **Therapeutic Outcome:** Decreased constipation

Uses: Short-term treatment of constipation, bowel or rectal preparation for surgery, examination

Dosage and routes
Adult: PO 10-15 mg in PM or AM; may use up to 30 mg for bowel or rec preparation; rec 10 mg; enema 1.25 oz
P ***Child <2 yr:*** Rec 5 mg
P ***Child >6 yr:*** PO 5-10 mg
P ***Child >12 yr:*** Rec 10 mg

Available forms: Enteric coated tabs 5 mg; rec supp 5, 10 mg

Side effects/adverse reactions

CNS: Muscle weakness
GI: *Nausea, vomiting, anorexia, cramps,* diarrhea, rectal burning (supp)
META: Protein-losing enteropathy, alkalosis, hypokalemia, ***tetany,*** electrolyte and fluid imbalances

Contraindications: Hypersensitivity, rectal fissures, abdominal pain, nausea, vomiting, appendicitis, acute surgical abdomen, ulcerated hemorrhoids, acute hepatitis, fecal impaction, intestinal/biliary tract obstruction

Precautions: Pregnancy **C**

Pharmacokinetics

Absorption	Poor
Distribution	Unknown
Metabolism	Liver, minimally
Excretion	Kidneys
Half-life	Unknown

Pharmacodynamics

	PO	REC
Onset	6-10 hr	15-60 min
Peak	Unknown	Unknown
Duration	Unknown	Unknown

Interactions
Drug/drug:

Drug classifications
Antacids: ↓ of enteric coating of drugs
H_2-blockers: ↑ gastric irritation

NURSING CONSIDERATIONS
Assessment

- Monitor blood, urine electrolytes if used often by patient; check I&O ratio to identify fluid loss
- Assess cramping, rectal bleeding, nausea, vomiting; if these symptoms occur, drug should be discontinued; identify cause of constipation; identify whether fluids, bulk, or exercise missing from lifestyle

Associated nursing diagnoses

- ✓ Constipation (uses)
- ✓ Diarrhea (side effects)
- ✓ Knowledge deficit (teaching)
- ✓ Noncompliance (teaching)

Implementation

PO route
- Give alone with water only for better absorption; do not take within 1 hr of antacids, milk
- Administer in AM or PM (oral dose)

Rectal route
- Lubricate before insertion, patient should retain for ½ hr

Patient/family education

- Discuss with the patient that adequate fluid and bulk consumption is necessary
- Advise patient that normal bowel movements do not always occur daily
- Teach patient not to use in presence of abdominal pain, nausea, vomiting; tell patient to notify prescriber if constipation unrelieved or if symptoms of electrolyte imbalance occur: muscle cramps, pain, weakness, dizziness, excessive thirst

Evaluation

Positive therapeutic outcome
- Decreased constipation within 3 days

bismuth subsalicylate

(bis'meth sub-sa-li'si-late)

Bismtrol, Pepto-Bismol, Pepto-Bismol Maximum Strength, Pink Bismuth

Func. class.: Antidiarrheal

Chem. class.: Salicylate

Pregnancy category **C**

Action: Inhibits prostaglandin synthesis responsible for GI hypermotility; stimulates absorption of fluid and electrolytes; antimicrobial, antisecretory effects

➡ **Therapeutic Outcome:** Absence of loose, watery stools

Uses: Diarrhea (cause undetermined); prevention of diarrhea when traveling

Dosage and routes

Adult: PO 30 ml or 2 tabs q30-60 min, not to exceed 8 doses for >2 days

P *Child 10-14 yr:* PO 15 ml

Available forms: Chewable tabs 262 mg; susp 262 mg/15 ml, 524 mg/15 ml

Side effects/adverse reactions

CNS: Confusion, twitching
EENT: Hearing loss, tinnitus, metallic taste, blue gums
GI: Increased fecal impaction (high doses), dark stools, constipation
HEMA: Increased bleeding time

P **Contraindications:** Child <3 yr; impaction, children, teens with flulike symptoms, hypersensitivity (aspirin)

Precautions: Anticoagulant G therapy, pregnancy **C**, elderly, lactation, gout, diabetes mellitus

Pharmacokinetics

Absorption	Salicylate >90%
Distribution	None
Metabolism	None
Excretion	Feces (unchanged)
Half-life	Unknown

Pharmacodynamics

	PO
Onset	1 hr
Peak	2 hr
Duration	4 hr

Interactions

Drug/drug:

Individual drugs

Aminosalicylic acid: ↑ side effects, ↑ toxicity
Aspirin: ↑ salicylate levels
Tetracycline: ↓ absorption

Drug classifications

Anticoagulants, oral: ↓ effect of anticoagulants

Lab test interferences

Interfere: Radiographic studies of GI system

NURSING CONSIDERATIONS

Assessment

- Monitor skin turgor; dehydration may occur in severe diarrhea; monitor electrolytes (potassium, sodium, chloride) if diarrhea is severe or continues long term
- Assess bowel pattern (frequency, consistency, shape,

volume, color) before drug therapy, after treatment; check weight, bowel sounds; identify factors contributing to diarrhea (bacteria, diet, medications, tube feedings)

Associated nursing diagnoses

- ✓ Diarrhea (uses)
- ✓ Constipation (adverse reactions)
- ✓ Knowledge deficit (teaching)

Implementation

PO route

• Shake susp before use; chewable tabs should not be swallowed whole

Patient/family education

• Teach patient to stop use if symptoms do not improve within 2 days or become worse, or if diarrhea is accompanied by high fever

• Teach patient to increase fluids for rehydration

• Tell patient to chew or dissolve chewable tabs in mouth; do not swallow whole; shake susp before using

• Tell patient to avoid other salicylates unless directed by prescriber; not to give to P children because of possibility of Reye's syndrome

• Tell patient that stools may turn gray; tongue may darken; impaction may occur in debilitated patients

Evaluation

Positive therapeutic outcome

• Decreased diarrhea

bisoprolol

(biss-op-proe'lol)

Zebeta

Func. class.: Antihypertensive

Chem. class.: β_1-blocker (selective)

Pregnancy category **B**

Action: Preferentially and competitively blocks stimulation of β_1-adrenergic receptor within cardiac muscle; produces negative chronotropic and inotropic activity (decreases rate of SA node discharge, increases recovery time), slows conduction of AV node, decreases heart rate, which decreases O_2 consumption in myocardium; decreases renin-aldosterone-angiotensin system; inhibits β_2-receptors in bronchial and vascular smooth muscle at high doses

➔ **Therapeutic Outcome:** Decreased B/P, heart rate

Uses: Mild to moderate hypertension

Investigational uses: Angina pectoris

Dosage and routes

Hypertension

Adult: PO 2.5-5 mg qd; may increase if necessary to 20 mg once daily; may need to reduce dose in presence of renal or hepatic impairment

Available forms: Tabs 5, 10 mg

Side effects/adverse reactions

CNS: Vertigo, headache, insomnia, fatigue, dizziness, mental changes, memory loss, hallucinations, depression, lethargy, drowsiness, strange dreams, catatonia, peripheral neuropathy
CV: ***Ventricular dysrhythmias, profound hypotension, bradycardia, CHF,*** cold extremities, postural hypotension, 2nd- or 3rd-degree heart block
EENT: Sore throat, dry burning eyes
ENDO: Increased hypoglycemic response to insulin
GI: Nausea, diarrhea, vomiting, mesenteric arterial thrombosis, ischemic colitis, flatulence, gastritis, gastric pain
GU: Impotence, decreased libido
HEMA: ***Agranulocytosis, thrombocytopenia,*** purpura, ***eosinophilia***
INTEG: Rash, fever, alopecia, pruritus, sweating
MISC: Facial swelling, weight gain, decreased exercise tolerance
MS: Joint pain, arthralgia
RESP: ***Bronchospasm,*** dyspnea, wheezing, cough, nasal stuffiness

Contraindications: Hypersensitivity to β-blockers, cardiogenic shock, heart block (2nd, 3rd degree), sinus bradycardia, CHF, cardiac failure

Precautions: Major surgery, P pregnancy **B**, lactation, children, diabetes mellitus, renal or hepatic disease, thyroid disease, COPD, asthma, well-compensated heart failure, aortic or mitral valve disease, peripheral vascular disease, myasthenia gravis

Pharmacokinetics

	PO
Absorption	Well absorbed
Distribution	Unknown; protein binding (30%)
Metabolism	Liver, inactive metabolites
Excretion	Urine, unchanged (50%)
Half-life	9-12 hr

Pharmacodynamics

Onset	Unknown
Peak	2-4 hr
Duration	24 hr

Interactions

Drug/drug:

Individual drugs

Alcohol: (large amounts) ↑ hypotension
Clonidine: Fatal reactions after discontinuing clonidine
Epinephrine: ↑ hypertension, then bradycardia
Flecainide: ↑ effects of both drugs
Haloperidol: ↑ effects of both drugs
Hydralazine: ↑ hypotension, bradycardia
Lidocaine: ↑ lidocaine toxicity
Quinidine: ↑ hypotension, bradycardia
Prazosin: ↑ hypotension, bradycardia
Theophylline: ↓ bronchodilatation

Drug classifications

Barbiturates: ↓ antihypertensive effects

Calcium channel blockers: ↑ hypotension
Contraceptives, oral: ↑ hypotension
Diuretics, loop: ↑ CV effects
MAOI: ↑ bradycardia
Penicillins: ↓ antihypertensive effects
Salicylates: ↓ antihypertensive effects
Sulfonylureas: ↓ hypoglycemic effect

Lab test interferences

Increase: AST (SGOT) and ALT (SGPT)
Interference: Glucose/insulin tolerance tests

NURSING CONSIDERATIONS

Assessment

- Monitor B/P during beginning treatment, periodically thereafter; pulse q4h: note rate, rhythm, quality; apical/radial pulse before administration; notify prescriber of any significant changes (pulse <50 bpm)
- Check for baselines in renal, liver function tests before therapy begins
- Assess for edema in feet, legs daily, monitor I&O, daily weight; check for jugular vein distention, rales bilaterally, dyspnea (CHF)
- Monitor skin turgor, dryness of mucous membranes for hydration status, especially G elderly

Associated nursing diagnoses

- ✓ Cardiac output, decreased (uses)
- ✓ Injury, risk for (side effects)
- ✓ Knowledge deficit (teaching)
- ✓ Noncompliance (teaching)

Implementation

PO route

- Give qd; give with food to prevent GI upset
- Store protected from light, moisture; place in cool environment

Patient/family education

- Teach patient not to discontinue drug abruptly; taper over 2 wk; may cause precipitate dysrhythmias if stopped abruptly
- Teach patient not to use OTC products containing α-adrenergic stimulants (such as nasal decongestants, cold preparations); to avoid alcohol, smoking and to limit sodium intake as prescribed
- Teach patient how to take pulse and B/P at home; advise when to notify prescriber
- Instruct patient to comply with weight control, dietary adjustments, modified exercise program
- Tell patient to carry/wear Medic Alert ID to identify drug being taken, allergies; tell patient drug controls symptoms but does not cure
- Caution patient to avoid hazardous activities if dizziness, drowsiness present
- Teach patient to take drug as prescribed, not to double doses, skip doses; take any missed doses as soon as remembered if at least 8 hr until next dose

Evaluation

Positive therapeutic outcome

- Decreased B/P in hypertension (after 1-2 wk)

Treatment of overdose: Lavage, **IV** atropine for bradycardia, **IV** theophylline for bronchospasm, digitalis, O_2, diuretic for cardiac failure, hemodialysis, **IV** glucose for hyperglycemia, **IV** diazepam (or phenytoin) for seizures

bitolterol

(bye-tol'te-role)

Tornalate

Func. class.: β_2-Adrenergic agonist; bronchodilator

Chem. class.: Acid ester of colterol

Pregnancy category **C**

Action: Causes bronchodilatation by action on β_2-receptors with increased synthesis of cyclic AMP; relaxes bronchial smooth muscle; inhibits mast cell degranulation; stimulates cilia to remove secretions with very little effect on heart rate

Therapeutic Outcome: Ability to breathe without difficulty

Uses: Asthma, bronchospasm

Dosage and routes

Inhaler

P ***Adult and child >12 yr:*** Inh 2 puffs; wait 1-3 min before 3rd puff if needed; not to exceed 3 inh q6h or 2 inh q4h

Nebulization

P ***Adult/child >12 yr:*** Inh 0.5 ml (1 mg) tid by intermittent flow or 1.25 mg tid by continuous flow

Available forms: Aerosol 0.37 mg/actuation, 0.2% neb sol

Side effects/adverse reactions

CNS: Tremors, anxiety, insomnia, headache, dizziness, stimulation, restlessness, hallucinations

CV: Palpitations, tachycardia, hypertension, angina, hypotension

EENT: Dry nose, irritation of nose and throat

GI: Heartburn, nausea, vomiting, anorexia

MS: Muscle cramps

RESP: ***Bronchospasm,*** dyspnea

Contraindications: Hypersensitivity to sympathomimetics

Precautions: Lactation, pregnancy **C**, cardiac disorders, hyperthyroidism, diabetes mellitus

Pharmacokinetics

Absorption	Unknown
Distribution	Unknown
Metabolism	Lungs to active metabolite
Excretion	Unknown
Half-life	Unknown

Pharmacodynamics

	INH
Onset	3-4 min
Peak	½-1 hr
Duration	5-8 hr

Interactions

Drug/drug:

Drug classifications

β-Adrenergic blockers: Block therapeutic effect
Bronchodilators, aerosol: ↑ action of bronchodilator
MAOI: ↑ chance of hypertensive crisis
Sympathomimetics: ↑ adrenergic side effects

NURSING CONSIDERATIONS

Assessment

- Monitor respiratory function: vital capacity, FEV, ABGs, lung sounds, heart rate, rhythm (baseline)
- Determine client's ability to self-medicate
- Monitor for evidence of allergic reactions; paradoxic bronchospasm; withhold dose; notify prescriber

Associated nursing diagnoses

☑ Impaired gas exchange (uses)
☑ Airway clearance, ineffective (uses)
☑ Knowledge deficit (teaching)

Implementation

Aerosol route

- Give after shaking, exhale, place mouthpiece in mouth, inhale slowly, hold breath, remove, exhale slowly; allow at least 1 min between inh
- Store in light-resistant container; do not expose to temp over 86° F (30° C)

Patient/family education

- Tell patient not to use OTC medications; extra stimulation may occur; to use this medication before other medications and allow at least 5 min between each; to prevent overstimulation
- Teach patient use of inhaler; review package insert with patient; to avoid getting aerosol in eyes; blurring may result; to wash inhaler in warm water daily and dry well; to avoid smoking, smoke-filled rooms, persons with respiratory tract infections
- Teach patient that paradoxic bronchospasm may occur and to stop drug immediately and notify prescriber; to limit caffeine products such as chocolate, coffee, tea, and colas
- Instruct patient on administration of dose; not to use more than prescribed; serious side effects may occur; if taking regularly and dose is missed, take when remembered; space other doses on new time schedule

Evaluation

Positive therapeutic outcome

- Absence of dyspnea, wheezing after 1 hr
- Improved airway exchange
- Improved ABGs

Treatment of overdose:

Administer a β_2-adrenergic blocker

bleomycin

(blee-oh-mye'sin)

Blenoxane

Func. class.: Antineoplastic, antibiotic

Chem. class.: Glycopeptide

Pregnancy category **D**

Action: Inhibits synthesis of DNA, RNA, protein; derived from *Streptomyces verticillus;* replication is decreased by binding to DNA, which causes strand splitting; phase specific in the G_2 and M phases; a nonvesicant

Therapeutic Outcome: Prevention of rapidly growing malignant cells

Uses: Cancer of head, neck, penis, cervix, vulva of squamous cell origin, Hodgkin's disease, lymphosarcoma, reticulum cell sarcoma, testicular carcinoma

Dosage and routes

Adult: SC/**IV**/IM 0.25-0.5 U/kg q1-2 wk or 10-20 U/m^2; then 1 U/day or 5 U/wk; may also be given intraarterially; do not exceed total dose, 400 U in lifetime

Available forms: Inj **IV**, SC, IM, IA, intralesional, intracavity 5 U

Side effects/adverse reactions

CNS: Fever, chills

CV: Hypotension, peripheral vasoconstriction

GI: Nausea, vomiting, anorexia, stomatitis, weight loss

HEMA: Hypotension, peripheral vasoconstriction

INTEG: Rash, hyperkeratosis, nail changes, alopecia, fever and chills

RESP: ***Fibrosis,*** pneumonitis, wheezing, ***pulmonary toxicity***

SYST: ***Anaphylaxis***

IDIOSYNCRATIC REACTION: Hypotension, confusion, fever, chills, wheezing

Contraindications: Hypersensitivity

Precautions: Renal, hepatic, respiratory disease, pregnancy **D**

Pharmacokinetics

Absorption	Well absorbed (IM, SC, intrapleural, intraperitoneal)
Distribution	Widely distributed
Metabolism	Liver, 30%
Excretion	Kidneys, unchanged (50%)
Half-life	2 hr; ↑ in renal disease

Pharmacodynamics

	SC/IM/IV
Onset	Unknown
Peak	Unknown
Duration	Unknown

Interactions

Drug/drug:

Individual drugs

Radiation: ↑ toxicity, bone marrow suppression

Drug classifications

Antineoplastics: ↑ toxicity, bone marrow suppression

B

NURSING CONSIDERATIONS

Assessment

- Assess buccal cavity q8h for dryness, sores or ulceration, white patches, oral pain, bleeding, dysphagia; obtain prescription for viscous lidocaine (Xylocaine)
- Assess symptoms indicating severe allergic reaction: rash, pruritus, urticaria, purpuric skin lesions, itching, flushing
- Monitor CBC, differential, platelet count weekly; withhold drug if WBC count is <4000/mm^3 or platelet count is <100,000/mm^3; notify prescriber of results if WBC <20,000/mm^3, platelets <150,000/mm^3
- Monitor temp q4h (may indicate beginning of infection)
- Monitor liver function tests before and during therapy (bilirubin, AST [SGOT], ALT [SGPT], LDH) as needed or monthly
- Assess for bleeding: hematuria, stool guaiac, bruising or petechiae, mucosa or orifices q8h; inflammation of mucosa, breaks in skin
- Identify dyspnea, rales, unproductive cough, chest pain, tachypnea
- Identify effects of alopecia on body image; discuss feelings about body changes; if edema in feet, joint pain, stomach pain, shaking present, prescriber should be notified; identify inflammation of mucosa, breaks in skin

Associated nursing diagnoses

- ✓ Injury, risk for (adverse reactions)
- ✓ Body image disturbance (adverse reactions)
- ✓ Infection, risk for (adverse reactions)
- ✓ Knowledge deficit (teaching)

Implementation

- Avoid contact with skin, very irritating; wash completely to remove
- Give fluids **IV** or PO before chemotherapy to hydrate patient
- Give antacid before oral agent; give drug after evening meal, before bedtime; give antiemetic 30-60 min before giving drug to prevent vomiting and prn and antibiotics for prophylaxis of infection
- Give in AM so drug can be eliminated before hs
- Provide liq diet: carbonated beverages; gelatin may be added if patient is not nauseated or vomiting
- Rinsing of mouth tid-qid with water, club soda; brushing of teeth bid-qid with soft brush or cotton-tipped applicators for stomatitis; use unwaxed dental floss

SC/IM route

- Reconstitute with 1-5 ml sterile water for inj; D_5W, 0.9% NaCl

IV **IV route**

- Drug should be prepared by experienced personnel using proper precautions
- Two test doses 2-5 U before initial dose; monitor for anaphylaxis
- Give by direct **IV** after reconstituting 15 U or less/5 ml or more of D_5W or 0.9% NaCl; give 15 U or less/10 min through Y-tube or 3-way

stopcock initial dose; monitor for anaphylaxis

Intermittent inf

• Administer after diluting 50-100 ml 0.9% NaCl, D_5W and giving at prescribed rate

Syringe compatibilities:

Cisplatin, cyclophosphamide, doxorubicin, droperidol, fluorouracil, furosemide, heparin, leucovorin, methotrexate, metoclopramide, mitomycin, vinblastine, vincristine

Y-site compatibilities:

Cisplatin, cyclophosphamide, doxorubicin, droperidol, fludarabine, fluorouracil, furosemide, heparin, leucovorin, melphalan, methotrexate, metoclopramide, mitomycin, ondansetron, paclitaxel, sargramostin, vinblastine, vincristine, vinorelbine

Additive incompatibilities:

Aminophylline, ascorbic acid inj, carbenicillin, cefazolin, cephalothin, diazepam, hydrocortisone sodium succinate, methotrexate, mitomycin, nafcillin, penicillin G sodium, terbutaline

Additive compatibilities:

Amikacin, cephapirin, dexamethasone sodium phosphate, diphenhydramine, fluorouracil, gentamicin, heparin, hydrocortisone sodium succinate, phenytoin, streptomycin, tobramycin, vincristine, vinblastine

Solution compatibilities:

D_5W, 0.9% NaCl

Patient/family education

• Teach patient to avoid use of products containing aspirin or ibuprofen, razors, commercial mouthwash; bleeding may occur; to report symptoms of bleeding (hematuria, tarry stools)

• Instruct patient to report signs of anemia (fatigue, headache, irritability, faintness, shortness of breath)

• Instruct patient to report any changes in breathing or coughing even several months after treatment; to avoid crowds and persons with respiratory tract or other infections

• Inform patient that hair may be lost during treatment; a wig or hairpiece may make patient feel better; new hair may be different in color, texture

• Caution patient not to have any vaccinations without the advice of the prescriber; serious reactions can occur

• Advise patient contraception is needed during treatment and for several months after completion of therapy

Evaluation

Positive therapeutic outcome

• Prevention of rapid division of malignant cells

bretylium 🗝

(bre-til'ee-um)

Bretylate ✦, bretylium tosylate, Bretylol

Func. class.: Antidysrhythmic (Class III)

Chem. class.: Quaternary ammonium compound

Pregnancy category C

Action: After a transient release of norepinephrine, inhibits further release by postganglionic nerve endings; prolongs action potential, duration, and effective refractory period

➔ **Therapeutic Outcome:** Absence of dysrhythmias

Uses: Serious ventricular tachycardia, cardioversion, ventricular fibrillation; for short-term use only

Dosage and routes

Severe ventricular fibrillation

Adult: **IV** bol 5 mg/kg; increase to 10 mg/kg repeated q15 min, up to 30 mg/kg; **IV** inf 1-2 mg/min or give 5-10 mg/kg over 10 min q6h (maintenance)

Ventricular dysrhythmias

Adult: **IV** inf 500 mg diluted in 50 ml D_5W or NS; infuse over 10-30 min; may repeat in 1 hr; maintain with 1-2 mg/min or 5-10 mg/kg over 10-30 min q6h; IM 5-10 mg/kg undiluted; repeat in 1-2 hr if needed; maintain with same dose q6-8h

Available forms: Inj **IV** 50 mg/ml; 1, 2, 4 mg/ml prefilled syringes

Side effects/adverse reactions

CNS: *Syncope, dizziness,* confusion, psychosis, anxiety

CV: ***Hypotension, postural hypotension, bradycardia,*** angina, PVCs, substernal pressure, transient hypertension, precipitation of angina

GI: *Nausea, vomiting*

RESP: ***Respiratory depression***

Contraindications: Hypersensitivity, digitalis toxicity, aortic stenosis, pulmonary hypertension, P children

Precautions: Renal disease, pregnancy **C**, lactation, P children

Pharmacokinetics

Absorption	Complete bioavailability (IV)
Distribution	Unknown
Metabolism	Not metabolized
Excretion	Kidneys, unchanged
Half-life	4-17 hr

Pharmacodynamics

	IV	IM
Onset	5 min	½-2 hr
Peak	Infusion's end	Unknown
Duration	6-24 hr	6-24 hr

Interactions

Drug/drug:

Individual drugs

Caffeine: ↓ effects of adenosine

Carbamazepine: ↑ heart block
Digoxin: ↑ digitalis toxicity
Dopamine: ↑ pressor effects
Norepinephrine: ↑ pressor effects

Drug classifications
Cardiac glycosides: ↑ toxicity

Lab test interferences
Increase: Liver function tests

NURSING CONSIDERATIONS
Assessment
- Monitor ECG continuously to determine drug effectiveness; measure PR, QRS, QT intervals; check for PVCs, other dysrhythmias; monitor B/P continuously for hypotension, hypertension; check for rebound hypertension after 1-2 hr

Associated nursing diagnoses
- ✓ Cardiac output, decreased (uses)
- ✓ Gas exchange, impaired (adverse reactions)
- ✓ Knowledge deficit (teaching)

Implementation
IM route
- Give in large muscle mass, rotate sites to prevent nerosis

IV **IV route**
Direct
- Give **IV** bol undiluted; give 6 mg or less over 1 min; if using an **IV** line, use port near insertion site, flush with normal saline (50 ml)

Intermittent inf
- Give by intermittent inf after diluting 500 mg/50 ml or more with 0.9% NaCl, D_5W, D_5/0.45% NaCl, D_5/0.9% NaCl, LR, ⅙ mol/L sodium lactate; run over >8 min

Cont inf
- Give by cont inf diluted in sol; give 1-2 mg/min; use inf site
- Store at room temp; sol should be clear

Additive compatibilities:
Aminophylline, calcium chloride, calcium gluconate, digoxine, dopamine, esmolol, regular insulin, lidocaine, potassium chloride, quinadine verapamil

Additive incompatibiliity:
Phenytoin

Y-site compatibilities:
Amrinone, dobutamine, famotidine, isoproterenol, ranitidine

Evaluation
Positive therapeutic outcome
- Decreased B/P, dysrhythmias, heart rate; normal sinus rhythm

bromocriptine
(broe-moe-krip'teen)
Parlodel
Func. class.: Antiparkinsonian agent; dopamine receptor agonist; ovulation stimulant
Chem. class.: Ergot alkaloid derivative
Pregnancy category **D**

Action: Inhibits prolactin release by activating postsynaptic dopamine receptors; activation of striatal dopamine receptors may be reason for improvement in Parkinson's disease

Therapeutic Outcome: Decreased involuntary movements in Parkinson's disease; decreased lactation; decreased hormone levels in acromegaly; absence of amenorrhea in hyperprolactinemia

Uses: Female infertility, adjunct with levodopa in Parkinson's disease, prevention of postpartum lactation, amenorrhea caused by hyperprolactinemia, acromegaly

Dosage and routes

Hyperprolactinemic indications

Adult: PO 1.25-2.5 mg with meals; may increase by 2.5 mg q3- 7 days; usual dosage 5-7.5 mg

Acromegaly

Adult: PO 1.25-2.5 mg/ day × 3 days hs; may increase by 1.25-2.5 mg q3-7 days; usual range 20-30 mg/day; max 100 mg/day

Postpartum lactation

Adult: PO 2.5 mg qd-tid with meal × 14 or 21 days

Parkinson's disease

Adult: PO 1.25 mg bid with meals; may increase q2-4 wk by 2.5 mg/day; not to exceed 100 mg/day

Available forms: Caps 5 mg; tabs 2.5 mg

Side effects/adverse reactions

CNS: Headache, depression, restlessness, anxiety, nervousness, confusion, ***convulsions,*** hallucinations, ***dizziness,*** fatigue, drowsiness, abnormal involuntary movements, psychosis

CV: ***Orthostatic hypotension,*** decreased B/P, palpitations, extrasystole, ***shock,*** dysrhythmias, bradycardia

EENT: Blurred vision, diplopia, burning eyes, nasal congestion

GI: Nausea, vomiting, anorexia, cramps, constipation, diarrhea, dry mouth, GI hemorrhage

GU: Frequency, retention, incontinence, diuresis

INTEG: Rash on face, arms, alopecia

Contraindications: Hypersensitivity to ergot, severe ischemic disease, pregnancy **D**, severe peripheral vascular disease

Precautions: Lactation, hepatic disease, renal disease, P children, pituitary tumors

Pharmacokinetics

Absorption	Poorly absorbed (PO)
Distribution	Unknown
Metabolism	Liver, completely
Excretion	85%-98% feces
Half-life	4 hr (initial); 50 hr (terminal)

Pharmacodynamics

	PO
Onset	½-1½ hr
Peak	1-3 hr
Duration	8-12 hr

Interactions

Drug/drug:

Individual drugs

Haloperidol: ↓ levels of bromocriptine
Levodopa: ↑ neurologic effects
Methyldopa: ↓ levels of bromocriptine
Reserpine: ↓ effects of bromocriptine

Drug classifications

Antihistamines: ↑ CNS depression
Antihypertensives: ↑ hypotension
Analgesics, opioid: ↑ CNS depression
Phenothiazines: ↓ levels of bromocriptine
Sedative/hypnotics: ↑ CNS depression
Antidepressants, tricyclics: ↓ levels of bromocriptine

Lab test interferences

Increase: Growth hormone, AST (SGOT), ALT (SGPT), CPK, BUN, uric acid, alkaline phosphatase, GGTP

NURSING CONSIDERATIONS

Assessment

- Assess symptoms of Parkinson's disease (extrapyramidal symptoms): shuffling gait, muscle rigidity, involuntary movements, pill rolling, muscle spasms, drooling before and during treatment
- Assess for symptoms of suppression of lactation: decreasing breast tenderness and discomfort, decreasing milk production
- Monitor B/P; establish baseline, compare with other readings; this drug decreases B/P; patient should remain recumbent for 2-4 hr after first dose; supervise ambulation

Associated nursing diagnoses

- ✓ Mobility, impaired (uses)
- ✓ Knowledge deficit (teaching)

Implementation

PO route

- With meals or milk to prevent GI symptoms; crush tab if patient has swallowing difficulty
- Give hs so dizziness, orthostatic hypotension do not occur
- Store at room temp in airtight container

Patient/family education

- Advise patient to change position slowly to prevent orthostatic hypotension
- Caution patient to use contraceptives during treatment with this drug; pregnancy may occur; to use methods other than oral contraceptives
- Teach patient that therapeutic effect for Parkinson's disease may take 2 mo: galactorrhea, amenorrhea
- Caution patient to avoid hazardous activity if dizziness, drowsiness occurs during treatment start-up
- Advise patient to avoid alcohol and OTC medication unless approved by prescriber
- Teach patients with acromegaly to notify prescriber immediately if severe headache, nausea, vomiting, blurred vision occur; indicates change in enlargement of tumor
- Teach patients using drug for lactation suppression that

treatment will last up to 3 wk and breast engorgement with milk production may occur after treatment is discontinued

Evaluation

Positive therapeutic outcome

- Parkinson's disease: decreased dyskinesia, decreased slow movements, decreased drooling
- Decreased breast engorgement with accompanied pain, tenderness
- Acromegly: decreased growth hormone levels

brompheniramine

(brome-fen-eer'a-meen)

Bromphen, brompheniramine, Codimal-A, Cophene-B, Dehist, Diamine T.D., Dimetane, Dimetane Extentabs, Histaject, Nasahist-B, ND-Stat, Oraminic II, Veltane

Func. class.: Antihistamine

Chem. class.: Alkylamine, H_1-receptor antagonist

Pregnancy category **B**

Action: Acts on blood vessels, GI, respiratory system by competing with histamine for H_1-receptor site; decreases allergic response by blocking histamine

Therapeutic Outcome: Absence of allergy symptoms and rhinitis

Uses: Allergy symptoms, rhinitis, allergic dermatoses, nasal allergies, hypersensitivity reactions including blood transfusion reactions, anaphylaxis

Dosage and routes

Adult: PO 4-8 mg tid-qid, not to exceed 36 mg/day; time rel 8-12 mg bid-tid, not to exceed 36 mg/day; IM/**IV**/SC 5-20 mg q6-12h, not to exceed 40 mg/day

P *Child >6 yr:* PO 2 mg tid-qid, not to exceed 12 mg/day; IM/**IV**/SC 0.5 mg/kg/day divided tid or qid

P *Child <6 yr:* 1 mg q4-6h (not to exceed 6 mg/day)

Available forms: Tabs 4, 8, 12 mg; time rel tabs 8, 12 mg; elix 2 mg/5 ml; inj IM/SC/**IV** 10, 100 mg/ml

Side effects/adverse reactions

CNS: Dizziness, drowsiness, poor coordination, fatigue, anxiety, euphoria, confusion, paresthesia, neuritis

CV: Hypotension, palpitations, tachycardia

EENT: Blurred vision, dilated pupils, tinnitus, nasal stuffiness, dry nose, throat, mouth

GI: Dry mouth, nausea, vomiting, anorexia, constipation, diarrhea

GU: Retention, dysuria, frequency, impotence

HEMA: Thrombocytopenia, agranulocytosis, hemolytic anemia

INTEG: Photosensitivity

RESP: Increased thick secretions, wheezing, chest tightness

Contraindications: Hypersensitivity to H_1-receptor antagonists, acute asthma attack, lower respiratory tract disease, child <6 yr

Precautions: Increased intraocular pressure, renal disease, cardiac disease, hypertension, bronchial asthma, seizure disorder, stenosed peptic ulcers, hyperthyroidism, prostatic hypertrophy, bladder neck obstruction, pregnancy **B**

Pharmacokinetics

Absorption	Well absorbed (PO, IM)
Distribution	Widely distributed; crosses blood-brain barrier
Metabolism	Liver, extensively
Excretion	Kidneys, metabolite; breast milk (minimal)
Half-life	12-34 hr

Pharmacodynamics

	PO	SC	IM	IV
Onset	15-30 min	30 min	30 min	Immediate
Peak	2-5 hr	Unknown	Unknown	Unknown
Duration	6-12 hr	8-12 hr	8-12 hr	8-12 hr

Interactions

Drug/drug:

Individual drugs

Alcohol: ↑ CNS depression

Drug classifications

CNS depressants: ↑ CNS depression

MAOI: ↑ anticholinergic effect

Narcotics: ↑ CNS depression

Sedative/hypnotics: ↑ CNS depression

Lab test interferences

False negative: Skin allergy tests (discontinue antihistamines before testing)

NURSING CONSIDERATIONS

Assessment

- Assess respiratory status: rate, rhythm, increase in bronchial secretions, wheezing, chest tightness; provide fluids to 2 L/day to decrease secretion thickness
- Monitor I&O ratio: be alert for urinary retention, frequency, dysuria, especially elderly; drug should be discontinued if these occur
- Monitor CBC during long-term therapy; blood dyscrasias may occur but are rare
- **IV** administration may result in rapid drop in B/P, sweating, dizziness, especially in elderly

Associated nursing diagnoses

- ✓ Airway clearance, ineffective (uses)
- ✓ Injury, risk for (side effects)
- ✓ Knowledge deficit (teaching)
- ✓ Noncompliance (teaching, overuse)

Implementation

PO route

- May give with food to prevent GI upset; absorption is not altered by food
- Store in tight, light-resistant container

IV route

- Give undiluted or dilute 10 mg/ml using 0.9% NaCl at a rate of 1 min or more
- May be further diluted in 0.9% NaCl, D_5W; give as intermittent inf at prescribed rate

Patient/family education

- Teach patient all aspects of drug use; to notify prescriber if confusion, sedation, hypotension occur; to avoid driving or other hazardous activity if drowsiness occurs; to avoid alcohol or other CNS depressants that may potentiate effect
- Instruct patient not to exceed recommended dosage; dysrhythmias may occur
- Teach patient hard candy, gum, frequent rinsing of mouth may be used for dryness

Evaluation

Positive therapeutic outcome

- Absence of running or congested nose, rashes

Treatment of overdose: Administer ipecac syrup or lavage, diazepam, vasopressors, barbiturates (short acting)

bumetanide

(byoo-met'a-nide)

Bumex

Func. class: Loop diuretic

Chem. class.: Sulfonamide derivative

Pregnancy category C

Action: Acts on the ascending loop of Henle in the kidney to inhibit the reabsorption of the electrolytes sodium and chloride, causing excretion of sodium, calcium, magnesium, chloride, water and some potassium; also decreases reabsorption of sodium and chloride and increases the excretion of potassium in the distal tubule of the kidney; responsible for antihypertensive effect and peripheral vasodilatation

➔ **Therapeutic Outcome:** Decreased edema in lung tissue and peripherally; decreased B/P

Uses: Edema in congestive heart failure, nephrotic syndrome, ascites caused by hepatic disease, hepatic cirrhosis

Investigational uses: May be used alone or as adjunct with antihypertensives such as spironolactone, triamterene

Dosage and routes

Adult: PO 0.5-2 mg qd; may give 2nd or 3rd dose at 4-5 hr intervals; not to exceed 20 mg/day; may be given on alternate days or intermittently; **IV**/IM 0.5-1 mg/day; may give 2nd or 3rd dose at 2-3 hr intervals; not to exceed 20 mg/day

Available forms: Tabs 0.5, 1, 2 mg; inj **IV**, IM 0.25 mg/ml

Side effects/adverse reactions

CNS: Headache, fatigue, weakness, vertigo, paresthesias

CV: *Orthostatic, hypotension,* chest pain, ECG changes, circulatory collapse

EENT: Ear pain, tinnitus, blurred vision

ELECT: *Hypokalemia, hypochlorsemic alkalosis, hypomagneemia, hyperuricemia, hypocalcemia, hyponatremia, metabolic alkalosis*

ENDO: *Hyperglycemia*
GI: *Nausea,* diarrhea, dry mouth, vomiting, anorexia, cramps, oral and gastric irritations, pancreatitis
GU: *Polyuria,* ***renal failure,*** *glycosuria*
HEMA: ***Thrombocytopenia, agranulocytosis, leukopenia, neutropenia, anemia***
INTEG: *Rash,* ***pruritus, purpura, urticaria***
MS: Cramps, stiffness

Contraindications: Hypersensitivity to sulfonamides, anuria, hypovolemia, lactation, electrolyte depletion

Precautions: Diabetes mellitus, dehydration, severe renal disease, pregnancy **C**

Pharmacokinetics

	PO/IM
Absorption	Rapidly, completely absorbed
	PO/IM/IV
Distribution	Crosses placenta
Metabolism	Liver (30%-40%)
Excretion	Breast milk, urine, feces
Half-life	1-1½ hr

Pharmacodynamics

	PO	IM	IV
Onset	½-1 hr	40 min	5 min
Peak	1-2 hr	Unknown	½ hr
Duration	4 hr	4 hr	2-3 hr

Interactions
Drug/drug:

Individual drugs
Alcohol: ↑ orthostatic hypotension
Cisplatin: ↑ risk of ototoxicity
Ethacrynic acid: Combination may cause ↑ chance of arrhythmias (do not use together)
Indomethacin: ↓ diuretic and antihypertensives effect of bumetanide
Lithium: ↓ renal clearance causing ↑ toxicity
Mezlocillin: ↑ hypokalemia
Probenecid: ↓ effect of bumetanide
Piperacillin: ↑ hypokalemia
Ticarcillin: ↑ hypokalemia

Drug classifications
Aminoglycosides: ↑ ototoxicity
Antihypertensives: ↑ antihypertensive effects
Digitalis glycosides: ↑ potassium loss with relating arrhythmias
Glucocorticoids: ↑ hypokalemia

NURSING CONSIDERATIONS
Assessment

- Assess patient for tinnitus, hearing loss, ear pain; periodic testing of hearing is needed when high doses of this drug are given by **IV** route
- Monitor for manifestations of hypokalemia; *Renal:* acidic urine, reduced urine osmolality, nocturia, polyuria, polydipsia; *CV:* hypotension, broad T wave, U wave, ectopy, tachycardia, weak pulse; *Neuro:* muscle weakness, altered LOC, drowsiness, apathy, lethargy, confusion, depression; *GI:* anorexia, nausea, cramps, constipation, distention, paralytic ileus; *Resp:* hypoventilation, respiratory muscle weakness
- Monitor for manifestations of hypocalcemia: *CNS:* personality changes, anxiety, disturbances, depression, psychosis;

GI: nausea, vomiting, constipation, abdominal pain from muscle spasm; *CV:* decreased contractility, decreased cardiac output, hypotension, lengthened ST segment, prolonged QT interval; *Integ:* scaling eczema, alopecia, hyperpigmentation; *Neuro:* tetany, muscle twitching, cramping, grimacing, seizure, altered deep tendon reflexes, spasm

• Monitor for manifestations of hypomagnesemia; *CNS:* agitation; *Neuro:* muscle twitching, paresthesias, hyperactive reflexes, positive Babinski's reflex, dysphagia, nystagmus, seizures, tetany; *GI:* nausea, vomiting, diarrhea, anorexia, abdominal distention; *CV:* ectopy, tachycardia, broad, flat, or inverted T waves, depressed ST segment, prolonged QT, decreased cardiac output, hypotension

• Monitor for manifestations of hyponatremia: *CV:* increased B/P, cold, clammy skin, hypovolemia or hypervolemia; *GI:* anorexia, nausea, vomiting, diarrhea, abdominal cramps; *Neuro:* lethargy, increased ICP, confusion, headache, seizures, coma, fatigue, tremors, hyperreflexia

• Monitor for manifestations of hyperchloremia: *Neuro:* weakness, lethargy, coma; *Resp:* deep rapid breathing

• Assess fluid volume status: I&O ratio and record, count or weigh diapers as appropriate, distended red veins, crackles in lung, color, quality and sp gr of urine, skin turgor, adequacy of pulses, moist mucous membranes, bilateral lung sounds, peripheral pitting edema; dehydration symptoms of decreasing output, thirst, hypotension, dry mouth and mucous membranes should be reported

• Monitor electrolytes: potassium, sodium, calcium, magnesium; also include BUN, blood pH, ABGs, uric acid, CBC, blood sugar

• Assess B/P before and during therapy with patient lying, standing, and sitting as appropriate; orthostatic hypotension can occur rapidly

Associated nursing diagnoses

✓ Altered urinary elimination (side effects)
✓ Fluid volume deficit (side effects)
✓ Fluid volume excess (uses)
✓ Knowledge deficit (teaching)

Implementation

• Give in AM to avoid interference with sleep

• Potassium replacement if potassium level is <3.0 mg/dl whole, or use oral solutions; drug may be crushed if patient is unable to swallow

PO route

• With food, if nausea occurs; absorption may be reduced

IV **IV route**

• Do not use solution that is yellow or has a precipitate or crystals

Direct IV

• Give undiluted through Y-tube on 3-way stopcock; give 20 mg or less/min

Intermittent inf

• May be added to NS, D_5W, $D_{10}W$, $D_{20}W$, invert sugar 10% in electrolyte #1, LR, sodium lactate ⅙ mol/L; use within 24

B

hr to ensure compatibility; give through Y-tube or 3-way stopcock; give at 4 mg/min or less; use infusion pump

Y-site incompatibilities:
Amsacrine, bleomycin sulfate, doxorubicin HCl, droperidol, esmolol HCl, fluconazole, gentamicin sulfate, metoclopramide HCl, milrinone, netilmicin sulfate, ondansetron HCl, quinidine gluconate, vinblastine sulfate, vincristine sulfate

Y-site compatibilities:
Amikacin sulfate, cisplatin, cyclophosphamide, dobutamine HCl, fumotidine, dintrate, fludarabine phosphate, fluorouracil, foscarnet sodium, heparin sodium, hydrocortisone sodium succinate, kanamycin sulfate, leucovorin calcium, methotrexate sodium, mitomycin, potassium chloride, tobramycin sulfate, tolazoline, vitamin B complex with C

Syringe incompatibilities:
Doxapram HCl, doxorubicin HCl, droperidol, metaclopramide HCl, milrinone

IV compatibilities:
Cisplatin, cyclophosphamide, fluorouracil, heparin sodium, leucovorin calcium, methotrexate sodium, mitomycin, vinblastine sulfate, vincristine sulfate

Additive compatibilities:
Amikacin sulfate, aminophylline, amiodarone, ampicillin, atropine, flumetanide, calcium gluconate, cefumandole nafate, cefuroxime sodium, cimetidine, cloxacillin, digoxin, epinephrine, heparin, isosorbide, kanamycin, lidocaine, morphine, nitroglycerin, ranitidine, sodium bicarbonate, tobramycin, verapamil

Additive incompatibilities:
Bleomycin sulfate, dobutamine, gentamicin sulfate, chlorpromazine HCl, diazepam, erythromycin lactobionate, isoproterenol HCl, meperidine HCl, metoclopramide HCl, netilmicin, opium alkaloids, prochlorperazine edisylate, tetracycline HCl

Patient/family education

- Teach patient to take the medication early in the day to prevent nocturia
- Instruct the patient to take with food or milk if GI symptoms of nausea and anorexia occur
- Teach patient to maintain weekly record of weight and notify prescriber of weight loss of >5 lb
- Caution the patient that this drug causes a loss of potassium so food rich in potassium should be added to the diet; refer to a dietician for assistance in planning
- Caution the patient not to exercise in hot weather or stand for prolonged periods since orthostatic hypotension will be enhanced
- Teach patient not to use alcohol or any OTC medications without prescriber's approval; serious drug reactions may occur
- Emphasize the need to contact prescriber immediately if

muscle cramps, weakness, nausea, dizziness, or numbness occurs
- Teach patient to take own B/P and pulse and record
- Caution the patient that orthostatic hypotension may occur; patient should rise slowly from sitting or reclining positions and lie down if dizziness occurs
- Teach patient to continue taking medication even if feeling better; this drug controls symptoms but does not cure the condition
- Advise the patient with hypertension to continue other medical treatment (exercise, weight loss, relaxation techniques, cessation of smoking)

Evaluation

Positive therapeutic outcome
- Decreased edema
- Decreased B/P
- Increased diuresis

buprenorphine

(byoo-pre-nor'feen)

Buprenex

Func. class.: Narcotic analgesic

Chem. class.: Opiate, thebaine derivative

Pregnancy category **C**

Controlled substance schedule **V**

Action: Inhibits ascending pain pathways in limbic system, thalamus, midbrain, hypothalamus by binding to opiate receptor sites; this alters pain perception and response; generalized CNS depression

Therapeutic Outcome: Relief of pain

Uses: Moderate to severe pain

B

Dosage and routes

Adult: IM/**IV** 0.3-0.6 mg q6h prn; may repeat dose after G ½ hr; reduce dosage in elderly

Available forms: Inj IM, **IV** 0.3 mg/ml (1 ml vials)

Side effects/adverse reactions

CNS: *Drowsiness, dizziness, confusion, headache, sedation, euphoria*

CV: Palpitations, bradycardia, change in B/P

EENT: Tinnitus, blurred vision, miosis, diplopia

GI: Nausea, vomiting, anorexia, constipation, cramps

GU: Increased urinary output, dysuria

INTEG: *Rash,* urticaria, bruising, flushing, diaphoresis, pruritus

RESP: ***Respiratory depression***

Contraindications: Hypersensitivity, addiction (narcotic)

Precautions: Addictive personality, pregnancy **C**, lactation, increased intracranial pressure, MI (acute), severe heart disease, respiratory depression, hepatic disease, renal disease

Pharmacokinetics	
Absorption	Well absorbed (IM)
Distribution	Crosses placenta
Metabolism	Liver, extensively
Excretion	Kidneys, breast milk
Half-life	2½-3½ hr

Pharmacodynamics

	IM	IV
Onset	10-15 min	Immediate
Peak	1 hr	5 min
Duration	4 hr	2-5 hr

Interactions

Drug/drug:

Individual drugs

Alcohol: ↑ respiratory depression, hypotension, sedation

Drug classifications

Antihistamines: ↑ respiratory depression, hypotension

CNS depressants: ↑ respiratory depression, hypotension

MAOI: Do not use 2 wk before alfentanil

Sedative/hypnotics: ↑ respiratory depression, hypotension

NURSING CONSIDERATIONS

Assessment

- Assess pain characteristics: location, intensity, type before medication administration and following treatment
- Monitor VS after parenteral route; note muscle rigidity, drug history, liver, kidney function tests, respiratory dysfunction: respiratory depression, character, rate, rhythm; notify prescriber if respirations are <10/min
- Monitor CNS changes: dizziness, drowsiness, hallucinations, euphoria, LOC, pupil reaction
- Monitor allergic reactions: rash, urticaria

Associated nursing diagnoses

- ✓ Pain (uses)
- ✓ Sensory-perceptual alteration: visual, auditory (adverse reactions)
- ✓ Breathing pattern, ineffective (adverse reactions)
- ✓ Knowledge deficit (teaching)

Implementation

- Give by inj (IM, **IV**), only with resuscitative equipment available; give slowly to prevent rigidity

IM route

- Give deep in large muscle mass; rotate sites of inj

IV **IV route**

- Give **IV** direct undiluted over 3-5 min; give slowly

Y-site compatibilities:
Melphalan, vinorelbine

Syringe compatibility:
Midazolam

Additive compatibilities:
Atropine, diphenhydramine, droperidol, glycopyrrolate, haloperidol, hydroxyzine, promethazine, scopolamine

Additive incompatibilities:
Diazepam, floxacillin, furosemide lorezepam

Patient/family education

- Instruct patient to report any symptoms of CNS changes, allergic reactions
- Caution patients to avoid CNS depressants: alcohol, sedative/hypnotics for at least 24 hr after taking this drug
- Discuss with patient that dizziness, drowsiness, and

confusion are common; to avoid getting up without assistance
- Discuss in detail all aspects of the drug
- Instruct patient to change position slowly to prevent orthostatic hypotension
- Teach patient to turn, cough, deep breathe after surgery to prevent atelectasis

Evaluation

Positive therapeutic outcome
- Relief of pain

Treatment of overdose: Narcan 0.2-0.8 **IV**, O_2, **IV** fluids, vasopressors

bupropion
(byoo-proe'pee-on)
Wellbutrin
Func. class.: Misc. antidepressant
Chem. class.: Amino ketone
Pregnancy category B

Action: Inhibits reuptake of dopamine, serotonin, norepinephrine

➔ **Therapeutic Outcome:** Decreased symptoms of depression after 2-3 wk

Uses: Depression

Dosage and routes

Adult: PO 100 mg bid initially, then increase after 3 days to 100 mg tid if needed; may increase after 1 mo to 150 mg tid

Available forms: Tabs 75, 100 mg

Side effects/adverse reactions

CNS: Headache, agitation, confusion, ***seizures,*** akathisia, delusions, insomnia, sedation, tremors
CV: Dysrhythmias, hypertension, palpitations, tachycardia, hypotension
EENT: Blurred vision, auditory disturbance
GI: Nausea, vomiting, dry mouth, increased appetite, constipation
GU: Impotence, frequency, retention
INTEG: Rash, pruritus, sweating

Contraindications: Hypersensitivity, seizure disorder, eating disorders

Precautions: Renal and hepatic disease, recent MI, cranial trauma, pregnancy **B**, lactation, P children

Pharmacokinetics

Absorption	Well absorbed; bioavailability poor
Distribution	Unknown
Metabolism	Liver extensively
Excretion	Kidneys
Half-life	14 hr

Pharmacodynamics

	PO
Onset	Up to 4 wk
Peak	Unknown
Duration	Unknown

Interactions

Drug/drug:

Individual drugs

Alcohol: ↑ risk of seizures
Cimetidine: ↑ levels, ↑ toxicity
Levodopa: ↑ adverse reactions
Phenytoin: ↑ toxicity

Drug classifications

Antihistamines: ↑ CNS depression
Barbiturates: ↑ effects
Benzodiazepines: ↑ risk of seizures
CNS depressants: ↑ effects
MAOI: Acute toxicity, convulsions
Phenothiazines: ↑ toxicity

Lab test interferences

Increase: Serum bilirubin, blood glucose, alkaline phosphatase
Decrease: VMA, 5-HIAA
False increase: Urinary catecholamines

NURSING CONSIDERATIONS

Assessment

- Monitor B/P (with patient lying, standing), pulse q4h; if systolic B/P drops 20 mm Hg hold drug, notify prescriber; take vital signs q4h in patients with cardiovascular disease
- Monitor blood studies: CBC, leukocytes, differential, cardiac enzymes if patient is receiving long-term therapy
- Monitor hepatic studies: AST (SGOT), ALT (SGPT), bilirubin if on long-term treatment
- Check weight weekly; appetite may increase with drug
- Assess ECG for flattening of T wave, bundle branch block, AV block, dysrhythmias in cardiac patients
- Assess for EPS primarily in elderly: rigidity, dystonia, akathisia
- Assess mental status: mood, sensorium, affect, suicidal tendencies; increase in psychiatric symptoms: depression, panic
- Monitor urinary retention, constipation; constipation is **P** more likely to occur in children **G** or elderly
- Identify alcohol consumption; if alcohol was consumed, hold dose

Associated nursing diagnoses

✓ Coping, ineffective individual (uses)
✓ Injury, risk for (side effects)
✓ Knowledge deficit (teaching)
✓ Noncompliance (teaching)

Implementation

PO route

- Give with food or milk for GI symptoms
- Store at room temp; do not freeze

Patient/family education

- Teach patient that therapeutic effects may take 2-3 wk
- Teach patient to use caution in driving or other activities requiring alertness because of drowsiness, dizziness, blurred vision; to avoid rising quickly from sitting to standing, **G** especially elderly
- Teach patient to avoid alcohol ingestion, obtain approval for other drugs
- Teach patient to increase fluids, bulk in diet if constipation, urinary retention occur, **G** especially elderly

- Teach patient to take gum, hard sugarless candy, or frequent sips of water for dry mouth

Evaluation

Positive therapeutic outcome

- Decrease in depression
- Absence of suicidal thoughts

Treatment of overdose: ECG monitoring, induce emesis, lavage, activated charcoal, administer anticonvulsant

buspirone

(byoo-spye'rone)

BuSpar

Func. class.: Antianxiety agent

Chem. class.: Azaspirodecanedione

Pregnancy category **B**

Action: Acts by inhibiting the action of serotonin (5-HT) by binding to serotonin and dopamine receptors; also increases norepinephrine metabolism

Therapeutic Outcome: Decreased anxiety

Uses: Management and short-term relief of anxiety disorders

Dosage and routes

Adult: PO 5 mg tid; may increase by 5 mg/day q2-3 days; not to exceed 60 mg/day

Available forms: Tabs 5, 10 mg

Side effects/adverse reactions

CNS: *Dizziness, headache, depression, stimulation, insomnia, nervousness, lightheadedness, numbness, paresthesia, incoordination, tremors,* excitement, involuntary movements, confusion, akathisia

CV: *Tachycardia, palpitations,* hypotension, hypertension, ***CVA, CHF, MI***

EENT: *Sore throat, tinnitus, blurred vision, nasal congestion,* red, itching eyes, change in taste, smell

GI: *Nausea, dry mouth, diarrhea, constipation,* flatulence, increased appetite, rectal bleeding

GU: Frequency, hesitancy, menstrual irregularity, change in libido

INTEG: *Rash,* edema, pruritus, alopecia, dry skin

MISC: *Sweating,* fatigue, weight gain, fever

MS: *Pain, weakness,* muscle cramps, spasms

RESP: Hyperventilation, chest congestion, shortness of breath

Contraindications: Hypersensitivity, child <18 yr

Precautions: Pregnancy **B**, lactation, elderly, impaired hepatic/renal function

Pharmacokinetics

Absorption	Rapidly absorbed
Distribution	Unknown
Metabolism	Liver, extensively
Excretion	Feces
Half-life	3 hr

Pharmacodynamics

	PO
Onset	Unknown
Peak	Unknown
Duration	Unknown

Interactions

Drug/drug:

Individual drugs

Alcohol: ↑ CNS depression
Trazodone: ↑ ALT (SGPT)

Drug classifications

MAOI: ↑ B/P
Psychotropics: ↑ CNS depression

NURSING CONSIDERATIONS

Assessment

- Assess anxiety reaction: inability to sleep, apprehension, dread, foreboding, or uneasiness related to unidentified source of danger
- Assess for previous drug dependence or tolerance; if patient is drug dependent or tolerant, amount of medication should be restricted
- Monitor B/P (lying, standing), pulse; if systolic B/P drops 20 mm Hg, hold drug, notify prescriber; check I&O; may indicate renal dysfunction
- Monitor mental status: mood, sensorium, affect, sleeping patterns, drowsiness, dizziness, suicidal tendencies

Associated nursing diagnoses

✓ Anxiety (uses)
✓ Knowledge deficit (teaching)
✓ Noncompliance (teaching)

Implementation

PO route

- Give with food or milk for GI symptoms; sugarless gum, hard candy, frequent sips of water for dry mouth

Patient/family education

- Teach patient that drug may be taken with food; if dose is missed take as soon as remembered; do not double doses
- Caution patient to avoid OTC preparations unless approved by the prescriber; to avoid alcohol ingestion and other psychotropic medications unless prescribed by prescriber; that 1-2 wk of therapy may be required before therapeutic effects occur
- Caution patient to avoid driving and activities requiring alertness, since drowsiness may occur; until medication response is known, tell patient that drowsiness may worsen at beginning of treatment
- Instruct patient not to discontinue medication abruptly after long-term use
- Advise patient to rise slowly or fainting may occur, especially in elderly [G]

Evaluation

Positive therapeutic outcome

- Increased well-being
- Decreased anxiety, restlessness, sleeplessness, dread

Treatment of overdose:

Gastric lavage, VS, supportive care

busulfan

(byoo-sul'fan)
Myleran
Func. class.: Antineoplastic alkylating agent
Chem. class.: Nitrosourea
Pregnancy category **D**

Action: Changes essential cellular ions to covalent bonding with resultant alkylation; this interferes with normal biologic function of DNA; activity is not phase specific; action is due to myelosuppression

Therapeutic Outcome: Prevention of rapid growth of malignant cells in chronic myelocytic leukemia

Uses: Chronic myelocytic leukemia

Dosage and routes

Adult: PO 4-12 mg/day initially until WBC levels fall to 10,000/mm^3; then drug is stopped until WBC levels rise over 50,000/mm^3; then 1-3 mg/day

Child: PO 0.06-0.12 mg/kg or 1.8-4.6 mg/m^2/day; dosage is titrated to maintain WBC levels at 20,000/mm^3

Available forms: Tabs 2 mg

Side effects/adverse reactions

GI: Nausea, vomiting, *diarrhea, weight loss*
GU: Impotence, sterility, amenorrhea, gynecomastia, ***renal toxicity,*** hyperuremia, adrenal insufficiency–like syndrome
HEMA: Thrombocytopenia, leukopenia, pancytopenia, severe bone marrow depression
INTEG: Dermatitis, hyperpigmentation, alopecia
RESP: Irreversible pulmonary fibrosis, pneumonitis
OTHER: Chromosomal aberrations

Contraindications: Radiation, chemotherapy, lactation, pregnancy **D** (3rd trimester), blastic phase of chronic myelocytic leukemia, hypersensitivity

Precautions: Childbearing age men and women, leukopenia, thrombocytopenia, anemia, hepatotoxicity, renal toxicity

Pharmacokinetics

Absorption	Rapidly absorbed (PO)
Distribution	Unknown; crosses placenta
Metabolism	Liver, extensively
Excretion	Kidneys, breast milk
Half-life	Unknown

Pharmacodynamics

	PO
Onset	Unknown
Peak	Unknown
Duration	Unknown

Interactions

Drug/drug:

Individual drugs

Radiation: ↑ toxicity, bone marrow suppression

Drug classifications

Antineoplastics: ↑ toxicity, bone marrow suppression

Lab test interferences

False positive: Breast, bladder, cervix, lung cytology tests

NURSING CONSIDERATIONS

Assessment

- Monitor CBC, differential, platelet count weekly; withhold drug if WBC is <4000 or platelet count is <75,000; notify prescriber of results if WBC <20,000/mm^3, platelets <150,000/mm^3
- Monitor pulmonary function tests, chest x-ray films before, during therapy; chest film should be obtained q2 wk during treatment; check for dyspnea, rales, unproductive cough, chest pain, tachypnea
- Assess for increased uric acid levels, swelling, joint pain primarily in extremities; patient should be well hydrated to prevent urate deposits
- Monitor renal function studies: BUN, serum uric acid, urine CrCl before, during therapy; I&O ratio; report fall in urine output of 30 ml/hr; check for decreased hyperuricemia
- Monitor for cold, fever, sore throat (may indicate beginning infection); identify edema in feet, joint or stomach pain, shaking; prescriber should be notified
- Assess for bleeding: hematuria, guaiac, bruising or petechiae, mucosa or orifices q8h; no rectal temps

Associated nursing diagnoses

- ✓ Injury, risk for (adverse reactions)
- ✓ Body image disturbance (adverse reactions)
- ✓ Infection, risk for (adverse reactions)
- ✓ Knowledge deficit (teaching)

Implementation

PO route

- Give 1 hr before or 2 hr pc to lessen nausea and vomiting or give antacid before oral agent; give drug after evening meal, before bedtime; antiemetic 30-60 min before giving drug to prevent vomiting
- Give either allopurinol or sodium bicarbonate to maintain uric acid levels, alkalinization of urine; increase fluid intake to 2-3 L/day to prevent urate deposits, calculus formation
- Administer antibiotics for prophylaxis of infection may be prescribed since infection potential is high
- Store in tight container

Patient/family education

- Teach patient to avoid use of products containing aspirin or ibuprofen, razors, commercial mouthwash since bleeding may occur; to report symptoms of bleeding (hematuria, tarry stools)
- Instruct patient to report signs of anemia (fatigue, headache, irritability, faintness, shortness of breath)
- Instruct patient to report any changes in breathing or coughing even several months after treatment; to avoid crowds and persons with respiratory tract or other infections
- Teach patient hair loss may occur; discuss the use of wigs or hair pieces

• Caution patient not to have any vaccinations without the advice of the prescriber; serious reactions can occur
• Advise patient contraception is needed during treatment and for several months after the completion of therapy

Evaluation

Positive therapeutic outcome
• Decreased leukocytes to normal limits
• Absence of sweating at night
• Increased appetite, increased weight

butoconazole
(byoo-toe-kon'ah-zole)
Femstat
Func. class.: Local antiinfective
Chem. class.: Antifungal
Pregnancy category **C**

Action: Binds sterols in fungal cell membrane, which increases membrane permeability, decreases osmotic resistance

Therapeutic Outcome: Fungistatic/fungicidal against susceptible organisms: *Candida* only

Uses: Vulvovaginal infections caused by *Candida* organisms

Dosage and routes
Adult: Intravaginal 1 applicatorful hs × 3 days (nonpregnant), × 6 days (2nd/3rd trimester pregnancy)

Available forms: Vaginal cream 2%

Side effects/adverse reactions
GU: Rash, stinging, *burning,* vulvovaginal itching, soreness, swelling, discharge, finger itching

Contraindications: Hypersensitivity

Precautions: Pregnancy **C**, lactation

Pharmacokinetics	
Absorption	Minimal
Distribution	Unknown
Metabolism	Liver
Excretion	Feces, kidneys
Half-life	Unknown

Pharmacodynamics	
Onset	Unknown
Peak	Unknown
Duration	Unknown

Interactions: None

NURSING CONSIDERATIONS

Assessment
• Check for allergic reaction: burning, stinging, itching, discharge, soreness

Associated nursing diagnoses
✓ Skin integrity, impaired (uses)
✓ Infection, risk for (uses)
✓ Knowledge deficit (teaching)

Implementation
Top route
• Administer 1 applicatorful QPM high into the vagina
• Store at room temp in dry place

Patient/family education

- Instruct patient in asepsis (hand washing) before, after each application
- Teach patient to apply with applicator only; to avoid use of any other vaginal product unless directed by prescriber; sanitary napkin may prevent soiling of undergarments
- Instruct patient to abstain from sexual intercourse until treatment is completed; reinfection and irritation may occur
- Instruct patient if symptoms persist to notify prescriber

Evaluation

Positive therapeutic outcome
- Decrease in itching or white discharge (vaginal)

butorphanol

(byoo-tor′fa-nole)
Stadol, Stadol NS
Func. class.: Narcotic analgesic
Chem. class.: Opiate
Pregnancy category **C**

Action: Inhibits ascending pain pathways in limbic system, thalamus, midbrain, hypothalamus by binding to opiate receptor sites; this alters pain perception and response

➡ Therapeutic Outcome: Relief of pain

Uses: Moderate to severe pain, analgesia during labor, sedation preoperatively

Investigational uses: Migraine headache, pain

Dosage and routes

Adult: IM 1-4 mg q3-4h prn; **IV** 0.5-2 mg q3-4h prn; nasal spray in 1 nostril; may give another in 1-1½ hr; may repeat q3-4h

Available forms: Inj IM, **IV** 1, 2 mg/ml, intranasal 10 mg/ml

Side effects/adverse reactions

CNS: Drowsiness, dizziness, confusion, headache, sedation, euphoria, weakness, hallucinations
CV: Palpitations, bradycardia, change in B/P
EENT: Tinnitus, blurred vision, miosis, diplopia
GI: Nausea, vomiting, anorexia, constipation, cramps
GU: Increased urinary output, dysuria, urinary retention
INTEG: Rash, urticaria, bruising, flushing, diaphoresis, pruritus
RESP: Respiratory depression, pulmonary hypertension

Contraindications: Hypersensitivity, addiction (narcotic), CHF, MI

Precautions: Addictive personality, pregnancy **C**, lactation, increased intracranial pressure, respiratory depression, hepatic disease, renal disease, P child <18 yr

Pharmacokinetics

Absorption	Well absorbed (IM, Nasal); complete (IV)
Distribution	Crosses placenta
Metabolism	Liver, extensively
Excretion	Feces (10%-15%); kidneys, unchanged (small amounts)
Half-life	3-4 hr

Pharmacodynamics

	IM	IV	NASAL
Onset	10-30 min	1 min	15 min
Peak	½ hr	5 min	1-2 hr
Duration	3-4 hr	2-4 hr	4-5 hr

Interactions

Drug/drug:

Individual drugs

Alcohol: ↑ respiratory depression, hypotension, sedation

Drug classifications

Antihistamines: ↑ respiratory depression, hypotension

CNS depressants: ↑ respiratory depression, hypotension

MAOI: Do not use 2 wk before alfentanil

Sedative/hypnotics: ↑ respiratory depression, hypotension

Lab test interferences

Increase: Amylase, lipase

NURSING CONSIDERATIONS

Assessment

- Monitor VS after parenteral route; note muscle rigidity, drug history, liver, kidney function tests, respiratory dysfunction: respiratory depression, character, rate, rhythm; notify prescriber if respirations are <10/min
- Monitor CNS changes: dizziness, drowsiness, hallucinations, euphoria, LOC, pupil reaction
- Monitor allergic reactions: rash, urticaria

Associated nursing diagnoses

✓ Pain (uses)
✓ Sensory-perceptual alteration: visual, auditory (adverse reactions)
✓ Injury, risk for (adverse reactions)
✓ Knowledge deficit (teaching)

Implementation

- Store in light resistant container at room temp

IM route

- Give deeply in large muscle mass; rotate injection sites

Intranasal

- Give 1 spray in nostril

IV **IV route**

- Give **IV** undiluted at a rate of ≤2 mg/>3-5 min; titrate to patient response

Syringe compatibilities:
Atropine, chlorpromazine, cimetidine, diphenhydramine, droperidol, fentanyl, hydroxyzine, meperidine, methotrimeprazine, metoclopramide, midazolam, morphine, pentazocine, perphenazine, prochlorperazine, promethazine, scopolamine, thiethylperazine

Syringe incompatibilities:
Dimenhydrinate, pentobarbital

Y-site compatibilities:
Enalaprilat, esmolol, fludarabine, melphalan, paclitaxel, sargramostim, vinorelbine

Patient/family education

- Instruct patient to report any symptoms of CNS changes, allergic reactions; to avoid CNS depressants: alcohol, sedative/hypnotics for at least 24 hr after taking this drug
- Discuss with patient that dizziness, drowsiness, and confusion are common; to avoid getting up without assistance
- Discuss in detail all aspects of the drug

Nasal route

- Teach patient to blow nose to clear both nostrils before using; remove clip and cover, prime before using until spray appears; pump must be reprimed q48h; close nostril with finger and spray once quickly; have patient sniff
- Patient should replace clip and cover after use; caution patient not to shake medication

Evaluation

Positive therapeutic outcome

- Pain relief

Treatment of overdose:

Narcan 0.2-0.8 **IV**, O_2, **IV** fluids, vasopressors

calcitonin (human)

(kal-si-toe'nin)

Cibacalcin, Miacalcin

Func. class.: Parathyroid agents (calcium regulator)

Chem. class.: Polypeptide hormone

Pregnancy category C

Action: Decreases bone resorption, blood calcium levels by direct action on bone, GI system, and kidney; increases deposits of calcium in bones; renal excretion of calcium occurs

Therapeutic Outcome: Lowered calcium level, decreasing symptoms of Paget's disease

Uses: Paget's disease

Dosage and routes

Adult: SC 0.5 mg/day initially; may require 0.5 mg bid × 6 mo, then decrease until symptoms reappear

Available forms: Inj (SC) 0.5 mg/vial

Side effects/adverse reactions

CNS: Headache, ***tetany,*** chills, weakness, dizziness
CV: Chest pressure
GI: Nausea, diarrhea, vomiting, anorexia, abdominal pain, salty taste, epigastric pain
GU: Diuresis
INTEG: Rash, flushing, pruritus of earlobes, edema of feet

MS: Swelling, tingling of hands
RESP: Dyspnea

Contraindications: Hypersensitivity

Precautions: Renal disease, children, lactation, osteogenic sarcoma, pregnancy **C**

Pharmacokinetics

Absorption	Completely absorbed (IM, SC)
Distribution	Unknown
Metabolism	Rapid; kidneys, tissue, blood
Excretion	Kidneys, inactive metabolite
Half-life	1 hr

Pharmacodynamics

	SC
Onset	15 min
Peak	4 hr
Duration	8-24 hr

Interactions: None

NURSING CONSIDERATIONS

Assessment

- Assess for GI symptoms, polyuria, flushing, head swelling, tingling, headache; may indicate hypercalcemia; nervousness, irritability, twitching, seizures, spasm, paresthesia indicate hypocalcemia during beginning of treatment
- Identify nutritional status; check diet for sources of vitamin D (milk, some seafood), calcium (dairy products, dark green vegetables), phosphates
- Monitor BUN, creatinine, uric acid, chloride, electrolytes, urine pH, urinary calcium, magnesium, phosphate, urinalysis (calcium should be kept at 9-10 mg/dl; vitamin D 50-135 IU/dl), alkaline phosphatase baseline and q3-6 mo; check urine sediment for casts throughout treatment
- Assess for increased drug level, since toxic reactions occur rapidly; have calcium chloride or gluconate on hand if calcium level drops too low; check for tetany

Associated nursing diagnoses

- ✓ Injury, risk for (adverse reactions)
- ✓ Pain, chronic (uses)
- ✓ Knowledge deficit (teaching)

Implementation

- Store at <77° F (25° C); protect from light

SC route

- Give by SC route only; rotate inj sites; use within 6 hr of reconstitution; give hs to minimize nausea, vomiting

Patient/family education

- Teach method of inj if patient will be responsible for self-medication
- Instruct patient to notify prescriber for hypercalcemic relapse: renal calculi, nausea, vomiting, thirst, lethargy, deep bone or flank pain
- Teach patient that warmth and flushing occur and last 1 hr
- Provide a low-calcium diet as prescribed (Paget's disease, hypercalcemia)
- Advise patients with osteoporosis to increase calcium and vitamin D in diet and to continue with moderate exercise to prevent continued bone loss

C

Evaluation

Positive therapeutic outcome
- Calcium levels 9-10 mg/dl
- Decreasing symptoms of Paget's disease, including pain
- Decreased bone loss in osteoporosis

calcitonin (salmon)
(kal-si-toe'nin)
Calcimar, Miacalcin
Func. class.: Parathyroid agents (calcium regulator)
Chem. class.: Polypeptide hormone
Pregnancy category **C**

Action: Decreases bone resorption, blood calcium levels by direct action on bone, GI system, and kidney; increases deposits of calcium in bones; renal excretion of calcium occurs

➡ **Therapeutic Outcome:** Lowered calcium level, decreasing symptoms of Paget's disease

Uses: Paget's disease, hypercalcemia, postmenopausal osteoporosis

Dosage and routes
Osteoporosis/Paget's disease
Adult: SC/IM 100 IU qd; maintenance for Paget's disease 50-100 IU qd or qod

Hypercalcemia
Adult: SC/IM 4-8 IU/kg q6-12h

Available forms: Inj SC/IM 200 IU/ml

Side effects/adverse reactions
CNS: Headache, flushing, *tetany*, chills, weakness, dizziness
GI: Nausea, diarrhea, vomiting, anorexia, abdominal pain, salty taste
GU: Diuresis
INTEG: Rash, pruritus of earlobes, edema of feet
MS: Swelling, tingling of hands

Contraindications: Hypersensitivity, P children, lactation

Precautions: Renal disease, osteoporosis, pernicious anemia, Zollinger-Ellison syndrome, pregnancy **C**

Pharmacokinetics

Absorption	Completely absorbed (IM, SC)
Distribution	Unknown
Metabolism	Rapid; kidneys, tissue, blood
Excretion	Kidneys, inactive metabolite
Half-life	Human 1 hr

Pharmacodynamics

	IM/SC
Onset	15 min
Peak	4 hr
Duration	8-24 hr

Interactions: None

NURSING CONSIDERATIONS
Assessment
- Assess for GI symptoms, polyuria, flushing, head swelling, tingling, headache; may indicate hypercalcemia; nervousness, irritability, twitching, seizures, spasm, paresthesia

indicate hypocalcemia during beginning of treatment
- Identify nutritional status; check diet for sources of vitamin D (milk, some seafood), calcium (dairy products, dark green vegetables), phosphates
- Monitor BUN, creatinine, uric acid, chloride, electrolytes, urine pH, urinary calcium, magnesium, phosphate, urinalysis (calcium should be kept at 9-10 mg/dl; vitamin D 50-135 IU/dl), alkaline phosphatase baseline and q3-6 mo; check urine sediment for casts throughout treatment
- Assess for increased drug level, since toxic reactions occur rapidly; have calcium chloride or gluconate on hand if calcium level drops too low; check for tetany

Associated nursing diagnoses

- ✓Injury, risk for (adverse reactions)
- ✓Pain, chronic (uses)
- ✓Knowledge deficit (teaching)

Implementation

- Store at <77° F (25° C); protect from light

SC route
- Give by SC route; rotate injection sites; use within 6 hr of reconstitution; give hs to minimize nausea, vomiting

IM route
- Rotate inj site; do not give >2 ml in one site

Patient/family education

- Teach method of injection if patient will be responsible for self-medication
- Instruct patient to notify prescriber for hypercalcemic relapse: renal calculi, nausea, vomiting, thirst, lethargy, deep bone or flank pain
- Teach patient that warmth and flushing occur and last 1 hr
- Provide a low calcium diet as prescribed (Paget's disease, hypercalcemia)
- Advise patients with osteoporosis to increase calcium and vitamin D in diet and to continue with moderate exercise to prevent continued bone loss

Evaluation

Positive therapeutic outcome
- Calcium levels 9-10 mg/dl
- Decreasing symptoms of Paget's disease including pain
- Decreased bone loss in osteoporosis

calcitriol (1,25-dihydroxycholecalciferol)

(kal-si-tree'ole)

Calcimar, Rocaltrol

Func. class.: Parathyroid agent (calcium regulator)

Chem. class.: Vitamin D hormone

Pregnancy category **C**

Action: Increases intestinal absorption of calcium, provides calcium for bones, increases renal tubular resorption of phosphate

➡ **Therapeutic Outcome:** Calcium at normal level

Uses: Hypocalcemia in chronic renal disease, hypoparathyroidism, pseudohypoparathyroidism

Dosage and routes

Hypocalcemia

Adult: PO 0.25 μg qd, may increase by 0.25 μg/day q4-8 wk; maintenance 0.25 μg qod-1 μg qd

Hypoparathyroidism/ pseudohypoparathyroidism

P *Adult and child >1 yr:* PO 0.25 μg qd; may be increased q2-4 wk; maintenance 0.25-2 μg qd

Available forms: Caps 0.25, 0.5 μg

Side effects/adverse reactions

CNS: Drowsiness, headache, vertigo, fever, lethargy
GI: Nausea, diarrhea, vomiting, jaundice, anorexia, dry mouth, constipation, cramps, metallic taste
GU: Polyuria, hypercalciuria, hyperphosphatemia, hematuria
MS: Myalgia, arthralgia, decreased bone development

Contraindications: Hypersensitivity, hyperphosphatemia, hypercalcemia, vitamin D toxicity

Precautions: Pregnancy **C**, renal calculi, lactation, CV disease

Pharmacokinetics

Absorption	Well absorbed
Distribution	To liver, crosses placenta
Metabolism	Liver
Excretion	Bile
Half-life	3-6 hr

Pharmacodynamics

	PO
Onset	2-6 hr
Peak	4 hr
Duration	Up to 5 days

Interactions: None

NURSING CONSIDERATIONS

Assessment

- Assess GI symptoms, polyuria, flushing, head swelling, tingling, headache; may indicate hypercalcemia
- Identify nutritional status; check diet for sources of vitamin D (milk, some seafood), calcium (dairy products, dark green vegetables), phosphates
- Monitor BUN, creatinine, uric acid, chloride, electrolytes, urine pH, urinary calcium, magnesium, phosphate, urinalysis (calcium should be kept at 9-10 mg/dl; vitamin D 50-135 IU/dl), alkaline phosphatase baseline and q3-6 mo
- Assess for increased drug level, since toxic reactions occur rapidly; have calcium chloride on hand if calcium level drops too low; check for tetany

Associated nursing diagnoses

- ✓ Injury, risk for (adverse reactions)
- ✓ Pain, chronic (uses)
- ✓ Knowledge deficit (teaching)

Implementation

PO route

- Give with meals for GI symptoms

Patient/family education

- Teach patient the symptoms of hypercalcemia and about foods rich in calcium
- Advise patient to avoid products with sodium: cured meats, dairy products, cold cuts, olives, beets, pickles, soups, meat tenderizers in chronic renal failure.
- Advise patient to avoid products with potassium: oranges, bananas, dried fruit, peas, dark green leafy vegetables, milk, melons, beans in chronic renal failure
- Advise patient to avoid OTC products containing calcium, potassium, or sodium in chronic renal failure
- Instruct patient to avoid all preparations containing Vit D
- Instruct patient to monitor weight weekly

Evaluation

Positive therapeutic outcome

- Calcium levels 9-10 mg/dl

calcium chloride/ calcium gluceptate/ calcium gluconate/ calcium lactate

Func. class.: Electrolyte replacement—calcium product

Pregnancy category C

Action: Cation needed for maintenance of nervous, muscular, skeletal systems, enzyme reactions, normal cardiac contractility, coagulation of blood; affects secretory activity of endocrine, exocrine glands

Therapeutic Outcome: Calcium at normal level, absence of increased magnesium, potassium

Uses: Prevention and treatment of hypocalcemia, hypermagnesemia, hypoparathyroidism, neonatal tetany, cardiac toxicity caused by hyperkalemia, lead colic, hyperphosphatemia, vitamin D deficiency

Dosage and routes

Calcium chloride

Adult: **IV** 500 mg-1 g q1-3 days as indicated by serum calcium levels; give at <1 ml/min; IAV 200-800 mg injected in ventricle of heart

P *Child:* **IV** 25 mg/kg over several min

Calcium gluceptate

Adult: **IV** 5-20 ml; IM 2-5 ml

P *Newborn:* 0.5 ml/100 ml of blood transfused

Calcium gluconate

Adult: PO 0.5-2 g bid-qid; **IV** 0.5-2 g at 0.5 ml/min (10% sol)

P *Child:* PO/**IV** 500 mg/kg/day in divided doses

Calcium lactate

Adult: PO 325 mg-1.3 g tid with meals

P *Child:* PO 500 mg/kg/day in divided doses

Available forms: Many; check product listings

Side effects/adverse reactions

CV: Shortened QT, heart block, hypotension, bradycardia, dysrythmias, ***cardiac arrest***
GI: Vomiting, nausea, constipation
HYPERCALCEMIA: Drowsiness, lethargy, muscle weakness, headache, constipation, ***coma,*** anorexia, nausea, vomiting, polyuria, thirst
INTEG: Pain, burning at **IV** site, severe venous thrombosis, necrosis, extravasation

Contraindications: Hypercalcemia, digitalis toxicity, ventricular fibrillation, renal calculi

Precautions: Pregnancy **C**, P lactation, children, renal disease, respiratory disease, cor pulmonale, digitalized patient, respiratory failure

Pharmacokinetics

Absorption	Complete bioavailability (IV)
Distribution	Readily extracellular; crosses placenta
Metabolism	Liver
Excretion	Feces (80%), kidney (20%), breast milk
Half-life	Unknown

Pharmacodynamics

	PO	IV
Onset	Unknown	Immediate
Peak	Unknown	Rapid
Duration	Unknown	½-1½ hr

Interactions

Drug/drug:

Individual drugs

Atenolol: ↓ effects of atenolol
Tetracycline: ↓ absorption of tetracycline (PO)
Verapamil: ↓ effects of verapamil

Drug classifications

Antacids: Milk-alkali syndrome (renal disease)
Cardiac glycosides: ↑ toxicity
Diuretics, thiazide: ↑ hypercalcemia
Fluoroquinolones: ↓ absorption of fluoroquinolones
Iron salts: ↓ absorption of iron

Drug/food: Calcium (dairy products): ↑ hypercalcemia

Lab test interferences

False decrease: Magnesium
Decrease: 17-OHCS

NURSING CONSIDERATIONS

Assessment

- Monitor ECG for decreased QT and T wave inversion: in hypercalcemia, drug should be reduced or discontinued
- Monitor calcium levels during treatment (9-10 mg/dl is normal level)
- Assess cardiac status: rate, rhythm, CVP, (PWP, PAWP if being monitored directly)

Associated nursing diagnoses

- ✓ Injury, risk for (uses, adverse reactions)
- ✓ Knowledge deficit (teaching)

Implementation

IV **IV route**

- Administer **IV** undiluted or diluted with equal amounts of 0.9% NaCl for inj to a 5% sol; give 0.5-1 ml/min

- Give through small-bore needle into large vein; if extravasation occurs, necrosis will result (**IV**); IM injection may cause severe burning, necrosis, and tissue sloughing; warm sol to body temp before administering
- Provide seizure precautions: padded side rails, decreased stimuli (noise, light); place airway suction equipment, padded mouth gag if calcium levels are low

PO route

- Give PO with or following meals to enhance absorption
- Store at room temp

Patient/family education

- Advise patient to remain recumbent 30 min after **IV** dose
- Caution patient to add food high in vitamin D content; to add calcium-rich foods to diet: dairy products, shellfish, dark green leafy vegetables; decrease oxalate-rich and zinc-rich foods: nuts, legumes, chocolate, spinach, soy
- Advise patient to prevent injuries, avoid immobilization

Evaluation

Positive therapeutic outcome

- Decreased twitching, paresthesias, muscle spasms
- Absence of tremors, convulsions, dysrhythmias, dyspnea, laryngospasm, negative Chvostek's sign, negative Trousseau's sign

calcium polycarbophil

(pol-i-kar'boe-fil)

Fiber Norm, Mitrolan

Func. class.: Laxative, bulk-forming

Pregnancy category **C**

C

Action: Attracts water, expands in intestine to increase peristalsis; also absorbs excess water in stool; decreases diarrhea

Therapeutic Outcome: Absence of constipation or diarrhea in irritable bowel syndrome

Uses: Constipation, irritable bowel syndrome (diarrhea), acute, nonspecific diarrhea

Dosage and routes

Adult: PO 1 g qd-qid prn, not to exceed 6 g/24 hr

P ***Child 6-12 yr:*** PO 500 mg bid prn, not to exceed 3 g/24 hr

P ***Child 3-6 yr:*** PO 500 mg bid prn, not to exceed 1.5 g/24 hr

Available forms: Chewable tabs 500, 625, 1250 mg

Side effects/adverse reactions

GI: ***Obstruction,*** abdominal distention, laxative dependency, flatus

Contraindications: Hypersensitivity, GI obstruction

Precautions: Pregnancy **C**

Pharmacokinetics

Absorption	None
Distribution	None
Excretion	Feces
Half-life	Not known

Pharmacodynamics

	PO
Onset	12-24 hr
Peak	1-3 days
Duration	Unknown

Interactions

Drug/drug:

Individual drugs

Tetracycline: ↓ absorption of tetracycline

NURSING CONSIDERATIONS

Assessment

- Monitor blood, urine electrolytes if used often by patient; check I&O ratio to identify fluid loss
- Assess cramping, rectal bleeding, nausea, vomiting; if these symptoms occur, drug should be discontinued; identify cause of constipation; identify whether fluids, bulk, or exercise is missing from lifestyle

Associated nursing diagnoses

✓ Constipation (uses)
✓ Diarrhea (side effects)
✓ Knowledge deficit (teaching)
✓ Noncompliance (teaching)

Implementation

PO route

- Give alone for better absorption; give after mixing with water immediately before use; administer with 8 oz water or juice followed by another 8 oz of fluid
- Administer in AM or PM

Patient/family education

- Discuss with the patient that adequate fluid consumption is necessary
- Teach patient that normal bowel movements do not always occur daily
- Teach patient not to use in presence of abdominal pain, nausea, vomiting; tell patient to notify prescriber if constipation unrelieved or if symptoms of electrolyte imbalance occur: muscle cramps, pain, weakness, dizziness, excessive thirst

Evaluation

Positive therapeutic outcome

- Decreased constipation within 3 days
- Decreased diarrhea in colitis within 1 wk

captopril 🔑

(kap'toe-pril)

Capoten

Func. class.: Antihypertensive

Chem. class.: Angiotensin-converting enzyme inhibitor

Pregnancy category C

Action: Selectively suppresses renin-angiotensin-aldosterone system; inhibits ACE; prevents conversion of angiotensin I to angiotensin II; results in dilatation of arterial, venous vessels

Therapeutic Outcome: Decreased B/P in hypertension; decreased preload, afterload in CHF

Uses: Hypertension, heart failure unresponsive to conventional therapy

Dosage and routes

Malignant hypertension

Adult: PO 25 mg increasing q2h until desired response; not to exceed 450 mg/day

Hypertension

Initial dose: 12.5 mg bid-tid; may increase to 50 mg bid-tid at 1-2 wk intervals; usual range 25-150 mg bid-tid; max 450 mg

CHF

Adult: PO 12.5 mg bid-tid given with a diuretic; may increase to 50 mg bid-tid; after 14 days may increase to 150 mg tid if needed

Available forms: Tabs 12.5, 25, 100 mg

Side effects/adverse reactions

CNS: Fever, chills
CV: Hypotension, postural hypotension
GI: Loss of taste
GU: Impotence, dysuria, nocturia, ***proteinuria, nephrotic syndrome, acute reversible renal failure,*** polyuria, oliguria, frequency
HEMA: Neutropenia
INTEG: Rash, ***angioedema***
META: Hyperkalemia
RESP: ***Bronchospasm,*** dyspnea, cough

Contraindications: Hypersensitivity, pregnancy **C**, lactation, P heart block, children, potassium-sparing diuretics, bilateral renal artery stenosis

Precautions: Dialysis patients, hypovolemia, leukemia, scleroderma, LE, blood dyscrasias, CHF, diabetes mellitus, renal disease, thyroid disease, COPD, asthma

Pharmacokinetics

Absorption	Well absorbed
Distribution	Widely distributed; crosses placenta
Metabolism	Liver (50%)
Excretion	Kidneys, unchanged (50%)
Half-life	1½-2 hr

Pharmacodynamics

	PO
Onset	¼-1 hr
Peak	1 hr
Duration	6-12 hr

Interactions

Drug/drug:

Individual drugs

Alcohol: ↑ hypotension (large amounts)
Allopurinol: ↑ hypersensitivity
Digoxin: ↑ serum levels
Indomethacin: ↓ antihypertensive effect
Lithium: ↑ serum levels
Tetracycline: ↓ absorption of tetracycline

Drug classifications

Antacids: ↓ absorption
Antihypertensives: ↑ hypotension
Diuretics: ↑ hypotension
Diuretics, potassium-sparing: ↑ toxicity

Potassium supplements: ↑ toxicity

Lab test interferences

False positive: Urine acetone

NURSING CONSIDERATIONS

Assessment

- Monitor blood studies: neutrophils, decreased platelets
- Monitor B/P, check for orthostatic hypotension, syncope; if changes occur, dosage change may be required
- Monitor renal studies: protein, BUN, creatinine; watch for increased levels that may indicate nephrotic syndrome and renal failure; monitor renal symptoms: polyuria, oliguria, frequency, dysuria
- Establish baselines in renal, liver function tests before therapy begins
- Check potassium levels throughout treatment, although hyperkalemia rarely occurs
- Check for edema in feet, legs daily; monitor weight daily
- Assess for allergic reactions: rash, fever, pruritus, urticaria; drug should be discontinued if antihistamines fail to help

Associated nursing diagnoses

✓ Cardiac output, decreased (uses)
✓ Injury, risk for (side effects)
✓ Knowledge deficit (teaching)
✓ Noncompliance (teaching)

Implementation

PO route

- Store in air-tight container at 86° F (30° C) or less
- Severe hypotension may occur after 1st dose of this medication; decreasing hypotension may be prevented by reducing or discontinuing diuretic therapy 3 days before beginning benzapril therapy
- Give **IV** inf of 0.9% NaCl (as ordered) to expand fluid volume if severe hypotension occurs

Patient/family education

- Caution patient not to discontinue drug abruptly; advise patient to tell all persons associated with care
- Teach patient not to use OTC products (cough, cold, allergy) unless directed by prescriber; serious side effects can occur; xanthines such as coffee, tea, chocolate, cola can prevent action of drug
- Teach patient importance of complying with dosage schedule, even if feeling better; to continue with medical regimen to decrease B/P: exercise, cessation of smoking, decreasing stress, diet modifications
- Emphasize the need to rise slowly to sitting or standing position to minimize orthostatic hypotension; not to exercise in hot weather or increased hypotension can occur
- Teach patient to notify prescriber of mouth sores, sore throat, fever, swelling of hands or feet, irregular heartbeat, chest pain, coughing, shortness of breath
- Caution patient to report excessive perspiration, dehydration, vomiting, diarrhea; may lead to fall in B/P
- Caution patient that drug may cause dizziness, fainting,

light-headedness; may occur during 1st few days of therapy; to avoid activities that may be hazardous
• Teach patient how to take B/P, and teach normal readings for age group; ensure patient takes regularly

Evaluation

Positive therapeutic outcome
• Decreased B/P in hypertension

Treatment of overdose: 0.9% NaCl **IV** infusion, hemodialysis

carbachol

(kar'ba-kole)

Isoptocarbachol, Miostat

Func. class.: Miotic, cholinergic

Pregnancy category **C**

Action: Contracts sphincter muscle of iris; causes spasms of ciliary muscle, deepening of anterior chamber

➔ **Therapeutic Outcome:** Reduction of intraocular pressure

Uses: Miosis in ocular surgery, glaucoma (open angle, narrow angle)

Dosage and routes

Ocular surgery

Adult: Instill 0.5 ml (intraocular) of 0.01% sol in anterior chamber of eye (done by physician) for miosis during surgery

Glaucoma

Adult: Instill 1-2 gtt (top) of 0.75%-3% sol into eye bid-tid

Available forms: 0.75%, 1.5%, 2.25%, 3.0% sol for top use; sol, powders for preparing sol for inj

Side effects/adverse reactions

CV:* *Marked hypotension, bradycardia, headache
EENT: Blurred vision, varying degrees of myopia, decreased visual acuity in dim light, slight conjunctival hyperemia, altered distance vision, decreased night vision, eyeache
GI: Nausea, vomiting, abdominal discomfort, diarrhea, salivation
RESP: Asthma attacks

Contraindications: Hypersensitivity; when miosis is undesirable; corneal abrasions

Precautions: Bradycardia, CAD, hyperthyroidism, asthma, pregnancy, obstruction of GI or urinary tract, peptic ulcer, parkinsonism, epilepsy, peritonitis

Pharmacokinetics

Absorption	Minimal
Distribution	Minimal
Metabolism	None
Excretion	Lacrimation
Half-life	Short

Pharmacokinetics

	OPHTHALMIC
Onset	10-20 min (miosis)
Peak	Unknown
Duration	4-8 hr

NURSING CONSIDERATIONS

Assessment

- Assess heart, respiratory rate, B/P; lung sounds, changes in respiratory rate; if these occur, notify prescriber

Associated nursing diagnoses

✓ Pain (uses)
✓ Sensory-perceptual alteration: visual (uses)
✓ Knowledge deficit (teaching)

Implementation

Ophthalmic route
- Use reconstituted sol immediately; discard unused portion

Patient/family education

- Teach patient to report change in vision, blurring, or loss of sight, trouble breathing, sweating, flushing
- Teach patient method of instillation, including pressure on lacrimal sac for 1 min, and not to touch dropper to eye; use demonstration, return demonstration
- Advise patient that blurred vision will decrease with repeated use of drug
- Caution patient not to drive during first few days of treatment; visual changes may occur including impaired night vision, eye and brow ache

Evaluation

Positive therapeutic outcome
- Decreasing intraocular pressure; miosis during ocular surgery

carbamazepine

(kar-ba-maz'e-peen)
Apo-Carbamazepine ✦, Epitol, Mazepine ✦, Tegretol
Func. class.: Anticonvulsant
Chem. class.: Iminostilbene derivative
Pregnancy category C

Action: Inhibits nerve impulses by limiting influx of sodium ions across cell membrane in motor cortex

➔ **Therapeutic Outcome:** Absence of seizures; decreased trigeminal neuralgia pain

Uses: Tonic-clonic, complex-partial, mixed seizures; trigeminal neuralgia

Investigational uses: Diabetes insipidus, bipolar disorder, neurogenic pain

Dosage and routes

Seizures

P ***Adult and child >12 yr:*** PO 200 mg bid; may be increased by 200 mg/day in divided doses q6-8h; maintenance 800-1200 mg/day; maximum 1200 mg/day; adjustment is needed to minimum dose to control seizures

P ***Child <12 yr:*** PO 10-20 mg/kg day in 2-3 divided doses

Trigeminal neuralgia

Adult: PO 100 mg/bid; may increase 100 mg q12h until pain subsides; not to exceed

1.2 g/day; maintenance is 200-400 mg bid

Available forms: Chewable tabs 100 mg; tabs 200 mg; oral susp 100 mg/5 ml; ext rel ✤ 200, 400 mg

Side effects/adverse reactions

CNS: Drowsiness, dizziness, confusion, fatigue, ***paralysis,*** headache, hallucinations
CV: Hypertension, CHF, hypotension, aggravation of CAD
EENT: Tinnitus, dry mouth, blurred vision, diplopia, nystagmus, conjunctivitis
GI: Nausea, constipation, diarrhea, anorexia, vomiting, abdominal pain, stomatitis, glossitis, increased liver enzymes, ***hepatitis***
GU: Frequency, retention, albuminuria, glycosuria, impotence
HEMA: Thrombocytopenia, agranulocytosis, leukocytosis, neutropenia, aplastic anemia, eosinophilia, increased pro-time
INTEG: Rash, ***Stevens-Johnson syndrome,*** urticaria
RESP: Pulmonary hypersensitivity (fever, dyspnea, pneumonitis)

Contraindications: Hypersensitivity to carbamazepine or tricyclic antidepressants, bone marrow depression, concomitant use of MAOIs

Precautions: Glaucoma, hepatic disease, renal disease, cardiac disease, psychosis, pregnancy **C**, lactation, P child <6 yr

Pharmacokinetics

Absorption	Slow; completely absorbed
Distribution	Widely distributed
Metabolism	Extensively, liver
Half-life	14-16 hr or more

Pharmacodynamics

	PO
Onset	2-4 day
Peak	4-8 hr
Duration	Unknown

Interactions

Drug/drug:

Individual drugs

Acetaminophen: ↑ metabolism, ↓ action
Doxycycline: ↓ half-life
Haloperidol: ↓ serum levels, ↓ therapeutic efficacy
Phenobarbital: ↑ effects
Phenytoin: ↑ and ↓ plasma levels, ↓ carbamazepine plasma levels
Lithium: ↑ CNS toxicity
Theophylline: ↓ effect of theophylline, carbamazepine
Valproic acid: ↓ plasma levels, ↑ half-life of carbamazepine

Drug classifications

Barbiturates: ↓ serum levels of carbamazepine
Nondepolarizing muscle relaxants: Resistance to or reversal of effects of these agents
Posterior pituitary hormones: Potentiates antidiuretic effects
Succinimides: ↓ plasma levels

Lab test interferences

Decrease: Thyroid function tests

NURSING CONSIDERATIONS

Assessment

- Monitor liver function tests (AST [SGOT], ALT [SGOT]) and urine function tests, BUN, urine protein periodically during treatments
- Check blood levels during treatment; therapeutic level 6-12 µg/ml
- Assess for blood dyscrasias: fever, sore throat, bruising, rash, jaundice, epistaxis (long-term treatment only)
- Assess seizure activity including type, location, duration, and character; provide seizure precaution

Associated nursing diagnoses

✓ Injury, risk for (side effects)
✓ Knowledge deficit (teaching)

Implementation

PO route
- Give with food for GI symptoms

Patient/family education

- Teach patient to carry Medic Alert ID stating patient's name, drugs taken, condition, prescriber's name, phone number
- Caution patient to avoid driving, other activities that require alertness until stabilized on medication
- Teach patient not to discontinue medication quickly after long-term use
- Teach patient to use a nonhormonal type of contraception to prevent harm to the fetus
- Advise patient to use sunscreen to prevent burns
- Teach patient to take exactly as prescribed, do not double or omit doses

Evaluation

Positive therapeutic outcome
- Decreased seizure activity

Treatment of overdose:
Lavage, vital signs

carbidopa-levodopa
(kar-bi-doe'pa lee-voe-doe'pa)
carbidopa/levodopa, Sinemet, Sinemet CR
Func. class.: Antiparkinsonism agent
Chem. class.: Catecholamine
Pregnancy category **C**

Action: Decarboxylation of levodopa to periphery is inhibited by carbidopa; more levodopa is made available for transport to brain and conversion to dopamine in the brain

➔ **Therapeutic Outcome:** Absence of involuntary movements

Uses: Parkinsonism

Dosage and routes

Adult: PO 3-6 tabs of 25 mg carbidopa/250 mg levodopa qd in divided doses, not to exceed 8 tabs/day; sus rel 1 tab bid at intervals of not less than 6 hr; usual dosage 2-8 tabs/day at intervals of 4-8 hr

Available forms: Tabs 10/100, 25/100, 25 mg carbidopa/250 mg levodopa; sus rel tabs 50 mg/200 mg (carbidopa/levodopa)

Side effects/adverse reactions

CNS: *Involuntary choreiform movements, hand tremors, fatigue, headache, anxiety, twitching, numbness, weakness, confusion, agitation, insomnia, nightmares,* psychosis, hallucination, hypomania, severe depression, dizziness
CV: *Orthostatic hypotension,* tachycardia, hypertension, palpitation
EENT: Blurred vision, diplopia, dilated pupils
GI: *Nausea, vomiting, anorexia, abdominal distress, dry mouth, flatulence, dysphagia, bitter taste, diarrhea, constipation*
HEMA: ***Hemolytic anemia, leukopenia, agranulocytosis***
INTEG: Rash, sweating, alopecia
MISC: Urinary retention, incontinence, weight change, dark urine

Contraindications: Hypersensitivity, narrow angle glaucoma, undiagnosed skin lesions

Precautions: Renal disease, cardiac disease, hepatic disease, respiratory disease, MI with dysrhythmias, convulsions, peptic ulcer, pregnancy **C**

Pharmacokinetics

Absorption	Well absorbed (PO); sus rel dose slow
Distribution	Widely distributed
Metabolism	Liver, extensively
Excretion	Kidneys, metabolites
Half-life	Levodopa (1 hr); carbidopa (1-2 hr)

Pharmacodynamics

	PO	PO-SUS REL
Onset	Unknown	Unknown
Peak	1 hr	2½ hr
Duration	6-24 hr	Unknown

Interactions

Drug/drug:

Individual drugs

Metoclopramide: ↑ effects of levodopa
Papaverine: ↓ effects of levodopa
Pyridoxine: ↓ effects of levodopa

Drug classifications

Antacids: ↑ effect of levodopa
Anticholinergics: ↓ effects of levodopa
Antidepressants, tricyclics: ↑ hypotension
Benzodiazepines: ↓ effects of levodopa
Hydantoins: ↓ effects of levodopa
MAOI: Hypertensive crisis

Lab test interferences

False positive: Urine ketones
False negative: Urine glucose
False increase: Uric acid, urine protein
Decrease: VMA, BUN, creatinine

NURSING CONSIDERATIONS

Assessment

- Monitor I&O ratio; retention commonly causes decreased urinary output, distention, frequency, incontinence; palpate bladder if retention occurs
- Assess for parkinsonism, shuffling gait, muscle rigidity, involuntary movements, pill rolling, muscle spasms, drooling before and during treatment
- Monitor for constipation, cramping, pain in abdomen, abdominal distention; increase fluids, bulk, exercise if this occurs
- Assess for tolerance over long-term therapy; dose may have to be increased or changed
- Assess for mental status: affect, mood, CNS depression, worsening of mental symptoms during early therapy

Associated nursing diagnoses

✓ Physical mobility, impaired (uses)
✓ Knowledge deficit (teaching)

Implementation

PO route

- Give drug until NPO before surgery; check with prescriber for continuing drug
- Adjust dosage depending on patient response
- Give with meals or pc to prevent GI symptoms; limit protein taken with drug
- Give only after MAOIs have been discontinued for 2 wk; if previously on levodopa, discontinue for at least 8 hr before change to levodopa-carbidopa
- Controlled-release tabs should be swallowed whole, not crushed or chewed

Patient/family education

- Teach patient to change positions slowly to prevent orthostatic hypotension
- Teach patient to report side effects: twitching, eye spasms, grimacing, protrusion of tongue, personality changes that indicate overdose
- Instruct patient to use drug exactly as prescribed; if drug is discontinued abruptly, parkinsonian crisis may occur; do not double doses; take missed dose as soon as remembered up to 2 hr before next dose
- Teach patient that urine, sweat may darken and is harmless
- Advise patient to use physical activities to maintain mobility and lessen spasms
- Instruct patient that OTC medications should not be used unless approved by prescriber
- Advise patient that drowsiness, dizziness are common; to avoid hazardous activities until response is known
- Explain that sips of water, hard candy, or gum may lessen dry mouth
- Teach patient to take with meals to prevent GI symptoms; to limit protein intake, which impairs drug's absorption

Evaluation

Positive therapeutic outcome

- Decrease in akathisia
- Improved mood
- Decreased involuntary movements

carboplatin

(kar'boe'pla-tin)
Paraplatin
Func. class.: Antineoplastic alkylating agent
Chem. class.: Platinum coordination compound
Pregnancy category **D**

Action: Produces interstrand DNA cross-links and to a lesser extent DNA-protein cross-links; activity is not cell cycle phase specific

➡ Therapeutic Outcome: Prevention of rapidly growing malignant cells

Uses: Palliative treatment of ovarian carcinoma recurrent after treatment with other antineoplastic agents, including cisplatin

Dosage and routes

(single agent)
Adult: **IV** inf 360 mg/m^2 given over 15 min on day 1 q4 wk; do not repeat single intermittent courses until neutrophil count is >2000/mm^3 and platelet count is >100,000/mm^3

Available forms: Inj 50, 150, 450 mg/vial

Side effects/adverse reactions

CNS: Convulsions, central neurotoxicity, peripheral neuropathy
CV: Cardiac abnormalities
EENT: Tinnitus, hearing loss, ***vestibular toxicity***
GI: Severe nausea, vomiting, diarrhea, weight loss
GU: Renal tubular damage, renal insufficiency, impotence, sterility, amenorrhea, gynecomastia
HEMA: Thrombocytopenia, leukopenia, pancytopenia, neutropenia, anemia, bleeding
INTEG: Alopecia, dermatitis, rash, erythema, pruritus, urticaria
META: Hypomagnesemia, hypocalcemia, hypokalemia, hyponatremia, hyperuremia
RESP: Mucositis

Contraindications: Hypersensitivity to this drug, platinum products, mannitol; severe bone marrow depression, significant bleeding, pregnancy **D**

Precautions: Radiation therapy with 1 mo, chemotherapy with 1 mo, lactation, liver disease

Pharmacokinetics

Absorption	Complete (IV)
Distribution	Unknown
Metabolism	Liver
Excretion	Kidneys
Half-life	Initial 1-2 hr; post-distribution 2½-6 hr; increased in renal disease

Pharmacodynamics

	IV
Onset	½ hr
Peak	Unknown
Duration	4-6 hr

Interactions

Drug/drug:

Individual drugs

Radiation: ↑ toxicity, bone marrow suppression

Drug classifications

Aminoglycosides: ↑ nephrotoxicity

Antineoplastics: ↑ toxicity, bone marrow suppression

Bone marrow–suppressing drugs: ↑ bone marrow suppression

Diuretics, loop: ↑ ototoxicity

Lab test interferences

False positive: Breast, bladder, cervix, lung, cytology tests

NURSING CONSIDERATIONS

Assessment

- Monitor CBC, differential, platelet count weekly; withhold drug if WBC count is <4000/mm^3 or platelet count is <100,000/mm^3; notify prescriber of results if WBC <20,000/mm^3, platelets <150,000/mm^3
- Monitor renal function studies: BUN, creatinine, serum uric acid, urine CrCl before and during therapy; I&O ratio; report fall in urine output to <30 ml/hr
- Monitor temp q4h (may indicate beginning of infection)
- Monitor liver function tests before and during therapy (bilirubin, AST [SGOT], ALT [SGPT], LDH) as needed or monthly; note yellowing of skin or sclera, dark urine, clay-colored stools, itchy skin, abdominal pain, fever, diarrhea
- Assess for bleeding: hematuria, stool guaiac, bruising or petechiae, mucosa or orifices q8h; inflammation of mucosa, breaks in skin
- Identify dyspnea, rales, unproductive cough, chest pain, tachypnea
- Identify effects of alopecia on body image; discuss feelings about body changes

Associated nursing diagnoses

- ✓ Injury, risk for (adverse reactions)
- ✓ Body image disturbance (adverse reactions)
- ✓ Infection, risk for (adverse reactions)
- ✓ Knowledge deficit (teaching)

Implementation

- Antiemetic 30-60 min before giving drug to prevent vomiting, and prn
- Administer antibiotics for prophylaxis of infection

IV **IV route**

- Give **IV** after diluting 10 mg/ml of sterile water for inj, D_5W, NS (10 mg/ml); then further dilute with the same sol 1-4 mg/ml; give over 15 min or more (intermittent inf)
- Give **IV** inf over 5-6 hr; do not use needles or **IV** administration sets containing aluminum; may cause precipitate
- Store protected from light at room temp; reconstituted sol are stable for 8 hr at room temp

Y-site compatibilities:

Fludarabine, melphalan, ondansetron, paclitaxel, sargramostim, vinorelbine

Additive compatibilities:
Ifosfamide, ifosfamide with etoposide

Additive incompatibilities:
Fluorouracil, mesna

Solution compatibilities:
D_5/0.2% NaCl, D_5/0.45% NaCl, D_5/0.9% NaCl, 0.9% NaCl, sterile water for inj

Solution incompatibility:
Sodium bicarbonate

Patient/family education

- Teach patient to avoid use of products containing aspirin or ibuprofen, razors, commercial mouthwash, since bleeding may occur; to report symptoms of bleeding (hematuria, tarry stools)
- Instruct patient to report signs of anemia (fatigue, headache, irritability, faintness, shortness of breath)
- Instruct patient to report any changes in breathing or coughing even several months after treatment; to avoid crowds and persons with respiratory tract or other infections
- Advise patient that hair may be lost during treatment; a wig or hairpiece may make patient feel better; new hair may be different in color, texture
- Caution patient not to have any vaccinations without the advice of the prescriber; serious reactions can occur
- Teach patient contraception is needed during treatment and for several months after the completion of therapy

Evaluation

Positive therapeutic outcome
- Prevention of rapid division of malignant cells

C

carboprost

(kar'boe-prost)
Hemabate,
Prostin/15M ✱
Func. class.: Oxytocic
Chem. class.: Prostaglandin
Pregnancy category C

Action: Stimulates uterine contractions, causing complete abortion in approximately 16 hr

➔ **Therapeutic Outcome:** Loss of fetus; decreased postpartum bleeding

Uses: Abortion between 13-20 wk gestation; postpartum hemorrhage

Dosage and routes

Adult: IM 250 μg, then 250 μg q1½-3½ hr, may increase to 500 μg if no response, not to exceed 12 mg total dose

Available forms: Inj IM 250 μg/ml carboprost

Side effects/adverse reactions

CNS: *Fever, chills,* headache
GI: *Nausea, vomiting, diarrhea*

Contraindications: Hypersensitivity, severe hepatic disease, severe renal disease, PID, respiratory disease, cardiac disease

Precautions: Asthma, anemia, jaundice, diabetes mellitus, convulsive disorders, past uterine surgery, pregnancy category **C**

Pharmacokinetics

Absorption	Well absorbed (nasal)
Distribution	Widely distributed (extracellular fluid)
Metabolism	Liver—rapidly
Excretion	Kidneys
Half-life	3-9 min

Pharmacodynamics

Onset	Unknown
Peak	16 hr
Duration	Unknown

Interactions

Drug/drug:

Drug classifications

Oxytocics: ↑ effects

NURSING CONSIDERATIONS

Assessment

- Monitor B/P, pulse; watch for change that may indicate hemorrhage
- Monitor respiratory rate, rhythm, depth; notify physician of abnormalities
- For length, duration of contraction; notify physician of contractions lasting over 1 min or absence of contractions
- Assess for incomplete abortion, pregnancy must be terminated by another method; drug is teratogenic

Associated nursing diagnoses

✓ Knowledge deficit (teaching)

Implementation

- Give IM in deep muscle mass; rotate injection sites if additional doses are given
- Have crash cart available on unit

Patient/family education

- Advise patient to report increased blood loss, abdominal cramps, increased temperature or foul-smelling lochia
- Teach methods of comfort control and pain control

Evaluation

Positive therapeutic outcome

- Loss of fetus

carisoprodol

(kar-i-soe-proe′dole)

carisoprodol, Rela, Sodol, Soma, Soprodol, Soridol

Func. class.: Skeletal muscle relaxant, central acting

Chem. class.: Meprobamate congener

Pregnancy category C

Action: Depresses CNS by blocking interneuronal activity in descending reticular formation of spinal cord, producing sedation

Therapeutic Outcome: Relaxation of skeletal muscles

Uses: Relieving pain, stiffness in musculoskeletal disorders

Dosage and routes

P ***Adult and child >12 yr:***
PO 350 mg tid-qid

Available forms: Tabs 350 mg

Side effects/adverse reactions

CNS: Dizziness, weakness, drowsiness, headache, tremor, depression, insomnia, ataxia, irritability
CV: Postural hypotension, tachycardia
EENT: Diplopia, temporary loss of vision
GI: Nausea, vomiting, hiccups, epigastric discomfort
INTEG: Rash, pruritus, fever, facial flushing

Contraindications: Hypersensitivity, P child <12 yr, intermittent porphyria

Precautions: Renal disease, hepatic disease, addictive personality, pregnancy **C**, elderly

Pharmacokinetics

Absorption	Well absorbed (PO)
Distribution	Crosses placenta
Metabolism	Liver, partially
Excretion	Kidney, unchanged; breast milk
Half-life	8 hr

Pharmacodynamics

	PO
Onset	½ hr
Peak	Unknown
Duration	4-6 hr

Interactions

Drug/drug:

Individual drugs

Alcohol: ↑ CNS depression

Drug classifications

Antidepressants, tricyclic: ↑ CNS depression
Barbiturates: ↑ CNS depression
Narcotics: ↑ CNS depression
Sedative/hypnotics: ↑ CNS depression

Lab test interferences

Increase: AST (SGOT), alkaline phosphatase, blood glucose

NURSING CONSIDERATIONS

Assessment

- Monitor ROM, atrophy, stiffness, and pain in muscles; assess throughout treatment
- Assess for idiosyncratic reaction with a few min or hr of administration (disorientation, restlessness, weakness, blurred vision); patient should be reassured that reaction is temporary.
- Check for allergic reactions: rash, fever

Associated nursing diagnoses

- ✓ Mobility, impaired uses
- ✓ Injury, risk for (adverse reactions)
- ✓ Knowledge deficit (teaching)

Implementation

PO route

- Give with meals for GI symptoms
- Have patient use gum, frequent sips of water for dry mouth

• Store in tight container at room temp

Patient/family education

• Caution patient not to take with alcohol, other CNS depressants
• Advise patient to avoid altering activities while taking this drug
• Caution patient to avoid hazardous activities if drowsiness or dizziness occurs
• Caution patient to avoid using OTC medication such as cough preparations, antihistamines, unless directed by prescriber

Evaluation

Positive therapeutic outcome
• Decreased pain, spasticity

Treatment of overdose: Induce emesis of conscious patient, lavage, dialysis

carmustine (BCNU)

(kar-mus'teen)
BiCNU, BCNU
Func. class.: Antineoplastic alkylating agent
Chem. class.: Nitrosourea
Pregnancy category **D**

Action: Alkylates DNA, RNA; inhibits enzymes that allow synthesis of amino acids in proteins; also responsible for cross-linking DNA strands; activity is not cell cycle phase specific

Therapeutic Outcome: Prevention of rapidly growing malignant cells

Uses: Brain tumors such as glioblastoma, medulloblastoma, astrocytoma; multiple myeloma, Hodgkin's disease, other lymphomas; GI, breast, bronchogenic and renal carcinomas

Dosage and routes

Adult: **IV** 75-100 mg/m^2 over 1-2 hr × 2 days or 200 mg/m^2 × 1 dose q6-8 wk; if leukocytes fall below 2000 or platelets below 75,000, only 50% of dose should be given

Available forms: Inj 100 mg

Side effects/adverse reactions

GI: Nausea, vomiting, anorexia, stomatitis, hepatotoxicity
GU: Azotemia, ***renal failure***
HEMA: Thrombocytopenia, leukopenia, myelosuppression, anemia
INTEG: Burning, hyperpigmentation at inj site, alopecia
RESP: Fibrosis, pulmonary infiltrate

Contraindications: Hypersensitivity, leukopenia, thrombocytopenia

Precautions: Pregnancy **D**

Pharmacokinetics

Absorption	Completely absorbed (IV)
Distribution	Readily penetrates CSF
Metabolism	Liver, rapid
Excretion	Kidneys, breast milk
Half-life	Unknown

Pharmacodynamics

	IV
Onset	Unknown
Peak	Unknown
Duration	Unknown

Interactions

Drug/drug:

Individual drugs

Phenytoin: ↑ metabolism, ↓ effect
Radiation: ↑ toxicity, bone marrow suppression

Drug classifications

Antineoplastics: ↑ toxicity, bone marrow suppression
Bone marrow–suppressing drugs: ↑ bone marrow suppression
Live vaccines: ↑ adverse reactions, ↓ antibody reaction

NURSING CONSIDERATIONS

Assessment

- Assess buccal cavity q8h for dryness, sores or ulceration, white patches, pain, bleeding, dysphagia; obtain prescription for viscous lidocaine (Xylocaine)
- Assess symptoms indicating severe allergic reaction: rash, pruritus, urticaria, purpuric skin lesions, itching, flushing; drug should be discontinued
- Monitor CBC, differential, platelet count weekly; withhold drug if WBC count is <4000/mm^3 or platelet count is <100,000/mm^3; notify prescriber of results if WBC <20,000/mm^3, platelets <150,000/mm^3
- Monitor renal function studies: BUN, creatinine, urine CrCl before and during therapy; I&O ratio; report fall in urine output to <30 ml/hr
- Monitor temp q4h (may indicate beginning of infection)
- Monitor liver function tests before and during therapy (bilirubin, AST [SGOT], ALT [SGPT], LDH) as needed or monthly; note yellowing of skin or sclera, dark urine, clay-colored stools, itchy skin, abdominal pain, fever, diarrhea; hepatoxicity can be serious and fatal
- Assess for bleeding: hematuria, stool guaiac, bruising or petechiae, mucosa or orifices q8h; inflammation of mucosa, breaks in skin
- Identify effects of alopecia on body image; discuss feelings about body changes

Associated nursing diagnoses

- ✓ Injury, risk for (adverse reactions)
- ✓ Body image disturbance (adverse reactions)
- ✓ Infection, risk for (adverse reactions)
- ✓ Knowledge deficit (teaching)

Implementation

IV route

- Administer after diluting 100 mg/3 ml ethyl alcohol (provided); then further dilute 27 ml sterile water for inj; then dilute with 100-500 ml 0.9% NaCl or D_5W; give over 1 hr or more; reduce rate if discomfort is felt

- Give fluids **IV** or PO before chemotherapy to hydrate patient
- Provide antiemetic 30-60 min before giving drug to prevent vomiting, and prn; antibiotics for prophylaxis of infection
- Provide liq diet (carbonated beverages); gelatin may be added if patient is not nauseated or vomiting

Additive incompatibility: Sodium bicarbonate

Y-site compatibilities: Fludarabine, melphalan, ondansetron, sargramostim, vinorelbine

Patient/family education

- Teach patient to avoid use of products containing aspirin or ibuprofen, razors, commercial mouthwash, since bleeding may occur; to report symptoms of bleeding (hematuria, tarry stools)
- Instruct patient to report signs of anemia (fatigue, headache, irritability, faintness, shortness of breath)
- Advise patient that hair may be lost during treatment; a wig or hair piece may make patient feel better; new hair may be different in color, texture
- Caution patient not to have any vaccinations without the advice of the prescriber; serious reactions can occur
- Advise patient contraception is needed during treatment and for several months after the completion of therapy; drug has teratogenic properties

Evaluation

Positive therapeutic outcome

- Prevention of rapid division of malignant cells

carteolol

(kar-tee'oe-lole)

Cartrol, Ocupress

Func.class.: Antihypertensive

Chem. class.: Nonselective β-blocker

Pregnancy category C

Action: Produces fall in B/P without reflex tachycardia or significant reduction in heart rate through mixture of alpha-blocking, beta-blocking effects and intrinsic sympathomimetic activity; elevated plasma renins are reduced; decreased intraoccual pressure in glaucoma and intraoccular hypertension

Therapeutic Outcome: Decreased B/P, heart rate; decreased intraoccular pressure

Uses: Mild to moderate hypertension

Dosage and routes

Adult: PO 2.5 mg tid initially; may gradually increase to desired response

Available forms: Tabs 2.5, 5, 10, mg; Oph sol 1%

C

Side effects/adverse reactions

CNS: Dizziness, mental changes, drowsiness, fatigue, headache, catatonia, depression, anxiety, nightmares, paresthesia, lethargy, insomnia, decreased concentration
CV: Orthostatic hypotension, ***bradycardia, CHF, chest pain, ventricular dysrhythmias, AV block, peripheral vascular insufficency,*** palpitations
EENT: Tinnitus, visual changes, sore throat, double vision, dry, burning eyes
GI: Nausea, vomiting, diarrhea, dry mouth, flatulence, constipation, anorexia
GU: Impotence, dysuria, ejaculatory failure, urinary retention
HEMA: Agranulocytosis, thrombocytopenic purpura (rare)
INTEG: Rash, alopecia, urticaria, pruritus, fever
MS: Joint pain, arthralgia, muscle cramps, pain
OTHER: Facial swelling, decreased exercise tolerance, weight change, Raynaud's disease
RESP: ***Bronchospasm,*** dyspnea, wheezing, nasal stuffiness, pharyngitis

Contraindications: Hypersensitivity to β-blockers, cardiogenic shock, heart block (2nd or 3rd degree), sinus bradycardia, CHF, bronchial asthma

Precautions: Major surgery, pregnancy **C**, lactation, diabetes mellitus, renal disease, thyroid disease, COPD, well-compensated heart failure, nonallergic bronchospasm

Pharmacokinetics

Absorption	80%-90%
Distribution	Unknown; protein binding 23%-30%
Metabolism	Liver to active metabolite
Excretion	Kidneys, unchanged (50%-75%)
Half-life	Carteolol (6-8 hr); metabolite (8-12 hr); ↑ renal disease

Pharmacodynamics

	PO	OPH
Onset	Unknown	Unknown
Peak	1-3 hr	Unknown
Duration	Unknown	Unknown

Interactions

Drug/drug:

Individual drugs

Alcohol: ↑ hypotension (large amounts)
Epinephrine: α-Adrenergic stimulation
Hydralazine: ↑ hypotension, bradycardia
Indomethacin: ↓ antihypertensive effect
Insulin: ↑ hypoglycemia
Prazosin: ↑ hypotension, bradycardia
Reserpine: ↑ hypotension, bradycardia
Thyroid: ↓ effectiveness of carteolol
Verapamil: ↑ myocardial depression

Drug classifications

Antihypertensives: ↑ hypertension
β_2-Agonists: ↓ bronchodilatation

Cardiac glycosides: ↑ bradycardia
Theophyllines: ↓ bronchodilatation

Lab test interferences

False increase: Urinary catecholamines

NURSING CONSIDERATIONS

Assessment

- Monitor B/P during beginning treatment, periodically thereafter; pulse q4h; note rate, rhythm, quality: apical/radial pulse before administration; notify prescriber of any significant changes (pulse <50 bpm)
- Check for baselines in renal, liver function tests before therapy begins
- Assess for edema in feet, legs daily; monitor I&O, daily weight; check for jugular vein distention and rales bilaterally, dyspnea (CHF)
- Monitor skin turgor, dryness of mucous membranes for hydration status, especially G elderly

Associated nursing diagnoses

- ✓ Cardiac output, decreased (uses)
- ✓ Injury, risk for (side effects)
- ✓ Knowledge deficit (teaching)
- ✓ Noncompliance (teaching)

Implementation

PO route

- Give ac, hs; tab may be crushed or swallowed whole; give with food to prevent GI upset; reduce dosage in renal dysfunction
- Store protected from light, moisture; placed in cool environment

Patient/family education

- Teach patient not to discontinue drug abruptly; taper over 2 wk; may cause precipitate dysrhythmias, hypertension if stopped abruptly
- Teach patient not to use OTC products containing α-adrenergic stimulants (such as nasal decongestants, cold preparations); to avoid alcohol, smoking and to limit sodium intake as prescribed
- Teach patient how to take pulse and B/P at home; advise when to notify prescriber
- Instruct patient to comply with weight control, dietary adjustments, modified exercise program
- Advise patient to carry/wear Medic Alert ID to identify drug being taken, allergies; tell patient drug controls symptoms but does not cure
- Caution patient to avoid hazardous activities if dizziness, drowsiness present
- Teach patient to report symptoms of CHF; difficult breathing, especially on exertion or when lying down, night cough, swelling of extremities or bradycardia, dizziness, confusion, depression, fever
- Teach patient to take drug as prescribed, not to double doses, skip doses; take any missed doses as soon as remembered if at least 4 hr until next dose

Evaluation

Positive therapeutic outcome

- Decreased B/P in hypertension (after 1-2 wk)

• Lessened intraocular pressure in glaucoma

Treatment of overdose: Lavage, **IV** atropine for bradycardia; **IV** theophylline for bronchospasm, digitalis, O_2, diuretic for cardiac failure; hemodialysis, **IV** glucose for hyperglycemia; **IV** diazepam (or phenytoin) for seizures

cascara sagrada/ cascara sagrada aromatic fluid extract/ cascara sagrada fluid extract

(kas-kar'a)

Func. class.: Laxative

Chem. class.: Anthraquinone

Pregnancy category **C**

Action: Direct chemical irritation in colon; increases propulsion of stool; increases fluid in colon

→ **Therapeutic Outcome:** Decreased constipation; removal of bowel contents before surgery or diagnostic tests

Uses: Constipation; bowel or rectal preparation for surgery or examination

Dosage and routes

Adult: PO 325 mg hs; fluid 1 ml qd; aromatic fluid 5 ml qd

P *Child 2-12 yr:* PO/fluid/ aromatic fluid ½ adult dose

P *Child <2 yr:* PO/fluid/ aromatic fluid ¼ adult dose

Available forms: Powder, tabs 325 mg; oral sol

Side effects/adverse reactions

GI: Nausea, vomiting, anorexia, cramps, diarrhea

META: Hypocalcemia, enteropathy, alkalosis, hypokalemia, ***tetany***

Contraindications: Hypersensitivity, GI bleeding, obstruction, CHF, lactation, abdominal pain, nausea/ vomiting, appendicitis, acute surgical abdomen, alcoholics (aromatic form)

Precautions: Pregnancy **C**

Pharmacokinetics

Absorption	Minimal
Distribution	Unknown
Metabolism	Liver, minimally
Excretion	Kidneys, feces
Half-life	Not known

Pharmacodynamics

	PO
Onset	6-12 hr
Peak	Unknown
Duration	Unknown

Interactions

Drug/drug:

Individual drugs

Digitalis: ↓ absorption

Nitrofurantoin: ↓ absorption

Drug classifications

Antibiotics: ↓ absorption

Oral anticoagulants: ↓ absorption

Salicylates: ↓ absorption

Tetracyclines: ↓ absorption

NURSING CONSIDERATIONS

Assessment

- Monitor blood, urine electrolytes if drug used often by patient; check I&O ratio to identify fluid loss
- Assess cramping, rectal bleeding, nausea, vomiting; if these symptoms occur, drug should be discontinued; identify cause of constipation; identify whether fluids, bulk, or exercise is missing from lifestyle

Associated nursing diagnoses

✓ Bowel elimination, altered: constipation (uses)
✓ Bowel elimination, altered: diarrhea (side effects)
✓ Knowledge deficit (teaching)
✓ Noncompliance (teaching)

Implementation

PO route

- Give alone with water only for better absorption; do not administer with food; do not take within 1 hr of antacids, milk, or cimetidine
- Give in AM or PM (oral dose); evacuation will occur 6-12 hr later

Patient/family education

- Discuss with the patient that adequate fluid consumption is necessary
- Teach patient that normal bowel movements do not always occur daily
- Teach patient not to use in presence of abdominal pain, nausea, vomiting; tell patient to notify prescriber if constipation unrelieved or if symptoms of electrolyte imbalance occur: muscle cramps, pain, weakness, dizziness, excessive thirst

Evaluation

Positive therapeutic outcome

- Decreased constipation in 6-12 hr
- Removal of bowel contents

cefaclor

(sef'a-klor)

Ceclor

Func. class.: Antibiotic

Chem. class.: Cephalosporin (2nd generation)

Pregnancy category **B**

Action: Inhibits bacterial cell wall synthesis, which renders cell wall osmotically unstable, leading to cell death

Uses: Upper and lower respiratory tract, urinary tract, skin infections; otitis media; increased bone, joint, gynecologic infections; septicemia

Therapeutic Outcome: Bactericidal effects for the following: gram-negative bacilli *Haemophilus influenzae, Escherichia coli, Proteus mirabilis, Klebsiella;* gram-positive organisms *Streptococcus pneumoniae, Staphylococcus,* Streptococci, beta-hemolytic; anaerobes, bacteroides sp.

Dosage and routes

Adult: PO 250-500 mg q8h, not to exceed 4 g/day

P ***Child >1 mo:*** PO 20-40 mg/kg/qd in divided doses q8h, not to exceed 1 g/day

Available forms: Caps 250, 500 mg; oral susp 125, 187, 250, 375 mg/5 ml

Side effects/adverse reactions

CNS: Headache, dizziness, weakness, paresthesia, fever, chills
GI: Nausea, vomiting, *diarrhea, anorexia,* pain, glossitis, bleeding; increased AST (SGOT), ALT (SGPT), bilirubin, LDH, alkaline phosphatase; abdominal pain, ***pseudomembranous colitis***
GU: Proteinuria, vaginitis, pruritus, candidiasis, increased BUN, ***nephrotoxicity, renal failure***
HEMA: Leukopenia, thrombocytopenia, agranulocytosis, anemia, ***neutropenia, lymphocytosis, eosinophilia, pancytopenia, hemolytic anemia***
INTEG: Rash, urticaria, dermatitis
RESP: Dyspnea
SYST: Anaphylaxis

Contraindications: Hypersensitivity to cephalosporins, P infants <1 mo

Precautions: Hypersensitivity to penicillins, pregnancy **B**, lactation, renal disease

Pharmacokinetics

Absorption	Well absorbed
Distribution	Widely distributed; crosses placenta
Metabolism	Not metabolized
Excretion	Unchanged by kidneys (60%-80%); enters breast milk
Half-life	36-54 min; increased in renal disease

Pharmacodynamics

	PO
Onset	15 min
Peak	½-1 hr

C

Interactions

Drug/drug:

Individual drugs

Probenecid: ↓ excretion of drug and increased blood levels
Sulfinpyrazone: ↑ toxicity
Vancomycin: ↑ toxicity

Drug classifications

Aminoglycosides: ↑ toxicity

Lab test interferences

Increase (false): Creatinine (serum urine), urinary 17-KS
False positive: Urinary protein, direct Coombs' test, urine glucose
Interference: Cross-matching

NURSING CONSIDERATIONS

Assessment

- Assess patient for previous sensitivity reaction to penicillins or other cephalosporins; cross-sensitivity between penicillins and cephalosporins is common
- Assess patient for signs and symptoms of infection including characteristics of wounds, sputum, urine, stool, WBC >10,000, earache, fever; obtain baseline information and during treatment
- Obtain C&S before beginning drug therapy to identify if correct treatment has been initiated
- Assess for allergic reactions: rash, urticaria, pruritus, chills, fever, joint pain; angioedema may occur a few days after therapy begins; epinephrine,

resuscitation equipment should be on unit for anaphylactic reaction
- Identify urine output; if decreasing, notify prescriber (may indicate nephrotoxicity); also check for increased BUN, creatinine
- Monitor blood studies: AST (SGOT), ALT (SGPT), CBC, Hct, bilirubin, LDH, alkaline phosphatase, Coombs' test monthly if patient is on long-term therapy
- Monitor electrolytes: potassium, sodium, chloride monthly if patient is on long-term therapy
- Assess bowel pattern qd; if severe diarrhea occurs, drug should be discontinued; may indicate pseudomembranous colitis
- Monitor for bleeding: ecchymosis, bleeding gums, hematuria, stool guaiac daily if on long-term therapy
- Assess for overgrowth of infection: perineal itching, fever, malaise, redness, pain, swelling, drainage, rash, diarrhea, change in cough, sputum

Associated nursing diagnoses

- ✓ Infection, risk for (uses)
- ✓ Diarrhea (side effects)
- ✓ Fluid volume deficit, risk for (side effects)
- ✓ Injury, risk for (side effects)
- ✓ Knowledge deficit (teaching)
- ✓ Noncompliance (teaching)

Implementation

PO route
- Give in even doses around the clock; if GI upset occurs, give with food; drug must be given for 10-14 days to ensure organism death and prevent superinfection
- Shake suspension

Patient/family education

- Teach patient to report sore throat, bruising, bleeding, joint pain; may indicate blood dyscrasias (rare)
- Advise patient to contact prescriber if vaginal itching, loose, foul-smelling stools, furry tongue occur; may indicate superinfection
- Instruct patient to take all medication prescribed for the length of time ordered
- Advise patient to notify prescriber of diarrhea with blood or pus, which may indicate pseudomembranous colitis

Evaluation

Positive therapeutic outcome
- Absence of signs/symptoms of infection (WBC <10,000, temp WNL, absence of red draining wounds, earache)
- Reported improvement in symptoms of infection

Treatment of anaphylaxis:

Epinephrine, antihistamines, resuscitate if needed

cefadroxil

(sef-a-drox'ill)

Cefadroxil, Duricef, Ultracef

Func. class.: Antibiotic

Chem. class.: Cephalosporin (1st generation)

Pregnancy category **B**

Action: Inhibits bacterial cell wall synthesis, rendering cell wall osmotically unstable, leading to cell death

Uses: Upper, lower respiratory tract, urinary tract, skin infections; otitis media; tonsillitis, pharyngitis; particularly for UTI

Therapeutic Outcome: Bactericidal effects for the following: gram-negative bacilli *Escherichia coli, Proteus mirabilis, Klebsiella (UTI only);* gram-positive organisms *Streptococcus pneumoniae, S. pyogenes, Staphylococcus aureus*

Dosage and routes

Adult: PO 1-2 g qd or q12h; give a loading dose of 1 g initially; dosage reduction indicated in renal impairment (CrCl <50 ml/min)

P *Child:* 30 mg/kg/day

Available forms: Caps 500 mg; tabs 1 g; oral susp 125, 250, 500 mg/5 ml

Side effects/adverse reactions

CNS: Headache, dizziness, weakness, paresthesia, fever, chills

GI: Nausea, vomiting, *diarrhea, anorexia,* pain, glossitis, bleeding; increased AST (SGOT), ALT (SGPT), bilirubin, LDH, alkaline phosphatase; abdominal pain, ***pseudomembranous colitis***

GU: Proteinuria, vaginitis, pruritus, candidiasis, increased BUN, ***nephrotoxicity, renal failure***

HEMA: Leukopenia, thrombocytopenia, agranulocytosis, anemia, ***neutropenia, lymphocytosis, eosinophilia, pancytopenia, hemolytic anemia***

INTEG: Rash, urticaria, dermatitis, ***anaphylaxis***

RESP: Dyspnea

Contraindications: Hypersensitivity to cephalosporins, P infants <1 mo

Precautions: Hypersensitivity to penicillins, pregnancy **B**, lactation, renal disease

Pharmacokinetics

Absorption	Well absorbed
Distribution	Widely distributed; crosses placenta
Metabolism	Not metabolized
Excretion	Unchanged by kidneys; enters breast milk
Half-life	1½-2 hr

Pharmacodynamics

	PO
Onset	Rapid
Peak	1½-2 hr

Interactions

Drug/drug:

Individual drugs

Probenecid: ↓ excretion of drug and ↑ blood levels

Vancomycin: ↑ toxicity

Drug classifications

Aminoglycosides: ↑ toxicity

Lab test interferences

Increase (false): Creatinine (serum urine), urinary 17-KS
False positive: Urinary protein, direct Coombs' test, urine glucose
Interference: Cross-matching

NURSING CONSIDERATIONS

Assessment

- Assess patient for previous sensitivity reaction to penicillins or other cephalosporins; cross-sensitivity between penicillins and cephalosporins is common
- Assess patient for signs and symptoms of infection including characteristics of wounds, sputum, urine, stool, WBC >10,000, earache, fever; obtain baseline information and during treatment
- Obtain C&S before beginning drug therapy to identify if correct treatment has been initiated
- Assess for allergic reactions: rash, urticaria, pruritus, chills, fever, joint pain; angioedema may occur a few days after therapy begins; epinephrine and resuscitation equipment should be available for anaphylactic reaction
- Identify urine output; if decreasing, notify prescriber (may indicate nephrotoxicity); also check for increased BUN, creatinine
- Monitor blood studies: AST (SGOT), ALT (SGPT), CBC, Hct, bilirubin, LDH, alkaline phosphatase, Coombs' test monthly if patient is on long-term therapy
- Monitor electrolytes: potassium, sodium, chloride monthly if patient is on long-term therapy
- Assess bowel pattern qd; if severe diarrhea occurs, drug should be discontinued; may indicate pseudomembranous colitis
- Monitor for bleeding: ecchymosis, bleeding gums, hematuria, stool guaiac daily if on long-term therapy
- Assess for superinfection: perineal itching, fever, malaise, redness, pain, swelling, drainage, rash, diarrhea, change in cough, sputum

Associated nursing diagnoses

- ✓ Infection, risk for (uses)
- ✓ Diarrhea (side effects)
- ✓ Fluid volume deficit, risk for (side effects)
- ✓ Injury, risk for (side effects)
- ✓ Knowledge deficit (teaching)
- ✓ Noncompliance (teaching)

Implementation

PO route

- Give in even doses around the clock; if GI upset occurs, give with food; drug must be given for 10-14 days to ensure organism death and prevent superinfection
- Shake suspension

Patient/family education

- Teach patient to report sore throat, bruising, bleeding, joint pain; may indicate blood dyscrasias (rare)
- Advise patient to contact prescriber if vaginal itching, loose, foul-smelling stools, furry tongue occur; may indicate superinfection

- Instruct patient to take all medication prescribed for the length of time ordered
- Advise patient to notify prescriber of diarrhea with blood or pus, which may indicate pseudomembranous colitis

Evaluation

Positive therapeutic outcome

- Absence of signs/symptoms of infection (WBC <10,000, temp WNL, absence of red draining wounds, earache)
- Reported improvement in symptoms of infection

Treatment of anaphylaxis: Epinephrine, antihistamines, resuscitate if needed

cefamandole

(sef-a-man'dole)

Mandol

Func. class.: Antibiotic

Chem. class.: Cephalosporin (2nd generation)

Pregnancy category **B**

Action: Inhibits bacterial cell wall synthesis, rendering cell wall osmotically unstable, leading to cell death

Uses: Upper, lower respiratory tract, urinary tract, skin infections; peritonitis, septicemia, surgical prophylaxis

Therapeutic Outcome: Bactericidal effects for the following: gram-negative anarobes *Bacteroides sp., clostridium sp., Fusobacterium sp., Peptococcus sp., Peptostreptococcus sp., Haemophilus influenzae, Escherichia coli, Proteus mirabilis, Klebsiella;* gram-positive organisms *S. pneumoniae, Streptococcus pyogenes, Staphylococcus aureus;* organisms *enterobacter sp., morganella morganii, proteus vulgaris, provencia rettgeris*

Dosage and routes

Adult: IM/**IV** 500 mg-1 g q4-8h; may give up to 2 g q4h for severe infections

P *Child >1 mo:* IM/**IV** 50-100 mg/kg/day in divided doses q4-8h, not to exceed adult dose

Dosage reduction indicated in renal impairment (CrCl <5 ml/min)

Available forms: Inj IM, **IV** 500 mg, 1, 2, 10 g; **IV** 1, 2 g

Side effects/adverse reactions

CNS: Headache, dizziness, weakness, paresthesia, fever, chills

GI: Nausea, vomiting, diarrhea, anorexia, pain, glossitis, bleeding; increased AST (SGOT), ALT (SGPT), bilirubin, LDH, alkaline phosphatase; abdominal pain, pseudomembranous colitis

GU: Proteinuria, vaginitis, pruritus, candidiasis, increased BUN, ***nephrotoxicity, renal failure***

HEMA: ***Leukopenia, thrombocytopenia, agranulocytosis,*** anemia, ***neutropenia, lymphocytosis, eosinophilia, pancytopenia, hemolytic anemia,*** bleeding, ***hypoprothrombinemia***

INTEG: Rash, urticaria, dermatitis, ***anaphylaxis***

RESP: Dyspnea

Contraindications: Hypersensitivity to cephalosporins, P infants <1 mo

Precautions: Hypersensitivity to penicillins, pregnancy **B**, lactation, renal disease

Pharmacokinetics

Absorption	Well absorbed
Distribution	Widely distributed; crosses placenta
Metabolism	Not metabolized
Excretion	Unchanged by kidneys (60%-80%); enters breast milk
Half-life	½-1½ hr

Pharmacodynamics

	IM	IV
Onset	Rapid	Immediate
Peak	½-2 hr	Infusion's end

Interactions

Drug/drug:

Individual drugs

Probenecid: ↓ excretion of drug and ↑ blood levels

Vancomycin: ↑ toxicity

Drug classifications

Aminoglycosides: ↑ toxicity

Anticoagulants: ↑ bleeding

Thrombolytics: ↑ bleeding

Lab test interferences

Increase (false): Urinary 17-KS

False positive: Urinary protein, direct Coombs', urine glucose

Interference: Cross-matching

NURSING CONSIDERATIONS

Assessment

- Assess patient for previous sensitivity reaction to penicillins or other cephalosporins; cross-sensitivity between penicillins and cephalosporins is common
- Assess patient for signs and symptoms of infection including characteristics of wounds, sputum, urine, stool, WBC >10,000, earache, fever; obtain baseline information and during treatment
- Obtain C&S before beginning drug therapy to identify if correct treatment has been initiated
- Assess for allergic reactions: rash, urticaria, pruritus, chills, fever, joint pain; angioedema may occur a few days after therapy begins; epinephrine and resuscitation equipment should be available for anaphylactic reaction
- Identify urine output; if decreasing, notify prescriber (may indicate nephrotoxicity); also check for increased BUN, creatinine
- Monitor blood studies: AST (SGOT), ALT (SGPT), CBC, Hct, bilirubin, LDH, alkaline phosphatase, Coombs' test monthly if patient is on long-term therapy
- Monitor electrolytes: potassium, sodium, chloride monthly if patient is on long-term therapy
- Assess bowel pattern qd; if severe diarrhea occurs, drug should be discontinued; may indicate pseudomembranous colitis
- Monitor for bleeding: ecchymosis, bleeding gums, hematuria, stool guaiac daily if on long-term therapy
- Assess for superinfection: perineal itching, fever, malaise, redness, pain, swelling, drainage, rash, diarrhea, change in cough, sputum

Associated nursing diagnoses

- ✓ Infection, risk for (uses)
- ✓ Injury, risk for (side effects)
- ✓ Diarrhea (side effects)
- ✓ Knowledge deficit (teaching)
- ✓ Noncompliance (teaching)

Implementation

IM route

• Reconstitute with 3 ml sterile or bacteriostatic water for inj, 0.9% NaCl, or 0.5%-2.0% lidocaine HCl; give deep in large muscle mass; massage; check for redness, abscess at inj site

IV **IV route**

• Check for irritation, extravasation, phlebitis daily; change site q72h

• Direct **IV**: Dilute each g of drug with 10 ml of D_5W, 0.9% NaCl, or sterile water for inj; give over 5 min

• For intermittent inf further dilute with 100 ml of D_5W, $D_{10}W$, D_5/0.25% NaCl, D_5/0.45% NaCl, D_5/0.9% NaCl, D_5 LR, 0.9% NaCl; give over 15-30 min; may be refrigerated up to 96 hr or 24 hr at room temp

• For cont inf dilute with 500-1000 ml of above solutions; give over prescribed rate

Y-*site incompatibilities:*

Amiodarone, hetastarch

Y-*site compatibilities:*

Acyclovir, cyclophosphamide, hydromorphone, magnesium sulfate, meperidine, morphine, perphenazine

Syringe incompatibilities:

Cimetidine, gentamicin, tobramycin

Syringe compatibility:

Heparin

Additive incompatibilities:

Aminoglycosides, calcium gluceptate, calcium gluconate, cimetidine, gentamicin

Additive compatibilities:

Clindamycin, floxacillin, furosemide, metronidazole, or verapamil

Patient/family education

• Teach patient to report sore throat, bruising, bleeding, joint pain; may indicate blood dyscrasias (rare)

• Advise patient to contact prescriber if vaginal itching, loose, foul-smelling stools, furry tongue occur; may indicate superinfection

• Instruct patient to take all medication prescribed for the length of time ordered

• Advise patient to notify prescriber of diarrhea with blood or pus, which may indicate pseudomembranous colitis

Evaluation

Positive therapeutic outcome

• Absence of signs/symptoms of infection (WBC <10,000, temp WNL, absence of red draining wounds, earache)

• Reported improvement in symptoms of infection

Treatment of anaphylaxis:

Epinephrine, antihistamines, resuscitate if needed

cefazolin

(sef-a'zoe-lin)

Ancef, cefazolin sodium, Kefzol, Zolicef

Func. class.: Antibiotic

Chem. class.: Cephalosporin (1st generation)

Pregnancy category **B**

Action: Inhibits bacterial cell wall synthesis, rendering cell wall osmotically unstable, leading to cell death

Uses: Upper, lower respiratory tract, urinary tract, skin infections; bone, joint, biliary, genital infections; endocarditis, surgical prophylaxis, septicemia

Therapeutic Outcome: Bactericidal effects for the following: gram-negative organisms *Enterobacter sp., Haemophilus influenzae, Escherichia coli, Proteus mirabilis, Klebsiella;* gram-positive organisms *Streptococcus pneumoniae, S. pyogenes, Staphlyococcus aureus*

Dosage and routes

Life-threatening infections

Adult: IM/**IV** 1-1.5 g q6h

P *Child >1 mo:* IM/**IV** 100 mg/kg in 3-4 equal doses

Mild/moderate infections

Adult: IM/**IV** 250-500 mg q8h

P *Child >1 mo:* IM/**IV** 25-50 mg/kg in 3-4 equal doses

Dosage reduction indicated in renal impairment (CrCl <54 ml/min)

Available forms: Inj IM, **IV**, 250, 500 mg, 1, 5, 10 g

Side effects/adverse reactions

CNS: Headache, dizziness, weakness, paresthesia, fever, chills

GI: Nausea, vomiting, *diarrhea, anorexia,* pain, glossitis, bleeding; increased AST (SGOT), ALT (SGPT), bilirubin, LDH, alkaline phosphatase; abdominal pain, oral candidiasis, ***pseudomembranous colitis***

GU: Proteinuria, vaginitis, pruritus, candidiasis, increased BUN, ***nephrotoxicity, renal failure***

HEMA: Leukopenia, thrombocytopenia, agranulocytosis, anemia, ***neutropenia, lymphocytosis, eosinophilia, pancytopenia, hemolytic anemia***

INTEG: Rash, urticaria, dermatitis, ***anaphylaxis***

Contraindications: Hypersensitivity to cephalosporins, infants <1 mo

Precautions: Hypersensitivity to penicillins, pregnancy **B**, lactation, renal disease

Pharmacokinetics

Absorption	Well absorbed
Distribution	Widely distributed; crosses placenta
Metabolism	Not metabolized
Excretion	Unchanged by kidneys; enters breast milk
Half-life	1½-2½ hr

Pharmacodynamics

	IM	IV
Onset	Rapid	10 min
Peak	1-2 hr	Infusion's end

Interactions

Drug/drug:

Individual drugs

Probenecid: ↓ excretion of drug and ↑ blood levels
Vancomycin: ↑ toxicity

Drug classifications

Aminoglycosides: ↑ toxicity, ↑ nephrotoxicity

Lab test interferences

Increase (false): Urinary 17-KS
False positive: Urinary protein, direct Coombs', urine glucose
Interference: Cross-matching

NURSING CONSIDERATIONS

Assessment

- Assess patient for previous sensitivity reaction to penicillins or other cephalosporins; cross-sensitivity between penicillins and cephalosporins is common
- Assess patient for signs and symptoms of infection including characteristics of wounds, sputum, urine, stool, WBC >10,000, earache, fever; obtain baseline information and during treatment
- Obtain C&S before beginning drug therapy to identify if correct treatment has been initiated
- Assess for allergic reactions: rash, urticaria, pruritus, chills, fever, joint pain; angioedema may occur a few days after therapy begins; epinephrine and resuscitation equipment should be available for anaphylactic reaction
- Identify urine output; if decreasing, notify prescriber (may indicate nephrotoxicity); also check for increased BUN, creatinine
- Monitor blood studies: AST (SGOT), ALT (SGPT), CBC, Hct, bilirubin, LDH, alkaline phosphatase, Coombs' test monthly if patient is on long-term therapy
- Monitor electrolytes: potassium, sodium, chloride monthly if patient is on long-term therapy
- Assess bowel pattern qd; if severe diarrhea occurs, drug should be discontinued; may indicate pseudomembranous colitis
- Monitor for bleeding: ecchymosis, bleeding gums, hematuria, stool guaiac daily if on long-term therapy
- Assess for overgrowth of infection: perineal itching, fever, malaise, redness, pain, swelling, drainage, rash, diarrhea, change in cough, sputum

Associated nursing diagnoses

- ✓ Infection, risk for (uses)
- ✓ Diarrhea (side effects)
- ✓ Injury, risk for (side effects)
- ✓ Knowledge deficit (teaching)
- ✓ Noncompliance (teaching)

Implementation

IM route

- Reconstitute 250-500 mg of drug with 2 ml sterile or bacteriostatic water for inj, or 0.9% NaCl; reconstitute 1 g of drug with 2.5 ml; give deep in large muscle mass, massage

IV route

- Check for irritation, extravasation, phlebitis daily, change site q72h
- For direct **IV** dilute in 10 ml of sterile water for injection; give over 5 min
- For intermittent inf dilute reconstituted sol (500 mg or 1 mg) in 50-100 ml D_5W, $D_{10}W$, D_5/0.25% NaCl, D_5/0.45% NaCl, D_5/0.9% NaCl, D_5/LR, or LR, 0.9% NaCl; give over 30-60 min; may be refrigerated up to 96 hr or stored 24 hr at room temp

Y-site incompatibilities:

Amiodarone, hetastarch, hydromorphone, idarubicin, vinorelbine tartrate

Y-site compatibilities:

Acyclovir, atracurium, calcium gluconate, cyclophosphamide, enalaprilat, esmolol, famotidine, fluconazole, fludarabine, foscarnet, labetalol, lidocaine, magnesium sulfate, melphalan, meperidine, morphine, multivitamins, ondansetron, perphenazine, pancuronium, regular insulin, sargramostim, vecuronium, vitamin B complex with C

Syringe incompatibilities:

Ascorbic acid injection, cimetidine, lidocaine, vitamin B complex with C

Syringe compatibilities:

Heparin, vitamin B complex

Additive incompatibilities:

Amikacin, amobarbital, bleomycin, calcium gluceptate, calcium gluconate, colistimethate, erythromycin, kanamycin, oxytetracycline, pentobarbital, polymyxin B, tetracycline

Additive compatibilities:

Aztreonam, cimetidine, clindamycin, metronidazole, verapamil

Patient/family education

- Teach patient to report sore throat, bruising, bleeding, joint pain; may indicate blood dyscrasias (rare)
- Advise patient to contact prescriber if vaginal itching, loose, foul-smelling stools, furry tongue occur; may indicate superinfection
- Advise patient to notify prescriber of diarrhea with blood or pus, which may indicate pseudomembranous colitis

Evaluation

Positive therapeutic outcome

- Absence of signs/symptoms of infection (WBC <10,000, temp WNL, absence of red draining wounds, earache)
- Reported improvement in symptoms of infection

Treatment of anaphylaxis: Epinephrine, antihistamines, resuscitate if needed

cefixime

(sef-ix'eem)

Suprax

Func. class: Broad-spectrum antibiotic

Chem. class: Cephalosporin (3rd generation)

Pregnancy category **B**

Action: Inhibits bacterial cell wall synthesis, rendering cell wall osmotically unstable, leading to cell death

Uses: Uncomplicated UTI, pharyngitis and tonsillitis, otitis media, acute bronchitis, and acute exacerbations of chronic bronchitis

Therapeutic Outcome: Bactericidal effects of the following: *Escherichia coli, Proteus mirabilis, Streptococcus pyogenes, Haemophilus influenzae, Moraxella catarrhalis, S. pneumoniae*

Dosage and routes

Adult: PO 400 mg qd as a single dose or 200 mg q12h

P *Child >50 kg or >12 years:* PO use adult dosage

P *Child <50 kg or <12 years:* PO 8 mg/kg/day as a single dose or 4 mg/kg/day q12h

Available forms: Tabs 200, 400 g: powder for oral susp 100 mg/5 ml

Side effects/adverse reactions

CNS: Headache, dizziness, paresthesia, fever, chills, lethargy, fatigue, confusion

GI: Nausea, vomiting, diarrhea, anorexia, pain, glossitis, bleeding; increased AST (SGOT), ALT (SGPT), bilirubin, LDH, alkaline phosphatase; heartburn, dysgeusia, flatulence, ***pseudomembranous colitis***

GU: ***Proteinuria,*** vaginitis, pruritus, increased BUN, ***nephrotoxicity, renal failure, pyuria, dysuria***

HEMA: ***Leukopenia, thrombocytopenia, agranulocytosis,*** anemia, ***neutropenia, lymphocytosis, eosinophilia, pancytopenia, hemolytic anemia***

INTEG: Rash, urticaria, ***exfoliative dermatitis***

RESP: ***Bronchospasm,*** dyspnea, tight chest

SYST: ***Anaphylaxis***

Contraindications: Hypersensitivity to cephalosporins, P infants <6 mo

Precautions: Hypersensitivity to penicillins, pregnancy **B**, lactation, renal disease

Pharmacokinetics

Absorption	40%-50% (PO—tab)
Distribution	Widely distributed
Metabolism	Not metabolized
Excretion	Kidneys, unchanged (50%); bile (10%); enters breast milk
Half-life	3-4 hr, increased in renal disease

Pharmacodynamics

	PO
Onset	15-30 min
Peak	1 hr

Interactions

Drug/drug:

Individual drugs

Probenecid: ↓ excretion of drug and ↑ blood levels
Vancomycin: ↑ toxicity

Drug classifications

Aminoglycosides: ↑ toxicity

Lab test interferences

Increase (false): Creatinine (serum urine), urinary 17-KS
False positive: Urinary protein, direct Coombs' test, urine glucose
Interference: Cross-matching

NURSING CONSIDERATIONS

Assessment

- Assess patient for previous sensitivity reaction to penicillins or other cephalosporins; cross-sensitivity between penicillins and cephalosporins is common
- Assess patient for signs and symptoms of infection including characteristics of wounds, sputum, urine, stool, WBC >10,000, earache, fever; obtain baseline information and during treatment
- Obtain C&S before beginning drug therapy to identify if correct treatment has been initiated
- Assess for allergic reactions: rash, urticaria, pruritus, chills, fever, joint pain; angioedema may occur a few days after therapy begins; epinephrine and resuscitation equipment should be available for anaphylactic reaction
- Identify urine output; if decreasing, notify prescriber (may indicate nephrotoxicity); also check for increased BUN, creatinine
- Monitor blood studies: AST (SGOT), ALT (SGPT), CBC, Hct, bilirubin, LDH, alkaline phosphatase, Coombs' test monthly if patient is on long-term therapy
- Monitor electrolytes: potassium, sodium, chloride monthly if patient is on long-term therapy
- Assess bowel pattern qd; if severe diarrhea occurs, drug should be discontinued; may indicate pseudomembranous colitis
- Monitor for bleeding: ecchymosis, bleeding gums, hematuria, stool guaiac daily if on long-term therapy
- Assess for overgrowth of infection: perineal itching, fever, malaise, redness, pain, swelling, drainage, rash, diarrhea, change in cough, sputum

Associated nursing diagnoses

- ✓ Infection, risk for (uses)
- ✓ Diarrhea (side effects)
- ✓ Injury, risk for (side effects)
- ✓ Knowledge deficit (teaching)
- ✓ Noncompliance (teaching)

Implementation

PO route

- Give in even doses around the clock; if GI upset occurs, give with food; drug must be given for 10-14 days to ensure organism death and prevent superinfection
- Shake suspension

Patient/family education

- Teach patient to report sore throat, bruising, bleeding,

joint pain; may indicate blood dyscrasias (rare)
- Advise patient to contact prescriber if vaginal itching, loose, foul-smelling stools, furry tongue occur; may indicate superinfection
- Instruct patient to take all medication prescribed for the length of time ordered
- Advise patient to notify prescriber of diarrhea with blood or pus, which may indicate pseudomembranous colitis

Evaluation

Positive therapeutic outcome
- Absence of signs/symptoms of infection (WBC <10,000, negative, temp WNL, absence of red draining wounds, earache)
- Reported improvement in symptoms of infection

Treatment of anaphylaxis: Epinephrine, antihistamines, resuscitate if needed

cefmetazole

(sef-met'a-zole)
Zefazone
Func. class.: Broad-spectrum antibiotic
Chem. class.: Cephalosporin (2nd generation)
Pregnancy category B

Action: Inhibits bacterial cell wall synthesis, rendering cell wall osmotically unstable, leading to cell death

Uses: Infections of lower respiratory tract, urinary tract, skin, bone; septicemia; intraabdominal infections

Therapeutic Outcome: Bactericidal effects for the following: anaerobes, including *Clostridium, Bacteroides sp., Fusobacterium sp.;* gram-negative organisms *Morganella morganii, Haemophilus influenzae, Escherichia coli, Proteus, Klebsiella, Bacteroides fragilis;* gram-positive organisms *Streptococcus pneumoniae, S. pyogenes, Staphylococcus aureus*

Dosage and routes

Adult: **IV** 1-8 g divided q6-12h × 5-14 days

Available forms: Powder for inj 1,2 g/vial

Side effects/adverse reactions

CNS: Headache, dizziness, paresthesia, fever, chills, lethargy, fatigue, confusion
GI: Nausea, vomiting, diarrhea, anorexia, pain, glossitis, bleeding; increased AST (SGOT), ALT (SGPT), bilirubin, LDH, alkaline phosphatase; heartburn, flatulence
GU: ***Proteinuria,*** vaginitis, pruritus, candidiasis, increased BUN, ***nephrotoxicity, renal failure***
HEMA: ***Leukopenia, thrombocytopenia, agranulocytosis,*** anemia, ***neutropenia, lymphocytosis, eosinophilia, pancytopenia, hemolytic anemia***
INTEG: Rash, urticaria, ***exfoliative dermatitis,*** thrombophlebitis ***angioedema,*** erythema, pruritus
SYST: ***Anaphylaxis***

Contraindications: Hypersensitivity to cephalosporins, P infants <1 mo

Precautions: Hypersensitivity to penicillins, pregnancy **B**, lactation, renal disease

Pharmacokinetics

Absorption	Complete
Distribution	Widely distributed; crosses placenta
Metabolism	Not metabolized
Excretion	Kidneys, unchanged (85%); enters breast milk
Half-life	½-2 hr; increased in renal disease

Pharmacodynamics

	IV
Onset	Rapid
Peak	Infusion's end

Interactions

Drug/drug:

Individual drugs

Alcohol: Disulfiram reaction if ingested within 48-72 hr of cephalosporin
Plicamycin: ↑ bleeding
Probenecid: ↓ excretion of drug and ↑ blood levels
Sulfinpyrazone: ↑ toxicity
Valproic acid: ↑ bleeding
Vancomycin: ↑ toxicity

Drug classifications

Aminoglycosides: ↑ toxicity
Anticoagulants: ↑ bleeding
Thrombolytics: ↑ bleeding

Lab test interferences

Increase (false): Creatinine (serum urine), urinary 17-KS
False positive: Urinary protein, direct Coombs' test, urine glucose
Interference: Cross-matching

NURSING CONSIDERATIONS

Assessment

- Assess patient for previous sensitivity reaction to penicillins or other cephalosporins; cross-sensitivity between penicillins and cephalosporins is common
- Assess patient for signs and symptoms of infection including characteristics of wounds, sputum, urine, stool, WBC >10,000, earache, fever; obtain baseline information and during treatment
- Obtain C&S before beginning drug therapy to identify if correct treatment has been initiated
- Assess for allergic reactions: rash, urticaria, pruritus, chills, fever, joint pain; angioedema may occur a few days after therapy begins; epinephrine and resuscitation equipment should be available for anaphylactic reaction
- Identify urine output; if decreasing, notify prescriber (may indicate nephrotoxicity); also check for increased BUN, creatinine
- Monitor blood studies: AST (SGOT), ALT (SGPT), CBC, Hct, bilirubin, LDH, alkaline phosphatase, Coombs' test monthly if patient is on long-term therapy
- Monitor electrolytes: potassium, sodium, chloride monthly if patient is on long-term therapy
- Assess bowel pattern qd; if severe diarrhea occurs, drug should be discontinued; may indicate pseudomembranous colitis
- Monitor for bleeding: ecchymosis, bleeding gums, hema-

turia, stool guaiac daily if on long-term therapy
- Assess for overgrowth of infection: perineal itching, fever, malaise, redness, pain, swelling, drainage, rash, diarrhea, change in cough, sputum

Associated nursing diagnoses

✓ Infection, risk for (uses)
✓ Diarrhea (side effects)
✓ Injury, risk for (side effects)
✓ Knowledge deficit (teaching)
✓ Noncompliance (teaching)

Implementation

IV route
- Check for irritation, extravasation, phlebitis daily; change site q72h
- For intermittent inf, reconstitute with sterile, bacteriostatic water for inj or 0.9% NaCl; may be further diluted with 0.9% NaCl, LR, D_5W (1-20 mg/ml); give over 30-60 min; may be refrigerated for 1 week or stored 24 hr at room temp

Patient/family education

- Teach patient to report sore throat, bruising, bleeding, joint pain, may indicate blood dyscrasias (rare)
- Advise patient to contact prescriber if vaginal itching, loose, foul-smelling stools, furry tongue occur; may indicate superinfection
- Advise patient to notify prescriber of diarrhea with blood or pus, which may indicate pseudomembranous colitis

Evaluation

Positive therapeutic outcome
- Absence of signs/symptoms of infection (WBC <10,000, temp WNL, absence of red draining wounds)
- Reported improvement in symptoms of infection

Treatment of anaphylaxis: Epinephrine, antihistamines, resuscitate if needed

cefonicid

(se-fon′i-sid)
Monocid
Func. class.: Antibiotic
Chem. class.: Cephalosporin (2nd generation)
Pregnancy category **B**

Action: Inhibits bacterial cell wall synthesis, rendering cell wall osmotically unstable, leading to cell death

Uses: Lower respiratory tract, urinary tract, skin, bone, joint infections; otitis media, peritonitis, septicemia, preoperative prophylaxis

Therapeutic Outcome: Bactericidal effects for the following: gram-negative organisms *Morganella morganii, Proteus valgaris, Providencia vettger, Haemophilus influenzae, Escherichia coli, Proteus mirabilis, Klebsiella;* gram-positive organisms *Streptococcus pneumoniae, S. pyogenes, Staphylococcus aureus*

Dosage and routes

Life-threatening infections

Adult: IM/**IV** bol or inf 1-2 g/24 hr; divide in 2 doses if giving 2 g

Dosage reduction indicated in renal impairment

Available forms: Inj IM, **IV**, 500 mg, 1, 10 g

Side effects/adverse reactions

CNS: Headache, dizziness, weakness, paresthesia, fever, chills
GI: Nausea, vomiting, diarrhea, anorexia, pain, glossitis, bleeding; increased AST (SGOT), ALT (SGPT), bilirubin, LDH, alkaline phosphatase; abdominal pain, ***Pseudomembranous colitis***
GU: Proteinuria, vaginitis, pruritus, candidiasis, increased BUN, ***nephrotoxicity, renal failure***
HEMA: Leukopenia, thrombocytopenia, agranulocytosis, anemia, ***neutropenia, lymphocytosis, eosinophilia, pancytopenia, hemolytic anemia***
INTEG: Rash, urticaria, dermatitis
SYST: ***Anaphylaxis***

Contraindications: Hypersensitivity to cephalosporins, P infants <1 mo

Precautions: Hypersensitivity to penicillins, pregnancy **B**, lactation, renal disease

Pharmacokinetics

Absorption	Well absorbed (IM)
Distribution	Widely distributed; crosses placenta
Metabolism	Not metabolized
Excretion	Kidneys, unchanged; enters breast milk
Half-life	4½ hr; increased in renal disease

Pharmacodynamics

	IM	IV
Onset	Rapid	5 min
Peak	1 hr	Infusion's end

Interactions

Drug/drug:

Individual drugs
Probenecid: ↓ excretion of drug and ↑ blood levels
Vancomycin: ↑ toxicity
Drug classifications
Aminoglycosides: ↑ toxicity

Lab test interferences

Increase (false): Creatinine (serum urine), urinary 17-KS
False positive: Urinary protein, direct Coombs' test, urine glucose
Interference: Cross-matching

NURSING CONSIDERATIONS

Assessment

- Assess patient for previous sensitivity reaction to penicillins or other cephalosporins; cross-sensitivity between penicillins and cephalosporins is common
- Assess patient for signs and symptoms of infection including characteristics of wounds, sputum, urine, stool, WBC >10,000, earache, fever; obtain baseline information and during treatment
- Obtain C&S before beginning drug therapy to identify if correct treatment has been initiated
- Assess for allergic reactions: rash, urticaria, pruritus, chills, fever, joint pain; angioedema may occur a few days after therapy begins; epinephrine and resuscitation equipment

should be available for anaphylactic reaction

- Identify urine output; if decreasing, notify prescriber (may indicate nephrotoxicity); also check for increased BUN, creatinine
- Monitor blood studies: AST (SGOT), ALT (SGPT), CBC, Hct, bilirubin, LDH, alkaline phosphatase, Coombs' test monthly if patient is on long-term therapy
- Monitor electrolytes: potassium, sodium, chloride monthly if patient is on long-term therapy
- Assess bowel pattern qd; if severe diarrhea occurs, drug should be discontinued; may indicate pseudomembranous colitis
- Monitor for bleeding: ecchymosis, bleeding gums, hematuria, stool guaiac daily if on long-term therapy
- Assess for overgrowth of infection: perineal itching, fever, malaise, redness, pain, swelling, drainage, rash, diarrhea, change in cough, sputum

Associated nursing diagnoses

- ✓ Infection, risk for (uses)
- ✓ Injury, risk for (side effects)
- ✓ Diarrhea (side effects)
- ✓ Knowledge deficit (teaching)
- ✓ Noncompliance (teaching)

Implementation

IM route

- Reconstitute 500 mg/2 ml of sterile water for inj (220 mg/ml) or 1000 mg/2.5 ml (325 mg/ml)
- Give deep in large muscle mass, massage

IV **IV route**

- Check for irritation, extravasation, phlebitis daily; change site q72h
- For direct **IV** give over 5 min
- For intermittent inf reconstituted sol should be further diluted in 50-100 ml D_5W, $D_{10}W$, D_5/LR, D_5/0.25% NaCl, D_5/0.45% NaCl, D_5/0.9% NaCl, 0.9% NaCl; or Ringer's, LR; give over 30 min may be refrigerated up to 96 hr or stored 24 hr at room temp

Y-site incompatibilities: Hetastarch, sargramostim

Y-site compatibility: Acyclovir

Additive incompatibility: Aminoglycosides

Additive compatibility: Clindamycin

Patient/family education

- Teach patient to report sore throat, bruising, bleeding, joint pain; may indicate blood dyscrasias (rare)
- Advise patient to contact prescriber if vaginal itching, loose, foul-smelling stools, furry tongue occur; may indicate superinfection
- Advise patient to notify prescriber of diarrhea with blood or pus, which may indicate pseudomembranous colitis

Evaluation

Positive therapeutic outcome

- Absence of signs/symptoms of infection (WBC <10,000, temp WNL, absence of red draining wounds, earache)

• Reported improvement in symptoms of infection

Treatment of anaphylaxis: Epinephrine, antihistamines, resuscitate if needed

cefoperazone
(sef-oh-per'a-zone)
Cefobid
Func. class.: Broad-spectrum antibiotic
Chem. class.: Cephalosporin (3rd generation)
Pregnancy category B

Action: Inhibits bacterial cell wall synthesis, rendering cell wall osmotically unstable, leading to cell death

Uses: Lower respiratory tract, urinary tract, skin, bone infections; bacterial septicemia, peritonitis, pelvic inflammatory disease (PID), endometritis

Therapeutic Outcome: Bactericidal effects for the following: gram-negative organisms *Acinetobacter molganella morganii, Neisseria gonorrhea, Proteus vulgarism;* gram positive organisms *Staphylococci, Streptococci, Streptococci* (beta-hemolytic), *Streptococci pneumoniae, Haemophilus influenzae, Escherichia coli, Proteus mirabilis, Klebsiella, Enterobacter, Serratia, Citrobacter, Providencia, Pseudomonas aeruginosa* anaerobes *Bacterioles, Clostridium, Eubacterium, Fusobacterium, Peptococcus, Peptostreptococcus*

Dosage and routes

Mild/moderate infections

Adult: IM/**IV** 1-2 g q12h or 2-4 g/day in divided doses q8-12h

Severe infections

Adult: IM/**IV** 6-12 g/day divided in 2-4 equal doses

Available forms: Inj IM, **IV**, 1, 2 g

Side effects/adverse reactions

CNS: Headache, dizziness, weakness, paresthesia, fever, chills
GI: Nausea, vomiting, diarrhea, anorexia, pain, glossitis, bleeding; increased AST (SGOT), ALT (SGPT), bilirubin, LDH, alkaline phosphatase; abdominal pain, ***pseudomembranous colitis***
GU: ***Proteinuria,*** vaginitis, pruritus, candidiasis, increased BUN, ***nephrotoxicity, renal failure***
HEMA: ***Leukopenia, thrombocytopenia, agranulocytosis,*** anemia, ***neutropenia, lymphocytosis, eosinophilia, pancytopenia, hemolytic anemia, bleeding, hypoprothrombinemia***
INTEG: Rash, urticaria, dermatitis
RESP: Dyspnea
SYST: ***Anaphylaxis***

Contraindications: Hypersensitivity to cephalosporins, P infants <1 mo

Precautions: Hypersensitivity to penicillins, pregnancy **B**, lactation, renal disease

Pharmacokinetics

Absorption	Well absorbed (IM)
Distribution	Widely distributed; crosses placenta
Metabolism	Not metabolized
Excretion	Bile; enters breast milk
Half-life	2 hr

Pharmacodynamics

	IM	IV
Onset	Rapid	5 min
Peak	1-2 hr	Infusion's end

Interactions

Drug/drug:

Individual drugs

Probenecid: ↓ excretion of drug and ↑ blood levels
Vancomycin: ↑ toxicity

Drug classifications

Aminoglycosides: ↑ toxicity
Anticoagulants: ↑ bleeding
Thrombolytics: ↑ bleeding

Lab test interferences

Increase (false): Creatinine (serum urine), urinary 17-KS
False positive: Urinary protein, direct Coombs' test, urine glucose
Interference: Cross-matching

NURSING CONSIDERATIONS

Assessment

- Assess patient for previous sensitivity reaction to penicillins or other cephalosporins; cross-sensitivity between penicillins and cephalosporins is common
- Assess patient for signs and symptoms of infection including characteristics of wounds, sputum, urine, stool, WBC >10,000, fever; obtain baseline information and during treatment
- Obtain C&S before beginning drug therapy to identify if correct treatment has been initiated
- Assess for allergic reactions: rash, urticaria, pruritus, chills, fever, joint pain; angioedema may occur a few days after therapy begins; epinephrine and resuscitation equipment should be available for anaphylactic reaction
- Identify urine output; if decreasing, notify prescriber (may indicate nephrotoxicity); also check for increased BUN, creatinine
- Monitor blood studies: AST (SGOT), ALT (SGPT), CBC, Hct, bilirubin, LDH, alkaline phosphatase, Coombs' test monthly if patient is on long-term therapy
- Monitor electrolytes: potassium, sodium, chloride monthly if patient is on long-term therapy
- Assess bowel pattern qd; if severe diarrhea occurs, drug should be discontinued; may indicate pseudomembranous colitis
- Monitor for bleeding: ecchymosis, bleeding gums, hematuria, stool guaiac daily if on long-term therapy
- Assess for overgrowth of infection: perineal itching, fever, malaise, redness, pain, swelling, drainage, rash, diarrhea, change in cough, sputum

Associated nursing diagnoses

- ✓ Infection, risk for (uses)
- ✓ Injury, risk for (side effects)
- ✓ Diarrhea (side effects)
- ✓ Knowledge deficit (teaching)

C

Implementation

IM route

- Reconstitute 1 g/2.8 ml of sterile or bacteriostatic water for inj, or 2 g/5.4 ml; may be diluted further with 1 ml or 1.8 ml of 2% lidocaine to prevent pain; give deep in large muscle mass, massage

IV **IV route**

- Check for irritation, extravasation, phlebitis daily; change site q72h
- For intermittent inf, reconstituted sol should be further diluted 1 g/20-40 ml of 0.9% NaCl, D_5W, D_5/0.9% NaCl, D_5/LR, or LR; give over 15-30 min; may be refrigerated up to 96 hr or stored 24 hr at room temp
- For cont inf, final concentration is 2-25 mg/ml give at prescribed rate

Y-site incompatibilities:
Gentamicin, hetastarch, labetalol, meperidine, ondansetron, perphenazine, sargramostim, tobramycin, vinorelbine tartrate

Y-site compatibilities:
Acyclovir, cyclophosphamide, enalaprilat, esmolol, famotidine, foscarnet, fludarabine, hydromorphone, magnesium sulfate, melphalan, morphine

Syringe incompatibility:
Doxapram

Syringe compatibility:
Heparin

Additive incompatibility:
Aminoglycosides

Additive compatibilities:
Cimetidine, clindamycin, furosemide

Patient/family education

- Teach patient to report sore throat, bruising, bleeding, joint pain, may indicate blood dyscrasias (rare)
- Advise patient to contact prescriber if vaginal itching, loose, foul-smelling stools, furry tongue occur; may indicate superinfection
- Advise patient to notify prescriber of diarrhea with blood or pus, which may indicate pseudomembranous colitis

Evaluation

Positive therapeutic outcome

- Absence of signs/symptoms of infection (WBC <10,000, temp WNL, absence of red draining wounds, pelvic pain)
- Reported improvement in symptoms of infection

Treatment of anaphylaxis: Epinephrine, antihistamines, resuscitate if needed

ceforanide

(sef-or'a-nide)

Precef

Func. class.: Broad-spectrum antibiotic
Chem. class.: Cephalosporin (2nd generation)

Pregnancy category B

Action: Inhibits bacterial cell wall synthesis, rendering cell wall osmotically unstable, leading to cell death

Uses: Lower respiratory tract, urinary tract, skin, bone infections; septicemia, endocarditis

Therapeutic Outcome: Bactericidal effects for the following: gram-negative organisms *Enterobacter, Moraxella catarrhalis, Neisseria gonorrhea, Providencia, Salmonella typhi, Haemophilus influenzae, Escherichia coli, Proteus mirabilis, Klebsiella;* gram-positive organisms *Streptococcus pneumoniae, Staphylococcus aureus* Streptococcus (beta-hemolytic); anaerobes *Bacteroides, Fusobacterium, Peptococcus, Peptostreptococcus*

Dosage and routes

Adult: IM/**IV** 0.5-1 g q12h

P *Child:* IM /**IV** 20-40 mg/kg/day in 2 equal doses q12h; dosage reduction indicated in renal impairment (CrCl <59 ml/min)

Available forms: Powder for inj IM, **IV** 500 mg, 1, 10 g

Side effects/adverse reactions

CNS: Headache, dizziness, weakness, paresthesia, fever, chills

GI: *Nausea, vomiting, diarrhea, anorexia,* pain, glossitis, bleeding; increased AST (SGOT), ALT (SGPT), bilirubin, LDH, alkaline phosphatase; abdominal pain

GU: Proteinuria, vaginitis, pruritus, increased BUN, ***nephrotoxicity, renal failure***

HEMA: Leukopenia, thrombocytopenia, agranulocytosis, anemia, ***neutropenia, lymphocytosis, eosinophilia, pancytopenia, hemolytic anemia***

INTEG: Rash, urticaria, dermatitis

RESP: Dyspnea

SYST: Anaphylaxis

Contraindications: Hypersensitivity to cephalosporins, P infants <1 mo

Precautions: Hypersensitivity to penicillins, pregnancy **B**, lactation, renal disease

Pharmacokinetics

Absorption	Well absorbed (IM)
Distribution	Widely distributed; crosses placenta
Metabolism	Not metabolized
Excretion	Kidneys, unchanged; enters breast milk
Half-life	2½-3 hr; increased in renal disease

Pharmacodynamics

	IM	IV
Onset	Rapid	Rapid
Peak	1 hr	2 hr

Interactions

Drug/drug:

Individual drugs

Probenecid: ↓ excretion of drug and ↑ blood levels

Vancomycin: ↑ toxicity

Drug classifications

Aminoglycosides: ↑ toxicity

Lab test interferences

Increase (false): Creatinine (serum urine), urinary 17-KS

False positive: Urinary protein, direct Coombs' test, urine glucose

Interference: Cross-matching

NURSING CONSIDERATIONS

Assessment

- Assess patient for previous sensitivity reaction to penicillins or other cephalosporins; cross-sensitivity between penicillins and cephalosporins is common
- Assess patient for signs and symptoms of infection including characteristics of wounds, sputum, urine, stool, WBC >10,000, fever; obtain baseline information and during treatment
- Obtain C&S before beginning drug therapy to identify if correct treatment has been initiated
- Assess for allergic reactions: rash, urticaria, pruritus, chills, fever, joint pain; angioedema may occur a few days after therapy begins; epinephrine and resuscitation equipment should be available for anaphylactic reaction
- Identify urine output; if decreasing, notify prescriber (may indicate nephrotoxicity); also check for increased BUN, creatinine
- Monitor blood studies: AST (SGOT), ALT (SGPT), CBC, Hct, bilirubin, LDH, alkaline phosphatase, Coombs' test monthly if patient is on long-term therapy
- Monitor electrolytes: potassium, sodium, chloride monthly if patient is on long-term therapy
- Assess bowel pattern qd; if severe diarrhea occurs, drug should be discontinued; may indicate pseudomembranous colitis
- Monitor for bleeding: ecchymosis, bleeding gums, hematuria, stool guaiac daily if on long-term therapy
- Assess for overgrowth of infection: perineal itching, fever, malaise, redness, pain, swelling, drainage, rash, diarrhea, change in cough, sputum

Associated nursing diagnoses

- ✓ Infection, risk for (uses)
- ✓ Diarrhea (side effects)
- ✓ Knowledge deficit (teaching)
- ✓ Noncompliance (teaching)
- ✓ Injury, risk for (side effects)

Implementation

IM route

- Reconstitute 500 mg/1.7 ml of sterile or bacteriostatic water for inj or 1 g/3.2; shake; give deep in large muscle mass, massage

IV **IV route**

- Check for irritation, extravasation, phlebitis daily; change site q72h
- For direct **IV** dilute 500 mg/5 ml or 1 g/10 ml of bacteriostatic water or 0.9% NaCl for inj; shake, give over 3-5 min
- For intermittent inf, further dilute 1 g/10 ml of 0.9% NaCl, D_5W, $D_{10}W$, D_5/0.25% NaCl, D_5/0.45% NaCl, D_5/LR, LR; give over 30 min; may be refrigerated up to 96 hr or stored 24 hr at room temp

Y-site compatibilities:

Acyclovir, cyclophosphamide, fludarabine, hydromorphone, magnesium sulfate, melphalan, meperidine, morphine, paclitaxel, ondansetron, perphenazine, sargramostim

Additive incompatibility: Aminoglycosides

Patient/family education

- Teach patient to report sore throat, bruising, bleeding, joint pain; may indicate blood dyscrasias (rare)
- Advise patient to contact physician if vaginal itching, loose, foul-smelling stools, furry tongue occur; may indicate superinfection
- Advise patient to notify physician of diarrhea with blood or pus, which may indicate pseudomembranous colitis

Evaluation

Positive therapeutic outcome

- Absence of signs/symptoms of infection (WBC <10,000, temp WNL, absence of red draining wounds)
- Reported improvement in symptoms of infection

Treatment of anaphylaxis: Epinephrine, antihistamines, resuscitate if needed

cefotetan

(sef'oh-tee-tan)

Cefotan

Func. class.: Broad-spectrum antibiotic

Chem. class.: Cephalosporin (2nd generation)

Pregnancy category **B**

Action: Inhibits bacterial cell wall synthesis, which renders cell osmotically unstable leading to cell death

Uses: Serious upper or lower respiratory tract, urinary tract, skin, gonococcal, intraabdominal infections; septicemia, meningitis

Therapeutic Outcome: Bactericidal effects for the following: gram-negative organisms *Haemophilus influenzae, Escherichia coli, Enterobacter aerogenes, Proteus mirabilis, Klebsiella, Morganella morganii, Proteis vulgaris, Providencia, Enterobacter, Salmonella, Shigella, Acinetobacter, Bacteroides fragilis, Neisseria, Serratia;* gram-positive organisms *Streptococcus pneumoniae, S. pyogenes, Staphylococcus aureus;* anaerobes *Bacteroides, Clostridium, Fusobacterium, Peptococcus, Peptostreptococcus*

Dosages and routes

Adult: **IV**/IM 1-2g q12h × 5-10 days

Perioperative prophylaxis

Adult: **IV** 1-2 g ½-1 hr before surgery

Available forms: Inj **IV**, IM

Side effects/adverse reactions

CNS: Headache, dizziness, weakness, paresthesia, fever, chills

GI: Nausea, vomiting, diarrhea, anorexia, pain, glossitis, bleeding; increased AST (SGOT), ALT (SGPT), bilirubin, LDH, alkaline phosphatase; *pseudomembranous colitis*

GU: Proteinuria, vaginitis, pruritus, candidiasis, increased BUN, *nephrotoxicity, renal failure*

HEMA: Leukopenia, thrombocytopenia, agranulocytosis, anemia, *neutropenia, lymphocytosis, eosinophilia, pancytopenia, hemolytic anemia*
INTEG: Rash, urticaria, dermatitis
RESP: Dyspnea
SYST: Anaphylaxis

Contraindications: Hypersensitivity to cephalosporins, P children

Precautions: Hypersensitivity to penicillins, pregnancy **B**, lactation, renal disease

Pharmacokinetics

Absorption	Well absorbed (IM)
Distribution	Widely distributed; crosses placenta
Metabolism	Not metabolized
Excretion	Kidneys, unchanged; enters breast milk
Half-life	5 hr; increased in renal disease

Pharmacodynamics

	IM	IV
Onset	Rapid	Immediate
Peak	1-3 hr	Infusion's end

Interactions

Drug/drug:

Individual drugs
Probenecid: ↓ excretion of drug and ↑ blood levels
Vancomycin: ↑ toxicity

Drug classifications
Aminoglycosides: ↑ toxicity
Anticoagulants: ↑ bleeding
Thrombolytics: ↑ bleeding

Lab test interferences

Increase (false): Creatinine (serum urine), urinary 17-KS
False positive: Urinary protein, direct Coombs' test, urine glucose
Interference: Cross-matching

NURSING CONSIDERATIONS

Assessment

- Assess patient for previous sensitivity reaction to penicillins or other cephalosporins; cross-sensitivity between penicillins and cephalosporins is common
- Assess patient for signs and symptoms of infection including characteristics of wounds, sputum, urine, stool, WBC >10,000, fever; obtain baseline information and during treatment
- Obtain C&S before beginning drug therapy to identify if correct treatment has been initiated
- Assess for allergic reactions: rash, urticaria, pruritus, chills, fever, joint pain; angioedema may occur a few days after therapy begins; epinephrine and resuscitation equipment should be available for anaphylactic reaction
- Identify urine output; if decreasing, notify prescriber (may indicate nephrotoxicity); also check for increased BUN, creatinine
- Monitor blood studies: AST (SGOT), ALT (SGPT), CBC, Hct, bilirubin, LDH, alkaline phosphatase, Coombs' test monthly if patient is on long-term therapy
- Monitor electrolytes: potassium, sodium, chloride monthly if patient is on long-term therapy
- Assess bowel pattern qd; if severe diarrhea occurs, drug should be discontinued; may

indicate pseudomembranous colitis.
- Monitor for bleeding: ecchymosis, bleeding gums, hematuria, stool guaiac daily if on long-term therapy
- Assess for overgrowth of infection: perineal itching, fever, malaise, redness, pain, swelling, drainage, rash, diarrhea, change in cough, sputum

Associated nursing diagnoses

- ✓ Infection, risk for (uses)
- ✓ Injury, risk for (side effects)
- ✓ Diarrhea (side effects)
- ✓ Knowledge deficit (teaching)

Implementation

IM route

- Reconstitute 1 g/2ml or 2 g/3 ml of sterile or bacteriostatic water for inj; may be diluted with 0.5% of 1% lidocaine to prevent pain; give deep in large muscle mass, massage

IV **IV route**

- Check for irritation, extravasation, phlebitis daily; change site q72h
- For direct **IV** dilute in 1 g/10 ml or more and give over 5 min
- For intermittent inf further dilute in 50-100 ml of 0.9% NaCl or D_5W; give over 3-5 min; discontinue primary line while running intermittent inf

Y-site compatibilities:

Famotidine, fluconazole, fludarabine, regular insulin, meperidine, morphine, sargramostim

Syringe incompatibility:

Doxapram

Additive incompatibilities:

Aminoglycosides, tetracyclines, heparin

Patient/family education

- Teach patient to report sore throat, bruising, bleeding, joint pain; may indicate blood dyscrasias (rare)
- Advise patient to contact prescriber if vaginal itching, loose, foul-smelling stools, furry tongue occur; may indicate superinfection
- Advise patient to notify prescriber of diarrhea with blood or pus, which may indicate pseudomembranous colitis

Evaluation

Positive therapeutic outcome

- Absence of signs/symptoms of infection (WBC <10,000, temp WNL, absence of red draining wounds)
- Reported improvement in symptoms of infection

Treatment of anaphylaxis:

Epinephrine, antihistamines, resuscitate if needed

cefoxitin

(se-fox'i-tin)

Mefoxin

Func. class.: Broad-spectrum antibiotic

Chem. class.: Cephalosporin (2nd generation)

Pregnancy category **B**

Action: Inhibits bacterial cell wall synthesis, rendering cell wall osmotically unstable, leading to cell death

Uses: Lower respiratory tract, urinary tract, skin, bone, gonococcal infections; septicemia, peritonitis

Therapeutic Outcome: Bactericidal effects for the following: gram-negative bacilli *Haemophilus influenzae, Escherichia coli, Proteus, Klebsiella, Providencia, Neisseria gonorrhoeae;* gram-positive organisms *Streptococcus pneumoniae, S. pyogenes, Staphylococcus aureus;* anaerobes including *Clostridium,* Bacteroides, Peptococcus, Peptostreptococcus

Dosage and routes

Adult: IM/**IV** 1-2 g q6-8h; dosage reduction indicated in renal impairment (CrCl <50 ml/min)

Uncomplicated gonorrhea

2 g IM as single dose with 1 g PO probenecid at same time

Severe infections

Adult: IM/**IV** 2 g q4h

Available forms: Powder for inj IM, **IV** 1, 2, 10 g

Side effects/adverse reactions

CNS: Headache, dizziness, weakness, paresthesia, fever, chills
GI: Nausea, vomiting, diarrhea, anorexia, pain, glossitis, bleeding; increased AST (SGOT), ALT (SGPT), bilirubin, LDH, alkaline phosphatase; abdominal pain
GU: Proteinuria, vaginitis, pruritus, candidiasis, increased BUN, ***nephrotoxicity, renal failure***
*HEMA: **Leukopenia, thrombocytopenia, agranulocytosis,*** anemia, ***neutropenia, lymphocytosis, eosinophilia, pancytopenia, hemolytic anemia***
INTEG: Rash, urticaria, dermatitis, thrombophlebitis
*SYST: **Anaphylaxis***

Contraindications: Hypersensitivity to cephalosporins; P infants <1 mo

Precautions: Hypersensitivity to penicillins, pregnancy **B**, lactation, renal disease

Pharmacokinetics

Absorption	Well absorbed (IM)
Distribution	Widely distributed; crosses placenta
Metabolism	Not metabolized
Excretion	Kidneys, unchanged; enters breast milk
Half-life	½-1 hr; increased in renal disease

Pharmacodynamics

	IM	IV
Onset	Rapid	Immediate
Peak	½ hr	Infusion's end

Interactions

Drug/drug:

Individual drugs
Probenecid: ↓ excretion of drug and ↑ blood levels
Vancomycin: ↑ toxicity
Drug classifications
Aminoglycosides: ↑ toxicity

Lab test interferences

Increase (false): Creatinine (serum urine), urinary 17-KS
False positive: Urinary protein, direct Coombs' test, urine glucose
Interference: Cross-matching

NURSING CONSIDERATIONS

Assessment

- Assess patient for previous sensitivity reaction to penicillins or other cephalosporins; cross-sensitivity between penicillins and cephalosporins is common
- Assess patient for signs and symptoms of infection including characteristics of wounds, sputum, urine, stool, WBC >10,000, fever; obtain baseline information and during treatment
- Obtain C&S before beginning drug therapy to identify if correct treatment has been initiated
- Assess for allergic reactions: rash, urticaria, pruritus, chills, fever, joint pain; angioedema may occur a few days after therapy begins; epinephrine and resuscitation equipment should be on unit for anaphylactic reaction
- Identify urine output; if decreasing, notify prescriber (may indicate nephrotoxicity); also check for increased BUN, creatinine
- Monitor blood studies: AST (SGOT), ALT (SGPT), CBC, Hct, bilirubin, LDH, alkaline phosphatase, Coombs' test monthly if patient is on long-term therapy
- Monitor electrolytes: potassium, sodium, chloride monthly if patient is on long-term therapy
- Assess bowel pattern qd; if severe diarrhea occurs, drug should be discontinued; may indicate pseudomembranous colitis
- Monitor for bleeding: ecchymosis, bleeding gums, hematuria, stool guaiac daily if on long-term therapy
- Assess for overgrowth of infection: perineal itching, fever, malaise, redness, pain, swelling, drainage, rash, diarrhea, change in cough, sputum

C

Associated nursing diagnoses

- ✓ Infection, risk for (uses)
- ✓ Injury, risk for (side effects)
- ✓ Diarrhea (side effects)
- ✓ Knowledge deficit (teaching)

Implementation

IM route

- Reconstitute 1 g/2 ml of sterile water for inj; may be diluted with 0.5% or 1% lidocaine to prevent pain; give deep in large muscle mass, massage

IV **IV route**

- Check for irritation, extravasation, phlebitis daily; change site q72h
- For direct **IV**, dilute 1 g/10 ml or 2 g/20 ml sterile water for inj; shake, let stand until clear; give over 3-5 min
- For intermittent inf further dilute with 50-100 ml of D_5W, $D_{10}W$, D_5/0.25% NaCl, D_5/0.45% NaCl, D_5/0.9% NaCl, 0.9% NaCl, D_5/LR, D_5/0.02%, sodium bicarbonate, Ringer's, or LR; give over 15-30 min
- For cont inf dilute in 500-1000 ml; give at prescribed rate

Y-site incompatibility:

Hetastarch

Y-site compatibilities:

Acyclovir, cyclophosphamide, famotidine, fluconazole, foscarnet, hydromorphone, magnesium sulfate, meperidine, morphine, ondansetron, perphenazine

Additive compatibilities:
Amikacin, cimetidine, clindamycin, gentamicin, kanamycin, multivitamins, sodium bicarbonate, tobramycin, verapamil, vitamin B complex with C

Additive incompatibility:
Aztreonam

Syringe compatibility:
Heparin

Patient/family education
- Teach patient to report sore throat, bruising, bleeding, joint pain; may indicate blood dyscrasias (rare)
- Advise patient to contact prescriber if vaginal itching, loose, foul-smelling stools, furry tongue occur; may indicate superinfection
- Advise patient to notify prescriber of diarrhea with blood or pus, which may indicate pseudomembranous colitis

Evaluation
Positive therapeutic outcome
- Absence of signs/symptoms of infection (WBC <10,000, temp WNL, absence of red draining wounds)
- Reported improvement in symptoms of infection

Treatment of anaphylaxis: Epinephrine, antihistamines, resuscitate if needed

cefpodoxime
(sef-poe-dox'eem)
Vantin
Func. class.: Antibiotic
Chem. class.: Cephalosporin (2nd generation)
Pregnancy category B

Action: Inhibits bacterial cell synthesis, which renders cell wall osmotically unstable, leading to cell death

Uses: Upper and lower respiratory tract, urinary tract, skin infections; otitis media, sexually transmitted diseases

➔ Therapeutic Outcome: Bactericidal effects for the following: gram-negative organisms *Neisseria gonorrhoeae, Haemophilus influenzae, Escherichia coli, Proteus mirabilis, Klebsiella;* gram-positive organisms *Streptococcus pneumoniae, S. pyogenes, Staphylococcus aureus*

Dosage and routes
P ***Adult and child ≥13 yr:***
Pneumonia: 200 mg q12h × 14 days

Uncomplicated gonorrhea: 200 mg single dose; skin and skin structure: 40 mg q12h × 7-14 days

Pharyngitis and tonsillitis: 100 mg q12h × 10 days

Uncomplicated UTI: 100 mg q12h × 7 days; dosing interval increased in presence of severe renal impairment

P *Child (6 mo-12 yr):*
Acute otitis media: 5 mg/kg q12h × 14 days; uncomplicated gonorrhea: 200 mg single dose; skin and skin structure: 400 mg q12h × 7-14 days

Pharyngitis and tonsillitis: 100 mg q12h (max 200 mg/dose or 400 mg/day) × 10 days

Pharyngitis/tonsillitis: 5 mg/kg q12h (max 100 mg/dose or 200 mg/day) × 10 days

Available forms: Tabs 100, 200 mg; granules for susp 50 mg/5 ml and 100 mg/5 ml

Side effects/adverse reactions

CNS: Headache, dizziness, lethargy, fatigue, paresthesia, fever, chills
GI: Nausea, vomiting, diarrhea, anorexia, pain, glossitis, bleeding; increased AST (SGOT), ALT (SGPT), bilirubin, LDH, alkaline phosphatase
GU: Proteinuria, vaginitis, pruritus, candidiasis, increased BUN, nephrotoxicity, renal failure
HEMA: Leukopenia, thrombocytopenia, agranulocytosis, anemia, neutropenia, lymphocytosis, eosinophilia, pancytopenia, hemolytic anemia
INTEG: Rash, urticaria, dermatitis
RESP: Dyspnea
SYST: ***Anaphylaxis***

Contraindications: Hypersensitivity to cephalosporins; P infants

Precautions: Hypersensitivity to penicillins, pregnancy **B**, lactation, renal disease

Pharmacokinetics

Absorption	Well absorbed (PO)
Distribution	Widely distributed; crosses placenta
Metabolism	Not metabolized
Excretion	Kidneys, unchanged; enters breast milk
Half-life	2-3 hr, increased in renal disease

Pharmacodynamics

	PO
Onset	Unknown
Peak	Unknown

Interactions

Drug/drug:

Individual drugs
Probenecid: ↓ excretion of drug and ↑ blood levels
Vancomycin: ↑ toxicity

Drug classifications
Aminoglycosides: ↑ toxicity
Anticoagulants: ↑ bleeding
Erythromycins: ↓ effects
Tetracyclines: ↓ effects
Thrombolytics: ↑ bleeding

Lab test interferences

Increase (false): Creatinine (serum urine), urinary 17-KS
False positive: Urinary protein, direct Coombs' test, urine glucose
Interference: Cross-matching

NURSING CONSIDERATIONS

Assessment

- Assess patient for previous sensitivity reaction to penicillins or other cephalosporins; cross-sensitivity between penicillins and cephalosporins is common
- Assess patient for signs and symptoms of infection including characteristics of wounds, sputum, urine, stool, WBC >10,000, earache, fever; obtain baseline information and during treatment
- Obtain C&S before beginning drug therapy to identify if correct treatment has been initiated
- Assess for allergic reactions: rash, urticaria, pruritus, chills, fever, joint pain; angioedema may occur a few days after therapy begins; epinephrine and resuscitation equipment should be available for anaphylactic reaction
- Identify urine output; if decreasing, notify prescriber (may indicate nephrotoxicity); also check for increased BUN, creatinine
- Monitor blood studies: AST (SGOT), ALT (SGPT), CBC, Hct, bilirubin, LDH, alkaline phosphatase, Coombs' test monthly if patient is on long-term therapy
- Monitor electrolytes: potassium, sodium, chloride monthly if patient is on long-term therapy
- Assess bowel pattern qd; if severe diarrhea occurs, drug should be discontinued; may indicate pseudomembranous colitis
- Monitor for bleeding: ecchymosis, bleeding gums, hematuria, stool guaiac daily if on long-term therapy
- Assess for overgrowth of infection: perineal itching, fever, malaise, redness, pain, swelling, drainage, rash, diarrhea, change in cough, sputum

Associated nursing diagnoses

- ✓ Infection, risk for (uses)
- ✓ Diarrhea (side effects)
- ✓ Injury, risk for (side effects)
- ✓ Knowledge deficit (teaching)
- ✓ Noncompliance (teaching)

Implementation

IM route

- Reconstitute 1 g/2 ml or 2 g/3 ml of sterile or bacteriostatic water for inj; may be diluted with 0.5% or 1% lidocaine to prevent pain; give deep in large muscle mass, massage

IV **IV route**

- Check for irritation, extravasation, phlebitis daily; change site q72h
- For direct **IV** dilute in 1 g/10 ml or more and give over 5 min
- For intermittent inf further dilute in 50-100 ml of 0.9% NaCl or D_5W; give over 3-5 min; discontinue primary line while running intermittent inf

Y-site compatibilities:

Famotidine, fluconazole, fludarabine, regular insulin, meperidine, morphine, sargramostim

Syringe incompatibility:

Doxapram

Additive incompatibility:

Aminoglycosides, tetracyclines, heparin

Patient/family education

- Teach patient to report sore throat, bruising, bleeding, joint pain; may indicate blood dyscrasias (rare)
- Advise patient to contact physician if vaginal itching, loose, foul-smelling stools, furry tongue occur; may indicate superinfection
- Advise patient to notify prescriber of diarrhea with blood or pus, which may indicate pseudomembranous colitis

Evaluation

Positive therapeutic outcome
- Absence of signs/symptoms of infection (WBC <10,000, temp WNL, absence of red draining wounds, earache)
- Reported improvement in symptoms of infection

Treatment of anaphylaxis: Epinephrine, antihistamines, resuscitate if needed

cefprozil
(sef-pro'zil)
Cefzil
Func. class.: Antibiotic
Chem. class.: Cephalosporin (2nd generation)
Pregnancy category B

Action: Inhibits bacterial cell synthesis, which renders cell wall osmotically unstable, leading to cell death

Uses: Upper and lower respiratory tract, urinary tract, skin infections; otitis media, sexually transmitted diseases

Therapeutic Outcome: Bactericidal effects for the following: gram-negative bacilli *Haemophilus influenzae, Escherichia coli;* gram-positive organisms *Streptococcus pneumoniae, S. pyogenes, Staphylococcus aureus*

Dosage and routes

Upper respiratory tract infections

Adult: PO 500 mg qd × 10 days

Child (6 mo-12 yr): PO 15mg/kg q12h × 10 days

Lower respiratory tract infections

Adult: PO 500 mg bid × 10 days

Skin/skin structure infections

Adult: PO 250-500mg q12h × 10 days

Available forms: Tabs 250, 500 mg; susp 125, 250 mg/5 ml

Side effects/adverse reactions

CNS: Headache, dizziness, lethargy, fatigue, paresthesia, fever, chills
GI: Nausea, vomiting, diarrhea, anorexia, pain, glossitis, bleeding; increased AST (SGOT), ALT (SGPT), bilirubin, LDH, alkaline phosphatase

GU: Proteinuria, vaginitis, pruritus, candidiasis, increased BUN, nephrotoxicity, renal failure
HEMA: ***Leukopenia, thrombocytopenia, agranulocytosis, anemia, neutropenia, lymphocytosis, eosinophilia, pancytopenia, hemolytic anemia***
INTEG: Rash, urticaria, dermatitis
RESP: Dyspnea
SYST: ***Anaphylaxis***

Contraindications: Hypersensitivity to cephalosporins; P infants

Precautions: Hypersensitivity to penicillins, pregnancy **B**, lactation, renal disease

Pharmacokinetics

Absorption	Well absorbed (PO)
Distribution	Widely distributed; crosses placenta
Metabolism	Not metabolized
Excretion	Kidneys, unchanged; enters breast milk
Half-life	1-1½ hr; increased in renal disease

Pharmacodynamics

	PO
Onset	Unknown
Peak	Unknown

Interactions
Drug/drug:
Individual drugs
Probenecid: ↓ excretion of drug and ↑ blood levels
Vancomycin: ↑ toxicity
Drug classifications
Aminoglycosides: ↑ toxicity
Anticoagulants: ↑ bleeding
Thrombolytics: ↑ bleeding

Lab test interferences
Increase (false): Creatinine (serum urine), urinary 17-KS
False positive: Urinary protein, direct Coombs' test, urine glucose
Interference: Cross-matching

NURSING CONSIDERATIONS
Assessment
- Assess patient for previous sensitivity reaction to penicillins or other cephalosporins; cross-sensitivity between penicillins and cephalosporins is common
- Assess patient for signs and symptoms of infection including characteristics of wounds, sputum, urine, stool, WBC >10,000, earache, fever; obtain baseline information and during treatment
- Obtain C&S before beginning drug therapy to identify if correct treatment has been initiated
- Assess for allergic reactions: rash, urticaria, pruritus, chills, fever, joint pain; angioedema may occur a few days after therapy begins; epinephrine and resuscitation equipment should be available for anaphylactic reaction
- Identify urine output; if decreasing, notify prescriber (may indicate nephrotoxicity); also check for increased BUN, creatinine
- Monitor blood studies: AST (SGOT), ALT (SGPT), CBC, Hct, bilirubin, LDH, alkaline phosphatase, Coombs' test monthly if patient is on long-term therapy
- Monitor electrolytes: potassium, sodium, chloride

monthly if patient is on long-term therapy
- Assess bowel pattern qd; if severe diarrhea occurs, drug should be discontinued; may indicate pseudomembranous colitis
- Monitor for bleeding: ecchymosis, bleeding gums, hematuria, stool guaiac daily if on long-term therapy
- Assess for overgrowth of infection: perineal itching, fever, malaise, redness, pain, swelling, drainage, rash, diarrhea, change in cough, sputum

Associated nursing diagnoses

✓ Infection, risk for (uses)
✓ Diarrhea (side effects)
✓ Injury, risk for (side effects)
✓ Knowledge deficit (teaching)
✓ Noncompliance (teaching)

Implementation

IM route
- Reconstitute 1 g/2 ml or 2 g/3 ml of sterile or bacteriostatic water for inj; may be diluted with 0.5% or 1% lidocaine to prevent pain; give deep in large muscle mass, massage

IV **IV** route
- Check for irritation, extravasation, phlebitis daily, change site q72h
- For direct **IV** dilute 1 g/10 ml or more and give over 5 min
- For intermittent inf further dilute in 50-100 ml of 0.9% NaCl or D_5W; give over 3-5 min; discontinue primary line while running intermittent infusion

Y-site compatibilities:

Famotidine, fluconazole, fludarabine, regular insulin, meperidine, morphine, sargramostim

Syringe incompatibility:

Doxapram

Additive incompatibilities:

Aminoglycosides, tetracyclines, heparin

Patient/family education

- Teach patient to report sore throat, bruising, bleeding, joint pain; may indicate blood dyscrasias (rare)
- Advise patient to contact prescriber if vaginal itching, loose, foul-smelling stools, furry tongue occur; may indicate superinfection
- Advise patient to notify prescriber of diarrhea with blood or pus, which may indicate pseudomembranous colitis

Evaluation

Positive therapeutic outcome
- Absence of signs/symptoms of infection (WBC <10,000, temp WNL, absence of red draining wounds, earache)
- Reported improvement in symptoms of infection

Treatment of anaphylaxis:

Epinephrine, antihistamines, resuscitate if needed

ceftazidime
(sef'ta-zi-deem)
Ceptaz, Fortaz, Pentacef, Tazicef, Tazidine
Func. class.: Broad-spectrum antibiotic
Chem. class.: Cephalosporin (3rd generation)
Pregnancy category B

Action: Inhibits bacterial cell wall synthesis, which renders cell osmotically unstable, leading to cell death

Uses: Serious upper or lower respiratory tract, urinary tract, skin, gonococcal, intraabdominal infections; septicemia, meningitis

Therapeutic Outcome: Bactericidal effects for the following: gram negative organisms: *Haemophilus influenzae, Escherichia coli, Enterobacter aerogenes, Proteus mirabilis, Klebsiella, Citrobacter, Enterobacter, Pseudomonas aeruginosa, Shigella, Acinetobacter, Bacteroides fragilis, Neisseria;* gram-positive organisms *Streptococcus pneumoniae, S. pyogenes, Staphylococcus aureus*

Dosage and routes
Adult: **IV**/IM 1 g q8-12h × 5-10 days
P ***Children:*** **IV** 30-50 mg/kg/day, not to exceed 6 g/day
P ***Neonates:*** **IV** 30 mg/kg q12h

Available forms: Inj **IV**, IM, 1, 2 g

Side effects/adverse reactions
CNS: Headache, dizziness, weakness, paresthesia, fever, chills
GI: Nausea, vomiting, diarrhea, anorexia, metallic taste, pain, glossitis, bleeding; increased AST (SGOT), ALT (SGPT), bilirubin, LDH, alkaline phosphatase; ***Pseudomembranous colitis***
GU: Proteinuria, vaginitis, pruritus, candidiasis, increased BUN, ***nephrotoxicity, renal failure***
HEMA: ***Leukopenia, thrombocytopenia, agranulocytosis,*** anemia, ***neutropenia, lymphocytosis, eosinophilia, pancytopenia, hemolytic anemia***
INTEG: Rash, urticaria, dermatitis
RESP: Dyspnea
SYST: ***Anaphylaxis***

Contraindications: Hypersensitivity to cephalosporins, P children

Precautions: Hypersensitivity to penicillins, pregnancy **B**, lactation, renal disease

Pharmacokinetics

Absorption	Well absorbed (IM)
Distribution	Widely distributed; crosses placenta
Metabolism	Not metabolized
Excretion	Kidneys, unchanged; enters breast milk
Half-life	½-1 hr; increased in renal disease

Pharmacodynamics

	IM	IV
Onset	Rapid	Immediate
Peak	1 hr	Infusion's end

Interactions

Drug/drug:

Individual drugs

Probenecid: ↓ excretion of drug and ↑ blood levels
Vancomycin: ↑ toxicity

Drug classifications

Aminoglycosides: ↑ toxicity
Erythromycins: ↓ effects
Tetracyclines: ↓ effects

Lab test interferences

Increase (false): Creatinine (serum urine), urinary 17-KS
False positive: Urinary protein, direct Coombs' test, urine glucose
Interference: Cross-matching

NURSING CONSIDERATIONS

Assessment

- Assess patient for previous sensitivity reaction to penicillins or other cephalosporins; cross-sensitivity between penicillins and cephalosporins is common
- Assess patient for signs and symptoms of infection including characteristics of wounds, sputum, urine, stool, WBC >10,000, temperature; obtain baseline information and during treatment
- Obtain C&S before beginning drug therapy to identify if correct treatment has been initiated
- Assess for allergic reactions: rash, urticaria, pruritus, chills, fever, joint pain; angioedema may occur a few days after therapy begins; epinephrine and resuscitation equipment should be available for anaphylactic reaction
- Identify urine output; if decreasing, notify prescriber (may indicate nephrotoxicity); also check for increased BUN, creatinine
- Monitor blood studies: AST (SGOT), ALT (SGPT), CBC, Hct, bilirubin, LDH, alkaline phosphatase, Coombs' test monthly if patient is on long-term therapy
- Monitor electrolytes: potassium, sodium, chloride monthly if patient is on long-term therapy
- Assess bowel pattern qd; if severe diarrhea occurs, drug should be discontinued; may indicate pseudomembranous colitis
- Monitor for bleeding: ecchymosis, bleeding gums, hematuria, stool guaiac daily if on long-term therapy
- Assess for overgrowth of infection: perineal itching, fever, malaise, redness, pain, swelling, drainage, rash, diarrhea, change in cough, sputum

Associated nursing diagnoses

- ✓ Infection, risk for (uses)
- ✓ Injury, risk for (side effects)
- ✓ Diarrhea (side effects)
- ✓ Knowledge deficit (teaching)

Implementation

IM route

- Reconstitute 500 mg/1.5 ml or 1 g/3 ml of sterile or bacteriostatic water for inj; may be diluted with 0.5% or 1% lidocaine to prevent pain; give deep in large muscle mass, massage

IV **IV route**

- Check for irritation, extravasation, phlebitis daily; change site q72h

• For direct **IV** dilute 500 mg/5 ml or 1 g/10 ml sterile water for inj; give over 3-5 min; do not use sol with benzyl alcohol for neonates
• For intermittent inf further dilute 1 g/10 ml or more 0.9% NaCl, D_5W, $D_{10}W$, D_5/0.25% NaCl, D_5/0.45% NaCl, D_5/0.9% NaCl, or LR; give over 30-60 min

Y-site incompatibilities:
Amsacrine, fluconazole, sargramostim, idarubicin

Y-site compatibilities:
Acyclovir, ciprofloxacin, enalaprilat, esmolol, fludarabine, foscarnet, hydromorphone, labetalol, meperidine, melphalan, morphine, ondansetron, paclitaxel, vinorelbine tartrate, zidovudine

Additive incompatibilities:
Aminoglycosides, sodium bicarbonate

Additive compatibilities:
Ciprofloxacin, clindamycin, metronidazole

Patient/family education
• Teach patient to report sore throat, bruising, bleeding, joint pain; may indicate blood dyscrasias (rare)
• Advise patient to contact prescriber if vaginal itching, loose, foul-smelling stools, furry tongue occur; may indicate superinfection
• Advise patient to notify prescriber of diarrhea with blood or pus, which may indicate pseudomembranous colitis

Evaluation
Positive therapeutic outcome
• Absence of signs/symptoms of infection (WBC <10,000, temp WNL, absence of red draining wounds, earache)
• Reported improvement in symptoms of infection

Treatment of anaphylaxis: Epinephrine, antihistamines, resuscitate if needed

ceftizoxime
(sef-ti-zox'eem)
Cefizox
Func. class.: Broad-spectrum antibiotic
Chem. class.: Cephalosporin (3rd generation)
Pregnancy category B

Action: Inhibits bacterial cell wall synthesis, which renders cell wall osmotically unstable, leading to cell death

Uses: Serious lower respiratory tract, urinary tract, skin, intraabdominal infections; septicemia, meningitis; bone, joint infections; pelvic inflammatory disease (PID) caused by *Neisseria gonorrhoeae*

Therapeutic Outcome: Bactericidal effects for the following: gram-negative organisms *Haemophilus influenzae, Escherichia coli, Enterobacter aerogenes, Proteus mirabilis, Klebsiella, Acinetobacter, Neisseriagonorrhea, Providencia rettgen, Pseudomonas aeruginosa, serratia Enterobacter;* gram-positive organisms *Strep-*

tococcus pneumoniae, S. pyogenes, Staphylococcus aureus; anarobes *Bacteroides, Peptococcus, Peptostreptococcus*

Dosage and routes

Adult: IM/**IV** 1-2 g q8-12h; may give up to 2 g q4h in life-threatening infections

Pelvic inflammatory disease

Adult: **IV** 2 g q8h; may increase to 2 g q4h in severe infections

Available forms: Inj 500 mg, 1, 2 g/100 ml piggyback, 50 ml/5% D_5

Side effects/adverse reactions

CNS: Headache, dizziness, paresthesia, fever
GI: Nausea, vomiting, diarrhea, anorexia, pain, glossitis, bleeding; increased AST (SGOT), ALT (SGPT), bilirubin, LDH, alkaline phosphatase; abdominal pain, ***pseudomembranous colitis***
GU: Proteinuria, vaginitis, pruritus, candidiasis
HEMA: Leukopenia, thrombocytopenia, agranulocytosis, anemia, ***neutropenia, eosinophilia, hemolytic anemia***
INTEG: Rash, urticaria, dermatitis
RESP: Dyspnea
SYST: Anaphylaxis

Contraindications: Hypersensitivity to cephalosporins, P infants <1 mo

Precautions: Hypersensitivity to penicillins, pregnancy **B**, lactation, renal disease

Pharmacokinetics

Absorption	Well absorbed (IM)
Distribution	Widely distributed; crosses placenta
Metabolism	Not metabolized
Excretion	Kidneys, unchanged; enters breast milk
Half-life	1½-2 hr; increased in renal disease

Pharmacodynamics

	IM	IV
Onset	Rapid	Immediate
Peak	1 hr	Infusion's end

Interactions

Drug/drug:

Individual drugs
Probenecid: ↓ excretion of drug and ↑ blood levels
Vancomycin: ↑ toxicity
Drug classifications
Aminoglycosides: ↑ toxicity

Lab test interferences

Increase (false): Creatinine (serum urine), urinary 17-KS
False positive: Urinary protein, direct Coombs' test, urine glucose
Interference: Cross-matching

NURSING CONSIDERATIONS

Assessment

- Assess patient for previous sensitivity reaction to penicillins or other cephalosporins; cross-sensitivity between penicillins and cephalosporins is common
- Assess patient for signs and symptoms of infection including characteristics of wounds, sputum, urine, stool, WBC >10,000, fever; obtain baseline information and during treatment

- Obtain C&S before beginning drug therapy to identify if correct treatment has been initiated
- Assess for allergic reactions: rash, urticaria, pruritus, chills, fever, joint pain; angioedema may occur a few days after therapy begins; epinephrine and resuscitation equipment should be on unit for anaphylactic reaction
- Identify urine output; if decreasing, notify prescriber (may indicate nephrotoxicity); also check for increased BUN, creatinine
- Monitor blood studies: AST (SGOT), ALT (SGPT), CBC, Hct, bilirubin, LDH, alkaline phosphatase, Coombs' test monthly if patient is on long-term therapy
- Monitor electrolytes: potassium, sodium, chloride monthly if patient is on long-term therapy
- Assess bowel pattern qd; if severe diarrhea occurs, drug should be discontinued; may indicate pseudomembranous colitis
- Monitor for bleeding: ecchymosis, bleeding gums, hematuria, stool guaiac daily if on long-term therapy
- Assess for overgrowth of infection: perineal itching, fever, malaise, redness, pain, swelling, drainage, rash, diarrhea, change in cough, sputum

Associated nursing diagnoses

✓ Infection, risk for (uses)
✓ Diarrhea (side effects)
✓ Injury, risk for (side effects)
✓ Knowledge deficit (teaching)
✓ Noncompliance (teaching)

Implementation

IM route

- Reconstitute 250 mg/0.9 ml, 500 mg/1.8 ml, 1 g/3.6 ml, 2 g/7.2 ml; may be diluted with 0.5% or 1% lidocaine to prevent pain; give deep in large muscle mass, massage

IV **IV route**

- Check for irritation, extravasation, phlebitis daily; change site q72h
- For intermittent inf reconstitute 250 mg/2.4 ml, 500 mg/4.8 ml, 1 gm/9.6 m/2 gm/19.2 ml sterile water for inj, D_5W, or 0.9% NaCl; do not use sol with benzyl alcohol P for neonates; may be further diluted in 50-100 ml D_5W, $D_{10}W$, 0.9% NaCl, or LR; give over 30-60 min

Y-site compatibilities:

Acyclovir, enalaprilat, esmolol, famotidine, fludarabine, foscarnet, hydromorphone, labetalol, melphalan, meperidine, morphine, ondansetron, sargramostim, vinorelbine tartrate

Additive incompatibility:

Aminoglycosides

Additive compatibility:

Clindamycin

Patient/family education

- Teach patient to report sore throat, bruising, bleeding, joint pain; may indicate blood dyscrasias (rare)
- Advise patient to contact prescriber if vaginal itching, loose, foul-smelling stools, furry tongue occur; may indicate superinfection

• Advise patient to notify prescriber of diarrhea with blood or pus, which may indicate pseudomembranous colitis

Evaluation

Positive therapeutic outcome
• Absence of signs/symptoms of infection (WBC <10,000, temp WNL, absence of red draining wounds)
• Reported improvement in symptoms of infection

Treatment of anaphylaxis: Epinephrine, antihistamines, resuscitate if needed

ceftriaxone

(sef-try-ax'one)
Rocephin
Func. class.: Broad spectrum antibiotic
Chem. class.: Cephalosporin (3rd generation)
Pregnancy category **B**

Action: Inhibits bacterial cell wall synthesis, which renders cell wall osmotically unstable, leading to cell death

Uses: Serious lower respiratory tract, urinary tract, skin, gonococcal, intraabdominal infections; septicemia, meningitis; bone, joint infections

Therapeutic Outcome: Bactericidal effects on the following: gram-negative organisms *Haemophilus influenzae, Escherichia coli, Enterobacter aerogenes, Proteus mirabilis, Klebsiella, Citrobacter, Enterobacter, Pseudomonas aeruginosa, Neisseria, Serratia;* gram-positive organisms *Streptococcus pneumoniae, S. pyogenes, Staphylococcus aureus;* anaerobes *Bacteroides*

C

Dosage and routes

Adult: IM/**IV** 1-2 g qd or in two equal doses

P *Child:* IM/**IV** 50-75 mg/kg/day in equal doses q12h

Uncomplicated gonorrhea:
250 mg IM as single dose

Dosage reduction may be indicated in severe renal impairment (CrCl <10 ml/min)

Meningitis

P *Adult and child:* IM/**IV** 100 mg/kg/day in equal doses q12h

Surgical prophylaxis

Adult: **IV** 1 g ½-2 hr preop

Available forms: Inj IM, **IV** 250, 500 mg, 1, 2, 10 g

Side effects/adverse reactions

CNS: Headache, dizziness, weakness, paresthesia, fever, chills

GI: Nausea, vomiting, diarrhea, anorexia, pain, glossitis, bleeding; increased AST (SGOT), ALT (SGPT), bilirubin, LDH, alkaline phosphatase; abdominal pain, ***pseudomembranous colitis***

GU: Proteinuria, vaginitis, pruritus, candidiasis, increased BUN, ***nephrotoxicity, renal failure***

HEMA: ***Leukopenia, thrombocytopenia, agranulocytosis,***

anemia, ***neutropenia, lymphocytosis, eosinophilia, pancytopenia, hemolytic anemia***
INTEG: Rash, urticaria, dermatitis
RESP: Dyspnea
SYST: ***Anaphylaxis***

Contraindications: Hypersensitivity to cephalosporins, P infants <1 mo

Precautions: Hypersensitivity to penicillins, pregnancy **B**, lactation, renal disease

Pharmacokinetics

Absorption	Well-absorbed
Distribution	Widely distributed; crosses placenta; enters CSF
Metabolism	Liver
Excretion	Kidneys, partly
Half-life	5-8 hr

Pharmacodynamics

	IM	IV
Onset	Rapid	Immediate
Peak	1 hr	Infusion's end

Interactions

Drug/drug:

Individual drugs

Probenecid: ↓ excretion of drug and ↑ blood levels
Vancomycin: ↑ toxicity

Drug classifications

Aminoglycosides: ↑ toxicity

Lab test interferences

Increase (false): Creatinine (serum urine), urinary 17-KS
False positive: Urinary protein, direct Coombs' test, urine glucose
Interference: Cross-matching

NURSING CONSIDERATIONS

Assessment

- Assess patient for previous sensitivity reaction to penicillins or other cephalosporins; cross-sensitivity between penicillins and cephalosporins is common
- Assess patient for signs and symptoms of infection including characteristics of wounds, sputum, urine, stool, WBC >10,000, fever; obtain baseline information and during treatment
- Obtain C&S before beginning drug therapy to identify if correct treatment has been initiated
- Assess for allergic reactions: rash, urticaria, pruritus, chills, fever, joint pain; angioedema may occur a few days after therapy begins; epinephrine and resuscitation equipment should be available for anaphylactic reaction
- Identify urine output; if decreasing, notify prescriber (may indicate nephrotoxicity); also check for increased BUN, creatinine
- Monitor blood studies: AST (SGOT), ALT (SGPT), CBC, Hct, bilirubin, LDH, alkaline phosphatase, Coombs' test monthly if patient is on long-term therapy
- Monitor electrolytes: potassium, sodium, chloride monthly if patient is on long-term therapy
- Assess bowel pattern qd; if severe diarrhea occurs, drug should be discontinued; may indicate pseudomembranous colitis
- Monitor for bleeding: ecchymosis, bleeding gums, hema-

turia, stool guaiac daily if on long-term therapy
- Assess for overgrowth of infection: perineal itching, fever, malaise, redness, pain, swelling, drainage, rash, diarrhea, change in cough, sputum

Associated nursing diagnoses

✓ Infection, risk for (uses)
✓ Injury, risk for (side effects)
✓ Diarrhea (side effects)
✓ Knowledge deficit (teaching)

Implementation

IM route
- Reconstitute 250 mg/0.9 ml, 500 mg/1.8 ml, 1 g/3.6 ml, 2 g/7.2 ml; may be diluted with 0.5% or 1% lidocaine to prevent pain; give deep in large muscle mass, massage

IV **IV route**
- Check for irritation, extravasation, phlebitis daily; change site q72h
- For intermittent inf reconstitute 250 mg/2.4 ml, 500 mg/4.8 ml, 1 g/9.6 ml/2 g/19.2 ml sterile water for inj, D_5W, 0.9% NaCl; do not use sol with benzyl alcohol for P neonates; may be further diluted in 50-100 ml D_5W, $D_{10}W$, 0.9% NaCl; or LR; give over 30-60 min

Y-*site incompatibilities:*

Amsacrine, fluconazole, vancomycin

Y-*site compatibilities:*

Acyclovir, fludarabine, foscarnet, melphalan, meperidine, morphine, paclitaxel, sargramostim, vinorelbine tartrate

Additive incompatibilities:

Aminoglycosides, clindamycin

Additive compatibilities:

Amino acids or sodium bicarbonate

Patient/family education

- Teach patient to report sore throat, bruising, bleeding, joint pain; may indicate blood dyscrasias (rare)
- Advise patient to contact prescriber if vaginal itching, loose, foul-smelling stools, furry tongue occur; may indicate superinfection
- Advise patient to notify prescriber of diarrhea with blood or pus, which may indicate pseudomembranous colitis

Evaluation

Positive therapeutic outcome
- Absence of signs/symptoms of infection (WBC <10,000, temp WNL, absence of red draining wounds)
- Reported improvement in symptoms of infection

Treatment of anaphylaxis:

Epinephrine, antihistamines, resuscitate if needed

cephalexin 🔑

(sef-a-lex'in)

Keftab, Biocef, Cefanex, cephalexin, Ceporex ♣, Keflet, Keflex, Novolexin ♣, Zartan

Func. class.: Antibiotic

Chem. class.: Cephalosporin (1st generation)

Pregnancy category B

Action: Inhibits bacterial cell wall synthesis, rendering cell wall osmotically unstable, leading to cell death

Uses: Upper, lower respiratory tract, urinary tract, skin, bone infections; otitis media

Therapeutic Outcome: Bactericidal effects of the following: gram-negative organisms *Haemophilus influenzae, Escherichia coli, Proteus mirabilis, Klebsiella;* gram-positive organisms *Streptococcus pneumoniae, S. pyogenes, Staphylococcus aureus*

Dosage and routes

Adult: PO 250-500 mg q6h

P *Child:* PO 25-50 mg/kg/day in 4 equal doses

Moderate skin infections

500 mg q12h

Severe infections

Adult: PO 500 mg-1 g q6h

P *Child:* PO 50-100 mg/kg/day in 4 equal doses

Dosage reduction indicated in renal impairment (CrCl <50 ml/min)

Available forms: Caps 250, 500 mg; tabs 250, 500, 1000 mg; pulvules 250 mg; oral susp 125, 250 mg/5 ml; pediatric susp 100 mg/5 ml

Side effects/adverse reactions

CNS: Headache, dizziness, weakness, paresthesia, fever, chills

GI: Nausea, vomiting, diarrhea, anorexia, pain, glossitis, bleeding; increased AST (SGOT), ALT (SGPT), bilirubin, LDH, alkaline phosphatase; abdominal pain, ***pseudomembranous colitis***

GU: Proteinuria, vaginitis, pruritus, candidiasis, increased BUN, ***nephrotoxicity, renal failure***

HEMA: Leukopenia, thrombocytopenia, agranulocytosis, anemia, ***neutropenia, lymphocytosis, eosinophilia, pancytopenia, hemolytic anemia***

INTEG: Rash, urticaria, dermatitis

RESP: Dyspnea

SYST: ***Anaphylaxis***

Contraindications: Hypersensitivity to cephalosporins, P infants <1 mo.

Precautions: Hypersensitivity to penicillins, pregnancy **B**, lactation, renal disease

C

Pharmacokinetics

Absorption	Well absorbed
Distribution	Widely distributed; crosses placenta
Metabolism	Not metabolized
Excretion	Kidneys, unchanged; enters breast milk
Half-life	½-1 hr; increased in renal disease

Pharmacodynamics

	PO
Onset	15-30 min
Peak	1 hr

Interactions

Drug/drug:

Individual drugs

Probenecid: ↓ excretion of drug and ↑ blood levels
Vancomycin: ↑ toxicity

Drug classifications

Aminoglycosides: ↑ toxicity, ↑ nephrotoxicity

Lab test interferences

Increase (false): Creatinine (serum urine), urinary 17-KS
False positive: Urinary protein, direct Coombs' test, urine glucose
Interference: Cross-matching

NURSING CONSIDERATIONS

Assessment

- Assess patient for previous sensitivity reaction to penicillins or other cephalosporins; cross-sensitivity between penicillins and cephalosporins is common
- Assess patient for signs and symptoms of infection including characteristics of wounds, sputum, urine, stool, WBC >10,000, earache, fever; obtain baseline information and during treatment
- Obtain C&S before beginning drug therapy to identify if correct treatment has been initiated
- Assess for allergic reactions: rash, urticaria, pruritus, chills, fever, joint pain; angioedema may occur a few days after therapy begins; epinephrine and resuscitation equipment should be available for anaphylactic reaction
- Identify urine output; if decreasing, notify prescriber (may indicate nephrotoxicity); also check for increased BUN, creatinine
- Monitor blood studies: AST (SGOT), ALT (SGPT), CBC, Hct, bilirubin, LDH, alkaline phosphatase, Coombs' test monthly if patient is on long-term therapy
- Monitor electrolytes: potassium, sodium, chloride monthly if patient is on long-term therapy
- Assess bowel pattern qd; if severe diarrhea occurs, drug should be discontinued; may indicate pseudomembranous colitis
- Monitor for bleeding: ecchymosis, bleeding gums, hematuria, stool guaiac daily if on long-term therapy
- Assess for overgrowth of infection: perineal itching, fever, malaise, redness, pain, swelling, drainage, rash, diarrhea, change in cough, sputum

Associated nursing diagnoses

✓ Infection, risk for (uses)
✓ Injury, risk for (side effects)

✓ Diarrhea (side effects)
✓ Knowledge deficit (teaching)
✓ Noncompliance (teaching)

Implementation

PO route

- Give in even doses around the clock; if GI upset occurs, give with food; drug must be taken for 10-14 days to ensure organism death and prevent superinfection
- Shake suspension

Patient/family education

- Teach patient to report sore throat, bruising, bleeding, joint pain; may indicate blood dyscrasias (rare)
- Advise patient to contact prescriber if vaginal itching, loose, foul-smelling stools, furry tongue occur; may indicate superinfection
- Instruct patient to take all medication prescribed for the length of time ordered
- Advise patient to notify prescriber of diarrhea with blood or pus, which may indicate pseudomembranous colitis

Evaluation

Positive therapeutic outcome

- Absence of signs/symptoms of infection (WBC <10,000, temp WNL, absence of red draining wounds, earache)
- Reported improvement in symptoms of infection

Treatment of anaphylaxis: Epinephrine, antihistamines, resuscitate if needed

cephalothin

(sef-a'loe-thin)
cephalothin sodium, Ceporacin ✦, Keflin Neutral
Func. class.: Broad-spectrum antibiotic
Chem. class.: Cephalosporin (1st generation)
Pregnancy category B

Action: Inhibits bacterial cell wall synthesis, rendering cell wall osmotically unstable and leading to cell death by binding to the cell wall membrane

Uses: Lower respiratory tract, urinary tract, skin and bone infections; septicemia, endocarditis, bacterial peritonitis

➡ Therapeutic Outcome: Bactericidal effects for the following: gram-negative bacilli *Haemophilus influenzae, Escherichia coli, Proteus mirabilis, Klebsiella, Salmonella, Shigella;* gram-positive organisms *Streptococcus pneumoniae, S. pyogenes, Staphylococcus aureus*

Dosage and routes

Adult: IM/**IV** 500 mg-1 g q4-6h

P ***Child:*** IM/**IV** 14-27 mg/kg q4h or 20-40 mg/kg q6h

Dosage reduction indicated in renal impairment (CrCl <50 ml/min)

Uncomplicated gonorrhea: 2 g IM as single dose

Severe infections
Adult: IM/**IV** 1-2 g q4h

Available forms: Powder for inj IM, **IV** 1, 2, 4, 10, 20 g; frozen **IV** 20, 30, 40 mg/ml

Side effects/adverse reactions

CNS: Headache, dizziness, weakness, paresthesia, fever, chills
GI: Nausea, vomiting, diarrhea, anorexia, pain, glossitis, bleeding; increased AST (SGOT), ALT (SGPT), bilirubin, LDH, alkaline phosphatase; abdominal pain, ***pseudomembranous colitis***
GU: ***Proteinuria,*** vaginitis, pruritus, candidiasis, increased BUN, ***nephrotoxicity, renal failure***
HEMA: ***Leukopenia, thrombocytopenia, agranulocytosis,*** anemia, ***neutropenia, lymphocytosis, eosinophilia, pancytopenia, hemolytic anemia***
INTEG: Rash, urticaria, dermatitis
RESP: Dyspnea
SYST: ***Anaphylaxis***

Contraindications: Hypersensitivity to cephalosporins

Precautions: Hypersensitivity to penicillins, pregnancy **B**, lactation, renal disease

Pharmacokinetics

Absorption	Well absorbed
Distribution	Widely distributed; crosses placenta
Metabolism	Not metabolized
Excretion	Kidneys, unchanged; enters breast milk
Half-life	½-1 hr

Pharmacodynamics

	IM	IV
Onset	Rapid	Immediate
Peak	½ hr	Infusion's end

Interactions
Drug/drug:
Individual drugs
Probenecid: ↓ excretion of drug and ↑ blood levels
Vancomycin: ↑ toxicity
Drug classifications
Aminoglycosides: ↑ toxicity, ↑ nephrotoxicity

Lab test interferences
Increase (false): Creatinine (serum urine), urinary 17-KS
False positive: Urinary protein, direct Coombs' test, urine glucose
Interference: Cross-matching

NURSING CONSIDERATIONS
Assessment
- Assess patient for previous sensitivity reaction to penicillins or other cephalosporins; cross-sensitivity between penicillins and cephalosporins is common
- Assess patient for signs and symptoms of infection including characteristics of wounds, sputum, urine, stool, WBC >10,000, fever; obtain baseline information and during treatment
- Obtain C&S before beginning drug therapy to identify if correct treatment has been initiated
- Assess for allergic reactions: rash, urticaria, pruritus, chills, fever, joint pain; angioedema may occur a few days after therapy begins; epinephrine

and resuscitation equipment should be available for anaphylactic reaction

- Identify urine output; if decreasing, notify prescriber (may indicate nephrotoxicity); also check for increased BUN, creatinine
- Monitor blood studies: AST (SGOT), ALT (SGPT), CBC, Hct, bilirubin, LDH, alkaline phosphatase, Coombs' test monthly if patient is on long-term therapy
- Monitor electrolytes: potassium, sodium, chloride monthly if patient is on long-term therapy
- Assess bowel pattern qd; if severe diarrhea occurs, drug should be discontinued; may indicate pseudomembranous colitis
- Monitor for bleeding: ecchymosis, bleeding gums, hematuria, stool guaiac daily if on long-term therapy
- Assess for overgrowth of infection: perineal itching, fever, malaise, redness, pain, swelling, drainage, rash, diarrhea, change in cough, sputum

Associated nursing diagnoses

- ✓ Infection, risk for (uses)
- ✓ Injury, risk for (side effects)
- ✓ Diarrhea (side effects)
- ✓ Knowledge deficit (teaching)

Implementation

IM route

- Reconstitute 1 g/4 ml sterile water for inj; give deep in large muscle mass and massage
- IM route not preferred; causes intense pain and induration

IV **IV route**

- Check for irritation, extravasation, phlebitis daily; change site q72h
- For direct **IV** dilute 1 g/10 ml or more sterile water for inj, D_5W, 0.9% NaCl; give over 3-5 min
- For intermittent inf, reconstitute 1-2 mg/50 ml sterile water for inj, D_5W, $D_{10}W$, D_5/LR, D_5/0.9% NaCl, 0.9% NaCl; may be further diluted in 50-100 ml D_5W, $D_{10}W$, 0.9% NaCl, or LR; give over 15-30 min
- For cont inf may be diluted in 500-1000 ml and run at prescribed rate; may use hydrocortisone 10-25 mg added to inf containing 4-6 g or more of cephalothin to decrease the incidence of thrombophlebitis

Y-site incompatibility:

Hetastarch

Y-site compatibilities:

Cyclophosphamide, famotidine, heparin, hydromorphone, magnesium sulfate, meperidine, morphine, multivitamins, perphenazine, potassium chloride, vitamin B complex with C

Syringe incompatibility:

Metoclopramide

Syringe compatibility:

Cimetidine

Additive incompatibilities:

Aminoglycosides, amikacin, aminophylline, amobarbital, bleomycin, calcium chloride, calcium gluceptate, calcium gluconate, colistimethate, diphenhydramine, doxorubicin, erythromycin, gentamicin, kanamycin, oxytetracycline, pentobarbital, penicillin G sodium, phenobarbital, polymyxin B, prochlorperazine, tetracycline

Additive compatibilities:
Ascorbic acid, chloramphenicol, clindamycin, fluorouracil, hydrocortisone sodium succinate, isoproterenol, magnesium sulfate, metaraminol bitartrate, methicillin, methotrexate, potassium chloride, prednisolone sodium phosphate, procaine, sodium bicarbonate

Patient/family education

- Teach patient to report sore throat, bruising, bleeding, joint pain; may indicate blood dyscrasias (rare)
- Advise patient to contact prescriber if vaginal itching, loose, foul-smelling stools, furry tongue occur; may indicate superinfection
- Advise patient to notify prescriber of diarrhea with blood or pus, which may indicate pseudomembranous colitis

Evaluation

Positive therapeutic outcome
- Absence of signs/symptoms of infection (WBC <10,000, temp WNL, absence of red draining wounds)
- Reported improvement in symptoms of infection

Treatment of anaphylaxis: Epinephrine, antihistamines, resuscitate if needed

cephapirin

(sef-a-pye'rin)
Cefadyl, cephapirin sodium
Func. class.: Broad spectrum antibiotic
Chem. class.: Cephalosporin (1st generation)
Pregnancy category **B**

Action: Inhibits bacterial cell wall synthesis, rendering cell wall osmotically unstable, leading to cell death

Uses: Lower respiratory tract, urinary tract, skin infections; septicemia, endocarditis, bacterial peritonitis

Therapeutic Outcome: Bactericidal effects for the following: gram-negative bacilli *Haemophilus influenzae, Escherichia coli, Proteus mirabilis, Klebsiella;* gram-positive organisms *Streptococcus pneumoniae, S. viridans, Staphylococcus aureus*

Dosage and routes

Adult: IM/**IV** 500 mg-1 g q4-6h
P *Child:* IM/**IV** 20-30 mg/kg, q6h

Dosage reduction indicated in renal impairment (CrCl <50 ml/min)

Available forms: Powder for inj IM, IV 500 mg, 1, 2, 20 g; IV only 1, 2, 4 g

Side effects/adverse reactions

CNS: Headache, dizziness, weakness, paresthesia, fever, chills
GI: Nausea, vomiting, diarrhea, anorexia, pain, glossitis, bleeding; increased AST (SGOT), ALT (SGPT), bilirubin, LDH, alkaline phosphatase; abdominal pain, ***pseudomembranous colitis***
GU: Proteinuria, vaginitis, pruritus, candidiasis, increased BUN, ***nephrotoxicity, renal failure***
HEMA: ***Leukopenia, thrombocytopenia, agranulocytosis,*** anemia, ***neutropenia, lymphocytosis, eosinophilia, pancytopenia, hemolytic anemia***
INTEG: Rash, urticaria, dermatitis
RESP: Dyspnea
SYST: ***Anaphylaxis***

Contraindications: Hypersensitivity to cephalosporins, P infants <1 mo

Precautions: Hypersensitivity to penicillins, pregnancy **B**, lactation, renal disease

Pharmacokinetics

Absorption	Well absorbed
Distribution	Widely distributed; crosses placenta
Metabolism	Not metabolized
Excretion	Kidneys, unchanged; enters breast milk
Half-life	½-1 hr

Pharmacodynamics

	IM	IV
Onset	Rapid	Immediate
Peak	½ hr	Infusion's end

Interactions

Drug/drug:

Individual drugs
Probenecid: ↓ excretion of drug and ↑ blood levels
Vancomycin: ↑ toxicity
Drug classifications
Aminoglycosides: ↑ toxicity

Lab test interferences

Increase (false): Creatinine (serum urine), urinary 17-KS
False positive: Urinary protein, direct Coombs' test, urine glucose
Interference: Cross-matching

NURSING CONSIDERATIONS

Assessment

- Assess patient for previous sensitivity reaction to penicillins or other cephalosporins; cross-sensitivity between penicillins and cephalosporins is common
- Assess patient for signs and symptoms of infection including characteristics of wounds, sputum, urine, stool, WBC >10,000, fever; obtain baseline information and during treatment
- Obtain C&S before beginning drug therapy to identify if correct treatment has been initiated
- Assess for allergic reactions: rash, urticaria, pruritus, chills, fever, joint pain; angioedema may occur a few days after therapy begins; epinephrine and resuscitation equipment should be available for anaphylactic reaction
- Identify urine output; if decreasing, notify prescriber (may indicate nephrotoxicity);

also check for increased BUN, creatinine
• Monitor blood studies: AST (SGOT), ALT (SGPT), CBC, Hct, bilirubin, LDH, alkaline phosphatase, Coombs' test monthly if patient is on long-term therapy
• Monitor electrolytes: potassium, sodium, chloride monthly if patient is on long-term therapy
• Assess bowel pattern qd; if severe diarrhea occurs, drug should be discontinued; may indicate pseudomembranous colitis
• Monitor for bleeding: ecchymosis, bleeding gums, hematuria, stool guaiac daily if on long-term therapy
• Assess for overgrowth of infection: perineal itching, fever, malaise, redness, pain, swelling, drainage, rash, diarrhea, change in cough, sputum

Associated nursing diagnoses

✓ Infection, risk for (uses)
✓ Injury, risk for (side effects)
✓ Diarrhea (side effects)
✓ Knowledge deficit (teaching)

Implementation

IM route
• Reconstitute 1-2 g/1-2 ml of sterile water for inj; give deep in large muscle mass and massage

IV **IV route**
• Check for irritation, extravasation, phlebitis daily; change site q72h
• For intermittent inf, reconstitute 250 mg/2.4 ml, 500 mg/4.8 ml, 1 g/9.6 ml, 2 gm/19.2 ml sterile water for inj, D_5W, 0.9% NaCl; do not use sol with benzyl alcohol for P neonates; may be further diluted in 50-100 ml D_5W, $D_{10}W$, 0.9% NaCl, or LR; give over 30-60 min

Y-site compatibilities:

Acyclovir, cyclophosphamide, famotidine, heparin, hydrocortisone sodium succinate, hydromorphone, magnesium sulfate, meperidine, morphine, multivitamins, perphenazine, potassium chloride, vitamin B complex with C

Additive incompatibilities:

Aminoglycosides, amikacin, ascorbic acid, epinephrine, gentamicin, kanamycin, mannitol, norepinephrine, oxytetracycline, phenytoin, tetracycline, thiopental

Additive compatibilities:

Bleomycin, calcium chloride, calcium gluconate, chloramphenicol, diphenhydramine, ergonovine maleate, heparin, hydrocortisone sodium phosphate, hydrocortisone sodium succinate, metaraminol bitartrate, oxacillin, penicillin G potassium, pentobarbital, phenobarbital, phytonadione, potassium chloride, sodium bicarbonate, succinylcholine, verapamil, warfarin, vitamin B complex

Patient/family education

• Teach patient to report sore throat, bruising, bleeding, joint pain; may indicate blood dyscrasias (rare)
• Advise patient to contact prescriber if vaginal itching, loose, foul-smelling stools,

furry tongue occur; may indicate superinfection
- Advise patient to notify prescriber of diarrhea with blood or pus, which may indicate pseudomembranous colitis

Evaluation

Positive therapeutic outcome
- Absence of signs/symptoms of infection (WBC <10,000, temp WNL, absence of red draining wounds)
- Reported improvement in symptoms of infection

Treatment of anaphylaxis: Epinephrine, antihistamines, resuscitate if needed

cephradine

(sef'ra-deen)

cephradine, Velosef

Func. class.: Antibiotic

Chem. class.: Cephalosporin (1st generation)

Pregnancy category B

Action: Inhibits bacterial cell wall synthesis, rendering cell wall osmotically unstable, leading to cell death

Uses: Serious respiratory tract, urinary tract, skin infections; otitis media

Therapeutic Outcome: Bactericidal effects for the following: gram-negative bacilli *Haemophilus influenzae, Escherichia coli, Proteus mirabilis, Klebsiella;* gram-positive organisms *Streptococcus pneumoniae, S. pyogenes, Staphylococcus aureus*

Dosage and routes

Adult: IM/**IV** 500 mg-1 g q4-6h; not to exceed 8 g/day; PO 250 mg-1 g q6-12h

P *Child >1 yr:* IM/**IV** 12-25 mg/kg q6h or 50-100 mg/kg/day q6h; PO 6-12 mg/kg q6h or 25-50 mg/kg/day q6-12h

Available forms: Powder for inj IM, **IV** 250, 500 mg, 1 g; caps 250, 500 mg; oral susp 125, 250 mg/5 ml

Side effects/adverse reactions

CNS: Headache, dizziness, weakness, paresthesia, fever, chills

GI: Nausea, vomiting, diarrhea, anorexia, pain, glossitis, bleeding; increased AST (SGOT), ALT (SGPT), bilirubin, LDH, alkaline phosphatase, abdominal pain, ***pseudomembranous colitis***

GU: Proteinuria, vaginitis, pruritus, candidiasis, increased BUN, ***nephrotoxicity, renal failure***

HEMA: ***Leukopenia, thrombocytopenia, agranulocytosis,*** anemia, ***neutropenia, lymphocytosis, eosinophilia, pancytopenia, hemolytic anemia***

INTEG: Rash, urticaria, dermatitis

RESP: Dyspnea

SYST: ***Anaphylaxis***

Contraindications: Hypersensitivity to cephalosporins, P infants <1 mo

Precautions: Hypersensitivity to penicillins, pregnancy **B**, lactation, renal disease

Pharmacokinetics

Absorption	Well absorbed
Distribution	Widely distributed; crosses placenta
Metabolism	Not metabolized
Excretion	Kidneys, unchanged; enters breast milk
Half-life	1-2 hr

Pharmacodynamics

	PO/IM	IV
Onset	Rapid	Immediate
Peak	1 hr	Infusion's end

Interactions

Drug/drug:

Individual drugs

Probenecid: ↓ excretion of drug and ↑ blood levels

Vancomycin: ↑ toxicity

Drug classifications

Aminoglycosides: ↑ toxicity

Lab test interferences

Increase (false): Creatinine (serum urine), urinary 17-KS

False positive: Urinary protein, direct Coombs' test, urine glucose

Interference: Cross-matching

NURSING CONSIDERATIONS

Assessment

- Assess patient for previous sensitivity reaction to penicillins or other cephalosporins; cross-sensitivity between penicillins and cephalosporins is common
- Assess patient for signs and symptoms of infection including characteristics of wounds, sputum, urine, stool, WBC >10,000, earache, fever; obtain baseline information and during treatment
- Obtain C&S before beginning drug therapy to identify if correct treatment has been initiated
- Assess for allergic reactions: rash, urticaria, pruritus, chills, fever, joint pain; angioedema may occur a few days after therapy begins; epinephrine and resuscitation equipment should be available for anaphylactic reaction
- Identify urine output; if decreasing, notify prescriber (may indicate nephrotoxicity); also check for increased BUN, creatinine
- Monitor blood studies: AST (SGOT), ALT (SGPT), CBC, Hct, bilirubin, LDH, alkaline phosphatase, Coombs' test monthly if patient is on long-term therapy
- Monitor electrolytes: potassium, sodium, chloride monthly if patient is on long-term therapy
- Assess bowel pattern qd; if severe diarrhea occurs, drug should be discontinued; may indicate pseudomembranous colitis
- Monitor for bleeding: ecchymosis, bleeding gums, hematuria, stool guaiac daily if on long-term therapy
- Assess for overgrowth of infection: perineal itching, fever, malaise, redness, pain, swelling, drainage, rash, diarrhea, change in cough, sputum

Associated nursing diagnoses

- ✓ Infection, risk for (uses)
- ✓ Diarrhea (side effects)
- ✓ Knowledge deficit (teaching)
- ✓ Noncompliance (teaching)(PO)
- ✓ Injury, risk for (side effects)

Implementation

PO route
• May be given with food for GI symptoms
• When giving susp, shake well; refrigerate unused portion

IM route
• Reconstitute 250 mg/1.2 ml, 500 mg/ml, 1 g/4 ml sterile or bacterostatic water for inj; give deep in large muscle mass, massage

IV **IV route**
• Check for irritation, extravasation, phlebitis daily; change q72h
• Direct **IV** route 250-500 mg/5 ml sterile water, 0.9% NaCl, D_5W, or 1 g/10 ml, 2 g/20 ml; give over 3-5 min
• For intermittent inf, dilute 1 g/10 ml or more sterile water for inj, D_5W, $D_{10}W$, or D_5/0.9% NaCl; give over 30-60 min

Additive incompatibilities:
Other antibiotics, calcium salts, D_5W, epinephrine, lidocaine, Ringer's or LR sol, Normosol-R, NaCl, TPN #61, tetracycline

Patient/family education

• Teach patient to report sore throat, bruising, bleeding, joint pain; may indicate blood dyscrasias (rare)
• Advise patient to contact prescriber if vaginal itching, loose, foul-smelling stools, furry tongue occur; may indicate superinfection
• Instruct patient to take all medication prescribed for the length of time ordered
• Advise patient to notify prescriber of diarrhea with blood or pus, which may indicate pseudomembranous colitis

Evaluation

Positive therapeutic outcome
• Absence of signs/symptoms of infection (WBC <10,000, temp WNL, absence of red draining wounds, earache)
• Reported improvement in symptoms of infection

Treatment of anaphylaxis: Epinephrine, antihistamines, resuscitate if needed

chloral hydrate
(klor'al hye'drate)
Aquachloral Supprettes, chloral hydrate, Noctec, Novochlorhydrate ✤
Func. class.: Sedative/hypnotic
Chem. class.: Chloral derivative

Pregnancy category C

Controlled substance schedule IV (USA), schedule F (Canada)

Action: Reduced to product trichloroethanol, which produces mild cerebral depression, causing sleep; generalized CNS depression

➔ **Therapeutic Outcome:** Ability to sleep, sedation

Uses: Sedation, insomnia, preoperative reduction of anxiety

Dosage and routes

Sedation

Adult: PO/rec 250 mg tid pc

P *Child:* PO 8 mg/kg tid, not to exceed 500 mg tid

Insomnia

Adult: PO/rec 500 mg-1g 30 min before hs

P *Child:* PO/rec 50 mg/kg in one dose

Available forms: Caps 250, 500 mg; syr 250, 500 mg/5 ml; supp 325, 500, 650 mg

Side effects/adverse reactions

CNS: Drowsiness, dizziness, stimulation, nightmares, ataxia, hangover (rare), lightheadedness, headache, paranoia

CV: Hypotension, dysrhythmias

GI: Nausea, vomiting, flatulence, diarrhea, unpleasant taste, ***gastric necrosis***

HEMA: Eosinophilia, leukopenia

INTEG: Rash, urticaria, angioedema, fever, purpura, eczema

RESP: Depression

Contraindications: Hypersensitivity to this drug or triclofos, severe renal disease, severe hepatic disease, GI disorders (oral forms), gastritis

Precautions: Severe cardiac disease, depression, suicidal individuals, asthma, intermittent porphyria, pregnancy **C**, lactation, elderly

Pharmacokinetics

Absorption	Well absorbed (PO, rec)
Distribution	Widely distributed; crosses placenta
Metabolism	Liver to trichloroethanol
Excretion	Kidneys (inactive metabolite), feces, breast milk
Half-life	8-10 hr; active metabolite

Pharmacodynamics

	PO	REC
Onset	½-1 hr	Slow
Peak	Unknown	Unknown
Duration	4-8 hr	4-6 hr

Interactions

Drug/drug:

Individual drugs

Alcohol: ↑ CNS depression

Fluoxetine: ↑ action

Furosemide: ↑ diaphoresis, flushing

Propoxyphene: ↑ action

Drug classification

Analgesics, opioid: ↑ CNS depression

Anticoagulants, oral: ↑ action of anticoagulants

Antidepressants: ↑ CNS depression

Antihistamines: ↑ CNS depression

Sedative/hypnotics: ↑ CNS depression

Lab test interferences

Interferences: Urine catecholamines, urinary 17-OHCS

False positive: Urine glucose (copper sulfate test)

NURSING CONSIDERATIONS

Assessment

- Assess patient's sleep pattern and note physical (sleep apnea,

obstructed airway, pain/discomfort, urinary frequency) and psychologic (fear, anxiety) circumstances that interrupt sleep
• Assess patient's bedtime routine, presleep cues/props
• Assess potential for abuse; this drug may lead to physical and psychologic dependency; amount of drug should be limited
• Monitor blood studies: Hct, Hgb, RBCs, serum folate (if on long-term therapy), protime in patients receiving anticoagulants since action of anticoagulant may be increased
• Monitor mental status: mood, sensorium, affect, memory (long, short)
• Monitor physical dependency: more frequent requests for medication, shakes, anxiety, pinpoint pupils
• Monitor respiratory dysfunction: respiratory depression, character, rate, rhythm; hold drug if respirations are <10/min or if pupils are dilated (rare)
• Assess for blood dyscrasias: fever, sore throat, bruising, rash, jaundice, epistaxis (rare)
• Assess previous history of substance abuse, cardiac disease, or gastritis

Associated nursing diagnoses

✓ Sleep pattern disturbance (uses)
✓ Anxiety (uses)
✓ Knowledge deficit (teaching)
✓ Noncompliance (teaching)

Implementation

General
• Regulate environmental stimuli (light, noise, temperature), remove foods and fluids that interfere with sleep
• Place side rails up after giving medication for hypnotic; remove cigarettes/matches from patient's environment to prevent fires

PO route
• Give ½-1 hr before hs for sleeplessness; give on empty stomach with full glass of water or juice for best absorption and to decrease corrosion (do not chew); after meals to decrease GI symptoms if used for sedation; dilute syr in 4 oz water or juice

Rectal route
• Store supp in dark container, in refrigerator; remove outer wrapper before insertion

Patient/family education

• Caution patient to avoid driving and other activities requiring alertness; to avoid alcohol ingestion or CNS depressants; serious CNS depression may result plus tachycardia, flushing, headache, hypotension
• Instruct patient not to discontinue medication quickly after long-term use; drug should be tapered over 1-2 wk; that effects may take 2 nights for benefits to be noticed; withdrawal symptoms include tremors, anxiety, hallucinations, delirium
• Teach patient alternate measures to improve sleep (reading, exercise several hours before hs, warm bath, warm milk, TV, self-hypnosis, deep breathing)
• Instruct the patient about factors that contribute to sleep

pattern disturbances (lifestyle, shift work, long work hours, environmental factors, frequent napping)
• Teach patient to take drug as prescribed, not to double doses

Evaluation

Positive therapeutic outcome
• Ability to sleep at night
• Decreased amount of early morning awakening if taking drug for insomnia
• Sedation

Treatment of overdose: Lavage, activated charcoal; monitor electrolytes, vital signs

chlorambucil

(klor-am'byoo-sil)
Leukeran
Func. class.: Antineoplastic alkylating agent
Chem. class.: Nitrogen mustard
Pregnancy category **D**

Action: Alkylates DNA, RNA; inhibits enzymes that allow synthesis of amino acids in proteins; activity is not cell cycle phase specific

➔ Therapeutic Outcome: Prevention of rapidly growing malignant cells

Uses: Chronic lymphocytic leukemia, Hodgkin's disease, other lymphomas, macroglobulinemia, nephrotic syndrome, breast carcinoma, choreocarcinoma, ovarian carcinoma

Dosage and routes

Adult: PO 0.1-0.2 mg/kg/day × 3-6 wk initially, then 2-6 mg/day; maintenance 0.2 mg/kg × 2-4 wk; course may be repeated at 2-4 wk intervals

P Child: PO 0.1-0.2 mg/kg/day in divided doses or 4.5 mg/m^2/day as 1 dose or in divided doses

Available forms: Tabs 2 mg

Side effects/adverse reactions

P ***CNS: Convulsions in children***
GI: Nausea, vomiting, diarrhea, weight loss, hepatoxicity, jaundice
GU: Hyperuremia
HEMA: Thrombocytopenia, leukopenia, pancytopenia (prolonged use), ***permanent bone marrow depression***
INTEG: Alopecia (rare), dermatitis, rash
RESP: Fibrosis, pneumonitis

Contraindications: Radiation therapy within 1 mo, chemotherapy within 1 mo, thrombocytopenia, smallpox vaccination, pregnancy (1st trimester) **D**

Precautions: ***Pneumococcus*** vaccination

Pharmacokinetics

Absorption	Rapidly, completely absorbed (PO)
Distribution	Crosses placenta
Metabolism	Liver, extensively
Excretion	Kidneys
Half-life	2 hr

Pharmacodynamics

	PO
Onset	Unknown
Peak	Unknown
Duration	Unknown

Interactions

Drug/drug:

Individual drugs

Radiation: ↑ toxicity, bone marrow suppression

Drug classifications

Antineoplastics: ↑ toxicity, bone marrow suppression

Bone marrow–suppressing drugs: ↑ bone marrow suppression

Live vaccines: ↑ adverse reactions, ↓ antibody reaction

Lab test interferences

Increase: Uric acid

NURSING CONSIDERATIONS

Assessment

- Monitor CBC, differential, platelet count weekly; withhold drug if WBC is <4000 or platelet count is <75,000; notify prescriber of results if WBC <20,000/mm^3, platelets <50,000/mm^3
- Monitor pulmonary function tests, chest x-ray films before, during therapy; chest film should be obtained q2 wk during treatment; check for dyspnea, rales, unproductive cough, chest pain, tachypnea
- Assess for increased uric acid levels, swelling, joint pain primarily in extremities; patient should be well hydrated to prevent urate deposits
- Monitor renal function studies: BUN, serum uric acid, urine CrCl before, during therapy; I&O ratio; report fall in urine output of 30 ml/hr; monitor for decreased hyperuricemia
- Monitor for cold, fever, sore throat (may indicate beginning infection); identify edema in feet, joint, stomach pain, shaking; prescriber should be notified
- Assess for bleeding: hematuria, guaiac, bruising or petechiae, mucosa or orifices q8h, no rec temp

Associated nursing diagnoses

- ☑ Injury, risk for (adverse reactions)
- ☑ Body image disturbance (adverse reactions)
- ☑ Infection, risk for (adverse reactions)
- ☑ Knowledge deficit (teaching)

Implementation

PO route

- Give 1 hr ac or 2 hr pc to lessen nausea and vomiting or antacid before oral agent, give drug after evening meal, before hs; antiemetic 30-60 min before giving drug to prevent vomiting
- Give either allopurinol or sodium bicarbonate to maintain uric acid levels, alkalinization of urine; increase fluid intake to 2-3 L/day to prevent urate deposits, calculus formation
- Use antibiotics for prophylaxis of infection may be prescribed, since infection potential is high
- Store in tight container

Patient/family education

- Teach patient to avoid use of products containing aspirin or ibuprofen, razors, commercial mouthwash, since bleeding may occur; to report symptoms of bleeding (hematuria, tarry stools)
- Instruct patient to report signs of anemia (fatigue, headache, irritability, faintness, shortness of breath)
- Instruct patient to report any changes in breathing or coughing even several mo after treatment; to avoid crowds and persons with respiratory tract or other infections
- Advise patient hair loss is common; discuss the use of wigs or hair pieces
- Caution patient not to have any vaccinations without the advice of the prescriber; serious reactions can occur
- Advise patient contraception is needed during treatment and for several months after the completion of therapy

Evaluation

Positive therapeutic outcome

- Decreased size of tumor
- Decreased spread of malignancy
- Improved blood values
- Absence of sweating at night
- Increased appetite, increased weight

C

chloramphenicol

(klor-am-fen′i-kole)

Ak-Chlor, Chloro-fab chlorophe, Econochlor, chloramphenicol, chloramphenicol sodium succinate, Chloromycetin Kapseals, Chloromycetin Sodium Succinate, Chloromycetin Palmitate, Novochlorocap ✤, Fenicol ✤, Ocu-Chlor, Ophthochlor Pentamycetin ✤, Sopamycetin ✤, Spectro-Chlor

Func. class.: Antibacterial/antirickettsial

Chem. class.: Dichloroacetic acid derivative

Pregnancy category C

Action: Binds to 50S ribosomal subunit, which interferes with or inhibits protein synthesis

➔ **Therapeutic Outcome:** Bacteriocital for *H. influenzae, S. typhi, Rickettsia, Neisseria,* mycloplasma

Uses: Meningitis, Bacterienia, Abdominal, skin, soft tissue infections; local infections of skin, ear, eye

Dosage and routes

Adult: PO/**IV** 12.5 mg/kg q6hr, not to exceed 4 g/day

P ***Children and infants >2 wk:*** **IV**/PO 12 mg/kg q6hr or 2.5 mg/kg q2hr

P ***Infants <2 wk and premature:*** **IV**/PO 6.25 mg/kg q6hr
P ***Adult and child:*** Ophth 1-2 gtt of sol or ointment q 3-6 mo; otic 2-3 gtt bid or tid; top 1% cream tid or qid
P ***Premature infants and neonates:*** **IV**/PO 25 mg/kg/day in divided doses q6hr

Available forms: Inj **IV** 100 mg/ml in 1 g vial; caps 250, 500 mg; oral susp 150 mg/5 ml; ophth ointment 10 mg/g; ophth sol 25 mg/15 ml, 5 mg/ml; top cream 1%, otic sol 0.5%

Side effects/adverse reactions

CNS: Headache, ***depression,*** confusion
CV: Gray syndrome in newborns: failure to feed, pallor, cyanosis, abdominal distention, irregular respiration, vasomotor collapse
EENT: Optic neuritis, blindness
GI: Nausea, vomiting, diarrhea, abdominal pain, xerostomia, glossitis, colitis, pruritus ani
HEMA: Anemia, bone marrow depression, thrombocytopenia, aplastic anemia, granulocytopenia, leukopenia (rare)
INTEG: Itching, urticaria, contact dermatitis, rash

Contraindications: Hypersensitivity, severe renal disease, severe hepatic disease, minor infections

Precautions: Hepatic disease, **P** renal disease, infants, children, bone marrow depression (drug-induced), pregnancy **C**, lactation

Pharmacokinetics

Absorption	Well (PO) Completely (IV)
Distribution	Wide
Metabolism	Liver
Excretion	Kidneys, unchanged
Half-life	1½-4 hr

Pharmacodynamics

	PO	IV	TOP	OPH	OTIC
Onset	15 min	Rapid	Unkn	Unkn	Unkn
Peak	1-2 hr	Inf end	Unkn	Unkn	Unkn

Interactions

Drug/drug:

Individual drugs
Chlorpromide: ↑ action of chlorpromide
Dicumarol: ↑ action of dicumarol
Folic acid: ↓ action of folic acid
Iron: ↑ action of iron
Phenobarbital: ↑ action of phenobarbital
Phenytoin: ↑ action of phenytoin
Tolubamide: ↑ action of tolubamide
Vitamin B_{12}: ↓ action of vitamin B_{12}
Drug classifications
Anticoagulants: ↑ prothrombin time
Barbiturates: ↑ levels of chloramphenicol
Penicillins: synergism

NURSING CONSIDERATIONS

Assessment

- Assess patient for previous sensitivity reaction to other antiinfectives; cross-sensitivity between penicillins and cephalosporins is common
- Assess patient for signs and symptoms of infection including characteristics of wounds, sputum, urine, stool, WBC >10,000, fever; obtain baseline information and during treatment
- Perform C&S testing before starting drug therapy to identify if correct treatment has been initiated
- Monitor blood studies: platelets q2 days, CBC
- Assess bowel pattern qd; if severe diarrhea occurs, drug should be discontinued
- Monitor for bleeding: ecchymosis, bleeding gums, hematuria, stool guaiac daily if on long-term therapy
- Assess for overgrowth of infection: perineal itching, fever, malaise, redness, pain, swelling, drainage, rash, diarrhea, change in cough, sputum

Associated nursing diagnoses

- ✓ Infection, risk for (uses)
- ✓ Diarrhea (adverse reaction)
- ✓ Injury, risk for (side effects)
- ✓ Knowledge deficit (teaching)
- ✓ Noncompliance (teaching)

Top route
- Wash hands, clean area to be treated with soap and water before application

Ophthalmic route
- Apply a small amount of ointment in lower lid
- Have patient tilt head back before application

Implementation

IV route
- Give after diluting 1 g/10 ml of sterile H_2O for inj or D_5W (10% sol); give over >1 min
- May be further diluted in 50-100 ml of D_5W; give through Y-tube, 3-way stopcock, or additive inf set; run over ½-1 hr reconstituted solution at room temp for up to 30 days

Syringe compatibility:

Heparin

Y-site incompatibility:

Fluconazole

Y-site compatibilities:

Acyclovir, cyclophosphamide, enalaprilat, esmolol, foscarnet, hydromorphone, labetalol, magnesium sulfate, meperidine, morphine, perphenazine

PO route
- Give oral form on empty stomach with full glass of water
- Store cap in airtight container at room temp

Patient/family education

- Teach patient all aspects of drug therapy; need to complete entire course of medication to ensure organism death (10-14 days); culture may be taken after complete course of medication
- Advise patient to report sore throat, fever, fatigue, unusual bleeding, or bruising; could indicate bone marrow depression (may occur weeks or months

after termination of drug)
- Tell patient that drug must be taken at regular intervals around clock to maintain blood levels

Evaluation

Positive therapeutic outcome
- Decreased symptoms of infection

chlordiazepoxide

(klor-dye-az-e-pox′ide)
Apo-Chlordiazepoxide ✱, chlordiazepoxide HCl, Libritabs, Librium, Medilium ✱, Mitran, Novopoxide ✱, Resposans-10, Solium ✱
Func. class.: Antianxiety
Chem. class.: Benzodiazepine
Pregnancy category **D**

Controlled substance schedule **IV**

Action: Potentiates the actions of GABA, an inhibitory neurotransmitter, especially in the limbic system reticular formation, which depresses the CNS

Therapeutic Outcome: Decreased anxiety, successful alcohol withdrawal, relaxation

Uses: Short-term management of anxiety, acute alcohol withdrawal, preoperative relaxation

Dosage and routes

Mild anxiety

Adult: PO 5-10 mg tid-qid

P ***Child >6 yr:*** 5 mg bid-qid, not to exceed 10 mg bid-tid

Severe anxiety

Adult: PO 20-25 mg tid-qid

Preoperatively

Adult: PO 5-10 mg tid-qid on day before surgery; IM 50-100 mg 1 hr before surgery

Alcohol withdrawal

Adult: PO/IM/**IV** 50-100 mg, not to exceed 300 mg/day

Available forms: Caps 5, 10, 25 mg; tabs 5, 10, 25 mg; powder for IM inj 100 mg

Side effects/adverse reactions

CNS: Dizziness, drowsiness, confusion, headache, anxiety, tremors, stimulation, fatigue, depression, insomnia, hallucinations
CV: Orthostatic hypotension, ***ECG changes, tachycardia,*** hypotension
EENT: Blurred vision, tinnitus, mydriasis
GI: Constipation, dry mouth, nausea, vomiting, anorexia, diarrhea
INTEG: Rash, dermatitis, itching

Contraindications: Hypersensitivity to benzodiazepines, narrow angle glaucoma, P psychosis, pregnancy **D**, child <18 yr

G **Precautions:** Elderly, debilitated, hepatic disease, renal disease

Pharmacokinetics

Absorption	Well absorbed (PO); slow, erratic (IM)
Distribution	Widely distributed; crosses placenta, blood-brain barrier
Metabolism	Liver extensively
Excretion	Kidneys, breast milk
Half-life	5-30 hr

Pharmacodynamics

	PO	IM	IV
Onset	30 min	15-30 min	1-5 min
Peak	½ hr	Unknown	Unknown
Duration	4-6 hr	Unknown	Up to 1 hr

Interactions

Drug/drug:

Individual drugs

Alcohol: ↑ CNS depression
Cimetidine: ↑ action of cimetidine
Disulfiram: ↑ action of disulfiram
Fluoxetine: ↑ action of fluoxetine
Isoniazid: ↑ action of isoniazid
Ketoconazole: ↑ action of ketoconazole
Levodopa: ↓ action of levodopa
Metoprolol: ↑ action of metoprolol
Propoxyphene: ↑ action of propoxyphene
Propranolol: ↑ action
Rifampin: ↓ action of chlordiazepoxide
Theophylline: ↓ sedative effects
Valproic acid: ↑ action of valproic acid

Drug classifications

Analgesics, opioid: ↑ CNS depression
Antidepressants: ↑ CNS depression
Antihistamines: ↑ CNS depression
Barbiturates: ↓ effect of chlordiazepoxide
Contraceptives, oral: ↑ effect of contraceptive

Lab test interferences

Increase: AST (SGOT)/ALT (SGPT), serum bilirubin
False increase: 17-OHCS
Decrease: RAIU

NURSING CONSIDERATIONS

Assessment

- Assess anxiety reaction: inability to sleep, apprehension, dread, foreboding, or uneasiness related to unidentified source of danger
- Assess for previous drug dependence or tolerance; if drug dependent or tolerant, amount of medication should be restricted
- Monitor B/P (with patient lying, standing), pulse; if systolic B/P drops 20 mm Hg, hold drug, notify prescriber
- Monitor blood studies: CBC during long-term therapy; blood dyscrasias have occurred rarely
- Monitor hepatic studies: AST (SGOT), ALT (SGPT), bilirubin, creatinine, LDH, alkaline phosphatase
- Monitor mental status: mood, sensorium, affect, sleeping patterns, drowsiness, dizziness, suicidal tendencies

Associated nursing diagnoses

- ✓ Anxiety (uses)
- ✓ Knowledge deficit (teaching)
- ✓ Noncompliance (teaching)

Implementation

PO route

• Give with food or milk for GI symptoms, crushed if patient unable to swallow medication whole; do not open capsules; provide sugarless gum, hard candy, frequent sips of water for dry mouth

IM route

• Reconstitute with diluent provided (2 ml); agitate slowly, do not shake; give deep in large muscle mass to prevent severe pain; do not use IM diluent for **IV** route

IV **IV route**

• Reconstitute 100 mg/5 ml sterile water for inj or 0.9% NaCl; give over at least 1 min to prevent cardiac arrest, apnea, bradycardia

Syringe incompatibility:

Benzquinamide

Y-*site compatibilities:*

Heparin, hydrocortisone sodium succinate, potassium chloride, Vitamin B with C

Solution compatibilities:

D_5W, Ringer's, 0.9% NaCl

Patient/family education

• Instruct patient that drug may be taken with food; if dose is missed take as soon as remembered; do not double doses

• Tell patient to avoid OTC preparations unless approved by prescriber; to avoid alcohol ingestion or other psychotropic medications unless directed by a prescriber

• Caution patient to avoid driving and activities requiring alertness, since drowsiness may occur; until medication response is known, tell patient that drowsiness may worsen at beginning of treatment

• Instruct patient not to discontinue medication abruptly after long-term use, drug should be tapered over 1 wk

• Caution patient to rise slowly or fainting may occur, especially in elderly G

Evaluation

Positive therapeutic outcome

• Increased well being

• Decreased anxiety, restlessness, sleeplessness, dread

• Successful alcohol withdrawal

Treatment of overdose:

Lavage, VS, supportive care

chloroquine ⊶

(klor'oh-kwin)

Aralen HCl, Aralen Phosphate, chloroquine phosphate, Novochloroquine ✤

Func. class.: Antimalarial

Chem. class.: Synthetic 4-aminoquinoline derivative

Pregnancy category **C**

Action: Inhibits parasite replications, transcription of DNA to RNA by forming complexes with DNA of parasite

➔ **Therapeutic Outcome:** Decreased symptoms of malaria, amebiasis

Uses: Malaria caused by *Plasmodium vivax, P. malariae, P. ovale, P. falciparum* (some strains), amebiasis

Dosage and routes

Malaria suppression

P ***Adult and child:*** PO 5 mg/kg/wk on same day of week, not to exceed 500 mg; treatment should begin 1-2 wk before exposure and for 8 wk after; if treatment begins after exposure, 600 mg for adult and 10 mg/kg for children in 2 divided doses 6 hr apart

Extraintestinal amebiasis

Adult: IM 200-250 mg qd (HCl) up to 12 days, then 1 g (phosphate) qd × 2 days, then 500 mg qd × 2-3 wk

P ***Child:*** IM/PO 10 mg/kg qd (HCl) × 2-3 wk, not to exceed 300 mg/day

Available forms: Tabs 250, 500 mg; inj IM 50 mg/ml

Side effects/adverse reactions

CNS: Headache, stimulation, fatigue, ***convulsion,*** psychosis

CV: Hypotension, heart block, asystole with syncope, ECG changes

EENT: Blurred vision, corneal changes, retinal changes, difficulty focusing, tinnitus, vertigo, deafness, photophobia, corneal edema

GI: Nausea, vomiting, anorexia, diarrhea, cramps

HEMA: Thrombocytopenia, agranulocytosis, hemolytic anemia, leukopenia

INTEG: Pruritus, pigmentary changes, skin eruptions, lichen planus–like eruptions, eczema, ***exfoliative dermatitis***

Contraindications: Hypersensitivity, retinal field changes, porphyria

Precautions: Pregnancy **C**, P children, blood dyscrasias, severe GI disease, neurologic disease, alcoholism, hepatic disease, G6PD deficiency, psoriasis, eczema, lactation, porphyria

Pharmacokinetics

Absorption	Well absorbed
Distribution	Widely
Metabolism	Liver
Excretion	Kidneys, feces
Half-life	3-5 days

Pharmacodynamics

	PO	IM
Onset	Rapid	Rapid
Peak	1-6 hr	45-60 min
Duration	6-8 hr	Unknown

Interactions

Drug/drug:

Individual drugs

Cimetidine: ↓ absorption

Kaolin: ↓ absorption

Drug classifications

Antacids, aluminum: ↓ absorption

NURSING CONSIDERATIONS

Assessment

- Monitor liver studies weekly: ALT (SGPT), AST (SGOT), bilirubin; renal status: before

exposure, monthly thereafter: BUN, creatinine, output, sp gr, urinalysis
• Assess mental status often: affect, mood, behavioral changes; psychosis may occur
• Assess hepatic status: decreased appetite, jaundice, dark urine, fatigue

Associated nursing diagnoses

- ✓ Infection, risk for (uses)
- ✓ Diarrhea (side effects)
- ✓ Knowledge deficit (teaching)
- ✓ Noncompliance (teaching)
- ✓ Injury, risk for (side effects)

Implementation

PO route
• Give with meals to decrease GI symptoms; better to take on empty stomach 1 hr ac or 2 hr pc
• Give antiemetic if vomiting occurs
• Give after C&S is completed; monthly to detect resistance
IM route
• Give IM after aspirating to prevent inj into bloodstream

Patient/family education

• Advise patient that compliance with dosage schedule, duration is necessary
• Instruct patient that scheduled appointments must be kept or relapse may occur
• Caution patient to avoid alcohol while taking drug
• Instruct diabetic to use blood glucose monitor to obtain correct result
• Teach patient to report weakness, fatigue, loss of appetite, nausea, vomiting, yellowing of skin or eyes, tingling/numbness of hands/feet
• Advise patient that urine may turn rust brown color
• Instruct patient to use sunglasses in bright sunlight to prevent photophobia

Evaluation

Positive therapeutic outcome
• Decreased symptoms of malaria

chlorothiazide

(klor-oh-thye'a-zide)
Diachlor, Diurigen, Diuril, Diuril Sodium
Func. class.: Diuretic, antihypertensive
Chem. class.: Thiazide; sulfonamide derivative
Pregnancy category **B**

Action: Acts on the distal tubule in the kidney, increasing excretion of sodium, water, chloride, magnesium, potassium and bicarbonate

➔ **Therapeutic Outcome:** Decreased BP, decreased edema in tissues, peripherally, diuresis

Uses: Edema in congestive heart failure, nephrotic syndrome; may be used alone or as adjunct with antihypertensives; also for edema in corticosteroids, estrogen therapy

Dosage and routes

Edema, hypertension
Adult: PO/**IV** 50 mg-2 g qd in 2 divided doses

Diuresis

P *Child >6 mo:* PO 20 mg/kg/day in 2 divided doses

P *Child <6 mo:* PO 30 mg/kg/day in 2 divided doses

Available forms: Tabs 250, 500 mg; oral susp 250 mg/5 ml; inj 500 mg

Side effects/adverse reactions

CNS: Drowsiness, paresthesia, anxiety, depression, headache, *dizziness, fatigue, weakness, fever*
CV: Irregular pulse, orthostatic hypotension, palpitations, volume depletion
EENT: Blurred vision
ELECT: Hypokalemia, hypercalcemia, hyponatremia, hypochloremia, hypophosphatemia, hypomagnesemia, hyperlipidemia
GI: Nausea, vomiting, anorexia, constipation, diarrhea, cramps, pancreatitis, GI irritation, ***hepatitis***
GU: Frequency, polyuria, ***uremia,*** glucosuria
HEMA: ***Aplastic anemia, hemolytic anemia, leukopenia, agranulocytosis, thrombocytopenia, neutropenia***
INTEG: Rash, urticaria, purpura, photosensitivity
META: Hyperglycemia, *hyperuricemia,* hypomagnesemia, increased creatinine, BUN

Contraindications: Hypersensitivity to thiazides or sulfonamides, anuria, renal decompensation, pregnancy **(B),** lactation

Precautions: Hypokalemia, renal disease, hepatic disease, gout, COPD, LE, diabetes mellitus, G elderly, hyperlipidemia

Pharmacokinetics

	PO
Absorption	GI tract (10%-20%)
Distribution	Extracellular spaces; crosses placenta
Metabolism	Liver
Excretion	Urine, unchanged; breast milk
Half-life	1-2 hr

Pharmacodynamics

	PO	IV
Onset	2 hr	15 min
Peak	4 hr	½ hr
Duration	6-12 hr	2 hr

Interactions

Drug/drug:

Individual drugs

Cholestyramine: ↓ absorption of chlorothiazide
Colestipol: ↓ absorption of chlorothiazide
Diazoxide: ↓ hyperglycemia, hyperuricemia, hypotension
Digitalis: ↑ toxicity
Indomethacin: ↓ hypotensive response
Lithium: ↑ toxicity
Mezlocillin: ↑ hypokalemia
Piperacillin: ↑ hypokalemia
Ticarcillin: ↑ hypokalemia

Drug classifications

Antidiabetics: ↓ effect of antidiabetic agent
Antihypertensives: ↑ antihypertensive effect
Nondepolarizing skeletal muscle relaxants: ↑ toxicity
Glucocorticoids: ↑ hypokalemia
Sulfonylureas: ↓ effect of sulfonylurea

Drug/food:

Food: ↑ absorption

Lab test interferences

False negative: Phentolamine and tyramine tests
Interfere: Urine steroid tests
Increase: BSP retention, calcium, amylase, parathyroid test
Decrease: PBI, PSP

NURSING CONSIDERATIONS

Assessment

- Assess glucose in urine if patient is diabetic
- Monitor improvement in CVP q8h
- Check for rashes, temp elevation qd
- Assess for confusion, especially in elderly; take safety precautions if needed
- Monitor manifestations of hypokalemia; *renal:* acidic urine, reduced urine, osmolality, nocturia; *CV:* hypotension, broad T wave, U wave, ectopy, tachycardia, weak pulse; *neuro:* muscle weakness, altered LOC, drowsiness, apathy, lethargy, confusion, depression; *GI:* anorexia, nausea, cramps, constipation, distention, paralytic ileus; *resp:* hypoventilation, respiratory muscle weakness
- Monitor for manifestations of hypomagnesemia; *CNS:* agitation, muscle twitching, paresthesias, hyperactive reflexes, positive Babinski reflex, dysphagia, nystagmus, seizures, tetany; *GI:* nausea, vomiting, diarrhea, anorexia, abdominal distention; *CV:* ectopy, tachycardia, broad, flat, or inverted T waves, depressed ST segment, prolonged QT, decreased cardiac output, hypotension
- Monitor for manifestations of hyponatremia: *CV:* increased BP, cold, clammy skin, hypovolemia or hypervolemia; *GI:* anorexia, nausea, vomiting, diarrhea, abdominal cramps; *neuro:* lethargy, increased ICP, confusion, headache, seizures, coma, fatigue, tremors, hyperreflexia
- Monitor for manifestations of hyperchloremia: *neuro:* weakness, lethargy, coma; *resp:* coma, deep rapid breathing
- Assess fluid volume status: I&O ratios and record, count or weigh diapers as appropriate, weight, distended red veins, crackles in lung, color, quality and sp gr of urine, skin turgor, adequacy of pulses, moist mucous membranes, bilateral lung sounds, peripheral pitting edema; dehydration symptoms of decreasing output, thirst, hypotension, dry mouth and mucous membranes should be reported
- Monitor electrolytes: potassium, sodium, calcium, magnesium; also include BUN, blood pH, ABGs, uric acid, CBC, blood sugar
- Assess BP before and during therapy with patient lying, standing, and sitting as appropriate; orthostatic hypotension can occur rapidly

Associated nursing diagnoses

- ✓ Altered urinary elimination (adverse reactions)
- ✓ Fluid volume deficit
- ✓ Fluid volume excess (uses)
- ✓ Knowledge deficit (teaching)

Implementation

- Give in AM to avoid interference with sleep
- Potassium replacement if potassium level is 3.0

- Give whole, or use oral sol; drug may be crushed if patient is unable to swallow

PO route

- Give with food; if nausea occurs, absorption may be increased

IV **IV route**

- Do not use solution that is yellow, has a precipitate, or crystals
- Administer **IV** after diluting 0.5 g/18 ml or more of sterile water for inj; may be diluted further with dextrose or NaCl: give over 5 min; sol is stable at room temp for 24 hr

Additive incompatibilities:

Blood, blood products, amikacin, chlorpromazine, codeine, hydralazine, insulin, levorphanol, methadone, morphine, multivitamins, norepinephrine, polymyxin B, procaine, prochlorperazine, promazine, promethazine, streptomycin, tetracycline, triflupromazine, vancomycin

Additive compatibilities:

Cimetidine, lidocaine, nafcillin, sodium bicarbonate

Patient/family education

- Teach patient to take the medication early in the day to prevent nocturia
- Instruct patient to take with food or milk if GI symptoms of nausea and anorexia occur
- Teach patient to maintain a weekly record of weight and notify prescriber of weight loss >5 lb
- Caution patient that this drug causes a loss of potassium, so food rich in potassium should be added to the diet; refer to a dietitian for assistance in planning
- Caution patient not to exercise in hot weather or stand for prolonged periods, since orthostatic hypotension will be enhanced; to use sunscreen to prevent burning
- Teach patient not to use alcohol or any OTC medications without prescriber's approval; serious drug reactions may occur
- Emphasize the need to contact prescriber immediately if muscle cramps, weakness, nausea, dizziness or numbness occurs
- Teach patient to take own BP and pulse and record
- Caution patient that orthostatic hypotension may occur; patient should rise slowly from sitting or reclining positions and lie down if dizziness occurs
- Teach patient to continue taking medication even if feeling better; this drug controls symptoms but does not cure the condition
- Advise the patient with hypertension to continue other medical treatment (exercise, weight loss, relaxation techniques, cessation of smoking)

Evaluation

Positive therapeutic outcome

- Decreased edema
- Decreased BP
- Increased diuresis

Treatment of overdose:

Lavage if taken orally, monitor electrolytes; administer dextrose in saline; monitor hydration, CV, renal status

chlorpheniramine

(klor-fen-eer'a-meen)
Aller-Chlor, Allergy, Chlo-Amine, Chlor-100, Chlorate, chlorpheniramine maleate, Chlor-Pro, Chlor-Pro 10, Chlorspan-12, Chlortab-B, Chlortab-4, Chlor-Trimeton, Chlor-Trimeton Repetabs, PediaCare Allergy Formula, Pfeiffer's Allergy, Phenetron, Telachlor, Teldrin
Func. class.: Antihistamine
Chem. class.: Alkylamine, H_1-receptor antagonist
Pregnancy category B

Action: Acts on blood vessels, GI, respiratory system by competing with histamine for H_1-receptor site; decreases allergic response by blocking histamine

Therapeutic Outcome: Absence of allergy symptoms and rhinitis

Uses: Allergy symptoms, rhinitis, allergic dermatoses, nasal allergies, hypersensitive reactions including blood transfusion reactions, anaphylaxis

Dosage and routes

Adult: PO 2-4 mg tid-qid, not to exceed 36 mg/day; time rel 8-12 mg bid-tid, not to exceed 36 mg/day; IM/**IV**/SC 5-40 mg/day

P ***Child 6-12 yr:*** PO 2 mg q4-6h, not to exceed 12 mg/day; sus rel 8 mg hs or qd; sus rel not recommended for child <6 yr

P ***Child 2-5 yr:*** PO 1 mg q4-6h, not to exceed 4 mg/day

Available forms: Chewable tabs 2 mg; tabs 4 mg; time-rel tabs 8, 12 mg; time-rel caps 8, 12 mg; syr 2 mg/5 ml; inj IM, SC, **IV** 10, 100 mg/ml

Side effects/adverse reactions

CNS: Dizziness, drowsiness, poor coordination, fatigue, anxiety, euphoria, confusion, paresthesia, neuritis
EENT: Blurred vision, dilated pupils, tinnitus, nasal stuffiness, dry nose, throat, mouth
GI: Dry mouth, nausea, anorexia, diarrhea
GU: Retention, dysuria, frequency
HEMA: Thrombocytopenia, agranulocytosis, hemolytic anemia
INTEG: Photosensitivity
RESP: Increased thick secretions, wheezing, chest tightness

Contraindications: Hypersensitivity to H_1-receptor antagonists, acute asthma attack, lower respiratory tract disease

Precautions: Increased intraocular pressure, renal disease, cardiac disease, hypertension, bronchial asthma, seizure disorder, stenosed peptic ulcers, hyperthyroidism, prostatic hypertrophy, bladder neck obstruction, pregnancy **B**, G elderly

Pharmacokinetics

Absorption	Well absorbed (PO, SC, IM, IV)
Distribution	Widely distributed; crosses blood-brain barrier
Metabolism	Liver, mostly
Excretion	Kidneys, metabolite; breast milk (minimal)
Half-life	12-15 hr

Pharmacodynamics

	PO	SC	IM	IV
Onset	15-30 min	Unknown	Unknown	Immediate
Peak	1-2 hr	Unknown	Unknown	Unknown
Duration	6-12 hr	6-12 hr	6-12 hr	6-12 hr

Interactions

Drug/drug:

Individual drugs

Alcohol: ↑ CNS depression
Atropine: ↑ anticholinergic reactions
Disopyramide: ↑ anticholinergic reactions
Haloperidol: ↑ anticholinergic reactions
Quinidine: ↑ anticholinergic reactions

Drug classifications

Antidepressants: ↑ anticholinergic reactions
Antihistamines: ↑ anticholinergic reactions
CNS depressants: ↑ CNS depression
MAOI: ↑ anticholinergic effect
Narcotics: ↑ CNS depression
Phenothiazines: ↑ anticholinergic reactions
Sedative/hypnotics: ↑ CNS depression

Lab test interferences

False negative: Skin allergy tests (discontinue antihistamines 3 days before testing)

NURSING CONSIDERATIONS

Assessment

- Assess respiratory status: rate, rhythm, increase in bronchial secretions, wheezing, chest tightness; provide fluids to 2 L/day to decrease secretion thickness
- Monitor I&O ratio: be alert for urinary retention, frequency, dysuria, especially G elderly; drug should be discontinued if these occur
- **IV** administration may result in rapid drop in B/P, sweating, G dizziness, especially in elderly

Associated nursing diagnoses

- ✓ Airway clearance, ineffective (uses)
- ✓ Injury, risk for (side effects)
- ✓ Knowledge deficit (teaching)
- ✓ Noncompliance (teaching, overuse)

Implementation

PO route

- May give with food to decrease GI upset; chewable tabs should be chewed and not swallowed whole; caps, time rel tabs should be swallowed whole; do not open or chew
- Store in tight, light-resistant container

SC/IM route

- Use only 20 mg/ml and 100 mg/ml strengths; does not need to be reconstituted or diluted

IV **IV route**
Give undiluted by direct **IV** (10 mg/ml strength only); administer 10 mg over 1 min or more

Additive incompatibilities:
Calcium chloride, kanamycin, norepinephrine, pentobarbital

Additive compatibility:
Amikacin

Patient/family education

- Teach all aspects of drug uses; to notify prescriber if confusion, sedation, hypotension occur; to avoid driving and other hazardous activity if drowsiness occurs; to avoid alcohol and other CNS depressants that may potentiate effect
- Teach patient not to exceed recommended dosage; dysrhythmias may occur
- Advise patient hard candy, gum, frequent rinsing of mouth may be used for dryness

Evaluation

Positive therapeutic outcome
- Absence of running or congested nose, rashes

Treatment of overdose:
Administer ipecac syrup or lavage, diazepam, vasopressors, barbiturates (short acting)

chlorpromazine 🔑
(klor-proe'ma-zeen)
chlorpromazine HCl, Chlorpromanyl ✦, Ormazine, Thorazine, Thorazine Spansules
Func. class.: Antipsychotic/neuroleptic
Chem. class.: Phenothiazine, aliphatic
Pregnancy category C

Action: Depress cerebral cortex, hypothalamus, limbic system, which control activity aggression; blocks neurotransmission produced by dopamine at synapse; exhibits a strong α-adrenergic, anticholinergic blocking action; mechanism for antipsychotic effects is unclear

→ **Therapeutic Outcome:** Decreased signs and symptoms of psychosis; control of nausea, vomiting, intractable hiccups, decreased anxiety preoperatively

Uses: Psychotic disorders, mania, schizophrenia, anxiety, intractable hiccups, nausea, vomiting, preoperative relaxation, acute intermittent porphyria, behavioral problems in
P children

Dosage and routes
Psychiatry
Adult: PO 10-50 mg q1-4h initially, then increase up to 2 g/day if necessary
Adult: IM 10-50 mg q1-4h
P *Child:* PO 0.25 mg/lb q4-6h or 0.5 mg/kg

P *Child:* IM 0.25 mg/lb q6-8h or 0.5 mg/kg

P *Child:* Rec 0.5 mg/lb q6-8h or 1 mg/kg

Nausea and vomiting

Adult: PO 10-25 mg q4-6h prn; IM 25-50 mg q3h prn; rec 50-100 mg q6-8h prn, not to exceed 400 mg/day

P *Child:* PO 0.25 mg/lb q4-6h prn, IM 0.25 mg/lb q6-8h prn not to exceed 40 mg/day (<5 yr) or 75 mg/day (5-12 yr); rec 0.5 mg/lb q6-8h prn

Adult: **IV** 25-50 mg qd-qid

P *Child:* **IV** 0.55 mg/kg q6-8h

Intractable hiccups

Adult: PO 25-50 mg tid-qid; IM 25-50 mg (used only if PO dose does not work); **IV** 25-50 mg in 500-1000 ml saline (only for severe hiccups)

Available forms: Tabs 10, 25, 50, 100, 200 mg; time rel caps 30, 75, 150, 200, 300 mg; syr 10 mg/5 ml; conc 30, 100 mg/ml; supp 25, 100 mg; inj IM, IV 25 mg/ml

Side effects/adverse reactions

CNS: ***Neuroleptic malignant syndrome,*** *extrapyramidal symptoms: pseudoparkinsonism, akathisia, dystonia, tardive dyskinesia,* seizures, *headache*

CV: Orthostatic hypotension, hypertension, ***cardiac arrest,*** ECG changes, ***tachycardia***

EENT: Blurred vision, glaucoma, dry eyes

GI: Dry mouth, nausea, vomiting, anorexia, constipation, diarrhea, jaundice, weight gain

GU: Urinary retention, urinary frequency, enuresis, impotence, amenorrhea, gynecomastia, breast engorgement

HEMA: Anemia, ***leukopenia, leukocytosis, agranulocytosis***

INTEG: Rash, photosensitivity, dermatitis

RESP: ***Laryngospasm,*** dyspnea, ***respiratory depression***

Contraindications: Hypersensitivity, circulatory collapse, liver damage, cerebral arteriosclerosis, coronary disease, severe hypertension/hypotension, blood dyscrasias, P coma, child <2 yr, brain damage, bone marrow depression, alcohol and barbiturate withdrawal

Precautions: Pregnancy **C,** lactation, seizure disorders, hypertension, hepatic disease, G cardiac disease, elderly

Pharmacokinetics

Absorption	Variable (PO); well absorbed (IM)
Distribution	Widely distributed; crosses placenta
Metabolism	Liver, GI mucosa extensively
Excretion	Kidneys
Half-life	30 hr

Pharmacodynamics

	PO	REC	IM	IV
Onset	½-1 hr	1-2 hr	Unkn	Rapid
Peak	Unkn	Unkn	Unkn	Unkn
Duration	4-6 hr*	3-4 hr	4-8 hr	Unkn

*Duration PO ext rel is 10-12 hr.

Interactions

Drug/drug:

Individual drugs

Alcohol: ↑ effects of both drugs, oversedation
Aluminum hydroxide: ↓ absorption
Bromocriptine: ↓ antiparkinsonian activity
Disopyramide: ↑ anticholinergic effects
Epinephrine: ↑ toxicity
Guanethidine: ↓ antihypertensive response
Levodopa: ↓ antiparkinsonian activity
Lithium: ↓ chlorpromazine levels, ↑ extrapyramidal symptoms, masking of lithium toxicity
Magnesium hydroxide: ↓ absorption
Norepinephrine: ↓ vasoresponse, ↑ toxicity
Phenobarbital: ↓ effectiveness, ↑ metabolism

Drug classifications

Antacids: ↓ absorption
Anticholinergics: ↑ anticholinergic effects
Antidepressants: ↑ CNS depression
Antidiarrheals, adsorbent: ↓ absorption
Antihistamines: ↑ CNS depression
Antihypertensives: ↑ hypotension
Antithyroid agents: ↑ agranulocytosis
Barbiturate anesthetics: ↑ CNS depression
β-Adrenergics: ↑ effects of both drugs
General anesthetics: ↑ CNS depression
MAOI: ↑ CNS depression
Narcotics: ↑ CNS depression
Sedative/hypnotics: ↑ CNS depression

Lab test interferences

Increase: Liver function tests, cardiac enzymes, cholesterol, blood glucose, prolactin, bilirubin, PBI, choline esterase I, alkaline phosphatase, leukocytes, granulocytes, platelets
Decrease: Hormones (blood and urine)
False positive: Pregnancy tests, PKU, urine bilirubin
False negative: Urinary steroids, 17-OHCS

NURSING CONSIDERATIONS

Assessment

- Assess mental status: orientation, mood, behavior, presence of hallucinations, and type before initial administration and monthly; this drug should significantly reduce psychotic behavior
- Check for swallowing of PO medication; check for hoarding or giving of medication to other patients
- Monitor I&O ratio; palpate bladder if low urinary output occurs, especially in elderly; urinalysis recommended before, during prolonged therapy
- Monitor bilirubin, CBC, liver function studies monthly
- Assess affect, orientation, LOC, reflexes, gait, coordination, sleep pattern disturbances
- Monitor B/P with patient sitting, standing, and lying; take pulse and respirations q4h during initial treatment; establish baseline before starting treatment; report drops of 30 mm Hg; obtain baseline ECG, Q wave, and T wave changes

- Check for dizziness, faintness, palpitations, tachycardia on rising; severe orthostatic hypotension is common
- Identify for neuroleptic malignant syndrome: hyperpyrexia, muscle rigidity, increased CPK, altered mental status; drug should be discontinued
- Assess for extrapyramidal symptoms including akathisia (inability to sit still, no pattern to movements), tardive dyskinesia (bizarre movements of the jaw, mouth, tongue, extremities), pseudoparkinsonism (rigidity, tremors, pill rolling, shuffling gate); an antiparkinsonian drug should be prescribed
- Assess for constipation, urinary retention daily; if these occur, increase bulk, water in diet

Associated nursing diagnoses

✓ Thought processes, altered (uses)
✓ Coping, ineffective individual (uses)
✓ Knowledge deficit (teaching)
✓ Noncompliance (teaching)

Implementation

PO route

- Give drug in liquid form mixed in glass of juice or cola if hoarding is suspected; decrease
- Give decreased dosage in elderly, since metabolism is slowed
- Give with full glass of water, milk; or give with food to decrease GI upset
- Store in tight, light-resistant container, oral sol in amber bottle

Rec route

- Give after placing in refrigerator for 30 min if too soft to insert; this route is used for nausea, vomiting, hiccups

IM route

- Inject in deep muscle mass; do not give SC; may be diluted with 0.9% NaCl, 2% procaine as prescribed; do not administer sol with a precipitate

IV **IV route**

- Give by direct **IV** by diluting with 0.9% NaCl to a concentration of 1 mg/1 ml; administer at a rate of 1 mg/2 min
- Give by cont inf after diluting 50 mg/500-1000 ml of D_5W, $D_{10}W$, 0.9% NaCl, 0.45% NaCl, LR, Ringer's or combinations (used for intractable hiccups)

Syringe incompatibilities:

Cimetidine, dimenhydrinate, heparin, pentobarbital, thiopental

Syringe compatibilities:

Atropine, butorphanol, diphenhydramine, doxapram, droperidol, fentanyl, glycopyrrolate, hydromorphone, hydroxyzine, meperidine, metoclopramide, midazolam, morphine, pentozocine, perphenazine, prochlorperazine, promazine, promethazine, scopolamine

Y-site compatibilities:

Heparin, hydrocortisone sodium succinate, ondansetron, potassium chloride

Additive incompatibilities:

Aminophylline, amphotericin B, ampicillin, chloramphenicol, chlorothiazide, methicillin, methohexital, penicillin G, phenobarbital

Additive compatibilities: Ascorbic acid, ethacrynate, netilmicin

Patient/family education

- Teach patient to use good oral hygiene; frequent rinsing of mouth, sugarless gum for dry mouth
- Caution patient to avoid hazardous activities until drug response is determined; dizziness, blurred vision may occur
- Inform patient that orthostatic hypotension occurs often and to rise from sitting or lying position gradually to remain lying down after IM injection for at least 30 min; tell patient to avoid hot tubs, hot showers, tub baths, since hypotension may occur; tell patient that in hot weather heat stroke may occur; take extra precautions to stay cool
- Advise patient to avoid abrupt withdrawal of this drug, or extrapyramidal symptoms may result; drug should be withdrawn slowly
- Teach patient to avoid OTC preparations (cough, hay fever, cold) unless approved by prescriber, since serious drug interactions may occur; avoid use with alcohol, CNS depressants, since increased drowsiness may occur
- Caution patient to use sunscreen and sunglasses to prevent burns
- Teach patient about extrapyramidal symptoms and necessity of meticulous oral hygiene, since oral candidiasis may occur
- Instruct patient to take antacids 2 hr before or after taking this drug
- Instruct patient to report sore throat, malaise, fever, bleeding, mouth sores; if these occur, CBC should be drawn and drug discontinued
- Teach that urine may turn pink or red

Evaluation

Positive therapeutic outcome

- Decrease in emotional excitement, hallucinations, delusions, paranoia
- Reorganization of patterns of thought, speech

Treatment of overdose: Lavage if orally ingested; provide airway, ***do not induce vomiting or use epinephrine***

chlorpropamide

(klor-proe′pa-mide)

Apo-chlorpropamide ✤, Chloronase ✤, Chlorpropamide, Diabinese, Novopropamide ✤

Func. class.: Antidiabetic, oral

Chem. class.: Sulfonylurea (1st generation)

Pregnancy category **C**

Action: Causes functioning β-cells in pancreas to release insulin, leading to drop in blood glucose levels; may improve insulin binding to insulin receptors or increase the number of insulin receptors with prolonged administration;

may also reduce basal hepatic glucose secretion; not effective if patient lacks functioning β-cells

Uses: Stable adult-onset diabetes mellitus (type II; NIDDM)

→ **Therapeutic Outcome:** Decreased blood glucose levels in diabetes mellitus

Dosage and routes

Adult: PO 100-250 mg qd initially, then 100-500 mg maintenance according to response; not to exceed 750 mg/day

Available forms: Tabs 100, 250 mg scored

Side effects/adverse reactions

CNS: Headache, weakness, dizziness, drowsiness, tinnitus, fatigue, vertigo
ENDO: Hypoglycemia, hyponatremia
GI: Hepatotoxicity, cholestatic jaundice, nausea, vomiting, diarrhea, heartburn
HEMA: Leukopenia, thrombocytopenia, agranulocytosis, aplastic anemia, pancytopenia, hemolytic anemia
INTEG: Rash, allergic reactions, pruritus, urticaria, eczema, photosensitivity, erythema

Contraindications: Hypersensitivity to sulfonylureas, P juvenile or brittle diabetes, pregnancy **C**, renal failure

G **Precautions:** Elderly, cardiac disease, thyroid disease, renal disease, hepatic disease, severe hypoglycemic reactions

Pharmacokinetics

Absorption	Well absorbed (PO)
Distribution	Bile
Metabolism	Liver to metabolites
Excretion	Kidneys, unchanged
Half life	36 hr

Pharmacodynamics

	PO
Onset	1 hr
Peak	3-6 hr
Duration	24 hr

Interactions

Drug/drug:

Individual drugs

Cimetidine: ↑ hypoglycemia
Chloramphenicol: ↑ hypoglycemia
Diazoxide: ↓ effect of both drugs
Guanethidine: ↑ hypoglycemia
Insulin: ↑ hypoglycemia
Methyldopa: ↑ hypoglycemia
Phenobarbital: ↓ action of chlorpropamide
Phenytoin: ↓ action of chlorpropamide
Rifampin: ↓ action of chlorpropamide

Drug classifications

Anticoagulants, oral: ↑ hypoglycemia
Calcium channel blockers: ↓ action of chlorpropamide
Corticosteroids: ↓ action of chlorpropamide
Diuretics, thiazide: ↓ action of chlorpropamide
Estrogens: ↓ action of chlorpropamide
MAOI: ↑ hypoglycemia
NSAIDs: ↑ hypoglycemia

Oral contraceptives: ↓ action of chlorpropamide
Phenothiazines: ↓ action of chlorpropamide
Salicylates: ↑ hypoglycemia
Sulfonamides: ↑ hypoglycemia
Sympathomimetics: ↓ action of chlorpropamide
Thyroid agents: ↓ action of chlorpropamide

NURSING CONSIDERATIONS

Assessment

- Assess for hypoglycemic reactions (sweating, weakness, dizziness, anxiety, tremors, hunger) and hyperglycemic reactions; can occur soon pc
- Monitor CBC (baseline, q3mo) during treatment; check liver function tests periodically (AST [SGOT], LDH) and renal studies (BUN, creatinine) during treatment

Associated nursing diagnoses

✓ Nutrition, altered: more than body requirements (uses)
✓ Nutrition altered: less than body requirements (adverse reactions)
✓ Knowledge deficit (teaching)
✓ Noncompliance (teaching)
✓ Injury, risk for physical (adverse reactions)

Implementation

- Conversion from other oral hypoglycemic agents or insulin dosage of <40 U/day may be made without gradual dosage change; patients taking insulin of >40 U/day convert gradually by receiving oral hypoglycemic and 50% of previous insulin dosage for 3-5 days; monitor serum or urine glucose and ketones tid during conversion

PO route

- Give drug 30 min before breakfast; if large dose is required, may be divided into two; give with meals to decrease GI upset and provide best absorption
- Give tabs crushed and mixed with meal or fluids for patients with difficulty swallowing
- Store in tight container in cool environment

Patient/family education

- Teach patient to check for symptoms of cholestatic jaundice: dark urine, pruritus, yellow sclera; if these occur, prescriber should be notified
- Teach patient to use capillary blood glucose test or Chemstrip tid
- Teach patient symptoms of hypoglycemia and hyperglycemia and what to do about each
- Instruct patient that drug must be continued daily; explain consequence of discontinuing drug abruptly
- Teach patient to take drug in morning to prevent hypoglycemic reactions at night
- Caution patient to avoid OTC medications unless they are prescribed
- Teach patient that diabetes is lifelong illness; that this drug is not a cure
- Teach patient that all food included in diet plan must be eaten to prevent hypoglycemia
- Advise patient to carry Medic Alert ID for emergency purposes; carry a glucagon emergency kit

Evaluation

Positive therapeutic outcome
- Decrease in polyuria, polydipsia, polyphagia; clear sensorium, absence of dizziness, stable gait

Treatment of overdose:
Glucose 25g **IV**, via dextrose 50% sol, 50 ml or 1 mg glucagon

chlorthalidone
Apo-Chlorthalidone ✤, Novothalidone ✤, Uridon ✤, Hygroton, Thalitone

Func. class.: Diuretic, antihypertensive

Chem. class.: Thiazide-like phthalimindine derivative

Pregnancy category **B**

Action: Acts on the distal tubule in the kidney, increasing excretion of sodium, water, chloride, magnesium, potassium, and bicarbonate

➾ **Therapeutic Outcome:** Decreased BP, decreased edema in lung tissues and peripherally, diuresis

Uses: Edema in congestive heart failure, nephrotic syndrome; may be used alone or as adjunct with antihypertensives; also for edema in corticosteroid estrogen therapy

Dosage and routes
Adult: PO 25-100 mg/day or 100 mg every other day or qd

P ***Child:*** PO 2 mg/kg 3 times a wk

Available forms: Tabs 15, 25, 50, 100 mg

Side effects/adverse reactions
CNS: Drowsiness, paresthesia, anxiety, depression, headache, *dizziness, fatigue, weakness,* fever

ELECT: Hypokalemia, hypercalcemia, hyponatremia, hypochloremia, hypomagnesemia

EENT: Blurred vision

GI: Nausea, vomiting, anorexia, constipation, diarrhea, cramps, pancreatitis, GI irritation, ***hepatitis***

GU: Frequency, polyuria, ***uremia,*** glucosuria

HEMA: Aplastic anemia, leukopenia, agranulocytosis, thrombocytopenia, neutropenia

INTEG: Rash, urticaria, purpura, photosensitivity

META: Hyperglycemia, hyperuricemia, increased creatinine, BUN

Contraindications: Hypersensitivity to thiazides or sulfonamides, anuria, renal decompensation, lactation

Precautions: Hypokalemia, renal disease, hepatic disease, gout, COPD, LE, diabetes G mellitus, elderly, pregnancy **B,** hyperlipidemia

Pharmacokinetics

	PO
Absorption	Well absorbed
Distribution	Extracellular spaces; crosses placenta
Metabolism	Liver
Excretion	Urine, unchanged (30%-60%)
Half-life	40 hr

Pharmacodynamics

	PO
Onset	2 hr
Peak	6 hr
Duration	24-72 hr

Interactions

Drug/drug:

Individual drugs

Cholestyramine: ↓ absorption of chlorothalidone
Colestipol: ↓ absorption of chlorothalidone
Diazoxide: ↓ hyperglycemia, hyperuricemia, hypotension
Digitalis: ↑ toxicity
Indomethacin: ↓ hypotensive response
Lithium: ↑ toxicity
Mezlocillin: ↑ hypokalemia
Piperacillin: ↑ hypokalemia
Ticarcillin: ↑ hypokalemia

Drug classifications

Antidiabetics: ↓ effect of antidiabetic agent
Antihypertensives: ↑ antihypertensive effect
Nitrates: ↑ hypotension
Nondepolarizing skeletal muscle relaxants: ↑ toxicity
Glucocorticoids: ↑ hypokalemia
Sulfonylureas: ↑ effect of sulfonylurea

Drug/food:

Food: ↑ absorption

Lab test interferences

Increase: BSP retention, triglycerides, calcium, amylase
Decrease: PBI, PSP

NURSING CONSIDERATIONS

Assessment

- Monitor manifestations of hypokalemia; *CV:* hypotension, broad T wave, U wave, ectopy, tachycardia, weak pulse; *GI:* anorexia, nausea, cramps, constipation, distention, paralytic ileus; *Neuro:* muscle weakness, altered LOC, drowsiness, apathy, lethargy, confusion, depression; *Renal:* acidic urine, reduced urine, osmolality, nocturia; *Resp:* hypoventilation, respiratory muscle weakness
- Monitor for manifestations of hypomagnesemia; *CNS:* agitation, muscle twitching, paresthesias, hyperactive reflexes, positive Babinski reflex, dysphagia, nystagmus seizures, tetany; *CV:* ectopy, tachycardia, broad, flat or inverted T waves, depressed ST segment, prolonged QT, decreased cardiac output, hypotension; *GI:* nausea, vomiting, diarrhea, anorexia, abdominal distention
- Monitor for manifestations of hyponatremia; *CV:* increased BP, cold, clammy skin, hypovolemia or hypervolemia; *GI:* anorexia, nausea, vomiting, diarrhea, abdominal cramps; *Neuro:* lethargy, increased ICP, confusion, headache, seizures, coma, fatigue, tremors, hyperreflexia

• Monitor for manifestations of hyperchloremia; *Neuro:* weakness, lethargy, coma; *Resp:* coma, deep rapid breathing
• Assess fluid volumes status: I&O ratios and record, count or weigh diapers as appropriate, weight, distended red veins, crackles in lung, color, quality and sp gr of urine, skin turgor, adequacy of pulses, moist mucous membranes, bilateral lung sounds, peripheral pitting edema; dehydration symptoms of decreasing output, thirst, hypotension, dry mouth, and mucous membranes should be reported
• Monitor electrolytes: potassium, sodium, calcium, magnesium; also include BUN, blood pH, ABGs, uric acid, CBC, blood sugar
• Assess BP before and during therapy with patient lying, standing, and sitting as appropriate; orthostatic hypotension can occur rapidly

Associated nursing diagnoses

✓ Altered urinary elimination (side effect)
✓ Fluid volume deficit (adverse reactions)
✓ Fluid volume excess (uses)
✓ Knowledge deficit (teaching)

Implementation

• Give in AM to avoid interference with sleep
• Provide potassium replacement if potassium level is 3.0 mg/dl; give whole, or use oral solutions lightly; drug may be crushed if patient is unable to swallow

PO route
• Give with food; if nausea occurs, may crush tab and mix with fluids or applesauce for swallowing

C

Patient/family education

General
• Teach patient to take the medication early in the day to prevent nocturia
• Instruct patient to take with food or milk if GI symptoms of nausea and anorexia occur
• Teach patient to maintain weekly record of weight and notify prescriber of weight loss >5 lb
• Caution patient that this drug causes a loss of potassium, so food rich in potassium should be added to the diet; refer to a dietician for assistance in planning
• Caution the patient not to exercise in hot weather or stand for prolonged periods, since orthostatic hypotension will be enhanced; to use sunscreen to prevent burns
• Teach patient not to use alcohol, or any OTC medications without prescriber's approval; serious drug reactions may occur
• Emphasize the need to contact prescriber immediately if muscle cramps, weakness, nausea, dizziness or numbness occurs
• Teach patient to take own BP and pulse and record
• Caution patient that orthostatic hypotension may occur; patient should rise slowly from sitting or reclining positions and lie down if dizziness occurs
• Teach patient to continue taking medication even if feel-

ing better; this drug controls symptoms but does not cure the condition
• Advise patient with hypertension to continue other medical treatment (exercise, weight loss, relaxation techniques, cessation of smoking)

Evaluation

Positive therapeutic outcome
• Decreased edema
• Decreased BP
• Increased diuresis

Treatment of overdose: Lavage if taken orally, monitor electrolytes; administer dextrose in saline; monitor hydration, CV, renal status

cholestyramine

(koe-less-tear'a-meen)
Cholybar, Questran, Questran Light
Func. class.: Antilipemic
Chem. class.: Bile acid sequestrant
Pregnancy catagory **C**

Action: Absorbs, combines with bile acids to form an insoluble complex that is excreted through feces; loss of bile acids lowers cholesterol levels

Therapeutic Outcome: Decreasing cholesterol levels and low-density lipoproteins, decreased pruritus

Uses: Primary hypercholesterolemia, pruritus associated with biliary obstruction, diarrhea caused by excess bile acid, digitalis toxicity, xanthomas

Dosage and routes

Adult: PO 4 g ac and hs, not to exceed 32 g/day
P *Child:* PO 240 mg/kg/day in 3 divided doses; administer with food or drink

Available forms: Powder 9 g

Side effects/adverse reactions

CNS: Headache, dizziness, drowsiness, vertigo, tinnitus
GI: Constipation, abdominal pain, nausea, fecal impaction, hemorrhoids, flatulence, vomiting, steatorrhea, peptic ulcer
HEMA: Decreased vitamin A, D, K, red cell folate content, ***hyperchloremic acidosis, bleeding,*** decreased pro-time
INTEG: Rash, irritation of perianal area, tongue, skin
MS: Muscle, joint pain

Contraindications: Hypersensitivity, biliary obstruction

Precautions: Pregnancy **C**, P lactation, children

Pharmacokinetics

Absorption	Not absorbed
Distribution	Not distributed
Metabolism	Not metabolized
Excretion	Binds with bile acids, feces
Half-life	Unknown

Pharmacodynamics

	PO
Onset	24-48 hr
Peak	1-3 wk
Duration	2-4 wk

Interactions

Drug/drug:

Individual drugs

Acetaminophen: ↓ absorption
Amiodarone: ↓ absorption
Methotrexate: ↓ absorption
Naproxen: ↓ absorption
Phenylbutazone: ↓ absorption
Piroxican: ↓ absorption
Propranolol: ↓ absorption
Thyroid: ↓ absorption
Ursodiol: ↓ absorption

Drug classifications

Anticoagulants, oral: ↓ absorption
Cardiac glycosides: ↓ absorption
Diuretics, thiazide: ↓ absorption
Vitamins A,D,E,K: ↓ absorption

Lab test interferences

Increase: Liver function studies, chlorine, PO_4

NURSING CONSIDERATIONS

Assessment

- Assess nutrition: fat, protein, carbohydrates, nutritional analysis should be completed by dietician
- Assess skin integrity after patient has been receiving drug; itching, pruritus often occur from bile deposits on skin
- Monitor cardiac glycoside level if both drugs are being administered; cardiac glycoside levels will be decreased
- Monitor for signs of vitamin A, D, E, K deficiency; serum cholesterol, triglyceride levels, electrolytes if on extended therapy
- Monitor bowel pattern daily; increase bulk, water in diet if constipation develops

Associated nursing diagnoses

✓ Constipation (adverse reactions)
✓ Knowledge deficit (teaching)
✓ Noncompliance (teaching)

Implementation

PO route

- Give drug ac, hs; give all other medications 1 hr before cholestyramine or 4 hr after cholestyramine to avoid poor absorption; do not take dry; mix drug with applesauce or stir into beverage (2-6 oz); let stand for 2 min
- Provide supplemental doses of vitamin A, D, E, K, if levels are low

Patient/family education

- Teach patient symptoms of hypoprothrombinemia: bleeding mucous membranes, dark tarry stools, hematuria, petechiae; report immediately
- Teach patient importance of compliance, since toxicity may result if doses are missed; not to discontinue suddenly
- Teach patient that risk factors should be decreased: high-fat diet, smoking, alcohol consumption, absence of exercise
- Have patient mix drug with 6 oz of milk, water, fruit juice; do not mix with carbonated beverages; rinse glass to make sure all medication is taken or may mix drug in applesauce; allow to stand for 2 min before mixing

Evaluation

Positive therapeutic outcome

- Decreased cholesterol level (hyperlipidemia)
- Decreased diarrhea, pruritus (excess bile acids)

choline salicylate

(koe'leen)

Arthropan, Teejel ♣

Func. class.: Nonnarcotic analgesic

Chem. class.: Salicylate

Pregnancy category **C**

Action: Blocks pain impulses in CNS that occur in response to inhibition of prostaglandin synthesis; antipyretic action results from inhibition of hypothalamic heat-regulating center to produce vasodilatation to allow heat dissipation

→ Therapeutic Outcome: Decreased pain, inflammation, fever

Uses: Mild to moderate pain or fever including arthritis, juvenile rheumatoid arthritis

Dosage and routes

Arthritis

P ***Adult and child >12 yrs:*** PO 870-1740 mg qid; max 6 times a day

Pain/fever

Adult: PO 870 mg q3-4h prn

P ***Child 3-6 yr:*** PO 105-210 mg q4h prn

Available forms: Liq 870 mg/5 ml

Side effects/adverse reactions

CNS: Stimulation, drowsiness, dizziness, confusion, ***convulsion***, headache, flushing, hallucinations, ***coma***

CV: Rapid pulse, pulmonary edema

EENT: Tinnitus, hearing loss

ENDO: Hypoglycemia, hyponatremia, hypokalemia

GI: *Nausea, vomiting, GI bleeding, diarrhea, heartburn,* anorexia, ***hepatitis***

HEMA: ***Thrombocytopenia, agranulocytosis, leukopenia, neutropenia, hemolytic anemia***, increased pro-time

INTEG: *Rash,* urticaria, bruising

RESP: Wheezing, hyperpnea

Contraindications: Hypersensitivity to salicylates, GI bleeding, bleeding disorders, P children <3 yr, vitamin K deficiency, children with flulike symptoms

Precautions: Anemia, hepatic disease, renal disease, Hodgkin's disease, pregnancy **C**, lactation

Pharmacokinetics

Absorption	Well absorbed
Distribution	Widely distributed; crosses placenta
Metabolism	Liver, extensively
Excretion	Kidney, active metabolites; breast milk
Half-life	2-3 hr (low doses); 30 hr (high doses)

Pharmacodynamics

	PO
Onset	15-30 min
Peak	1-3 hr
Duration	3-6 hr

Interactions

Drug/drug:

Individual drugs

Alcohol: ↑ bleeding
Cefamandole: ↑ bleeding
Furosemide: ↑ toxic effects
Heparin: ↑ bleeding
Insulin: ↑ effects
Methotrexate: ↑ effects
PABA: ↑ toxic effects
Phenytoin: ↑ effects
Plicamycin: ↑ bleeding
Probenecid: ↓ effects
Spironolactone: ↓ effects
Sulfinpyrazone: ↓ effects
Valproic acid: ↑ effects, ↑ bleeding
Vancomycin: ↑ ototoxicity

Drug classifications

Antacids: ↓ effects of choline salicylate
Anticoagulants: ↑ effects
Carbonic anhydrase inhibitors: ↑ toxic effects
NSAIDs: ↑ gastric ulcers
Penicillins: ↑ effects
Salicylates: ↓ blood sugar levels
Steroids: ↓ effects of choline salicylate, ↑ gastric ulcers
Sulfonylamides: ↓ effects
Urinary acidifiers: ↑ salicylate levels
Urinary alkalizers: ↓ effects of choline salicylate

Lab test interferences

Increase: Coagulation studies, liver function studies, serum uric acid, amylase, CO_2, urinary protein
Decrease: Serum potassium, PBI, cholesterol
Interfere: Urine catecholamines, pregnancy test, urine glucose tests (Clinistix, Tes-Tape)

C

NURSING CONSIDERATIONS

Assessment

• Monitor pain: location, duration, type, intensity, prior to dose and 1 hr after
• Monitor musculoskeletal status: ROM before dose
• Identify fever, length of time and related symptoms
• Monitor liver function studies: AST (SGOT), ALT (SGPT), bilirubin, creatinine if patient is on long-term therapy
• Monitor renal function studies: BUN, urine creatinine if patient is on long-term therapy
• Monitor blood studies: CBC, Hct, Hgb, pro-time if patient is on long-term therapy
• Check I&O ratio; decreasing output may indicate renal failure (long-term therapy)
• Assess hepatotoxicity: dark urine, clay-colored stools, yellowing of the skin and sclera, itching, abdominal pain, fever, diarrhea if patient is on long-term therapy
• Assess for allergic reactions: rash, urticaria; if these occur, drug may have to be discontinued
• Assess for ototoxicity: tinnitus, ringing, roaring in ears; audiometric testing needed before, after long-term therapy
• Assess for visual changes: blurring, halos; corneal, retinal damage
• Check edema in feet, ankles, legs

• Identify prior drug history; there are many drug interactions

Associated nursing diagnoses

✓ Pain (uses)
✓ Mobility, impaired physical (uses)
✓ Knowledge deficit (teaching)
✓ Injury, risk for (side effects)

Implementation

PO route

• Administer to patient crushed or whole
• Give with food or milk to decrease gastric symptoms; give 30 min ac or 2 hr pc; absorption may be slowed
• Give antacids 1-2 hr after enteric products

Patient/family education

• Teach patient to report any symptoms of hepatotoxicity, renal toxicity, visual changes, ototoxicity, allergic reactions, bleeding (long-term therapy)
• Advise patient to take with 8 oz of water and sit upright for 30 min after dose
• Caution patient not to exceed recommended dosage; acute poisoning may result
• Caution patient to read label on other OTC drugs; many contain aspirin products
• Inform patient that the therapeutic response takes 2 wk (arthritis)
• Teach patient to report tinnitus, confusion, diarrhea, sweating, hyperventilation
• Caution patient to avoid alcohol ingestion; GI bleeding may occur
• Teach patient that patients who have allergies may develop allergic reactions
• Caution patient to avoid buffered or effervescent products
• Teach patient not to give to P children; Reye's syndrome may develop

Evaluation

Positive therapeutic outcome

• Decreased pain
• Decreased inflammation
• Decreased fever
• Increased mobility

Treatment of overdose: Lavage, activated charcoal, monitor electrolytes, VS

ciclopirox (topical)

(sye-kloe-peer'ox)

Loprox

Func. class.: Local antiinfective

Chem. class.: Antifungal

Pregnancy category **B**

Action: Interferes with fungal cell membrane, which increases permeability, leaking of cell nutrients

➔ **Therapeutic Outcome:** Fungistatic/fungicidal against susceptible organisms causing tinea pedis, tinea cruris, tinea corporis, tinea versicolor

Uses: Tinea cruris, tinea corporis, tinea pedis, tinea versicolor, cutaneous candidiasis

Dosage and routes

P *Adult and child >10 yr:* Top rub into affected area bid for 2 wks

Available forms: Cream, lotion 1%

Side effects/adverse reactions

INTEG: Rash, urticaria, stinging, burning, pruritus, pain

Contraindications: Hypersensitivity

Precautions: Pregnancy **B**, P lactation, child <10 yr

Pharmacokinetics

Absorption	Minimal
Distribution	Unknown
Metabolism	Liver
Excretion	Feces, kidneys
Half-life	2 hr

Pharmacodynamics

Onset	Unknown
Peak	Unknown
Duration	Unknown

Interactions: None

NURSING CONSIDERATIONS

Assessment

- Assess skin for fungal infections: peeling, dryness, itching before and throughout treatment
- Monitor for allergic reaction: burning, stinging, swelling, redness, dermatitis, rash; drug should be discontinued, antihistamines (mild reaction)

Associated nursing diagnoses

- ✓ Skin integrity, impaired (uses)
- ✓ Infection, risk for (uses)
- ✓ Knowledge deficit (teaching)

Implementation

Top route

- Apply enough medication to cover lesions completely
- Clean with soap, water before each application; dry well
- Store at room temp in dry place

Patient/family education

- Tell patient to apply with glove to prevent further infection; not to cover with occlusive dressings
- Teach patient proper hygiene: hand-washing technique, nail care, use of concomitant top agents if prescribed
- Advise patient to avoid use of OTC creams, ointments, lotions unless directed
- Teach patient to use hand washing before, after each application
- Teach patient to change socks and shoes once a day during treatment of tinea pedis
- Instruct patient to report to prescriber if infection persists or returns or if blisters, burning, oozing, swelling occurs

Evaluation

Positive therapeutic outcome

- Decrease in size, number of lesions

cimetidine 🔑
(sye-met'i-deen)
Apo-Cimetidine ♣, Novocimetine ♣, Peptol ♣, Tagamet
Func. class.: H_2-receptor antagonist
Chem. class.: Imidazole derivative
Pregnancy category **B**

Action: Inhibits histamine at H_2-receptor site in the gastric parietal cells, which inhibits gastric acid secretion

➡ **Therapeutic Outcome:** Healing of duodenal or gastric ulcers; prevention of duodenal ulcers; decreases symptoms of gastroesophageal reflux disease (GERD) and Zollinger-Ellison syndrome

Uses: Short-term treatment of duodenal and gastric ulcers and maintenance; management of GERD and Zollinger-Ellison syndrome

Investigational uses: Prevention of aspiration pneumonitis, stress ulcers, upper GI bleeding

Dosage and routes

Treatment of active ulcers

P *Adult and child:* PO 300 mg qid with meals, hs × 8 wk or 400 mg bid, 800 mg hs; after 8 wk give hs dose only; **IV** bol 300 mg/20 ml 0.9% NaCl over 1-2 min q6h; **IV** inf 300 mg/50 ml D_5W over 15-20 min; IM 300 mg q6h, not to exceed 2400 mg

Prophylaxis of duodenal ulcer

P *Adult and child >16 yr:* 400 mg hs

GERD

Adult: PO 800-1600 mg/day in divided doses

Hypersecretory conditions (Zollinger-Ellison syndrome)

Adult: PO/IM/**IV** 300-600 mg q6h; may increase to 12 g/day if needed

Upper GI bleeding prophylaxis

Adult: **IV** 50 mg/hr; lowered in renal disease

Aspiration pneumonitis prophylaxis

Adult: IM/**IV** 300 mg IM 1 hr before anesthesia, then 300 mg **IV** q4h until patient is alert

Available forms: Tabs 200, 300, 400, 800 mg; liq 300 mg/5 ml; inj **IV** 300 mg/2 ml, 300 mg/50 ml 0.9% NaCl

Side effects/adverse reactions

CNS: Confusion, headache, depression, dizziness, anxiety, weakness, psychosis, tremors, ***convulsions***
CV: Bradycardia, tachycardia
GI: Diarrhea, abdominal cramps, ***paralytic ileus, jaundice***
GU: Gynecomastia, galactorrhea, impotence, increase in BUN, creatinine
HEMA: Agranulocytosis, thrombocytopenia, neutropenia, aplastic anemia, increase in pro-time

INTEG: Urticaria, rash, alopecia, sweating, flushing, ***exfoliative dermatitis***

Contraindications:
Hypersensitivity

Precautions:
Pregnancy **B**, P lactation, child <16 yr, organic brain syndrome, hepatic dis- G ease, renal disease, elderly

Pharmacokinetics

Absorption	Well absorbed (PO, IM); completely absorbed (IV)
Distribution	Widely distributed; crosses placenta
Metabolism	Liver (30%)
Excretion	Kidneys, unchanged (70%); breast milk
Half-life	1½-2 hr; increased in renal disease

Pharmacodynamics

	PO	IV/IM
Onset	½ hr	10 min
Peak	45-90 min	½ hr
Duration	4-5 hr	4-5 hr

Interactions
Drug/drug:
Individual drugs
Indomethacin: ↓ absorption of cimetidine
Ketoconazole: ↓ absorption of cimetidine
Lidocaine: ↑ toxicity
Metoprolol: ↑ toxicity
Procainamide: ↑ toxicity
Propranolol: ↑ toxicity
Quinidine: ↑ toxicity
Tocainamide: ↓ absorption of tocainamide
Drug classifications
Antacids: ↓ absorption of cimetidine
Anticoagulants, oral: ↑ toxicity
Antidepressants, tricyclic: ↑ toxicity
Benzodiazepines: ↑ toxicity
Iron salts: ↓ absorption of iron salts
Phenytoins: ↑ toxicity
Tetracyclines: ↓ absorption of tetracyclines
Theophyllines: ↑ toxicity

Drug/smoking:
↓ effectiveness

Lab test interferences
Increase: Alkaline phosphatase, AST (SGOT), creatinine
False positive: Gastric bleeding test, skin allergy tests

NURSING CONSIDERATIONS
Assessment
- Assess patient with ulcers or suspected ulcers: epigastric or abdominal pain, hematemesis, occult blood in stools, blood in gastric aspirate before and/or throughout treatment; monitor gastric pH (5 should be maintained)
- Monitor I&O ratio, BUN, creatinine, CBC with differential monthly

Associated nursing diagnoses
✓ Pain (uses)
✓ Knowledge deficit (teaching)

Implementation
PO route
- Give with meals for lengthened drug effect; antacids 1 hr before or 1 hr after cimetidine

IV route

- Give by direct **IV** after diluting 300 mg/20 ml of normal saline for inj; give over 2 min or more
- Give intermittent **IV** by diluting 300 mg/50 ml of D_5W; run over 15-20 min
- Give by cont inf after using total daily dose (900 mg) diluted in 100-1000 ml D_5W given over 24 hr
- Store diluted sol at room temp up to 48 hr

Syringe compatibilities:

Atropine, butorphanol, cephalothin, diazepam, diphenhydramine, doxapram, droperidol, fentanyl, glycopyrrolate, heparin, hydromorphone, hydroxyzine, lorazepam, meperidine, midazolam, morphine, nafcillin, nalbuphine, penicillin GT sodium, pentazocine, perphenazine, prochlorperazine, promazine, promethazine, scopolamine, sodium acetate, NaCl, sodium lactate, sterile water

Syringe incompatibilities:

Cefamandole, cefazolin, chlorpromazine, pentobarbital, secobarbital

Y-site compatibilities:

Acyclovir, aminophylline, amrinone, atracurium, enalaprilat, esmolol, foscarnet, haloperidol heparin, hetastarch, idarubicin, labetalol, melphalan, ondansetron, paclitaxel, pancuronium, tolazoline, vecuronium, vinorelbine, zidovudine

Y-site incompatibility:

Amsacrine

Additive compatibilities:

Acetazolamide, amikacin, aminophylline, cefoxitin, chlorothiazide, clindamycin, colistimethate, dexamethasone, digoxin, epinephrine, erythromycin, ethacrynate, furosemide, gentamicin, insulin, isoproterenol, lidocaine, lincomycin, metaraminol bitartrate, methylprednisolone, norepinephrine, penicillin G potassium, phytonadione, polymyxin B, potassium chloride, protamine sulfate, quinidine, sodium nitroprusside, tetracycline, verapamil, vitamin B complex

Additive incompatibility:

Amphotericin B

Patient/family education

- Advise patient that any gynecomastia or impotence that develops is reversible after treatment is discontinued
- Caution patient to avoid driving, other hazardous activities until stabilized on this medication; drowsiness or dizziness may occur
- Advise patient to avoid black pepper, caffeine, alcohol, harsh spices, extremes in temp of food; tell patient to avoid OTC preparations: aspirin, cough, cold preparations; condition may worsen
- Advise patient that smoking decreases the effectiveness of the drug; smoking cessation should be considered
- Teach patient that drug must be continued for prescribed time to be effective and taken exactly as prescribed; doses are not to be doubled; to take

missed dose when remembered up to 1 hr before next dose

- Instruct patient to report bruising, fatigue, malaise; blood dyscrasias may occur
- Have patient report to prescriber immediately any diarrhea, black tarry stools, sore throat, rash, dizziness, confusion, rash, or delirium

Evaluation

Positive therapeutic outcome

- Decreased pain in abdomen
- Healing of ulcers
- Absence of gastroesophageal reflex

ciprofloxacin

(sip-ro-floks'a-sin)

Ciloxin Cipro, Cipro IV

Func. class.: Urinary antiinfectives

Chem. class.: Fluoroquinolone antibacterial

Pregnancy category **C**

Action: Interferes with conversion of intermediate DNA fragments into high-molecular-weight DNA in bacteria; DNA gyrase inhibitor

Therapeutic Outcome: Bactericidal action against the following: gram-positive organisms *Staphylococcus epidermidis,* methicillin-resistant strains of *S. aureus, Streptococcus pyogenes, S. pneumoniae;* gram-negative organisms *Escherichia coli, Klebsiella* species, *Enterobacter, Salmonella, Shigella, Proteus vulgaris, Providencia stuartii, P. retgerii, Morganella morganii, Pseudomonas aeruginosa, Serratia, Haemophilus, Acinetobacter, Neisseria gonorrhoeae meningitidis, Branhamella catarrhalis, Yersinia, Vibrio, Brucella, Campylobacter, Aeromonas*

Uses: Adult urinary tract infections (including complicated); lower respiratory, skin, bone, joint infections; infectious diarrhea; conjunctivitis, corneal ulcers (ophthalmic)

Dosage and routes

Uncomplicated urinary tract infections

Adult: PO 250 mg q12h; **IV** 200 mg q12h

Complicated/severe urinary tract infections

Adult: PO 500 mg q12h; **IV** 400 mg q12h

Respiratory, bone, skin, joint infections

Adult: PO 500 mg q12h

Corneal ulcers, conjunctivitis

Adult: Ophth i-ii gtts q15-30 min, then i-ii gtts 4-6 times daily

Available forms: Tabs 250, 500, 750, mg; **IV** 200 mg/100 ml D_5, 400 mg/200 ml D_5; 200, 400 mg vial; oph sol

Side effects/adverse reactions

CNS: Headache, dizziness, fatigue, insomnia, depression, restlessness

GI: Nausea, constipation, increased ALT (SGPT), AST

(SGOT), flatulence, insomnia, heartburn, vomiting, diarrhea, oral candidiasis, dysphagia
INTEG: Rash, pruritus, urticaria, photosensitivity, flushing, fever, chills
MS: Blurred vision, tinnitus

Contraindications: Hypersensitivity to quinolones

Precautions: Pregnancy **C**, P lactation, children, renal disease

Pharmacokinetics

Absorption	Well absorbed (75%) (PO)
Distribution	Widely distributed
Metabolism	Liver (15%)
Excretion	Kidneys (40%-50%)
Half-life	3-4 hr; increased in renal disease

Pharmacodynamics

	PO	IV
Onset	Rapid	Immediate
Peak	1 hr	Infusion's end

Interactions

Drug/drug:

Individual drugs
Caffeine: ↓ effect of ciprofloxacin
Cyclosporine: ↑ nephrotoxicity
Nitrofurantoin: ↓ effectiveness
Probenecid: ↑ blood levels
Sucralfate: ↓ absorption of ciprofloxacin
Theophylline: ↑ toxicity
Warfarin: ↑ warfarin effect
Zinc sulfate: ↓ absorption of ciprofloxacin

Drug classifications
Antacids: ↓ absorption of ciprofloxacin
Anticoagulants, oral: ↑ effect of anticoagulants
Antineoplastics: ↓ ciprofloxacin levels
Iron salts: ↓ absorption of ciprofloxacin

Lab test interferences

Increase: AST (SGOT), ALT (SGPT), BUN, creatinine, alkaline phosphatase

NURSING CONSIDERATIONS

Assessment

- Assess patient for previous sensitivity reaction
- Assess patient for signs and symptoms of infection including characteristics of wounds, sputum, urine, stool, WBC >10,000, fever; obtain baseline information before and during treatment
- Obtain C&S before beginning drug therapy to identify if correct treatment has been initiated
- Assess for allergic reactions: rash, urticaria, pruritus, chills, fever, joint pain; may occur a few days after therapy begins; epinephrine and resuscitation equipment should be available for anaphylactic reaction
- Identify urine output; if decreasing, notify prescriber (may indicate nephrotoxicity); also check for increased BUN, creatinine
- Monitor blood studies: AST (SGOT), ALT (SGPT), CBC, Hct, bilirubin, LDH, alkaline phosphatase, Coombs' test monthly if patient is on long-term therapy

- Monitor electrolytes: potassium, sodium, chloride monthly if patient is on long-term therapy
- Assess bowel pattern qd; if severe diarrhea occurs, drug should be discontinued
- Monitor for bleeding: ecchymosis, bleeding gums, hematuria, stool guaiac daily if on long-term therapy
- Assess for overgrowth of infection: perineal itching, fever, malaise, redness, pain, swelling, drainage, rash, diarrhea, change in cough, sputum

Associated nursing diagnoses

✓ Infection, risk for (uses)
✓ Diarrhea (side effects)
✓ Injury, risk for (side effects)
✓ Knowledge deficit (teaching)
✓ Noncompliance (teaching)

Implementation

PO route
- Give around the clock to maintain proper blood levels

IV **IV route**
- Check for irritation, extravasation, phlebitis daily
- For intermittent inf, dilute to 1-2 mg/ml of D_5W, 0.9% NaCl; give over 60 min; it will remain stable under refrigeration for 2 wks

Y-site incompatibilities:
Heparin, mezlocillin

Y-site compatibilities:
Aztreonam, ceftazidime, heparin, piperacillin, tobramycin

Additive compatibilities:
Amikacin, aztreonam, ceftazidime, gentamicin, metronidazole, piperacillin, tobramycin

Additive incompatibilities:
Aminophylline, amoxicillin, clindamycin, floxacillin, mezlocillin

Syringe compatibility:
Heparin

Patient/family education

- Teach patient to report sore throat, bruising, bleeding, joint pain; may indicate blood dyscrasias (rare)
- Advise patient to contact prescriber if vaginal itching, loose, foul-smelling stools, furry tongue occur; may indicate superinfection; report itching, rash, pruritus, urticaria
- Instruct patient to take all medication prescribed for the length of time ordered; drug must be taken around the clock to maintain blood levels; do not give medication to others
- Advise patient to notify prescriber of diarrhea with blood or pus

Evaluation

Positive therapeutic outcome
- Absence of signs/symptoms of infection (WBC <10,000, temp WNL, absence of red draining wounds)
- Reported improvement in symptoms of infection

cisapride

(siss'a-pride)

Propulsid

Func. class.: Cholinergic, gastrointestinal (antireflex)

Pregnancy category C

Action: Enhances response to acetylcholine at the myenteric plexus; the strength of esophageal and sphincter pressure are increased

Therapeutic Outcome: Absence of heartburn

Uses: Treatment of heartburn associated with gastroesophageal reflux

Dosage and routes

Adult: PO 10 mg qid at least 15 min ac and hs; may increase to 20 mg; elderly may need higher dosage

Available forms: Tabs 10 mg

Side effects/adverse reactions

CNS: Headache, sleeplessness, anxiety, nervousness, pain, fever

GI: Constipation, nausea, anorexia, abdominal pain, flatulence, dyspepsia

GU: UTI, frequency

INTEG: Pruritus, rash

Contraindications: Hypersensitivity; GI hemorrhage, obstruction, perforation

Precautions: Pregnancy **C**, lactation, children, elderly

Pharmacokinetics

Absorption	Rapidly absorbed PO
Distribution	Unknown
Metabolism	Liver, extensively
Excretion	Breast milk, kidneys
Half-life	6-12 hr

Pharmacodynamics

	PO
Onset	½-1 hr
Peak	1 hr
Duration	Unknown

Interactions

Drug/drug:

Individual drugs

Alcohol: ↑ sedation

Cimetidine: ↑ levels of cisapride

Digoxin: ↑ or ↓ effects

Ranitidine: GI absorption is increased

Warfarin: ↑ effects of warfarin

Drug classifications

Anticholinergics: ↓ effects of cisapride

Anticonvulsants: ↑ drug effects

Benzodiazepines: ↑ sedation

NURSING CONSIDERATIONS

Assessment

- Assess patient for GI complaints: nausea, vomiting, anorexia, constipation; check for decreasing heartburn

Associated nursing diagnoses

- ✓ Pain, acute (uses)
- ✓ Pain, chronic (uses)
- ✓ Knowledge deficit (teaching)

Implementation

PO route
- Give before meals for better absorption and hs

Patient/family education

- Advise patient to avoid alcohol and other CNS depressants that will enhance sedating properties of this drug
- Warn patient to take exactly as prescribed

Evaluation

Positive therapeutic outcome
- Absence of heartburn

cisplatin

(sis'pla-tin)

Platinol, Platinol-AQ

Func. class.: Antineoplastic alkylating agent

Chem. class.: Inorganic heavy metal

Pregnancy category **D**

Action: Alkylates DNA, RNA; inhibits enzymes that allow synthesis of amino acids in proteins; activity is not cell cycle phase specific

➔ Therapeutic Outcome: Prevention of rapidly growing malignant cells

Uses: Advanced bladder cancer; adjunctive in metastatic testicular cancer and metastatic ovarian cancer; head, neck, esophageal, prostatic, lung and cervical cancer; lymphoma

Dosage and routes

Testicular cancer

Adult: **IV** 20 mg/m^2 qd × 5 days, repeat q3 wk for 3 cycles or more, depending on response

Bladder cancer

Adult: **IV** 50-70 mg/m^2 q3-4 wk

Ovarian cancer

Adult: **IV** 100 mg/m^2 q4 wk or 50 mg/m^2 q3 wk with doxorubicin therapy; mix with 2 L of NaCl and 37.5 g mannitol over 6 hr

Available forms: Inj **IV** 10, 50 mg

Side effects/adverse reactions

CNS: ***Convulsions,*** peripheral neuropathy
CV: Cardiac abnormalities
EENT: Tinnitus, hearing loss, vestibular toxicity
GI: Severe nausea, vomiting, diarrhea, weight loss
GU: ***Renal tubular damage,*** renal insufficiency, impotence, sterility, amenorrhea, gynecomastia, hyperuremia
HEMA: ***Thrombocytopenia, leukopenia, pancytopenia***
INTEG: Alopecia, dermatitis
META: Hypomagnesemia, hypocalcemia, hypokalemia, hypophosphatemia
RESP: ***Fibrosis***
SYST: ***Hypersensitivity reaction***

Contraindications: Radiation therapy within 1 mo, chemotherapy within 1 mo, thrombocytopenia, smallpox vaccination

Precautions: Pneumococcal vaccination, pregnancy **D**

Pharmacokinetics

Absorption	Complete bioavailability
Distribution	Widely distributed
Metabolism	Liver
Excretion	Kidneys
Half-life	30 hr

Pharmacodynamics

	IV
Onset	Unknown
Peak	Unknown
Duration	Unknown

Interactions

Drug/drug:

Individual drugs

Radiation: ↑ toxicity, bone marrow suppression

Drug classifications

Aminoglycosides: ↑ nephrotoxicity

Antineoplastics: ↑ toxicity, bone marrow suppression

Bone marrow–suppressing drugs: ↑ bone marrow suppression

Diuretics, loop: ↑ ototoxicity

Lab test interferences

False positive: Breast, bladder, cervix, lung, cytology tests

NURSING CONSIDERATIONS

Assessment

- Monitor CBC, differential, platelet count weekly; withhold drug if WBC count is <4000/mm^3 or platelet count is <100,000/mm^3; notify prescriber of results if WBC <20,000/mm^3, platelets <150,000/mm^3
- Monitor renal function studies: BUN, creatinine, serum uric acid, urine CrCl before and during therapy; I&O ratio; report fall in urine output to <30 ml/hr
- Monitor temp q4h (may indicate beginning of infection)
- Monitor liver function tests before and during therapy (bilirubin, AST [SGOT], ALT [SGPT], LDH) as needed or monthly; note yellowing of skin or sclera, dark urine, clay-colored stools, itchy skin, abdominal pain, fever, diarrhea
- Assess for increased uric acid levels, swelling, joint pain primarily in extremities; patient should be well hydrated to prevent urate deposits
- Assess for bleeding: hematuria, stool guaiac, bruising or petechiae, mucosa or orifices q8h; note inflammation of mucosa, breaks in skin
- Identify dyspnea, rales, unproductive cough, chest pain, tachypnea
- Identify effects of alopecia on body image; discuss feelings about body changes
- Identify edema in feet, joint pain, stomach pain, shaking; prescriber should be notified

Associated nursing diagnoses

- ✓ Injury, risk for (adverse reactions)
- ✓ Body image disturbance (adverse reactions)
- ✓ Infection, risk for (adverse reactions)
- ✓ Knowledge deficit (teaching)

Implementation

- Hydrate patient with 1-2 L of fluids over 8-12 hr before treatment
- Give epinephrine for hypersensitivity reaction; antiemetic 30-60 min before giving drug to prevent vomiting, and prn; allopurinol or sodium bicarbonate to maintain uric acid level, alkalinization of urine; antibiotics for prophylaxis of infection; diuretic (furosemide 40 mg **IV**) or mannitol after infusion

IV **IV route**

- After diluting 10 mg/10 ml or 50 mg/50 ml sterile water for inj; withdraw prescribed dose, dilute ½ dose with 1000 ml D_5 0.2 NaCl or D_5 0.45 NaCl with 37.5 g mannitol; **IV** inf is given over 3-4 hr; use a 0.45 μm filter; total dose 2000 ml over 6-8 hr; check site for irritation, phlebitis; do not use equipment containing aluminum

Y-site compatibilities:

Bleomycin, cyclophosphamide, doxapram, doxorubicin, droperidol, fludarabine, fluorouracil, furosemide, heparin, leucovorin, melphalan, methotrexate, metoclopramide, mitomycin, ondansetron, paclitaxel, sargramostim, vinblastine, vincristine, vinorelbine

Syringe compatibilities:

Bleomycin, cyclophosphamide, doxapram, doxorubicin, droperidol, fluorouracil, furosemide, heparin, leucovorin, methotrexate, metoclopramide, mitomycin, vinblastine, vincristine

Additive incompatibilities:

Fluorouracil, mesna, thiotepa

Additive compatibilities:

Cyclophosphamide with etoposide, etoposide, etoposide with floxuridine, floxuridine, floxuridine with leucovorin calcium, hydroxyzine, ifosfamide, ifosfamide with etoposide, leucovorin, magnesium sulfate, mannitol

Solution incompatibilities:

Sodium bicarbonate 5%, 0.1% NaCl, water

Solution compatibilities:

D_5/0.225% NaCl, D_5/0.45% NaCl, D_5/0.9% NaCl, D_5/0.45% NaCl with mannitol 1.875%, D_5/0.33% NaCl with mannitol 1.875%, D_5/0.33% NaCl with KCl 20 mEq and mannitol 1.875%, 0.9% NaCl, 0.45% NaCl, 0.3% NaCl, 0.225% NaCl, water

Patient/family education

- Teach patient to avoid use of products containing aspirin or ibuprofen, razors, commercial mouthwash, since bleeding may occur; to report symptoms of bleeding (hematuria, tarry stools)
- Instruct patient to report signs of anemia (fatigue, headache, irritability, faintness, shortness of breath)
- Instruct patient to report any changes in breathing or coughing even several months after treatment; to avoid crowds and persons with respiratory tract or other infections
- Advise patient that hair may be lost during treatment; a wig

or hair piece may make patient feel better; new hair may be different in color, texture
- Tell patient not to have any vaccinations without the advice of the prescriber; serious reactions can occur
- Caution patient contraception is needed during treatment and for several months after the completion of therapy

Evaluation

Positive therapeutic outcome
- Prevention of rapid division of malignant cells

clarithromycin
(clare-i-thro-mye'sin)
Biaxin
Func. class.: Antibacterial
Chem. class.: Macrolide antibiotic
Pregnancy category **C**

Action: Binds to 5OS ribosomal subunits of susceptible bacteria and suppresses protein synthesis

Therapeutic Outcome: Bactericidal action against the following: *Streptococcus pneumoniae, Mycoplasma pneumoniae, Corynebacterium diphtheriae, Bordetella pertussis, Listeria monocytogenes, Haemophilus influnzae, S. pyogenes, Staphylococcus aureus*

Uses: Mild to moderate infections of the upper respiratory tract, lower respiratory tract; uncomplicated skin and skin structure infections

Dosage and routes

Adult: PO 250-500 mg bid × 7-14 days

Available forms: Tabs 250, 500 mg

Side effects/adverse reactions

GI: Nausea, vomiting, diarrhea, ***hepatotoxicity,*** abdominal pain, stomatitis, heartburn, anorexia, abnormal taste
GU: Vaginitis, moniliasis
INTEG: Rash, urticaria, pruritus
MISC: Headache

Contraindications: Hypersensitivity

Precautions: Pregnancy **C**, lactation, hepatic/renal disease

Pharmacokinetics	
Absorption	50% (PO)
Distribution	Widely distributed
Metabolism	Liver
Excretion	Kidneys, unchanged (20%-30%)
Half-life	4-6 hr

Pharmacodynamics	PO
Onset	Unknown
Peak	2 hr

Interactions

Drug/drug:

Bromocriptine: ↑ effects of bromocriptine
Carbamazepine: ↑ toxicity, from ↑ levels of carbamazepine
Clindamycin: ↓ action of clindamycin

Cyclosporine: ↑ effects of cyclosporine
Digoxin: ↑ blood levels of digoxin
Disopyramide: ↑ effects of disopyramide
Theophylline: ↑ toxicity from ↑ levels of theophylline
Triazolam: ↑ effects of triazolam

Drug classifications

Oral anticoagulants: ↑ effects of oral anticoagulants
Penicillins: ↑ or ↓ action of penicillins

Lab test interferences

False increase: 17-OHCS/17-KS, AST (SGOT), ALT (SGPT)
Decrease: Folate assay

NURSING CONSIDERATIONS

Assessment

- Assess patient for signs and symptoms of infection including characteristics of wounds, sputum, urine, stool, WBC >10,000, earache, fever; obtain baseline information before and during treatment
- Obtain C&S before beginning drug therapy to identify if correct treatment has been initiated
- Monitor blood studies: AST (SGOT), ALT (SGPT), CBC, Hct, bilirubin, LDH, alkaline phosphatase, Coombs' test monthly if patient is on long-term therapy
- Assess bowel pattern qd; if severe diarrhea occurs, drug should be discontinued
- Assess for overgrowth of infection: perineal itching, fever, malaise, redness, pain, swelling, drainage, rash, diarrhea, change in cough, sputum

Associated nursing diagnoses

✓ Infection, risk for (uses)
✓ Diarrhea (side effects)
✓ Knowledge deficit (teaching)
✓ Noncompliance (teaching)

Implementation

PO route

- Give in equal doses in each 24-hr period to maintain proper blood levels

Patient/family education

- Advise patient to contact physician if vaginal itching, loose, foul-smelling stools, furry tongue occur; may indicate superinfection
- Instruct patient to take all medication prescribed for the length of time ordered

Evaluation

Positive therapeutic outcome

- Absence of signs/symptoms of infection (WBC <10,000, temp WNL, absence of red draining wounds)
- Reported improvement in symptoms of infection

clemastine

(klem'as-teen)

Tavist, Tavist-1

Func. class.: Antihistamine

Chem. class.: Ethanolamine derivative, H_1-receptor antagonist

Pregnancy category **B**

Action: Acts on blood vessels, GI, respiratory system by competing with histamine for H_1-receptor site; decreases allergic response by blocking histamine

Therapeutic Outcome: Absence of allergy symptoms and rhinitis

Uses: Allergy symptoms, rhinitis, allergic dermatoses, nasal allergies, hypersensitive reactions including blood transfusion reactions, anaphylaxis

Dosage and routes

P *Adult and child >12 yr:* PO 1.34-2.68 mg bid-tid, not to exceed 8.04 mg/day

Available forms: Tabs 1.34, 2.68 mg; syr 0.67 mg/ml

Side effects/adverse reactions

CNS: Dizziness, drowsiness, poor coordination, fatigue, anxiety, euphoria, confusion, paresthesia, neuritis, paradoxic excitement (child) P

CV: Hypotension, palpitations, tachycardia

EENT: Blurred vision, dilated pupils, tinnitus, nasal stuffiness, dry nose, throat, *mouth*

GI: Constipation, dry mouth, nausea, vomiting, anorexia, diarrhea

GU: Retention, dysuria, frequency

HEMA: Thrombocytopenia, agranulocytosis, hemolytic anemia

INTEG: Rash, urticaria, photosensitivity, sweating

RESP: Increased thick secretions, wheezing, chest tightness

Contraindications: Hypersensitivity to H_1-receptor antagonists, acute asthma attack, lower respiratory tract disease

Precautions: Increased intraocular pressure, renal disease, cardiac disease, hypertension, bronchial asthma, seizure disorder, stenosed peptic ulcers, hyperthyroidism, prostatic hypertrophy, bladder neck obstruction, pregnancy **B**, G elderly

Pharmacokinetics

Absorption	Well absorbed (PO)
Distribution	Widely distributed
Metabolism	Liver, extensively
Excretion	Kidneys, breast milk (high)
Half-life	Unknown

Pharmacodynamics

	PO
Onset	15-60 min
Peak	1-2 hr
Duration	12 hr

Interactions

Drug/drug:

Individual drugs

Alcohol: ↑ CNS depression

Drug classifications

CNS depressants: ↑ CNS depression
MAOI: ↑ anticholinergic effect
Narcotics: ↑ CNS depression
Sedative/hypnotics: ↑ CNS depression

Lab test interferences

False negative: Skin allergy tests (discontinue antihistamines 3 days before testing)

NURSING CONSIDERATIONS

Assessment

- Assess respiratory status: rate, rhythm, increase in bronchial secretions, wheezing, chest tightness; provide fluids to 2 L/day to decrease secretion thickness
- Monitor I&O ratio: be alert for urinary retention, frequency, dysuria, especially G elderly; drug should be discontinued if these occur

Associated nursing diagnoses

- ✓ Airway clearance, ineffective (uses)
- ✓ Injury, risk for (side effects)
- ✓ Knowledge deficit (teaching)
- ✓ Noncompliance (teaching, overuse)

Implementation

PO route

- May give with food to decrease GI upset
- Store in tight, light-resistant container

Patient/family education

- Teach all aspects of drug uses; to notify prescriber if confusion, sedation, hypotension occur; to avoid driving and other hazardous activity if drowsiness occurs; to avoid alcohol and other CNS depressants that may potentiate effect
- Instruct patient to take 1 hr ac or 2 hr pc to facilitate absorption
- Caution patient not to exceed recommended dosage; dysrhythmias may occur
- Teach patient hard candy, gum, frequent rinsing of mouth may be used for dryness
- Tell patient if EENT or CNS symptoms occur (blurred vision, severe dry mouth, throat, confusion, dizziness, poor coordination, euphoria), prescriber should be notified

Evaluation

Positive therapeutic outcome

- Absence of running or congested nose, rashes

Treatment of overdose:

Administer ipecac syrup or lavage, diazepam, vasopressors, barbiturates (short acting)

clindamycin

(klin-da-mye'sin)

Cleocin HCl, clindamycin HCl, Dalacin C ✤, Cleocin Pediatric, Cleocin phosphate, clindamycin phosphate

Func. class.: Antibacterial macrolide

Chem. class.: Lincomycin derivative

Pregnancy category **B**

Action: Binds to 50S subunit of bacterial ribosomes; suppresses protein synthesis

➡ **Therapeutic Outcome:** Absence of infection

Uses: Infections caused by staphylococci, streptococci, pneumococci, *Rickettsia, Fusobacterium, Actinomyces, Peptococcus, Clostridium*

Dosage and routes

Adults: PO 150-450 mg q6hr; IM/**IV** 300 mg q6-12hr, not to exceed 4800 mg/day

PID: Adult **IV** 600 mg qid plus gentamicin

Vaginal route

Adult: 5 g applicatorful at bedtime × 1 wk

Topical route

Adult: Sol 1% apply bid

P ***Child >1 mo:*** PO 20-40 mg/kg/day in divided doses q6-8hr, IM/**IV** 15-40 mg/kg/day in divided doses q6-8hr in 3-4 equal doses

Available forms: Inj 150-300 mg/ml; caps 75, 150, 300 mg; oral sol 75 mg/ml; top 1% lotion, soap, solution, gel; vag 2% cream

Side effects/adverse reactions

EENT: Rash, urticaria, pruritus, erythema, pain, abscess at injection site

GI: *Nausea, vomiting, abdominal pain, diarrhea,* ***pseudomembranous colitis,*** *anorexia, weight loss*

GU: Increased AST (SGOT), ALT (SGPT), bilirubin, alk phosphatase, jaundice, *vaginitis,* urinary frequency

HEMA: *Leukopenia, eosinophilia, agranulocytosis, thrombocytopenia, polyarthritis*

Contraindications: Hypersensitivity to this drug or lincomycin, ulcerative colitis/enteritis, infants <1 mo

Precautions: Renal disease, G liver disease, GI disease, elderly, pregnancy **B**, lactation, tartrazine sensitivity

Pharmacokinetics

Absorption	Well absorbed (PO, IM), minimal (top)
Distribution	Widely distributed; crosses placenta
Metabolism	Liver, extensively
Excretion	Kidneys, breast milk
Half-life	2½ hr

Pharmacodynamics

	PO	IM	IV	TOP	VAG
Onset	Rapid	Rapid	Rapid	Rapid	Rapid
Peak	½-1 hr	1½ hr	Infusions end	Unknown	Unknown

Interactions

Drug/drug:

Individual drugs

Chloramphenicol: ↓ action of chloramphenicol
Erythromicin: ↓ action of erythromicin

Drug classifications

Nondepolarizing muscle relaxants: ↑ neuromuscular blockade

Lab test interferences

Increase: Alk phosphatase, bilirubin, CPK, AST (SGOT), ALT (SGPT)

NURSING CONSIDERATIONS

Assessment

- Assess any patient with compromised renal system; drug is excreted slowly in poor renal system function; toxicity may occur rapidly
- Assess patient for signs and symptoms of infection including characteristics of wounds, sputum, urine, stool, WBC >10,000, fever; obtain baseline information before and during treatment
- Complete culture and sensitivity testing before beginning drug therapy; this will identify if correct treatment has been initiated
- Assess for allergic reactions: rash, urticaria, pruritus, chills, fever, joint pain; may occur a few days after therapy begins—epinephrine and resuscitation equipment should be available in case of an anaphylactic reaction
- Identify urine output; if decreasing, notify prescriber (may indicate nephrotoxicity); also look for increased BUN and creatinine levels
- Monitor blood studies: AST (SGOT), ALT (SGPT), CBC, Hct, bilirubin, LDH, alk phosphatase, Coombs' test monthly if patient is on long-term therapy
- Monitor electrolytes: potassium, sodium, chloride monthly if patient is on long-term therapy
- Assess bowel pattern qd; if severe diarrhea occurs, drug should be discontinued; may indicate pseudomembranous colitis
- Monitor for bleeding: ecchymosis, bleeding gums, hematuria, stool guaiac daily if on long-term therapy
- Assess for overgrowth of infection: perineal itching, fever, malaise, redness, pain, swelling, drainage, rash, diarrhea, change in cough, sputum

Associated nursing diagnoses

✓ Infection, risk for (uses)
✓ Diarrhea (adverse reactions)
✓ Injury, risk for (adverse reaction)
✓ Knowledge deficit (teaching)
✓ Noncompliance (teaching)

Implementation

PO route

- Give with 8 oz of water; give with meals for GI symptoms
- Shake liquids well
- Do not refrigerate oral preparations; stable at room temperature for 2 wks

IM route

- If more than 600 mg must be given, divide into two injections

- Give deeply in large muscle mass; rotate sites

IV route

- Give by infusion only; do not administer bolus dose; dilute 300 mg or more/50 ml or more of D_5W, NS
- May be further diluted in greater amounts of D_5W, 0.9% NaCl and given as a cont inf in acute pelvic inflammatory disease (PID); give first dose 10 mg/min over ½ hr, then 0.75 mg/min; increased rates may be used to keep serum blood levels higher; run over >10 min; no more than 120 mg in a 1 hr inf

Syringe compatibilities:

Amikacin, aztreonam, gentamicin, heparin

Syringe incompatibility:

Tobramycin

Y-site incompatibility:

Idarubicin

Y-site compatibilities:

Cyclophosphamide, enalaprilat, esmolol, foscarnet, hydromorphone, labetolol, magnesium sulfate, melphalan, meperidine, morphine, multivitamins, odansetron, perphenazine, vinorelbine, zidovudine

Additive incompatibility:

Ciprofloxacin

Top route

- Avoid contact with eyes, mucous membranes, and open cuts during topical application; if accidental contact occurs, rinse with cool water
- Wash affected areas with warm water and soap, rinse, pat dry before application

Patient/family education

- Tell patient to take oral drug with full glass of water; may take with food if GI symptoms occur; antiperistaltic drugs may worsen diarrhea
- Teach patient aspects of drug therapy: need to complete entire course of medication to ensure organism death (10-14 days); culture may be taken after medication course has been completed
- Advise patient to report sore throat, fever, fatigue; may indicate superimposed infection
- Advise patient that drug must be taken at equal intervals around clock to maintain blood levels

Evaluation

Positive therapeutic outcome

- Decreased temperature, negative C&S

Treatment of hypersensitivity: Withdraw drug; maintain airway; administer epinephrine, aminophylline, O_2, **IV** corticosteroids

clioquinol

(klee-oh-kwee'nole)

Vioform

Func.class.: Local anti-infective

Chem. class.: Halogenated hydroxyquinoline

Pregnancy category **C**

Action: Increases cell membrane permeability in susceptible organisms by binding sterols; decreases potassium, sodium, and nutrients in cell

Therapeutic Outcome: Fungistatic/fungicidal against susceptible organisms: tinea pedis, tinea cruris, tinea corporis, tinea versicolor

Uses: Cutaneous infections: athletes's foot, eczema, and other fungal infections

Dosage and routes

Top: Apply to affected area bid or tid × 7 days only

Available forms: Cream 3%; oint 3%

Side effect/adverse reactions

INTEG: Rash, urticaria, stinging, burning, dry skin, pruritus, contact dermatitis, erythema, redness, staining of hair and skin

Contraindications: Hypersensitivity to iodine, chloroxine

Precautions: Pregnancy **C**, varicella, viral skin conditions, deep or puncture wounds, serious burns

Pharmacokinetics

Absorption	Rapid
Distribution	Unknown
Metabolism	Liver
Excretion	Unknown
Half-life	Unknown

Pharmacodynamics

Onset	Unknown
Peak	Unknown
Duration	Unknown

Interactions: None

NURSING CONSIDERATIONS

Assessment

- Assess skin for fungal infections: peeling, dryness, itching before and throughout treatment
- Monitor for allergic reaction: burning, stinging, swelling, redness, dermatitis, rash; drug should be discontinued; antihistamines (mild reaction) given

Associated nursing diagnoses

- ✓ Skin integrity, impaired (uses)
- ✓ Infection, risk for (uses)
- ✓ Knowledge deficit (teaching)

Implementation

Top route

- Use enough medication to cover lesions completely
- Apply after cleansing with soap, water before each application; dry well
- Store at room temp in dry place

Patient/family education

- Teach patient to apply with glove to prevent further infection; not to cover with occlusive dressings
- Teach patient proper hygiene: hand-washing technique, nail care, use of concomitant top agents if prescribed
- Instruct patient to avoid use of OTC creams, ointments, lotions unless directed
- Advise patient to change socks and shoes once a day during treatment of tinea pedis
- Instruct patient to report to prescriber if infection persists or returns or if blisters, burning, oozing, swelling develops
- Caution patient to avoid alcohol, since nausea, vomiting, hypertension may occur

Evaluation

Positive therapeutic outcome

- Decrease in size, number of lesions

clobetasol

(klo-bet'a-sol)

Temovate

Func. class.: Topical corticosteroid

Chem. class.: Synthetic fluorinated agent, group I potency

Pregnancy category C

Action: Antipruritic, anti-inflammatory

Therapeutic Outcome: Decreased inflammatory skin disorders

Uses: Psoriasis, eczema, contact dermatitis, pruritus; usually reserved for severe dermatoses that have not responded to less potent formulation

Dosage and routes

P *Adult and child:* Apply to affected area bid

Available forms: Oint 0.05%; cream 0.05%

Side effects/adverse reactions

INTEG: Burning, dryness, itching, irritation, acne, folliculitis, hypertrichosis, perioral dermatitis, hypopigmentation, atrophy, striae, miliaria, allergic contact dermatitis, secondary infection

Contraindications: Hypersensitivity to corticosteroids, fungal infections

Precautions: Pregnancy **C**, lactation, viral infections, bacterial infections

Pharmacokinetics	
Absorption	Minimal
Distribution	Not distributed
Metabolism	None
Excretion	None
Half-life	Unknown

Pharmacodynamics	
Onset	Unknown
Peak	Unknown
Duration	Unknown

Interactions: None

NURSING CONSIDERATIONS

Assessment

- Monitor temp; if fever develops, drug should be discontinued
- Assess for syst absorption: increased temp, inflammation, irritation

Associated nursing diagnoses

- ✓ Infection, risk for (adverse reactions)
- ✓ Knowledge deficit (teaching)
- ✓ Noncompliance (teaching)

Implementation

Top route

- Apply only to affected areas; do not get in eyes
- Leave area uncovered or lightly covered; occlusive dressing is not recommended; syst absorption may occur
- Apply only to dermatoses; do not use on weeping, denuded, or infected area
- Cleanse area before application of drug
- Treat for a few days after area has cleared
- Store at room temp

Patient/family education

- Caution patient to avoid sunlight on affected area; burns may occur
- Teach patient to limit treatment to 14 days using <50 g/wk

Evaluation

Positive therapeutic outcome

- Absence of severe itching, patches on skin, flaking

clocortolone

(klo-kort′o-lone)

Cloderm

Func. class.: Topical corticosteroid

Chem. class.: Synthetic fluorinated agent, group IV potency

Pregnancy category **C**

C

Action: Antipruritic, antiinflammatory

➔ **Therapeutic Outcome:** Decreased inflammatory skin disorders

Uses: Psoriasis, eczema, contact dermatitis, pruritus

Dosage and routes

P *Adult and child:* Apply to affected area tid or qid

Available forms: Cream 0.1%

Side effects/adverse reactions

INTEG: Burning, dryness, itching, irritation, acne, folliculitis, hypertrichosis, perioral dermatitis, hypopigmentation, atrophy, striae, miliaria, allergic contact dermatitis, secondary infection

Contraindications: Hypersensitivity to corticosteroids, fungal infections

Precautions: Pregnancy **C**, lactation, viral infections, bacterial infections

Pharmacokinetics

Absorption	Minimal; syst absorption on large areas
Distribution	Site only
Metabolism	Not metabolized
Excretion	Not excreted
Half-life	Unknown

Pharmacodynamics

	TOP
Onset	Up to 1 hr
Peak	Up to several days
Duration	Up to several days

Interactions: None

NURSING CONSIDERATIONS

Assessment

- Monitor temp, worsening of condition; if fever develops drug should be discontinued
- Monitor for systemic absorption: increased temp, inflammation, irritation

Associated nursing diagnoses

✓ Skin integrity, impairment (uses)
✓ Infection, risk for (adverse reactions)
✓ Knowledge deficit (teaching)

Implementation

Top route

- Apply only to affected areas; do not get in eyes; apply medication, then cover with occlusive dressing (only if prescribed), seal to normal skin, changed q12h; systemic absorption may occur; apply only to dermatoses; do not use on weeping, denuded, or infected area
- Cleanse area before application of drug
- Treat for a few days after area has cleared
- Store at room temp

Patient/family education

- Caution patient to avoid sunlight on affected area; burns may occur
- Advise patient to discontinue drug, notify prescriber if local irritation or fever develops

Evaluation

Positive therapeutic outcome

- Absence of severe itching, patches on skin, flaking

clofazimine

(kloe-faz′i-meen)

Lamprene

Func. class.: Leprostatic

Pregnancy category **C**

Action: Inhibits mycobacterial growth, binds to mycobacterial DNA; exerts antiinflammatory properties in controlling leprosy reactions

Uses: Lepromatous leprosy, dapsone-resistant leprosy, lepromatous leprosy complicated by erythema nodosum leprosum

➡ **Therapeutic Outcome:** Decreased infection of leprosy

Dosage and routes

Erythema nodosum leprosum

Adult: PO 100-200 mg qd × 3 mo, then taper dosage to 100 mg when disease is controlled; do not exceed 200 mg/day

Dapsone-resistant leprosy
Adult: PO 100 mg/day in combination with at least one other antileprosy drug × 3 yr, then 100 mg qd clofazimine only

Available forms: Caps 50, 100 mg

Side effects/adverse reactions

CNS: Dizziness, headache, fatigue, drowsiness
EENT: Pigmentation of cornea and conjunctiva, drying, burning, itching, irritation
GI: Diarrhea, nausea, vomiting, abdominal pain, intolerance, ***GI bleeding, obstruction,*** anorexia, constipation, ***hepatitis,*** jaundice
INTEG: Pink or brown discoloration, dryness, pruritus, rash, photosensitivity, acne, monilial cheilosis
MISC: Discolored urine, feces, sputum, sweat

Precautions: Pregnancy **C**, P lactation, children, abdominal pain, diarrhea, depression

Pharmacokinetics

Absorption	Partially
Distribution	Crosses placenta
Metabolism	Liver
Excretion	Feces, bile
Half-life	70 days

Pharmacodynamics

	PO
Onset	Unknown
Peak	Unknown
Duration	Unknown

Interactions

Drug/drug:

Individual drugs
Alcohol: ↑ toxicity
Carbamazepine: ↑ toxicity
Cycloserine: ↑ toxicity
Ethionamide: ↑ toxicity
Rifampin: ↑ toxicity

Drug classifications
Antacids, aluminum: ↓ absorption

NURSING CONSIDERATIONS

Assessment

- Perform liver studies weekly: ALT (SGPT), AST (SGOT), bilirubin
- Monitor renal status: before initiation of therapy, then monthly: BUN, creatinine, output, sp gr, urinalysis
- Assess mental status often: affect, mood, behavioral changes; psychosis may occur
- Monitor hepatic status: decreased appetite, jaundice, dark urine, fatigue

Associated nursing diagnoses

✓ Infection, risk for (uses)
✓ Diarrhea (side effects)
✓ Injury, risk for (side effects)
✓ Knowledge deficit (teaching)

Implementation

PO route

- Give with meals to decrease GI symptoms
- Provide antiemetic if vomiting occurs

Patient/family education

- Teach patient that compliance with dosage schedule, duration is necessary

- Teach patient that scheduled appointments must be kept or relapse may occur
- Caution patient to avoid alcohol while taking drug
- Teach diabetic patients to use blood glucose monitor to obtain correct result
- Advise patient to report weakness, fatigue, loss of appetite, nausea, vomiting, yellowing of skin or eyes, tingling/numbness of hands/feet

Evaluation

Positive therapeutic outcome
- Decreased symptoms of leprosy

clomiphene

(kloe'mi-feen)

Clomid, clomiphene citrate, Milophene, Serophene

Func. class.: Ovulation stimulant

Chem. class.: Nonsteroidal antiestrogenic

Pregnancy category **X**

Action: Increases LH, FSH release from the pituitary, which increase maturation of ovarian follicle, ovulation, development of corpus luteum

Therapeutic Outcome: Pregnancy

Uses: Female infertility (ovulatory failure)

Dosage and routes

Adult: PO 50-100 mg qd × 5 days or 50-100 mg qd beginning on day 5 of cycle; may be repeated until conception occurs or 3 cycles of therapy have been completed

Available forms: Tabs 50 mg

Side effects/adverse reactions

CNS: ***Headache, depression,*** restlessness, anxiety, nervousness, fatigue, insomnia, dizziness, flushing

CV: Vasomotor flushing, phlebitis, deep vein thrombosis

EENT: Blurred vision, diplopia, photophobia

GI: ***Nausea, vomiting, constipation,*** abdominal pain, bloating

GU: Polyuria, frequency, birth defects, spontaneous abortions, multiple ovulation, breast pain, oliguria, abnormal uterine bleeding

INTEG: ***Rash, dermatitis,*** urticaria, alopecia

Contraindications: Hypersensitivity, pregnancy **X**, hepatic disease, undiagnosed vaginal bleeding

Precautions: Hypertension, depression, convulsions, diabetes mellitus

Pharmacokinetics

Absorption	Well distributed
Distribution	Unknown
Metabolism	Liver, extensively
Excretion	Feces
Half-life	5 days

Pharmacodynamics

	PO
Onset	Unknown
Peak	Unknown
Duration	Unknown

Interactions: None

Lab test interferences

Increase: FSH/LH, BSP, thyroxine, TBG

NURSING CONSIDERATIONS

Assessment

- Determine liver function tests before therapy: AST (SGOT), ALT (SGPT), alkaline phosphatase
- Monitor serum progesterone, urinary excretion of pregnanediol to identify occurrence of ovulation
- Pelvic examination should be done to determine ovarian size, cervical condition
- Endometrial biopsy may be done in women over 35 to rule out endometrial carcinoma

Associated nursing diagnoses

✓ Sexual dysfunction (uses)
✓ Knowledge deficit (teaching)

Implementation

PO route

- Give after discontinuing estrogen therapy
- Give at same time qd to maintain drug level; begin on 5th day of menstrual cycle

Patient/family education

- Advise patient that multiple births are common after drug is taken
- Instruct patient to notify prescriber if low abdominal pain occurs; may indicate ovarian cyst, cyst rupture
- Teach patient if dose is missed, double at next time; if more than one dose is missed, call prescriber
- Instruct patient that response usually occurs 4-10 days after last day of treatment
- Teach patient method for taking, recording basal body temp to determine whether ovulation has occurred; if ovulation can be determined (there is a slight decrease in temp, then a sharp increase for ovulation), to attempt coitus 3 days before and qod until after ovulation
- Teach patient if pregnancy is suspected, to notify prescriber immediately

Evaluation

Positive therapeutic outcome

- Fertility

clomipramine

(klom-ip′ra-meen)

Anafranil

Func. class.: Tricyclic antidepressant

Chem. class.: Tertiary amine

Pregnancy category **C**

Action: Potent inhibitor of serotonin uptake; also increases dopamine metabolism

Uses: Depression, dysphoria, anxiety, agoraphobia and other phobias, obsessive-compulsive disorder

Therapeutic Outcome: Decreased signs and symptoms of obsessive-compulsive disorder, decreased depression

Dosage and routes

Obsessive-compulsive disorder

Adult: PO 25 mg hs; increase gradually over 4 wk to a dosage of 75-300 mg/day in divided doses

P *Child 10-18 yr:* PO 25-50 mg/day gradually increased; not to exceed 200 mg/day

Depression

Adult: PO 50-150 mg/day in a single or divided dose

Anxiety/agoraphobia

Adult: PO 25-75 mg/day

Available forms: Caps 25, 50, 75 mg

Side effects/adverse reactions

*CNS: Dizziness, tremors, **mania, seizures,*** aggressiveness
CV: Hypotension, tachycardia, ***cardiac arrest***
ENDO: Galactorrhea, hyperprolactinemia
GI: Constipation, dry mouth, nausea, dyspepsia
GU: Delayed ejaculation, anorgasmy, retention
HEMA: Agranulocytosis, neutropenia, pancytopenia
INTEG: Diaphoresis
META: Hyponatremia

Contraindications: Hypersensitivity

Precautions: Seizures, suicidal patients, G elderly, pregnancy **C**

Pharmacokinetics

Absorption	Well absorbed
Distribution	Widely distributed
Metabolism	Liver, extensively
Excretion	Kidneys, breast milk
Half-life	21 hr parent compound; 36 hr metabolite

Pharmacodynamics

	PO
Onset	Unknown
Peak	Unknown
Duration	Unknown

Interactions

Drug/drug:

Individual drugs

Alcohol: ↑ CNS depression
Cimetidine: ↑ levels, ↑ toxicity
Clonidine: Severe hypertension; avoid use
Disulfiram: Delirium
Fluoxetine: ↑ levels, ↑ toxicity
Guanethidine: ↓ effects

Drug classifications

MAOI: Hypertensive crisis, convulsions
Barbiturates: ↑ effects
Benzodiazepines: ↑ effects
CNS depressants: ↑ effects
Sympathomimetics, indirect-acting: ↓ effects
Oral contraceptives: ↑ effects, toxicity

Drug/smoking:

↑ metabolism, ↓ effects

Lab test interferences

Increase: Serum bilirubin, blood glucose, alkaline phosphatase

Decrease: VMA, 5-HIAA
False increase: Urinary catecholamines

NURSING CONSIDERATIONS
Assessment

- Monitor B/P (with patient lying, standing), pulse q4h; if systolic B/P drops 20 mm Hg hold drug, notify prescriber; take vital signs q4h in patients with cardiovascular disease
- Monitor blood studies: CBC, leukocytes, differential, cardiac enzymes if patient is receiving long-term therapy
- Monitor hepatic studies: AST (SGOT), ALT (SGPT), bilirubin
- Check weight weekly; appetite may increase with drug
- Assess ECG for flattening of T wave, bundle branch block, AV block, dysrhythmias in cardiac patients
- Assess for EPS primarily in G elderly: rigidity, dystonia, akathisia
- Assess mental status: mood, sensorium, affect, suicidal tendencies; increase in psychiatric symptoms: depression, panic
- Monitor urinary retention, constipation; constipation is P more likely to occur in children G or elderly
- Assess for withdrawal symptoms: headache, nausea, vomiting, muscle pain, weakness; do not usually occur unless drug was discontinued abruptly
- Identify alcohol consumption; if alcohol is consumed, hold dose until morning

Associated nursing diagnoses

- ✓ Coping, ineffective individual (uses)
- ✓ Injury, risk for physical (side effects)
- ✓ Knowledge deficit (teaching)
- ✓ Noncompliance (teaching)

Implementation

PO route

- Give with food or milk for GI symptoms
- Store at room temp; do not freeze

Patient/family education

- Teach patient that therapeutic effects may take 2-3 wk
- Teach patient to use caution in driving or other activities requiring alertness because of drowsiness, dizziness, blurred vision; to avoid rising quickly from sitting to standing, espe- G cially elderly
- Teach patient to avoid alcohol ingestion, other CNS depressants
- Teach patient not to discontinue medication quickly after long-term use: may cause nausea, headache, malaise
- Teach patient to wear sunscreen or large hat, since photosensitivity occurs
- Teach patient to increase fluids, bulk in diet if constipation, urinary retention occur, G especially elderly
- Teach patient to take gum, hard sugarless candy, or frequent sips of water for dry mouth

Evaluation

Positive therapeutic outcome

- Decrease in depression
- Absence of suicidal thoughts

Treatment of overdose: ECG monitoring, induce emesis, lavage, activated charcoal, administer anticonvulsant

clonazepam
(kloe-na'zi-pam)

Klonopin, Rivotril ✦

Func. class.: Anticonvulsant

Chem. class.: Benzodiazepine derivative

Pregnancy category C

Controlled substance schedule IV

Action: Inhibits spike, wave formation in absence seizures (petit mal), decreases amplitude, frequency, duration, spread of discharge in minor motor seizures

Uses: Absence, atypical absence, akinetic, myoclonic seizures

⇒ Therapeutic Outcome: Decreased frequency, severity of seizures

Dosage and routes

Adult: PO not to exceed 1.5 mg/day in 3 divided doses; may be increased 0.5-1 mg q3 days until desired response; not to exceed 20 mg/day

P ***Child <10 yr or 30 kg:*** PO 0.01-0.03 mg/kg/day in divided doses q8h, not to exceed 0.05 mg/kg/day; may be increased 0.25-0.5 mg q3 days until desired response; not to exceed 0.1-0.2 mg/kg/day

Available forms: Tabs 0.5, 1, 2 mg

Side effects/adverse reactions

CNS: Drowsiness, dizziness, confusion, behavioral changes, tremors, insomnia, headache, suicidal tendencies, slurred speech

CV: Palpitations, bradycardia

EENT: Increased salivation, nystagmus, diplopia, abnormal eye movements

GI: Nausea, constipation, polyphagia, anorexia, xerostomia, diarrhea, gastritis, sore gums

GU: Dysuria, enuresis, nocturia, retention

HEMA: Thrombocytopenia, leukocytosis, eosinophilia

INTEG: Rash, alopecia, hirsutism

RESP: Respiratory depression, dyspnea, congestion

Contraindications: Hypersensitivity to benzodiazepines, acute narrow-angle glaucoma

Precautions: Open angle glaucoma, chronic respiratory disease, pregnancy **C**, renal/ G hepatic disease, elderly

Pharmacokinetics	
Absorption	Well absorbed
Distribution	Crosses blood-brain barrier, placenta
Metabolism	Liver
Excretion	Kidneys
Half life	18-50 hr

Pharmacodynamics

	PO
Onset	½-1 hr
Peak	1-2 hr
Duration	6-12 hr

Interactions
Drug/drug:
Individual drugs
Alcohol: ↑ CNS depression
Carbamazepine: ↓ effectiveness
Cimetidine: ↓ metabolism, ↑ action
Disulfiram: ↓ metabolism, ↑ action
Fluoxetine: ↓ metabolism, ↑ action
Isoniazid: ↓ metabolism, ↑ action
Ketoconazole: ↓ metabolism, ↑ action
Levodopa: ↓ effectiveness
Metoprolol: ↓ metabolism, ↑ action
Phenytoin: ↑ levels, ↓ clonazepam levels
Propranolol: ↓ metabolism, ↑ action
Propoxyphene: ↓ metabolism, ↑ action
Valproic acid: ↑ seizures
Drug classifications
Antidepressants: ↑ CNS depression
Anticonvulsants: ↑ CNS depression
Antihistamines: ↑ CNS depression
Barbiturates: ↑ CNS depression; ↓ effect of clonazepam
General anesthetics: ↑ CNS depression
Hypnotics: ↑ CNS depression
Oral contraceptives: ↓ metabolism, ↑ action
Narcotics: ↑ CNS depression
Sedatives: ↑ CNS depression

Lab test interferences
Increase: AST (SGOT), alkaline phosphatase

C

NURSING CONSIDERATIONS
Assessment
- Assess mental status: mood, sensorium, affect, memory (long, short), especially elderly G
- Assess for blood dyscrasias: fever, sore throat, bruising, rash, jaundice, epistaxis (long-term treatment only)
- Assess seizure activity including type, location, duration, and character; provide seizure precaution
- Assess renal studies: urinalysis, BUN, urine creatinine
- Monitor blood studies: RBC, Hct, Hgb, reticulocyte counts weekly for 4wk then monthly
- Monitor hepatic studies: ALT (SGPT), AST (SGOT), bilirubin, creatinine
- Monitor drug levels during initial treatment
- Assess for signs of physical withdrawal if medication suddenly discontinued
- Assess eye problems: need for ophthalmic examinations before, during, after treatment (slit lamp, fundoscopy, tonometry
- Assess allergic reaction: red raised rash; if this occurs, drug should be discontinued
- Monitor for toxicity: bone marrow depression, nausea, vomiting, ataxia, diplopia, cardiovascular collapse

Associated nursing diagnoses

✓ Injury, risk for (side effects)
✓ Knowledge deficit (teaching)

Implementation

PO route

• Give on empty stomach for best absorption

Patient/family education

• Teach patient to carry ID card or Medic Alert bracelet stating patient's name, drugs taken, condition, physician's name, phone number
• Caution patient to avoid driving, other activities that require alertness
• Caution patient to avoid alcohol ingestion or CNS depressants; increased sedation may occur
• Teach patient not to discontinue medication quickly after long-term use; taper off over several weeks

Evaluation

Positive therapeutic outcome

• Decreased seizure activity

Treatment of overdose: Lavage, activated charcoal, VS, monitor electrolytes

clonidine

(klon'i-deen)

Catapres, Catapres-TTS, clonidine HCl, Dixarit ✦

Func. class.: Antihypertensive

Chem. class.: Central α-adrenergic agonist

Pregnancy category C

Action: Inhibits sympathetic vasomotor center in CNS, which reduces impulses in sympathetic nervous system; B/P, pulse rate, cardiac output decrease

Therapeutic Outcome: Decreased B/P in hypertension

Uses: Mild to moderate hypertension; used alone or in combination

Investigational uses: Narcotic withdrawal, prevention of vascular headaches, treatment of menopausal symptoms, dysmenorrhea, attention deficit disorder

Dosage and routes

Hypertension

Adult: PO/trans 0.1 mg bid, then increase by 0.1 mg/day or 0.2 mg/day until desired response; range 0.2-0.8 mg/day in divided doses

Opioid withdrawal

Adult: PO 0.3-1.2 mg/day; decreased dosage given over several days

Available forms: Tabs 0.1, 0.2, 0.3 mg; trans sys 2.5, 5,

7.5 mg delivering 0.1, 0.2, 0.3 mg/24 hr, respectively

Side effects/adverse reactions

CNS: *Drowsiness, sedation, headache, fatigue,* nightmares, insomnia, mental changes, anxiety, depression, hallucinations, delirium
CV: *Orthostatic hypotension, palpitations,* **CHF,** ECG abnormalities
EENT: Taste change, parotid pain
ENDO: Hyperglycemia
GI: *Nausea, vomiting, malaise,* constipation, dry mouth
GU: Impotence, dysuria, *nocturia,* gynecomastia
INTEG: *Rash,* alopecia, facial pallor, pruritus, hives, edema, burning papules, excoriation (trans patches)
MS: Muscle, joint pain, leg cramps

Contraindications:
Hypersensitivity

Precautions:
MI (recent), diabetes mellitus, chronic renal failure, Raynaud's disease, thyroid disease, depression, P COPD, child <12 (patches), asthma, pregnancy **C**, lactation, G elderly

Pharmacokinetics

Absorption	Well absorbed (PO, trans)
Distribution	Widely distributed; crosses blood-brain barrier
Metabolism	Liver, extensively
Excretion	Kidneys, unchanged (30%)
Half-life	12-16 hr

Pharmacodynamics

	PO	TRANS
Onset	½-1 hr	3 days
Peak	2-4 hr	Unknown
Duration	8 hr	8 hr (after removal)

Interactions
Drug/drug:
Individual drugs
Alcohol: ↑ CNS depression
Drug classifications
Amphetamines: ↓ hypotensive effects
Anesthetics: ↑ CNS depression
Antidepressants, tricyclic: ↓ hypotensive effects
β-Blockers: ↑ bradycardia
Cardiac glycosides: ↑ bradycardia
Diuretics: ↑ hypotensive effects
Hypnotics: ↑ CNS depression
Narcotics: ↑ CNS depression
Nitrates: ↑ hypotensive effects
Sedatives: ↑ CNS depression

Lab test interferences
Increase: Blood glucose
Decrease: VMA, catecholamines, aldosterone

NURSING CONSIDERATIONS
Assessment
- Perform blood studies: neutrophils, decreased platelets
- Perform renal studies: protein, BUN, creatinine; watch for increased levels that may indicate nephrotic syndrome: polyuria, oliguria, frequency
- Monitor baselines in renal, liver function tests before therapy begins; check potassium levels, although hyperkalemia rarely occurs

• Check dipstick of urine for protein qd in first morning specimen; if protein is increased, a 24-hr urinary protein should be collected
• Monitor B/P, pulse if the drug is being used for hypertension; notify prescriber of changes
• Assess for narcotic withdrawal in patients receiving the drug for opioid withdrawal, including fever, diarrhea, nausea, vomiting, cramps, insomnia, shivering, dilated pupils, weakness
• Check for edema in feet, legs daily; monitor I&O; check for decreasing output
• Note allergic reaction: rash, fever, pruritus, urticaria; drug should be discontinued if antihistamines fail to help
• Note allergic reaction from patches: rash, urticaria, angioedema; should not continue to use
• Assess for symptoms of CHF: edema, dyspnea, wet rales, B/P, weight gain
• Monitor for retinal degeneration: periodic eye exam

Associated nursing diagnoses

✓ Injury, potential for physical (side effects)
✓ Knowledge deficit (teaching)
✓ Noncompliance (teaching)

Implementation

PO route
• PO: give last dose at hs
Trans route
• Apply patch weekly; remove old patch and wash off residue; aply to site without hair; best absorption over chest or upper arm; rotate sites with each application; clean site before application; apply firmly, especially around edges
• Store patches in cool environment, tabs in tight container

Patient/family education

• Instruct patient not to discontinue drug abruptly, or withdrawal symptoms may occur: anxiety, increased B/P, headache, insomnia, increased pulse, tremors, nausea, sweating
• Caution patient not to use OTC (cough, cold, or allergy) products unless directed by prescriber
• Caution patient to avoid sunlight or wear sunscreen, protective clothing if in sunlight; photosensitivity may occur
• Teach patient to comply with dosage schedule even if feeling better; drug controls symptoms, does not cure
• Caution patient to change position slowly, to rise slowly to sitting or standing position to minimize orthostatic hypotension, especially elderly [G]
• Instruct patient to notify physician of mouth sores, sore throat, fever, swelling of hands or feet, irregular heartbeat, chest pain, signs of angioedema, increased weight
• Teach patient about excessive perspiration, dehydration, vomiting; diarrhea may lead to fall in B/P; consult prescriber if these occur
• Tell patient that drug may cause dizziness, fainting; lightheadedness may occur during 1st few days of therapy; use

hard candy, saliva product, or frequent rinsing of mouth for dry mouth

- Advise patient that compliance is necessary; not to skip or stop drug unless directed by prescriber
- Teach patient that drug may cause skin rash or impaired perspiration
- Teach patient that response may take 2-3 days if drug is given trans; instruct on administration of patch; return demonstration
- Teach patient to avoid hazardous activities, since drug may cause drowsiness, dizziness
- Teach patient to administer 1 hr ac

Evaluation

Positive therapeutic outcome

- Decrease in B/P in hypertension
- Decrease in withdrawal symptoms
- Decrease in vascular headaches
- Decrease in dysmenorrhea
- Decrease in menopausal symptoms

Treatment of overdose: Supportive treatment; administer tolazoline, atropine, dopamine prn

clorazepate

(klor-az'e-pate)

clorazepate dipotassium, Gen-Xene, Tranxene, Tranxene-SD, Tranxene-SD Half Strength

Func. class.: Antianxiety

Chem. class.: Benzodiazepine

Pregnancy category **D**

Controlled substance schedule **IV**

Action: Potentiates the actions of GABA, especially in limbic system, reticular formation has anticonvulsant effects

Therapeutic Outcome: Decreased anxiety, restlessness, insomnia

Uses: Anxiety, acute alcohol withdrawal, adjunct in seizure disorders

Dosage and routes

Anxiety

Adult: PO 15-60 mg/day

Alcohol withdrawal

Adult: PO 30 mg then day 1, 30-60 mg in divided doses; day 2, 45-90 mg in divided doses; day 3, 22.5-45 mg in divided doses; day 4, 15-30 mg in divided doses; then reduce daily dose to 7.5-15 mg

Seizure disorders

P *Adult and child >12 yr:* PO 7.5 mg tid; may increase by 7.5 mg/wk or less, not to exceed 90 mg/day

P Child 9-12 yr:
PO 7.5 mg bid; may increase by 7.5 mg/wk or less, not to exceed 60 mg/day

Available forms: Caps 3.75, 7.5, 15 mg; tabs 3.75, 7.5, 15 mg; single-dose tab 11.25, 22.5 mg

Side effects/adverse reactions

CNS: Dizziness, drowsiness, confusion, headache, anxiety, tremors, stimulation, fatigue, depression, insomnia, hallucinations, lethargy
CV: Orthostatic hypotension, ***ECG changes, tachycardia,*** hypotension
EENT: Blurred vision, tinnitus, mydriasis
GI: Constipation, dry mouth, nausea, vomiting, anorexia, diarrhea
INTEG: Rash, dermatitis, itching

Contraindications: Hypersensitivity to benzodiazepines, narrow angle glaucoma, psychosis, pregnancy **D**, P child <18 yr

G **Precautions:** Elderly, debilitated, hepatic disease, renal disease

Pharmacokinetics

Absorption	Well absorbed
Distribution	Widely distributed; crosses placenta
Metabolism	Liver
Excretion	Kidneys, breast milk
Half-life	30-100 hr

Pharmacodynamics

	PO
Onset	15 min
Peak	1-2 hr
Duration	4-6 hr

Interactions

Drug/drug:

Individual drugs
Alcohol: ↑ effects of clorazepate
Cimetidine: ↑ effects of clorazepate
Disulfiram: ↑ effects of clorazepate
Valproic acid: ↓ effects of clorazepate
Drug classifications
CNS depressants: ↑ effects of clorazepate
MAOI: ↑ effects of clorazepate
Oral contraceptives: ↑ effects of clorazepate

Lab test interferences

Increase: AST (SGOT)/ALT (SGPT), serum bilirubin
Decrease: RAIU
False increase: 17-OHCS

NURSING CONSIDERATIONS

Assessment

- Monitor B/P (with patient lying, standing), pulse; if systolic B/P drops 20 mm Hg, hold drug, notify prescriber
- Monitor blood studies: CBC during long-term therapy; blood dyscrasias have occurred rarely
- Monitor hepatic studies: AST (SGOT), ALT (SGPT), bilirubin, creatinine, LDH, alkaline phosphatase
- Monitor I&O; may indicate renal dysfunction

- Monitor mental status: mood, sensorium, affect, sleeping pattern, drowsiness, dizziness, physical dependency; withdrawal symptoms: headache, nausea, vomiting, muscle pain, weakness after long-term use; suicidal tendencies

Associated nursing diagnoses

- ✓ Coping, ineffective individual (uses)
- ✓ Knowledge deficit (teaching)
- ✓ Noncompliance (teaching)

Implementation

PO route

- Give with food or milk for GI symptoms
- Use sugarless gum, hard candy, frequent sips of water for dry mouth
- Check to see PO medication has been swallowed

Patient/family education

- Teach patient that drug may be taken with food
- Teach patient not to use for everyday stress or longer than 4 mo, unless directed by a prescriber; not to take more than prescribed amount; may be habit forming
- Caution patient to avoid OTC preparations unless approved by a prescriber
- Caution patient to avoid driving, activities that require alertness; drowsiness may occur, especially in elderly
- Advise patient to avoid alcohol ingestion or other psychotropic medications, unless prescribed
- Advise patient not to discontinue medication abruptly after long-term use
- Advise patient to rise slowly or fainting may occur
- Teach patient that drowsiness may worsen at beginning of treatment

Evaluation

Positive therapeutic outcome

- Decreased anxiety, restlessness
- Decreased seizure activity

Treatment of overdose: Lavage, VS, supportive care, flumazenil

clotrimazole

(kloe-trim'a-zole)

Canesten ✤, Clotimaderm ✤, FemCare, Gyne-Lotrimin, Lotrimin, Lotrimin AF, Mycelex, Mycelex OTC, Mycelex-G, Mycelex-7, Mycelex Troches, Mycelex Twin Pack, Myclo ✤, Neozol ✤

Func. class.: Local antiinfective

Chem. class.: Imidazole derivative

Pregnancy category **B**

Action: Interferes with fungal DNA replication; binds sterols in fungal cell membrane, which increases permeability, leaking of cell nutrients; fungicidal

Therapeutic Outcome: Fungistatic/fungicidal against susceptible organisms: *Candida,* tinea pedis, tinea cruris, tinea corporis, tinea versicolor

Uses: Tinea pedis, tinea cruris, tinea corporis, tinea versicolor, *C. albicans* infection of the vagina, vulva, throat, mouth

Dosage and routes

P ***Adult and child:*** Top rub into affected area bid × 1-4 wk; loz dissolve in mouth 5 times/day × 2 wk; intravag 1 applicator/1 tab × 1-2 wk hs; oral troches 10 mg 5 times/day × 14 days

Available forms: Cream 1%; sol 1%; lotion 1%; vag tabs 100, 500 mg; vag cream 1%; troches 10 mg

Side effects/adverse reactions

INTEG: Rash, urticaria, stinging, burning, peeling, blistering, skin fissures
OTHER: Abdominal cramps, bloating, urinary frequency, dyspareunia

Contraindications: Hypersensitivity

Precautions: Pregnancy **B**, lactation

Pharmacokinetics	
Absorption	Minimal
Distribution	Unknown
Metabolism	Liver
Excretion	Feces, kidneys
Half-life	Unknown

Pharmacodynamics	
Onset	Unknown
Peak	Unknown
Duration	Unknown

Interactions: None

NURSING CONSIDERATIONS

Assessment

- Monitor for allergic reaction: burning, stinging, itching, discharge, soreness
- Assess skin for fungal infections: peeling, dryness, itching before and throughout treatment
- Monitor for allergic reaction: dermatitis, rash; drug should be discontinued, antihistamines (mild reaction)

Associated nursing diagnoses

- ✓ Skin integrity, impaired (uses)
- ✓ Infection, risk (uses)
- ✓ Knowledge deficit (teaching)

Implementation

Top route

- Administer 1 applicatorful every night high into the vagina
- Apply to affected, surrounding area; do not cover with occlusive dressings
- Store below 30° C (86° F)

Patient/family education

- Teach patient proper hygiene: hand-washing technique, nail care, use of concomitant top agents if prescribed
- Advise patient to wear cotton clothing; to use clean towel, dry well; to avoid contact of affected areas with mucous membranes; to avoid covering affected areas unless directed to by prescriber
- Instruct patient to report excessive itching, burning
- Teach patient how to apply: massage cream into affected area and surrounding skin in AM, PM; effects observed within

1 wk, continue 1-2 wk after symptoms decrease; wash hands after application

- Teach patient to apply with applicator only; to avoid use of any other vaginal product unless directed by prescriber; sanitary napkin may prevent soiling of undergarments
- Advise patient to abstain from sexual intercourse until treatment is completed; reinfection and irritation may occur
- Instruct patient to notify prescriber if symptoms persist

Evaluation

Positive therapeutic outcome

- Decrease in size, number of lesions
- Decrease in itching or white patches around vulva

cloxacillin

(klox-a-sill'in)

Apo Cloxi ✤, Bactopen ✤, cloxacillin sodium, Cloxapen, Novocloxin ✤, Orbenin ✤, Tegopen

Func. class.: Broad-spectrum antibiotic

Chem. class.: Penicillinase-resistant penicillin

Pregnancy category **B**

Action: Interferes with cell wall replication of susceptible organisms; the cell wall, rendered osmotically unstable, swells, bursts from osmotic pressure

Uses: Penicillinase-producing staphylococci, streptococci; respiratory tract, skin, skin structure infections; sinusitis

Therapeutic Outcome: Bactericidal effects for the following: gram-positive cocci *Staphylococcus aureus, S. epidermis, penicillinase-producing staphylococci*

Dosage and routes

Adult: PO 1-4 g/day in divided doses q6h or 250 mg-1 g q6h

P *Child:* PO 50-100 mg/kg in divided doses q6h

Available forms: Caps 250, 500 mg; powder for oral susp 125 mg/5 ml

Side effects/adverse reactions

CNS: Lethargy, hallucinations, anxiety, depression, muscle twitching, ***coma, convulsions***

GI: Nausea, vomiting, diarrhea, increased AST (SGOT), ALT (SGPT), abdominal pain, glossitis, ***pseudomembranous*** colitis

GU: Oliguria, proteinuria, hematuria, *vaginitis, moniliasis,* ***glomerulonephritis***

HEMA: Anemia, increased bleeding time, ***bone marrow depression, granulocytopenia***

SYST: Anaphylaxis

Contraindications: Hypersensitivity to penicillins; P neonates

Precautions: Pregnancy **B**, hypersensitivity to cephalosporins

Pharmacokinetics

Absorption	Moderate (35%-60%)
Distribution	Widely distributed; crosses placenta
Metabolism	Liver (up to 22%)
Excretion	Breast milk; kidneys, unchanged (30%-45%)
Half-life	0.5-1.1 hr, increased in hepatic/renal disease

Pharmacodynamics

	PO
Onset	½ hr
Peak	½-2 hr

Interactions

Drug/drug:

Individual drugs

Probenecid: ↑ cloxacillin levels, ↓ renal excretion

Drug classifications

Oral anticoagulants: ↑ anticoagulant effects

Drug/food:

Food, carbonated drinks, citrus fruit juices: ↓ absorption

Lab test interferences

False positive: Urine glucose, urine protein

NURSING CONSIDERATIONS

Assessment

- Assess patient for previous sensitivity reaction to penicillins or other cephalosporins; cross-sensitivity between penicillins and cephalosporins is common
- Assess patient for signs and symptoms of infection including characteristics of wounds, sputum, urine, stool, WBC >10,000, fever; obtain baseline information and during treatment
- Obtain C&S before beginning drug therapy to identify if correct treatment has been initiated
- Assess for allergic reactions: rash, urticaria, pruritus, chills, fever, joint pain may occur a few days after therapy begins; epinephrine and resuscitation equipment should be available for anaphylactic reaction
- Identify urine output; if decreasing, notify prescriber (may indicate nephrotoxicity); also check for increased BUN, creatinine
- Monitor blood studies: AST (SGOT), ALT (SGPT), CBC, Hct, bilirubin, LDH, alkaline phosphatase, Coombs' test monthly if patient is on long-term therapy
- Monitor electrolytes: potassium, sodium, chloride monthly if patient is on long-term therapy
- Assess bowel pattern qd; if severe diarrhea occurs, drug should be discontinued; may indicate pseudomembranous colitis
- Monitor for bleeding: ecchymosis, bleeding gums, hematuria, stool guaiac daily if on long-term therapy
- Assess for overgrowth of infection: perineal itching, fever, malaise, redness, pain, swelling, drainage, rash, diarrhea, change in cough, sputum

Associated nursing diagnoses

- ✓ Infection, risk for (uses)
- ✓ Diarrhea (side effects)
- ✓ Injury, risk for (side effects)

✓ Knowledge deficit (teaching)
✓ Noncompliance (teaching)

Implementation

PO route

- Give in even doses around the clock; if GI upset occurs, give with food; drug must be given for 10-14 days to ensure organism death and prevent superinfection; store in airtight container
- Shake susp; store in refrigerator for 2 wk, 1 wk at room temp

Patient/family education

- Teach patient to report sore throat, bruising, bleeding, joint pain; may indicate blood dyscrasis (rare)
- Advise patient to contact prescriber if vaginal itching, loose, foul-smelling stools, furry tongue occur; may indicate superinfection
- Instruct patient to take all medications prescribed for the length of time ordered
- Advise patient to notify prescriber of diarrhea with blood or pus, which may indicate pseudomembranous colitis

Evaluation

Positive therapeutic outcome

- Absence of signs/symptoms of infection (WBC <10,000, temp WNL, absence of red draining wounds)
- Reported improvement in symptoms of infection

Treatment of anaphylaxis: Withdraw drug, maintain airway, administer epinephrine, aminophylline, O_2, **IV** corticosteroids

clozapine

(kloe'za-peen)

Clozaril

Func. class.: Antipsychotic
Chem. class.: Tricyclic dibenzodiazepine derivative

Pregnancy category B

C

Action: Interferes with dopamine receptor binding with lack of extrapyramidal symptoms and tardive dyskinesia; also acts as an adrenergic, cholinergic, histaminergic, serotonergic antagonist

➔ **Therapeutic Outcome:** Decreased psychotic behavior

Uses: Management of psychotic symptoms in schizophrenic patients for whom other antipsychotics have failed

Dosage and routes

Adult: PO 25 mg qd or bid; may increase by 25-50 mg/day; normal range 300-450 mg/day after 2 wk; do not increase dosage more than 2 times/wk; do not exceed 900 mg/day; use lowest dosage to control symptoms

Available forms: Tabs 25, 100 mg

Side effects/adverse reactions

CNS: Sedation, salivation, dizziness, headache, tremors, sleep problems, akinesia, fever, ***seizures,*** *sweating, akathisia, confusion, fatigue, insomnia, depression, slurred speech,*

*anxiety, **neuroleptic malignant syndrome***
CV: Tachycardia, hypotension, hypertension, chest pain, ECG changes
GI: Drooling or excessive salivation, constipation, nausea, abdominal discomfort, vomiting, diarrhea, anorexia
GU: Urinary abnormalities, incontinence, ejaculation dysfunction, frequency, urgency, retention
HEMA: Leukopenia, neutropenia, agranulocytosis, eosinophilia
MS: Weakness; pain in back, neck, legs; spasm
RESP: Dyspnea, nasal congestion, throat discomfort

Contraindications: Hypersensitivity, myeloproliferative disorders, severe granulocytopenia, CNS depression, coma, narrow angle glaucoma

Precautions: Pregnancy **B**, P lactation, children <16, hepatic, renal, cardiac disease, seizures, prostatic enlargement, G elderly

Pharmacokinetics

Absorption	Well absorbed
Distribution	Widely distributed; crosses blood-brain barrier, placenta; 95% bound to plasma proteins
Metabolism	Liver
Excretion	Kidneys, feces (metabolites)
Half-life	8-12 hr

Pharmacodynamics

	PO
Onset	Unknown
Peak	Steady state 2½ hr
Duration	4-12 hr

Interactions
Drug/drug:
Individual drugs
Alcohol: ↑ effects of both drugs, oversedation
Digoxin: ↑ plasma concentration of digoxin
Warfarin: ↑ plasma concentrations
Drug classifications
Antacids: ↓ absorption
Anticholinergics: ↑ anticholinergic effects
Antidepressants: ↑ CNS depression
Antihistamines: ↑ CNS depression
Antihypertensives: ↑ hypotension
Antineoplastics: ↑ bone marrow suppression

Lab test interferences
Increase: Liver function tests, cardiac enzymes, cholesterol, blood glucose, prolactin, bilirubin, PBI, cholinesterase, ^{131}I
False positive: Pregnancy tests, PKU
False negative: Urinary steroids, 17-OHCS

NURSING CONSIDERATIONS
Assessment
- Assess mental status: orientation, mood, behavior, presence of hallucinations, and type before initial administration and monthly; this drug should significantly reduce psychotic behavior
- Check for swallowing of PO medication; check for hoarding or giving of medication to other patients
- Monitor I&O ratio, palpate bladder if low urinary output G occurs, especially in elderly;

urinalysis recommended before, during prolonged therapy
• Monitor bilirubin, CBC, liver function studies monthly
• Assess affect, orientation, LOC, reflexes, gait, coordination, sleep pattern disturbances
• Monitor B/P with patient sitting, standing, and lying; take pulse and respirations q4h during initial treatment; establish baseline before starting treatment; report drops of 30 mm Hg
• Check for dizziness, faintness, palpitations, tachycardia on rising
• Identify for neuroleptic malignant syndrome: hyperpyrexia, muscle rigidity, increased CPK, altered mental status; drug should be discontinued
• Assess for extrapyramidal symptoms including akathisia (inability to sit still, no pattern to movements), tardive dyskinesia (bizarre movements of the jaw, mouth, tongue, extremities), pseudoparkinsonism (rigidity, tremors, pill rolling, shuffling gate)
• Assess for constipation, urinary retention daily; if these occur, increase bulk, water in diet

Associated nursing diagnoses

✓ Thought processes, altered (uses)
✓ Coping, ineffective individual (uses)
✓ Knowledge deficit (teaching)
✓ Noncompliance (teaching)

Implementation

PO route

G • Decrease dosage in elderly since metabolism is slowed
• Give with full glass of water, milk; or give with food to decrease GI upset
• Store in tight, light-resistant container; oral sol in amber bottle

C

Patient/family education

• Teach patient to use good oral hygiene; frequent rinsing of mouth, sugarless gum for dry mouth
• Caution patient to avoid hazardous activities until drug response is determined
• Inform patient that orthostatic hypotension occurs often and to rise from sitting or lying position gradually
• Caution patient to avoid hot tubs, hot showers, tub baths, since hypotension may occur
• Teach patient to avoid OTC preparations (cough, hay fever, cold) unless approved by prescriber, since serious drug interactions may occur; avoid use with alcohol, CNS depressants; increased drowsiness may occur
• Teach patient about extrapyramidal symptoms and necessity of meticulous oral hygiene, since oral candidiasis may occur
• Teach patient to report sore throat, malaise, fever, bleeding, mouth sores; if these occur, CBC should be drawn and drug discontinued
• Advise patient that in hot weather, heat stroke may occur; take extra precautions to stay cool

Evaluation

Positive therapeutic outcome
• Decrease in emotional excitement, hallucinations, delusions, paranoia

• Reorganization of patterns of thought, speech

Treatment of anaphylaxis: Withdraw drug, maintain airway

codeine 🔑
(koe'deen)
Paveral ✤, Codeine
Narcotic analgesics
Func. class.: Opiate, phenanthrene derivative
Pregnancy category C
Controlled substance schedule II, III, IV, V (depends on route)

Action: Depresses pain impulse transmission at the spinal cord level by interacting with opioid receptors

➔ **Therapeutic Outcome:** Pain relief, decreased cough, decreased diarrhea depending on route

Uses: Moderate to severe pain, nonproductive cough

Investigational uses: Diarrhea

Dosage and routes

Pain

Adult: PO 15-60 mg q4h prn; IM/SC 15-60 mg q4h prn

P *Child:* PO 3 mg/kg/day in divided doses q4h prn

Cough

Adult: PO 10-20 mg q4-6h, not to exceed 120 mg/day

P *Child:* PO 1-1.5 mg/kg/day in 4 divided doses, not to exceed 60 mg/day

Diarrhea

Adult: PO 30 mg; may repeat qid prn

Available forms: Inj 15, 30, 60 mg/ml; tabs 15, 30, 60 mg; oral sol 10mg/5 ml ✤, 15 mg/5 ml

Side effects/adverse reactions

CNS: Drowsiness, sedation, dizziness, agitation, dependency, lethargy, restlessness
CV: Bradycardia, palpitations, orthostatic hypotension, tachycardia
GI: Nausea, vomiting, anorexia, constipation
GU: Urinary retention
INTEG: Flushing, rash, urticaria
RESP: Respiratory depression, respiratory paralysis

Contraindications: Hypersensitivity to opiates, respiratory depression, increased intracranial pressure, seizure disorders, severe respiratory disorders

G **Precautions:** Elderly, cardiac dysrhythmias, pregnancy **C**

Pharmacokinetics

Absorption	Complete (IM)
Distribution	Widely distributed; crosses placenta
Metabolism	Liver, extensively
Excretion	Kidneys (up to 15%), breast milk
Half-life	2½-4 hr

Pharmacodynamics

	PO	IM	SC
Onset	30-45 min	15-30 min	15-30 min
Peak	1-2 hr	30-60 min	Unknown
Duration	4 hr	4 hr	4 hr

Interactions

Drug/drug:

Individual drugs

Alcohol: ↑ respiratory depression, hypotension, ↑ sedation
Nalbuphine: ↓ analgesia
Pentazocine: ↓ analgesia

Drug classifications

Antihistamines: ↑ respiratory depression, hypotension
CNS depressants: ↑ respiratory depression, hypotension
MAOI: Use with caution
Phenothiazines: ↑ respiratory depression, hypotension
Sedative/hypnotics: ↑ respiratory depression, hypotension

Lab test interferences

Increase: Amylase, lipase

NURSING CONSIDERATIONS

Assessment

- Assess pain: intensity, type, aleviating factors
- Monitor VS after parenteral route; note muscle rigidity, drug history, liver, kidney function tests, respiratory dysfunction: respiratory depression, character, rate, rhythm; notify prescriber if respirations are <10/min
- Monitor CNS changes: dizziness, drowsiness, hallucinations, euphoria, LOC, pupil reaction
- Monitor allergic reactions: rash, urticaria

Associated nursing diagnoses

- ✓ Pain (uses)
- ✓ Sensory perceptual alteration: visual, auditory (adverse reactions)
- ✓ Breathing pattern, ineffective (adverse reactions)
- ✓ Knowledge deficit (teaching)

Implementation

- Give with antiemetic if nausea, vomiting occur
- Administer when pain is beginning to return, determine dosage interval by patient response; continuous dosing of medication is more effective given prn; explain analgesic effect
- Medication should be slowly withdrawn after long-term use to prevent withdrawal symptoms
- Store in light-resistant container at room temp

PO route

- May be given with food or milk to lessen GI upset

IM/SC route

- Do not give if cloudy, or a precipitate has formed

Syringe compatibilities:

Glycopyrrolate, hydroxyzine

Additive incompatibilities:

Aminophylline, amobarbital, chlorothiazide, heparin, methicillin, pentobarbital, phenobarbital, phenytoin, secobarbital, thiopental

Patient/family education

- Teach patient to report any symptoms of CNS changes, allergic reactions; to avoid CNS depressants: alcohol,

C

sedative/hypnotics for at least 24 hr after taking this drug
- Discuss with patient that dizziness, drowsiness, and confusion are common, to avoid getting up without assistance
- Discuss in detail all aspects of the drug

Evaluation

Positive therapeutic outcome
- Decreased pain
- Decreased cough

Treatment of overdose: Narcan 0.2-0.8 **IV**, O_2, **IV** fluids, vasopressors

colchicine

(kol'chi-seen)
Func. class.: Antigout agent
Chem. class.: Colchicum autumnale alkaloid
Pregnancy category **C**

Action: Inhibits microtubule formation of lactic acid in leukocytes, which decreases phagocytosis and inflammation in joints

Therapeutic Outcome: Decreased pain, inflammation of joints

Uses: Gout, gouty arthritis (prevention, treatment); to arrest progression of neurologic disability in multiple sclerosis

Dosage and routes

Prevention

Adult: PO 0.5-1.8 mg qd depending on severity; **IV** 0.5-1 mg qd-bid

Treatment

Adult: PO 0.5-1.2 mg, then 0.5-1.2 mg q1h, until pain decreases or side effects occur; **IV** 2 mg, then 0.5 mg q6h, not to exceed 4 mg/24 hr

Available forms: Tabs 0.5, 0.6 mg; inj **IV** 1 mg/2 ml

Side effects/adverse reactions

GI: Nausea, vomiting, anorexia, malaise, metallic taste, cramps, peptic ulcer, diarrhea
GU: Hematuria, oliguria, renal damage
HEMA: Agranulocytosis, thrombocytopenia, aplastic anemia, pancytopenia
INTEG: Chills, dermatitis, pruritus, purpura, erythema
MISC: Myopathy, alopecia, reversible azoospermia, peripheral neuritis

Contraindications: Hypersensitivity; serious GI, renal, hepatic, cardiac disorders; blood dyscrasias

Precautions: Severe renal disease, blood dyscrasias, pregnancy **C**, hepatic disease, G elderly, lactation, P children

Pharmacokinetics

Absorption	Well absorbed
Distribution	WBCs
Metabolism	Deacetylates in liver
Excretion	Feces (metabolites/active drug)
Half-life	20 min

Pharmacodynamics

	PO
Onset	Unknown
Peak	½-2 hr
Duration	Unknown

Interactions

Drug/drug:

Individual drugs

Vitamin B_{12}: ↓ action of vitamin B_{12}

Drug classifications

Acidifiers: ↓ action of colchicine

Alkalinizers: ↑ action of colchicine

CNS depressants: ↑ action of CNS depressants

Sympathomimetics: ↑ action of sympathomimetics

Lab test interferences

Increase: Alkaline phosphatase, AST (SGOT)/ALT (SGPT)

False positive: RBC, Hgb

NURSING CONSIDERATIONS

Assessment

- Assess pain and mobility of joints
- Monitor I&O ratio; observe for decrease in urinary output; CBC, platelets, reticulocytes before, during therapy (q 3 mo): Coombs' test to determine Coomb's negative hemolytic anemia

Associated nursing diagnoses

✓ Pain, chronic (uses)
✓ Immobility, impaired (uses)
✓ Knowledge deficit (teaching)

C

Implementation

PO route

- Give on empty stomach (1 hr ac or 2 hr pc) for better absorption

IV **IV route**

- Give **IV** undiluted or diluted 1 mg/10-20 ml normal saline or sterile water for inj; give over 2-5 min

Patient/family education

- Teach patient to increase fluids to 3-4 L/day
- Caution patient to avoid alcohol, OTC preparations that contain alcohol; skin rashes have occurred
- Instruct patient to report any pain, redness, or hard area, usually in legs
- Teach patient importance of complying with medical regimen; bone marrow depression may occur

Evaluation

Positive therapeutic outcome

- Decreased stone formation on x-ray
- Decreased pain in kidney region
- Absence of hematuria
- Decreased pain in joints

colestipol
(koe-les'ti-pole)
Colestid
Func. class.: Antilipemic
Chem. class.: Bile sequestrant, resin exchange agent
Pregnancy category B

Action: Absorbs, combines with bile acids to form an insoluble complex that is excreted through feces; loss of bile acids lowers cholesterol levels

Therapeutic Outcome: Decreasing cholesterol levels and low-density lipoproteins, decreased pruritus

Uses: Primary hypercholesterolemia, xanthomas, digitalis toxicity, pruritus due to biliary obstruction, diarrhea due to bile acids

Dosage and routes
Adult: PO 15-30 g/day in 2-4 divided doses

Available forms: Granules 5 g packets

Side effects/adverse reactions
GI: Constipation, abdominal pain, nausea, fecal impaction, hemorrhoids, flatulence, vomiting, steatorrhea, peptic ulcer
HEMA: Decreased vitamin A, D, E, K, red folate content; ***hyperchloremic acidosis,*** bleeding, decreased pro-time
INTEG: Rash, irritation of perianal area, tongue, skin

Contraindications: Hypersensitivity, biliary obstruction

Precautions: Pregnancy **B**, P lactation, children , bleeding disorders

Pharmacokinetics

Absorption	Not absorbed
Distribution	Not distributed
Metabolism	Not metabolized
Excretion	Binds with bile acids, feces
Half-life	Unknown

Pharmacodynamics

	PO
Onset	Unknown
Peak	Unknown
Duration	Unknown

Interactions
Drug/drug:
Individual drugs
Acetaminophen: ↓ absorption of acetominophen
Amiodarone: ↓ absorption of amiodarone
Methotrexate: ↓ absorption of methotrexate
Naproxen: ↓ absorption of naproxen
Phenylbutazone: ↓ absorption of phenylbutazone
Piroxicam: ↓ absorption of piroxicam
Propranolol: ↓ absorption of propanolol
Thyroid: ↓ absorption of thyroid
Ursodiol: ↓ absorption of ursodiol

Drug classifications

Anticoagulants, oral: ↓ absorption
Cardiac glycosides: ↓ absorption
Diuretics, thiazide: ↓ absorption
Vitamins A,D,E,K: ↓ absorption

Lab test interferences

Increase: Liver function studies, Cl, PO_4

NURSING CONSIDERATIONS

Assessment

- Assess nutrition: fat, protein, carbohydrates; nutritional analysis should be completed by dietician
- Assess skin integrity after patient has been receiving drug; itching, pruritus often occur from bile deposits on skin
- Monitor cardiac glycoside level, if both drugs are being administered; cardiac glycoside levels will be decreased
- Monitor for signs of vitamin A, D, E, K deficiency; check serum cholesterol, triglyceride levels, electrolytes if on extended therapy
- Monitor bowel pattern daily; increase bulk, water in diet if constipation develops

Associated nursing diagnoses

✓ Constipation (adverse reactions)
✓ Knowledge deficit (teaching)
✓ Noncompliance (teaching)

Implementation

PO route

- Give drug ac, hs; give all other medications 1 hr before or 4 hr after colestipol to avoid poor absorption; give drug mixed with applesauce or stirred into beverage (2-6 oz); do not take dry, let stand for 2 min
- Provide supplemental doses of vitamins A, D, E, K, if levels are low

Patient/family education

- Teach patient symptoms of hypoprothrombinemia: bleeding mucous membranes, dark tarry stools, hematuria, petechiae; report immediately
- Teach patient importance of compliance, since toxicity may result if doses are missed; not to discontinue suddenly
- Teach patient that risk factors should be decreased: high-fat diet, smoking, alcohol consumption, absence of exercise
- Tell patient to mix drug with 6 oz of milk, water, fruit juice; may be mixed with carbonated beverages; rinse glass to make sure all medication is taken or may mix drug in applesauce; allow to stand for 2 min before mixing

Evaluation

Positive therapeutic outcome

- Decreased cholesterol level (hyperlipidemia)
- Decreased diarrhea, pruritus (excess bile acids)

colfosceril
(kohl-foss'sir-ill)
Exosurf Neonatal
Func. class.: Synthetic lung surfactant
Chem. class.: Dipalmitoylphosphatidylcholine (DPPC)
Pregnancy category **N/A**

Action: Surfactant maintains lung inflation and prevents collapse by lowering surface tension

➡ **Therapeutic Outcome:** Ability to breathe without assistance

Uses: Treatment of respiratory distress syndrome (RDS) in premature infants

Dosage and routes
Prophylactic treatment
Endotracheally: 5 ml/kg as soon as possible after birth and repeat doses 12 and 24 hr later P to infants remaining on mechanical ventilation

Rescue treatment
Endotracheally: Administer in two half doses of 5 ml/kg doses; give initial dose after treatment of RDS, then second dose in 12 hr

Available forms: 10 ml/vial with sterile water for inj and 5 endotracheal tube adapters

Side effects/adverse reactions
RESP: Apnea, pulmonary hemorrhage, pulmonary air leak, congenital pneumonia
SYST: Nonpulmonary fatal infections

Precautions: Congenital anomalies, prophylactic treatment

Pharmacokinetics

Absorption	Unknown
Distribution	All lobes, alveolar spaces, distal airways
Metabolism	90% of alveolar phospholipids are recycled
Excretion	Unknown
Half-life	Alveolar-12 hr

Pharmacodynamics

Onset	Immediate
Peak	Unknown
Duration	12 hr

Interactions: None

NURSING CONSIDERATIONS
Assessment
- Assess respiratory rate, rhythm, character; chest expansion, color, transcutaneous saturation, ABGs
- Monitor endotracheal tube placement before dosing; for apnea after endotracheal administration
- Check for reflux of drug into the endotracheal tube during administration; stop drug administration if this occurs, and, if needed, increase peak inspiratory pressure on the ventilator by 4-5 cm H_2O until tube is cleared

Associated nursing diagnoses
✓ Impaired gas exchange (uses)
✓ Breathing patterns ineffective (uses)

Implementation

Endo route

- P • Infants should be suctioned before administration
- P • Give after selecting an adapter size that corresponds to the diameter of the endotracheal tube, insert the adapter into the tube by twisting, connect the breathing circuit to the adapter, remove the cap from the adapter sideport, and attach the syringe to the sideport; after dose is completed, remove the syringe and recap the sideport
- P • Administer after reconstituting each vial with 8 ml preservative-free sterile water for inj, fill a 10-12 ml syringe with 8 ml preservative-free sterile water for inj, using an 18-19 G needle; allow the vacuum in the vial to draw the liquid into the vial; aspirate the 8 ml out of the vial into the syringe while maintaining the vacuum and then release the syringe plunger; repeat the aspiration and release until adequately mixed; draw the dose required into the syringe from below the froth in the vial; do not use if large particles are present
- Administer by endotracheal administration only by persons P trained in neonatal intubation and ventilation
- P • Provide reduction in peak ventilator inspiratory pressures immediately if chest expansion improves substantially after dose
- Provide reduction in FIO_2 in small, repeated steps when P infant becomes pink and transcutaneous oxygen saturation is in excess of 95%; oxygen saturation should remain between 90% and 95%
- Perform suctioning of all P infants before administration to prevent mucous plugging; if endotracheal tube obstruction is suspected, remove the obstruction and replace tube immediately
- Store at room temp in dry place

Evaluation

Positive therapeutic outcome

- Decreased respiratory distress

C

corticotropin

(kor-ti-koe-troe'pin)

ACTH, Acthar, corticotropin, ACTH-40, ACTH-80, Duracton ✦, H.P. Acthar Gel

Func. class.: Pituitary hormone

Chem. class.: Adrenocorticotropic hormone

Pregnancy category **C**

Action: Stimulates adrenal cortex to produce, secrete corticosterone, cortisol; suppresses adrenal function (chronic use); potent mineralocorticoid

➔ **Therapeutic Outcome:** Increased production of adrenal steroids in adrenal insufficiency

Uses: Testing adrenocortical function, treatment of adrenal insufficiency caused by administration of corticosteroids (long term), multiple sclerosis

Dosage and routes

Testing of adrenocortical function

Adult: IM/SC up to 80 U in divided doses; **IV** 10-25 U in 500 ml D_5W given over 8 hr

Inflammation

Adult: SC/IM 40 U in 4 divided doses (aqueous) or 40 U q12-24h (gel/repository form)

Available forms: Inj 25, 40 U/vial; repository inj IM, SC 40, 80/ml

Side effects/adverse reactions

CNS: ***Convulsions,*** dizziness, euphoria, insomnia, headache, mood swings, behavioral changes, depression, psychosis
EENT: Cataracts, glaucoma
ENDO: Cushingoid symptoms, diabetes mellitus, antibody formation, growth retardation in children, menstrual irregularities
GI: Nausea, vomiting, ***peptic ulcer perforation,*** pancreatitis, distention, ulcerative esophagitis
GU: Water, sodium retention, hypokalemia
INTEG: *Impaired wound healing,* rash, urticaria, hirsutism, petechiae, ecchymoses, sweating, acne, hyperpigmentation
MS: Weakness, osteoporosis, compression fractures, muscle atrophy, steroid myopathy, myalgia, arthralgia

Contraindications: Hypersensitivity, scleroderma, osteoporosis, CHF, peptic ulcer disease, hypertension, systemic fungal infections, smallpox vaccination, recent surgery, ocular herpes simplex, primary adrenocortical insufficiency/hyperfunction

Precautions: Pregnancy **C**, lactation, latent TB, hepatic disease, hypothyroiditis, childbearing-age women, psychiatric diagnosis, myasthenia gravis, acute gouty arthritis

Pharmacokinetics

Absorption	Rapidly absorbed (IM, SC)
Distribution	Widely distributed to tissues
Metabolism	Unknown
Excretion	Unknown
Half-life	<20 min

Pharmacodynamics

	IM (gelatin repository)	IV
Onset	Unknown	Unknown
Peak	3-12 hr	1 hr
Duration	Up to 3 days	Unknown

Interactions

Drug/drug:

Individual drugs

Amphotericin B: ↑ hypokalemia
Insulin: ↑ need for insulin
Mezlocillin: ↑ hypokalemia
Phenobarbital: ↓ effectiveness of corticotropin
Phenytoin: ↓ effectiveness of corticotropin
Piperacillin: ↑ hypokalemia
Rifampin: ↓ effectiveness of corticotropin
Ticarcillin: ↑ hypokalemia

Drug classifications

Diuretics, potassium depleting: ↑ hypokalemia
Live virus vaccines: ↓ antibody reactions
Oral contraceptive: Blocked metabolism of corticotropin

NURSING CONSIDERATIONS

Assessment

- Monitor I&O ratio, weight weekly; report gain over 5 lb/wk
- Obtain 2-hr postprandial chest x-ray, serum potassium, 17-KS, 17-OHCS, cortisol, during long-term treatment
- Assess for dependent edema, moon face, pulmonary edema, cerebral edema; monitor baseline ECG, B/P, chest x-ray, GTT, pulse
- Assess for increased stress in patient's life that may require increased corticosteroids; assess for infection which drug may mask
- Assess for mental status: affect, mood, increased aggressiveness, irritability; a change in mental status may require decreased steroids; changes can be extreme
- P Identify growth rate of child; growth suppression may occur frequently
- Identify hypoadrenalism in P neonates if drug was given during pregnancy
- Identify allergic reaction: rash, urticaria, fever, nausea, vomiting, dyspnea; drug should be discontinued immediately; administer epinephrine 1 : 1000

Associated nursing diagnoses

- ✓ Infection, risk for (adverse reactions)
- ✓ Injury, risk for (adverse reactions)
- ✓ Knowledge deficit (teaching)

Implementation

- Give diet with decreased sodium, increased potassium for dependent edema; increase protein in diet for nitrogen loss before giving; give deep IM using 21 G needle, massage, rotate sites; injection is painful
- Store unused portion in refrigerator; use within 24 hr

IV route

- Give by direct **IV**: give over 2 min; dilute 25 U/1 ml sterile water or normal saline or 40 U/2 ml
- Give by intermittent inf: dilute 10-25 U/500 ml D_5W, 0.9% NaCl, D_5/0.9% NaCl, or LR; give over 8 hr; or 40 U/12-48 hr
- Store unused portion in refrigerator; use within 24 hr

Additive incompatibilities:

Aminophylline, sodium bicarbonate

Additive compatibilities:

Calcium gluconate, chloramphenicol, cytarabine, dimenhydrinate, erythromycin gluceptate, heparin, hydrocortisone sodium succinate, methicillin, norepinephrine, oxytetracycline, penicillin G potassium, potassium chloride, tetracycline, vancomycin

Patient/family education

- Caution patient to avoid vaccinations during drug treatment; tell patient to notify anyone involved in medical or dental care that this drug is being taken
- Teach patient to maintain adequate hydration up to 2 L/day unless contraindicated
- Advise patient to avoid OTC products: salicylates, products with alcohol
- Teach patient not to discontinue medication abruptly; adrenal crisis may occur; drug should be tapered off over several wk; teach patient that drug does not cure condition, only decreases symptoms
- Teach patient to wear Medic Alert ID specifying steroid therapy
- Instruct patient to notify prescriber of infection: increased temp, sore throat, muscular pain

Evaluation

Positive therapeutic outcome
- Absence of inflammation, pain
- Increased muscle strength in multiple sclerosis

cortisone

(kor'ti-sone)
Cortone
Func. class.: Corticosteroid, synthetic
Chem. class.: Short-acting glucocorticoid
Pregnancy category C

Action: Decreases inflammation by suppression of migration of polymorphonuclear leukocytes, fibroblasts, reversal of increased capillary permeability, and lysosomal stabilization; suppresses adrenal function with long-term use

Therapeutic Outcome: Replacement of cortisol in adrenal insufficiency

Uses: Inflammation, severe allergy, adrenal insufficiency, collagen disorders, respiratory and dermatologic disorders

Dosage and routes

Adult: PO/IM 25-300 mg qd or q2 days, titrated to patient response

Available forms: Tabs 5, 10, 25 mg; inj 50 mg/ml

Side effects/adverse reactions

CNS: Depression, flushing, sweating, headache, mood changes
*CV: Hypertension, **circulatory collapse, thrombophlebitis, embolism,*** tachycardia, ***necrotizing angiitis, CHF,*** edema

EENT: Fungal infections, increased intraocular pressure, blurred vision
GI: Diarrhea, nausea, abdominal distention, ***GI hemorrhage,*** increased appetite, ***pancreatitis***
HEMA: ***Thrombocytopenia***
INTEG: Acne, poor wound healing, ecchymosis, bruising, petechiae
MS: Fractures, osteoporosis, weakness

Contraindications: Psychosis, hypersensitivity, idiopathic thrombocytopenia, acute glomerulonephritis, amebiasis, fungal infections, nonasthmatic bronchial disease, P child <2 yr, AIDS, TB

Precautions: Pregnancy **C**, diabetes mellitus, glaucoma, osteoporosis, seizure disorders, ulcerative colitis, CHF, myasthenia gravis, renal disease, esophagitis, peptic ulcer

Pharmacokinetics

Absorption	Slowly IM
Distribution	Widely, crosses placenta
Metabolism	Liver
Excretion	Unknown
Half-life	½ hr

Pharmacodynamics

	PO	IM
Onset	Unknown	Unknown
Peak	2 hr	20-48 hr
Duration	1½ days	1½ days

Interactions
Drug/drug:
Individual drugs
Amphotericin B: ↑ hypokalemia
Insulin: ↑ need for insulin
Mezlocillin: ↑ hypokalemia
Phenobarbital: ↓ effectiveness of cortisone
Phenytoin: ↓ effectiveness of cortisone
Drug classifications
Contraceptives, oral: Blocked metabolism of cortisone

Lab test interferences
Increase: Cholesterol, sodium, blood glucose, uric acid, calcium, urine glucose
Decrease: Calcium, potassium, T_4, T_3, thyroid ^{131}I uptake test, urine 17-OHCS, 17-KS, PBI
False negative: Skin allergy tests

NURSING CONSIDERATIONS
Assessment
- Assess for adrenal insufficiency symptoms: weakness, nausea, vomiting, confusion, anxiety, restlessness, decreased B/P, weight loss; check before and during treatment
- Monitor potassium, blood sugar, urine glucose for patient on long-term therapy; hypokalemia and hyperglycemia can occur
- Check B/P, pulse q4h; notify prescriber if chest pain occurs
- Monitor I&O ratio and weight daily; be alert for decreasing urinary output and increasing edema with bilateral rales, dyspnea, weight gain
- Monitor plasma cortisol levels during long-term therapy (normal level: 138-635 nmol/L if drawn at 8 AM)
- Assess for symptoms of infection: increased temp,

WBC even after withdrawal of medication; drug masks symptoms of infection
- Monitor for potassium depletion: paresthesias, fatigue, nausea, vomiting, depression, polyuria, dysrhythmias, weakness, edema, hypertension, cardiac symptoms, weight daily; notify prescriber of weekly gain >5 lb
- Assess for mental changes: affect, mood, behavioral changes, aggression; depression, psychoses may occur

Associated nursing diagnoses

- ✓ Infection, risk for (adverse reactions)
- ✓ Injury, risk for (adverse reactions)
- ✓ Knowledge deficit (teaching)

Implementation

IM route
- Give after shaking susp (parenteral); titrate dose; use lowest effective dosage
- Give IM inj deep in large muscle mass; rotate sites; avoid deltoid; use a 21 G needle
- Administer in 1 dose in AM to prevent adrenal suppression; avoid SC administration; damage may be done to tissue; do not give **IV**

PO route
- Administer with food or milk to decrease GI symptoms

Patient/family education

- Advise patient that ID as steroid user should be carried at all times
- Instruct patient to notify prescriber if therapeutic response decreases; dosage adjustment may be needed; teach not to discontinue this medication abruptly or adrenal crisis can result; teach all aspects of drug usage, including cushingoid symptoms
- Caution patient to avoid OTC products: salicylates, potassium, alcohol in cough products, cold preparations unless directed by prescriber
- Teach patient symptoms of adrenal insufficiency: nausea, anorexia, fatigue, dizziness, dyspnea, weakness, joint pain, tarry stools, bruising, blurred vision
- Advise patient to avoid persons with known infections; report probable infection rapidly; drug masks infection
- Caution patient that diet modification is necessary if on long-term treatment: increased calcium, potassium, and protein; also low sodium and carbohydrates

Evaluation

Positive therapeutic outcome
- Ease of respirations, decreased inflammation

cosyntropin

(koe-sin-troe'pin)

Cortrosyn, Synacthen, Tetracosactrin

Func. class.: Pituitary hormone

Chem. class.: Synthetic polypeptide

Pregnancy category C

Action: Stimulates adrenal cortex to produce, secrete corticosterone, cortisol; suppresses adrenal function (chronic use); potent mineralocorticoid

Therapeutic Outcome: Increased production of adrenal steroids

Uses: Testing adrenocortical function

Dosage and routes

Adult and child >2 yr: IM/**IV** 0.25-1 mg between blood sampling

Child <2 yr: IM/**IV** 0.125 mg

Available forms: Inj 0.25 mg/vial

Side effects/adverse reactions

INTEG: Rash urticaria, pruritus, flushing
SYST: ***Anaphylaxis***

Contraindications: Hypersensitivity

Precautions: Pregnancy **C**

Pharmacokinetics

Absorption	Rapidly absorbed
Distribution	Widely distributed to tissues
Metabolism	Unknown
Excretion	Unknown
Half-life	15 min

Pharmacodynamics

Onset	5 min
Peak	1 hr
Duration	2-4 hr

Interactions

Drug/drug:

Drug classifications

Estrogens: Blocks metabolism
Glucocorticoids: Altered test results

NURSING CONSIDERATIONS

Assessment

- Identify allergic reaction: rash, urticaria, fever, nausea, vomiting, dyspnea; drug should be discontinued immediately; administer epinephrine 1 : 1000

Associated nursing diagnosis

Knowledge deficit (teaching)

Implementation

- Store at room temp for 24 hr or refrigerate for 3 wk

IV route

Direct IV

- Give after reconstituting 250 μg/1 ml 0.9% NaCl over 2 min

Intermittent inf

Further dilute in D_5W or normal saline; run 40 μg/hr over 4-8 hr as an inf; remains stable for 12 hr at room temp

Patient/family education

- Explain that drug is used for determining type of adrenocortical insufficiency

Evaluation

Positive therapeutic outcome

- Diagnosis of adrenocortical insufficiency (primary, secondary)

cyclobenzaprine
(sye-kloe-ben'za-preen)
cyclobenzaprine HCl, Cycloflex, Flexeril
Func. class.: Skeletal muscle relaxant, central acting
Chem. class.: Tricyclic amine salt
Pregnancy category **B**

Action: Unknown; may be related to antidepressant effects

Therapeutic Outcome: Relaxation of skeletal muscle

Uses: Adjunct for relief of muscle spasm and pain in musculoskeletal conditions

Dosage and routes
Adult: PO 10 mg tid × 1 wk, not to exceed 60 mg/day × 3 wk

Available forms: Tabs 10 mg

Side effects/adverse reactions
CNS: ***Dizziness, weakness, drowsiness,*** headache, tremor, depression, insomnia, confusion, paresthesia
CV: Postural hypotension, tachycardia, dysrhythmias
EENT: Diplopia, temporary loss of vision
GI: ***Nausea,*** vomiting, hiccups, dry mouth
GU: Urinary retention, frequency, change in libido
INTEG: Rash, pruritus, fever, facial flushing, sweating

Contraindications: Acute recovery phase of MI, dysrhythmias, heart block, CHF, P hypersensitivity, child <12 yr, intermittent porphyria, thyroid disease

Precautions: Renal disease, hepatic disease, addictive personality, pregnancy **B**, G elderly

Pharmacokinetics

Distribution	Well
Metabolism	Liver, partially
Excretion	Kidney (unchanged)
Half-life	1-3 days

Pharmacodynamics

	PO
Onset	1 hr
Peak	3-8 hr
Duration	12-24 hr

Interactions
Drug/drug:
Individual drugs
Alcohol: ↑ CNS depression
Drug classifications
Antidepressants, tricyclic: ↑ CNS depression
Antihistamines: ↑ CNS depression
Barbiturates: ↑ CNS depression
MAOI: Do not use within 14 days
Narcotics: ↑ CNS depression
Sedative/hypnotics: ↑ CNS depression

NURSING CONSIDERATIONS
Assessment
- Monitor ECG in epileptic patients; poor seizure control has occurred in patients taking this drug

- Check for allergic reactions: rash, fever, respiratory distress
- Check for severe weakness, numbness, in extremities
- Assess for CNS depression: dizziness, drowsiness, psychiatric symptoms

Associated nursing diagnoses

- ✓ Physical mobility, impaired uses
- ✓ Injury, risk for (adverse reactions)
- ✓ Knowledge deficit (teaching)

Implementation

PO route

- Give with meals for GI symptoms
- Store in airtight container at room temp

Patient/family education

- Teach patient not to discontinue medication quickly; insomnia, nausea, headache, spasticity, tachycardia will occur; drug should be tapered off over 1-2 wk
- Caution patient not to take with alcohol, other CNS depressants
- Advise to avoid altering activities while taking this drug
- Caution patient to avoid hazardous activities if drowsiness/dizziness occurs
- Caution patient to avoid using OTC medication: cough preparations, antihistamines, unless directed by prescriber
- Teach patient to use gum, frequent sips of water for dry mouth

Evaluation

Positive therapeutic outcome

- Decreased pain, spasticity; muscle spasms of acute, painful musculoskeletal conditions are generally short term; long-term therapy is seldom warranted

Treatment of overdose:

Empty stomach with emesis, gastric lavage, then administer activated charcoal; use anticonvulsants if indicated; monitor cardiac function

cyclophosphamide

(sye-kloe-foss'fa-mide)

Cytoxan, Neosar, Procytox ✦

Func. class.: Antineoplastic alkylating agent

Chem. class.: Nitrogen mustard

Pregnancy category **D**

Action: Alkylates DNA, RNA; inhibits enzymes that allow synthesis of amino acids in proteins; is also responsible for cross-linking DNA strands; activity is not cell cycle phase specific

Therapeutic Outcome: Prevention of rapidly growing malignant cells

Uses: Hodgkin's disease, lymphomas, leukemia, multiple myeloma, neuroblastoma, retinoblastoma, Ewing's sarcoma, cancer of female reproductive tract, lung, prostate

Dosage and routes

Adult: PO initially 1-5 mg/kg over 2-5 days; maintenance 1-5 mg/kg; **IV** initially 40-50 mg/kg in divided doses over 2-5 days; maintenance 10-15 mg/kg q7-10 days, or 3-5 mg/kg q3 days

P *Child:* PO/**IV** 2-8 mg/kg or 60-250 mg/m^2 in divided doses × 6 or more days; maintenance **IV** 10-15 mg/kg q7-10 days or 30 mg/kg q3-4 wk; or PO 2-5 mg/kg 2×/wk dose should be reduced by half when bone marrow depression occurs

Available forms: Powder for inj **IV** 100, 200, 500 mg, 1, 2 g; tabs 25, 50 mg

Side effects/adverse reactions

CNS: Headache, dizziness
CV: ***Cardiotoxicity*** (high doses)
ENDO: Syndrome of inappropriate antidiuretic hormone (SIADH)
GI: Nausea, vomiting, diarrhea, weight loss, colitis, ***hepatotoxicity***
GU: ***Hemorrhagic cystitis, hematuria, neoplasms, amenorrhea, azoospermia, sterility, ovarian fibrosis***
HEMA: ***Thrombocytopenia, leukopenia, pancytopenia, myelosuppression***
INTEG: Alopecia, dermatitis
RESP: ***Fibrosis***

Contraindications: Lactation, pregnancy **D**

Precautions: Radiation therapy

Pharmacokinetics

Absorption	Well absorbed (PO)
Distribution	Widely distributed; crosses placenta, blood-brain barrier (50%)
Metabolism	Liver to active drug
Excretion	Kidneys, unchanged (30%)
Half-life	4-6½ hr

Pharmacodynamics

	PO/IV
Onset	Unknown
Peak	Unknown
Duration	Unknown

Interactions

Drug/drug:

Individual drugs
Allopurinol: ↑ bone marrow suppression
Doxorubicin: ↑ cardiotoxicity
Phenobarbital: ↑ toxicity
Radiation: ↑ toxicity, bone marrow suppression
Rifampin: ↑ toxicity, bone marrow suppression
Succinylcholine: ↑ neuromuscular blockade

Drug classifications
Aminoglycosides: ↑ nephrotoxicity
Anticoagulants, oral: ↑ bleeding
Antineoplastics: ↑ toxicity, bone marrow suppression
Bone marrow–suppressing drugs: ↑ bone marrow suppression
Diuretics, loop: ↑ ototoxicity
Live virus vaccines: ↓ antibody reaction

Lab test interferences

Increase: Uric acid
False positive: Pap test

False negative: PPD, mumps trichophytin, *Candida*
Decrease: Pseudocholinesterase

NURSING CONSIDERATIONS

Assessment

- Assess symptoms indicating severe allergic reaction: rash, pruritus, urticaria, purpuric skin lesions, itching, flushing
- Assess for tachypnea, ECG changes, dyspnea, edema, fatigue
- Monitor CBC, differential, platelet count weekly; withhold drug if WBC count is <4000/mm^3 or platelet count is <75,000/mm^3; notify prescriber of results
- Monitor renal function studies: BUN, creatinine, serum uric acid, urine CrCl before and during therapy; I&O ratio; report fall in urine output to <30 ml/hr
- Monitor temp q4h (may indicate beginning of infection)
- Monitor liver function tests before and during therapy (bilirubin, AST [SGOT], ALT [SGPT], LDH) as needed or monthly; note yellowing of skin or sclera, dark urine, clay-colored stools, itchy skin, abdominal pain, fever, diarrhea
- Assess for bleeding: hematuria, stool guaiac, bruising or petechiae, mucosa or orifices q8h
- Identify dyspnea, rales, unproductive cough, chest pain, tachypnea
- Identify effects of alopecia on body image; discuss feelings about body changes
- Identify edema in feet, joint pain, stomach pain, shaking; prescriber should be notified
- Identify inflammation of mucosa, breaks in skin

Associated nursing diagnoses

- ✓ Injury, risk for (adverse reactions)
- ✓ Body image disturbance (adverse reactions)
- ✓ Infection, risk for (adverse reactions)
- ✓ Knowledge deficit (teaching)

Implementation

- Give fluids **IV** or PO before chemotherapy to hydrate patient
- Give antacid before oral agent, pc PM, before hs; antiemetic 30-60 min before giving drug to prevent vomiting, and prn; antibiotics for prophylaxis of infection
- Give top or syst analgesics for pain; give in AM so drug can be eliminated before hs

IV route

- Give **IV** after diluting 100 mg/5 ml of sterile or bacteriostatic water; shake; let stand until clear; may be further diluted in up to 250 ml D_5 0.9% NaCl, D_5/0.9% NaCl, 0.45% NaCl, LR, Ringer's; give 100 mg or less/min through 3-way stopcock of glucose or saline inf

• Use 21, 23, 25 G needle; check site for irritation, phlebitis

Y-site compatibilities:

Amikacin, ampicillin, azlocillin, bleomycin, cefamandole, cefazolin, cefoperazone, ceforanide, cefotaxime, cefoxitin, cefuroxime, cephalothin, cephapirin, chloramphenicol sodium succinate, cisplatin, clindamycin, doxorubicin, doxycycline, droperidol, erythromycin lactobionate, fludarabine, fluorouracil, furosemide, gentamicin, heparin, idarubicin, kanamycin, leucovorin, melphalan, methotrexate, metoclopramide, metronidazole, mezlocillin, mihocycline, mitomycin, moxalactam, nafcillin, ondansetron, oxacillin, paclitaxel, penicillin G potassium, piperacillin, sargramostim, tetracycline, ticarcillin, ticarcillin-clavulanic, tobramycin, trimethoprim-sulfamethoxazole, vancomycin, vinblastine, vincristine, vinorelbine

Syringe compatibilities:

Bleomycin, cisplatin, doxapram, doxorubicin, droperidol, fluorouracil, furosemide, heparin, leucovorin, metoclopramide, methotrexate, mitomycin, mitoxantrone, vinblastine, vincristine

Additive compatibilities:

Cisplatin with etoposide, hydroxyzine, methotrexate, methotrexate with fluorouracil

Solution compatibilities:

Amino acids 4.25%/D_{25}, D_5/0.9% NaCl, D_5W, 0.9% NaCl

Patient/family education

• Teach patient to avoid use of products containing aspirin or ibuprofen, razors, commercial mouthwash, since bleeding may occur; to report symptoms of bleeding (hematuria, tarry stools)
• Instruct patient to report signs of anemia (fatigue, headache, irritability, faintness, shortness of breath)
• Teach patient to report any changes in breathing or coughing even several months after treatment
• Advise patient that hair may be lost during treatment; a wig or hair piece may make patient feel better; new hair may be different in color, texture
• Teach patient not to have any vaccinations without the advice of the prescriber; serious reactions can occur
• Advise patient contraception is needed during treatment and for several months after the completion of therapy

Evaluation

Positive therapeutic outcome
• Prevention of rapid division of malignant cells
• Increased appetite, increased weight

cyclosporine

(sye-kloe-spor'een)
Ciclosporin, Cyclosporin A, Sandimmune
Func. class.: Immunosuppressant
Chem. class.: Fungus-derived peptide
Pregnancy category **C**

Action: Produces immunosuppression by inhibiting T lymphocytes

Therapeutic Outcome: Absence of transplant rejection

Uses: Organ transplants to prevent rejection

Dosage and routes

Adult and child: PO 15 mg/kg several hours before surgery, daily for 2 wk; reduce dosage by 2.5 mg/kg/wk to 5-10 mg/kg/day; **IV** 5-6 mg/kg several hours before surgery; daily, switch to PO form as soon as possible

Available forms: Oral sol 100 mg/ml; inj IV 50 mg/ml

Side effects/adverse reactions

CNS: Tremors, headache
GI: Nausea, vomiting, diarrhea, *oral Candida, gum hyperplasia,* ***hepatotoxicity,*** pancreatitis
GU: Albuminuria, hematuria, proteinuria, renal failure
INTEG: Rash, acne, *hirsutism*

Contraindications: Hypersensitivity

Precautions: Severe renal disease, severe hepatic disease, pregnancy **C**

Pharmacokinetics

Absorption	Poorly absorbed (PO)
Distribution	Crosses placenta
Metabolism	Liver to mercaptopurine
Excretion	Kidney, minimal
Half-life	Biphasic 1.2 hr, 25 hr

Pharmacodynamics

	PO
Onset	Unknown
Peak	4 hr
Duration	Unknown

Interactions

Drug/drug:

Individual drugs
Amphotericin B: ↑ action of cyclosporine
Cimetidine: ↑ action of cyclosporine
Ketoconazole: ↑ action of cyclosporine
Phenytoin: ↓ action of cyclosporine
Ritampin: ↓ action of cyclosporine

NURSING CONSIDERATIONS

Assessment

- Monitor renal studies: BUN, creatinine at least monthly during treatment, 3 mo after treatment
- Monitor liver function studies: alk phosphatase, AST, ALT, bilirubin
- Monitor drug blood levels during treatment
- Assess for hepatotoxicity: dark urine, jaundice, itching,

light-colored stools; drug should be discontinued

Associated nursing diagnoses

- ✓ Mobility, impaired (uses)
- ✓ Infection, risk for (uses)
- ✓ Knowledge deficit (teaching)

Implementation

PO route

- Give with meals for GI upset or drug placed in chocolate milk
- Give with oral antifungal for *Candida* infections

IV **IV route**

- Give IV after diluting each 50 mg/20-100 ml of normal saline or D_5W; run over 2-6 hr; use an infusion pump, glass inf bottles only
- Give for several days before transplant surgery
- Give with corticosteroids

Patient/family education

- Advise patient to report fever, rash, severe diarrhea, chills, sore throat, fatigue, since serious infections may occur; also to report clay-colored stools, cramping (may indicate hepatotoxicity)
- Caution patient to use contraceptive measures during treatment and for 12 wk after ending therapy; drug is teratogenic
- Caution patient to avoid crowds and persons with known infections to reduce risk of infection

Evaluation

Positive therapeutic outcome

- Absence of graft rejection

cyproheptadine

(si-proe-hep'ta-deen)
cyproheptadine HCl,
Periactin, Vimicon ✦
Func. class.: Antihistamine, H_1-receptor antagonist
Chem. class.: Piperidine
Pregnancy category **B**

Action: Acts on blood vessels, GI, respiratory system by competing with histamine for H_1-receptor site; decreases allergic response by blocking histamine; blocks serotonin to increase appetite and relieve vascular headaches

➔ **Therapeutic Outcome:** Absence of allergy symptoms and rhinitis

Uses: Allergy symptoms, rhinitis, pruritus, cold urticaria

Investigational uses: Appetite stimulant, management of vascular headache

Dosage and routes

Adult: PO 4 mg tid-qid, not to exceed 0.5 mg/kg/day

P ***Child 7-14 yr:*** PO 4 mg bid-tid, not to exceed 16 mg/day

P ***Child 2-6 yr:*** PO 2 mg bid-tid, not to exceed 12 mg/day

Available forms: Tabs 4 mg; syr 2 mg/5 ml

Side effects/adverse reactions

CNS: Dizziness, drowsiness, poor coordination, fatigue,

anxiety, euphoria, confusion, paresthesia, neuritis
CV: Hypotension, palpitations, tachycardia
EENT: Blurred vision, dilated pupils; tinnitus; nasal stuffiness; dry nose, throat, mouth
GI: Constipation, dry mouth, nausea, vomiting, anorexia, diarrhea, weight gain
GU: Retention, dysuria, frequency, increased appetite
INTEG: Rash, urticaria, photosensitivity
RESP: Increased thick secretions, wheezing, chest tightness

Contraindications: Hypersensitivity to H_1-receptor antagonist, acute asthma attack, lower respiratory tract disease

Precautions: Increased intraocular pressure, renal disease, cardiac disease, hypertension, bronchial asthma, seizure disorder, stenosed peptic ulcers, hyperthyroidism, prostatic hypertrophy, bladder neck obstruction, pregnancy **B**, G elderly

Pharmacokinetics

Absorption	Well absorbed (PO)
Distribution	Unknown
Metabolism	Liver, complete
Excretion	Kidneys
Half-life	Unknown

Pharmacodynamics

	PO
Onset	15-60 min
Peak	1-2 hr
Duration	8 hr

Interactions

Drug/drug:

Individual drugs
Alcohol: ↑ CNS depression

Drug classifications
CNS depressants: ↑ CNS depression
MAOI: ↑ anticholinergic effect
Narcotics: ↑ CNS depression
Sedative/hypnotics: ↑ CNS depression

Lab test interferences

False negative: Skin allergy tests (discontinue antihistamine 3 days before testing)

NURSING CONSIDERATIONS

Assessment

- Assess respiratory status: rate, rhythm, increase in bronchial secretions, wheezing, chest tightness; provide fluids to 2 L/day to decrease secretion thickness
- Monitor I&O ratio: be alert for urinary retention, frequency, dysuria, especially G elderly; drug should be discontinued if these occur; monitor food intake, weight if using as an appetite stimulant

Associated nursing diagnoses

✓ Airway clearance, ineffective (uses)
✓ Injury, risk for (side effects)
✓ Knowledge deficit (teaching)
✓ Noncompliance (teaching, overuse)

Implementation

PO route
- May give with food to decrease GI upset
- Syrup may be used for patients with difficulty swallowing or P children

• Store in tight, light-resistant container

Patient/family education

• Teach all aspects of drug uses; tell patient to notify prescriber if confusion, sedation, hypotension occur; to avoid driving and other hazardous activity if drowsiness occurs; to avoid alcohol and other CNS depressants that may potentiate effect
• Caution patient not to exceed recommended dosage; dysrhythmias may occur
• Teach patient hard candy, gum, frequent rinsing of mouth may be used for dryness

Evaluation

Positive therapeutic outcome
• Absence of running or congested nose, rashes

Treatment of overdose: Administer ipecac syrup or lavage, diazepam, vasopressors, barbiturates (short acting)

cytarabine

(sye-tare'a-been)
cytarabine, Cytosar ✤, Cytosar-U, Tarabine PFS
Func. class.: Antineoplastic, antimetabolite
Chem. class.: Pyrimidine nucleoside
Pregnancy category **C**

Action: Competes with physiologic substrate of DNA synthesis, thus interfering with cell replication in the S phase of the cell cycle (before mitosis)

➡ Therapeutic Outcome: Prevention of rapidly growing malignant cells

Uses: Acute myelocytic leukemia, acute lymphocytic leukemia, chronic myelocytic leukemia, and in combination for non-Hodgkin's lymphomas in P children

Dosage and routes

Acute myelocytic leukemia

Adult: **IV** inf 200 mg/m^2/day × 5 days; intrathecal 30 mg/m^2 q4 days, then another dose every 1-4 days × 4 days

In combination

P *Child:* **IV** inf 100 mg/m^2/day × 5-10 days

Available forms: Inj IV, intrathecal 100, 500 mg, 1, 2 g

Side effects/adverse reactions

CNS: Neuritis, dizziness, headache, personality changes, ataxia, mechanical dysphasia, ***coma***
CV: Chest pain, ***cardiopathy***
CYTARABINE SYNDROME: Fever, myalgia, bone pain, chest pain, rash, conjunctivitis, malaise (6-12 hr after administration)
EENT: Sore throat, conjunctivitis
GI: Nausea, vomiting, anorexia, diarrhea, stomatitis, ***hepatotoxicity,*** abdominal pain, hematemesis, ***GI hemorrhage***
GU: Urinary retention, ***renal failure, hyperuricemia***
HEMA: Thrombophlebitis, bleeding, ***thrombocytopenia,***

leukopenia, myelosuppression, anemia
INTEG: *Rash, fever,* freckling, cellulitis
RESP: Pneumonia, dyspnea

Contraindications: Hypersensitivity, infants, pregnancy (1st trimester)

Precautions: Renal disease, hepatic disease, pregnancy **C**

Pharmacokinetics

Absorption	Complete (IV)
Distribution	Widely distributed; crosses blood-brain barrier, placenta
Metabolism	Liver, extensively
Excretion	Kidneys
Half-life	1-3 hr

Pharmacodynamics

	IV
Onset	Unknown
Peak	Unknown
Duration	Unknown

Interactions

Drug/drug:

Individual drugs

Cyclophosphamide: ↑ cardiotoxicity, CHF
Radiation: ↑ toxicity, bone marrow suppression

Drug classifications

Antineoplastics: ↑ toxicity, bone marrow suppression

NURSING CONSIDERATIONS

Assessment

- Assess buccal cavity q8h for dryness, sores or ulceration, white patches, pain, bleeding, dysphagia; obtain prescription for viscous lidocaine (Xylocaine)
- Assess symptoms indicating severe allergic reaction: rash, pruritus, urticaria, purpuric skin lesions, itching, flushing
- Assess tachypnea, dyspnea, edema, fatigue; identify dyspnea, rales, unproductive cough, chest pain, tachypnea
- Monitor CBC, differential, platelet count weekly; withhold drug if WBC count is <4000/mm^3 or platelet count is <75,000/mm^3
- Assess for increased uric acid levels, swelling, joint pain primarily in extremities; patient should be well hydrated to prevent urate deposits
- Monitor renal function studies: BUN, creatinine, serum uric acid, urine CrCl before and during therapy; I&O ratio; report fall in urine output to <30 ml/hr
- Monitor temp q4h (may indicate beginning of infection)
- Monitor liver function tests before and during therapy (bilirubin, AST [SGOT], ALT [SGPT], LDH) as needed or monthly; note yellowing of skin or sclera, dark urine, clay-colored stools, itchy skin, abdominal pain, fever, diarrhea
- Assess for bleeding: hematuria, stool guaiac, bruising or petechiae, mucosa or orifices q8h
- Identify edema in feet, joint pain, stomach pain, shaking; prescriber should be notified
- Identify inflammation of mucosa, breaks in skin

Associated nursing diagnoses

✓ Injury, risk for (adverse reactions)

C

✓ Body image disturbance (adverse reactions)
✓ Infection, risk for (adverse reactions)
✓ Knowledge deficit (teaching)

Implementation

- Avoid contact with skin; very irritating; wash completely to remove
- Give fluids **IV** or PO before chemotherapy to hydrate patient
- Give antiemetic 30-60 min before giving drug to prevent vomiting, and prn; antibiotics for prophylaxis of infection
- Give top or syst analgesics for pain
- Give in AM so drug can be eliminated before hs
- Provide liquid diet: carbonated beverages; gelatin may be added if patient is not nauseated or vomiting
- Provide rinsing of mouth tid-qid with water, club soda; brushing of teeth bid-qid with soft brush or cotton-tipped applicators for stomatitis; use unwaxed dental floss

IV **IV route**

- Give **IV** direct after diluting 100 mg/5 ml of sterile water for inj; give by direct IV over 1-3 min through free-flowing tubing

IV inf

- May be further diluted in 50-100 ml normal saline or D_5W and given over 30 min to 24 hr depending on dosage

Syringe compatibility:
Metoclopramide

Y-site compatibilities:
Amsacrine, fludarabine, ondansetron, sargramostim

Additive incompatibilities:
Carbenicillin, fluorouracil, heparin, regular insulin, nafcillin, oxacillin, penicillin G sodium

Additive compatibilities:
Corticotropin, daunorubicin with etoposide, hydroxyzine, lincomycin, methotrexate, potassium chloride, prednisolone, sodium bicarbonate, vincristine

Solution compatibilities:
Amino acids, 4.25%/D_{25}, D_5/LR, D_5/0.2% NaCl, D_5/0.9% NaCl, D_{10}/0.9% NaCl, D_5W, invert sugar 10% in electrolyte #1, Ringer's LR, 0.9% NaCl, sodium lactate 1/6 mol/L, TPN #57

Intrathecal route

- Reconstitute with 0.9% NaCl (preservative free) or other compatible sol; to prevent contamination use immediately; discard unused portions if any

SC/IM route

- Reconstitute 100 mg/5 ml or 500 mg/10 ml with bacteriostatic water for inj with benzyl alcohol 0.9%; do not use sol with precipitate; stable for 48 hr

Patient/family education

- Advise patient that contraceptive measures are recommended during therapy
- Teach patient to avoid use of products containing aspirin or ibuprofen, razors, commercial mouthwash, since bleeding may occur; to report symptoms of bleeding (hematuria, tarry stools)

• Advise patient to report signs of anemia (fatigue, headache, irritability, faintness, shortness of breath)
• Instruct patient to report any changes in breathing or coughing even several months after treatment; to avoid crowds and persons with respiratory tract or other infections
• Caution patient not to have any vaccinations without the advice of the prescriber; serious reactions can occur

Evaluation

Positive therapeutic outcome
• Prevention of rapid division of malignant cells

dacarbazine (DTIC)

(da-kar'ba-zeen)
DTIC-Dome, DTIC ♣
Func. class.: Antineoplastic misc agent
Chem. class.: Imidazole
Pregnancy category **C**

Action: Alkylates DNA, RNA; inhibits enzymes that allow synthesis of amino acids in proteins; also responsible for cross-linking DNA strands; activity is not cell cycle phase specific

➡ **Therapeutic Outcome:** Prevention of rapidly growing malignant cells

Uses: Hodgkin's disease, sarcomas, neuroblastoma, malignant melanoma

Investigational uses: Metastatic sarcoma

Dosage and routes

Adult: **IV** 2-4.5 mg/kg or 70-160 mg/m^2 qd × 10 days; repeat q4 wk depending on response or 250 mg/m^2 qd × 5 days; repeat q3 wk

Available forms: Inj **IV** 100, 200 mg

Side effects/adverse reactions

CNS: Facial paresthesia, flushing, fever, malaise
GI: Nausea, anorexia, vomiting, ***hepatotoxicity***
HEMA: ***Thrombocytopenia, leukopenia,*** anemia
INTEG: Alopecia, dermatitis, pain at inj site

Contraindications: Lactation

Precautions: Radiation therapy, pregnancy (1st trimester) **C**

Pharmacokinetics

Absorption	Complete bioavailability (IV)
Distribution	Widely distributed; concentrates in liver
Metabolism	Liver (50%, 5% protein bound)
Excretion	Kidneys, unchanged (50%)
Half-life	Initial 35 min, terminal 5 hr

Pharmacodynamics

	IV
Onset	Unknown
Peak	Unknown
Duration	Unknown

Interactions

Drug/drug:

Individual drugs

Phenobarbital: ↑ toxicity
Phenytoin: ↑ metabolism, ↓ effect
Radiation: ↑ toxicity, bone marrow suppression

Drug classifications

Aminoglycosides: ↑ nephrotoxicity
Antineoplastics: ↑ toxicity, bone marrow suppression
Bone marrow–suppressing drugs: ↑ bone marrow suppression
Diuretics, loop: ↑ ototoxicity
Live vaccines: ↑ adverse reactions, ↓ antibody reaction

NURSING CONSIDERATIONS

Assessment

- Assess symptoms indicating severe allergic reaction: rash, pruritus, urticaria, purpuric skin lesions, itching, flushing; drug should be discontinued
- Monitor CBC, differential, platelet count weekly; withhold drug if WBC count is <4000/mm^3 or platelet count is <100,000/mm^3
- Monitor renal function studies: BUN, creatinine, urine CrCl before and during therapy; I&O ratio; report fall in urine output to <30 ml/hr
- Monitor temp q4h (may indicate beginning of infection)
- Monitor liver function tests before and during therapy (bilirubin, AST [SGOT], ALT [SGPT], LDH) as needed or monthly; note yellowing of skin or sclera, dark urine, clay-colored stools, itchy skin, abdominal pain, fever, diarrhea; hepatoxicity can be serious and fatal
- Assess for bleeding: hematuria, stool guaiac, bruising or petechiae, mucosa or orifices q8h; check for inflammation of mucosa, breaks in skin
- Identify effects of alopecia on body image; discuss feelings about body changes

Associated nursing diagnoses

- ✓ Injury, risk for (adverse reactions)
- ✓ Body image disturbance (adverse reactions)
- ✓ Infection, risk for (adverse reactions)
- ✓ Knowledge deficit (teaching)

Implementation

- Give fluids **IV** or PO before chemotherapy to hydrate patient
- Give antiemetic 30-60 min before giving drug to prevent vomiting, and prn; antibiotics for prophylaxis of infection
- Provide liquid diet: carbonated beverages; gelatin may be added if patient is not nauseated or vomiting

IV **IV route**

- After diluting 100 mg/9.9 ml of sterile water for inj (10 mg/ml), give by direct **IV** over 1 min through Y-tube or 3-way stopcock
- May be further diluted in 50-250 ml of D_5W or normal saline for inj and given over 30 min
- Watch for extravasation; give 3-5 ml of mixture of 4 ml sodium thiosulfate 10% plus 5 ml sterile water SC as prescribed

Y-site compatibilities:
Fludarabine, melphalan, ondansetron, sargramostim, paclitaxel, vinorelbine

Additive incompatibilities:
Hydrocortisone sodium succinate, cysteine

Additive compatibilities:
Bleomycin, carmustine, cyclophosphamide, cytarabine, dactinomycin, doxorubicin, fluorouracil, mercaptopurine, methotrexate, vinblastine

Patient/family education
- Teach patient to avoid use of products containing aspirin or ibuprofen, razors, commercial mouthwash, since bleeding may occur; to report symptoms of bleeding (hematuria, tarry stools)
- Instruct patient to report signs of anemia (fatigue, headache, irritability, faintness, shortness of breath)
- Advise patient that hair may be lost during treatment; a wig or hair piece may make patient feel better; new hair may be different in color, texture
- Caution patient not to have any vaccinations without the advice of prescriber; serious reactions can occur
- Advise patient contraception is needed during treatment and for several months after the completion of therapy; drug has teratogenic properties

Evaluation
Positive therapeutic outcome
- Prevention of rapid division of malignant cells

dactinomycin
(dak-ti-noe-mye'sin)
actinomycin D, Cosmegen
Func. class.: Antineoplastic, antibiotic
Pregnancy category **C**

D

Action: Inhibits DNA, RNA, protein synthesis; derived from *Streptomyces parvulus;* replication is decreased by binding to DNA, which causes strand splitting; cell cycle nonspecific; a vesicant

Therapeutic Outcome: Prevention of rapidly growing malignant cells, immunosuppression

Uses: Sarcomas, melanomas, trophoblastic tumors in women, testicular cancer, Wilms' tumor, rhabdomyosarcoma

Dosage and routes
Adult: **IV** 500 μg/m²/day × 5 days; stop drug for 2-4 wk; then repeat cycle

P *Child:* **IV** 15 μg/kg/day × 5 days, not to exceed 500 μg/day; stop drug until bone marrow recovery, then repeat cycle

Available forms: Inj **IV** 0.5 mg/vial

Side effects/adverse reactions
CNS: Malaise, fatigue, lethargy, fever

EENT: Cheilitis, dysphagia, esophagitis
GI: ***Nausea, vomiting, anorexia, stomatitis, hepatotoxicity,*** abdominal pain, diarrhea
HEMA: Thrombocytopenia, leukopenia, aplastic anemia
INTEG: *Rash,* alopecia, pain at inj site, folliculitis, acne, desquamation, ***extravasation***
MS: Myalgia

Contraindications: Hypersensitivity, herpes infections, child <6 months P

Precautions: Renal disease, hepatic disease, pregnancy **C**, lactation, bone marrow depression

Pharmacokinetics

Absorption	Complete bioavailability
Distribution	Widely distributed; crosses placenta
Metabolism	Unknown
Excretion	Bile; feces, unchanged (50%); kidneys (10%)
Half-life	36 hr

Pharmacodynamics

	IV
Onset	Unknown
Peak	Unknown
Duration	Unknown

Interactions
Drug/drug:
Individual drugs
Radiation: ↑ toxicity, bone marrow suppression
Drug classifications
Antineoplastics: ↑ toxicity, bone marrow suppression
Bone marrow–suppressing drugs: ↑ bone marrow suppression
Live virus vaccines: ↓ antibody reaction

Lab test interferences
Increase: Uric acid

NURSING CONSIDERATIONS
Assessment
- Assess buccal cavity q8h for dryness, sores or ulceration, white patches, pain, bleeding, dysphagia; obtain prescription for viscous lidocaine (Xylocaine)
- Assess symptoms indicating severe allergic reaction: rash, pruritus, urticaria, purpuric skin lesions, itching, flushing; drug should be discontinued
- Monitor CBC, differential, platelet count weekly; withhold drug if WBC count is <4000/mm^3 or platelet count is <100,000/mm^3; notify prescriber of results if WBC <20,000/mm^3, platelets <150,000/mm^3
- Monitor renal function studies: BUN, creatinine, serum uric acid, urine CrCl before and during therapy; I&O ratio; report fall in urine output to <30 ml/hr
- Monitor temp q4h (may indicate beginning of infection)
- Monitor liver function tests before and during therapy (bilirubin, AST [SGOT], ALT [SGPT], LDH) as needed or monthly; note yellowing of skin or sclera, dark urine, clay-colored stools, itchy skin, abdominal pain, fever, diarrhea
- Assess for bleeding: hematuria, stool guaiac, bruising or petechiae, mucosa or orifices q8h; check for inflammation of mucosa, breaks in skin

- Identify effects of alopecia on body image; discuss feelings about body changes

Associated nursing diagnoses

- ✓ Injury, high risk for (adverse reactions)
- ✓ Body image disturbance (adverse reactions)
- ✓ Oral mucous membranes, altered (adverse reactions)
- ✓ Infection, high risk for (adverse reactions)
- ✓ Knowledge deficit (teaching)

Implementation

- Provide antacid before oral agent; give drug pc PM, before hs; antiemetic 30-60 mins before giving drug to prevent vomiting, and prn; antibiotics for prophylaxis of infection
- Provide liquid diet: carbonated beverages; gelatin may be added if patient is not nauseated or vomiting
- Help patient rinse mouth tid-qid with water, club soda, brush teeth bid-qid with soft brush or cotton-tipped applicators for stomatitis, use unwaxed dental floss

IV **IV route**

- Drug should be prepared by experienced personnel using proper precautions
- Give after diluting 0.5 mg/ 1.1 ml of sterile water for inj without preservative; use 2.2 ml (0.25 mg/ml), give by direct **IV** at 0.5 mg or less/min through Y-tube or 3 way stopcock of inf in progress

Intermittent inf

- May be further diluted in 50 ml D_5W or normal saline for inf; run over 10/15 min
- Give hydrocortisone, sodium thiosulfate to infiltration area, and ice compress after stopping inf
- Store in darkness in cool environment

D

Y-site compatibilities:

Fludarabine, ondansetron, sargramostim

Patient/family education

- Teach patient to avoid use of products containing aspirin or ibuprofen, razors, commercial mouthwash, since bleeding may occur; to report symptoms of bleeding (hematuria, tarry stools)
- Instruct patient to report signs of anemia (fatigue, headache, irritability, faintness, shortness of breath)
- Advise patient that hair may be lost during treatment; a wig or hair piece may make patient feel better; new hair may be different in color, texture
- Caution patient not to have any vaccinations without the advice of the prescriber, serious reactions can occur
- Advise patient contraception is needed during treatment and for several months after the completion of therapy

Evaluation

Positive therapeutic outcome

- Prevention of rapid division of malignant cells

danazol

(da'na-zole)

Cyclomen ♣, danazol, Danocrine

Func. class.: Androgen, hormone

Chem. class.: α-Ethinyl testosterone derivative

Pregnancy category **C**

Action: Atrophy of endometrial tissue; decreases FSH, LH, which are controlled by pituitary; this leads to amenorrhea/anovulation; has weak androgen, anabolic activity

→ Therapeutic Outcome: Decreased pain and nodules/fibrocystic breast disease; correction in hereditary angioedema; atrophy of endometrial tissue (ectopic)

Uses: Endometriosis, prevention of hereditary angioedema, fibrocystic breast disease

Dosage and routes

Endometriosis

Adult: PO initial dose 500 mg bid, then decrease to 400 mg bid × 3-9 mo

Fibrocystic breast disease

Adult: PO 100-400 mg qd in 2 divided doses × 2-6 mo

Hereditary angioedema

Adult: PO 200 mg bid-tid until desired response, then decrease dose to 100 mg at 1-3 mo intervals

Available forms: Caps 50, 100, 200 mg

Side effects/adverse reactions

CNS: Dizziness, headache, fatigue, tremors, paresthesias, flushing, sweating, anxiety, lability, insomnia, carpal tunnel syndrome

CV: Increased B/P

EENT: Conjunctival edema, nasal congestion

ENDO: Abnormal GTT

GI: Nausea, vomiting, constipation, weight gain, ***cholestatic jaundice***

GU: Hematuria, amenorrhea, atrophic vaginitis, decreased libido, decreased breast size, clitoral hypertrophy, testicular atrophy

INTEG: Rash, acneiform lesions, oily hair and skin, flushing, sweating, acne vulgaris, alopecia, hirsutism

MS: Cramps, spasms

Contraindications: Severe renal disease, severe cardiac disease, severe hepatic disease, hypersensitivity, genital bleeding (abnormal)

Precautions: Migraine headaches, seizure disorders, pregnancy **C**

Pharmacokinetics

Absorption	GI absorption
Distribution	Unknown
Metabolism	Liver
Excretion	Kidneys
Half-life	4½ hr

Pharmacodynamics

	PO
Onset	Unknown
Peak	Unknown
Duration	Unknown

Interactions

Drug/drug:

Individual drugs

Cyclosporine: ↑ risk of toxicity
Insulin: ↓ effects of insulin
Oxyphenbutazone: ↑ effects of oxyphenbutazone

Drug classifications

Adrenal steroids: ↑ edema
Anticoagulants: ↑ pro-time
Oral hypoglycemics: ↑ effects of hypoglycemics

Lab test interferences

Increase: Cholesterol
Decrease: Cholesterol, T_4, T_3, thyroid ^{131}I uptake test, 17-KS, PBI
Interferences: GTT

NURSING CONSIDERATIONS

Assessment

- Assess for lower abdominal (endometrial) pain before and throughout treatment to identify if treatment is effective
- Monitor potassium, blood sugar, urine glucose while patient is on long-term therapy
- Assess breast for fibrocystic nodules; check for pain, tenderness before therapy and throughout to identify if treatment is effective
- Monitor weight daily; notify prescriber if weekly weight gain is >5 lb; I&O ratio; be alert for decreasing urinary output, increasing edema, hypertension, cardiac symptoms, jaundice
- Assess for mental status: affect, mood, behavioral changes, aggression, sleep disorders, depression; change may be extreme
- Assess for signs of virilization: deepening of voice, decreased libido, facial hair (may not be reversible)

Associated nursing diagnoses

✓ Infection, risk for (adverse reactions)
✓ Injury, risk for (adverse reactions)
✓ Knowledge deficit (teaching)

Implementation

- Store in airtight container at room temp
- Provide ROM exercise for patients who are immobile

PO route

- Give with food or milk to decrease GI symptoms

Patient/family education

- Teach patient to notify prescriber if therapeutic response decreases; advise that endometriosis tends to recur after drug is discontinued; not to discontinue medication abruptly but to taper over several weeks
- Advise patient that alternate contraceptive measures are needed during treatment; amenorrhea may occur with higher dosages
- Teach patient to report menstrual irregularities; that amenorrhea usually occurs but menstruation resumes 2-3 mo after termination of therapy; that drug should induce anovulation; reversible within 60-90 days after drug is discontinued
- Teach patient about routine breast self-exam technique, to report any increase in nodule size

D

- Instruct patient to report masculinization: deepening voice, facial hair growth, body hair growth

Evaluation

Positive therapeutic outcome
- Decreased pain in endometriosis
- Decreased size, pain in fibrocystic breast disease
- Decreased signs of angioedema (hereditary)

dantrolene
(dan'troe-leen)
Dantrium, Dantrium Intravenous
Func. class.: Skeletal muscle relaxant, direct acting
Chem. class.: Hydantoin
Pregnancy category **C**

Action: Interferes with intracellular release from the sarcoplasmic reticulum of calcium necessary to initiate contraction; slows catabolism in malignant hyperthermia

Therapeutic Outcome: Decreased muscle spasticity; absence of malignant hyperthermia

Uses: Spasticity in multiple sclerosis, stroke, spinal cord injury, cerebral palsy, prevention and treatment of malignant hyperthermia

Dosage and routes

Spasticity

Adult: PO 25 mg/day; may increase by 25-100 mg bid-qid, not to exceed 400 mg/day × 1 wk

P *Child:* PO 1 mg/kg/day given in divided doses bid-tid; may increase gradually, not to exceed 100 mg qid

Malignant hyperthermia

P *Adult and child:* **IV** 1 mg/kg; may repeat to total dose of 10 mg/kg; PO 4-8 mg/kg/day in 4 divided doses × 3 days to prevent further hyperthermia

Prevention of malignant hyperthermia

P *Adult and child:* PO 4-8 mg/kg/day in 3-4 divided doses × 1-2 days before procedures; give last dose 4 hr preoperatively

Available forms: Caps 25, 50, 100 mg; powder for inj **IV** 20 mg/vial

Side effects/adverse reactions

CNS: ***Dizziness, weakness, fatigue, drowsiness,*** headache, disorientation, insomnia, paresthesias, tremors
CV: Hypotension, chest pain, palpitations
EENT: Nasal congestion, blurred vision, mydriasis
GI: ***Nausea,*** constipation, vomiting, increased AST (SGOT) and alkaline phosphatase, abdominal pain, dry mouth, anorexia, hepatitis
GU: Urinary frequency, nocturia, impotence, crystalluria

HEMA: Eosinophilia
INTEG: Rash, pruritus, photosensitivity

Contraindications: Hypersensitivity, compromised pulmonary function, active hepatic disease, impaired myocardial function

Precautions: Peptic ulcer disease, renal disease, hepatic disease, stroke, seizure disorder, diabetes mellitus, pregnancy **C**, G elderly

Pharmacokinetics

Absorption	PO (30%-35%)
Distribution	Unknown
Metabolism	Liver, extensively
Excretion	Kidney
Half-life	9 hr

Pharmacodynamics

	PO	IV
Onset	Unknown	Immediate
Peak	5 hr	5 hr
Duration	Dose related	Dose related

Interactions

Drug/drug:

Individual drugs
Alcohol: ↑ CNS depression
Verapamil: ↑ hyperkalemia

Drug classifications
Antidepressants, tricyclic: ↑ CNS depression
Antihistamines: ↑ CNS depression
Barbiturates: ↑ CNS depression
Estrogens: ↑ hepatotoxicity
Narcotics: ↑ CNS depression
Sedative/hypnotics: ↑ CNS depression

NURSING CONSIDERATIONS

Assessment

- Monitor I&O ratio; check for urinary retention, frequency, hesitancy, especially G elderly
- Monitor ECG in epileptic patients; poor seizure control has occurred with patients taking this drug; assess for increased seizure activity in epilepsy patient
- Monitor hepatic function by frequent determination of AST (SGOT), ALT (SGPT), renal function studies, CBC
- Assess for allergic reactions: rash, fever, respiratory distress
- Monitor for severe weakness, numbness in extremities
- Assess for CNS depression: dizziness, drowsiness, psychiatric symptoms
- Assess for signs of hepatotoxicity: jaundice, yellow sclera, pain in abdomen, nausea, fever; drug should be discontinued if these signs and symptoms occur

Associated nursing diagnoses

- ✓ Pain, chronic (uses)
- ✓ Physical mobility, impaired (uses)
- ✓ Injury, risk for (adverse reactions)
- ✓ Knowledge deficit (teaching)

Implementation

PO route

- Give with meals for GI symptoms; capsules may be opened and mixed with liquid; patient should drink after mixing
- Store in airtight container at room temp

IV route
- Administer **IV** after reconstituting 20 mg/60 ml sterile water for inj without bacteriostatic agent (333 μg/ml); shake until clear; give by rapid **IV** push through Y-tube or 3-way stopcock; follow by prescribed doses immediately; assess site for extravasation, phlebitis
- Protect diluted sol from light; use reconstituted sol within 6 hr

Patient/family education
- Notify prescriber of abdominal pain, jaundiced sclera, clay-colored stools, change in color of urine; rash, itching occur
- Caution patient not to take with alcohol, other CNS depressants; severe CNS depression can occur; avoid using OTC medication: cough preparations, antihistamines, unless directed by prescriber
- Tell patient that if improvement does not occur within 6 wk, prescriber may discontinue
- Advise patient to avoid altering activities while taking this drug
- Caution patient to avoid hazardous activities if drowsiness, dizziness, blurred vision occurs; wait several days to identify patient response to medication
- Teach patient to use sunscreen, protective clothing for photosensitivity
- Instruct patient to take medication as prescribed; do not double doses; take dose if missed within 1 hr of scheduled time

Evaluation
Positive therapeutic outcome
- Decreased pain, spasticity
- Absence or decreased symptoms of malignant hyperthermia

Treatment of overdose: Induce emesis of conscious patient; lavage, dialysis

daunorubicin
(daw-noe-roo'bi-sin)
Cerubidine
Func. class.: Antineoplastic, antibiotic
Chem. class.: Anthracycline glycoside
Pregnancy category **D**

Action: Inhibits DNA synthesis, primarily; derived from *Streptomyces coeruleorubidus;* replication is decreased by binding to DNA, which causes strand splitting; cell cycle specific (S phase); a vesicant

Therapeutic Outcome: Prevention of rapidly growing malignant cells; immunosuppression

Uses: Myelogenous, monocytic leukemia, acute nonlymphocytic leukemia, Ewing's sarcoma, Wilms' tumor, neuroblastoma, rhabdomyosarcoma

Dosage and routes
Single agent
Adult: **IV** 60 mg/m^2/day × 3-5 day q4 wk

In combination
Adult: **IV** 45 mg/m^2/day × 3 days, then 2 days of subsequent courses with cytosine arabinoside

Available forms: Inj **IV** 20 mg powder/vial

Side effects/adverse reactions

CNS: Fever, chills
CV: ***Dysrhythmias, CHF, pericarditis, myocarditis,*** peripheral edema
GI: Nausea, vomiting, anorexia, mucositis, ***hepatotoxicity***
GU: Impotence, sterility, amenorrhea, gynecomastia, hyperuricemia
HEMA: ***Thrombocytopenia, leukopenia, anemia***
INTEG: Rash, ***extravasation,*** dermatitis, reversible alopecia, cellulitis, thrombophlebitis at inj site

Contraindications: Hypersensitivity, pregnancy (1st trimester) **D**, lactation, syst infections, cardiac disease

Precautions: Renal, hepatic disease, gout, bone marrow depression

Pharmacokinetics

Absorption	Complete (IV)
Distribution	Widely distributed; crosses placenta
Metabolism	Liver, extensively
Excretion	Biliary (40%-50%)
Half-life	18½ hr

Pharmacodynamics

	IV
Onset	Unknown
Peak	Unknown
Diuretic	Unknown

D

Interactions

Drug/drug:
Individual drugs
Cyclophosphamide: ↑ cardiotoxicity, CHF
Radiation: ↑ toxicity, bone marrow suppression
Drug classifications
Antineoplastics: ↑ toxicity, bone marrow suppression

Lab test interferences

Increase: Uric acid

NURSING CONSIDERATIONS

Assessment

- Assess buccal cavity q8h for dryness, sores or ulceration, white patches, pain, bleeding, dysphagia; obtain prescription for viscous lidocaine (Xylocaine)
- Assess symptoms indicating severe allergic reaction: rash, pruritus, urticaria, purpuric skin lesions, itching, flushing; drug should be discontinued
- Assess tachypnea, ECG changes, dyspnea, edema, fatigue
- Monitor CBC, differential, platelet count weekly; withhold drug if WBC count is <4000/mm^3 or platelet count is <100,000/mm^3; notify prescriber of results if WBC <20,000/mm^3, platelets <150,000/mm^3
- Assess for increased uric acid levels, swelling, joint pain primarily in extremities; patient

should be well hydrated to prevent urate deposits

- Monitor renal function studies: BUN, creatinine, serum uric acid, urine CrCl before and during therapy; I&O ratio; report fall in urine output to <30 ml/hr
- Monitor temp q4h (may indicate beginning of infection)
- Monitor liver function tests before and during therapy (bilirubin, AST [SGOT], ALT [SGPT], LDH) as needed or monthly; note yellowing of skin or sclera, dark urine, clay-colored stools, itchy skin, abdominal pain, fever, diarrhea; hepatoxicity can be severe
- Assess for bleeding: hematuria, stool guaiac, bruising or petechiae, mucosa or orifices q8h; check for inflammation of mucosa, breaks in skin
- Identify effects of alopecia on body image; discuss feelings about body changes

Associated nursing diagnoses

- ✓ Injury, risk for (adverse reactions)
- ✓ Cardiac output, decreased (adverse reactions)
- ✓ Body image disturbance (adverse reactions)
- ✓ Infection, risk for (adverse reactions)
- ✓ Knowledge deficit (teaching)

Implementation

- Avoid contact with skin; very irritating; wash completely to remove
- Give fluids **IV** or PO before chemotherapy to hydrate patient; give antiemetic 30-60 min before giving drug to prevent vomiting, and prn; antibiotics for prophylaxis of infection
- Provide liquid diet: carbonated beverages; gelatin may be added if patient is not nauseated or vomiting
- Help patient rinse mouth tid-qid with water, club soda, brush teeth bid-qid with soft brush or cotton-tipped applicators for stomatitis, use unwaxed dental floss

IV IV route

- Drug should be prepared by experienced personnel using proper precautions
- Give **IV** after diluting 20 mg/4 ml sterile water for inj (5 mg/ml); rotate; further dilute in 10-15 ml normal saline; give over 3-5 min by direct IV through Y-tube or 3-way stopcock of inf of D_5W or 0.9% NaCl

Intermittent inf route

- Dilute further in 50-100 ml 0.9% NaCl, LR, D_5W; give over 15 min (50 ml), 30 min (100 ml)

Y-site incompatibility:

Fludarabine

Y-site compatibilities:

Ondansetron, melphalan, vinorelbine

Additive incompatibilities:

Dexamethasone, heparin

Additive compatibilities:

Cytarabine with etoposide, hydrocortisone sodium succinate; not recommended for admixing

Solution compatibilities:
$D_{3.3}$/0.3% NaCl, D_5W, Normosol R, Ringer's, 0.9% NaCl

Patient/family education

- Teach patient to avoid use of products containing aspirin or ibuprofen, razors, commercial mouthwash, since bleeding may occur; to report symptoms of bleeding (hematuria, tarry stools)
- Instruct patient to report signs of anemia (fatigue, headache, irritability, faintness, shortness of breath)
- Advise patient that hair may be lost during treatment; a wig or hair piece may make patient feel better; new hair may be different in color, texture
- Caution patient not to have any vaccinations without the advice of the prescriber; serious reactions can occur
- Advise patient contraception is needed during treatment and for several months after the completion of therapy

Evaluation

Positive therapeutic outcome
- Prevention of rapid division of malignant cells

deferoxamine

(de-fer-ox'a-meen)
Desferal
Func. class.: Heavy metal antagonist
Chem. class.: Chelating agent
Pregnancy category **C**

D

Action: Binds iron ions (ferric ions) to form water-soluble complex that is removed by kidneys

Therapeutic Outcome: Excretion of excess iron and aluminum

Uses: Acute, chronic iron intoxication, hemochromatosis, hemosiderosis

Dosage and routes

Acute iron toxicity

P *Adult and child:* IM/**IV** 1 g; then 500 mg q4h × 2 doses; then 500 mg q4-12h × 2 doses, not to exceed 15 mg/kg/hr or 6 g/24 hr

Chronic iron toxicity

P *Adult and child:* IM 500 mg-1 g/day plus **IV** inf 2 g given by separate line with each blood transfusion, not to exceed 15 mg/kg/hr or 6 g/24 hr; SC 1-2 g over 8-24 hr by SC infusion pump

Available forms: Powder for inj 500 mg/vial

Side effects/adverse reactions

CNS: Flushing, shock following rapid IV administration

CV: Hypotension, tachycardia
EENT: Blurred vision, cataracts, decreased healing, ***ototoxicity***
GI: Diarrhea, abdominal cramps
GU: Dysuria, pyelonephritis, red urine
INTEG: Urticaria, erythema, pruritus, pain at inj site, fever
MS: Leg cramps
SYST: ***Anaphylaxis***

Contraindications: Hypersensitivity, anuria, severe renal disease

Precautions: Pregnancy **C**, P lactation; child <3 yr

Pharmacokinetics

Absorption	Well absorbed (IM, SC); completely absorbed (IV)
Distribution	Widely distributed
Metabolism	Plasma enzymes
Excretion	Kidneys, unchanged; chelated, excess iron removed by feces and bile (33%-35%)
Half-life	1 hr

Pharmacodynamics

	SC/IM/IV
Onset	Unknown
Peak	Unknown
Duration	Unknown

Interactions: None

NURSING CONSIDERATIONS

Assessment

- Assess for poisoning: type of iron agent, time, amount ingested acute or chronic
- Assess for acute iron toxicity: acute early symptoms (nausea, vomiting, abdominal cramping, bloody diarrhea); acute late symptoms (metabolic acidosis, coma, shock)
- Assess vision and hearing periodically; ototoxicity may occur
- Check VS during **IV** administration; watch for dropping B/P, urine color (urine may turn red), rash, urticaria; if these occur, drug should be discontinued; resuscitation equipment should be available for anaphylaxis
- Monitor I&O, renal function studies: BUN, creatinine, CrCl, serum iron levels

Associated nursing diagnoses

✓ Poisoning (uses)
✓ Knowledge deficit (teaching)

Implementation

IV **IV route**

- Give **IV** (used for shock) after diluting 500 mg/2 ml water for inj; when dissolved, must be further diluted with D_5W, LR, or 0.9% NaCl; run at <15 mg/kg/hr; 2 g/1000 ml usually given over 24 hr; to be used only for short time; IM is preferred route
- Administer only when epinephrine 1:1000 is available for anaphylaxis

IM route

- Give IM after diluting with 2 ml sterile water for inj per 500 mg of drug; rotate inj sites; give deep in large muscle mass; rotate sites

SC route

- Use abdominal SC tissue by inf pump for 8-24 hr/treatment; use only for chronic iron toxicity

Patient/family education

- Teach patient that urine may turn red; this is not blood but iron excretion
- Caution patient to avoid vitamin C preparations including multivitamins unless approved by prescriber
- Instruct patient that tests are required after treatment for chronic iron toxicity including blood, hearing, and eye tests; stress the importance of follow-up

Evaluation

Positive therapeutic outcome

- Decreased symptoms of heavy metal intoxication

desmopressin

(des-moe-press′in)

Concentraid, DDAVP

Func. class.: Pituitary hormone

Chem. class.: Synthetic antidiuretic hormone

Pregnancy category **B**

Action: Promotes reabsorption of water by action on renal tubular epithelium in the kidney; causes smooth muscle constriction and increase in plasma factor VIII levels, which increases platelet aggregation resulting in vasopressor effect; similar to vasopressor

Therapeutic Outcome: Prevention of nocturnal enuresis, decreased bleeding in hemophilia A, von Willebrand's disease type 1, control and stabilization of water in diabetes insipidus

Uses: Hemophilia A, von Willebrand's disease type 1, nonnephrogenic diabetes insipidus, symptoms of polyuria/polydipsia caused by pituitary dysfunction, nocturnal enuresis

D

Dosage and routes

Diabetes insipidus

Adult: Intranasal 0.1-0.4 mg qd in divided doses (1-4 sprays with pump) **IV**/SC 0.2-0.4 mg qd in two divided doses

P *Child 3 mo to 12 yr:* Intranasal 0.05-0.3 mg qd or in divided doses bid

Hemophilia/von Willebrand's disease

P *Adult and child:* **IV** 0.3 µg/kg in NaCl over 15-30 min; may repeat if needed

Nocturnal enuresis (primary)

P *Child 6 yr or more:* 10 µg in each nostril at hs

Available forms: Intranasal 0.01 mg/ml, inj **IV**, SC 4 µg/ml

Side effects/adverse reactions

CNS: Drowsiness, headache, lethargy, flushing
CV: Increased B/P
EENT: Nasal irritation, congestion, rhinitis
GI: Nausea, heartburn, cramps
GU: Vulval pain

Contraindications: Hypersensitivity, nephrogenic diabetes insipidus

Precautions: Pregnancy **B**, CAD, lactation, hypertension

Pharmacokinetics

Absorption	Nasal (up to 20%)
Distribution	Unknown
Metabolism	Unknown
Excretion	Unknown; breast milk
Half-life	8 min (initial), 76 min (terminal)

Pharmacodynamics

	INTRANASAL	IV/SC
Onset	1 hr	Rapid
Peak	1-2 hr	15-30 min
Duration	8-20 hr	3 hr

Interactions

Drug/drug:

Individual drugs

Alcohol: ↓ response of desmopressin
Carbamazepine: ↑ response of desmopressin
Chlorpropamide: ↑ response of desmopressin
Clofibrate: ↑ response of desmopressin
Demeclocycline: ↓ response of desmopressin
Epinephrine (large doses): ↓ response of desmopressin
Heparin: ↓ response of desmopressin
Lithium: ↓ response of desmopressin
Norepinephrine: ↓ response of desmopressin

NURSING CONSIDERATIONS

Assessment

- Monitor I&O ratio, urine osmolality, sp gr, weight daily; check for edema in extremities; if water retention is severe, diuretic may be prescribed; check pulse, B/P when giving drug **IV** or SC
- Assess for water intoxication: lethargy, behavioral changes, disorientation, neuromuscular excitability, dehydration, poor skin turgor, severe thirst, dry skin, tachycardia
- Assess intranasal use: nausea, congestion, cramps, headache; usually decreased with decreased dosage
- Monitor for enuresis during treatment (nocturnal enuresis)

Associated nursing diagnoses

- ✓ Fluid volume deficit (uses)
- ✓ Fluid volume excess (side effects)
- ✓ Knowledge deficit (teaching)

Implementation

- Store in refrigerator or cool environment

IV IV route

Direct IV

- Give undiluted over 1 min in diabetes insipidus or **IV** for hemophilia

Intermittent inf

- Give single dose diluted in 50 ml of 0.9% NaCl (adult and child >10 kg); a single dose/10 ml as an **IV** inf over 15-30 min in von Willebrand's disease or hemophilia A

Patient/family education

- Use demonstration, return demonstration to teach technique for nasal instillation: draw medication into tube, insert tube into nostril to instill drug and blow on other end to deliver sol into nasal cavity; rinse after use
- Teach patient to notify prescriber of dyspnea, vomiting,

cramping, drowsiness, headache, nasal congestion
• Caution patient to avoid OTC products (cough, hay fever), since these preparations may contain epinephrine and decrease drug response; do not use with alcohol
• Advise patient to wear Medic Alert ID or other identification specifying disease and medication used
• Advise patient if dose is missed, take when remembered up to 1 hr before next dose; do not double doses

Evaluation

Positive therapeutic outcome
• Absence of severe thirst
• Decreased urine output, osmolality
• Absence of bleeding (hemophilia)

desonide

(dess'oh-nide)

DesOwen, Tridesilon

Func. class.: Topical corticosteroid

Chem. class.: Synthetic nonfluorinated agent, group IV potency

Pregnancy category **C**

Action: Antipruritic, anti-inflammatory

Therapeutic Outcome: Decreased inflammatory skin disorders

Uses: Psoriasis, eczema, contact dermatitis, pruritus; usually reserved for severe dermatoses that have not responded to less potent formulation

Dosage and routes

P *Adult and child:* Apply to affected area bid-tid

Available forms: Cream 0.05%; oint 0.05%

Side effects/adverse reactions

INTEG: Burning, dryness, itching, irritation, acne, folliculitis, hypertrichosis, perioral dermatitis, hypopigmentation, atrophy, striae, miliaria, allergic contact dermatitis, secondary infection

Contraindications: Hypersensitivity to corticosteroids, fungal infections

Precautions: Pregnancy **C**, lactation, viral infections, bacterial infections

Pharmacokinetics

Absorption	Minimal; systemic absorption on large areas
Distribution	Site only
Metabolism	Not metabolized
Excretion	Not excreted
Half-life	Unknown

Pharmacodynamics

	TOP
Onset	Up to 1 hr
Peak	Unknown
Duration	Unknown

Interactions: None

NURSING CONSIDERATIONS

Assessment

- Monitor temp; if fever develops, drug should be discontinued
- Assess for systemic absorption: increased temp, inflammation, irritation

Associated nursing diagnoses

- ✓ Infection, risk for (adverse reactions)
- ✓ Knowledge deficit (teaching)
- ✓ Noncompliance (teaching)

Implementation

Top route

- Apply only to affected areas; do not get in eyes
- Leave area uncovered or lightly covered; occlusive dressing is not recommended; syst absorption may occur
- Apply only to dermatoses; do not use on weeping, denuded, or infected area
- Cleanse affected area before application of drug
- Treat for a few days after area has cleared
- Store at room temp

Patient/family education

- Caution patient to avoid sunlight on affected area; burns may occur
- Instruct patient to limit treatment to 14 days using <50 g/wk

Evaluation

Positive therapeutic outcome

- Absence of severe itching, patches on skin, flaking

dextroamphetamine

(dex-troe-am-fet'a-meen)

Dexedrine, Dexedrine Spansules, dextroamphetamine sulfate, Ferndex, Oxydess II, Spancap #1

Func. class.: Cerebral stimulant

Chem. class.: Amphetamine

Pregnancy category C

Controlled substance schedule II

Action: Increases release of norepinephrine, dopamine in cerebral cortex to reticular activating system

➔ Therapeutic Outcome: Increased alertness, decreased fatigue, ability to stay awake (narcolepsy); increased attention span, decreased hyperactivity (ADHD)

Uses: Narcolepsy, attention deficit disorder with hyperactivity

Dosage and routes

Narcolepsy

Adult: PO 5-60 mg qd in divided doses

P ***Child >12 yr:*** PO 10 mg qd increasing by 10 mg/day at weekly intervals

P ***Child 6-12 yr:*** PO 5 mg qd increasing by 5 mg/wk (max 60 mg/day)

ADHD

P *Child >6 yr:* PO 5 mg qd-bid increasing by 5 mg/day at weekly intervals

P *Child 3-6 yr:* PO 2.5 mg qd increasing by 2.5 mg/day at weekly intervals

Available forms: Tabs 5, 10 mg; sus rel caps 5, 10, 15 mg; elix 5 mg/5 ml

Side effects/adverse reactions

CNS: Hyperactivity, insomnia, restlessness, talkativeness, dizziness, headache, chills, stimulation, dysphoria, irritability, aggressiveness, tremor, dependence, addiction
CV: Palpitations, tachycardia, hypertension, decrease in heart rate, dysrhythmias
GI: Anorexia, dry mouth, diarrhea, constipation, weight loss, metallic taste
GU: Impotence, change in libido
INTEG: Urticaria

Contraindications: Hypersensitivity to sympathomimetic amines, hyperthyroidism, hypertension, glaucoma, severe arteriosclerosis, drug abuse, cardiovascular disease, anxiety

Precautions: Gilles de la Tourette's disorder, pregnancy C, lactation, P child <3 yr

Pharmacokinetics

Absorption	Well absorbed (PO)
Distribution	Widely distributed; crosses placenta
Metabolism	Liver
Excretion	Kidneys, pH dependent: increased pH, increased reabsorption
Half-life	10-30 hr; increased when urine is alkaline

Pharmacodynamics

	PO
Onset	½ hr
Peak	1-3 hr
Duration	4-10 hr

Interactions

Drug/drug:

Individual drugs

Acetazolamide: ↓ excretion, ↑ effect
Ammonium chloride: ↓ effect
Ascorbic acid: ↓ effect
Meperidine: Hypertensive crisis
Sodium bicarbonate: ↓ excretion, ↑ effect
Thyroid: ↑ effects

Drug classifications

Antidepressants, tricyclics: ↑ dysrhythmias
β-Blockers: ↑ hypertension
Cardiac glycosides: ↑ dysrhythmias
MAOI: Hypertensive crisis
Sympathomimetics: ↑ effect

NURSING CONSIDERATIONS

Assessment

- Monitor VS, B/P, since this drug may reverse antihypertensives; check patients with cardiac disease more often for increased B/P
- Monitor CBC, urinalysis; for diabetic patients monitor

blood sugar, urine sugar; insulin changes may be required, since eating will decrease
- Monitor height and weight q3 mo since growth rate in P children may be decreased; appetite is suppressed so weight loss is common during the first few months of treatment
- Monitor mental status: mood, sensorium, affect, stimulation, insomnia; aggressiveness may occur; depression with crying spells may occur after drug has worn off
- Assess for physical dependency; should not be used for extended time except in ADHD; dosage should be decreased gradually to prevent withdrawal symptoms
- Assess for narcoleptic symptoms before medication and after; ability to stay awake should increase significantly
- P In children or adults with ADHD, monitor for improved organizational skills, attention span, attending to tasks, impulse control, socialization, and ability to get along better with others
- Assess for withdrawal symptoms: headache, nausea, vomiting, muscle pain, weakness; drug tolerance develops after long-term use; dosage should not be increased if tolerance develops; this medication has a high abuse potential

Associated nursing diagnoses

✓ Thought processes, altered (uses, adverse reactions)
✓ Coping, impaired individual (uses)
✓ Family coping, impaired individual (uses)
✓ Knowledge deficit (teaching)

Implementation

PO route
- Give at least 6 hr before hs to avoid sleeplessness; titrate to patient's response; lowest dosage should be used to control symptoms
- Give gum, hard candy, frequent sips of water for dry mouth at beginning of treatment; these symptoms tend to lessen with time

Patient/family education

- Advise patient to decrease caffeine consumption (coffee, tea, cola, chocolate), which may increase irritability and stimulation; to avoid OTC preparations unless approved by prescriber; to avoid alcohol ingestion; these may cause serious drug interactions
- Caution patient to taper off drug over several weeks, or depression, increased sleeping, lethargy may occur
- Caution patient to avoid hazardous activities until patient is stabilized on medication
- Instruct patient not to double doses if medication is missed; prescriber may suggest drug holidays (ADHD) during the school year to assess progress and determine continued drug necessity
- Instruct patient/family to notify prescriber if significant side effects occur: tremors, insomnia, palpitations, restlessness, drug changes may be needed

- Inform patient that if dry mouth occurs to use frequent sips of water, sugarless gum, hard candy during beginning therapy; dry mouth lessens with continued treatment
- Advise patient to get needed rest; patients will feel more tired at end of day; to give last dose at least 6 hr before hs to avoid insomnia

Evaluation

Positive therapeutic outcome

- Decreased activity in ADHD
- Absence of sleeping during day in narcolepsy

Treatment of overdose: Administer fluids, hemodialysis, peritoneal dialysis, antihypertensives for increased B/P; ammonium chloride for increased excretion

dextromethorphan

(dex-troe-meth-or'fan)

Balminil DM ✦, Benylin DM, Broncho-Grippol-DM ✦, Children's Hold, Delsym, Dextromethorphan, DM Syrup ✦, Hold DM, Koffex ✦, Neo-DM ✦, Ornex-DM ✦, Pertussin, Pertussin ES, Robidex ✦, Robitussin Cough Calmers, Robitussin Pediatric, Sedatuss ✦, St. Joseph Cough Suppressant, Sucrets Cough Control, Suppress, Trocal, Vicks Formula 44

Func. class.: Antitussive, nonnarcotic

Chem. class.: Levorphanol derivative

Pregnancy category C

Action: Depresses cough center in medulla by direct effect related to levorphanol

Therapeutic Outcome: Absence of cough

Uses: Nonproductive cough carried by minor respiratory tract infections or irritants that might be inhaled

Dosage and routes

Adult: PO 10-20 mg q4h, or 30 mg q6-8h, not to exceed 120 mg/day; sus rel liq 60 mg bid, not to exceed 120 mg/day

Child 6-12 yr: PO 5-10 mg q4h; sus rel lip 30 mg bid, not to exceed 60 mg/day

P *Child 2-6 yr:* PO 2.5-5 mg q4h, or 7.5 mg q6-8h, not to exceed 30 mg/day

Available forms: Loz 2.5, 5 mg; sol 3.5. 5, 7.5, 10, 15 mg/5 ml, syr 15 mg/15 ml, 10 mg/5 ml; sus action liq 30 mg/5 ml

Side effects/adverse reactions

CNS: Dizziness

GI: Nausea

Contraindications: Hypersensitivity, asthma/emphysema, productive cough

Precautions: Nausea/vomiting, increased temp, persistent headache, pregnancy **C**

Pharmacokinetics

Absorption	Rapid (PO); slow (sus rel)
Distribution	Unknown
Metabolism	Liver
Excretion	Kidneys
Half-life	Unknown

Pharmacodynamics

	PO	PO-SUS
Onset	15-30 min	Unknown
Peak	Unknown	Unknown
Duration	3-6 hr	12 hr

Interactions

Drug/drug:

Alcohol: ↑ CNS depression

Drug classifications

Analgesics: ↑ CNS depression

Antihistamines: ↑ CNS depression

Antidepressants: ↑ CNS depression

MAOI: ↑ hypotension, hyperpyrexia

NURSING CONSIDERATIONS

Assessment

- Assess cough: type, frequency, character including sputum; provide adequate hydration to 2 L/day to decrease viscosity of secretions

Associated nursing diagnoses

✓ Airway clearance, ineffective (uses)

✓ Knowledge deficit (teaching)

Implementation

PO route

- Administer decreased dosage G to elderly patients; their metabolism may be slowed; do not provide water within 30 min of administration because it dilutes drug
- Shake sus before administration

Patient/family education

- Caution patient to avoid driving or other hazardous activities stabilized on this medication; may cause drowsiness, dizziness in some individuals
- Advise patient to avoid smoking, smoke-filled rooms, perfumes, dust, environmental pollutants, cleaners, which increase cough; may use gum, hard candy to prevent dry cough
- Advise patient to avoid alcohol or other CNS depressants while taking this medication; drowsiness will be increased
- Caution patient that any cough lasting over a few days

should be assessed by prescriber

Evaluation

Positive therapeutic outcome
- Absence of dry, irritating cough

dextrose (D-glucose)

Glucose, Glutose, Insta-Glucose, Insulin Reaction

Func. class.: Caloric agent

Pregnancy category **D**

Action: Needed for adequate utilization of amino acids; decreases protein, nitrogen loss; prevents ketosis

Therapeutic Outcome: Provides calories, prevents severe hypoglycemia

Uses: Increases intake of calories; increases fluids in patients unable to take adequate fluids, calories orally; 2.5%-11.5% forms provide calories, increased hydration; 20%-70% forms used to treat severe hypoglycemia

Investigational uses: Varicose veins, acute alcohol intoxication

Dosage and routes

P *Adult and child:* **IV**, depends on individual requirements

Available forms: Inj **IV** 2.5%, 5%, 10%, 20%, 40%, 50%, 60%, 70%; oral gel 40%; chewable tabs 5 g

Side effects/adverse reactions

CNS: Confusion, ***loss of consciousness,*** dizziness
CV: Hypertension, ***CHF, pulmonary edema***
ENDO: Hyperglycemia, rebound hypoglycemia, hyperosmolar syndrome, hyperglycemic nonketotic syndrome
GU: Glycosuria, osmotic diuresis
INTEG: Chills, flushing, warm feeling, rash, urticaria, extravasation necrosis

Contraindications: Hyperglycemia, delirium tremens, hemorrhage (cranial/spinal), CHF

Precautions: Renal, liver, cardiac disease, diabetes mellitus

Pharmacokinetics

Absorption	Well absorbed (PO); completely absorbed (IV)
Distribution	Widely distributed
Metabolism	Unknown
Excretion	Unknown
Half-life	Unknown

Pharmacodynamics

	IV	PO
Onset	Immediate	Rapid
Peak	Immediate	Rapid
Duration	Immediate	Rapid

Interactions

Drug/drug:

Insulin: ↑ need for insulin

Drug classifications

Corticosteroids: Cautiously administer fluids

Hypoglycemics, oral: ↑ need for hypoglycemic

NURSING CONSIDERATIONS

Assessment

- Assess I&O, skin turgor, edema, electrolytes (potassium, sodium, calcium, chloride, magnesium), blood glucose, ammonia, phosphate
- Monitor inj site for extravasation: redness along vein, edema at site, necrosis, pain, hard tender area; site should be changed immediately
- Monitor temp q4h for increased fever, indicating infection; if infection suspected, inf is discontinued and tubing, bottle, catheter tip cultured
- Monitor serum glucose in patients receiving hypertonic glucose 5% and over
- Assess nutritional status: calorie count by dietician; GI system function

Associated nursing diagnoses

- ✓ Nutrition: less than body requirements (uses)
- ✓ Fluid volume excess (adverse reactions)
- ✓ Knowledge deficit (teaching)

Implementation

PO route

- Oral glucose preparations (gel, chewable tabs) are to be used for conscious patients only; serum blood glucose should be monitored after first oral dose; if glucose has not increased by 20 mg/100 ml in 20-30 min, dose should be repeated and serum glucose checked again

IV **IV route**

- Give only protein (4%) and dextrose (up to 12.5%) via peripheral vein; stronger sol requires central **IV** administration
- May be given undiluted via prepared sol; give 10% sol (5 ml/15 sec), 20% sol (1000 ml/3 hr or more), 50% sol (500 ml/30-60 min); too rapid **IV** administration may cause fluid overload and hyperglycemia
- After changing **IV** catheter, change dressing q24h with aseptic technique

Patient/family education

- Teach patient reason for dextrose infusion
- Provide literature and information on when and how to use oral products for hypoglycemia
- Review hypoglycemia/hyperglycemia symptoms
- Review blood glucose monitoring procedure

Evaluation

Positive therapeutic outcome

- Increased weight
- Blood glucose level at normal limits for patient
- Adequate hydration

dezocine
(dez'oh-seen)
Dalgan
Func. class.: Narcotic agonist-antagonist analgesic
Chem. class.: Opioid, synthetic
Pregnancy category **C**

Action: Inhibits ascending pain pathways in limbic system, thalamus, midbrain, hypothalamus by binding to opiate receptor sites, which alters pain perception and response

Therapeutic Outcome: Relief of moderate, severe pain

Uses: Moderate to severe pain

Dosage and routes
Adult: IM 5-20 mg q3-6h, not to exceed 120 mg/day; **IV** 2.5-10 mg q2-4h

Available forms: Inj 5, 10, 15 mg single-dose vials, multiple dose 10 mg/ml

Side effects/adverse reactions
CNS: Drowsiness, dizziness, confusion, sedation, anxiety, headache, depression, delirium, sleep disturbances, dependency
CV: Hypotension, pulse irregularity, hypertension, chest pain, pallor, edema, thrombophlebitis
EENT: Blurred vision, slurred speech, diplopia
GI: Nausea, vomiting, anorexia, constipation, cramps, abdominal pain, dry mouth, diarrhea
GU: Urinary frequency, hesitancy, retention
INTEG: Inj site reactions, pruritus, rash, swelling, chills
RESP: ***Respiratory depression,*** hiccups

Contraindications: Hypersensitivity

Precautions: Addictive personality, pregnancy **C**, lactation, increased intracranial pressure, respiratory depression, hepatic disease, renal disease, P child <18 yr, G elderly, biliary surgery, COPD, sulfite sensitivity

Pharmacokinetics
Absorption	Completely absorbed (IM, IV)
Distribution	Not known
Metabolism	Liver, extensively
Excretion	Kidneys
Half-life	1½-7 hr

Pharmacodynamics
	IM	IV
Onset	½ hr	10 min
Peak	1-2 hr	30 min
Duration	2-4 hr	2-4 hr

Interactions
Drug/drug:
Individual drugs
Alcohol: ↑ respiratory depression, hypotension, sedation
Cimetidine: ↑ recovery
Erythromycin: ↑ recovery
Nalbuphine: ↓ analgesia
Pentazocine: ↓ analgesia

Drug classifications
Antihistamines: ↑ respiratory depression, hypotension
CNS depressants: ↑ respiratory depression, hypotension
MAOI: Do not use 2 wk before dezocine
Phenothiazines: ↑ respiratory depression, hypotension
Sedative/hypnotics: ↑ respiratory depression, hypotension

NURSING CONSIDERATIONS

Assessment

- Assess respiratory status: respiratory depression, character, rate, rhythm; notify prescriber if respirations are <12/min; note CV status, bradycardia, syncope; monitor ECG continuously
- Assess pain: location, intensity, duration, alleviating factors

Associated nursing diagnoses

- ✓ Pain (uses)
- ✓ Sensory-perceptual alteration: visual, auditory (adverse reactions)
- ✓ Breathing pattern, ineffective (adverse reactions)
- ✓ Knowledge deficit (teaching) (preoperatively)

Implementation

IM route

- Give deeply in large muscle mass; rotate sites; do not give SC

IV **IV route**

- Give undiluted ≤5 mg over 2-3 min

Patient/family education

- Caution patients to avoid CNS depressants: alcohol, sedative/hypnotics for at least 24 hr after taking this drug
- Discuss with patient that dizziness, drowsiness, and confusion are common; to avoid getting up without assistance
- Advise patient to make position changes to lessen orthostatic hypotension

Evaluation

Positive therapeutic outcome

- Decreased pain perception

Treatment of overdose: Narcan 0.2-0.8 **IV**, O_2, **IV** fluids, vasopressors

diazepam 🗝

(dye-az'e-pam)
diazepam, diazepam Intensol, D-Tran ✤, E-Pam ✤, Meval ✤, Novodipam ✤, Stress-Pam ✤, Valium, Valrelease, Vazepam, Vivol ✤, Zetran

Func. class.: Antianxiety
Chem. class.: Benzodiazepine

Pregnancy category **D**
Controlled substance schedule **IV**

Action: Potentiates the actions of GABA, especially in limbic system, reticular formation; enhances presympathetic inhibition, inhibits spinal polysynaptic afferent paths

➡ **Therapeutic Outcome:** Decreased anxiety, restlessness, insomnia

Uses: Anxiety, acute alcohol withdrawal, adjunct in seizure disorders; preoperative skeletal muscle relaxation

Dosage and routes

Anxiety/convulsive disorders

Adult: PO 2-10 mg tid-qid; ext rel 15-30 mg qd

P *Child >6 mo:* PO 1-2.5 mg tid-qid

Tetanic muscle spasms

P *Child <5 yr:* IM/**IV** 5-10 mg q3-4h prn

P *Infants >30 days:* IM/**IV** 1-2 mg q3-4h prn

Status epilepticus

Adult: **IV** bol 5-20 mg, 2 mg/min; may repeat q5-10 min, not to exceed 60 mg; may repeat in 30 min if seizures reappear

P *Child:* **IV** bol 0.1-0.3 mg/kg (1 mg/min over 3 min); may repeat q15 min × 2 doses

Available forms: Tabs 2, 5, 10 mg; ext rel caps 15 mg, IM/**IV** inj

Side effects/adverse reactions

CNS: Dizziness, drowsiness, confusion, headache, anxiety, tremors, stimulation, fatigue, depression, insomnia, hallucinations

CV: Orthostatic hypotension, ***ECG changes, tachycardia,*** hypotension

EENT: Blurred vision, tinnitus, mydriasis

GI: Constipation, dry mouth, nausea, vomiting, anorexia, diarrhea

INTEG: Rash, dermatitis, itching

Contraindications: Hypersensitivity to benzodiazepines, narrow angle glaucoma, psychosis, pregnancy **D**

G **Precautions:** Elderly, debilitated, hepatic disease, renal disease

Pharmacokinetics

Absorption	Rapid (PO); erratic (IM)
Distribution	Widely distributed; crosses blood-brain barrier, placenta
Metabolism	Liver, extensively
Excretion	Kidneys, breast milk
Half-life	20-80 hr

Pharmacodynamics

	PO	IM	IV
Onset	½ hr	15 min	5 min
Peak	1-2 hr	½-1½ hr	15 min
Duration	2-3 hr	1-1½ hr	15 min

Interactions

Drug/drug:

Individual drugs

Alcohol: ↑ CNS depression

Cimetidine: ↓ effect of diazepam

Disulfiram: ↓ effect of diazepam

Rifampin: ↓ effect of diazepam

Valproic acid: ↓ effect of diazepam

Drug classifications

CNS depressants: ↑ CNS depression

Narcotic analgesics: ↓ effects of diazepam

Oral contraceptives: ↓ effects of diazepam

Lab test interferences

Increase: AST (SGOT)/ALT (SGPT), serum bilirubin
False increase: 17-OHCS
Decrease: RAIU

NURSING CONSIDERATIONS

Assessment

- Assess degree of anxiety; what precipitates anxiety and whether drug controls symptoms; other signs of anxiety: dilated pupils, inability to sleep, restlessness, inability to focus
- Assess for alcohol withdrawal symptoms, including hallucinations (visual, auditory), delirium, irritability, agitation, fine to coarse tremors
- Monitor B/P (with patient lying, standing), pulse, respiratory rate; if systolic B/P drops 20 mm Hg, hold drug, notify prescriber; monitor respirations q5-15 min if given **IV**
- Monitor blood studies: CBC during long-term therapy; blood dyscrasias have occurred (rarely)
- Monitor for seizure control; type, duration and intensity of convulsions; what precipitates seizures
- Monitor hepatic studies: AST (SGOT), ALT (SGPT), bilirubin, creatinine, LDH, alkaline phosphatase
- Assess mental status: mood, sensorium, affect, sleeping pattern, drowsiness, dizziness, suicidal tendencies and ability of drug to control these symptoms; check for tolerance, withdrawal symptoms: headache, nausea, vomiting, muscle pain, weakness after long-term use

Associated nursing diagnoses

- ✓ Anxiety (uses)
- ✓ Injury, risk of (uses, adverse reactions)
- ✓ Coping, ineffective individual (uses)
- ✓ Knowledge deficit (teaching)
- ✓ Noncompliance (teaching)

Implementation

PO route

- Give with food or milk for GI symptoms; crush tab if patient is unable to swallow medication whole; do not crush ext rel caps; use sugarless gum, hard candy, frequent sips of water for dry mouth
- Reduce narcotic dosage by ⅓ if given concomitantly with diazepam
- Check to see PO medication has been swallowed

IV **IV route**

- Administer **IV** into large vein; do not dilute or mix with any other drug; give **IV** 5 mg or less/1 min or total dose P over 3 min or more (children, infants); cont inf is not recommended
- Check **IV** site for thrombosis or phlebitis, which may occur rapidly

Y-*site incompatibilities:*

Hydromorphone, fluconazole foscarnate, heparin, pancuronium, potassium chloride, vecuronium, vitamin B with C

Y-*site compatibilities:*

Dobutamine, nafcillin, quinidine

Syringe incompatibilities:
Benzquinamide, doxapram, glycopyrrolate, heparin, nalbuphine

Syringe compatibility:
Cimetidine

Patient/family education

- Advise patient that drug may be taken with food; that drug is not to be used for everyday stress or used longer than 4 mo unless directed by prescriber; take no more than prescribed amount; may be habit forming
- Caution patient to avoid OTC preparations unless approved by a prescriber; to avoid alcohol, other psychotropic medications unless prescribed; not to discontinue medication abruptly after long-term use
- Inform patient to avoid driving, activities that require alertness; drowsiness may occur; to rise slowly or fainting G may occur, especially in elderly
- Inform patient that drowsiness may worsen at beginning of treatment

Evaluation

Positive therapeutic outcome
- Decreased anxiety, restlessness, insomnia

Treatment of overdose: Lavage, VS, supportive care

diazoxide

(dye-az-ox'ide)
Hyperstat, Proglycem
Func. class.: Hyperglycemic
Chem. class.: Vasodilator
Pregnancy category **C**

Action: Decreases release of insulin from β-cells in pancreas, resulting in an increase in blood glucose; relaxes vascular smooth muscle (peripheral arterioles)

Therapeutic Outcome: Decreased B/P, increased blood glucose

Uses: Hypoglycemia caused by hyperinsulinism; emergency treatment of hypertension

Dosage and routes

Hypoglycemia

P *Adult and child:* PO 3-8 mg/kg/day in 2-3 divided doses q8-12h

P *Infants and neonates:* PO 8-15 mg/kg/day in 2-3 divided doses 8-12h

Hypertension

P *Adult and child:* **IV** 1-3 mg/kg q5-15 min; max 150 mg/dose

Available forms: Caps 50 mg; oral susp 50 mg/ml; inj 15 mg/ml, 300 mg/20 ml

Side effects/adverse reactions

CNS: Headache, weakness, malaise, anxiety, dizziness, insomnia, paresthesia

CV: Tachycardia, palpitations, hypotension, transient hypertension
EENT: Diplopia, cataracts, ring scotoma, subconjunctival hemorrhage, lacrimation
GI: Nausea, vomiting, anorexia, abdominal pain, transient loss of taste, diarrhea
GU: Reversible nephrotic syndrome, decreased urinary output, hematuria
HEMA: ***Thrombocytopenia, leukopenia,*** eosinophilia, decreased Hgb, Hct
INTEG: Increased hair growth or loss of scalp hair, rash, dermatitis, herpes
META: Hyperuricemia, sodium/fluid retention, ketoacidosis, hyperglycemia, azotemia

Contraindications: Hypersensitivity to this drug or thiazides, functional hypoglycemia

Precautions: Pregnancy **C**, lactation, renal disease, diabetes mellitus, CV disease, gout

Pharmacokinetics

Absorption	Well absorbed (PO); completely absorbed (IV)
Distribution	Crosses blood-brain barrier, placenta
Metabolism	Liver (50%)
Excretion	Kidney, unchanged (50%)
Half-life	20-36 hr

Pharmacodynamics

	PO	IV
Onset	1 hr	1-2 min
Peak	8-12 hr	5 min
Duration	8 hr	3-12 hr

Interactions

Drug/drug:

Individual drugs

Coumadin: ↑ effects
Estrogen/progesterone: ↑ hyperglycemia
Guanethidine: ↑ effects
Phenytoin: ↑ hyperglycemia
Warfarin: ↑ effects

Drug classifications

Antihypertensives: ↑ effects
Corticosteroids: ↑ hyperglycemia
Diuretics: ↑ hyperglycemia

NURSING CONSIDERATIONS

Assessment

- Assess for allergies to sulfonamide; cross-sensitivity may occur
- Assess B/P q5 min for 2 hr, then q1h for 2 hr, then q4h; pulse, jugular venous distention q4h
- Monitor electrolytes, blood studies: potassium, sodium, chloride, carbon dioxide, CBC, serum glucose
- Monitor weight daily, I&O; edema in feet, legs daily; check skin turgor, dryness of mucous membranes for hydration status
- Assess for rales, dyspnea, orthopnea; peripheral edema, fatigue, weight gain, jugular vein distention (congestive heart failure)
- Assess for signs of hyperglycemia: acetone breath, increased urinary output, severe thirst, lethargy, dizziness

Associated nursing diagnoses

✓ Cardiac output, decreased (adverse reactions)

- ✓ Injury, risk for (side effects)
- ✓ Knowledge deficit (teaching)

Implementation

PO route

- Shake susp before using
- Store protected from light and heat

IV **IV route**

- Give by direct **IV** over 30 sec or less; may repeat q5-15 min until desired response; do not administer dark solution
- Give to patient in recumbent position; keep in that position for 1 hr after

Syringe compatibility:
Heparin

Y-site incompatibilities:
Hydralazine, propranolol

Evaluation

Positive therapeutic outcome

- Decreased B/P in hypertension

Treatment of overdose: Administer levarterenol, dopamine, or norepinephrine for hypotension, dialysis

dibucaine (topical)

(dye'byoo-kane)

dibucaine, Nupercainal

Func. class.: Topical anesthetic

Chem. class.: Amide

Pregnancy category **C**

Action: Inhibits conduction of nerve impulses from sensory nerves

➔ **Therapeutic Outcome:** Decreasing inflammation, itching

Uses: Oral irritation, sore throat, toothache, cold sore, canker sore, sunburn, minor cuts, insect bites, pain, itching

Dosage and routes

P *Adult and child:* Top apply qid as needed; rec insert tid and after each BM

Available forms: Cream 0.5%; rec or top oint 1%

Side effects/adverse reactions

INTEG: Rash, irritation, sensitization

Contraindications: Hypersensitivity, P infants <1 yr, application to large areas

P **Precautions:** Child <6 yr, sepsis, pregnancy **C**, denuded skin

Pharmacokinetics

Absorption	Poorly absorbed
Distribution	Unknown
Metabolism	Plasma, liver cholinesterase
Excretion	Unknown
Half-life	Unknown

Pharmacodynamics

	TOP
Onset	1 min
Peak	Unknown
Duration	½-1 hr

Interactions: None

NURSING CONSIDERATIONS

Assessment

- Assess pain: location, duration, characteristics before and after administration
- Assess for infection: redness, drainage, inflammation; this drug should not be used until infection is treated

Associated nursing diagnoses

✓ Pain (uses)
✓ Knowledge deficit (teaching)

Implementation

Top route
- Apply to gums as needed for teething pain; rub on gums with finger or cotton swab

Spray route
- Use by spraying in the back of the throat
- Store in tight, light-resistant container; do not freeze, puncture, or incinerate aerosol container

Patient/family education

- Caution patient to avoid contact with eyes
- Instruct patient not to use for prolonged periods: use for <1 wk; if condition remains, prescriber should be contacted

Evaluation

Positive therapeutic outcome
- Absence of redness, swelling, pain of affected area

diclofenac

(dye-kloe'fen-ak)

Voltaren, Voltaren SR ✱

Func. class.: Nonsteroidal antiinflammatory

Chem. class.: Phenylacetic acid

Pregnancy category B

Action: Inhibits prostaglandin synthesis by decreasing enzyme needed for biosynthesis; analgesic, antiinflammatory, antipyretic properties

➔ **Therapeutic Outcome:** Decreased pain, inflammation

Uses: Acute, chronic rheumatoid arthritis, osteoarthritis, ankylosing spondylitis; ophthalmic: to decrease inflammation after cataract extraction

Dosage and routes

Osteoarthritis

Adult: PO 100-125 mg/day in 2-3 divided doses; after therapeutic response occurs, decrease to least amount to control symptoms

Rheumatoid arthritis

Adult: PO 150-200 mg/day in 2-4 divided doses; after therapeutic response decrease to lowest amount to control symptoms

Ankylosing spondylitis

Adult: PO 100-125 mg/day in 4-5 divided doses; give 25 mg qid and 25 mg hs if needed

After cataract surgery

Adult: Ophth i gtt of 0.1% sol qid × 2 wk beginning 24 hr after surgery

Available forms: Enteric coated tabs 25, 50, 75 mg; ext rel tabs 75, 100 mg; ophth sol 1%

Side effects/adverse reactions

CNS: Dizziness, drowsiness, fatigue, tremors, confusion, insomnia, anxiety, depression, nervousness, paresthesia, muscle weakness

CV: **CHF**, tachycardia, peripheral edema, palpitations, dysrhythmias, hypotension, hypertension, fluid retention

EENT: Tinnitus, hearing loss, blurred vision

GI: Nausea, anorexia, vomiting, diarrhea, ***jaundice, cholestatic hepatitis,*** constipation, flatulence, cramps, dry mouth, peptic ulcer, GI bleeding

GU: Nephrotoxicity: dysuria, hematuria, oliguria, azotemia, cystitis, UTI

HEMA: Blood dyscrasias, epistaxis, bruising

INTEG: Purpura, rash, pruritus, sweating, erythema, petechiae, photosensitivity, alopecia

RESP: Dyspnea, hemoptysis, pharyngitis, ***bronchospasm, laryngeal edema,*** rhinitis, shortness of breath

Contraindications: Hypersensitivity to aspirin, iodides, other NSAIDs, asthma

Precautions: Pregnancy **B** 1st, 2nd trimester, lactation, **P** children, bleeding disorders, GI disorders, cardiac disorders, hypersensitivity to other antiinflammatory agents

Pharmacokinetics

Absorption	Well absorbed (PO, ophth)
Distribution	Crosses placenta; 90% bound to plasma proteins
Metabolism	Liver (50%)
Excretion	Breast milk
Half-life	1-2 hr

Pharmacodynamics

	PO	OPHTH
Onset	Unknown	Unknown
Peak	2-3 hr	Unknown
Duration	Unknown	Unknown

Interactions

Drug/drug:

Individual drugs

Acetaminophen (long-term use): ↑ renal reactions

Alcohol: ↑ adverse reactions

Aspirin: ↓ effectiveness, ↑ adverse reactions

Coumarin: ↑ anticoagulant effects

Digoxin: ↑ toxicity, ↑ levels

Insulin: ↓ insulin effect

Lithium: ↑ toxicity

Methotrexate: ↑ toxicity

Phenytoin: ↑ toxicity

Probenecid: ↑ toxicity

Sulfonylurea: ↑ toxicity

Drug classifications

Anticoagulants: ↑ risk of bleeding

Antihypertensives: ↓ effect of antihypertensives

Antineoplastics: ↑ risk of hematologic toxicity

ß-Blockers: ↑ antihypertension

Cephalosporins: ↑ risk of bleeding

Glucocorticoids: ↑ adverse reactions
Hypoglycemics: ↓ hypoglycemic effect
Diuretics: ↓ effectiveness of diuretics
NSAIDs: ↑ adverse reactions
Potassium supplements: ↑ adverse reactions
Radiation: ↑ risk of hematologic toxicity
Sulfonamides: ↑ toxicity

NURSING CONSIDERATIONS

Assessment

- Assess for pain of rheumatoid arthritis, osteoarthritis, ankylosing spondylitis; check ROM, inflammation of joints, characteristics of pain
- Assess ophth patients for pain, inflammation, redness, swelling
- Monitor blood counts during therapy; watch for decreasing platelets; if low, therapy may need to be discontinued, restarted after hematologic recovery; and for blood dyscrasias (thrombocytopenia): bruising, fatigue, bleeding, poor healing

Associated nursing diagnoses

✓ Pain (uses)
✓ Mobility, impaired physical (uses)
✓ Injury, risk for (side effects)
✓ Knowledge deficit (teaching)

Implementation

PO route
- Administer with food or milk to decrease gastric symptoms; do not crush, dissolve or chew enteric coated or sus rel caps

Ophth route
- Administer with patient recumbent or tilting head back; pull down on lower lid; when conjunctival sac is exposed, instill 1 drop; wait a few minutes before instilling other drops

Patient/family education

- Teach patient that drug must be continued for prescribed time to be effective; to avoid aspirin, alcoholic beverages
- Caution patient to report bleeding, bruising, fatigue, malaise, since blood dyscrasia do occur
- Instruct patient to use caution when driving; drowsiness, dizziness may occur
- Teach patient to take with a full glass of water to enhance absorption; do not crush, break, or chew

Evaluation

Positive therapeutic outcome
- Decreased pain in arthritic conditions
- Decreased inflammation in arthritic conditions
- Decreased ocular irritation

dicloxacillin

(dye-klox-a-sill'in)

dicloxacillin sodium, Dycill, Dynapen, Pathocil

Func. class.: Broad-spectrum antibiotic

Chem. class.: Penicillinase-resistant penicillin

Pregnancy category B

Action: Interferes with cell wall replication of susceptible organisms; osmotically unstable cell wall swells, bursts from osmotic pressure

Uses: Penicillinase-producing staphylococci, streptococci; respiratory tract, skin, skin structure infections; sinusitis

Therapeutic Outcome: Bactericidal effects for the following: gram-positive cocci *Staphylococcus aureus, Streptococcus pyogenes, S. viridans, S. faecalis, S. bovis, S. pneumoniae;* infections caused by penicillinase-producing *Staphylococcus* organisms

Dosage and routes

Adult: PO 0.5-4 g/day in divided doses q6h

P *Child:* PO 12.5-25 mg/kg in divided doses q6h, max 4 g/d

Available forms: Caps 125, 250, 500 mg; powder for oral susp 62.5 mg/5 ml

Side effects/adverse reactions

CNS: Lethargy, hallucinations, anxiety, depression, twitching, ***coma, convulsions***

GI: Nausea, vomiting, diarrhea, increased AST (SGOT), ALT (SGPT), abdominal pain, glossitis, pseudomembranous colitis

GU: Oliguria, proteinuria, hematuria, vaginitis, moniliasis, glomerulonephritis

HEMA: Anemia, increased bleeding time, ***bone marrow depression, granulocytopenia***

SYST: Anaphylaxis

Contraindications: Hypersensitivity to penicillins; neonates

Precautions: Hypersensitivity to cephalosporins, pregnancy **B**

Pharmacokinetics

Absorption	Rapid, incomplete (35%-75%)
Distribution	Widely distributed; crosses placenta
Metabolism	Liver (6%-10%)
Excretion	Kidneys, unchanged (60%); breast milk
Half-life	½-1 hr, increased in hepatic renal disease

Pharmacodynamics

	PO
Onset	½ hr
Peak	½-2 hr

Interactions

Drug/drug:

Individual drugs

Probenecid: ↑ dicloxacillin levels, ↓ renal excretion

Drug classifications

Oral anticoagulants: ↑ anticoagulant effects

Drug/food:

Food, carbonated drinks, citrus fruit juices: ↓ absorption

Lab test interferences

False positive: Urine glucose, urine protein

NURSING CONSIDERATIONS

Assessment

- Assess patient for previous sensitivity reaction to penicillins or other cephalosporins; cross-sensitivity between penicillins and cephalosporins is common.
- Assess patient for signs and symptoms of infection including characteristics of wounds, sputum, urine, stool, WBC >10,000, fever; obtain baseline information and during treatment
- Obtain C&S before beginning drug therapy to identify if correct treatment has been initiated
- Assess for allergic reactions: rash, urticaria, pruritus, chills, fever, joint pain may occur a few days after therapy begins; epinephrine and resuscitation equipment should be available for anaphylactic reaction
- Identify urine output; if decreasing, notify prescriber (may indicate nephrotoxicity); check for increased BUN, creatinine
- Monitor blood studies: AST (SGOT), ALT (SGPT), CBC, Hct, bilirubin, LDH, alkaline phosphatase, Coombs' test monthly if patient is on long-term therapy
- Monitor electrolytes: potassium, sodium, chloride monthly if patient is on long-term therapy
- Assess bowel pattern qd; if severe diarrhea occurs, drug should be discontinued; may indicate pseudomembranous colitis
- Monitor for bleeding: ecchymosis, bleeding gums, hematuria, stool guaiac daily if on long-term therapy
- Assess for overgrowth of infection: perineal itching, fever, malaise, redness, pain, swelling, drainage, rash, diarrhea, change in cough, sputum

Associated nursing diagnoses

- ✓ Infection, risk for (uses)
- ✓ Diarrhea (side effects)
- ✓ Knowledge deficit (teaching)
- ✓ Noncompliance (teaching)
- ✓ Injury, risk for (side effects)

Implementation

PO route

- Give in even doses around the clock; if GI upset occurs, give with food; drug must be given for 10-14 days to ensure organism death and prevent superinfection; store in airtight container
- Shake susp; store in refrigerator for 2 wk or 1 wk at room temp

Patient/family education

- Teach patient to report sore throat, bruising, bleeding, joint pain; may indicate blood dyscrasias (rare)
- Advise patient to contact prescriber if vaginal itching, loose, foul-smelling stools, furry tongue occur; may indicate superinfection
- Instruct patient to take all medication prescribed for the length of time ordered
- Advise patient to notify prescriber of diarrhea with blood or pus, which may indicate pseudomembranous colitis

Evaluation

Positive therapeutic outcome
- Absence of signs/symptoms of infection (WBC <10,000, temp WNL, absence of red draining wounds)
- Reported improvement in symptoms of infection

Treatment of anaphylaxis:
Withdraw drug, maintain airway, administer epinephrine, aminophylline, O_2, **IV** corticosteroids

didanosine (ddI, dideoxyinosine)
(dye-dan'o-seen)
Videx, DDL, dideoxyinosine
Func. class.: Antiviral
Chem. class.: Synthetic purine nucleoside of deoxyadenosine
Pregnancy category **B**

Action: Nucleoside analog incorporating into cellular DNA by viral reverse transcriptase, thereby terminating the cellular DNA chain that prevents viral replication

Therapeutic Outcome: Antiviral against the retroviruses, primarily HIV

Uses: Advanced HIV, or AIDS, infections in adults and P children who have been unable to use zidovudine or who have not responded to treatment

Dosage and routes
Adult: >75 kg, PO 300 mg tabs or 375 mg buffered powder bid; 50-74 kg, 200 mg tabs or 250 mg buffered powder bid; 35-49 kg, 125 mg tabs or 167 mg buffered powder bid

P *Child:* 1.1-1.4 m^2, PO 100 mg tabs or 125 mg pedi powder bid; 0.8-1 m^2, 75 mg tabs or 94 mg pedi powder bid; 0.5-0.7 m^2, 50 mg tabs or 62 mg pedi powder bid; <0.4 m^2, 25 mg tabs or 31 mg pedi powder bid

Available forms: Buffered chewable/dispersable tabs 25, 50, 100, 150 mg; buffered powder for oral sol 100, 167, 250, 375 mg; pedi powder for oral sol 2, 4 g

Side effects/adverse reactions
CNS: Peripheral neuropathy, seizures, confusion, anxiety, hypertonia, abnormal thinking, asthenia, insomnia, *CNS depression,* pain, dizziness, chills, fever
CV: Hypertension, vasodilatation, dysrhythmia, syncope, CHF, palpitations
EENT: Ear pain, otitis, photophobia, visual impairment
GI: Pancreatitis, diarrhea, nausea, vomiting, abdominal pain, constipation, stomatitis, dyspepsia, liver abnormalities, flatulence, taste perversion, dry mouth, oral thrush, melena, increased ALT (SGPT), AST (SGOT), alkaline phosphatase, amylase
GU: Increased bilirubin, uric acid

HEMA: ***Leukopenia, granulocytopenia, thrombocytopenia, anemia***
INTEG: Rash, pruritus, alopecia, ecchymosis, hemorrhage, petechiae, sweating
MS: Myalgia, arthritis, myopathy, muscular atrophy
RESP: Cough, pneumonia, dyspnea, asthma, epistaxis, hypoventilation, sinusitis

Contraindications: Hypersensitivity

Precautions: Renal, hepatic disease, pregnancy **B,** lactation, P children, sodium-restricted diets, elevated amylase, preexistent peripheral neuropathy

Pharmacokinetics

Absorption	Rapidly absorbed (up to 40%)
Distribution	Unknown
Metabolism	Not metabolized
Excretion	Kidneys (55%)
Half-life	0.8-1.6 hr, shorter in children

Pharmacodynamics

	PO
Onset	Unknown
Peak	Up to 1 hr
Duration	Unknown

Interactions

Drug/drug:

Individual drugs

Atropine: ↑ anticholinergic effects
Dapsone: ↓ absorption of dapsone
Disopyramide:↑ anticholinergic effects
Ketoconazole: ↓ absorption of ketoconazole
Quinidine: ↑ anticholinergic effects

Drug classifications

Antidepressants, tricyclic: ↑ anticholinergic effects
Antihistamines: ↑ anticholinergic effects
Fluoroquinolones: ↓ absorption of fluoroquinolones
Phenothiazines: ↑ anticholinergic effects
Tetracyclines: ↓ absorption of tetracyclines

Drug/food: ↓ absorption when used with food

NURSING CONSIDERATIONS

Assessment

- Assess for peripheral neuropathy: tingling or pain in hands and feet, distal numbness; if these occur during therapy drug may be decreased or discontinued
- Assess for pancreatitis: abdominal pain, nausea, vomiting, elevated liver enzymes; drug should be discontinued, since condition can be fatal
- P Assess children by dilated retinal examination q6mo to rule out retinal depigmentation
- Monitor CBC, differential, platelet count monthly; withhold drug if WBC is <4000 or platelet count is <75,000; notify prescriber of results
- Monitor renal function studies: BUN, serum uric acid, urine CrCl before, during therapy; these may be elevated throughout treatment
- Monitor temp q4h; may indicate beginning infection
- Monitor liver function tests before, during therapy (bilirubin, AST (SGOT), ALT (SGPT), amylase, alkaline

phosphatase) as needed or monthly

Associated nursing diagnoses

- ✓ Infection, risk for (uses)
- ✓ Injury, risk for (adverse reactions)
- ✓ Knowledge deficit (teaching)

Implementation

PO route

- Give on empty stomach, 1 hr ac or 2 hr pc, q12h; food decreases effectiveness of drug
- Patient should chew tabs; may be crushed and mixed with water
- P • Ped powder for oral sol should be prepared in the pharmacy; shake before using
- Packets for oral sol must be mixed with ½ glass of water; stir until dissolved

Patient/family education

- Advise patient to take on empty stomach; not to take dapsone at same time as DDL; to use exactly as prescribed
- Instruct patient to report signs of infection: increased temp, sore throat, flu symptoms; to avoid crowds and those with known infections
- Instruct patient to report signs of anemia: fatigue, headache, faintness, shortness of breath, irritability
- Instruct patient to report bleeding; avoid use of razors and commercial mouthwash
- Advise patient that hair may be lost during therapy; a wig or hair piece may make patient feel better (rare)
- Caution patient to avoid OTC products and other medications without approval of prescriber
- Teach patient not to have any sexual contact without use of a condom; needles should not be shared; blood from infected individual should not come in contact with another's mucous membranes

Evaluation

Positive therapeutic outcome

- Absence of opportunistic infection, symptoms of HIV

dienestrol

(dye-en-ess'trole)

D V, Ortho Dienestrol

Func. class.: Estrogen

Chem. class.: Nonsteroidal synthetic estrogen

Pregnancy category **X**

Action: Needed for adequate functioning of female reproductive system and maintenance of secondary sex characteristics; it affects release of pituitary gonadotropins, inhibits ovulation, promotes adequate calcium use in bone structures; reduces cholesterol, protein synthesis, sodium, and water

➡ Therapeutic Outcome: Decreased vaginal, vulval itching, dryness, redness, inflammation in postmenopausal women

Uses: Atrophic vaginitis, kraurosis vulvae

Dosage and routes

Adult: Vag cream 1-2 applications qd × 2 wk, then ½ dose × 2 wk, then 1 application

Available forms: Vag cream 0.01%

Side effects/adverse reactions

CNS: Dizziness, headache, migraines, depression
CV: Hypotension, thrombophlebitis, edema, ***thromboembolism, stroke, pulmonary embolism, MI***
EENT: Contact lens intolerance, increased myopia, astigmatism
GI: Nausea, vomiting, diarrhea, anorexia, pancreatitis, cramps, constipation, increased appetite, increased weight, ***cholestatic jaundice***
GU: Amenorrhea, cervical erosion, breakthrough bleeding, dysmenorrhea, vaginal candidiasis, breast changes
INTEG: Rash, urticaria, acne, hirsutism, alopecia, oily skin, seborrhea, purpura, melasma
META: Folic acid deficiency, hypercalcemia, hyperglycemia

Contraindications: Breast cancer, thromboembolic disorders, reproductive cancer, genital bleeding (abnormal, undiagnosed), pregnancy **X**

Precautions: Hypertension, asthma, blood dyscrasias, gallbladder disease, CHF, diabetes mellitus, bone disease, depression, migraine headache, convulsive disorders, hepatic disease, renal disease, family history of cancer of the breast or reproductive tract

Pharmacokinetics

Absorption	Through mucous membranes
Distribution	Widely distributed, crosses placenta
Metabolism	Liver
Excretion	Kidneys
Half-life	Unknown

Pharmacodynamics

Onset	Unknown
Peak	Unknown
Duration	Unknown

Interactions

Drug/drug:

Individual drugs
Phenylbutazone: ↓ action of phenylbutazone
Rifampin: ↓ action of rifampin
Drug classifications
Anticoagulants: ↓ action of anticoagulants
Anticonvulsants: ↓ action of chlorotrianisene
Antidepressants, tricyclic: ↑ toxicity
Barbiturates: ↓ action of dienestrol
Corticosteroids: ↑ action of corticosteroids
Oral hypoglycemics: ↓ action of hypoglycemics

NURSING CONSIDERATIONS

Assessment

• Monitor urine glucose in patient with diabetes; increased urine glucose may occur
• Monitor weight daily; notify prescriber if weekly weight gain is >5 lb; if increased, diuretic may be ordered; monitor I&O ratio; be alert for decreasing

urinary output and increasing edema; check for hypertension, cardiac symptoms, jaundice
• Monitor B/P q4h; watch for increase caused by water and sodium retention
• Obtain liver function studies, including AST (SGOT), ALT (SGPT), bilirubin, alkaline phosphatase
• Assess mental status: affect, mood and behavioral changes, aggression, occur frequently

Associated nursing diagnoses

✓ Sexual dysfunction (uses)
✓ Injury, risk for physical (side effects)
✓ Knowledge deficit (teaching)

Implementation

Vag route
• Use at bedtime for better absorption

Patient/family education

• Teach patient how to fill applicator and insert cream; patient should lie down for 30 min after application; use of a sanitary napkin is recommended
• Instruct patient to weigh weekly, report gain >5 lb; demonstrate how to check for peripheral edema
• Advise female patient to report breast lumps, vaginal bleeding, edema, jaundice, dark urine, clay-colored stools, dyspnea, headache, blurred vision, abdominal pain, numbness, stiffness, or pain in legs, chest; male to report impotence or gynecomastia
• Caution patient to check with prescriber before using OTC drugs
• Instruct patient to stop using drug and report to prescriber if pregnancy is suspected

Evaluation

Positive therapeutic outcome
• Decreased signs and symptoms of atrophic vaginitis including itching, inflammation, redness

diethylstilbestrol

(dye-eth-il-stil-bess′trole)
DES, diethylstilbestrol, Honvol ✱, Stilphostrol
Func. class.: Estrogen
Chem. class.: Nonsteroidal synthetic estrogen
Pregnancy category X

Action: Needed for adequate functioning of female reproductive system; it affects release of pituitary gonadotropins, inhibits ovulation, promotes adequate calcium use in bone structures; responsible for maintenance of water and secondary sex characteristics; lowers cholesterol, retention of water and sodium

Therapeutic Outcome: Decreased vaginal, vulval itching, dryness, redness, inflammation; decreased spread of malignant cells

Uses: Postmenopausal breast cancer, prostatic cancer

Dosage and routes

Prostatic cancer

Adult: PO 1-3 mg qd, then 1 mg qd; PO 50-200 mg tid (diphosphate); IM 5 mg 2 times/wk, then 4 mg 2 times/wk; **IV** 0.25-1 g qd × 5 days, then 1-2 times/wk

Breast cancer (postmenopausal)

Adult: PO 15 mg qd

Available forms: Tabs 1, 5 mg; diethylstilbestrol diphosphate tabs 50 mg; inj 0.25 g

Side effects/adverse reactions

CNS: Dizziness, headache, migraines, depression
CV: Hypotension, thrombophlebitis, edema, ***thromboembolism, stroke, pulmonary embolism, MI***
EENT: Contact lens intolerance, increased myopia, astigmatism
GI: Nausea, vomiting, diarrhea, anorexia, pancreatitis, cramps, constipation, increased appetite, increased weight, ***cholestatic jaundice***
GU: Amenorrhea, cervical erosion, breakthrough bleeding, dysmenorrhea, vaginal candidiasis, breast changes, *gynecomastia, testicular atrophy, impotence*
INTEG: Rash, urticaria, acne, hirsutism, alopecia, oily skin, seborrhea, purpura, melasma
META: Folic acid deficiency, hypercalcemia, hyperglycemia

Contraindications: Breast cancer, thromboembolic disorders, reproductive cancer, genital bleeding (abnormal, undiagnosed), pregnancy **X**

Precautions: Hypertension, asthma, blood dyscrasias, gallbladder disease, CHF, diabetes mellitus, bone disease–blocking agents

Pharmacokinetics

Absorption	Well absorbed
Distribution	Widely distributed; crosses placenta
Metabolism	Liver
Excretion	Kidneys
Half-life	Unknown

Pharmacodynamics

	PO/IV
Onset	Unknown
Peak	Unknown
Duration	Unknown

Interactions

Drug/drug:

Individual drugs

Phenylbutazone: ↓ action of phenylbutazone
Rifampin: ↓ action of diethylstilbestrol

Drug classifications

Anticoagulants: ↓ action of anticoagulants
Antidepressants, tricyclic: ↑ toxicity
Barbiturates: ↓ action of diethylstilbestrol
Corticosteroids: ↑ action of diethylstilbestrol
Oral hypoglycemics: ↓ action of hypoglycemics

Lab test interferences

Increase: BSP retention test, PBI, T_4, serum sodium, platelet aggregation, thyroxine-binding globulin (TBG), pro-

thrombin, factors VII, VIII, IX, X, triglycerides
Decrease: Serum folate, serum triglyceride, T_3 resin uptake test, GTT, antithrombin III, pregnanediol, metyrapone test
False positive: LE prep, ANA

NURSING CONSIDERATIONS

Assessment

- Monitor urine glucose in patient with diabetes; increased urine glucose may occur; check weight daily; notify prescriber if weekly weight gain is >5 lb; if increased, diuretic may be ordered; monitor I&O ratio; be alert for decreasing urinary output and increasing edema
- Monitor B/P q4h; watch for increase caused by water and sodium retention; check liver function studies, including AST (SGOT), ALT (SGPT), bilirubin, alkaline phosphatase
- Assess edema, hypertension, cardiac symptoms, jaundice
- Assess mental status: affect, mood, behavioral changes, aggression

Associated nursing diagnoses

✓ Sexual dysfunction (uses)
✓ Injury, risk for physical (teaching)

Implementation

PO route
- Give titrated dosage; provide food or milk to decrease GI symptoms
- Give in one dose in AM for prostatic cancer

IV **IV route**
- Give IV after diluting in 300 mg of dextrose or saline inj; give at a rate of 1-2 ml/min × 15 min; may increase rate to complete inf 1 hr after starting

Patient/family education

- Instruct patient to weigh weekly, report gain >5 lb
- Teach female patient to report breast lumps, vaginal bleeding, edema, jaundice, dark urine, clay-colored stools, dyspnea, headache, blurred vision, abdominal pain, numbness, stiffness, or pain in legs, chest pain; male to report impotence or gynecomastia
- Advise patient to check with prescriber before using OTC drugs; to take medication as prescribed; do not double doses; if dose is missed take as soon as remembered

Evaluation

Positive therapeutic outcome
- Decrease in tumor size in prostatic cancer, breast cancer

digitoxin

(di-ji-tox'in)
Crystodigin, digitoxin
Func. class.: Antidysrhythmic, cardiac glycoside, cardiotonic
Chem. class.: Digitalis preparation
Pregnancy category **C**

Action: Acts by increased influx of calcium ions from extracellular to intracellular cytoplasm, increasing force of contraction and cardiac output; decreases conduction velocity through AV node; prolongs effective refractory period

⇒ **Therapeutic Outcome:** Positive inotropic and negative chronotropic effect

Uses: Rapid digitalization in CHF, atrial fibrillation, atrial flutter, atrial tachycardia

Dosage and routes

P ***Adult and child >12 yr:*** PO 1.2-1.6 initially; give in divided doses over 24 hr; then 150 μg qd

Maintenance dose: 10% initial dose

Available forms: Tabs 50, 100, 150, 200 μg

Side effects/adverse reactions

CNS: Headache, drowsiness, apathy, confusion, disorientation, fatigue, depression, hallucinations
CV: Dysrhythmias, hypotension, bradycardia, AV block
EENT: Blurred vision, yellow-green halos, photophobia, diplopia
GI: Nausea, vomiting, anorexia, abdominal pain, diarrhea
MS: Muscular weakness

Contraindications: Hypersensitivity to digitalis, ventricular fibrillation, ventricular tachycardia, carotid sinus syndrome, 2nd- or 3rd-degree heart block

Precautions: Hepatic disease, acute MI, AV block, hypokalemia, hypomagnesemia, sinus node disease, lactation, severe respiratory disease, hypothyroidism, G elderly, pregnancy C

Pharmacokinetics

Absorption	Complete (PO)
Distribution	Widely distributed
Metabolism	Liver
Excretion	Kidneys
Half-life	5-7 days

Pharmacodynamics

	PO
Onset	½-2 hr
Peak	4-12 hr
Duration	14-21 days

Interactions

Drug/drug:

Individual drugs
Amiodarone: ↑ levels of digitoxin
Colestipol: ↓ effects
Cholestyramine: ↓ effects
Diltiazem: ↑ levels of digitoxin
Phenylbutazone: ↓ effects
Piperacillin: ↑ hypokalemia
Quinidine: ↑ toxicity
Rifampin: ↓ effects
Spironolactone: ↑ blood levels
Succinylcholine: ↑ toxicity
Thyroid: ↓ level of digitoxin
Ticarcillin: ↑ hypokalemia
Drug classifications
Adrenergics: ↑ toxicity
Barbiturates: ↓ effects
Diuretics, thiazide: ↑ hypokalemia
Hydantoins: ↓ effects
Thioamines: ↑ toxicity

Lab test interferences

Increase: CPK

NURSING CONSIDERATIONS

Assessment

- Check apical pulse for 1 min before giving drug; if pulse <60 in adult or <90 in an

P infant, take again in 1 hr; if <60 in adult, call prescriber; note rate, rhythm, character

- Monitor electrolytes: potassium, sodium, chloride, magnesium, calcium; renal function studies: BUN, creatinine; blood studies: ALT (SGPT), AST (SGOT), bilirubin, Hct, Hgb before initiating treatment and periodically thereafter
- Monitor I&O ratio, daily weight; check skin turgor, lung sounds, peripheral edema
- Monitor drug levels (therapeutic level 20-35 ng/ml)

Associated nursing diagnoses

✓ Cardiac output, decreased (uses)
✓ Impaired gas exchange (adverse reactions)
✓ Knowledge deficit (teaching)

Implementation

PO route

- Give PO with or without food; tabs may be crushed and mixed with food/fluids for swallowing difficulty
- Give potassium supplements if ordered for potassium levels <3 mEq/L, or give foods high in potassium: bananas, orange juice

Patient/family education

- Instruct patient not to stop drug abruptly; teach all aspects of drug; to take exactly as ordered; to keep tabs in container protected from light
- Teach patient to avoid OTC medications, since many adverse drug interactions may occur; do not take antacid or cold products at same time
- Emphasize the importance of notifying prescriber of any loss of appetite, lower stomach pain, diarrhea, weakness, drowsiness, headache, blurred or yellow vision, rash, depression, toxicity
- Teach patient toxic symptoms of this drug and when to notify prescriber
- Advise patient to report shortness of breath, difficulty breathing, weight gain, edema, persistent cough
- Advise patient to carry ID with diagnosis and medication used

Evaluation

Positive therapeutic outcome

- Decreased weight, edema, pulse, respiration, rales
- Increased urine output
- Serum digitoxin level (20-35 ng/ml)

Treatment of overdose:

Discontinue drug; administer potassium; monitor ECG, administer an adrenergic blocking agent, digoxin immune Fab

digoxin 🔑

(di-jox'in)

digoxin, Lanoxicaps, Lanoxin, Novodigoxin ✦

Func. class.: Antidysrhythmic, cardiac glycoside

Chem. class.: Digitalis preparation

Pregnancy category C

Action: Inhibits sodium-potassium ATPase, which makes more calcium available for contractile proteins, resulting in increased cardiac output

D

Therapeutic Outcome: Decreased edema, pulse, respiration, rales

Uses: Rapid digitalization in CHF, atrial fibrillation, atrial flutter, atrial tachycardia; cardiogenic shock, paroxysmal atrial tachycardia

Dosage and routes

Adult: **IV** 0.5 mg given over >5 min; then PO 0.125-0.5 mg qd in divided doses q4-6h as needed

G *Elderly:* PO 0.125 mg qd maintenance

P *Child >2 yr:* PO 0.02-0.04 mg/kg divided q8h over 24 hr; maintenance 0.006-0.012 mg/kg qd in divided doses q12h; **IV** loading dose 0.015-0.035 mg/kg over >5 min

P *Child 1 mo-2 yr:* **IV** 0.03-0.05 mg/kg in divided doses over >5 min q48h; change to PO as soon as possible; PO 0.035-0.06 mg/kg divided in 3 doses over 24 hr; maintenance 0.01-0.02 mg/kg in divided doses q12h

P *Neonates:* **IV** loading dose 0.02-0.03 mg/kg over >5 min in divided doses q4-8h; change to PO as soon as possible; PO loading dose 0.035 mg/kg divided q8h over 24 hr; maintenance 0.01 mg/kg in divided doses q12h

P *Premature infants:* **IV** 0.015-0.025 mg/kg divided in 3 doses over 24 hr, given over >5 min; maintenance 0.003-0.009 mg/kg in divided doses q12h

Available forms: Caps 50, 100, 200 μg; elix 50 μg/ml; tabs 125, 250, 500 μg; inj 100, 250 μg/ml; pedi inj 10 μg/ml

Side effects/adverse reactions

CNS: Headache, drowsiness, apathy, confusion, disorientation, fatigue, depression, hallucinations
CV: ***Dysrhythmias, hypotension,*** bradycardia, ***AV block***
EENT: Blurred vision, yellow-green halos, photophobia, diplopia
GI: Nausea, vomiting, anorexia, abdominal pain, diarrhea

Contraindications: Hypersensitivity to digitalis, ventricular fibrillation, ventricular tachycardia, carotid sinus syndrome, 2nd- or 3rd-degree heart block

Precautions: Renal disease, acute MI, AV block, severe respiratory disease, hypothyroidism, G elderly, pregnancy **C**, sinus nodal disease, lactation, hypokalemia

Pharmacokinetics

Absorption	
Distribution	Widely distributed; 20%-25% protein bound
Metabolism	Liver, small amount; also intestinal bacteria
Excretion	Urine
Half-life	1½ days

Pharmacodynamics

	PO	IV
Onset	½-1½ hr	5-30 min
Peak	2-6 hr	1-5 hr
Duration	After steady state	6-8 days

Interactions

Drug/drug:

Amiodarone: ↑ digoxin levels, bradycardia
Amphotericin B: ↑ hypokalemia, toxicity
Calcium IV: ↑ risk of fatal dysrhythmias, digoxin toxicity
Carbaicillin: ↑ hypokalemia
Charcoal: ↓ levels of digoxin by absorption
Piperallin: ↑ hypokalemia
Propafenone: ↑ digoxin levels, toxicity
Quinidine: ↑ toxicity, digoxin levels
Rifampin: ↓ digoxin effects
Spironolactone: ↑ blood levels of digoxin
Succinylcholine: ↑ toxicity
Thyroid: ↓ level of digitoxin
Ticarcillin: ↑ hypokalemia
Verapamil: ↑ blood levels

Drug classifications

Adrenergics: ↑ toxicity
Antacids: ↓ digoxin absorption
Barbiturates: ↓ effects
Beta-blockers: ↑ bradycardia
Calcium channel blockers: ↑ digoxin levels, toxicity
Corticosteroids: ↑ hypokalemia, toxicity
Diuretics, thiazide: ↑ hypokalemia, toxicity
Hydantoins: ↓ effects of digoxin
Thioamines: ↑ toxicity

Lab test interferences

Increase: CPK

NURSING CONSIDERATIONS

Assessment

• Assess and document apical pulse for 1 min before giving drug; if pulse for 1 min before giving drug; if pulse <60 in P adult or <90 in an infant or is significantly different, take again in 1 hr; if <60 in adult, call prescriber; note rate, rhythm, character

• Monitor electrolytes: potassium, sodium, chloride, magnesium, calcium; renal function studies: BUN, creatinine; other blood studies: ALT (SGPT), AST (SGOT), bilirubin, Hct, Hgb drug levels (therapeutic level 0.5-2 ng/ml) before initiating treatment and periodically thereafter

• Monitor I&O ratio, daily weights; monitor turgor, lung sounds, edema

• Monitor cardiac status: apical pulse, character, rate, rhythm; resolution of atrial dysrhythmias by ECG; if tachydysrhythmia develops, hold drug; delay cardioversion while drug levels are determined

• Monitor ECG continuously during parenteral loading doses and for patients with suspected toxicity; provide hemodynamic monitoring for patients with heart failure or administer multiple cardiac drugs

Associated nursing diagnoses

✓ Cardiac output, decreased (uses)
✓ Impaired gas exchange (adverse reactions)
✓ Knowledge deficit (teaching)

Implementation

• Do not give at same time as antacids or other drugs that decrease absorption

PO route

• Give PO with or without food; may crush tabs

D

- Give potassium supplements if ordered for potassium levels <3, or give foods high in potassium: bananas, orange juice

IV **IV route**

- Give **IV** undiluted or 1 ml of drug/4 ml sterile water, D_5, or NS; give over >5 min through Y-tube or 3-way stopcock; during digitalization close monitoring is necessary
- Store protected from light

Y-site compatibilities:

Amrinone, famotidine, meperidine, milrinone, morphine, potassium chloride, vitamin B with C

Y-site incompatibilities:

Fluconazole, foscarnet

Additive compatibilities:

Bretylium, cimetidine, floxacillin, furosemide, lidocaine, verapamil

Additive incompatibility:

Dobutamine

Syringe compatibility:

Heparin, milrinone

Syringe incompatibility:

Doxapram

Patient/family education

- Caution patient to avoid OTC medications including cough, cold, allergy preparations, antacids, since many adverse drug interactions may occur; do not take antacid at same time
- Instruct patient to notify prescriber of any loss of appetite, lower stomach pain, diarrhea, weakness, drowsiness, headache, blurred or yellow-green vision, rash, depression; teach toxic symptoms of this drug and when to notify prescriber
- Advise patient to maintain a sodium-restricted diet as ordered; to take potassium supplements as ordered to prevent toxicity
- Instruct patient to report shortness of breath, difficulty breathing, weight gain, edema, persistent cough
- Teach patient purpose of drug is to regulate the heart's functioning
- Teach patient that as outpatient to check and record pulse for 1 min before taking dose; if there is a change of >15 bpm from usual pulse, prescriber should be notified
- Teach patient to take medication at the same time each day, take missed doses within 12 hr; do not double doses; notify prescriber if doses are missed for 2 days or more
- Advise patient to carry ID describing dosage and reason for digoxin

Evaluation

Positive therapeutic outcome

- Decreased weight, edema, pulse, respiration, rales
- Increased urine output
- Serum digoxin level 0.5-2 ng/ml

Treatment of overdose:

Discontinue drug, administer potassium, monitor ECG, administer an adrenergic blocking agent, digoxin immune Fab

digoxin immune Fab (ovine)

(di-jox′in)
Digibind
Func. class.: Antidote, digoxin specific
Pregnancy category **C**

Action: Antibody fragments bind to free digoxin to reverse digoxin toxicity by not allowing digoxin to bind to sites of action

Therapeutic Outcome: Correction of digoxin toxicity

Uses: Reversal of life-threatening digoxin or digitoxin toxicity, including severe bradycardia, ventricular tachycardia/fibrillation, severe hypertension

Dosage and routes

Digoxin toxicity

Adult: **IV** dose (mg) = Dose ingested (mg) x 0.8 x 66.7; if ingested amount is unknown, give 800 mg **IV**; if digoxin liquid caps or digoxin used, do not multiply ingested dose by 0.8

Available forms: Inj 40 mg/vial (binds 0.6 mg digoxin or digitoxin)

Side effects/adverse reactions

CV: Worsening of CHF, *ventricular rate increase,* ***atrial fibrillation,*** *low cardiac output*
INTEG: Hypersensitivity, allergic reactions, facial swelling, redness
META: Hypokalemia
RESP: Impaired respiratory function, rapid respiratory rate

Contraindications: Mild digoxin toxicity, hypersensitivity

Precautions: Children, lactation, cardiac disease, renal disease, pregnancy **C**

Pharmacokinetics

Absorption	Complete (IV)
Distribution	Widely distributed into plasma, interstitial fluids
Metabolism	Unknown
Excretion	Kidneys
Half-life	Biphasic (14-20 hr); increased in renal disease

Pharmacodynamics

	IV
Onset	30 mins (variable)
Peak	Unknown
Duration	Unknown

Lab test interferences

Interfere: Immunoassay (digoxin)

Interactions

Drug/drug:

Digitoxin: ↓ effect of digitoxin
Digoxin: ↓ effect of digoxin
Lanatoside C: ↓ effect of lanatoside

NURSING CONSIDERATIONS

Assessment

- Assess for hypokalemia: ST depression, flat T waves, presence of U wave, ventricular dysrhythmias

- Obtain information on previous allergies: previous exposure to sheep (ovine) proteins; scratch test may be performed before use of this product; hypersensitive reactions are more common in persons with previous exposure
- Monitor vital signs before, throughout, and after infusion
- Monitor heart rate, B/P q10 min during inf and after it is complete until stabilized; hemodynamic monitoring is used for unstable or hypotensive patients; check potassium levels until toxicity is resolved
- Assess for oxygen or perfusion deficit: hypotension, chest pain, dizziness, loss of consciousness
- Assess respiratory status: auscultate lung fields for bibasilar crackles in patients with advanced CHF

Associated nursing diagnoses

✓ Injury, risk for (uses)
✓ Knowledge deficit (teaching)

Implementation

IV IV route

- Give after diluting 40 mg/4 ml of sterile water (10 mg/ml), mix gently; may be further diluted with 0.9% NaCl; sol should be clear, colorless
- Give by bol if cardiac arrest is imminent or **IV** over 30 min using a 0.22 μm filter
- Store reconstituted sol for up to 4 hr in refrigerator

Patient/family education

- Teach that purpose of medication is to bind excess digoxin and reduce high blood levels
- Instruct patients to report fever, chills, itching, sweating, dyspnea
- Advise other prescribers that this medication has been used previously

Evaluation

Positive therapeutic outcome

- Correction of digoxin toxicity
- Digoxin blood levels 0.5-2 ng/ml

dihydrotachysterol

(dye-hye-droe-tak-iss'ter-ole)

DHT, DHT Intensol, Hytakerol

Func. class.: Parathyroid agent (calcium regulator)

Chem. class.: Vitamin D analog

Pregnancy category **C**

Action: Increases intestinal absorption of calcium, increases renal tubular absorption of phosphorus; is able to regulate calcium levels by regulation of calcitonin, parathyroid hormone

Therapeutic Outcome: Prevention of continued calcium loss in bones

Uses: Renal osteodystrophy, hypoparathyroidism, pseudohypoparathyroidism, familial hypophosphatemia, postoperative tetany

Investigational uses: Renal osteodystrophy

Dosage and routes

Hypophosphatemia

P ***Adult and child:*** PO 0.5-2 mg qd; maintenance 0.3-1.5 mg qd

Hypoparathyroidism/ pseudohypoparathyroidism

Adult: PO 0.8-2.4 mg qd × 4 days, maintenance 0.2-2 mg qd regulated by serum calcium levels

P ***Child:*** PO 1-5 mg qd 1 wk; maintenance 0.2-1 mg qd regulated by serum calcium levels

Renal osteodystrophy

Adult: PO 0.1-0.25 mg qd, then 0.2-1 mg/day

Available forms: Tab 0.125, 0.2, 0.4 mg; cap 0.125 mg; oral sol 0.2, 0.25 mg/5 ml

Side effects/adverse reactions

CNS: Drowsiness, headache, vertigo, fever, lethargy
EENT: Tinnitus
GI: Nausea, diarrhea, vomiting, jaundice, anorexia, dry mouth, constipation, cramps, metallic taste
GU: ***Polyuria,*** hypercalciuria, hyperphosphatemia, ***hematuria***
MS: Myalgia, arthralgia, decreased bone development

Contraindications: Hypersensitivity, renal disease, hyperphosphatemia, hypercalcemia

Precautions: Pregnancy **C,** renal calculi, lactation, CV disease

Pharmacokinetics

Absorption	Well absorbed (PO)
Distribution	Liver, fat
Metabolism	Liver
Excretion	Feces (inactive, active metabolites)
Half-life	Unknown

D

Pharmacodynamics

	PO
Onset	2 wk
Peak	2 wk
Duration	2 wk

Interactions

Drug/drug:

Individual drugs

Cholestyramine: ↓ absorption dihydrotachysterol
Colestipol: ↓ absorption of dihydrotachysterol
Mineral oil: ↓ absorption of dihydrotachysterol
Phenytoin: ↓ effect of dihydrotachysterol
Verapamil: ↑ dysrhythmias

Drug classifications

Barbiturates: ↓ effect of dihydrotachysterol
Calcium supplements: ↑ hypercalcemia
Cardiac glycosides: ↑ dysrhythmias
Corticosteroids: ↓ effect of dihydrotachysterol
Diuretics, thiazide: ↑ hypercalcemia

Lab test interferences

False increase: Cholesterol

NURSING CONSIDERATIONS

Assessment

- Monitor BUN, urinary calcium, AST (SGOT), ALT (SGPT), cholesterol, alkaline

phosphatase, creatinine, uric acid, chloride, magnesium, electrolytes, urine pH, phosphate; may increase calcium; should be kept at 9-10 mg/dl; keep vitamin D at 50-135 IU/dl, phosphate at 70 mg/dl; these tests should be checked before and throughout treatment
• Monitor for increased blood level, since toxic reaction may occur rapidly
• Monitor for dry mouth, metallic taste, polyuria, bone pain, muscle weakness, headache, fatigue, tinnitus, change in LOC, irregular pulse, dysrhythmias, increased respirations, anorexia, nausea, vomiting, cramps, diarrhea, constipation; may indicate hypercalcemia; if these occur, discontinue drug, give laxatives, low-calcium diet
• Monitor renal status: decreased urinary output (oliguria, anuria), edema in extremities, weight gain >5 lb, periorbital edema
• Assess nutritional status; check diet for sources of vitamin D (milk, some seafood), calcium (dairy products, dark green vegetables); phosphates (dairy products) must be avoided

Associated nursing diagnoses

✓ Nutrition: Less than body requirements (uses)
✓ Knowledge deficit (teaching)

Implementation

PO route
• May be increased q4 wk depending on blood level; give with meals for GI symptoms
• Store in tight, light-resistant containers at room temp
• Restrict sodium, potassium if required
• Restriction of fluids may be required for chronic renal failure

Patient/family education

• Teach symptoms of hypercalcemia and when to report symptoms to prescriber
• Teach patient about foods rich in calcium, vitamin D; provide list of calcium-rich foods; renal failure patients are given a renal diet
• Caution patient not to double doses, take exactly as prescribed

Evaluation

Positive therapeutic outcome
• Prevention of bone deficiencies
• Calcium, phosphorus at normal levels

diltiazem

(dil-tye′a-zem)
Apo-Diltiaz ✦, Cardizem, Cardizem SR, Cardizem CD, diltiazem, Dilacor-XR
Antianginal
Func. class.: Calcium channel blocker, antianginal
Chem. class.: Benzodiazepine
Pregnancy category **C**

Action: Inhibits calcium ion influx across cell membrane during cardiac depolarization, produces relaxation of coronary vascular smooth muscle, dilates coronary arteries, slows SA/AV node conduction times, dilates peripheral arteries

Therapeutic Outcome: Decreased angina pectoris, dysrhythmias, B/P

Uses

Oral: Angina pectoris due to coronary insufficiency, hypertension, vasospasm

Parenteral: Atrial fibrillation, flutter

Dosage and routes

Adult: PO 30 mg qid, increasing dose gradually to 180-360 mg/day in divided doses or 60-120 mg bid; may increase to 240-360 mg/day

Adult **IV**: 0.25 mg/kg over bol 2 min initially, then 0.35 mg/kg may be given after 15 min; if no response, may give cont inf 5-15 mg/hr for up to 24 hr

Adult: PO 180-240 mg (Cardizem CD) qd

Available forms: Tab 30, 60, 90, 120 mg; sus rel 60, 90, 120, 150 mg; inj **IV** 5 mg/ml (5, 10 ml)

Side effects/adverse reactions

CNS: Headache, fatigue, drowsiness, dizziness, depression, weakness, insomnia, tremor, paresthesia

CV: Dysrhythmia, edema, ***CHF:*** bradycardia, hypotension, palpitations, heart block, peripheral edema, angina

GI: Nausea, vomiting, diarrhea, gastric upset, constipation, increased liver function studies

GU: Nocturia, polyuria, ***acute renal failure***

INTEG: Rash, pruritus, flushing, photosensitivity

Contraindications: Sick sinus syndrome, 2nd- or 3rd-degree heart block, hypotension less than 90 mm Hg systolic, acute MI, pulmonary congestion

Precautions: CHF, hypotension, hepatic injury, pregnancy P C, lactation, children, renal disease

Pharmacokinetics

Absorption	Well absorbed
Distribution	Not known
Metabolism	Liver, extensively
Excretion	Metabolites (96%)
Half-life	3½-9 hr

Pharmacodynamics

	PO	PO–SUS REL	IV
Onset	½ hr	Unknown	Unknown
Peak	2-3 hr	Unknown	Unknown
Duration	6-8 hr	12 hr	Unknown

Interactions

Drug/drug:

Individual drugs

Alcohol: ↑ hypotension

Carbamazepine: ↑ toxicity

Digoxin: ↑ digoxin levels, bradycardia, CHF

Phenobarbital: ↓ effectiveness

Phenytoin: ↓ effectiveness

Propranolol: ↑ toxicity

Drug classifications

Antihypertensives: ↑ hypotension

β-Adrenergic blockers: ↑ bradycardia, CHF
Nitrates: ↑ nitrates

NURSING CONSIDERATIONS

Assessment

- Monitor blood levels (therapeutic levels: 0.025-0.1 μg/ml)
- Assess fluid volume status: I&O ratio and record, weight, distended red veins, crackles in lung, color, quality, and sp gr of urine, skin turgor, adequacy of pulses, moist mucous membranes, bilateral lung sounds, peripheral pitting edema; dehydration symptoms of decreasing output, thirst, hypotension, dry mouth and mucous membranes should be reported
- Monitor B/P and pulse, PCWP, CVP often during infusion; if B/P drops 30 mm Hg, stop inf and call prescriber
- Monitor ALT (SGOT), AST (SGPT), bilirubin daily; if these are elevated, hepatotoxicity is suspected
- If platelets are <150,000/mm^3, drug is usually discontinued and another drug started
- Assess for extravasation: change site q48h

Associated nursing diagnoses

✓ Cardiac output, decreased (uses)
✓ Knowledge deficit (teaching)

Implementation

PO route

- Give with meals for GI symptoms; may be crushed and mixed with food/fluids for swallowing difficulty; do not chew or crush sus rel caps
- Store in airtight container at room temp

IV **IV route**

- Give direct **IV** undiluted over 2 min
- For continuous inf dilute 125 mg/100 ml, (1.25 mg/ml) or 250 mg/250 ml, (1 mg/ml) or 250 mg/500 ml (0.5 mg/ml) of D_5W, 0.9% NaCl, D_5/0.45% NaCl; give 10 mg/hr; may increase by 5 mg/hr to 15 mg/hr; may continue inf up to 24 hr

Patient/family education

- Caution patient to avoid hazardous activities until stabilized on drug and dizziness is no longer a problem
- Instruct patient to limit caffeine consumption; to avoid alcohol and OTC drugs unless directed by prescriber
- Tell patient to comply in all areas of medical regimen; diet, exercise, stress reduction, drug therapy; to notify prescriber of irregular heart beat, shortness of breath, swelling of feet and hands, pronounced dizziness, constipation, nausea, hypotension
- Teach patient to use as directed even if feeling better; may be taken with other cardiovascular drugs (nitrates, β-blockers)

Evaluation

Positive therapeutic outcome

- Decreased anginal pain
- Decreased B/P
- Absence of dysrhythmias

Treatment of overdose:

Defibrillation, atropine for AV block, vasopressor for hypotension

dimenhydrinate
(dye-men-hye'dri-nate)
Calm-X, dimenhydrinate, Dimentabs, Dinate, Dommanate, Dramamine, Dramanate, Dramocen, Dramoject, Dymenate, Gravol ♣, Hydrate, Marmine, Nauseal ♣, Nauseatol ♣, Nico-Vert, Novodimenate ♣, Travamine ♣, Triptone Caplets, Wehamine
Func. class.: Antiemetic, antihistamine, anticholinergic
Chem. class.: H_1-receptor antagonist, ethanolamine derivative
Pregnancy category **B**

Action: Vestibular stimulator is decreased; anticholinergic, antiemetic, antihistamine response

➔ **Therapeutic Outcome:** Absence of motion sickness

Uses: Motion sickness, nausea, vomiting

Dosage and routes

Adult: PO 50-100 mg q4h; rec 100 mg qd or bid; IM/**IV** 50 mg as needed

P *Child:* IM/PO 5 mg/kg divided in 4 equal doses

Available forms: Tab 50 mg; inj 50 mg/ml; liq 12.5 mg/4 ml; supp 50, 100 mg; chew tab 50 mg; cap 50 mg

Side effects/adverse reactions

CNS: *Drowsiness,* restlessness, headache, dizziness, insomnia, confusion, nervousness, tingling, vertigo; hallucinations and ***convulsions*** in young children P

CV: Hypertension, hypotension, palpitations

EENT: Dry mouth, blurred vision, diplopia, nasal congestion, photosensitivity

GI: Nausea, anorexia, diarrhea, vomiting, constipation

INTEG: Rash, urticaria, fever, chills, flushing

Contraindications: Hypersensitivity to narcotics, shock

P G **Precautions:** Children, cardiac dysrhythmias, elderly, asthma, pregnancy **B,** prostatic hypertrophy, bladder neck obstruction, narrow angle glaucoma, stenosing peptic ulcer, pyloroduodenal obstruction

Pharmacokinetics

Absorption	Well absorbed (PO, IM)
Distribution	Unknown; crosses placenta
Metabolism	Liver
Excretion	Kidneys, breast milk
Half-life	Unknown

Pharmacodynamics

	PO	IM	IV
Onset	15-60 min	30 min	Immediate
Peak	1-2 hr	1-2 hr	Unknown
Duration	4-6 hr	4-6 hr	4-6 hr

Interactions

Drug/drug:

Individual drugs

Alcohol: ↑ CNS depression
Atropine: ↑ anticholinergic reactions
Disopyramide: ↑ anticholinergic reactions
Haloperidol: ↑ anticholinergic reactions
Quinidine: ↑ anticholinergic reactions

Drug classifications

Antidepressants: ↑ anticholinergic reactions
Antihistamines: ↑ anticholinergic reactions
CNS depressants: ↑ CNS depression
MAO inhibitors: ↑ anticholinergic effect
Narcotics: ↑ CNS depression
Phenothiazines: ↑ anticholinergic reactions
Sedative/hypnotics: ↑ CNS depression

Lab test interferences

False negative: Skin allergy tests (discontinue antihistamines 3 days before testing)

NURSING CONSIDERATIONS

Assessment

• Assess for signs of toxicity to other drugs or masking of symptoms of disease (brain tumor, intestinal obstruction); monitor GI symptoms including nausea, vomiting, abdominal pain, increased bowel sounds

• Monitor VS, B/P; check patients with cardiac disease more often

• Monitor I&O; check for dehydration (poor skin turgor, increased sp gr, tachycardia, severe thirst) especially in the G elderly

Associated nursing diagnoses

✓ Injury, risk for (side effects)
✓ Knowledge deficit (teaching)

Implementation

PO route

• Tab may be swallowed whole, chewed, or allowed to dissolve; give 1-2 hr before activity that may cause motion sickness; use measuring device for liq for correct dosing

IM route

• Give IM injection in large muscle mass; aspirate to avoid IV administration; massage

IV **IV route**

• Give **IV** directly after diluting 50 mg/10 ml or NaCl inj; give 50 mg or less over 2 min

Syringe incompatibilities:

Butorphanol, chlorpromazine, glycopyrrolate, hydroxyzine, midazolam, pentobarbital, prochlorperazine, promazine, promethazine, thiopental

Syringe compatibilities:

Atropine, diphenhydramine, droperidol, fentanyl, heparin, meperidine, metoclopramide, morphine, pentazocine, perphenazine, ranitidine, scopolamine

Y-site incompatibilities:

Aminophylline, heparin, hydrocortisone sodium succinate, hydroxyzine, phenobarbital, phenytoin, prednisolone, prochlorperazine, promazine, promethazine

Additive compatibilities:

Amikacin, calcium gluconate, chloramphenicol, corticotropin, erythromycin, heparin, hydroxyzine, methicillin, norepinephrine, oxytetracycline, penicillin G potassium, pentobarbital, phenobarbital, potassium chloride, prochlorperazine, vancomycin, vitamin B with C

Additive incompatibilities:

Tetracycline, thiopental

Patient/family education

- Teach all aspects of drug uses; to notify prescriber if confusion, sedation, hypotension occur; to avoid driving and other hazardous activity if drowsiness occurs; to avoid alcohol and other CNS depressants that may potentiate effect
- Tell patient not to exceed recommended dosage
- Inform patient hard candy, gum, frequent rinsing of mouth may be used for dryness
- Advise patient that a false negative result may occur with skin testing; these procedures should not be scheduled until 4 days after discontinuing use
- Caution patient to avoid hazardous activities, activities requiring alertness; dizziness may occur; instruct patient to request assistance with ambulation
- Caution patient to avoid alcohol, other CNS depressants when taking this medication; response will be increased

Evaluation

Positive therapeutic outcome

- Absence of motion sickness
- Absence of nausea, vomiting

dimercaprol

(dye-mer-cap′role)

BAL in Oil, British Anti-Lewisite ✤, **Dimercaptopropanol**

Func. class.: Heavy metal antagonist

Chem. class.: Chelating agent (dithiol compound)

Pregnancy category **D**

Action: Binds ions from arsenic, gold, mercury, lead, copper to form water-soluble complex removed by kidneys

➡ **Therapeutic Outcome:** Excretion of heavy metals and prevention of damage and death

Uses: Arsenic, gold, mercury, lead poisoning; adjunct in severe lead poisoning with encephalopathy

Dosage and routes

Severe gold/arsenic poisoning

Adult: IM 3 mg/kg q4h x 2 days; then qid x 1 day; then bid x 10 days

Mild gold/arsenic poisoning

Adult: IM 2.5 mg/kg qid x 2 days; then bid x 1 day; then qd x 10 days

Acute lead poisoning

Adult: IM 4 mg/kg; then q4h with edetate calcium disodium 12.5 mg/kg IM; not to exceed 5 mg/kg/dose

Mercury poisoning

Adult: IM 5 mg/kg; then 2.5 mg/kg/day or bid x 10 days

Available forms: Inj IM 100 mg/ml

Side effects/adverse reactions

CNS: Headache, paresthesia, anxiety, tremors, ***convulsions, shock***
CV: Hypertension, tachycardia
EENT: Rhinorrhea, throat pain or constriction, lacrimation
GI: Nausea, vomiting, salivation
GU: Burning sensation in penis, ***nephrotoxicity***
INTEG: Urticaria, erythema, pruritus, pain at inj site, fever, burning of lips, mouth, throat
SYST: ***Anaphylaxis,*** metabolic acidosis

Contraindications: Hypersensitivity, anuria, hepatic insufficiency, poisoning with other metals, severe renal disease, P child <3 yr, pregnancy **D**

Precautions: Hypertension, lactation G6PD deficiency

Pharmacokinetics

Absorption	Well absorbed (IM)
Distribution	Widely distributed
Metabolism	Liver (50%)
Excretion	Unknown
Half-life	Unknown

Pharmacodynamics

Onset	Unknown
Peak	Unknown
Duration	4 hr

Lab test interferences

Decreased: ^{131}I uptake

Interactions

Drug/drug:

Individual drugs
Cadmium: ↑ toxicity
Iron: ↑ toxicity
Selenium: ↑ toxicity
Uranium: ↑ toxicity
Urine alkalinizers: ↓ nephrotoxicity

Drug/food:

Alkalinergics: ↓ nephrotoxicity

NURSING CONSIDERATIONS

Assessment

- Assess for poisoning: type of agent, time ingested, amount ingested
- Assess for acute toxicity: gold, lead, arsenic
- Check B/P, pulse, tachycardia may occur
- Monitor I&O, kidney function studies: BUN, creatinine, CrCl, serum iron levels
- Assess for allergic reactions: rash, urticaria; if these occur, drug should be discontinued
- Check temperature q4hr; P drug may cause fever in children, as well as burning sensation of mouth, lips, eyes, thoat

Associated nursing diagnoses

✓ Poisoning (uses)
✓ Knowledge deficit (teaching)

Implementation

• Give within 2 hr of ingestion; have antihistamine available for allergic reaction
• Wash hands immediately if sol comes in contact with skin; dermatitis can occur

IM route

• Rotate inj sites; give deeply in large muscle mass

Patient/family education

• Explain all aspects of drug administration including purpose for medication
• Advise patient to notify prescriber of adverse reactions: constriction in throat, burning of lips, mouth; tell patient that IM route is painful

Evaluation

Positive therapeutic outcome

• Decreased symptoms of heavy metal intoxication

dinoprostone

(dye-noe-prost′one)

Prostin E_2

Func. class.: Oxytocic, abortifacient

Chem. class.: Prostaglandin E_2

Pregnancy category N/A

Action: Stimulates uterine contractions similar to labor by myometrium stimulation, causing abortion; acts within 30 hr for complete abortion; GI smooth muscle stimulation, effacement, dilatation of the cervix

Therapeutic Outcome: Beginning of labor, fetal expulsion

Uses: Abortion during 2nd trimester, benign hydatidiform mole, expulsion of uterine contents in fetal deaths to 28 wk, missed abortion, cervical effacement and dilatation in term pregnancy when they have not occurred spontaneously

Dosage and routes

Adult: Vag supp 20 mg; repeat q3-5h until abortion occurs; max dose is 240 mg

Available forms: Vag supp 20 mg; gel 0.5 mg/3 g (prefilled syringe)

Side effects/adverse reactions

CNS: *Headache,* dizziness, chills, fever
CV: Hypotension
EENT: Blurred vision
GI: *Nausea, vomiting, diarrhea*
GU: Vaginitis, vaginal pain, vulvitis, vaginismus
INTEG: Rash, skin color changes
MS: *Leg cramps, joint swelling,* weakness

Contraindications: Hypersensitivity, uterine fibrosis, cervical stenosis, pelvic surgery, pelvic inflammatory disease (PID), respiratory disease

Precautions: Hepatic disease, renal disease, cardiac disease, asthma, anemia, jaundice, diabetes mellitus, convulsive disorders, hypertension, hypotension

Pharmacokinetics

Absorption	Rapidly absorbed
Distribution	Unknown
Metabolism	Enzymes
Excretion	Kidneys
Half-life	Unknown

Pharmacodynamics

	GEL	SUPP
Onset	Rapid	10 min
Peak	30-45 min	Unknown
Duration	Unknown	2-3 hr

Interactions

Drug/drug:

Individual drugs

Oxytocin: ↑ effect

NURSING CONSIDERATIONS

Assessment

- Assess dilatation and effacement of the cervix, uterine contractions, fetal heart tones; watch for contractions lasting over 1 min, hypertonus, fetal distress; drug should be slowed or discontinued
- Assess for fever that occurs approximately 30 min following supp insertion (abortion)
- Monitor for nausea, vomiting, diarrhea; these may require medication
- Assess for hypersensitive reaction: dyspnea, rash, chest discomfort
- Assess respiratory rate, rhythm, depth; notify prescriber of abnormalities, in pulse, B/P
- Check vaginal discharge; itching, irritation indicates vaginal infection

Associated nursing diagnoses

- ✓ Injury, high risk for (side effects)
- ✓ Knowledge deficit (teaching)

Implementation

Supp

- Warm suppository by running warm water over package; insert high in vagina, wear gloves to prevent absorption; have patient recumbent for at least 10 min

Gel

- Do not allow to come in contact with skin; use soap and water to wash after use
- Gel should be at room temp
- Place patient in dorsal or lithotomy position to insert gel into cervical canal; remove catheter; discard all items after use; keep supine 15-30 min

Patient/family education

- Teach patient all aspects of treatment including purpose of medication and expected results
- Tell patient that gel may produce warmth in her vagina
- Caution patient that if contractions are longer than 1 min to notify nurse or prescriber
- Advise patient to notify prescriber of cramping, pain, increased bleeding, chills, increased temp, or foul-smelling discharge; these symptoms may indicate uterine infection

Evaluation

Positive therapeutic outcome

- Progression of labor
- Abortion

diphenhydramine

(dye-fen-hye'dra-meen)

Allerdryl ♣, AllerMax, Banophen, Belix, Bena-D 10, Bena-D 50, Benadryl, Benadryl 25, Benadryl Kapseals, Benahist 10, Benahist 50, Ben-Allergin-50, Benoject, Benoject-10, Benoject-50, Benylin Cough, Bydramine, Compoz, Dermamycin, Diahist, Diphenacen-50, Diphen Cough, Diphenhist, diphenhydramine HCl, Dormarex 2, Dormin, Dyrexin, Genahist, Hydramine, Hydramyn, Hyrexin-50, Insomnal ♣, Nidryl, Nordryl, Nordryl Cough, Nytol, Phendry, Scot-Tussin Allergy, Silphen Cough, Sleep-Eze 3, Sleepinal, Sominex 2, Sominex Caplets, Tusstat, Twilite, Uni-Bent Cough, Wehdryl

Func. class.: Antihistamine, antitussive

Chem. class.: Ethanolamine derivative, H_1-receptor antagonist

Pregnancy category C

Action: Acts on blood vessels, GI, respiratory system by competing with histamine for H_1-receptor site; decreases allergic response by blocking histamine; causes increased heart rate, vasodilatation, secretions

Therapeutic Outcome: Absence of allergy symptoms and rhinitis, decreased dystonic symptoms, absence of motion sickness, absence of cough, ability to sleep

Uses: Allergy symptoms, rhinitis, motion sickness, antiparkinsonism, nighttime sedation, infant colic, nonproductive cough, anaphylaxis, nasal allergies, allergic dermatoses, dystonic reactions

Dosage and routes

Adult: PO 25-50 mg q4-6h, not to exceed 400 mg/day; IM/**IV** 10-50 mg, not to exceed 400 mg/day

P *Child >12 kg:* PO/IM/**IV** 5 mg/kg/day in 4 divided doses, not to exceed 300 mg/day

Available forms: Cap 25, 50 mg; tab 25, 50 mg; elix 12.5 mg/5 ml; syr 12.5 mg/5 ml; inj IM, **IV** 50 mg/ml; cream 1, 2%; lotion 1%

Side effects/adverse reactions

CNS: Dizziness, drowsiness, poor coordination, fatigue, anxiety, euphoria, confusion, paresthesia, neuritis

EENT: Blurred vision, dilated pupils, tinnitus, nasal stuffiness, dry nose, throat, mouth

GI: Dry mouth, nausea, anorexia, diarrhea

GU: Retention, dysuria, frequency

HEMA: Thrombocytopenia, agranulocytosis, hemolytic anemia

INTEG: Photosensitivity

RESP: Increased thick secretions, wheezing, chest tightness

Contraindications:
Hypersensitivity to H_1-receptor antagonist, acute asthma attack, lower respiratory tract disease

Precautions:
Increased intraocular pressure, renal disease, cardiac disease, hypertension, bronchial asthma, seizure disorder, stenosed peptic ulcers, hyperthyroidism, prostatic hypertrophy, bladder neck obstruction, pregnancy **C**

Pharmacokinetics

Absorption	Well absorbed (PO, IM); minimally absorbed (top); completely absorbed (IV)
Distribution	Widely distributed; crosses placenta
Metabolism	Liver (95%)
Excretion	Kidneys, breast milk
Half-life	2½-7 hr

Pharmacodynamics

	PO	IM	IV
Onset	15-60 min	30 min	Immediate
Peak	1-4 hr	1-4 hr	Unknown
Duration	4-8 hr	4-8 hr	4-8 hr

Interactions

Drug/drug:

Individual drugs
Alcohol: ↑ CNS depression
Disopyramide: ↑ anticholinergic response
Quinidine: ↑ anticholinergic response

Drug classifications
Antidepressants, tricyclic: ↑ anticholinergic response
CNS depressants: ↑ CNS depression
MAOI: ↑ anticholinergic effect
Narcotics: ↑ CNS depression
Sedative/hypnotics: ↑ CNS depression

Lab test interferences

False negative: Skin allergy tests (discontinue antihistamines 3 days before testing)

NURSING CONSIDERATIONS

Assessment

- Assess respiratory status: rate, rhythm, increase in bronchial secretions, wheezing, chest tightness; provide fluids to 2 L/day to decrease secretion thickness
- Monitor I&O ratio: be alert for urinary retention, frequency, dysuria, especially G elderly; drug should be discontinued if these occur
- Monitor CBC during long-term therapy; blood dyscrasias may occur but are rare
- If giving for dystonic reactions, assess type of involuntary movements and evaluate response to this medication
- Assess cough characteristics including type, frequency, thickness of secretions and evaluate response to this medication if using for cough

Associated nursing diagnoses

- ✓ Injury, risk for (side effects)
- ✓ Sleep pattern disturbance (uses)
- ✓ Knowledge deficit (teaching)

Implementation

- Give 20 min before hs if using for sleep aid

PO route

- Give with meals if GI symptoms occur; absorption may be slightly decreased; cap may be opened and drug mixed with food/fluids for patients with swallowing difficulties

IM route

- Give IM injection in large muscle mass; aspirate to avoid **IV** administration; rotate sites

IV **IV route**

- Give **IV** undiluted 25 mg/min; may be diluted with 0.9% NaCl, D_5W, $D_{10}W$, 0.45% NaCl, D_5/0.9% NaCl, D_5/0.45% NaCl, D_5/0.25% NaCl, LR, Ringer's, give 25 mg/min or less

Syringe incompatibilities:

Pentobarbital, phenytoin, thiopental

Syringe compatibilities:

Atropine, butorphanol, chlorpromazine, cimetidine, dimenhydrinate, droperidol, fentanyl, glycopyrrolate, hydromorphone, hydroxyzine, meperidine, metoclopromide, midazolam, morphine, nalbuphine, pentazocine, perphenazine, prochloperazine, promazine, promethazine, ranitidine, scopolamine

Y-*site compatibilities:*

Acyclovir, amsacrine, fluconazole, fludarabine, heparine, meperidine, ondansetron, sargramostium, idarubicin, melphalan, paclitaxel, vinorelbine

Y-*site incompatibility:*

Foscarnet

Additive compatibilities:

Amikacin, aminophylline, bleomycin, cephaparin, erythromycin, methyldopate, nafcillin, netilmicin, methicillin, penicillin G potassium, polymyxin B, tetracycline, vitamin B with C

Additive incompatibilities:

Amobarbital, cephalothin, thiopental

Patient/family education

- Tell patient that a false-negative result may occur with skin testing; these procedures should not be scheduled until 3 days after discontinuing use
- Caution patient to avoid hazardous activities and activities requiring alertness, since dizziness may occur; instruct patient to request assistance with ambulation
- Advise patient to avoid alcohol, other depressants; CNS depression may occur
- Teach all aspects of drug uses; to notify prescriber if confusion, sedation, hypotension occur; to avoid driving and other hazardous activity if drowsiness occurs; to avoid alcohol or other CNS depressants that may potentiate effect
- Teach patient hard candy, gum, frequent rinsing of mouth may be used for dryness

Evaluation

Positive therapeutic outcome

- Absence of motion sickness
- Absence of nausea, vomiting
- Ability to sleep
- Absence of cough
- Decrease in involuntary movements

D

Treatment of overdose:

- Administer ipecac syrup or lavage, diazepam, vasopressors, barbiturates (short acting)

diphenoxylate with atropine/difenoxin with atropine

(dye-fen-ox′i-late)

Diphenatol, Lofene, Logen, Lomanate, Lomotil, Lonox, Lo-Trop, Motofen, Nor-mil

Func. class.: Antidiarrheal

Chem. class.: Phenylpiperidine derivative, opiate agonist

Pregnancy category C

Controlled substance schedule V (diphenoxylate/atropine); IV (difenoxin/atropine)

Action: Inhibits gastric motility by acting on mucosal receptors responsible for peristalsis; related to narcotic analgesics as adjunct

Therapeutic Outcome: Decreased loose stools

Uses: Diarrhea (cause undetermined)

Dosage and routes

Adult: PO 2.5-5 mg qid, titrated to patient response

P ***Child 2-12 yr:*** PO 0.3-0.4 mg/kg/day in divided doses

Available forms: Tab 2.5 mg diphenoxylate/0.025 mg atropine; tab 1 mg difenoxin/0.025 mg atropine; liq 2.5 mg diphenoxylate/0.025 mg atropine/5 ml

Side effects/adverse reactions

CNS: Drowsiness, headache, sedation, depression, weakness, lethargy, flushing, hyperthermia
CV: Tachycardia
EENT: Blurred vision, nystagmus, mydriasis
GI: ***Nausea, vomiting,*** abdominal pain, glossitis, colitis
GU: Urine retention
INTEG: Rash, urticaria, pruritus, ***angioneurotic edema***

Contraindications: Hypersensitivity, severe liver disease, pseudomembranous entero-
P colitis, glaucoma, child <2 yr, electrolyte imbalances

Precautions: Hepatic disease, renal disease, ulcerative colitis,
G pregnancy **C**, lactation, elderly

Pharmacokinetics

Absorption	Well absorbed (PO)
Distribution	Unknown
Metabolism	Liver, active metabolite
Excretion	Kidneys
Half-life	2½ hr

Pharmacodynamics

	PO
Onset	45-60 min
Peak	2 hr
Duration	3-4 hr

Interactions

Drug/drug:

Individual drugs

Alcohol: ↑ action of alcohol
Disopyramide: ↑ anticholinergic effect

Drug classifications

Anticholinergics: ↑ anticholinergic effect
Antidepressants, tricyclic: ↑ anticholinergic effect
Antihistamines: ↑ CNS depression
Barbiturates: ↑ action of barbiturates
CNS depressants: ↑ action of CNS depressants
MAOI: Hypertensive crisis; do not use together
Narcotics: ↑ action of narcotics
Sedative/hypnotics: ↑ CNS depression

NURSING CONSIDERATIONS

Assessment

- Monitor electrolytes (potassium, sodium, chloride) if on long-term therapy; fluid status, skin turgor
- Assess bowel pattern before, during treatment; check for rebound constipation after termination of medication; check bowel sounds
- Check response after 48 hr; if no response, drug should be discontinued and other treatment initiated
- Assess for abdominal distention and toxic megacolon, which may occur in ulcerative colitis

Associated nursing diagnoses

- ✓ Diarrhea (uses)
- ✓ Constipation (adverse reactions)
- ✓ Knowledge deficit (teaching)
- ✓ Noncompliance (teaching)

Implementation

PO route

- Give for 48 hr only; tabs may be given with food, crushed and mixed with fluids; liq should be measured accurately

Patient/family education

- Advise patient to avoid alcohol and OTC products unless directed by prescriber; may cause increased CNS depression
- Caution patient not to exceed recommended dosage; that drug may be habit forming
- Advise patient that drug may cause drowsiness; to avoid hazardous activities until response to drug is determined
- Teach patient that dry mouth can be decreased by frequent sips of water, hard candy, sugarless gum

Evaluation

Positive therapeutic outcome

- Decreased diarrhea

dipyridamole

(dye-peer-id'a-mole)
Apo-Dipyridamole ✦, dipyridamole, Persantine, Persantine IV
Func. class.: Coronary vasodilator, antiplatelet agent
Chem. class.: Nonnitrate
Pregnancy category **B**

Action: Inhibits adenosine uptake, which produces coronary vasodilatation; increases oxygen saturation in coronary tissues, coronary blood flow; acts on small vessels with little effect on vascular resistance; may increase development of collateral circulation; decreased platelet aggregation by the inhibition of phosphodiesterases (enzymes)

➔ **Therapeutic Outcome:** Inhibition of platelet aggregation; absence of ischemic attacks, reinfarction

Uses: Prevention of transient ischemic attacks, inhibition of platelet adhesion to prevent myocardial reinfarction, thromboembolism, with warfarin in prosthetic heart valves, prevention of coronary bypass graft occlusion with aspirin; possibly effective for long-term therapy of chronic angina pectoris

Dosage and routes

Transient ischemic attacks

Adult: PO 50 mg tid, 1 hr ac, not to exceed 400 mg qd

Inhibition of platelet adhesion

Adult: PO 50-75 mg qid in combination with aspirin or warfarin

Available forms: Tab 25, 50, 75 mg; **IV**

Side effects/adverse reactions

CNS: Headache, dizziness, weakness, fainting, syncope
CV: Postural hypotension
GI: Nausea, vomiting, anorexia, diarrhea
INTEG: Rash, flushing

Contraindications: Hypersensitivity, hypotension

Precautions: Pregnancy **B**

Pharmacokinetics

Absorption	30%-50% (PO)
Distribution	Widely distributed; crosses placenta
Metabolism	Liver
Excretion	Bile, undergoes enterohepatic recirculation; enters breast milk
Half-life	10 hr

Pharmacodynamics

	PO	IV
Onset	Unknown	Unknown
Peak	2½ hr	6 min
Duration	6 hr	½ hr
Therapeutic effect	Several mo	

Interactions

Drug/drug:

Individual drugs

Aspirin: ↑ antiplatelet effect
Coumadin: ↑ bleeding
Theophylline: ↓ effects of disopyramide (thallium)

Drug classifications
Anticoagulants: ↑ risk of bleeding
NSAIDs: ↑ risk of bleeding
Thrombolytics: ↑ risk of bleeding

NURSING CONSIDERATIONS

Assessment

- Monitor B/P, pulse baseline and during treatment until stable; take B/P with patient lying, standing; orthostatic hypotension is common
- Assess cardiac status: chest pain, what aggravates or ameliorates condition
- If using by **IV** route, monitor vital signs before, during, and after infusion; monitor for chest pain, bronchospasm; use ECG for identifying dysrhythmias; use aminophylline up to 250 mg **IV** for bronchospasm and chest pain if chest pain is unrelieved with the 250 mg dose of aminophylline; give SL dose of nitroglycerin

Associated nursing diagnoses

✓ Cardiac output, decreased (uses)
✓ Pain (uses)
✓ Knowledge deficit (teaching)

Implementation

PO route

- Give with 8 oz of water; to improve absorption give on an empty stomach; if GI symptoms occur may give with meals
- Tabs may be crushed, mixed with food or fluids for swallowing difficulty or swallowed whole
- Store at room temp

IV **IV Intermittent inf**

- Give by **IV** after diluting each 5 mg/2 ml or more in D_5W, 0.45% NaCl, or 0.9% NaCl 20-50 ml should be given; give over 4 min; do not give undiluted

Patient/family education

- Teach patient that this medication is not a cure; that drug may have to be taken continuously in evenly spaced doses only as directed; if a dose is missed, take one when remembered up to 4 hr; do not double doses
- Inform patient that it is necessary to quit smoking to prevent excessive vasoconstriction
- Advise patient to rise slowly from sitting or lying down to prevent orthostatic hypotension
- Caution patient not to use alcohol or OTC medication unless approved by prescriber
- Caution patient to avoid hazardous activities until stabilized on medication; dizziness may occur

Evaluation

Positive therapeutic outcome

- Absence of reinfarction, ischemic attacks

Treatment of overdose:

Administer **IV** phenylephrine

disopyramide
(dye-soe-peer'a-mide)
disopyramide, Napamide, Norpace, Norpace CR, Rhythmodan
Func. class.: Antidysrhythmic (Class IA)
Chem. class.: Nonnitrate
Pregnancy category C

Action: Prolongs action potential duration and effective refractory period; reduces disparity in refractory between normal and infarcted myocardium; prevents increased myocardial excitability and conduction contractility

Therapeutic Outcome: Prevention of supraventricular dysrhythmias

Uses: PVCs, ventricular tachycardia, supraventricular tachycardia, atrial flutter, fibrillation

Investigational uses: Supraventricular tachycardia (prevention, treatment)

Dosage and routes

Adult: PO 100-200 mg q6h; in renal dysfunction 100 mg q6h; sus rel cap 200 mg q12h

P *Child 12-18 yr:* PO 6-15 mg/kg/day, in divided doses q6h

P *Child 4-12 yr:* PO 10-15 mg/kg/day in divided doses q6h

P *Child 1-4 yr:* PO 10-20 mg/kg/day in divided doses q6h

P *Child <1 yr:* PO 10-30 mg/kg/day, in divided doses q6h

Available forms: Cap 100, 150 mg (as phosphate); sus rel cap 100, 150 mg

Side effects/adverse reactions

CNS: Headache, dizziness, psychosis, fatigue, depression, paresthesias, anxiety, insomnia
CV: Hypotension, bradycardia, angina, PVCs, tachycardia, increases in QRS and QT segments, ***cardiac arrest,*** edema, weight gain, AV block, ***CHF,*** syncope, chest pain
GI: Dry mouth, constipation, nausea, anorexia, flatulence, diarrhea, vomiting
GU: Retention, hesitancy, impotence, urinary frequency, urgency
EENT: Blurred vision, dry nose, throat, eyes, narrow angle glaucoma
HEMA: ***Thrombocytopenia, agranulocytosis,*** anemia (rare), decreased Hgb, Hct
INTEG: Rash, pruritus, urticaria
META: Hypoglycemia
MS: Weakness, pain in extremities

Contraindications: Hypersensitivity, 2nd- or 3rd-degree heart block, cardiogenic shock, CHF (uncompensated), sick sinus syndrome, QT prolongation

Precautions: Pregnancy **C,** lactation, diabetes mellitus, P renal disease, children, hepatic disease, myasthenia gravis, narrow angle glaucoma, cardiomyopathy, conduction abnormalities

Pharmacokinetics

Absorption	Well absorbed
Distribution	Widely distributed
Metabolism	Liver
Excretion	Kidneys
Half-life	4-10 hr

Pharmacodynamics

	PO	PO–SUS REL
Onset	½-3½ hr	Unknown
Peak	2 hr	Unknown
Duration	1½-8 hr	12 hr

Interactions

Drug/drug:

Individual drugs

Flecainide: ↑ levels, toxicity
Lidocaine: Bradycardia, arrest
Mexiletine: ↑ levels, toxicity
Phenytoin: ↑ blood levels, toxicity
Procainamide: ↑ levels, toxicity
Quinidine: ↑ levels, toxicity
Rifampin: ↓ disopyramide levels
Warfarin: ↑ level, bleeding

Drug classifications

Anticoagulants: ↓ prothrombin time
Antidysrhythmics: Widening of QRS or QRT
β Blockers: ↑ dysrhythmias, arrest

Lab test interferences

Increase: CPK

NURSING CONSIDERATIONS

Assessment

- Assess respiratory status: auscultate lung fields for bibasilar crackles in patients with advanced CHF
- Monitor I&O ratio and electrolytes: (potassium, sodium, chloride); watch for decreasing urinary output, possible retention
- Monitor liver function studies: AST (SGOT), ALT (SGPT), bilirubin, alkaline phosphatase
- Monitor ECG to determine drug effectiveness, measure PR, QRS, QT intervals; check for PVCs, other dysrhythmias; monitor B/P for hypotension; check for prolonged widening QT intervals, QRS complex; if QT or QRS increase by 50% or more, withhold next dose, notify prescriber
- Monitor for dehydration or hypovolemia
- Monitor for CNS symptoms: psychosis, numbness, depression; if these occur, drug should be discontinued

Associated nursing diagnoses

- ✓ Cardiac output, decreased (uses)
- ✓ Knowledge deficit (teaching)

Implementation

PO route

- Do not crush or break sus rel caps
- Give 1 hr ac or 2 hr pc
- If changing from regular release to sus rel cap, give sus rel 6 hr after last dose of regular release

Patient/family education

- Teach patient to report side effects immediately to prescriber; to take exactly as prescribed; if dose is missed take when remembered if within 3-4 hr of next dose; do not double doses
- Teach patient to complete

follow-up appointment with prescriber including pulmonary function studies, chest x-ray
• Instruct patient that dry mouth may be relieved by frequent sips of water, hard candy, sugarless gum
• Caution patient to make position changes from lying to standing slowly to prevent orthostatic hypotension

Evaluation

Positive therapeutic outcome
• Decreased PVCs, ventricular tachycardia

Treatment of overdose: Administer O_2, artificial ventilation, ECG; administer dopamine for circulatory depression; administer diazepam or thiopental for convulsions, isoproterenol

disulfiram
(dye-sul′fi-ram)
Antabuse, disulfiram
Func. class.: Alcohol deterrent
Chem. class.: Aldehyde dehydrogenase inhibitor
Pregnancy category **X**

Action: Blocks oxidation of alcohol at acetaldehyde stage; accumulation of acetaldehyde produces the disulfiram-alcohol reaction

Therapeutic Outcome: Disulfiram reaction when alcohol is ingested

Uses: Chronic alcoholism (as adjunct)

Dosage and routes

Adult: PO 250-500 mg qd × 1-2 wk, then 125-500 mg qd until fully socially recovered

Available forms: Tab 250, 500 mg

Side effects/adverse reactions

CNS: Headache, drowsiness, restlessness, dizziness, fatigue, tremors, psychosis, neuritis, sweating, ***convulsions, death,*** peripheral neuropathy
GI: Nausea, vomiting, anorexia, severe thirst, ***hepatotoxicity,*** metallic, garliclike aftertaste
INTEG: Rash, dermatitis, urticaria
Disulfiram reaction: Alcohol reaction: flushing, throbbing headache, respiratory difficulty, nausea, vomiting, sweating, thirst, chest pain, palpitations, dyspnea, hyperventilation, tachycardia, confusion, CV collapse, MI, CHF, convulsions, death

Contraindications: Hypersensitivity, alcohol intoxication, psychoses, CV disease, pregnancy **X**

Precautions: Hypothyroidism, hepatic disease, diabetes mellitus, seizure disorders, nephritis, cerebral damage

Pharmacokinetics

Absorption	Well absorbed
Distribution	Fat
Metabolism	Liver, oxidized
Excretion	Feces (unchanged)
Half-life	4-10 hr

Pharmacodynamics

	PO
Onset	10 min
Peak	Unknown
Duration	Unknown

Interactions

Drug/drug:

Individual drugs

Alcohol: Disulfiram reaction
Diazepam: ↑ effects of diazepam
Isoniazid: ↑ effects of isoniazid
Metronidazole: Psychosis
Paraldehyde: ↑ effects of paraldehyde
Phenytoin: ↑ effects of phenytoin

Drug classifications

Antidepressants, tricyclic: ↑ effect of antidepressants

Lab test interferences

Increase: Cholesterol
Decrease: ^{131}I uptake, PBI, VMA

NURSING CONSIDERATIONS

Assessment

- Monitor liver function studies q2 wk during therapy: AST (SGOT), ALT (SGPT); these may be elevated
- Monitor CBC, SMA q3-6 mo to detect any abnormality, including increased cholesterol q6 months during treatment
- Assess mental status: affect, mood, drug history, ability to follow treatment, abstain from alcohol
- Assess for signs of hepatotoxicity: jaundice, dark urine, clay-colored stools, abdominal pain

Associated nursing diagnoses

✓ Coping, ineffective individual (uses)
✓ Noncompliance (teaching)
✓ Knowledge deficit (teaching)

D

Implementation

PO route

- Give only with patient's knowledge; do not give to intoxicated individuals; check other medication for alcohol content
- Give once per day in AM or hs if drowsiness occurs
- Give only after patient has not been drinking for >12 hr
- Tab may be crushed and mixed with beverages

Patient/family education

- Teach patient effect of this drug if alcohol is taken; written consent for disulfiram therapy should be obtained
- Caution patient that shaving lotions, creams, lotions, cough preparations, skin products must be checked for alcohol content; even in small amount, alcohol can produce a reaction; tolerance will not develop if treatment is prolonged
- Teach patient that disulfiram reaction may occur for 2 wk after last dose; to carry ID listing disulfiram therapy
- Teach patient that tabs can be crushed, mixed with beverage
- Advise patient to avoid driving and hazardous tasks if drowsiness occurs
- Caution patient that disulfiram reaction can be fatal; occurs 15 min after drinking and may last several hr

• Give patient written instructions and symptoms of alcohol-antabuse reaction (nausea, vomiting, flushing, dyspnea, sweating, convulsions, weakness, blurred vision, chest pain, confusion, dizziness, pounding heartbeat, loss of consciousness, heart attack, death)

Evaluation

Positive therapeutic outcome
• Prevention of alcohol intake

Treatment of overdose: **IV** vitamin C, ephedrine sulfate, antihistamines, O_2

dobutamine

(doe-byoo'ta-meen)
Dobutrex
Func. class.: Adrenergic direct-acting β_1-agonist, inotropic agent
Chem. class.: Catecholamine
Pregnancy category C

Action: Causes increased contractility, increased coronary blood flow and heart rate by acting on β_1-receptors in heart

Therapeutic Outcome: Cardiac output increased with decreased fatigue and dyspnea

Uses: Cardiac surgery, refractory heart failure

Investigational uses: Cardiogenic shock in children [P]

Dosage and routes

Adult: **IV** inf 2.5-10 μg/kg/min; may increase to 40 μg/kg/min if needed

Available forms: Inj 250 mg vial; **IV**

Side effects/adverse reactions

CNS: *Anxiety*, headache, dizziness
CV: Palpitations, tachycardia, hypertension, PVCs, angina
GI: Heartburn, nausea, vomiting
MS: Muscle cramps (leg)

Contraindications: Hypersensitivity, idiopathic hypertropic subaortic stenosis

Precautions: Pregnancy **C**, [P] lactation, children, hypertension

Pharmacokinetics

Absorption	Complete (IV)
Distribution	Unknown
Metabolism	Liver
Excretion	Kidney
Half-life	2 min

Pharmacodynamics

	IV
Onset	1-5 min
Peak	10 min
Duration	<10 min

Interactions

Drug/drug:

Individual drugs
Bretylium: ↑ dysrhythmias
Disopyramide: ↑ hypotension
Guanethidine: ↑ pressor response
Oxytocin: ↑ dysrhythmias

Phenytoin: ↑ hypotension, bradycardia

Drug classifications

Anesthetics: ↑ dysrhythmias
Antidepressants, tricyclic: ↑ pressor response
Antihypertensives: ↑ hypotension
β-Blockers: ↑ pressor response
Cardiac glycosides: ↑ inotropic effect
MAOI: ↑ dysrhythmias

NURSING CONSIDERATIONS

Assessment

- Assess for hypovolemia; if present, correct before beginning treatment with dobutamine; avoid use in patients with atrial fibrillation before digitalization
- Monitor ECG for dysrhythmias, ischemia during treatment; some patients may not need continuous ECG monitoring; also monitor PCWP, CVP, CO_2, urinary output; notify prescriber if <30 ml hr
- Assess for heart failure: bibasilar crackles, S_3 gallop, dyspnea, neck vein distention in patients with cardiomyopathy or CHF
- Assess for oxygenation or perfusion deficit: decreased B/P, chest pain, dizziness, loss of consciousness
- Monitor B/P and pulse q5 min during inf; if B/P drops 30 mm Hg, stop inf and call prescriber
- Monitor ALT (SGOT), AST (SGPT), bilirubin daily

Associated nursing diagnoses

✓ Cardiac output, decreased (uses)

✓ Knowledge deficit (teaching)

Implementation

IV **IV route**

- Reconstitute 250 mg/10 ml of D_5W or sterile water for inj; may add another 10 ml to dissolve completely if needed, then dilute in 50 ml or more D_5W, 0.9% NaCl, 0.45% NaCl, D_5/0.45% NaCl, D_5/0.9% NaCl, D_5/LR, LR; titrate to patient response; use inf pump for correct dose

Syringe incompatibility:

Doxapran

Syringe compatibilities:

Heparin, ranitidine

Y-site compatibilities:

Amrinone, atracurium, bretylium, calcium chloride, calcium gluconate, diazepam, dilitazem, dopamine, enalaprilat, famotidine, haloperidol, insulin, lidocaine, magnesium sulfate, nitroglycerin, pancuronium, potassium chloride, ranitidine, sodium nitroprusside, streptokinase, tolazoline, vecuronium, verapamil, zidovudine

Y-site incompatibilities:

Acyclovir, alteplase, aminophylline, foscarnet, phytonadione

Additive compatibilities:

Atropine, dopamine, epinephrine, hydralazine, indomethazin, isoproterenol, lidocaine, meperidine, metaraminol bitartrate, morphine, nitroglycerin, norepinephrine, phenotolamine, phenylephrine, procainamide, propranolol, ranitidine

Additive incompatibilities:

Acyclovir, aminophylline, bumetanide, calcium gluconate, diazepam, digoxin, furosemide, insulin, magnesium sulfate, phenytoin, potassium phosphate, sodium bicarbonate

Patient/family education

- Teach patient reason for medication and expected results, reason for all monitoring and procedures
- Advise patient to report all side effects

Evaluation

Positive therapeutic outcome

- Increased cardiac output
- Decreased PCWP, adequate CVP
- Decreased dyspnea, fatigue, edema, ECG

Treatment of overdose:

Discontinue drug, support circulation

docusate calcium/ docusate potassium/ docusate sodium

(dok'yoo-sate)

DC Softgels, docusate calcium, Pro-Cal-Sof, Sulfalax Calcium, Surfak/ Dialose, Diocto-K, Kasof/ Colace, Correctol Extra Gentle, Diocto, Dioeze, Disonate, docusate sodium, DOK, DOS Softgel, Doxinate, D-S-S, Modane Soft, Regulex SS, Regutol

Func. class.: Laxative, emollient

Chem. class.: Anionic surfactant

Pregnancy category C

Action: Increases water, fat penetration in intestine; allows for easier passage of stool; increases electrolyte, water secretion in colon

Therapeutic Outcome: Passage of softened stool, absence of constipation

Uses: To soften stools, prevent constipation, soften fecal impaction (rec route)

Dosage and routes

Adult: PO 50-300 mg qd (docusate sodium) or 240 mg (docusate calcium or docusate potassium) prn; enema 5 ml (docusate sodium)

P ***Child >12 yr:*** Enema 2 ml (docusate sodium)

P ***Child 6-12 yr:*** PO 40-120 mg qd (docusate sodium)

P *Child 3-6 yr:* PO 20-60 mg qd (docusate sodium)
P *Child <3 yr:* PO 10-40 mg qd (docusate sodium)

Available forms: Cap 50, 100, 240, 250, 300 mg; tab 50, 100 mg; oral sol 10, 50 mg/ml, 16.7, 20 mg/ml, enema conc 18 g/100 ml
Docusate calcium: cap 50, 240 mg
Docusate potassium: cap 100, 240 mg
Docusate sodium: cap 50, 100, 240, 250 mg
Tab 100 mg; syr 50, 60 mg/15 ml; liq 150 mg/15 ml; sol 50 ml/ml; enema 283 mg/3.9 g cap

Side effects/adverse reactions

EENT: Bitter taste, throat irritation
GI: Nausea, anorexia, cramps, diarrhea
INTEG: Rash

Contraindications: Hypersensitivity, obstruction, fecal impaction, nausea/vomiting

Precautions: Pregnancy **C**

Pharmacokinetics

Absorption	Minimal (PO)
Distribution	Unknown
Metabolism	Not metabolized
Excretion	Bile
Half-life	Unknown

Pharmacodynamics

	PO	REC
Onset	24-72 hr	4-6 hr
Peak	Unknown	Unknown
Duration	Unknown	Unknown

Interactions: None

NURSING CONSIDERATIONS

Assessment

- Assess cramping, rectal bleeding, nausea, vomiting; if these symptoms occur, drug should be discontinued; identify cause of constipation; identify whether fluids, bulk, or exercise is missing from lifestyle

Associated nursing diagnoses

✓ Bowel elimination, altered: constipation (uses)
✓ Bowel elimination, altered; diarrhea (side effects)
✓ Knowledge deficit (teaching)
✓ Noncompliance (teaching)

Implementation

PO route
- Dilute oral sol in juice or other fluid to disguise taste
- Give tabs or caps with 8 oz of liq; give on empty stomach for increased absorption, results

Patient/family education

- Discuss with patient that adequate fluid consumption is as necessary as bulk, exercise for adequate bowel function
- Teach patient that normal bowel movements do not always occur daily
- Advise patient not to use in presence of abdominal pain, nausea, vomiting; tell patient to notify prescriber if unrelieved constipation or if symptoms of electrolyte imbalance occur: muscle cramps, pain, weakness, dizziness, excessive thirst

• Caution patients with heart disease to avoid using the Valsalva maneuver to expedite evacuation

Evaluation

Positive therapeutic outcome
• Decreased constipation within 3 days

dopamine

(doe'pa-meen)
Dopastat, dopamine HCl, Intropin, Revimine ♣
Func. class.: Agonist, vasopressor, inotropic agent
Chem. class.: Catecholamine
Pregnancy category **C**

Action: Causes increased cardiac output; acts on α-receptors, causing vasoconstriction in blood vessels; when low doses are administered, causes renal and mesenteric vasodilatation

➔ **Therapeutic Outcome:** Increased B/P, cardiac output

Uses: Shock; to increase perfusion; hypotension

Dosage and routes

Adult: **IV** inf 2-5 μg/kg/min, not to exceed 50 μg/kg/min; titrate to patient's response

Available forms: Inj 0.8, 1.6, 40, 80, 160 mg/ml

Side effects/adverse reactions

CNS: *Headache*
CV: *Palpitations, tachycardia, hypertension, ectopic beats, angina, wide QRS complex,* peripheral vasoconstriction
GI: *Nausea, vomiting, diarrhea*
INTEG: Necrosis, tissue sloughing with extravasation, ***gangrene***
RESP: Dyspnea

Contraindications: Hypersensitivity, ventricular fibrillation, tachydysrhythmias, pheochromocytoma

Precautions: Pregnancy **C,** lactation, arterial embolism, peripheral vascular disease

Pharmacokinetics

Absorption	Complete (IV)
Distribution	Widely
Metabolism	Liver
Excretion	Kidney
Half-life	2 min

Pharmacodynamics

	IV
Onset	2-5 min
Peak	Unknown
Duration	<10 min

Interactions

Drug/drug:

Individual drugs
Phenytoin: ↑ hypotension, bradycardia
Drug classifications
Anesthetics: ↑ dysrhythmias
Antidepressants, tricyclic: ↑ pressor response
β-Blockers: ↓ cardiac response

Cardiac glycosides: ↑ inotropic effect
MAOIs: ↑ hypertension (severe)

NURSING CONSIDERATIONS

Assessment

- Monitor ECG for dysrhythmias, ischemia during treatment; some patients may not need continuous ECG monitoring; also monitor PCWP, CVP, CO_2, urinary output; notify prescriber if <30 ml/hr
- Assess for heart failure: bibasilar crackles, S_3 gallop, dyspnea, neck vein distention in patients with cardiomyopathy or CHF
- Assess for oxygenation or perfusion deficit: decreased B/P, chest pain, dizziness, loss of consciousness
- Monitor B/P and pulse q5 min during inf; if B/P drops 30 mm Hg, stop inf and call prescriber
- Check for extravasation: change site q48h

Associated nursing diagnoses

✓ Cardiac output, decreased (uses)
✓ Tissue perfusion, altered (uses)
✓ Fluid volume excess (uses)
✓ Knowledge deficit (teaching)

Implementation

IV **IV route**

- Give by continuous inf; dilute 200-400 mg/250-500 ml D_5W, 0.9% NaCl, D_5/LR, D_5/0.45% NaCl, D_5/0.9% NaCl, LR; do not use discolored sol; sol is stable for 24 hr; give 0.5-5 μg/kg/min; may increase by 1-4 μg/kg/min q15-30 min until desired patient response; use inf pump

Y-site incompatibilities:

Acyclovir, alteplase, indomethacin sodium trihydrate

Y-site compatibilities:

Amrinone, atracurium, diltiazem, dobutamine, esmolol, famotidine, foscarnet, haloperidol, heparin, hydrocortisone sodium succinate, labetalol, lidocaine, meperidine, morphine, nitroglycerin, pancuronium, potassium chloride, ranitidine, sodium nitroprusside, streptokinase, tolazoline, vecuronium, verapamil, vitamin B with C, zidovudine

Patient/family education

- Teach patient reason for medication, expected results, reason for all monitoring, and procedures
- Advise patient to report all side effects

Evaluation

Positive therapeutic outcome

- Increased cardiac output

Treatment of overdose:

Discontinue drug, support circulation

dorzolamide

(door-zol'a-mide)
Truscopt
Func. class.: Carbonic anhydrase inhibitor
Pregnancy category **B**

Action: Converted to epinephrine, which decreases aqueous production and increases outflow

➔ **Therapeutic Outcome:** Lessening of intraocular pressure

Uses: Open-angle glaucoma, ocular hypertension

Dosage and routes

Adult: Instill 1 gtt q8-12h in each eye

Available forms: Sol 2%

Side effects/adverse reactions

CNS: Headache
CV: Hypertension, tachycardia, dysrhythmias
EENT: Burning, stinging
GI: Bitter taste

Contraindications: Hypersensitivity

Precautions: Pregnancy **B,** P lactation, children, aphakia, hypersensitivity to carbonic anhydrase inhibitors, sulfonamides, thiazide diuretics, ocular inhibitors, hepatic and renal insufficiency

Pharmacokinetics

Absorption	Unknown
Distribution	Unknown
Metabolism	Unknown
Excretion	Unknown
Half-life	Unknown

Pharmacodynamics

Onset	Unknown
Peak	2 hr
Duration	8-12 hr

Interactions: None

NURSING CONSIDERATIONS

Assessment

- Monitor ophth exams and intraocular pressure readings
- Monitor blood counts, liver, renal function tests and serum electrolytes during long-term treatment

Associated nursing diagnoses

✓ Sensory-perceptual alteration: visual (uses)
✓ Knowledge deficit (teaching)

Implementation

Ophthalmic route

- Store at room temp away from light

Patient/family education

- Teach patient how to instill drops
- Advise patient that drug may cause burning, itching, blurring, dryness of eye area

Evaluation

Positive therapeutic response

- Absence of increased intraocular pressure

doxacurium

(dox'a-cure-ee-yum)

Nuromax

Func. class.: Neuromuscular blocker (nondepolarizing)

Pregnancy category **C**

Action: Inhibits transmission of nerve impulses by binding with cholinergic receptor sites, antagonizing action of acetylcholine; no analgesic response

➔ **Therapeutic Outcome:** Paralysis of all skeletal muscles

Uses: Facilitation of endotracheal intubation, skeletal muscle relaxation during mechanical ventilation, surgery, or general anesthesia

Dosage and routes

Adult: **IV** 0.05 mg/kg; 0.08 mg/kg is used for prolonged neuromuscular blockade; maintenance 0.025 mg/kg

P *Child:* 2-12 yr **IV** 0.03-0.05 mg/kg; may increase for maintenance dose

Available forms: Inj 1 mg/ml

Side effects/adverse reactions

CV: ***Decreased B/P, ventricular fibrillation, MI, cardiovascular accident***
EENT: Diplopia
INTEG: Rash, urticaria
RESP: ***Prolonged apnea, bronchospasm, wheezing, respiratory depression***
MS: *Weakness,* prolonged skeletal muscle relaxation, ***paralysis***

Contraindications: Hypersensitivity

Precautions: Pregnancy **C,** renal hepatic disease, lactation, P children <3 mo, fluid and electrolyte imbalances, neuromuscular disease, respiratory disease, obesity, G elderly, severe burns

Pharmacokinetics

Absorption	Complete (IV)
Distribution	Unknown
Metabolism	Unknown
Excretion	Kidneys, bile, unchanged
Half-life	½-2 hr; increased in renal transplant patient

Pharmacodynamics

	IV
Onset	Up to 5 min
Peak	Unknown
Duration	1½ hr

Interactions

Drug/drug:

Individual drugs

Clindamycin: ↑ paralysis length and intensity
Colistin: ↑ paralysis length and intensity
Lidocaine: ↑ paralysis length and intensity
Lithium: ↑ paralysis length and intensity
Magnesium: ↑ paralysis length and intensity
Polymyxin B: ↑ paralysis length and intensity
Procainamide: ↑ paralysis length and intensity

Quinidine: ↑ paralysis length and intensity
Succinylcholine: ↑ paralysis length and intensity

Drug classifications

Aminoglycosides: ↑ paralysis length and intensity
β-Blockers: ↑ paralysis length and intensity
Diuretics, potassium-losing: ↑ paralysis length and intensity
General anesthesia: ↑ paralysis length and intensity

NURSING CONSIDERATIONS

Assessment

- Monitor for electrolyte imbalances (potassium, magnesium) before drug is used; electrolyte imbalances may lead to increased action of this drug
- Monitor vital signs (B/P, pulse, respirations, airway) until fully recovered; rate, depth, pattern of respirations, strength of hand grip; patient should be intubated before use
- Monitor recovery: decreased paralysis of face, diaphragm, leg, arm, rest of body; residual weakness and respiratory problems may occur during recovery period
- Monitor allergic reactions: rash, fever, respiratory distress, pruritus; drug should be discontinued

Associated nursing diagnoses

✓ Breathing pattern, ineffective (uses)
✓ Communication, impaired verbal (adverse reactions)
✓ Anxiety (adverse reactions)
✓ Knowledge deficit (teaching)

Implementation

IV **IV route**

- Anesthesiologist uses peripheral nerve stimulator to determine neuromuscular blockade; deep tendon reflexes should be monitored during extended periods
- Give direct **IV** undiluted over 1 min, or diluted in 10-50 ml of D_5W, ½ NaCl or NS and give as an infusion at prescribed rate (only by qualified person, usually an anesthesiologist); do not administer IM
- Further dilute in D_5W, 0.9% NaCl, D_5/0.9% NaCl q15-25 min (intermittent inf)
- Maintenance is given q20-45 min after 1st dose (cont inf); titrate to patient response
- Store in light-resistant area

Solution compatibilities:

LR, D_5/LR, D_5/0.9% NaCl

Patient/family education

- Provide reassurance if communication is difficult during recovery from neuromuscular blockade
- Provide explanation to patients regarding all procedures or treatments; patient will remain conscious if anesthesia is not given also

Evaluation

Positive therapeutic outcome

- Paralysis of jaw, eyelid, head, neck, rest of body as evaluated by peripheral nerve stimulator

Treatment of overdose:

Administer edrophonium or neostigmine, atropine; monitor VS; may require mechanical ventilation

doxapram
(dox'a-pram)
Dopram
Func. class.: Analeptic (respiratory/cerebral stimulant)
Pregnancy category **B**

Action: Respiratory stimulation through activation of peripheral carotid chemoreceptor in low dosages; with higher dosages medullary respiratory centers are stimulated, producing general CNS stimulation

Therapeutic Outcome: Ease of breathing, ABGs at normal limits

Uses: COPD, postanesthesia CNS and respiratory stimulation, prevention of acute hypercapnia, drug-induced CNS depression

Dosage and routes

Postanesthesia stimulation

Adult: **IV** inj 0.5-1 mg/kg, not to exceed 1.5 mg/kg total as a single inj; **IV** inf 250 mg in 250 ml sol, not to exceed 4 mg/kg; run at 1-3 mg/min

Drug-induced CNS depression

Adult: **IV** priming **IV** dose of 2 mg/kg, repeated in 5 min; repeat q1-2h until patient awakens; **IV** inf priming dose 2 mg/kg at 1-3 mg/min, not to exceed 3 g/day

COPD (Hypercapnia)

Adult: **IV** inf 1-2 mg/min, not to exceed 3 mg/min for no longer than 2 hr

Available forms: Inj **IV** 20 mg/ml

D

Side effects/adverse reactions

CNS: Convulsions (clonus/generalized), *headache,* restlessness, dizziness, confusion, paresthesias, flushing, sweating, bilateral Babinski's sign, rigidity, depression
CV: Chest pain, hypertension, change in heart rate, lowered T waves, tachycardia, arrhythmias
EENT: Pupil dilation, sneezing
GI: Nausea, vomiting, diarrhea, hiccups
GU: Retention, incontinence
INTEG: Pruritus, irritation at inj site
RESP: Laryngospasm, bronchospasm, rebound hypoventilation, dyspnea, cough, tachypnea, hiccups

Contraindications: Hypersensitivity, seizure disorders, severe hypertension, severe bronchial asthma, severe dyspnea, severe cardiac disorders, pneumothorax, pulmonary embolism, severe respiratory disease, P newborns

Precautions: Bronchial asthma, pheochromocytoma, severe tachycardia, dysrhythmias, pregnancy **B,** hypertension, lactation, P children

Pharmacokinetics

Absorption	Complete (IV)
Distribution	Unknown
Metabolism	Liver
Excretion	Kidneys, metabolites
Half-life	2.5-4 hr

Pharmacodynamics

	IV
Onset	20-40 sec
Peak	1-2 min
Duration	5-10 min

Interactions

Drug/drug:

Individual drugs

Cyclopropone: ↑ dysrhythmias
Enflurane: ↑ dysrhythmias
Halothane: ↑ dysrhythmias

Drug classifications

MAOI: ↑ hypertension
Skeletal muscle relaxants: May mask the effects of skeletal muscle relaxants
Sympathomimetics: Synergistic pressor effect

NURSING CONSIDERATIONS

Assessment

- Monitor B/P, heart rate, deep tendon reflexes, level of consciousness, ABGs before administration q30 min; check for Po_2, Pco_2, O_2 saturation during treatment
- Monitor ECG; watch for hypertension, increased pulse, increased pulmonary artery pressures
- Monitor for hypertension: dysrhythmias, tachycardia, dyspnea, skeletal muscle hyperactivity; may indicate overdosage; discontinue if these occur
- Assess for respiratory stimulation: increased respiratory rate, depth, abnormal rhythm; check for patent airway; elevate head of bed to 45 degrees or higher, position patient on side
- Check for extravasation: redness, inflammation, pain; may cause phlebitis; change **IV** site q48h

Associated nursing diagnoses

- ✓ Breathing pattern, ineffective (uses)
- ✓ Impaired gas exchange (uses)
- ✓ Knowledge deficit (teaching)

Implementation

IV route

- May give by **IV** diluted with equal parts of sterile water for inj; may be diluted 250 mg/250 ml (1 mg/ml) of D_5W, $D_{10}W$ (dilute 400 mg/180 ml of compatible IV sol [2 mg/ml]) and run as inf over 2 hr
- Give **IV** undiluted over 5 min; **IV** inf at 1-3 mg/min; adjust for desired respiratory response, using inf pump **IV**; if an inf is used after initial dose, start at 1-3 mg/min; adjust for desired respiratory response, using inf pump **IV**; if an inf is used after initial dose, start at 1-3 mg/min depending on patient response; D/C after 2 hr; wait 1-2 hr and repeat
- Give only after adequate airway is established; ensure O_2, **IV** barbiturates, resuscitative equipment available
- Discontinue inf if side effects occur; narrow margin of safety

Syringe compatibilities:

Amikacin, bumetadine, chlorpromazine, cimetidine, cisplatin, cyclophosphamide, deslanoside, dopamine, doxycycline, epinephrine, hydroxyzine, imipramine, isoniazid, lincomycin, methotrexate, netilmicin, phytonadione, pyridoxine, terbutaline, thiamine, tobramycin, vincristine

Syringe incompatibilities:

Aminophylline, ascorbic acid, cefoperazone, cefotaxime, cefotetan, cefuroxime, dexamethasone, diazepam, digoxin, dobutamine, folic acid, furosemide, hydrocortisone, ketamine, methylprednisolone, minocycline, thiopental, ticarcillin

Patient/family education

- Teach all aspects of drug, purpose, expected reactions
- Caution patient if difficulty breathing or shortness of breath occurs to notify nurse or prescriber

Evaluation

Positive therapeutic outcome

- Increased breathing capacity
- ABGs WNL for patient

Treatment of overdose:

Lavage, activated charcoal; monitor electrolytes, VS; diazepam for seizures; discontinue inf

doxazosin

(dox-ay'zoe-sin)

Cardura

Func. class.: Peripheral α-adrenergic blocker, antihypertensive

Chem. class.: Quinazoline

Pregnancy category **B**

D

Action: Peripheral blood vessels are dilated, peripheral resistance lowered; reduction in B/P results from α-adrenergic receptors being blocked

➔ **Therapeutic Outcome:** Decreased B/P

Uses: Hypertension alone or as an adjunct

Dosage and routes

Adult: PO 1 mg qd, increasing up to 16 mg qd if required; usual range 4-16 mg/day

Available forms: Tab 1, 2, 4, 8, mg

Side effects/adverse reactions

CNS: Dizziness, headache, drowsiness, anxiety, depression, vertigo, weakness, fatigue, asthenia

CV: Palpitations, orthostatic hypotension, tachycardia, edema, dysrhythmias, chest pain

EENT: Epistaxis, tinnitus, dry mouth, red sclera, pharyngitis, rhinitis

GI: Nausea, vomiting, diarrhea, constipation, abdominal pain

GU: Incontinence, polyuria

Contraindications: : Hypersensitivity to quinazolines

Precautions: Pregnancy **B,** P children, lactation, hepatic disease

Pharmacokinetics

Absorption	Well absorbed
Distribution	Not known; 98% plasma protein bound
Metabolism	Liver, extensively (<63%)
Excretion	Kidneys
Half-life	22 hr

Pharmacodynamics

	PO
Onset	2 hr
Peak	2-6 hr
Duration	6-12 hr

Interactions
Drug/drug:
Drug classifications
Beta-blockers: ↑ postural hypotension

Lab test interferences
False positive: Urine acetone

NURSING CONSIDERATIONS
Assessment
- Monitor B/P, orthostatic hypotension, syncope; check for edema in feet, legs daily; I&O; monitor for weight daily; notify prescriber of changes
- Assess for orthostatic hypotension; tell patient to rise slowly from sitting or lying position

Associated nursing diagnoses
- ✓ Cardiac output, decreased (uses)
- ✓ Injury, potential for physical (side effects)
- ✓ Knowledge deficit (teaching)
- ✓ Noncompliance (teaching)

Implementation
PO route
- Store in tight container at 86° F (30° C) or less
- May be used in combination with other antihypertensives
- May be given with food to prevent GI symptoms

Patient/family education
- Teach patient not to discontinue drug abruptly; emphasize the importance of complying with dosage schedule, even if feeling better; if dose is missed take as soon as remembered; take at same time each day
- Teach patient not to use OTC products (cough, cold, allergy) unless directed by prescriber; also to avoid large amounts of caffeine
- Emphasize the need to rise slowly to sitting or standing position to minimize orthostatic hypotension
- Teach patient to notify prescriber of mouth sores, sore throat, fever, swelling of hands or feet, irregular heartbeat, chest pain
- Caution patient to report excessive perspiration, dehydration, vomiting, diarrhea; may lead to fall in B/P
- Caution patient that drug may cause dizziness, fainting, lightheadedness; may occur during 1st few days of therapy; to avoid hazardous activities

• Teach patient how to take B/P, and normal readings for age group; to take B/P q7 days

Evaluation

Positive therapeutic outcome
• Decreased B/P in hypertension

Treatment of overdose: Administer volume expanders or vasopressors; discontinue drug; place in supine position

doxepin
(dox'e-pin)
doxepin HCl, Sinequan, Sinequan Concentrate, Triadapin ♣
Func. class.: Antidepressant, tricyclic; antianxiety
Chem. class.: Dibenzoxepin, tertiary amine
Pregnancy category **C**

Action: Blocks reuptake of norepinephrine, serotonin into nerve endings, increasing action of norepinephrine, serotonin in nerve cells; has anticholinergic effects

Therapeutic Outcome: Decreased symptoms of depression after 2-3 wk

Uses: Major depression, anxiety

Investigational uses: Chronic pain management

Dosage and routes
Adult: PO 50-75 mg/day in divided doses; may increase to 300 mg/day or may give daily dose hs

Available forms: Cap 10, 25, 50, 75, 100, 150 mg; oral conc 10 mg/ml

Side effects/adverse reactions
CNS: Dizziness, drowsiness, confusion, headache, anxiety, tremors, stimulation, weakness, insomnia, nightmares, extrapyramidal symptoms G (elderly), increased psychiatric symptoms, paresthesia
CV: Orthostatic hypotension, ECG changes, tachycardia, ***hypertension,*** palpitations
EENT: Blurred vision, tinnitus, mydriasis, ophthalmoplegia, glossitis
GI: Diarrhea, dry mouth, nausea, vomiting, ***paralytic ileus,*** increased appetite, cramps, epigastric distress, jaundice, ***hepatitis,*** stomatitis, constipation
GU: Retention, ***acute renal failure***
HEMA: ***Agranulocytosis, thrombocytopenia, eosinophilia, leukopenia***
INTEG: Rash, urticaria, sweating, pruritus, photosensitivity

Contraindications: Hypersensitivity to tricyclic antidepressants, urinary retention, narrow angle glaucoma, prostatic hypertrophy

Precautions: Suicidal patients, G elderly, pregnancy **C**

Pharmacokinetics

Absorption	Well absorbed
Distribution	Widely distributed; crosses placenta
Metabolism	Liver, extensively
Excretion	Kidneys, breast milk
Half-life	8-24 hr

Pharmacodynamics

	PO
Onset	Unknown
Peak	Unknown
Duration	Unknown

Interactions

Drug/drug:

Individual drugs

Alcohol: ↑ CNS depression
Cimetidine: ↑ levels, toxicity
Clonidine: Severe hypotension; avoid use
Disulfiram: Organic brain syndrome
Fluoxetine: ↑ levels, toxicity
Guanethidine: ↓ effects of guanethidine

Drug classifications

Analgesics: ↑ CNS depression
Anticholinergics: ↑ side effects
Antihistamines: ↑ CNS depression
Antihypertensives: May block antihypertensive effect
Barbiturates: ↑ effects
Benzodiazepines: ↑ effects
CNS depressants: ↑ effects
MAOI: Hypertensive crisis, convulsions
Oral contraceptives: ↑ effects, toxicity
Phenothiazines: ↑ toxicity
Sedative/hypnotics: ↑ CNS depression
Sympathomimetics, indirect acting: ↓ effects

Drug/smoking:

↑ metabolism, ↓ effects

Lab test interferences

Increase: Serum bilirubin, blood glucose, alkaline phosphatase
Decrease: VMA, 5-HIAA, blood glucose
False increase: Urinary catecholamines

NURSING CONSIDERATIONS

Assessment

- Monitor B/P (with patient lying, standing), pulse q4h; if systolic B/P drops 20 mm Hg, hold drug, notify prescriber; take vs q4h in patients with cardiovascular disease
- Monitor blood studies: CBC, leukocytes, differential, cardiac enzymes if patient is receiving long-term therapy
- Monitor hepatic studies: AST (SGOT), ALT (SGPT), bilirubin
- Check weight weekly; appetite may increase with drug
- Assess ECG for flattening of T wave, bundle branch block, AV block, dysrhythmias in cardiac patients
- Assess for extrapyramidal G symptoms primarily in elderly: rigidity, dystonia, akathisia
- Assess mental status: mood, sensorium, affect, suicidal tendencies; increase in psychiatric symptoms: depression, panic
- Monitor urinary retention, constipation; constipation is P more likely to occur in children G or elderly
- Assess for withdrawal symptoms: headache, nausea, vomiting, muscle pain, weakness; do not usually occur

unless drug was discontinued abruptly
• Identify alcohol consumption; if alcohol is consumed, hold dose until AM

Associated nursing diagnoses

✓ Coping, ineffective individual (uses)
✓ Injury, risk for (side effects)
✓ Knowledge deficit (teaching)

Implementation

PO route
• Give with food or milk for GI symptoms; dilute concentrate with fruit juice, water, milk to disguise taste
• Give dosage hs if oversedation occurs during day; may take entire dose hs; elderly may not tolerate once/day dosing
• Store at room temp; do not freeze

Patient/family education

• Tell patient that therapeutic effects may take 2-3 wk; to use caution in driving and other activities requiring alertness because of drowsiness, dizziness, blurred vision
• Advise patient to avoid rising quickly from sitting to standing, especially elderly
• Teach patient to avoid alcohol ingestion, other CNS depressants; not to discontinue medication quickly after long-term use: may cause nausea, headache, malaise
• Teach patient to wear sunscreen or large hat, since photosensitivity occurs
• Teach patient to increase fluids, bulk in diet if constipation, urinary retention occur, especially elderly; to take gum, hard sugarless candy, or frequent sips of water for dry mouth

Evaluation

Positive therapeutic outcome
• Decrease in depression
• Absence of suicidal thoughts

Treatment of overdose:

ECG monitoring, induce emesis, lavage, activated charcoal, administer anticonvulsant

doxorubicin

(dox-oh-roo'bi-sin)
Adriamycin, Adriamycin PFS, Adriamycin RDF, doxorubicin HCl, Rubex
Func. class.: Antineoplastic, antibiotic
Chem. class.: Anthracycline glycoside
Pregnancy category **D**

Action: Inhibits DNA synthesis primarily; derived from *Streptomyces peucetius;* replication is decreased by binding to DNA, which causes strand splitting; active throughout entire cell cycle; a vesicant

Therapeutic Outcome: Prevention of rapidly growing malignant cells

Uses: Wilms' tumor; bladder, breast, cervical, head, neck, liver, lung, ovarian, prostatic, stomach, testicular, thyroid cancer; Hodgkin's disease; acute lymphoblastic leukemia; myeloblastic leukemia;

neuroblastomas; lymphomas; sarcomas

Dosage and routes

Adult: 60-75 mg/m² q3 wk, or 30 mg/m² on days 1-3 of 4-wk cycle, not to exceed 550 mg/m² cumulative dose

Available forms: Inj **IV** 10, 20, 50 mg

Side effects/adverse reactions

CV: Increased B/P, ***sinus tachycardia, PVCs,*** chest pain, ***bradycardia, extrasystole***
GI: Nausea, vomiting, anorexia, mucositis, ***hepatotoxicity***
GU: Impotence, sterility, amenorrhea, gynecomastia, hyperuricemia
HEMA: ***Thrombocytopenia, leukopenia, anemia***
INTEG: *Rash, necrosis at inj site,* dermatitis, reversible alopecia, cellulitis, thrombophlebitis at inj site

Contraindications: Hypersensitivity, pregnancy (1st trimester) **D,** lactation, systemic infections

Precautions: Renal, hepatic, cardiac disease, gout, bone marrow depression (severe)

Pharmacokinetics

Absorption	Complete bioavailability
Distribution	Widely distributed; crosses placenta
Metabolism	Liver, extensively
Excretion	Bile (40%-50%)
Half-life	12 min; 3½ hr; 29⅔ hr

Pharmacodynamics

	IV
Onset	Unknown
Peak	Unknown
Duration	Unknown

Interactions

Drug/drug:

Individual drugs

Cyclophosphamide: ↑ cardiotoxicity, CHF
Mercaptopurine: ↑ liver disorders, hepatitis
Radiation: ↑ toxicity, bone marrow suppression

Drug classifications

Antineoplastics: ↑ toxicity, bone marrow suppression
Live virus vaccines: ↑ adverse reactions, ↓ antibody response

Lab test interferences

Increase: Uric acid

NURSING CONSIDERATIONS

Assessment

- Monitor ECG; watch for ST-T wave changes, low QRS and T; possible dysrhythmias (sinus tachycardia, heart block, PVCs) may occur
- Assess buccal cavity q8h for dryness, sores or ulceration, white patches, pain, bleeding, dysphagia; obtain prescription for viscous lidocaine (Xylocaine)
- Assess symptoms indicating severe allergic reaction: rash, pruritus, urticaria, purpuric skin lesions, itching, flushing; drug should be discontinued
- Assess tachypnea, ECG changes, dyspnea, edema, fatigue
- Monitor CBC, differential, platelet count weekly; withhold

drug if WBC count is <4000/ mm^3 or platelet count is <100,000/mm^3; notify prescriber of results if WBC <20,000/mm^3, platelets <150,000/mm^3

- Assess for increased uric acid levels, swelling, joint pain, primarily extremities; patient should be well hydrated to prevent urate deposits
- Monitor renal function studies: BUN, creatinine, serum uric acid, urine CrCl before and during therapy; I&O ratio; report fall in urine output to <30 ml/hr
- Monitor temp q4h (may indicate beginning of infection)
- Monitor liver function tests before and during therapy (bilirubin, AST [SGOT], ALT [SGPT], LDH) as needed or monthly; note yellowing of skin or sclera, dark urine, clay-colored stools, itchy skin, abdominal pain, fever, diarrhea
- Assess for bleeding: hematuria, stool guaiac, bruising or petechiae, mucosa or orifices q8h; inflammation of mucosa, breaks in skin
- Identify effects of alopecia on body image; discuss feelings about body changes

Associated nursing diagnoses

- ✓ Injury, risk for (adverse reactions)
- ✓ Body image disturbance (adverse reactions)
- ✓ Infection, risk for (adverse reactions)
- ✓ Knowledge deficit (teaching)

Implementation

- Avoid contact with skin; very irritating; wash completely to remove; give fluids **IV** or PO before chemotherapy to hydrate patient
- Give antiemetic 30-60 min before giving drug to prevent vomiting and prn; give antibiotics for prophylaxis of infection
- Provide liq diet: carbonated beverages; gelatin may be added if patient is not nauseated or vomiting
- Help patient to rinse mouth tid-qid with water or club soda, brush teeth bid-qid with soft brush or cotton-tipped applicators for stomatitis, use unwaxed dental floss

IV route

- Drug should be prepared by experienced personnel using proper precautions
- Give **IV** after diluting 10 mg/5 ml of NaCl for inj; another 5 ml of diluent/10 mg is recommended; shake; give over 3-5 min; give through Y-tube or 3-way stopcock through free-flowing D_5 inf or NS
- Use hydrocortisone, dexamethasone, or sodium bicarbonate (1 mEq/1 ml) for extravasation: apply ice compress

Syringe compatibilities:

Bleomycin, cisplatin, cyclophosphamide, droperidol, fluorouracil, leucovorin calcium, methotrexate, metoclopramide, mitomycin, vincristine

Syringe compatibilities:

Furosemide, heparin

Y-site compatibilities:

Bleomycin, cisplatin, cyclophosphamide, droperidol, fluorouracil, leucovorin calcium, methotrexate, metoclopramide, mitomycin, vinblastine, vincristine

Y-site incompatibilities:

Furosemide, heparin

Additive incompatibilities:

Aminophylline, cephalothin, dexamethasone, diazepam, fluorouracil, hydrocortisone

Patient/family education

- Tell patient that urine and other body fluids may be red-orange for 48 hr; contraceptive measures are recommended during therapy; drug is teratogenic to fetus
- Advise patient to avoid use of products containing aspirin or ibuprofen, razors, commercial mouthwash, since bleeding may occur; to report symptoms of bleeding (hematuria, tarry stools)
- Instruct patient to report signs of anemia (fatigue, headache, irritability, faintness, shortness of breath)
- Inform patient that hair may be lost during treatment; a wig or hair piece may make patient feel better; new hair may be different in color, texture
- Caution patient not to have any vaccinations without the advice of the prescriber; serious reactions can occur

Evaluation

Positive therapeutic outcome

- Prevention of rapid division of malignant cells

doxycycline

(dox-i-sye'kleen)

Apo-Doxy ✦, Doryx, Doxy 100, Doxy 200, Doxy-Caps, Doxychel Hyclate, Doxycin ✦, doxycycline, Monodox, Novodoxyclin ✦, Vibramycin, Vibramycin IV, Vibra-Tabs, Vovox

Func. class.: Broad-spectrum antibiotic/antiinfective

Chem. class.: Tetracycline

Pregnancy category **D**

Action: Inhibits protein synthesis, phosphorylation in microorganisms by binding to 30S ribosomal subunits, reversibly binding to 50S ribosomal subunits; bacteriostatic

→ Therapeutic Outcome: Bactericidal action against the following: gram-positive pathogens *Bacillus anthracis, Clostridium perfringens, C. tetani, Listeria monocytogenes, Nocardia, Propionibacterium acnes, Actinomyces israelii;* gram-negative pathogens *Haemophilus influenzae, Legionella pneumophila, Yersinia enterocolitica, V. pestis, Neisseria gonorrhoeae, N. meningitidis, Mycoplasma, Chlamydia, Rickettsia*

Uses: Syphilis, gonorrhea, lymphogranuloma venereum, uncommon gram-negative-positive organisms, malaria prophylaxis

Investigational uses: Traveler's diarrhea, Lyme disease, prevention of chronic bronchitis

Dosage and routes

Adult: PO 100 mg q12h on day 1, then 100 mg/day; **IV** 200 mg in 1-2 inf on day 1, then 100-200 mg/day

P *Child >8 yr:* PO/**IV** 4.4 mg/kg/day in divided doses q12h on day 1, then 2.2-4.4 mg/kg/day

Gonorrhea

Adult: Uncomplicated, PO 200 mg, then 100 mg hs and 100 mg bid × 3 days or 300 mg, then 300 mg in 1 hr; disseminated, 100 mg PO bid × at least 7 days

Chlamydia trachomatis

Adult: PO 100 mg bid × 7days

Syphilis

Adult: PO 300 mg/day in divided doses × 10 days

Available forms: Tab 50, 100 mg; cap 50, 100 mg; syr 50 mg/ml; powder for inj **IV** 100, 200 mg; powder for oral susp 25 mg/5 ml

Side effects/adverse reactions

CNS: Fever
CV: Pericarditis
EENT: Dysphagia, glossitis, decreased calcification of deciduous teeth, oral candidiasis
GI: *Nausea, abdominal pain, vomiting, diarrhea,* anorexia, enterocolitis, ***hepatotoxicity,*** flatulence, abdominal cramps, gastric burning, stomatitis
GU: *Increased BUN*
HEMA: ***Eosinophilia, neutropenia, thrombocytopenia, hemolytic anemia***
INTEG: Rash, urticaria, photosensitivity, increased pigmentation, ***exfoliative dermatitis,*** pruritus, ***angioedema***

Contraindications: Hypersensitivity to tetracyclines, children <8 yr, pregnancy **D**

Precautions: Hepatic disease, lactation

Pharmacokinetics

Absorption	Well absorbed
Distribution	Widely distributed, crosses placenta
Metabolism	Some hepatic recycling
Excretion	Bile, feces; kidneys unchanged (20%-40%)
Half-life	15-22 hr; increased in severe renal disease

Pharmacodynamics

	PO	IV
Onset	1½-4 hr	Immediate
Peak	1.5-4 hr	Infusion's end

Interactions

Drug/drug:

Calcium: Forms chelates, ↓ absorption
Carbamazepine: ↑ effect of carbamazepine
Iron: Forms chelates, ↓ absorption
Magnesium: Forms chelates, ↓ absorption
Phenytoin: ↓ effect of doxycycline

Drug classifications
Anticoagulants, oral: ↑ effect of anticoagulants
Barbiturates: ↓ effect of doxycycline
Contraceptives, oral: ↓ effect of oral contraceptive

Drug/food: ↓ absorption with dairy products

Lab test interferences

Increase (false): Urinary catecholamines, ALT (SGOT), AST (SGPT)
False negative: urine glucose

NURSING CONSIDERATIONS

Assessment

- Assess patient for previous sensitivity reaction
- Assess patient for signs and symptoms of infection including characteristics of wounds, sputum, urine, stool, WBC >10,000, fever; obtain baseline information before and during treatment
- Obtain C&S before beginning drug therapy to identify if correct treatment has been initiated
- Assess for allergic reactions: rash, urticaria, pruritus, chills, fever, joint pain; angioedema may occur a few days after therapy begins
- Assess bowel pattern daily; if severe diarrhea occurs, drug should be discontinued
- Monitor for bleeding: ecchymosis, bleeding gums, hematuria, stool guaiac daily if on long-term therapy; blood dyscrasias may occur
- Assess for overgrowth of infection: perineal itching, fever, malaise, redness, pain, swelling, drainage, rash, diarrhea, change in cough, sputum

Associated nursing diagnoses

- ✓ Infection, risk for (uses)
- ✓ Diarrhea (side effects)
- ✓ Injury, risk for (side effects)
- ✓ Knowledge deficit (teaching)
- ✓ Noncompliance (teaching)

Implementation

PO route

- Give around the clock to maintain proper blood levels; give with food to increase absorption of drug; do not give within 3 hr of other agents; drug actions may occur
- Give with 8 oz of water, 1 hr before hs to prevent ulceration
- Shake liq preparation well before giving; use calibrated device for proper dosing
- Do not give with iron, calcium, magnesium products or antacids, which decrease absorption and form insoluble chelate

IV **IV route**

- Check for irritation, extravasation, phlebitis daily; change site q72h
- For intermittent inf, dilute each 100 mg/10 ml 0.9% NaCl, sterile water for inj; further dilute in at least 100 ml 0.9% NaCl, D_5W, Ringer's, LR, D_5/LR protect from direct light; give over 1-4 hr

Y-site incompatibility:

Hetastarch

Y-site compatibilities:

Acyclovir, amiodarone, cyclophosphamide, hydromorphone, magnesium sulfate, melphalan, meperidine, morphine, ondansetron, perphenazine, sargramostim, vinorelbine

Additive compatibility:
Ranitidine

Syringe compatibility:
Doxapram

Patient/family education

- Teach patient to report sore throat, bruising, bleeding, joint pain; may indicate blood dyscrasias (rare)
- Advise patient to contact prescriber if vaginal itching, loose, foul-smelling stools, furry tongue occur; may indicate superinfection; report itching, rash, pruritus, urticaria
- Instruct patient to take all medication prescribed for the length of time ordered; drug must be taken around the clock to maintain blood levels; do not give medication to others
- Advise patient to notify prescriber of diarrhea with blood or pus

Evaluation

Positive therapeutic outcome
- Absence of signs/symptoms of infection (WBC <10,000, temp WNL, absence of red draining wounds)
- Reported improvement in symptoms of infection

droperidol
(droe-per′i-dole)
Droperidol, Inapsine
Func. class.: Neuroleptic, tranquilizer, antiemetic
Chem. class.: Butyrophenone derivative
Pregnancy category **C**

D

Action: Acts on CNS at subcortical levels, producing tranquilization, sleep; antiemetic

➔ **Therapeutic Outcome:** Maintenance of anesthesia

Uses: Premedication for surgery; induction, maintenance in general anesthesia; postoperatively for nausea and vomiting

Dosage and routes

Induction
Adult: **IV**/IM 0.22-0.275 mg/kg given with analgesic or general anesthetic; may give 1.25-2.5 mg additionally
P *Child 2-12 yr:* **IV**/IM 88-165 µg/kg, titrated to response needed

Premedication
Adult: IM/**IV** 2.5-10 mg ½-1 hr before surgery
P *Child 2-12 yr:* IM/**IV** 88-165 µg/kg

Maintaining general anesthesia
Adult: **IV** 1.25-2.5 mg

Regional anesthesia adjunct
Adult: IM/**IV** 2.5-5 mg

Diagnostic procedures without general anesthesia

Adult: IM 2.5-10 mg ½-1 hr before procedure; 1.25-2.5 mg may be needed additionally

Available forms: Inj 2.5 mg/ml

Side effects/adverse reactions

CNS: Dystonia, akathisia, flexion of arms, fine tremors, dizziness, anxiety, drowsiness, restlessness, hallucinations, depression
CV: Tachycardia, hypotension
EENT: Upward rotation of eyes, oculogyric crisis
INTEG: Chills, facial sweating, shivering
RESP: Laryngospasm, bronchospasm

Contraindications: Hyper-
P sensitivity, child <2 yr, pregnancy **C**

G **Precautions:** Elderly, cardiovascular disease (hypotension, bradydysrhythmias), renal disease, liver disease, Parkinson's disease

Pharmacokinetics

Absorption	Well absorbed (IM)
Distribution	Crosses blood-brain barrier, placenta
Metabolism	Liver
Excretion	Kidneys, unchanged (10%)
Half-life	Unknown

Pharmacodynamics

	IM/IV
Onset	3-10 min
Peak	30 min
Duration	3-6 hr

Interactions

Drug/drug:

Individual drugs

Alcohol: ↑ CNS depression
Lithium: ↑ side effects of lithium

Drug classifications

Amphetamines: ↓ effects of amphetamines
Anticholinergics: ↓ effects of anticholinergics
Anticoagulants: ↓ effects of anticoagulants
Anticonvulsants: ↓ effects of anticonvulsants
Antiparkinsonian agents: ↓ effects of antiparkinsonian agents
Antipsychotics: ↑ CNS depression
Barbiturates: ↑ CNS depression
CNS depressants: ↑ CNS depression
Narcotics: ↑ CNS depression

NURSING CONSIDERATIONS

Assessment

- Check VS q10 min during **IV** administration, q30 min after IM dose; for increasing heart rate or decreasing B/P, notify prescriber at once; do not place patient in Trendelenburg's position, or sympathetic blockade may occur, causing respiratory arrest
- Assess extrapyramidal reactions: dystonia, akathisia, extended neck, restlessness, tremors; if these occur, an anticholinergic should be given
- If given for nausea or vomiting, monitor for significant loss of fluids, bowel sounds before and during administration

Associated nursing diagnoses

✓ Injury, risk for (adverse reactions)
✓ Knowledge deficit (teaching)

Implementation

IM route
- Give deeply in large muscle mass

IV **IV route**
- Give direct **IV** undiluted; give through Y-tube or 3-way stopcock at 10 mg or less/min; titrate to patient response
- Intermittent inf may be given by adding dose to 250 ml LR, D_5W, 0.9% NaCl; give slowly
- Give anticholinergics (benztropine, diphenhydramine) for extrapyramidal reaction
- Give only with crash cart, resuscitative equipment nearby

Syringe compatibilities:

Atropine, bleomycin, butorphanol, chlorpromazine, cimetidine, cisplatin, cyclophosphamide, dimenhydrinate, diphenhydramine, doxorubicin, fentanyl, glycopyrrolate, hydroxyzine, meperidine, metoclopramide, midazolam, mitomycin, morphine, nalbuphine, pentazocine, perphenazine, prochlorperazine, promazine, promethazine, scopolamine, vinblastine, vincristine

Syringe incompatibilities:

Fluorouracil, furosemide, heparin, leucovorin calcium, methotrexate, pentobarbital

Y-site compatibilities:

Bleomycin, buprenorphine, cisplatin, cyclophosphamide, doxorubicin, hydrocortisone sodium succinate, metoclopramide, mitomycin, ondansetron, potassium chloride, vinblastine, vincristine, vitamin B with C

Y-site incompatibilities:

Fluorouracil, foscarnet, furosemide, leucovorin calcium, methotrexate, nafcillin

Additive incompatibility:

Barbiturates

Patient/family education

- Advise patient that orthostatic hypotension is common; to rise from lying or sitting position slowly
- Caution patient that drowsiness may occur; to call for assistance for ambulation

Evaluation

Positive therapeutic outcome
- Decreased anxiety
- Absence of vomiting during and after surgery

dyphylline

(dye'fi-lin)

Dilor, Dyflex-200, Dyflex-400, Dylline, dyphylline, Lufyllin, Lufyllin-400, Neothylline, Protophylline ✤

Func. class.: Bronchodilator, phosphodiesterase inhibitor

Chem. class.: Xanthine, ethylenediamide

Pregnancy category **C**

Action: Relaxes smooth muscle of respiratory system by blocking phosphodiesterase, which increases cyclic AMP; cyclic AMP results in positive inotropic, chronotropic effects, bronchodilatation, stimulation of CNS

➡ **Therapeutic Outcome:** Bronchodilatation with ease of breathing

Uses: Bronchial asthma, bronchospasm in chronic bronchitis, COPD

Dosage and routes

Adult: PO 200-800 mg q6h; IM 250-500 mg q6h injected slowly

Available forms: Tab 200, 400 mg; elix 100, 160 mg/15 ml; inj IM 250 mg/ml

Side effects/adverse reactions

CNS: Anxiety, restlessness, insomnia, dizziness, ***convulsions,*** headache, lightheadedness, muscle twitching

CV: Palpitations, sinus tachycardia, hypotension, flushing, dysrhythmias

GI: Nausea, vomiting, anorexia, dyspepsia, epigastric pain

INTEG: Flushing, urticaria

OTHER: Fever, dehydration, ***albuminuria,*** hyperglycemia

RESP: Tachypnea

Contraindications: Hypersensitivity to xanthines, tachydysrhythmias

G **Precautions:** Elderly, CHF, cor pulmonale, hepatic disease, active peptic ulcer disease, diabetes mellitus, hyperthyroidism, hypertension, P children, renal disease, pregnancy **C,** glaucoma

Pharmacokinetics

Absorption	Well absorbed (PO)
Distribution	Unknown
Metabolism	Liver
Excretion	Kidneys (85%)
Half-life	2 hr; increased in renal disease

Pharmacodynamics

	PO	IM
Onset	Unknown	Unknown
Peak	1 hr	Unknown
Duration	6 hr	Unknown

Interactions

Drug/drug:

Individual drugs

Cimetidine: ↓ metabolism, ↑ toxicity

Ketamine: Do not use together; seizures may occur

Drug classifications

Barbiturates: ↓ effect of dyphylline

β-Adrenergic blockers: ↓ metabolism, ↑ toxicity
Benzodiazapines: ↓ sedative effect
Sympathomimetics: ↑ CNS, CV adverse reactions

Drug/smoking:
↑ metabolism, ↓ effect

Drug/food:
Caffeinated foods (cola, coffee, tea, chocolate): ↑ CNS, CV, adverse reactions

NURSING CONSIDERATIONS
Assessment
- Monitor dyphylline blood levels (therapeutic level is <20 μg/ml); toxicity may occur with small increase above 20 μg/ml, especially elderly; determine whether theophylline was given recently (24 hr)
- Monitor I&O; an increase in diuresis occurs; dehydration may result in elderly or children
- Assess respiratory rate, rhythm, depth; before and during treatment auscultate lung fields bilaterally; notify prescriber of abnormalities
- Assess for allergic reactions: rash, urticaria; if these occur, drug should be discontinued

Associated nursing diagnoses
- ✓ Injury, high risk for (uses, adverse reactions)
- ✓ Airway clearance, ineffective (uses)
- ✓ Activity intolerance (uses)
- ✓ Knowledge deficit (teaching)

Implementation
PO route
- Give 1 hr ac and 2 hr pc to increase absorption; elix should be measured accurately

IM route
- Inject slowly; do not give by **IV** route; do not administer if cloudy or a precipitate occurs

Patient/family education
- Teach patient to take doses as prescribed, not to skip doses or double dose; patient should check OTC medications and current prescription medications for ephedrine, which increases CNS stimulation; tell patient not to drink alcohol or caffeine products (tea, coffee, chocolate, colas) or cardiovascular effects may occur
- Advise patient to avoid hazardous activities; dizziness may occur
- Caution patient if GI upset occurs, to take drug with 8 oz water; avoid food, since absorption may be decreased
- Teach patient to notify prescriber of change in smoking habit; a change in dosage may be required
- Instruct patient to report nausea, vomiting, insomnia, tachycardia, dysrhythmias, convulsions, or restlessness; can indicate toxicity
- Teach patient to increase fluids to 2 L/day to decrease viscosity of secretions

Evaluation
Positive therapeutic outcome
- Decreased dyspnea
- Clear lung fields bilaterally

echothiophate
(ek-oh-thye'oh-fate)
ecostigmine iodide, Phospholine Iodide
Func. class.: Miotic
Chem. class.: Cholinesterase inhibitor, irreversible
Pregnancy category **C**

Action: Prevents breakdown of neurotransmitter acetylcholine, which then accumulates, causing enhancement and prolongation of its physiologic effects

Therapeutic Outcome: Increased outflow of aqueous humor

Uses: Glaucoma (open angle), accommodative esotropia, treatment of obstructed aqueous outflow; extremely effective in control of chronic wide angle glaucoma, aphakic glaucoma, congenital glaucoma

Dosage and routes
P ***Adult and child:*** Instill 1 gtt of 0.03%, or 0.125% sol qd in conjunctival sac, not to exceed 1 gtt bid

Available forms: Powder for reconstitution, 1.5 mg (0.03%), 3 mg (0.06%), 6.25 mg (0.125%), 12.5 mg (0.25%) with 5 ml diluent

Side effects/adverse reactions
CV: Hypotension, bradycardia, ***cardiac arrest***
EENT: *Blurred vision; stinging; burning; lacrimation;* lid muscle twitching; conjunctival, ciliary redness; browache; headache; induced myopia; iris cysts; hyperemia; hyphema
GI: Nausea, vomiting, abdominal cramps, diarrhea
GU: Frequency
INTEG: Sweating, pallor, cyanosis
RESP: ***Bronchospasm***

Contraindications: Hypersensitivity, ureitis

Precautions: Asthma, bradycardia, parkinsonism, peptic ulcer, pregnancy **C**

Pharmacokinetics

Absorption	Minimal
Distribution	None
Metabolism	None
Excretion	None
Half-life	Unknown

Pharmacodynamics

	OPHTH
Onset	4-8 hr
Peak	Unknown
Duration	1-4 wk

Interactions
Drug/drug:
Individual drugs
Succinylcholine: ↑ neuroblockade

NURSING CONSIDERATIONS
Assessment
• Assess specific condition being treated; watch for ability to see, presence of pain, inflammation
• Assess history of patient's previous/current conditions (e.g., asthma, cardiac), possible

sensitivity, contraindications, drug interactions

Associated nursing diagnoses

- ✓ Sensory-perceptual alteration: visual (uses)
- ✓ Infection, risk for (uses)
- ✓ Knowledge deficit (teaching)

Implementation

Ophth route

- Give after checking vial for concentration; give immediately after reconstituting; discard unused portion
- Give after reconstituting powder with diluent provided
- Have patient recumbent before putting drops in the eyes; patient should tilt head back, pull down on lower lid; place drop in sac created; patient should close lids and roll eyes to distribute drug. Wash hands before and after administration

Patient/family education

- Explain why patient is receiving medication; patient, family should fully know regimen as well as name of medication
- Advise patient to report change in vision, blurring or loss of sight, trouble breathing, sweating, flushing
- Teach patient method of instillation, not to touch dropper to eye; use demonstration, return demonstration
- Advise patient that long-term therapy may be required and that blurred vision will decrease with repeated use of drug
- Caution patient that visual ability will be decreased at night; instruct patient not to drive

Evaluation

Positive therapeutic outcome

- Decreased outflow of aqueous humor in eye

E

econazole (topical)

(e-kone'a-zole)

Spectazole

Func. class.: Local antiinfective

Chem. class.: Imidazole derivative, antifungal

Pregnancy category **C**

Action: Interferes with fungal cell membrane, which increases permeability, causing leakage of cell nutrients

➔ **Therapeutic Outcome:** Fungistatic/fungicidal against organisms: tinea pedis, tinea cruris, tinea corporis, tinea versicolor

Uses: Tinea pedis, tinea cruris, tinea corporis, tinea versicolor, cutaneous candidiasis

Dosage and routes

P *Adult and child:* Top apply to affected area bid-qid depending on condition

Available forms: Cream 1%

Side effects/adverse reactions

INTEG: Rash, urticaria, stinging, burning, pruritus

Contraindications:
Hypersensitivity

Precautions: Pregnancy **C**, lactation

Pharmacokinetics

Absorption	Minimal
Distribution	Unknown
Metabolism	Liver
Excretion	Feces, kidneys
Half-life	2-3 days

Pharmacodynamics

Onset	Unknown
Peak	Unknown
Duration	Unknown

Interactions: None

NURSING CONSIDERATIONS
Assessment
- Assess skin for fungal infections: peeling, dryness, itching before and throughout treatment
- Monitor for allergic reaction: burning, stinging, swelling, redness, dermatitis, rash; drug should be discontinued, antihistamines (mild reaction)

Associated nursing diagnoses
- ✓ Skin integrity, impaired (uses)
- ✓ Infection, risk for (uses)
- ✓ Knowledge deficit (teaching)

Implementation
Top route
- Apply enough medication to cover lesions completely
- Apply after cleansing with soap and water; dry well
- Store at room temp in dry place

Patient/family education
- Teach patient to apply while wearing glove to prevent further infection; not to cover with occlusive dressings
- Teach patient that long-term therapy may be needed to clear infection (2 wk-6 mo depending on organism); compliance is needed even after feeling better
- Teach patient proper hygiene: hand-washing technique, nail care, use of concomitant top agents if prescribed
- Warn patient to avoid use of OTC creams, ointments, lotions unless directed
- Caution patient to use asepsis (hand washing) before, after each application
- Advise patient to change socks and shoes once a day during treatment of tinea pedis
- Advise patient to report to health care provider if infection persists or returns; if blisters, burning, oozing, or swelling occurs

Evaluation
Positive therapeutic outcome
- Decrease in size, number of lesions

edetate calcium disodium

(ed'e-tate)

calcium disodium versenate, calcium EDTA, edathamil calcium disodium, sodium chloride edetate

Func. class.: Heavy metal antagonist; antidote

Chem. class.: Chelating agent

Pregnancy category **C**

Action: Binds ions of lead by displacement of calcium to form a water-soluble complex that is removed by kidneys

Therapeutic Outcome: Decreased lead levels, absence of toxicity

Uses: Lead poisoning, acute lead encephalopathy

Dosage and routes

Acute lead encephalopathy

P ***Adult and child:*** 1.5 g/m^2/day × 3-5 days, with dimercaprol; may be given again after 4 days off drug

Lead poisoning

Adult: **IV** 1 g/250-500 ml D_5W or 0.9% NaCl over 1-2 hr or q12h × 3-5 days; may repeat after 2 days; not to exceed 50 mg/kg/day; may be given as a continuous inf over 8-24 hr

Adult: IM 35 mg/kg bid

P ***Child:*** IM 35 mg/kg/day in divided doses q8-12h, not to exceed 50 mg/kg/day; may give for 3-5 days, off 4 days before next course

Available forms: Inj 200 mg/ml

Side effects/adverse reactions

CNS: *Headache, paresthesia,* numbness

CV: Hypotension, dysrhythmias, thrombophlebitis

EENT: Nasal congestion, sneezing

GI: Vomiting, *diarrhea, abdominal cramps, anorexia,* cheilosis, histamine-like reaction with GI distress

GU: ***Hematuria, renal tubular necrosis, proteinuria***

INTEG: Urticaria, erythema, pruritus, pain at injection site, fever, cheilosis

MS: *Leg cramps,* myalgia, arthralgia, weakness

Contraindications: Hypersensitivity, anuria, poisoning of other metals, severe renal P disease, child <3 yr

Precautions: Hypertension, pregnancy **C**, lactation, gout, active TB

Pharmacokinetics

Absorption	Well absorbed (IM), complete (IV)
Distribution	Extracellular fluid
Metabolism	Not metabolized
Excretion	Kidneys, unchanged; lead complex
Half-life	IV 20-60 min, IM 1½ hr

Pharmacodynamics

	IM	IV
Onset	Unknown	Unknown
Peak	Unknown	Unknown
Duration	Unknown	Unknown

Interactions: None

NURSING CONSIDERATIONS

Assessment

- Assess patient's VS, B/P, pulse, respirations; weigh daily
- Monitor I&O, kidney function studies, BUN, creatinine, CrCl; watch for decreasing urine output
- Assess neuro status: watch for paresthesias, beginning convulsions
- Monitor urine: pH, albumin, casts, blood, coproporphyrins, calcium
- Assess for febrile reactions that may occur 4-8 hr following drug therapy
- Monitor for cardiac abnormalities: dysrhythmias, hypotension, tachycardia
- Assess for allergic reactions (rash, urticaria); if these occur, drug should be discontinued

Associated nursing diagnoses

✓ Poisoning, risk for (uses)
✓ Injury, risk for (uses, adverse reactions)
✓ Knowledge deficit (teaching)

Implementation

IV route

- Give by intermitent inf after diluting 5 ml EDTA/250-500 ml D_5W or 0.9% NaCl; give over 1 hr in less severe lead toxicity and over 2 hr in severe lead toxicity
- Cont inf may be given over 8-24 hr

Additive incompatibilities: Amphotericin B, hydralazine

Additive compatibility: Netilmicin

IM route

- Give by IM 1 ml procaine HCl 1% per 1 ml of drug; rotate inj sites, administer deeply in large muscle mass

Patient/family education

- Explain reason for medication and expected results
- Provide a referral to health department to assess lead levels in home or work place

Evaluation

Positive therapeutic outcome

- Decreased symptoms of lead intoxication
- Decreased lead level <50 μg/dl

Treatment of overdose: IV calcium salt

edrophonium

(ed-roe-fone'ee-yum)
Enlon, Reversol, Tensilon
Func. class.: Cholinergics, anticholinesterase
Chem. class.: Quaternary ammonium compound
Pregnancy category **C**

Action: Inhibits destruction of acetylcholine, which increases concentration at sites where acetylcholine is released; this facilitates transmission of impulses across myoneural junction

Therapeutic Outcome: Reversal of nondepolarizing neuromuscular blockers; absence of difficulty with muscular function in myasthenia gravis

Uses: Diagnosis of myasthenia gravis; curare antagonist; differentiation of myasthenic crisis from cholinergic crisis; reversal of nondepolarizing neuromuscular blockers

Dosage and routes

Tensilon test (Myasthenia Gravis Diagnosis)

Adult: **IV** 1-2 mg over 15-30 sec, then 8 mg if no response; IM: 10 mg; if cholinergic reaction occurs, retest after ½ hr with 2 mg IM

P *Child >34 kg:* **IV** 2 mg; if no response in 45 sec, then 1 mg q45 sec, not to exceed 10 mg; IM 5 mg

P *Child <34 kg:* **IV** 1 mg; if no response in 45 sec, then 1 mg q45 sec, not to exceed 5 mg;IM 2 mg

P *Infant:* **IV** 0.5 mg

Reversal of nondepolarizing neuromuscular blockers

Adult: **IV** 10 mg over 30-45 sec, may repeat, not to exceed 40 mg

Differentiation of myasthenic crisis from cholinergic crisis

Adult: **IV** 1 mg, if no response in 1 min, may repeat

Available forms: Inj 10 mg/ml

Side effects/adverse reactions

CNS: Dizziness, headache, sweating, weakness, ***convulsions,*** uncoordination, ***paralysis,*** drowsiness, ***loss of consciousness***

CV: Tachycardia, dysrhythmias, bradycardia, hypotension, AV block, ECG changes, ***cardiac arrest,*** syncope

EENT: Miosis, blurred vision, lacrimation, visual changes

GI: *Nausea, diarrhea, vomiting, cramps, increased salivary and gastric secretions, dysphagia, increased peristalsis*

GU: Frequency, incontinence, urgency

INTEG: Rash, urticaria

RESP: ***Respiratory depression, bronchospasm, constriction, laryngospasm, respiratory arrest,*** dyspnea

Contraindications: Obstruction of intestine, renal system, hypersensitivity

Precautions: Seizure disorders, bronchial asthma, coronary occlusion, hyperthyroidism, dysrhythmias, peptic ulcer, megacolon, poor GI motility, pregnancy **C**, bradycardia, hypotension

Pharmacokinetics

Absorption	Unknown
Distribution	Unknown
Metabolism	Unknown
Excretion	Unknown
Half-life	Unknown

Pharmacodynamics

	IM	IV
Onset	2-10 min	30-60 sec
Peak	Unknown	Unknown
Duration	12-45 min	6-25 min

Interactions

Drug/drug:

Drug classifications
Anticholinergics: ↓ effect of edrophonium

NURSING CONSIDERATIONS

Assessment

- Assess vital signs, respiration during test
- Monitor diabetic patient carefully—this drug lowers blood glucose

Associated nursing diagnoses

✓ Breathing pattern, ineffective (uses)
✓ Knowledge deficit (teaching)

Implementation

IV **IV route**

- Administer undiluted 2 mg or less over 15-30 sec, or give as continuous inf in myasthenia crisis
- Give only after ensuring that atropine sulfate is available for cholinergic crisis
- Give only after all other cholinergics have been discontinued
- Store at room temp

Y-site compatibilities:

Heparin, hydrocortisone, potassium chloride, vitamin B with C

Patient/family education

- Instruct patient to wear Medic Alert ID specifying myasthenia gravis and drugs taken

Evaluation

Positive therapeutic outcome

- Increased muscle strength, hand grasp; improved gait; absence of labored breathing (if severe)

Treatment of overdose: Respiratory support, atropine 1-4 mg (**IV**)

enalapril/enalaprilat

(e-nal'april/e-nal-a-pril-at)

Vasotec, Vasotec IV

Func. class.: Antihypertensive

Chem. class.: Angiotensin-converting enzyme inhibitor

Pregnancy category **C**

Action: Selectively suppresses renin-angiotensin-aldosterone system; inhibits ACE; prevents conversion of angiotensin I to angiotensin II, resulting in dilatation of arterial and venous vessels

➔ **Therapeutic Outcome:** Decreased B/P in hypertension; decreased preload, afterload in CHF

Uses: Hypertension, CHF, alone or in combination

Dosage and routes

Adult: PO 5 mg/day, may increase or decrease to desired response; range 10-40 mg/day

Hypertension

Adult: **IV** 1.25 mg q6h over 5 min

Patients on diuretics

Adult: **IV** 0.625 mg over 5 min, may give additional doses of 1.25 mg q6h

Renal impairment

Adult: **IV** 1.25 mg q6h with CrCl <3 mg/dl or 0.625 mg if CrCl >3 mg/dl

Available forms: Tabs 2.5, 5, 10, 20 mg, inj 1.25 mg/ml

Side effects/adverse reactions

CNS: Insomnia, dizziness, paresthesias, headache, fatigue, anxiety
CV: Hypotension, chest pain, tachycardia, dysrhythmias
EENT: Tinnitus, visual changes, sore throat, double vision, dry burning eyes
GI: Nausea, vomiting, colitis, cramps, diarrhea, constipation, flatulence, dry mouth, loss of taste
GU: ***Proteinuria, renal failure,*** increased frequency of polyuria or oliguria
HEMA: ***Agranulocytosis, neutropenia***
INTEG: Rash, purpura, alopecia, hyperhidrosis
META: Hyperkalemia
RESP: Dyspnea, cough, rales, angioedema

Contraindications: Pregnancy **C**, lactation

Precautions: Renal disease, hyperkalemia

Pharmacokinetics

Absorption	Well absorbed (PO), complete (IV)
Distribution	Unknown
Metabolism	Liver (active metabolite—enalaprilat)
Excretion	Kidneys (60%—enalaprilat, 20%—enalapril)
Half-life	Enalaprilat 11 hr, increased in renal disease

Pharmacodynamics

	PO	IV
Onset	1 hr	15 min
Peak	4-6 hr	1-4 hr
Duration	24 hr	6 hr

Interactions

Drug/drug:

Individual drugs

Alcohol: ↑ hypotension (large amounts)
Allopurinol: ↑ hypersensitivity
Digoxin: ↑ serum levels
Hydralazine: ↑ toxicity
Indomethacin: ↓ antihypertensive effect
Lithium: ↑ serum levels
Prazosin: ↑ toxicity

Drug classifications

Adrenergic blockers: ↑ hypotension
Antacids: ↓ absorption
Antihypertensives: ↑ hypotension
Diuretics: ↑ hypotension
Diuretics, potassium-sparing: ↑ toxicity
Ganglionic blockers: ↑ hypotension
Potassium supplements: ↑ toxicity
Sympathomimetics: ↑ toxicity

Lab test interferences

Interference: Glucose/insulin tolerance tests

NURSING CONSIDERATIONS

Assessment

- Monitor blood studies: neutrophils, decreased platelets
- Monitor B/P, orthostatic hypotension, syncope; if changes occur dosage change may be required
- Monitor renal studies: protein, BUN, creatinine; increased levels may indicate nephrotic syndrome and renal failure
- Monitor renal symptoms: polyuria, oliguria, frequency, dysuria
- Establish baselines in renal, liver function tests before therapy begins
- Check potassium levels throughout treatment, although hyperkalemia rarely occurs
- Check for edema in feet, legs daily
- Assess for allergic reactions: rash, fever, pruritus, urticaria; drug should be discontinued if antihistamines fail to help

Associated nursing diagnoses

✓ Cardiac output, decreased (uses)
✓ Injury, potential for (adverse reactions)
✓ Knowledge deficit (teaching)
✓ Noncompliance (teaching)

Implementation

PO route

- Store in air-tight container at 86° F (30° C) or less
- Severe hypotension may occur after 1st dose of this medication; decreased hypotension may be prevented by reducing or discontinuing diuretic therapy 3 days before beginning benazepril therapy
- Give by **IV** inf of 0.9% NaCl (as ordered) to expand fluid volume if severe hypotension occurs

IV **IV route**

- Give **IV** direct over 5 min
- Dilute in 50 ml 0.9% NaCl, D_5W, D_5/0.9% NaCl, D_5/LR; diluted solution may be used for 24 hr

Y-site compatibilities:
Amikacin, aminophylline, ampicillin, ampicillin/sulbactam, aztreonam, butorphanol, calcium gluconate, cefazolin, cefoperazone, ceftazidime, ceftizoxime, chloramphenicol, cimetidine, clindamycin, erythromycin lactobionate, esmolol, famotidine, fentanyl, ganciclovir, gentamicin, heparin, hetastarch, hydrocortisone sodium succinate, labetalol, lidocaine, magnesium sulfate, melphalan, methylprednisolone sodium succinate, metronidazole, morphine, nafcillin, penicillin G, potassium, phenobarbital, piperacillin, potassium chloride, potassium phosphate, ranitidine, sodium acetate, tobramycin, trimethoprim/sulfamethoxazole, vancomycin, vinorelbine

Y-site incompatibilities:
Amphotericin B, phenytoin

Patient/family education

- Advise patient not to discontinue drug abruptly; advise patient to tell all persons associated with his care
- Teach patient not to use OTC products (cough, cold, allergy medications) unless directed by

physician; serious side effects can occur. Xanthines, such as coffee, tea, chocolate, cola can prevent action of drug
• Instruct patient on the importance of complying with dosage schedule, even if feeling better; to continue with medical regimen to decrease B/P: exercise, cessation of smoking, decreasing stress, diet modifications
• Emphasize the need to rise slowly to sitting or standing position to minimize orthostatic hypotension; not to exercise in hot weather, which can cause increased hypotension
• Advise patient to notify prescriber of mouth sores, sore throat, fever, swelling of hands or feet, irregular heartbeat, chest pain, coughing, shortness of breath
• Caution patient to report excessive perspiration, dehydration, vomiting, diarrhea; may lead to fall in B/P
• Caution patient that drug may cause dizziness, fainting, light-headedness; may occur during 1st few days of therapy; to avoid activities that may be hazardous
• Teach patient how to take B/P, and normal readings for age group

Evaluation

Positive therapeutic outcome
• Decreased B/P in hypertension

Treatment of overdose:

Lavage, **IV** atropine for bradycardia, **IV** theophylline for bronchospasm, digitalis, O_2, diuretic for cardiac failure, hemodialysis

enoxacin

(en-ox'a-sin)
Penetrex
Func. class.: Antiinfective
Chem. class.: Fluoroquinolone
Pregnancy category **C**

E

Action: Interferes with conversion of intermediate DNA fragments into high–molecular-weight DNA in bacteria; DNAgyrase inhibitor

➔ Therapeutic Outcome: Bactericidal against the following organisms: staphylococci, *Enterobacter* sp, *Escherichia coli, Klebsiella* sp, *Neisseria gonorrhea, Pseudomonas aeruginosa*

Uses: Uncomplicated urethral or cervical gonorrhea, uncomplicated and complicated urinary tract infections (UTI)

Dosage and routes

Gonorrhea

Adult: PO 400 mg as a single dose

Uncomplicated UTI

Adult: PO 200 mg bid × 7 days

Complicated UTI

Adult: PO 400 mg bid × 14 days

Available forms: Tabs 200, 400 mg

Side effects/adverse reactions

CNS: Dizziness, headache, fatigue, somnolence, depression, insomnia, anxiety
EENT: Visual disturbances, dizziness
GI: Diarrhea, nausea, vomiting, anorexia, flatulence, heartburn, abdominal pain, dry mouth, increased AST (SGOT), ALT (SGPT)
INTEG: Rash, pruritus, photosensitivity

Contraindications: Hypersensitivity to quinolones

P G **Precautions:** Pregnancy **C**, lactation, children, elderly, renal disease, seizure disorders

Pharmacokinetics

Absorption	Well absorbed
Distribution	Widely
Metabolism	Liver 20%
Excretion	Kidneys 50%-80%
Half-life	3-6 hr, increased in renal disease

Pharmacodynamics

	PO
Onset	Unknown
Peak	Unknown

Interactions

Drug/drug:

Bismuth subsalicylate: ↓ enoxacin level
Caffeine: ↓ effect of enoxacin
Cyclosporine: ↑ nephrotoxicity
Digoxin: ↑ digoxin levels
Nitrofurantoin: ↓ effectiveness
Probenecid: ↑ blood levels
Sucralfate: ↓ absorption of enoxacin
Theophylline: ↑ toxicity
Warfarin: ↑ warfarin effect
Zinc sulfate: ↓ absorption of enoxacin

NURSING CONSIDERATIONS

Assessment

- Assess patient for previous sensitivity reaction to quinolones
- Assess patient for signs and symptoms of infection including WBC >10,000, hematuria, foul-smelling urine; obtain baseline information before and during treatment
- Complete C&S testing before beginning drug therapy; this will identify if correct treatment has been initiated
- Assess for allergic reactions: rash, urticaria, pruritus
- Identify urine output; also monitor increases in BUN, creatinine
- Monitor blood studies: AST (SGOT), ALT (SGPT)

Associated nursing diagnoses

✓ Infection, risk for (uses)
✓ Diarrhea (adverse reactions)
✓ Knowledge deficit (teaching)
✓ Noncompliance (teaching)

Implementation

PO route

- Give 1 hr ac or 2 hr pc to maintain proper blood levels
- Give with 8 oz of water, 1 hr before hs to prevent ulceration
- Do not give with iron products or antacids, which will decrease absorption; should not be given 4 hr before or 2 hr after medication

Patient/family education

- Instruct patient to increase fluids to 3L/day to prevent crystallization in the kidney
- Instruct patient to report itching, rash, pruritus, urticaria
- Instruct patient to take all medication prescribed for the length of time ordered; drug must be taken as ordered
- Advise patient to limit intake of alkaline foods and drugs: milk, dairy products, peanuts, vegetables, alkaline antacids, sodium bicarbonate

Evaluation

Positive therapeutic outcome

- Reported improvement in symptoms of infection
- Negative C&S test results

enoxaparin

(ee-nox'a-par-in)

Lovenox

Func. class.: Antithrombotic

Chem. class.: Unfractionated porcine heparin (low-molecular heparin)

Pregnancy category **C**

Action: Prevents conversion of fibrinogen to fibrin and prothrombin to thrombin by enhancing inhibitory effects of antithrombin III; produces higher ratio of anti-factor Xa to anti-factor IIa

➡ **Therapeutic Outcome:** Prevention of deep vein thrombosis

Uses: Prevention of deep vein thrombosis, pulmonary emboli in hip and knee replacement

Dosage and routes

Adult: SC 30 mg bid immediately after surgery; continue to administer until deep vein thrombosis is no longer a threat (7-14 days)

Available forms: Inj 30 mg/0.3 ml (prefilled syringes)

Side effects/adverse reactions

CNS: Fever, confusion
GI: Nausea
GU: Edema, peripheral edema
HEMA: Hypochromic anemia, thrombocytopenia, bleeding
INTEG: Ecchymosis

Contraindications: Hypersensitivity to this drug, heparin, or pork; hemophilia; leukemia with bleeding; peptic ulcer disease; thrombocytopenic purpura

Precautions: Alcoholism, G elderly, pregnancy **C**, hepatic disease (severe), renal disease (severe), blood dyscrasias, severe hypertension, subacute bacterial endocarditis, acute nephritis, lactation, P children

Pharmacokinetics

Absorption	Well absorbed (SC)
Distribution	Unknown
Metabolism	Unknown
Excretion	Unknown
Half-life	4½ hr

Pharmacodynamics

Onset	Unknown
Peak	Unknown
Duration	Unknown

Interactions

Drug/drug:

Drug classifications

Anticoagulants: ↑ bleeding
Nonsteroidal antiinflammatories: ↑ bleeding
Salicylates: ↑ bleeding

Lab test interferences

Increase: T_3 uptake
Decrease: Uric acid

NURSING CONSIDERATIONS

Assessment

- Monitor blood studies (Hct, occult blood in stools) q3mo; partial pro-time, which should be 1½-2 × control; PTT; often done qd; APTT, ACT; platelet count q2-3 days; thrombocytopenia may occur
- Assess patient for bleeding gums, petechiae, ecchymosis, black tarry stools, hematuria, epistaxis, decrease in B/P; indicate bleeding and possible hemorrhage; notify prescriber immediately

Associated nursing diagnoses

- ✓ Injury, risk for (uses, adverse reactions)
- ✓ Tissue perfusion, altered (uses)
- ✓ Knowledge deficit (teaching)

Implementation

SC route

- Give at same time each day to maintain steady blood levels
- Administer SC deeply; do not give IM; sol is clear to yellow; do not use sol with precipitate; rotate sites; apply gentle pressure for 1 min

Patient/family education

- Warn patient to avoid OTC preparations unless directed by prescriber because they could cause serious drug interactions
- Instruct patient to use soft-bristled toothbrush to avoid bleeding gums; to avoid contact sports; to use electric razor; to avoid IM inj
- Advise patient to report any signs of bleeding, bruising: gums, under skin, urine, stools

Evaluation

Positive therapeutic outcome

- Absence of deep vein thrombosis

ephedrine

(e-fed'rin)

ephedrine, ephedrine sulfate, Neorespin, Kondon's Nasal Jelly, Pretz-D

Func. class.: Adrenergic, mixed direct and indirect effects; bronchodilator, nasal decongestant, vasopressor

Chem. class.: Phenylisopropylamine

Pregnancy category C

Action: Increases contractility and heart rate by acting on β-receptors in the heart; also acts on α-receptors, causing vasoconstriction in blood vessels

➡ Therapeutic Outcome: Decreased nasal congestion, bronchodilation, stimulation, increased B/P

Uses: Shock; increased perfusion; hypotension, bronchodilation; nasal congestion; orthostatic hypotension, depression, narcolepsy; vasopressor

Dosage and routes

Adult: IM/SC 25-50 mg, not to exceed 150 mg/24 hr
IV 10-25 mg, not to exceed 150 mg/24 hr

P *Child:* SC/**IV** 3 mg/kg/day or 100 mg/m^2/day in divided doses q4-6h

Bronchodilator

Adult: PO 25-50 mg bid-qid, not to exceed 400 mg/day; IM/SC 12½-25 mg

P *Child:* PO 2-3 mg/kg/day or 100 mg/m^2/day in 4-6 divided doses

Nasal decongestant

P *Adult and child >6 yr:* Nasal i-ii sprays in each nostril prn q4hr for <3-4 days

Stimulation

Adult: PO 25-50 mg q3-4 hr prn

P *Child:* PO 3 mg/kg/day or 100 mg/m^2/day in 4-6 divided doses

Orthostatic hypotension

Adult: PO 25 mg qd-qid

P *Child:* PO 3 mg/kg/day in 4-6 divided doses

Available forms: Inj 25, 50 mg/ml; cap 25, 50 mg; syr, 20 mg/5 ml; nasal spray 0.25% nasal drops 0.5%; nasal jelly 1%

Side effects/adverse reactions

CNS: Tremors, anxiety, insomnia, headache, dizziness, confusion, hallucinations, ***convulsions, CNS depression***
CV: Palpitations, tachycardia, hypertension, chest pain, ***dysrhythmias***
EENT: Rebound congestion (nasal)
GI: Anorexia, nausea, vomiting
GU: Dysuria, urinary retention
RESP: Dyspnea

Contraindications: Hypersensitivity to sympathomimetics, angle-closure glaucoma

Precautions: Pregnancy **C**, cardiac disorders, hyperthyroidism, diabetes mellitus, prostatic hypertrophy

Pharmacokinetics

Absorption	Well absorbed (PO/IM/SC) complete (IV)
Distribution	Unknown
Metabolism	Liver
Excretion	Kidneys—unchanged
Half-life	3-5 hr

Pharmacodynamics

	PO	SC	IM	IV	NASAL
Onset	¼-1 hr	Unkn	15-30 min	5 min	Unkn
Peak	Unkn	Unkn	Unkn	Unkn	Unkn
Duration	2-4 hr	1 hr	1 hr	2 hr	6 hr

Interactions

Drug/drug:

Drug classifications

Antidepressants, tricyclics: ↓ effect of vasopressor
Anesthetics, halothane: Increased dysrhythmias
Beta-adrenergic blockers: Blocks therapeutic effect
Bronchodilators, aerosol: ↑ action of bronchodilator
MAOI: ↑ chance of hypertensive crisis
Oxytoxics: ↑ severe hypertension
Sympathomimetics: ↑ adrenergic side effects

NURSING CONSIDERATIONS

Assessment

- Monitor respiratory function: vital capacity, forced expiratory volume, ABGs, lung sounds, heart rate, baseline rhythm (bronchodilator)
- Monitor for evidence of allergic reactions; paradoxical bronchospasm; withhold dose; notify prescriber
- Monitor ECG, B/P, pulse, q5 min when using **IV** route (shock)
- Assess nasal congestion to identify factors contributing to ongoing congestion (nasal use)
- Assess mental status and sleeping patterns; mood, sensorium, ability to stay awake

Associated nursing diagnoses

✓ Airway clearance, ineffective (uses)
✓ Gas exchange impaired (uses)
✓ Sleep pattern disturbance (uses)
✓ Knowledge deficit (teaching)

Implementation

PO route

- Administer several hr (up to 6 hr) before hs to prevent sleeplessness

IV **IV route**

- Give **IV** directly undiluted using 3-way stopcock or Y-site; give 10 mg/min or less
- Use clear sol without precipitate; unused sol should be discarded

Solution compatibilities:

0.9% NaCl, 0.45% NaCl, D5W, D10W, Ringers, LR, ionosol

Patient/family education

- Advise patient to avoid use of OTC medications—extra stimulation may occur, and not to use alcohol

Evaluation

Positive therapeutic outcome

- Increased B/P (vasopressor)
- Ability to stay awake (absence of narcolepsy) or improved mood (absence of depression)
- Absence of bronchospasm
- Decreased nasal congestion

Treatment of overdose:

Administer a B_2-adrenergic blocker

epinephrine

(ep-i-nef'rin)

Adrenalin Chloride, Adrenalin Chloride Solution, AsthmaHaler, Asthma Nefrin, Bronitin Mist, Bronkaid Mist, Dysne-Inhal, epinephrine, Epinal, Epitrate, Eppy/N, Glaucon, epinephrine HCl, Epinephrine Pediatric, EpiPen Jr., Medihaler-Epi, micronefrin, Nephron Inhalant, Primatene Mist, S-2 Inhalant, Sus-Phrine, Vaponefrin

Func. class.: Adrenergic, bronchodilator, cardiac stimulant

Chem. class.: Catecholamine

Pregnancy category **C**

Action: β_1- and β_2-agonist causing increased levels of cyclic AMP producing bronchodilation, cardiac, and CNS stimulation; large doses cause vasoconstriction; small doses can cause vasodilation via β_2-vascular receptors

Therapeutic Outcome: Vasoconstrictor, cardiac stimulator, bronchodilator, decreased aqueous humor

Uses: Acute asthmatic attacks, hemostasis, bronchospasm, anaphylaxis, allergic reactions, cardiac arrest, adjunct in anesthesia

Dosage and routes

Asthma

P *Adult and child:* Inh 1-2 puffs of 1:100 or 2.25% racemic q15 min

Bronchodilator (parenteral epinephrine solution)

Adult: SC 0.2-0.5 mg, q20 min-4 hr max/mg/dose

Anaphylactic shock/vasopressor

Adult: SC/IM 0.5, repeat q5 min if needed, then **IV** 0.1-0.25 mg, repeat q5-15 min or infusion 1 mg/min, increase to 4 mg/min

P *Child:* SC/IM/**IV** 10 μg/kg, repeat q5-15 min, up to 0.3 mg

Anaphylactic reaction

Adult: SC/IM 0.2-0.5 mg, repeat q10-15 min, not to exceed 1 mg/dose

P *Child:* SC 0.01 mg/kg, repeat q15min × 2 doses, then q4h as needed, up to 0.5 mg/dose

Bronchodilator

P *Adult and child:* Inh 1-2 inh of 1:100 or 2.25% racepineprine - 0.2 mg/dose, may repeat q3h

Adult: Ophth: 1 gtt qd or bid

Cardiac arrest

Adult: IC, **IV**, endotracheal 0.1-1 mg repeat q5 min prn

P *Child:* IC, **IV**, endotracheal 5-10 μg q5 min, may use 0.1 μ/kg/min **IV** inf after initial dose

Available forms: Aerosol 0.16 mg/spray, 0.2 mg/spray, 0.25 mg/spray, inj 1:1000 (1 mg/ml), 1:200 (5 mg/ml), 0.01 mg/ml (1:100,000), 0.1 mg/ml (1:10,000), 0.5 mg/ml (1:2,000); IM, **IV**, SC; sol for nebulization 1:100, 1.25% 2.25% (base)

Side effects/adverse reactions

CNS: Tremors, anxiety, insomnia, headache, dizziness, confusion, hallucinations, ***cerebral hemorrhage***
CV: Palpitations, tachycardia, hypertension, *dysrhythmias,* increased T wave
GI: Anorexia, nausea, vomiting
GU: Urinary retention, hesitancy
RESP: Dyspnea

Contraindications: Hypersensitivity to sympathomimetics, narrow angle glaucoma

Precautions: Pregnancy **C**, cardiac disorders, hyperthyroidism, diabetes mellitus, prostatic hypertrophy, G elderly, lactation

Pharmacokinetics

Absorption	Well absorbed (PO), complete (IV)
Distribution	Unknown, crosses placenta
Metabolism	Liver
Excretion	Breast milk
Half-life	Unknown

Pharmacodynamics

	SC	IM	IV	INH	OPTH
Onset	3-5 min	5-10 min	immediate	1 min	½-1 hr
Peak	Unknown	Unknown	Unknown	Unknown	Unknown
Duration	1-4 hr	1-4 hr	Unknown	1-4 hr	24 hr

Interactions

Drug/drug:

Drug classifications
Anesthetics, general: ↑ dysrythmias
Antidepressants, tricyclics: ↑ pressor response
Beta-adrenergic blockers: Block therapeutic effect
Bronchodilators, aerosol: ↑ action of bronchodilator
Cardiac glycosides: ↑ dysrhythmias
Insulin: ↑ need for insulin in diabetics
Lithium: ↓ effect of epinephrine
Methyldopa: ↑ pressor response
MAOI: ↑ chance of hypertensive crisis
Other Sympathomimetics: ↑ adrenergic side effects, additive effects

NURSING CONSIDERATIONS

Assessment

- Monitor respiratory function: vital capacity, forced expiratory volume, ABGs, lung sounds, heart rate, rhythm (baseline); amount, color of sputum
- Monitor ECG during administration continuously, if B/P increases, drug should be decreased; check B/P, pulse q5min after parenteral route; CVP, PCWP

- Check inj site for tissue sloughing; if this occurs, administer phentolamine mixed with 0.9% NaCl
- Monitor for evidence of allergic reactions; paradoxical bronchospasm; withhold dose; notify prescriber

Associated nursing diagnoses

- ✓ Airway clearance, ineffective (uses)
- ✓ Gas exchange impaired (uses)
- ✓ Cardiac output, decreased (uses)
- ✓ Sensory-perceptual alteration, visual (uses) (ophth)
- ✓ Knowledge deficit (teaching)

Implementation

IV **IV route**

- Give after diluting 1 mg of 1:1000 sol/10 ml or more; 0.9% NaCl yields 1:10,000 sol, give 1 mg/min
- Give by continuous inf after further diluting in 0.9% NaCl, D5W, D10W, D5/LR, LR—give via 3-way stopcock; for Y-site, use inf pump

Y-site incompatibility:
Ampicillin

Y-site compatibilities:
Amrinone, atracurium, calcium chloride, calcium gluconate, famotidine, heparin, hydrocortisone sodium succinate, pancuronium, phytonadione, potassium chloride, vecuronium, vitamin B with C

Syringe compatibilities:
Doxapram, heparin, milrinone

Additive compatibilities:
Amikacin, cimetidine, dobutamide, floxacillin, furosemide, metaraminol, verapamil

Additive incompatibilities:
Aminophylline, mephentermine, sodium bicarbonate, warfarin

SC/IM route

- Rotate inj sites, massage well, do not use gluteal (IM) site
- Shake suspension before using

Inh route

- Use 2.25% sol diluted in nebulizer/respirator
- 10 gtt of a 1% sol should be placed in nebulizer

Endotracheal route

- Only used in intubated patient; use **IV** dose that should be injected by endotracheal tube into bronchi

Patient/family education

- Tell patient not to use OTC medications; extra stimulation may occur; to use this medication before other medications and allow at least 5 min between each, to prevent overstimulation
- Teach patient that paradoxical bronchospasm may occur and to stop drug immediately and notify health care provider; to limit caffeine products such as chocolate, coffee, tea, and colas
- Patient should rinse mouth after inh
- Patient should report blurred vision, irritation with ophth preparations

Evaluation

Positive therapeutic outcome
- Absence of dyspnea, wheezing
- Improved airway exchange, improved ABGs
- Decreased aqueous humor
- Stabilization of heart rate and cardiac output

Treatment of overdose: Administer a B_2-adrenergic blocker

epoetin alfa

(ee-poe'e-tin al'fa)

rHU-EPO, Eprex ♣, Erythropoietin

Func. class.: Hormone

Chem. class.: Amino acid polypeptide

Pregnancy category C

Action: Erythropoietin is one factor controlling rate of red cell production; drug is developed by recombinant DNA technology

➡ Therapeutic Outcome: Decreased anemia with increased RBCs

Uses: Anemia caused by reduction endogenous erythropoietin production, primarily end-stage renal disease; to correct hemostatic defect in uremia; anemia caused by AZT (zidovudine) treatment in HIV-positive patients; anemia caused by chemotherapy

Dosage and routes

Anemia secondary to chemotherapy

Adult: SC 150 U/kg 3×/wk, may increase after 2 mo up to 300 U/kg 3×/wk

Anemia in chronic renal failure

Adult: SC/**IV** 50-100 U/kg 3×/wk, then adjust dose by 25 U/kg/dose to maintain appropriate Hct

Anemia secondary to zidovudine treatment

Adult: SC/**IV** 100 U/kg 3×/wk × 2 mo; may increase by 50-100 U/kg q1-2 mo, up to 300 U/kg 3×/wk

Available forms: 2000, 3000, 4000, 10,000 U/ml

Side effects/adverse reactions

CNS: ***Seizures,*** coldness, sweating

CV: *Hypertension,* ***hypertensive encephalopathy***

MS: Bone pain

Contraindications: Hypersensitivity to albumin, severe hypertension, erythropoietin levels of >200 mU/ml

Precautions: Pregnancy **C**

Pharmacokinetics	
Absorption	Well absorbed (SC), completely absorbed (IV)
Distribution	Unknown
Metabolism	Unknown
Excretion	Unknown
Half-life	5-14 hr

Pharmacodynamics

	SC/IV
Onset	Unknown
Peak	Unknown
Duration	Unknown
Increased RBC count	1-2 wk

Interactions: None

NURSING CONSIDERATIONS

Assessment

- Monitor renal studies: urinalysis, protein, blood, BUN, creatinine; I&O; report drop in output to <50 ml/hr
- Monitor blood studies: reticulocyte count weekly; check for symptoms of anemia: fatigue, pallor, dyspnea
- Assess for CNS symptoms: coldness, sweating
- Assess CV status: B/P before and during treatment; hypertension may occur rapidly leading to hypertension encephalopathy
- Assess patient during hemodialysis for bruits, thrills of shunts; drug prevents severe anemia in chronic renal failure; clotting may need to be treated with increased anticoagulant
- Monitor serum iron levels, ferritin, transferrin levels; iron therapy may be needed to prevent recurring anemia
- Monitor blood studies: BUN, creatinine, uric acid, platelets, WBC, phosphorus, potassium, bleeding time. Hct, Hgb, RBCs, reticulocytes should be checked in chronic renal failure

Associated nursing diagnoses

- ✓ Fatigue (uses)
- ✓ Activity intolerance (uses)
- ✓ Knowledge deficit (teaching)

Implementation

IV route

- Administer by direct route at end of dialysis by venous line

SC route

- Give by SC route in patients not using dialysis

Patient/family education

- Teach patients with renal disease to include high-iron and low-potassium foods in their diets (meat, dark green leafy vegetables, eggs, enriched breads)
- Teach patient the reason for treatment, expected results
- Advise patient to use contraception (pregnancy may occur)

Evaluation

Positive therapeutic outcome

- Increased appetite
- Enhanced sense of well-being
- Increase in reticulocyte count in 1-2 wk

ergonovine

(er-goe-noe'veen)

Ergometrine, ergotrate maleate

Func. class.: Oxytocic

Chem. class.: Ergot alkaloid

Pregnancy category **N/A**

Action: Stimulates uterine and vascular smooth muscle contractions, decreases bleeding

Therapeutic Outcome: Uterine contraction, decreases bleeding

Uses: Treatment of postpartum or postabortion hemorrhage

Investigational uses: To induce a coronary artery spasm

Dosage and routes

Oxytoxic

Adult: IM 0.2 mg q2-4h, not to exceed 5 doses; **IV** 0.2 mg given over 1 min; PO 0.2-0.4 mg q6-12h × 2-7 days after initial IM or **IV** dose

Induced coronary artery spasm

Adult: **IV** 50 mg q5 min up to 400 μg or until chest pain occurs

Available forms: Inj 0.2 mg/ml; tab 0.2 mg

Side effects/adverse reactions

CNS: *Headache, dizziness,* fainting
CV: Hypertension, chest pain
EENT: Tinnitus
GI: *Nausea, vomiting*
GU: Cramping
INTEG: Sweating
RESP: Dyspnea

Contraindications: Hypersensitivity to ergot medication, augmentation of labor, before delivery of placenta, spontaneous abortion (threatened), pelvic inflammatory disease (PID)

Precautions: Hepatic disease, renal disease, cardiac disease, asthma, anemia, convulsive disorders, hypertension, glaucoma, obliterative vascular disease

Pharmacokinetics

Absorption	Well absorbed (PO, IM), completely absorbed (IV)
Distribution	Unknown
Metabolism	Liver
Excretion	Kidneys
Half-life	Unknown

Pharmacodynamics

	PO	IM	IV
Onset	5-25 min	2-5 min	Immediate
Peak	Unknown	Unknown	Unknown
Duration	3 hr	3 hr	45 min

Interactions

Drug/drug:

Drug classifications

Ergots: ↑ hypertension
Sympathomimetics: ↑ hypertension

NURSING CONSIDERATIONS

Assessment

- Monitor B/P, pulse; watch for change that may indicate hemorrhage; check respiratory rate, rhythm, depth; notify prescriber of abnormalities
- Assess fundal tone, nonphasic contractions; check for relaxation or severe cramping
- Assess for ergotism or overdose: nausea, vomiting, weakness, muscular pain, insensitivity to cold, paresthesia of extremities; drug should be decreased or inf discontinued
- Before administering ergonovine, calcium levels

should be checked; if hypocalcemia is present, correction should be made to increase effectiveness of this drug
• Monitor prolactin levels and decreased breast milk production

Associated nursing diagnoses

✓ Tissue perfusion, decreased (uses)
✓ Injury, risk for (adverse reactions)
✓ Knowledge deficit (teaching)

Implementation

PO route
• Tablets may be swallowed whole or used SL
• Give for a limited time during postpartum, usually 2 days is sufficient
IM route
• Contractions begin in 2-5 min, drug is given q2-4h for contractions to continue; give deeply in large muscle mass; rotate inj sites if additional doses are given
IV **IV route**
• Give **IV** directly after dilution with 5 ml of 0.9% NaCl, give over >1 min through Y-site of free-running **IV** of 0.9% NaCl or D_5W

Patient/family education

• Advise patient to report increased blood loss, increased temp or foul-smelling lochia
• Inform patient that cramping is normal—pad count should be done to determine amount of bleeding
• Tell patient not to smoke during treatment to prevent excessive vasoconstriction

Evaluation

Positive therapeutic outcome
• Absence of severe bleeding

Treatment of overdose:
Stop drug; give vasodilators, heparin, dextran

E

ergotamine

(er-got'a-meen)
Ergostat, Ergomar ✱, Gynergen ✱, Medihaler Ergotamine ✱
Func. class.: α-adrenergic blocker, vascular headache suppressant
Chem. class.: Ergot alkaloid-amino acid
Pregnancy category **X**

Action: Constricts smooth muscle in peripheral, cranial blood vessels, relaxes uterine muscle; blocks serotonin release

➔ **Therapeutic Outcome:** Absence of headache

Uses: Vascular headache (migraine, histamine, cluster)

Dosage and routes

Adult: 2 mg, then 1-2 mg qh or q½h for SL, not to exceed 6 mg/day or 10 mg/wk; inh 1 puff, may repeat in 5 min, not to exceed 6/24 hr

Available forms: SL tab 2 mg; tab 1 mg

Side effects/adverse reactions

CNS: Numbness in fingers, toes, headache, weakness

CV: Transient tachycardia, chest pain, bradycardia, edema, claudication, increase or decrease in B/P
GI: Nausea, vomiting
MS: Muscle pain

Contraindications: Hypersensitivity to ergot preparations, occlusion (peripheral, vascular), CAD, hepatic disease, renal disease, peptic ulcer, hypertension, pregnancy **X**

Precautions: Lactation, P children, anemia

Pharmacokinetics

Absorption	Erratic (PO), poor (SL), rapidly (SC, IM)
Distribution	Crosses blood-brain barrier
Metabolism	Liver—extensively
Excretion	Kidneys, (metabolites)
Half-life	Biphasic 2.7 hr, 21 hr

Pharmacodynamics

	PO	SL
Onset	1-2 hr	Unknown
Peak	½-3 hr	Unknown
Duration	Unknown	Unknown

Interactions

Drug/drug:

Individual drugs
Methysergide: ↑ effect
Sumatriptan: ↑ vasoconstriction

Drug classifications
Antiinfectives (macrolide): ↑ vasoconstriction
Ergots: ↑ hypertension
Oral contraceptives: ↑ vasoconstriction
Sympathomimetics: ↑ hypertension

NURSING CONSIDERATIONS

Assessment

- Assess characteristics of pain: duration, intensity, location, frequency, alleviating factors; also identify if halos, nausea, vomiting, blurred vision occur with headache. Assess before and during treatment
- Assess for ergotism or overdose: nausea, vomiting, weakness, muscular pain, insensitivity to cold, paresthesia of extremities; drug should be decreased or infusion discontinued
- Check for hypertension: B/P, pulse, monitor all peripheral pulses; if hypertension occurs, notify prescriber. Also, check for tachycardia or bradycardia

Associated nursing diagnoses

✓ Pain, acute (uses)
✓ Injury, risk for (adverse reactions)
✓ Knowledge deficit (teaching)

Implementation

SL route

- Have patient place tab under tongue; patient should not chew, crush, or swallow SL tab
- Patient should not drink, eat, or smoke until tab has dissolved

Patient/family education

- Caution patient not to smoke during treatment to prevent excessive vasoconstriction
- Advise patient to avoid alcohol or OTC medications unless approved by prescriber
- Tell patient to inform prescriber if pregnancy occurs

Treatment of overdose: Stop drug, give vasodilators, heparin, dextran

erythromycin base, erythromycin estolate, erythromycin ethylsuccinate, erythromycin gluceptate, erythromycin lactobionate, erythromycin stearate

(eh-rith-roe-mye'sin)

Apo Erythro-El ✦, Erybid ✦, E-Base, E-Mycin, ERYC, Ery-Tab, erythromycin, erythromycin base, Erythromycin Filmtabs, Novorythro ✦, PCE Dispertab, Robimycin Robitabs/Erythromid ✦, erythromycin estolate, Ilosone, Ilosone Pulvules/ E.E.S. 200, E.E.S. 400, Eryped, Ery Ped Drops, Eryped 200, Eryped 400, erythromycin ethylsuccinate, erythromycin lactobionate, Ilotycin Gluceptate

Func. class.: Antibacterial
Chem. class.: Macrolide antibiotic

Pregnancy category C

Action: Binds to 50S ribosomal subunits of susceptible bacteria and suppresses protein synthesis

Therapeutic Outcome: Bactericidal action against the following organisms: *N. gonorrhoeae, D. pneumoniae, M. pneumoniae, C. diphtheriae, B. pertussis, B. burgdorferi, L. monocytogenes;* syphilis, Legionnaire's disease; *C. trachomatis; H. influenzae,* streptococci, staphylocci; gram-positive bacilli: Clostridium, Corynebacterium; gram-negative pathogens: *Neisseria, Haemophilus influenzae,* Legionella pneumophila, mycoplasma, and chlamydia trachomatis, Entamoeba histolytica

Uses: Mild to moderate respiratory tract, skin, soft tissue infections

Dosage and routes

Soft tissue infections

Adult: PO 250-500 mg q6h (base, estolate, stearate); PO 400-800 mg q6h (ethylsuccinate); **IV** inf 15-20 mg/kg/day (lactobionate)

Child: PO 30-50 mg/kg/day in divided doses q6h (salts); **IV** 15-20 mg/kg/day in divided doses q4-6h (lactobionate)

N. gonorrhoeae/PID

Adult: **IV** 500 mg q6h × 3 days (gluceptate, lactobionate), then PO 250 mg (base, estolate, stearate) or 400 mg (ethylsuccinate) q6h × 1 wk

Syphilis

Adult: PO 20 g in divided doses over 15 days (base, estolate, stearate)

Chlamydia

Adult: PO 500 mg q6h × 1 wk or 250 mg qid × 2 wk

P *Infant:* PO 50 mg/kg/day in 4 divided doses × 3 wk or more

P *Newborn:* PO 50 mg/kg/day in 4 divided doses × 2 wk or more

Intestinal amebiasis

Adult: PO 250 mg q6h × 10-14 days (base, estolate, stearate)

P *Child:* PO 30-50 mg/kg/day in divided doses q6h × 10-14 days (base, estolate, stearate)

Available forms: Base: tab, enteric-coated 250, 333, 500 mg; tab film-coated 250, 500 mg; cap, enteric-coated 125, 250 mg; estolate: tab chewable 125, 250 mg; tab 500 mg; cap 125, 250 mg; drops 100 mg/ml; susp 125, 250 mg/5 ml; stearate: tab, film-coated 250, 500 mg; ethylsuccinate: tab, chewable 200, 100 mg/2.5 ml, 200, 400 mg/5 ml; susp 200, 400 mg powder for susp, 100 mg/2.5 ml, 200, and 400 mg/5 ml powder for inj; 500 mg and 1 g (lactobionate), 250 mg, 500 mg, 1 g (as gluceptate)

Side effects/adverse reactions

EENT: Hearing loss, tinnitus
GI: *Nausea, vomiting, diarrhea,* ***hepatotoxicity,*** abdominal pain, stomatitis, heartburn, anorexia, pruritus ani
GU: *Vaginitis, moniliasis*
INTEG: Rash, urticaria, pruritus, thrombophlebitis (**IV** site)

Contraindications: Hypersensitivity

Precautions: Pregnancy **C**, hepatic disease, lactation

Pharmacokinetics

Absorption	Well absorbed (PO), minimally absorbed (Top, Ophth)
Distribution	Widely distributed; minimally distributed (CSF); crosses placenta
Metabolism	Liver, partially
Excretion	Bile, unchanged; kidneys (minimal), unchanged
Half-life	1-3 hr

Pharmacodynamics

	PO	IV
Onset	1 hr	Rapid
Peak	4 hr	Infusion's end

Interactions

Drug/drug:

Individual drugs
Alfentanil: ↑ toxicity
Bromocriptine: ↑ toxicity
Carbamazepine: ↑ toxicity, from ↑ levels
Clindamycin: ↓ action of clindamycin
Cyclosporine: ↑ toxicity
Digoxin: ↑ blood levels of digoxin
Disopyramide: ↑ toxicity
Methylprednisolone: ↑ toxicity
Theophylline: ↑ toxicity from ↑ levels
Triazolam: ↑ effects of triazolam

Drug classifications
Antihistamines: ↑ levels of antihistamine
Ergots: ↑ ergotism

Oral anticoagulants: ↑ effects of oral anticoagulants
Penicillins: ↑ or ↓ action of penicillins

Lab test interferences

False increase: 17-OHCS/17-KS, AST (SGOT)/ALT (SGPT)
Decrease: Folate assay

NURSING CONSIDERATIONS

Assessment

- Assess patient for previous sensitivity reaction
- Assess patient for signs and symptoms of infection including characteristics of wounds, sputum, urine, stool, WBC >10,000, earache, fever. Obtain baseline information before and during treatment.
- Obtain C&S test results before beginning drug therapy to identify if correct treatment has been initiated.
- Assess for allergic reactions: rash, urticaria may occur a few days after therapy begins.
- Identify urine output; if decreasing, notify prescriber (may indicate nephrotoxicity). Also, monitor increases in BUN, creatinine.
- Monitor blood studies: AST (SGOT), ALT (SGPT), CBC, Hct, bilirubin, LDH, alk phosphatase, Coombs' test monthly if patient is on long-term therapy.
- Monitor electrolytes: potassium, sodium, chloride monthly if patient is on long-term therapy.
- Assess bowel pattern qd; if severe diarrhea occurs, drug should be discontinued.
- Assess for overgrowth of infection: perineal itching, fever, malaise, redness, pain, swelling, drainage, rash, diarrhea, change in cough, sputum.

Associated nursing diagnoses

- ✓ Infection, risk for (uses)
- ✓ Diarrhea (adverse reactions)
- ✓ Knowledge deficit (teaching)
- ✓ Noncompliance (teaching)
- ✓ Injury, risk for (adverse reactions)

Implementation

PO route

- Give around the clock on an empty stomach, at least 1 hr ac or 2 hr pc. May be taken with food if GI upset occurs. Do not take with juices. Take dose with a full glass of water: use calibrated measuring device for drops or susp. Shake well.
- Chewable tab may be crushed or chewed, not swallowed whole.
- Do not open, crush, or chew time-release cap or tab, enteric-coated tab may be given

IV **IV route**

- Add 10 ml of sterile water for inj without preservatives to 250- or 500-mg vials and 20 ml to 1-g vial. Sol is stable for 1 wk after reconstitution if refrigerated
- Intermittent inf: dilute further in 100-250 ml of 0.9% NaCl or D_5W
- Give over 20-60 min to avoid phlebitis. Assess for pain along vein; slow inf if pain occurs; apply ice to site and notify prescriber if unable to relieve pain
- Continuous inf: May also be administered as an infusion in a dilution of 1 g/l of 0.9% NaCl, D_5W, over 4 hr

E

Additive compatibilities:
Calcium gluconate, corticotropin, dimenhydrinate, heparin, hydrocortisone sodium succinate, methicillin, penicillin G potassium, potassium chloride, sodium bicarbonate

Additive incompatibilities:
Aminophylline, cephapirin, pentobarbital, secobarbital, streptomycin, tetracycline

Syringe incompatibility:
Heparin

Erythromycin lactobionate
Additive incompatibilities:
Cephalothin, colistimethate, floxacillin, furosemide, heparin, metaraminol, metoclopramide, tetracycline, vitamin B with C

Additive compatibilities:
Aminophylline, ampicillin, cimetidine, diphenhydramine, hydrocortisone sodium succinate, lidocaine, methicillin, penicillin G potassium, penicillin G sodium, pentobarbital, polymyxin B, potassium chloride, prednisolone sodium phosphate, prochlorperazine, promazine, sodium bicarbonate, sodium iodide, verapamil

Syringe incompatibilities:
Ampicillin, heparin

Syringe compatibility:
Methicillin

Y-site incompatibility:
Fluconazole

Y-site compatibilities:
Acyclovir, amiodarone, cyclophosphamide, enalaprilat, esmolol, famotidine, foscarnet, hydromorphone, idarubicin, labetol, magnesium sulfate, merperidine, morphine, multivitamins, perphenazine, vitamin B with C, zidovudine

Patient/family education

- Teach patient to report sore throat, bruising, bleeding, joint pain—may indicate blood dyscrasias (rare)
- Advise patient to contact prescriber if vaginal itching, loose, foul-smelling stools, furry tongue occur—may indicate superimposed infection
- Instruct patient to take all medication prescribed for the length of time ordered

Evaluation

Positive therapeutic outcome
- Absence of signs/symptoms of infection (WBC <10,000, temp WNL, absence of red, draining wounds, earache)
- Reported improvement in symptoms of infection

Treatment of overdose:
Withdraw drug, maintain airway, administer epinephrine, aminophylline, O_2, **IV** corticosteroids

esmolol

(ess'moe-lol)

Brevibloc

Func. class.: β-adrenergic blocker (antidysrhythmic II)

Pregnancy category **C**

Action: Competitively blocks stimulation of β_1-adrenergic receptors in the myocardium; produces negative chronotropic, inotropic activity (decreases rate of SA node discharge, increases recovery time), slows conduction of AV node, decreases heart rate, decreases O_2 consumption in myocardium; also decreases renin-aldosterone-angiotensin system at high doses; inhibits β_2-receptors in bronchial system slightly

➔ Therapeutic Outcome: Decreased supraventricular tachycardia

Uses: Supraventricular tachycardias, noncompensatory tachycardia, hypertensive crisis

Dosage and routes

Adult: **IV** loading dose—500 μg/kg/min over 1 min; maintenance—50 μg/kg/min for 4 min; may repeat q5 min, increasing maintenance inf by 50 μg/kg/min (max of 200 μg/kg/min); titrate to patient response

Available forms: Inj 10 mg, 250 mg/ml

Side effects/adverse reactions

CNS: Confusion, lightheadedness, paresthesia, somnolence, fever, dizziness, fatigue, headache, depression, anxiety

CV: Hypotension, bradycardia, chest pain, peripheral ischemia, shortness of breath, CHF, conduction disturbances

GI: *Nausea,* vomiting, anorexia, gastric pain, flatulence, constipation, heartburn, bloating

GU: Urinary retention, impotence, dysuria

INTEG: *Induration, inflammation at site,* discoloration, edema, erythema, burning pallor, flushing, rash, pruritus, dry skin, alopecia

RESP: ***Bronchospasm,*** dyspnea, cough, wheezing, nasal stuffiness

Contraindications: 2nd- or 3rd-degree heart block, cardiogenic shock, CHF, cardiac failure, hypersensitivity

Precautions: Hypotension, pregnancy **C**, peripheral vascular disease, diabetes, hypoglycemia, thyrotoxicosis, renal disease, lactation

Pharmacokinetics

Absorption	Complete (IV)
Distribution	Unknown
Metabolism	Liver
Excretion	Kidneys
Half-life	9 min

Pharmacodynamics

	IV
Onset	Rapid
Peak	Unknown
Duration	1-2 min

Interactions

Drug/drug:

Individual drugs

Alcohol: ↑ hypotension (large amounts)
Epinephrine: Alpha-adrenergic stimulation
Hydralazine: ↑ hypotension, bradycardia
Phenytoin (IV): ↑ myocardial depression
Prazosin: ↑ hypotension, bradycardia
Thyroid: ↓ effectiveness
Verapamil: ↑ myocardial depression

Drug classifications

Antihypertensives: ↑ hypertension
β_2 agonists: ↓ bronchodilation
Cardiac glycosides: ↑ bradycardia
Nitrates: ↑ hypotension
Theophyllines: ↓ bronchodilation

Drug/smoking:

↑ tachycardia

Lab test interferences

Increase: Liver function tests

NURSING CONSIDERATIONS

Assessment

- Monitor B/P during beginning treatment, periodically thereafter; pulse q4hr; note rate, rhythm, quality; apical/radial pulse before administration; notify prescriber of any significant changes (pulse <50 bpm)
- Check for baselines in renal, liver function tests before therapy begins
- Assess for edema in feet, legs daily, monitor I&O, daily weight; check for jugular vein distention, rales bilaterally, dyspnea (CHF)
- Monitor skin turgor, dryness of mucous membranes for hydration status, especially G elderly

Associated nursing diagnoses

- ✓ Cardiac output, decreased (uses)
- ✓ Injury, risk for (adverse reactions)
- ✓ Knowledge deficit (teaching)
- ✓ Noncompliance (teaching)

Implementation

IV route

- Give by intermittent inf after diluting 5 g/500 ml D_5W, 0.9% NaCl, D_5/0.45% NaCl, D_5/LR, D_5/0.9% NaCl, 0.45% NaCl, LR, (10 mg/ml)
- Give loading dose over 1 min, then maintenance dose over 4 min, may repeat loading dose q5 min with increased maintenance dose; maintenance should not be >200 mcg/kg/min and be administered up to 48 hr; dosage should be tapered at a rate of 25 µg/kg/min
- Store at room temp for 24 hr; sol should be clear

Y-site compatibilities:

Amikacin, aminophylline, ampicillin, atracurium, butorphanol, calcium chloride, cefazolin, cefoperazone, ceftazidime, ceftizoxime, chloramphenicol, cimetidine, clindamycin, co-trimoxazole, dopamine, enalaprilat, erythromycin lactobionate, famotidine, fentanyl, gentamicin, heparin, hydrocortisone sodium succinate, magnesium sulfate, methyldopate, metronidazole, morphine sulfate, nafcillin, pancuronium, penicillin G potassium, phenytoin, piperacillin, polymyxin B, potassium chloride, potassium phosphate, ranitidine, sodium acetate, streptomycin, tobramycin, vancomycin, vecuronium

Y-site compatibility:
Furosemide

Additive compatibilities:
Aminophylline, bretyllium, heparin

Additive incompatibilities:
Diazepam, procainamide, sodium bicarbonate, thiopental

Patient/family education

- Teach patient need for medication and expected results
- Caution patient to rise slowly to prevent orthostatic hypotension

Evaluation

Positive therapeutic outcome
- Absence of dysrhythmias

Treatment of overdose:
Defibrillation, vasopressor for hypotension

estazolam
(ess-taz'oh-lam)
ProSom
Func. class.: Sedative-hypnotic
Chem. class.: Benzodiazepine derivative
Pregnancy category X
Controlled substance schedule IV

Action: Produces CNS depression at the limbic, thalamic, hypothalamic levels of the CNS; may be mediated by neurotransmitter γ-aminobutyric acid (GABA); results are sedation, hypnosis, skeletal muscle activity, anxiolytic action

Therapeutic Outcome: Ability to sleep, relaxation

Uses: Insomnia (short-term)

Dosage and routes
Adult: PO 1-2 mg hs

Available forms: Tab 1, 2 mg

Side effects/adverse reactions
CNS: Lethargy, drowsiness, daytime sedation, dizziness, confusion, light-headedness, headache, anxiety, irritability, weakness, tremors, depression, lack of coordination
CV: Chest pain, pulse changes, palpitations, tachycardia
GI: Nausea, vomiting, diarrhea, heartburn, abdominal pain, constipation, anorexia, taste alteration

HEMA: ***Leukopenia, granulocytopenia (rare)***
INTEG: Dermatitis, allergy, sweating, flushing, pruritus
MISC: Joint pain, respiratory congestion, dependency

Contraindications: Hypersensitivity to benzodiazepines, pregnancy **X**, sleep apnea

Precautions: Hepatic disease, renal disease, suicidal individuals, drug abuse, G elderly, psy-P chosis, child <18, lactation, depression, **pulmonary insufficiency**

Pharmacokinetics

Absorption	Well absorbed (PO)
Distribution	Crosses blood-brain barrier, placenta
Metabolism	Liver
Excretion	Kidneys, feces, breast milk
Half-life	10-24 hr

Pharmacodynamics

	PO
Onset	15-45 min
Peak	1½-2 hr
Duration	7-8 hr

Interactions

Drug/drug:

Individual drugs
Alcohol: ↑ CNS depression
Cimetidine: ↑ action
Disulfiram: ↑ action
Fluoxetine: ↑ action
Isoniazid: ↑ action
Ketoconazole: ↑ action
Levodopa: ↓ action of levodopa
Metoprolol: ↑ action
Propoxyphene: ↑ action
Propranolol: ↑ action
Rifampin: ↓ action of chlordiazepoxide
Theophylline: ↓ sedative effects
Valproic acid: ↑ action

Drug classifications
Analgesics, opioid: ↑ CNS depression
Antidepressants: ↑ CNS depression
Antihistamines: ↑ CNS depression
Barbiturates: ↓ effect of chlordiazepoxide
Contraceptives: ↑ effect
MAOI: ↑ CNS depression

NURSING CONSIDERATIONS

Assessment

- Assess patient's sleep pattern and note physical circumstances that interrupt sleep (sleep apnea, obstructed airway, pain/discomfort, urinary frequency) and psychologic (fear, anxiety); patient's bedtime routine, pre-sleep cues/props
- Identify potential for abuse; this drug may lend to physical and psychologic dependency; amount of drug should be limited
- Monitor blood studies: Hct, Hgb, RBCs, serum folate (if on long-term therapy) protime in patients receiving anticoagulants because action of anticoagulant may be increased
- Assess patient's mental status: mood, sensorium, affect, memory (long-term, short-term); for physical dependency: more frequent requests for medication, shakes, anxiety, pinpoint pupils

Associated nursing diagnoses

✓ Sleep pattern disturbance
✓ Knowledge deficit (teaching)
✓ Noncompliance (teaching)

Implementation

PO route

- Give ½-1 hr before hs for sleeplessness; on empty stomach for fast onset, but may be taken with food if GI symptoms occur
- Store in air-tight container in cool environment

Patient/family education

- Advise patient to avoid driving or other activities requiring alertness; to avoid alcohol ingestion or CNS depressants; serious CNS depression may result plus tachycardia, flushing, headache, hypotension
- Provide patient with alternate measures to improve sleep (reading, exercise several hr before hs, warm bath, warm milk, TV, self-hypnosis, deep breathing)
- Inform patient that hangover G is common in elderly but less common than with barbiturates
- Teach patient symptoms of withdrawal: nausea, vomiting, anxiety, hallucinations, insomnia, tachycardia, fever, cramps, tremors, seizures
- Advise patient to watch for allergic reaction (rash) and to discontinue drug if rash occurs

Evaluation

Positive therapeutic outcome

- Ability to sleep at night
- Decreased amount of early AM awakenings

estradiol/estradiol cypionate/estradiol valerate/estradiol transdermal system

(ess-tra-dye'ole)

Cypionate, depGynogen, Depo Estradiol, Depogen, Dura-Estrin, Estra-D, Estradiol Cypionate, Estro-Cyp, Estroject-L.A., Estronol-LA/Estrace, Esaderm/Deladiol-40, Delestrogen, Dioval 40, Dioval XX, Duragen-10, Duragen-20, Duragen-40, Estradiol Valerate, Estra-L 20, Estra-L 40, Gynogen L.A. "10", Gynbogen L.A. "20", Gynogen L.A. "40", L.A.E. 20, Valergen 10, Valergen 20, Valergen 40/Estrace, Estraderm TTS

Func. class.: Estrogen
Chem. class.: Nonsteroidal synthetic estrogen

Pregnancy category **X**

Action: Needed for adequate functioning of female reproductive system; affects release of pituitary gonadatropins, inhibits ovulation, adequate calcium use in bone structure

➔ **Therapeutic Outcome:** Decreased tumor size in prostatic cancer; increased estrogen levels in menopause, female hypogonadism

Uses: Menopause, breast cancer, prostatic cancer, atrophic vaginitis, kraurosis vulvae, hypogonadism, castration, primary ovarian failure, prevention of osteoporosis

Dosage and routes

Menopause/hypogonadism/castration/ovarian failure

Adult: PO 1-2 mg qd 3 wk on, 1 wk off or 5 days on, 2 days off; IM 0.2-1 mg qwk

Prostatic cancer

Adult: PO 1-2 mg qd 3 wk on, 1 wk off or 5 days on, 2 days off; IM 0.2-1 mg qwk

Breast cancer

Adult: PO 10 mg tid × 3 mo or longer

Atropic vaginitis

Adult: Vag cream 2-4 g qd × 1-2 wk, then 1 g 1-3 ×/wk

Kraurosis vulvae

Adult: IM 1-1.5 mg 1-2 ×/wk

Available forms: Extradiol tab 1,2 mg; cypionate inj IM 5 mg/ml; valerate inj IM 10,20,40 mg/ml; transderm 0.05 mg/24-hr release rate, 0.1 mg/24-hr release rate; vag cream 100 μg/g

Side effects/adverse reactions

CNS: Dizziness, headache, migraine, depression
CV: Hypotension, thrombophlebitis, edema, ***thromboembolism, stroke, pulmonary embolism, myocardial infarction***
EENT: Contact lens intolerance, increased myopia, astigmatism
GI: *Nausea,* vomiting, diarrhea, anorexia, pancreatitis, cramps, constipation, increased appetite, increased weight, ***cholestatic jaundice***
GU: Amenorrhea, cervical erosion, breakthrough bleeding, dysmenorrhea, vaginal candidiasis, breast changes, *gynecomastia, testicular atrophy, impotence*
INTEG: Rash, urticaria, acne, hirsutism, alopecia, oily skin, seborrhea, purpura, melasma
META: Folic acid deficiency, hypercalcemia, hyperglycemia

Contraindications: Breast cancer, thromboembolic disorders, reproductive cancer, genital bleeding (abnormal, undiagnosed), pregnancy **X**

Precautions: Hypertension, asthma, blood dyscrasias, gallbladder disease, CHF, diabetes mellitus, bone disease, depression, migraine headache, convulsive disorders, hepatic disease, renal disease, family history of cancer of breast or reproductive tract

Pharmacokinetics

Absorption	Well absorbed
Distribution	Widely distributed, crosses placenta
Metabolism	Unknown
Excretion	Unknown
Half-life	Unknown

Pharmacodynamics

	PO	IM	IV
Onset	Rapid	Slow	Rapid
Peak	Unknown	Unknown	Unknown
Duration	Unknown	Unknown	Unknown

Interactions

Drug/drug:

Drug classifications

Anticoagulants: ↓ action of anticoagulants
Antidepressants, tricyclics: ↑ toxicity
Barbiturates: ↓ action of chlorotrianisene
Corticosteroids: ↑ action of corticosteroids
Oral hypoglycemics: ↓ action of hypoglycemics

Lab test interferences

Increase: BSP retention test; PBI; T_4; serum sodium; platelet aggregation; thyroxine-binding globulin (TBS); prothrombin; factors VII, VIII, IX, X; triglycerides
Decrease: Serum folate, serum triglyceride, T_3 resin uptake test, glucose tolerance test, antithrombin III, pregnanediol, metyrapone test
False positive: LE prep, antinuclear antibodies

NURSING CONSIDERATIONS

Assessment

- Monitor blood glucose in patient with diabetes; increased urine glucose may occur
- Monitor B/P q4h; watch for increase caused by water and sodium retention
- Monitor I&O ratio; be alert for decreasing urinary output and increasing edema; monitor weight daily; notify prescriber if weekly weight gain is >5 lb; if increased, diuretic may be ordered
- Obtain liver function studies, including AST (SGOT), ALT (SGPT), bilirubin, alk phosphatase
- Assess edema, hypertension, cardiac symptoms, jaundice
- Assess mental status: affect, mood, behavioral changes, aggression; depression may occur, drug may need to be discontinued

Associated nursing diagnoses

✓ Sexual dysfunction (uses)
✓ Injury, risk for (adverse reactions)

Implementation

PO route

- Give titrated dose, use lowest effective dose
- Give with food or milk to decrease GI symptoms

IM route

- Administer deeply in large muscle mass; drug is painful
- Rotate syringe to mix oil and medication

Trans route

- Apply to area free of hair to ensure adhesion
- Start trans dose 7 days before last PO dose if routes are to be changed

Vag route

- Place cream in applicator by attaching tube to applicator; squeeze cream into tube to mark; insert with patient reclining
- Applicator should be washed after each use

Patient/family education

- Tell patient to take exactly as prescribed; do not double doses
- Advise patient that increased weight gain and symptoms of fluid retention should be reported to prescriber: edema of feet, ankles, sacral area; abnor-

mal vaginal bleeding; breast lumps; hepatic disease (dark urine, clay-colored stools, jaundice of skin, sclera, pruritus)

• Caution patient that thromboembolic symptoms should be reported: tenderness in legs, chest pain, dyspnea, headaches, blurred vision
• Inform patient to use sunscreen and protective clothing because sunburns may occur
• Advise patient to stop smoking—smokers have a greater chance of thromboembolic disorder
• Tell patient to use a nonhormonal birth control, and to notify prescriber if pregnancy is suspected

Evaluation

Positive therapeutic outcome
• Reversal of menopausal symptoms
• Decrease in tumor size in prostatic or breast cancer
• Decrease in itching, inflammation of vagina
• Absence of symptoms of osteoporosis

estramustine

(ess-tra-muss'teen)
Emcyt
Func. class.: Antineoplastic
Chem. class.: Hormone, alkylating agent
Pregnancy category D

Action: Combination drug consisting of nitrogen mustard/estrogen; estrogen is a carrier for the nitrogen mustard into estrogen-dependent tissue; acts like a weak alkylating agent; decreases serum testosterone levels

Therapeutic Outcome: Prevention of rapidly growing malignant cells

Uses: Metastatic prostate cancer (palliative treatment only)

Dosage and routes

Adult: PO 10-16 mg/kg in 3-4 divided doses/day; treatment may continue for 3 mo; 600 mg/m^2/day in 3 divided doses

Available forms: Cap 140 mg

Side effects/adverse reactions

CNS: Headache, anxiety, seizures, insomnia, mood swings
CV: ***Myocardial infarction,*** hypertension, ***CHF, CVA***
GI: *Nausea, vomiting, anorexia,* ***hepatotoxicity***
GU: ***Renal failure,*** impotence, gynecomastia
HEMA: ***Anemia,*** thrombocytopenia, leukopenia
INTEG: *Rash,* urticaria, pruritus, flushing, alopecia
RESP: Dyspnea, ***emboli,*** hoarseness

Contraindications: Hypersensitivity to estradiol, thromboembolic disorders, pregnancy **D**

Precautions: Edema, hepatic disease, CVA, MI, seizures, hypertension, diabetes mellitus

Pharmacokinetics

Absorption	Well absorbed (PO)
Distribution	Prostatic area
Metabolism	Liver
Excretion	Bile, feces
Half-life	20 hr (terminal)

Pharmacodynamics

	PO
Onset	1-2 hr
Peak	1-2 hr
Duration	1-2 hr

Interactions

Drug/drug:

Drug classifications

Calcium supplements: Blocked absorption

Live virus vaccines: ↑ adverse reactions

Drug/food:

Calcium (dairy foods): Blocked absorption

Drug/smoking:

↑ cardiotoxicity

NURSING CONSIDERATIONS

Assessment

- Assess symptoms indicating severe allergic reaction: rash, pruritus, urticaria, purpuric skin lesions, itching, flushing
- Monitor temp q4h (may indicate beginning of infection)
- Monitor liver function tests before and during therapy (bilirubin, AST [SGOT], ALT [SGPT], LDH) as needed or monthly; yellowing of skin, sclera, dark urine, clay-colored stools, itchy skin, abdominal pain, fever, diarrhea; renal function studies: BUN, urine CrCl, electrolytes before and during therapy
- Assess patient for bleeding: hematuria, stool guaiac, bruising or petechiae, mucosa or orifices q8h; inflammation of mucosa, breaks in skin

Associated nursing diagnoses

- ✓ Injury, risk for (adverse reactions)
- ✓ Body image disturbance (adverse reactions)
- ✓ Infection, risk for (adverse reactions)
- ✓ Knowledge deficit (teaching)

Implementation

PO route

- Give in divided doses over 1-3 mo; administer with water 1 hr ac or 2 hr pc; give antiemetic if nausea, vomiting, or anorexia become severe; do not give with calcium-rich products or antacids with calcium

Patient/family education

- Teach patient to avoid use of products containing aspirin or ibuprofen, razors, commercial mouthwash—bleeding may occur; to report symptoms of bleeding (hematuria, tarry stools)
- Instruct patient to report signs of anemia, (fatigue, headache, irritability, faintness, shortness of breath)

• Caution patient that contraception is needed during treatment and several mo after
• Teach patient to watch for pain, swelling, redness, tenderness, change in vision and chest pain; should be reported immediately to prescriber (thromboembolic disorders)

Evaluation

Positive therapeutic outcome
• Prevention of rapid division of malignant cells

estrogenic substances, conjugated 🔑

C.E.S ✦, conjugated estrogens, Conjugated Estrogens C.S.D. ✦, Premarin, Premarin Intravenous

Func. class.: Estrogen hormone

Chem. class.: Nonsteroidal synthetic estrogen

Pregnancy category X

Action: Needed for adequate functioning of female reproductive system; affects release of pituitary gonadotropins; inhibits ovulation; promotes adequate calcium use in bone structures

➡ **Therapeutic Outcome:** Decreased tumor size in prostatic cancer; increased estrogen levels in menopause, female hypogonadism

Uses: Menopause, breast cancer, prostatic cancer, abnormal uterine bleeding, hypogonadism, castration, primary ovarian failure, osteoporosis

Dosage and routes

Menopause

Adult: PO 0.3-1.25 mg qd 3 wk on, 1 wk off

Osteoporosis

Adult: PO 0.625 mg qd or in a cycle

Atrophic vaginitis

Adult: Vag 2-4g cream qd × 21 days, off 7 days, repeat

Prostatic cancer

Adult: PO 1.25-2.5 mg tid

Breast cancer

Adult: PO 10 mg tid × 3 mo or longer

Abnormal uterine bleeding

IV *Adult:* **IV**/IM 25 mg, repeat in 6-12 hr

Ovariectomy/primary ovarian failure

Adult: PO 1.25 mg qd 3 wk on, 1 wk off

Hypogonadism

Adult: PO 2.5 mg bid-tid × 20 days/mo

Available forms: Tab 0.3, 0.625, 0.9, 1.25, 2.5 mg; inj 25 mg/vial; vag cream 0.625 mg/g

Side effects/adverse reactions

CNS: Dizziness, headache, migraine, depression
CV: Hypotension, thrombophlebitis, edema, ***throm-***

boembolism, stroke, pulmonary embolism, MI
EENT: Contact lens intolerance, increased myopia, astigmatism
GI: Nausea, vomiting, diarrhea, anorexia, pancreatitis, cramps, constipation, increased appetite, increased weight, ***cholestatic jaundice***
GU: Amenorrhea, cervical erosion, breakthrough bleeding, dysmenorrhea, vaginal candidiasis, breast changes, *gynecomastia, testicular atrophy, impotence*
INTEG: Rash, urticaria, acne, hirsutism, alopecia, oily skin, seborrhea, purpura, melasma
META: Folic acid deficiency, hypercalcemia, hyperglycemia

Contraindications: Breast cancer, thromboembolic disorders, reproductive cancer, genital bleeding (abnormal, undiagnosed), pregnancy **X**, lactation

Precautions: Hypertension, asthma, blood dyscrasias, gallbladder disease, CHF, diabetes mellitus, bone disease, depression, migraine headache, convulsive disorders, hepatic disease, renal disease, family history of cancer of breast or reproductive tract

Pharmacokinetics

Absorption	Well absorbed (PO), completely absorbed (IV)
Distribution	Widely distributed, crosses placenta
Metabolism	Liver—exclusively; hepatic recirculation
Excretion	Kidney
Half-life	Unknown

Pharmacodynamics

	PO	IM	IV
Onset	Rapid	Slow	Immediate
Peak	Unknown	Unknown	Unknown
Duration	Unknown	Unknown	Unknown

E

Interactions
Drug/drug:
Individual drugs
Phenylbutazone: ↓ action of phenylbutazone
Rifampin: ↓ action of phenylbutazone
Drug classifications
Anticoagulants: ↓ action of anticoagulants
Anticonvulsants: ↓ action of chlorotrianisene
Antidepressants, tricyclics: ↑ toxicity
Barbiturates: ↓ action of chlorotrianisene
Corticosteroids: ↑ action of corticosteroids
Oral hypoglycemics: ↓ action of hypoglycemics

Lab test interferences
Increase: BSP retention test; PBI, T_4; serum sodium; platelet aggressability; thyroxine-binding globulin (TBG); prothrombin; factors VII, VIII, IX, X; triglycerides
Decrease: Serum folate, serum triglyceride, T_3 resin uptake test, glucose tolerance test, antithrombin III, pregnanediol, metyrapone test
False positive: LE prep, antinuclear antibodies

NURSING CONSIDERATIONS

Assessment

- Monitor blood glucose in patient with diabetes; increased urine glucose may occur
- Monitor B/P q4h; watch for increase caused by water and sodium retention
- Monitor I&O ratio; be alert for decreasing urinary output and increasing edema; monitor weight daily; notify prescriber if weekly weight gain is >5 lb; if increased, diuretic may be ordered
- Obtain liver function studies, including AST (SGOT), ALT (SGPT), bilirubin, alk phosphatase
- Assess edema, hypertension, cardiac symptoms, jaundice
- Assess mental status: affect, mood, behavioral changes, aggression; depression may occur, drug may need to be discontinued

Associated nursing diagnoses

✓ Sexual dysfunction (uses)
✓ Injury, risk for (adverse reactions)

Implementation

PO route

- Give titrated dose, use lowest effective dose
- Give in one dose in AM for prostatic cancer, vaginitis, hypogonadism
- Give with food or milk to decrease GI symptoms

IM route

- Reconstitute after withdrawing at least 5 ml of air from container and inject sterile diluent on vial side, rotate to dissolve
- Give IM injection deeply in large muscle

IV **IV route**

- Direct **IV**: Reconstitute as for IM, inject into distal port of running **IV** line of D_5W, 0.9% NaCl, LR, at a rate of 5 mg/min or less

Vag route

- Place cream in applicator by attaching tube to applicator, squeeze cream into tube to mark, insert with patient recumbent
- Applicator should be washed after each use

Patient/family education

- Caution patient to take exactly as prescribed and not to double doses
- Advise patient that increased weight gain and symptoms of fluid retention should be reported to prescriber: edema of feet, ankles, sacral area; abnormal vaginal bleeding; breast lumps; hepatic disease (dark urine, clay-colored stools, jaundice of skin, sclera, pruritus)
- Caution patient that thromboembolic symptoms should be reported: tenderness in legs, chest pain, dyspnea, headaches, blurred vision
- Inform patient that sunburns may occur and to use sunscreen and protective clothing
- Advise patient to stop smoking because smoking increases the chance of developing a thromboembolic disorder
- Tell patient to use a nonhormonal birth control, and to notify prescriber if pregnancy is suspected

Evaluation

Positive therapeutic outcome
- Reversal of menopause symptoms
- Decrease in tumor size in prostatic, breast cancer
- Decrease in itching, inflammation of vagina
- Absence of symptoms of osteoporosis

ethambutol

(e-tham'byoo-tole)

Etibi ✱, Myambutol

Func. class.: Antitubercular

Chem. class.: Diisopropylethylene diamide derivative

Pregnancy category **D**

Action: Inhibits RNA synthesis, decreases tubercle bacilli replication

Therapeutic Outcome: Resolution of TB infection

Uses: Pulmonary tuberculosis, as an adjunct of other mycobacterial infections

Dosage and routes

P *Adult and child >13 yr:* PO 15-25 mg/kg/day as a single dose

Retreatment

P *Adult and child >13 yr:* PO 25 mg/kg/day as single dose × 2 mo with at least 1 other drug, then decrease to 15 mg/kg/day as single dose

Available forms: Tab 100, 400 mg

Side effects/adverse reactions

CNS: Headache, confusion, fever, malaise, dizziness, disorientation, hallucinations
EENT: Blurred vision, optic neuritis, photophobia, decreased visual acuity
GI: Abdominal distress, anorexia, nausea, vomiting
INTEG: Dermatitis, pruritis
META: Elevated uric acid, acute gout, liver function impairment
MISC: *Thrombocytopenia,* joint pain, bloody sputum

Contraindications: Hypersensitivity, optic neuritis, P child <13 yr; pregnancy **D**

Precautions: Renal disease, diabetic retinopathy, cataracts, ocular defects, hepatic and hematopoietic disorders

Pharmacokinetics

Absorption	Rapidly absorbed (PO)
Distribution	Widely distributed, crosses blood-brain barrier, placenta
Metabolism	Liver
Excretion	Kidneys—unchanged
Half-life	3 hr, increased in liver, kidney disease

Pharmacodynamics

	PO
Onset	Rapid
Peak	2-4 hr

Interactions

Drug/drug:

Individual drugs

Cisplatin: ↑ renal toxicity

Drug classifications

Antacids, aluminum: ↓ absorption

NURSING CONSIDERATIONS

Assessment

- Obtain C&S tests including sputum tests before initiating treatment; monitor q mo to detect resistance
- Monitor liver studies qwk: ALT (SGPT), AST (SGOT), bilirubin; renal studies: before, qmo: BUN, creatinine, output, specific gravity, urinalysis, uric acid
- Assess patient's mental status often: affect, mood, behavioral changes; psychosis may occur with hallucinations, confusion
- Assess patient's hepatic status: decreased appetite, jaundice, dark urine, fatigue
- Assess patient for visual disturbance that may indicate optic neuritis: blurred vision, change in color perception may lend to blindness

Associated nursing diagnoses

- ✓ Infection, risk for (uses)
- ✓ Diarrhea (adverse reactions)
- ✓ Sensory-perceptual alterations (adverse reactions)
- ✓ Knowledge deficit (teaching)
- ✓ Noncompliance (teaching)

Implementation

PO route

- Give with meals to decrease GI symptoms, at same time each day to maintain blood level
- Give antiemetic if vomiting occurs

Patient/family education

- Advise patient that compliance with dosage schedule and duration is necessary to eradicate disease; to keep scheduled appointments including ophthalmic appointments or relapse may occur
- Caution patient to report weakness, fatigue, loss of appetite, nausea, vomiting, yellowing of skin or eyes, tingling/numbness of hands/feet, weight gain, or decreased urine output
- Caution patient to inform prescriber if pregnancy is suspected

Evaluation

Positive therapeutic outcome

- Decreased symptoms of TB

ethosuximide

(eth-oh-sux'i-mide)

Zarontin

Func. class.: Anticonvulsant

Chem. class.: Succinimide

Pregnancy category **C**

Action: Inhibits spike and wave formation in absence seizures (petit mal); decreases amplitude, frequency, duration, spread of discharge in minor motor seizures

➡ Therapeutic Outcome: Decreased seizure activity

Uses: Absence seizures, partial seizures, tonic-clonic seizures

Dosage and routes

P ***Adult and child >6 yr:*** PO 250 mg bid initially; may increase by 250 mg q4-7d, not to exceed 1.5 g/day

P ***Child 3-6 yr:*** PO 250 mg/day or 125 mg bid; may increase by 250 mg q4-7d, not to exceed 1.5 g/day

Available forms: Cap 250 mg, syr 250 mg/5 ml

Side effects/adverse reactions

CNS: Drowsiness, dizziness, fatigue, euphoria, lethargy, anxiety, aggressiveness, irritability, depression, insomnia, headache
EENT: Myopia, blurred vision
GI: Nausea, vomiting, heartburn, anorexia, diarrhea, abdominal pain, cramps, constipation, hiccups, weight loss, gum hypertrophy, tongue swelling
GU: Vaginal bleeding; pink, brown urine
HEMA: ***Agranulocytosis, aplastic anemia, thrombocytopenia, leukocytosis, eosinophilia, pancytopenia***
INTEG: Urticaria, pruritic erythema, hirsutism, **Stevens-Johnson syndrome**

Contraindications: Hypersensitivity to succinimide derivatives

Precautions: Lactation, pregnancy **C**, hepatic disease, renal disease

Pharmacokinetics

Absorption	Rapidly, completely absorbed
Distribution	Body water
Metabolism	Liver
Excretion	Kidneys, 10% unchanged
Half-life	Adult—60 hr; child—24-30 hr

E

Pharmacodynamics

	PO
Onset	Several hr, days
Peak	1-7 days
Duration	Days
Steady state	4-7 days

Interactions

Drug/drug:

Individual drugs
Alcohol: ↑ CNS depression
Phenytoin: ↑ metabolism, ↓ effectiveness

Drug classification
Antidepressants: ↑ CNS depression, decreased seizure threshold
Antihistamines: ↑ CNS depression
MAOI: ↓ seizure threshold
Narcotics: ↑ CNS depression
Phenothiazines: ↓ seizure threshold
Sedative/hypnotics: ↑ CNS depression

NURSING CONSIDERATIONS

Assessment

- Monitor drug level: therapeutic level 30-50 μg/ml
- Assess blood studies; CBC platelets q2 wk until stabilized, then qmo × 12, then q3 mo
- Assess mental status: mood, sensorium, affect, memory (long, short)

• Assess respiratory depression: rate, depth, character
• Assess blood dyscrasias: fever, sore throat, bruising, rash, jaundice

Associated nursing diagnoses

✓ Injury, risk for (adverse reactions)
✓ Knowledge deficit (teaching)

Implementation

PO route
• Administer on empty stomach for best absorption

Patient/family education

• Teach patient to carry ID card or Medic-Alert bracelet stating patient's name, drugs taken, condition, prescriber's name, phone number
• Caution patient to avoid driving, other activities that require alertness; to avoid alcohol ingestion and CNS depressants because increased sedation may occur
• Advise patient not to discontinue medication abruptly after long-term use; absence seizures may occur
• Inform patient that drug must be taken as prescribed; not to double doses because serious reactions may occur; may take drug within 4 hr if missed
• Advise patient to notify prescriber of hepatic symptoms, blood dyscrasia (fatigue, fever, sore throat, bruises, rash)
• Caution patient to notify prescriber if pregnancy is anticipated or suspected
• Inform patient that urine may become pink or brown

Evaluation

Positive therapeutic outcome
• Decreased seizure activity

Treatment of overdose: Lavage, activated charcoal, warming blanket, vital signs; monitor electrolytes

etidronate

(eh-tin-droe'nate)
Didronel, Didronel IV
Func. class.: Parathyroid agent (calcium regulator)
Chem. class.: Diphosphate
Pregnancy category **B**

Action: Decreases bone resorption and new bone development (accretion)

Therapeutic Outcome: Decreased bone reabsorption, calcium levels WNL

Uses: Paget's disease, heterotopic ossification, hypercalcemia of malignancy

Dosage and routes

Paget's disease
Adult: PO 5-10 mg/kg/day 2 hr ac with water, not to exceed 20 mg/kg/day, max 6 mo or 11-20 mg/kg/day for max of 3 mo

Heterotropic ossification
Adult: PO 20 mg/kg qd × 2 wk, then 10 mg/kg/day for 10 wk, total 12 wk

Hypercalcemia
Adult: **IV** 7.5 mg/kg/day × 3 days, then 20 mg/kg/day (PO)

Heterotropic ossification/hip replacement

Adult: PO 20 mg/kg/day × 4 wk before and 3 mo after surgery

Available forms: Tab 200, 400 mg; inj 300 mg/6 ml

Side effects/adverse reactions

GI: Nausea, diarrhea
GU: Nephrotoxicity
MS: Bone pain, hypocalcemia, decreased mineralization of nonaffected bones

Contraindications: Pathologic fractures, children, colitis, severe renal disease with creatinine >5 mg/dl

Precautions: Pregnancy **B**, renal disease, lactation, restricted Vit D/Ca

Pharmacokinetics

Absorption	Poorly absorbed (PO), completely absorbed (IV)
Distribution	50% bond to crystals in osteogenesis
Metabolism	None
Excretion	Feces (unabsorbed), kidney (unchanged)
Half-life	5-7 hr; in bone >3 mo

Pharmacodynamics

	PO	IV
Onset	4 wk	24 hr
Peak	Unknown	3-4 days
Duration	Up to 1 yr	10-12 days

Interactions

Drug/drug:

Drug classifications

Antacids: ↓ absorption of etidronate

Mineral supplements with magnesium, calcium, or aluminum: ↓ absorption of etidronate

Individual drugs

Didanosine: ↓ absorption of etidronate

Calcitonin: ↑ effect of calcitonin

Drug/food:

Dairy products: ↓ absorption of etidronate

NURSING CONSIDERATIONS

Assessment

- Assess for GI symptoms, polyuria, flushing, head swelling, tingling, headache—may indicate hypercalcemia; nervousness, irritability, twitching, seizures, spasm, paresthesia indicates hypocalcemia at start of treatment
- Identify nutritional status; evaluate diet for sources of vitamin D (milk, some seafood), calcium (dairy products, dark green vegetables), phosphates
- Monitor BUN, creatinine, uric acid, chloride, electrolytes, urine pH, urinary calcium, magnesium, phosphate, urinalysis (calcium should be kept at 9-10 mg/dl) albumin, alk phosphatase baseline and q3-6 mo; check urine sediment for casts throughout treatment
- Assess for increased drug level—toxic reactions occur rapidly; have calcium chloride or gluconate on hand if calcium level drops too low; check for tetany

Associated nursing diagnoses

✓ Injury, risk for (adverse reactions)
✓ Pain, chronic (uses)
✓ Knowledge deficit (teaching)

Implementation

PO route

• Administer on empty stomach to improve absorption (2 hr ac)

IV route

• Used in hypercalcemias—give by intermittent inf after diluting 300 mg/250 ml or more 0.9% NaCl; run over 2-3 hr

Patient/family education

• Teach method of inj if patient will be responsible for self-medication
• Caution patient to notify prescriber of hypercalcemic relapse: renal calculi, nausea, vomiting, thirst, lethargy, deep bone or flank pain
• Teach patient that warmth and flushing occur and last 1 hr
• Teach patient to follow a low-calcium diet as prescribed (Paget's disease, hypercalcemia)
• Advise patient to notify prescriber of diarrhea, nausea; dose may be divided to lessen these symptoms
• Inform patient that metallic taste may occur with **IV** dosing

Evaluation

Positive therapeutic outcome

• Calcium levels 9-10 mg/dl
• Decreasing symptoms of Paget's disease including pain
• Decreased bone loss in osteoporosis

etodolac

(e-toe-doe'lak)

Lodine

Func. class.: Nonsteroidal antiinflammatory, nonnarcotic analgesic

Pregnancy category C

Action: Inhibits prostaglandin synthesis by decreasing enzyme needed for biosynthesis; analgesic, antiinflammatory properties

Therapeutic Outcome: Decreased pain, inflammation

Uses: Mild to moderate pain, osteoarthritis

Dosage and routes

Osteoarthritis

Adult: PO 800-1200 mg/day in divided doses to 600-1200 mg/day in divided doses; do not exceed 1200 mg/day; patients <60 kg not to exceed 20 mg/kg

Analgesia

Adult: PO 200-400 mg q6-8h prn for acute pain; do not exceed 1200 mg/day; patients 60 kg, not to exceed 20 mg/kg

Available forms: Cap 200, 300 mg

Side effects/adverse reactions

CNS: Dizziness, headache, drowsiness, fatigue, tremors, confusion, insomnia, anxiety, depression, light-headedness, vertigo
CV: Tachycardia, peripheral edema, fluid retention, palpitations, dysrhythmias, CHF
EENT: Tinnitus, hearing loss, blurred vision
GI: *Nausea, anorexia,* vomiting, diarrhea, jaundice, ***cholestatic hepatitis,*** constipation, flatulence, cramps, dry mouth, peptic ulcer, dyspepsia, ***GI bleeding***
GU: ***Nephrotoxicity: dysuria, hematuria, oliguria, azotemia, cystitis, UTI***
HEMA: ***Blood dyscrasias,*** epistaxis, bruising
INTEG: Erythema, urticaria, purpura, rash, pruritus, sweating

Contraindications:

Hypersensitivity; patients in whom aspirin, iodides, or other NSAIDs have produced asthma, rhinitis, urticaria, nasal polyps, angioedema, bronchospasm

Precautions:

Pregnancy **C**; P lactation; children, bleeding; G GI, cardiac disorders; elderly; renal, hepatic disorders

Pharmacokinetics

Absorption	Well absorbed (PO)
Distribution	Highly bound to plasma protein
Metabolism	Unknown
Excretion	Unknown
Half-life	7 hr

Pharmacodynamics

	PO
Onset	½ hr
Peak	1-2 hr
Duration	4-12 hr

E

Interactions

Drug/drug:

Individual drugs

Acetaminophen (long-term use): ↑ renal reactions
Alcohol: ↑ adverse reactions
Aspirin: ↓ effectiveness, ↑ adverse reactions
Coumarin: ↑ anticoagulant effects
Digoxin: ↑ toxicity, ↑ levels
Insulin: ↓ insulin effect
Lithium: ↑ toxicity
Methotrexate: ↑ toxicity
Phenytoin: ↑ toxicity
Probenecid: ↑ toxicity
Sulfonylurea: ↑ toxicity

Drug classifications

Anticoagulants: ↑ risk of bleeding
Antihypertensives: ↓ effect of antihypertensives
Antineoplastics: ↑ risk of hematologic toxicity
β-blockers: ↑ antihypertension
Cephalosporins: ↑ risk of bleeding
Diuretics: ↓ effectiveness of diuretics
Glucocorticoids: ↑ adverse reactions
Hypoglycemics: ↓ hypoglycemic effect
Nonsteroidal antiinflammatories: ↑ adverse reactions
Potassium supplements: ↑ adverse reactions
Radiation: ↑ risk of hematologic toxicity
Sulfonamides: ↑ toxicity

NURSING CONSIDERATIONS

Assessment

- Monitor blood counts during therapy; watch for decreasing platelets; if low, therapy may need to be discontinued, then restarted after hematologic recovery; watch for blood dyscrasia (thrombocytopenia): bruising, fatigue, bleeding, poor healing

Associated nursing diagnoses

✓ Pain (uses)
✓ Mobility, impaired physical mobility (uses)
✓ Knowledge deficit (teaching)
✓ Injury, risk for (adverse reactions)

Implementation

PO route

- Administer with food or milk to decrease gastric symptoms. Food will slow absorption slightly, will not decrease absorption.

Patient / family education

- Inform patient that drug must be continued for prescribed time to be effective; to avoid aspirin, alcoholic beverages
- Caution patient to report bleeding, bruising, fatigue, malaise because blood dyscrasias can occur
- Instruct patient to use caution when driving; drowsiness, dizziness may occur
- Teach patient to take with a full glass of water to enhance absorption; do not crush, break, or chew medication

Evaluation

Positive therapeutic outcome

- Decreased pain
- Decreased inflammation
- Increased mobility

etoposide (VP-16)

(e-toe'poe-side)

VePesid

Func. class.: Antineoplastic
Chem. class.: Semisynthetic podophyllotoxin

Pregnancy category **D**

Action: Inhibits mitotic activity through metaphase to mitosis; also inhibits cells from entering mitosis, depresses DNA, RNA synthesis

➡ **Therapeutic Outcome:** Prevention of rapid growth of malignant cells

Uses: Leukemias, lung, testicular cancer, lymphomas, neuroblastoma, melanoma, ovarian cancer; being investigated for use in leukemia, lymphoma

Dosage and routes

Adult: **IV** 45-75 mg/m^2/day × 3-5 days given q3-5 wk or 200-250 mg/m^2/wk, or 125-140 mg/m^2/day 3 × wk, q5 wk

Available forms: Inj 20 mg/ml, cap 50 mg

Side effects/adverse reactions

CNS: Headache, *fever*
CV: *Hypotension*

GI: *Nausea, vomiting, anorexia,* ***hepatotoxicity***
GU: Nephrotoxicity
HEMA: Thrombocytopenia, leukopenia, myelosuppression, anemia
INTEG: *Rash, alopecia,* phlebitis at **IV** site
RESP: Bronchospasm

Contraindications: Hypersensitivity, bone marrow depression, severe hepatic disease, severe renal disease, bacterial infection, pregnancy **D**

Precautions: Renal disease, hepatic disease, lactation, P children, gout

Pharmacokinetics

Absorption	Variably absorbed
Distribution	Rapidly absorbed, 97% protein binding, crosses placenta
Metabolism	Liver—some
Excretion	Kidneys, unchanged 50%, breast milk
Half-life	3 hr initially, 15 hr terminally

Pharmacodynamics

	PO/IV
Onset	Unknown
Peak	Unknown
Duration	Unknown

Interactions
Drug/drug:
Individual drugs
Radiation: ↑ toxicity, bone marrow suppression
Drug classifications
Antineoplastics: ↑ toxicity, bone marrow suppression
Live virus vaccines: ↑ adverse reactions

NURSING CONSIDERATIONS
Assessment
- Monitor B/P, (baseline and q15 min) during administration
- Monitor CBC, differential, platelet count weekly; withhold drug if WBC is <4000 or platelet count is <75,000; notify prescriber of results—recovery will take 3 wk
- Monitor renal function studies: BUN, urine CrCl before, during therapy; I&O ratio; report fall in urine output of 30 ml/hr; for decreased hyperuricemia
- Monitor for cold, fever, sore throat (may indicate beginning infection); notify prescriber if these occur
- Assess for bleeding: hematuria, guaiac, bruising or petechiae, mucosa or orifices q8h: no rectal temp; avoid IM inj; use pressure to venipuncture sites
- Identify nutritional status: an antiemetic may need to be prescribed
- Assess for symptoms indicating severe allergic reactions: rash, pruritus, urticaria, itching, flushing, bronchospasm, hypotension; epinephrine and crash cart should be nearby

Associated nursing diagnoses
- ✓ Injury, risk for (adverse reactions)
- ✓ Body image disturbance (adverse reactions)
- ✓ Infection, risk for (adverse reactions)
- ✓ Knowledge deficit (teaching)

Implementation

PO route
- Cap need to be refrigerated

IV route
- Give by intermittent inf
- Sol should be prepared by qualified personnel and only under controlled conditions
- Use Luer Loc tubing to prevent leakage; do not let sol come in contact with skin—if contact occurs, wash well with soap and water
- Give after diluting 100 mg/250 ml or more D_5W or NaCl to a concentration of 0.2-0.4 mg/ml; infuse over 30-60 min
- Give hyaluronidase 150 U/ml to 1 ml NaCl to infiltration area; ice compress for treatment of vesicant activity

Y-site compatibilities:

Ondansetron, fludarabine, sargramostim, melphalan, paclitaxel

Y-site incompatibility:

Idarubicin

Additive compatibilities:

Cisplatin, floxuridine, fluorouracil, ifosfamide

Patient/family education

- Teach patient to avoid use of products containing aspirin or ibuprofen, razors, commercial mouthwash because bleeding may occur; to report symptoms of bleeding (hematuria, tarry stools)
- Instruct patient to report signs of anemia (fatigue, headache, irritability, faintness, shortness of breath)
- Teach patient to report any changes in breathing or coughing even several months after treatment
- Advise patient that contraception will be necessary during treatment because teratogenesis may occur
- Caution patient that hair loss may occur during treatment; a wig or hairpiece may make patient feel better; new hair will be different in color, texture
- Advise patient to avoid vaccinations during treatment because serious reactions may occur
- Teach patient to report signs/symptoms of infection; fever, chills, sore throat. Patient should avoid crowds and persons with known infections

Evaluation

Positive therapeutic outcome
- Decreased spread of malignant, leukemic cells

etretinate

(e-tret'inate)

Tegison

Func. class.: Systemic antipsoriatic

Chem. class.: Retinol derivative

Pregnancy category **X**

Action: Unknown; drug is related to retinol

Therapeutic Outcome: Decrease in size and number of lesions

Uses: Severe recalcitrant psoriasis including erythrodermic and generalized pustular types

Dosage and routes

Adult: PO 0.75-1 mg/kg/day in divided doses, not to exceed 1.5 mg/kg/day; maintenance dose 0.5-0.75 mg/kg/day generally beginning after 8-16 wk of therapy

Available forms: Cap 10, 25 mg

Side effects/adverse reactions

CNS: Fatigue, headache, dizziness, fever, pain, anxiety, amnesia, depression
CV: Edema, ***CV obstruction, atrial fibrillation,*** chest pain, coagulation disorders
EENT: Eye irritation, eye pain, double vision, change in lacrimation; earache, otitis externa, dry nose, eyes, mouth; nosebleed, chelitis, sore tongue
GI: Anorexia, abdominal pain, nausea, ***hepatitis,*** constipation, diarrhea, flatulence, weight loss
GU: WBC in urine, ***proteinuria,*** glycosuria, *increased BUN, creatinine,* ***hematuria,*** *casts,* ***acetonuria, hemoglobinuria, dysuria***
INTEG: Alopecia; peeling of palms, soles, fingertips; itching; rash; dryness; red scaling on face; bruising; sunburn; pyogenic granuloma; paronychia; onycholysis; perspiration change, nail changes
META: Increase or decrease in potassium, calcium, P, sodium, chloride
MS: Hyperostosis, bone pain, cramps, myalgia, gout, hypertonia
RESP: Dyspnea, cough

Contraindications: Pregnancy **X**

Precautions: Lactation, children, hepatic disease, diabetes, obesity

P

Pharmacokinetics

Absorption	Well absorbed (PO)
Distribution	Stored in fatty tissue, crosses placenta, 99% protein binding
Metabolism	Liver (extensively)
Excretion	Kidney (metabolite)
Half-life	Terminal 120 days

Pharmacodynamics

	PO
Onset	4-6 wk
Peak	4-9 mo
Duration	Years

Interactions

Drug/drug:

Individual drugs

Vitamin D: ↑ toxicity

Drug classifications

Abrasives: ↑ irritation
Desquamating agents: ↑ irritation
Tetracyclines: ↑ pseudotumor cerebri

Drug/food:

↑ absorption with food (fatty)

NURSING CONSIDERATIONS

Assessment

- Assess patient for pseudotumor cerebri: headache, nausea, vomiting, visual problems, papilledema

• Monitor hepatic studies: AST (SGOT), ALT (SGPT), LDH, q1-2 wk × 3 mo, q1-3 mo thereafter because hepatotoxicity may occur
• Assess patient for visual problems: blurring, decreased night vision, poor visual acuity; drug should be discontinued and ophthalmologist consulted
• Check lipids (cholesterol, triglycerides, HDL) before, q1-2 wk during treatment; after discontinuing treatment, lipids will return to normal
• Monitor blood and renal studies: CBC (Hct, Hgh, platelets, WBC); urinalysis, BUN, creatinine (may be increased); urine may show protein, glucose, acetone, blood; electrolytes may be increased or decreased (sodium, potassium, calcium, phosphate)

Associated nursing diagnoses

✓ Body image disturbance (uses)
✓ Injury, risk for (adverse reactions)
✓ Knowledge deficit (teaching)

Implementation

PO route
• Give with food (fatty) to increase absorption

Patient/family education

• Advise patient to take with food to enhance absorption
• Caution patient not to use during pregnancy; contraception must be used for 1 mo before or after therapy; teratogenic effects are longlasting
• Caution patient not to take vitamin A supplements because increased vitamin A levels may occur and to avoid alcohol and fatty diet or lipid levels will increase
• Inform patient that contact lens intolerance is common; glasses may need to be used
• Advise patient to use gum, hard candy, or frequent sips of water to prevent dry mouth, and to prevent burns by using sunscreen or protective clothing
• Inform patient that blurred vision, change in color perception, joint pain, jaundice, cramping should be reported to prescriber

Evaluation

Positive therapeutic outcome
• Decrease in scaling, itching, amount of psoriasis

factor IX complex (human)/factor IX (human)

Konyne 80, Proplex T, Proplex SX-T, Profilnine Heat-Treated/Alphanine, Alpha Nine SD, Mononine

Func. class.: Hemostatic
Chem. class.: Factors II, VII, IX, X

Pregnancy category **C**

Action: Causes an increase in blood levels of clotting factors II, VII, IX, X; factor IX (human) has IX activity only

Therapeutic Outcome: Replacement of factors II, VII, IX, X

Uses: Hemophilia B (Christmas disease), factor IX deficiency, anticoagulant reversal, control of bleeding in patients with factor VIII inhibitors; reversal of overdose of anticoagulants in emergencies

Dosage and routes

Bleeding in hemophilia A and inhibitors of factor VIII

P ***Adult/child:*** 75 U/kg, repeat in 12 hr

Bleeding in hemophilia B

P ***Adult/child:*** Give to establish 25% of normal Factor IX activity or 60-75 U/kg/day then 10-20 U/kg/day × 1 wk

Prophylaxis of bleeding in hemophilia B

P ***Adult/child:*** 10-20 U/kg/day × 1 wk

Reversal of oral anticoagulant

P ***Adult/child:*** 15 U/kg

Factor VII deficiency (use Proplex T)

P ***Adult/child:*** 0.5 U/kg × body weight (kg) × desired factor IX increase (in % of normal). Repeat q4-6h if needed

Factor IX (human) AlphaNine, AlphaNine SD (minor to moderate hemorrhage)

P ***Adult/child:*** Give amount to increase plasma Factor IX level to 20%-30%

Serious hemorrhage

P ***Adult/child:*** Give amount to increase plasma Factor IX level to 30%-50% given as daily inf

Mononine

Minor hemorrhage

P ***Adult/child:*** Give amount to increase plasma Factor IX level to 15%-25% (20-30 U/kg), may repeat in 24 hr

Major trauma

P ***Adult/child:*** Give amount to increase plasma Factor IX level to 25%-50% (75 U/kg) q18-30 h for up to 10 days

Available forms: Inj (number of units noted on label)

Side effects/adverse reactions

CNS: Headache, dizziness, malaise, paresthesia, *lethargy, chills, fever, flushing*
CV: Hypotension, tachycardia, *MI,* ***venous thrombosis, pulmonary embolism***
EENT: Tinnitus, eyelid swelling
GI: Nausea, vomiting, abdominal cramps, jaundice, ***viral hepatitis***
HEMA: ***Thrombosis, hemolysis, AIDS, DIC***
INTEG: Rash, flushing, *urticaria*
RESP: ***Bronchospasm***

Contraindications: Hypersensitivity, hepatic disease, DIC, elective surgery, mild factor IX deficiency

Precautions: Neonates/ P infants, pregnancy **C**

F

Pharmacokinetics

Absorption	40% (PO), complete (IV)
Distribution	Unknown
Metabolism	Rapidly cleared from plasma, liver 30%
Excretion	70% unchanged—kidneys
Half-life	24 hr

Pharmacodynamics

	IV
Onset	Unknown
Peak	Unknown
Duration	Unknown

Interactions

Drug/drug:

Individual drugs

Aminocaproic acid: ↑ risk of thrombosis; do not use together

NURSING CONSIDERATIONS

Assesment

- Monitor blood studies (coagulation factors assays by % normal: 5% prevents spontaneous hemorrhage, 30%-50% for surgery, 80%-100% for severe hemorrhage); check for bleeding q15-30 min, immobilize and apply ice to affected joints
- Monitor for increased B/P, pulse
- Monitor I&O; if urine becomes orange or red, notify prescriber
- Assess for allergic or pyrogenic reaction: fever, chills, rash, itching; slow inf rate if not severe
- Assess for DIC: bleeding, ecchymosis, hypersensitivity, changes in coagulation tests

Associated nursing diagnoses

- ✓ Injury, risk for (uses)
- ✓ Tissue perfusion, altered (uses)
- ✓ Knowledge deficit (teaching)

Implementation

IV **IV route**

- Give **IV** after warming to room temp 3 ml/min or less, with plastic syringe only; do not admix
- Give after dilution with provided diluent, 50 U/ml or 25 U/ml; give so as not to exceed 10 ml/min; decrease rate if fever, headache, flushing, tingling occur
- Give after crossmatch is completed if patient has blood type A, B, AB, to determine incompatibility with factor
- Store reconstituted sol for 3 hr at room temp or up to 2 yr if refrigerated (powder); check expiration date

Patient/family education

- Advise patient to report any signs of bleeding: gums, under skin, urine, stools, emesis
- Caution patient about risk of viral hepatitis, AIDS; that immunization for hepatitis B may be given first; to be tested q2-3 mo for HIV
- Tell patient to carry ID identifying disease and treatment; avoid salicylates, to inform other health professionals about condition

Evaluation

Positive therapeutic outcome

- Prevention of hemorrhage

famciclovir

(fam-sye-klo'vir)
Famvir
Func. class.: Antiviral
Chem. class.: Guanosine nucleoside
Pregnancy category **B**

Action: Inhibits DNA polymerase and viral DNS synthesis by the conversion of this guanosine nucleoside to penciclovir

Therapeutic Outcome: Decreasing size and number of lesions

Uses: Treatment of acute herpes zoster, genital herpes

Dosage and routes

Adult: PO 500 mg q8h; in renal disease if creatinine clearance is ≥ 60 ml/min/1.73 m^2 (500 mg q8h); if 40-59 ml/min/1.73 m^2 (500 mg q12h); if 20-39 ml/min/1.73 m^2 (500 mg q24h)

Available forms: Tab 500 mg

Side effects/adverse reactions

CNS: Headache, fatigue
GI: Nausea, vomiting, diarrhea, constipation, abdominal pain
GU: Decreased sperm count
INTEG: Pruritis
MS: Back pain
RESP: Pharyngitis, sinusitis

Contraindications: Hypersensitivity to this drug or penciclovir

Precautions: Renal disease, pregnancy **B**, hypersensitivity to acyclovir, ganciclovir

Pharmacokinetics

Absorption	Well absorbed (PO)
Distribution	Unknown
Metabolism	Intestinal tissue, blood, liver
Excretion	Breast milk, kidney, bile
Half-life	3 hr

Pharmacodynamics

	PO
Onset	Unknown
Peak	1 hr
Duration	8 hr

Interactions: None known

NURSING CONSIDERATIONS

Assessment

- Assess amount and distribution of lesions; also burning, itching, or pain (early symptoms of herpes infection)
- Monitor renal function studies: urine CrCl, BUN before and during treatment if patient has decreased renal function; dose may need to be lowered
- Monitor bowel pattern before, during treatment; diarrhea may occur

Associated nursing diagnoses

- ✓ Infection, risk for (uses)
- ✓ Knowledge deficit (teaching)

Implementation

- Give with or without meals; absorption does not appear to be lowered when taken with food

Patient/family education

- Teach patient how to recognize signs of beginning infection
- Teach patient how to prevent the spread of infection to others
- Teach patient reason for medication and expected results

Evaluation

Positive therapeutic outcome
- Decreased size and spread of lesions

famotodine
(fa-moe'to-deen)
Pepcid, Pepcid IV
Func. class.: H_2 histamine receptor antagonist, antiulcer agent
Pregnancy category **B**

Action: Inhibits histamine at H_2 receptor site in gastric parietal cells, which inhibits gastric acid secretion

Therapeutic Outcome: Healing of duodenal ulcers or gastric ulcers; prevention of duodenal ulcers; decreases symptoms of GERD or Zollinger-Ellison syndrome

Uses: Short-term treatment of active duodenal ulcer, maintenance therapy for duodenal ulcer, Zollinger-Ellison syndrome, multiple endocrine adenomas, gastric ulcers

Dosage and routes

Duodenal ulcer

Adult: PO 40 mg qd hs × 4-8 wk, then 20 mg qd hs if needed (maintenance); **IV** 20 mg q12h if unable to take PO

Hypersecretory conditions

Adult: PO 20 mg q6h; may give 160 mg q6h if needed; **IV** 20 mg q12h if unable to take PO

Available forms: Tab 20, 40 mg; powder for oral susp 40 mg/5 ml; inj 10 mg/ml

Side effects/adverse reactions

CNS: ***Headache, dizziness,*** paresthesia, ***seizure,*** depression, anxiety, somnolence, insomnia, fever
EENT: Taste change, tinnitus, orbital edema
GI: ***Constipation,*** nausea, vomiting, anorexia, cramps, abnormal liver enzymes
HEMA: ***Thrombocytopenia***
INTEG: Rash
MS: Myalgia, arthralgia
RESP: ***Bronchospasm***

Contraindications: Hypersensitivity

Precautions: Pregnancy **B**, P lactation, children, severe renal disease, severe hepatic function, G elderly

Pharmacokinetics

Absorption	50% absorbed (PO)
Distribution	Plasma, protein binding (15%-20%)
Metabolism	Liver (30% active metabolizing)
Excretion	Kidneys (70%)
Half-life	2½-3½ hr

Pharmacodynamics

	PO	IV
Onset	30-60 min	Immediate
Peak	1-3 hr	½-3 hr
Duration	6-12 hr	6-12 hr

Interactions

Drug/drug:

Individual drugs

Ketoconazole: ↓ absorption of ketoconazole

Drug classifications

Antacids: ↓ absorption of famotodine

NURSING CONSIDERATIONS

Assessment

- Assess patient with ulcers or suspected ulcers: epigastric, abdominal pain, hematemesis, occult blood in stools, blood in gastric, aspirate prior to treatment—throughout treatment, monitor gastric pH (5 should be maintained)
- Monitor I&O ratio, BUN, creatinine, CBC with differential monthly

Associated nursing diagnoses

✓ Pain (uses)
✓ Knowledge deficit (teaching)

Implementation

PO route

- Give antacids 1 hr before or 2 hr after famotodine; may be given with foods or liq
- Administer oral susp after shaking well; discard unused sol after 1 mo

IV **IV route**

- Give **IV** direct after diluting 2 ml of drug (10 mg/ml) in 0.9% NaCl to total volume of 5-10 ml; inject over 2 min to prevent hypotension
- Administer **IV** intermittent inf after diluting 20 mg of drug in 100 ml of LR, 0.9% NaCl, D_5W, $D_{10}W$; run over 15-30 min
- Store in cool environment (oral); **IV** solution is stable for 48 hr at room temp; do not use discolored sol

F

Y-site compatibilities:

Aminophylline, ampicillin, ampicillin/sulbactam, amrinone, atropine, bretylium, calcium gluconate, cefazolin, cefoperazone, cefotaxime, cefotetan, cefoxitin, ceftazidime, ceftizoxime, cefuroxime, cephalotin, cephapirin, dexamethasone, dextran 40, digoxin, dobutamine, dopamine, enalaprilat, epinephrine, erythromycin lactobionate, esmolol, folic acid, furosemide, gentamicin, haloperidol, heparin, hydrocortisone sodium succinate, imipenem/cilastatin, insulin, isoproterenol, labetalol, lidocaine, magnesium sulfate, melphalan, methylprednisolone, metoclopramide, mezlocillin, nitroglycerin, norepinephrine, ondansetron, oxacillin, paclitaxel, perphenazine, phenylephrine, phenytoin, phytonadione, piperacillin, potassium chloride, potassium phosphate, procainamide, sodium bicarbonate, sodium nitroprusside, theophylline, thiamine, ticarcillin, verapamil

Patient/family education

- Caution patient to avoid driving, other hazardous activities until stabilized on this medication; dizziness may occur

• Advise patient to avoid black pepper, caffeine, alcohol, harsh spices, extremes in temperature of food; tell patient to avoid OTC preparations: aspirin, cough, cold preparations; condition may worsen
• Tell patient that smoking decreases the effectiveness of the drug; that smoking cessation should be considered
• Instruct patient that drug must be continued for prescribed time to be effective and taken exactly as prescribed; doses are not to be doubled; to take missed dose when remembered up to 1 hr before next dose
• Tell patient to report bruising, fatigue, malaise; blood dyscrasias may occur
• Tell patient to report diarrhea, black tarry stools, sore throat, rash, dizziness, confusion, rash, or delirium to prescriber immediately

Evaluation

Positive therapeutic outcome
• Decreased pain in abdomen
• Healing of ulcers

fat emulsions

(fat ee-mul'shuns)
Intralipid 10%, Intralipid 20%, Liposyn II 10%, Liposyn II 20%, Liposyn III 10%, Liposyn III 20%, Soyacal 20%
Func. class.: Caloric
Chem. class.: Fatty acid, long chain
Pregnancy category **C**

Action: Needed for energy, heat production; consists of neutral triglycerides, primarily unsaturated fatty acids

Therapeutic Outcome: Increased available calories and fatty acids

Uses: Increase calorie intake, prevent fatty acid deficiency

Dosage and routes

Deficiency
P ***Adult and child:*** **IV** 8%-10% of required calorie intake (intralipid)

Adjunct to TPN
Adult: **IV** 1 ml/min over 15-30 min (10%) or 0.5 ml/min over 15-30 min (20%); may increase to 500 ml over 4-8 hr if no adverse reactions occur; not to exceed 2.5 g/kg
P ***Child:*** **IV** 0.1 ml/min over 10-15 min (10%) or 0.05 ml/min over 10-15 min (20%); may increase to 1 g/kg over 4 hr if no adverse reactions occur; not to exceed 4 g/kg

Prevention of deficiency

Adult: **IV** 500 ml 2 × wk (10%), given 1 ml/min for 30 min, not to exceed 500 ml over 6 hr

P *Child:* **IV** 5-10 ml/kg/day (10%), given 0.1 ml/min for 30 min, not to exceed 100 ml/hr

Available forms: 10% (50, 100, 200, 250, 500 ml), 20% (50, 100, 200, 250, 500 ml)

Side effects/adverse reactions

CNS: Dizziness, headache, drowsiness, focal seizures
CV: ***Shock***
GI: Nausea, vomiting, ***hepatomegaly***
HEMA: ***Hyperlipemia, hypercoagulation, thrombocytopenia, leukopenia, leukocytosis***
RESP: Dyspnea, ***fat in lung tissue***

Contraindications: Hypersensitivity, hyperlipemia, lipid necrosis, acute pancreatitis accompanied by hyperlipemia, hyperbilirubinemia of the P newborn

Precautions: Severe liver disease, diabetes mellitus, thrombocytopenia, gastric ulcers, premature, term P newborns, pregnancy **C**, sepsis

Pharmacokinetics

Absorption	Completely absorbed (IV)
Distribution	Intravascular space
Metabolism	Conversion to triglycerides, to free fatty acids
Excretion	Unknown
Half-life	Unknown

Pharmacodynamics

	IV
Onset	Unknown
Peak	Unknown
Duration	Unknown

Interactions: None

NURSING CONSIDERATIONS

Assessment

- Monitor triglycerides, free fatty acid levels, platelet counts daily to prevent fat overload, thrombocytopenia
- Monitor liver function studies: AST (SGOT), ALT (SGPT); Hct, Hgb—notify prescriber if abnormal
- Assess nutritional status: calorie count by dietician; monitor weight daily

Associated nursing diagnoses

✓ Nutrition, less than body requirements (uses)
✓ Knowledge deficit (teaching)

Implementation

IV **IV route**

- Administer using inf pump at prescribed rate; do not use in-line filter sized for lipid emulsion; clogging will occur
- Do not use mixed sol that look oily or are not separated; discard unused sol
- Change **IV** tubing at each inf: infection may occur with old tubing
- Give by intermittent inf at a rate of 10% sol (1 ml/min); 20% sol (0.5 ml/min) initially for 15-30 min; may be increased to 10% sol (120 ml/hr) or 20% sol (62.5 ml/hr) if no adverse reactions occur; do

not give more than 500 ml during the first day. Children should be given 10% (0.1 mg/ml) or 20% (0.05 ml/min) initially for 15-30 min, may be increased 1 g/kg/4hr, do not give more than 10% (100 ml/hr) or 20% (50 ml/hr)

Y-*site compatibilities:*

Aldesleukin, ampicillin, cefamandole, cefazolin, cefoxitin, cephapirin, clindamycin, digoxin, dopamine, erythromycin lactobionate, furosemide, gentamicin, isoproterenol, lidocaine, kanamycin, norepinephrine, oxacillin, penicillin G potassium, ticarcillin, tobramycin

Y-*site incompatibilities:*

Amikacin, tetracycline

Additive compatibilities:

INTRALIPID with FreAmine II 8.5%, FreAmine III 8.5%, Travasol without electrolytes 8.5% and 10%, or Dextrose Injection 10% and 70%, nizatidine

Patient/family education

- Teach patient reason for use of lipids and expected results

Evaluation

Positive therapeutic outcome
- Increased weight
- Fatty acids at adequate levels

felbamate

(fell-ba'mate)

Felbatol

Func. class.: Anticonvulsant

Chem. class.: Carbamate derivative

Pregnancy category C

Action: Mechanism of action unknown; may increase seizure threshold; has weak inhibitory effects on GABA-receptor and benzodiazinepine-receptor binding

Therapeutic Outcome: Absence of seizures

Uses: Partial seizures, with or without generalization in adults; partial and generalized seizures in children with Lennox-Gastaut syndrome

Dosage and routes

Adjunctive therapy

Adult: PO add 1.2 g/day in 3-4 divided doses; reduce other anticonvulsants (valproic acid, phenytoin, carbamazepine, and derivatives) by 20% to control plasma concentrations; may increase felbamate in 1.2 g/day increments qwk, up to 3.6 g/day

Monotherapy

Adult: PO 1.2 g/day in 3-4 divided doses; titrate with close supervision; increase dose in 600-mg increments q2wk to 3.6 g/day if needed

Lennox-Gastaut syndrome

P ***Child (2-14 yr):*** PO add 15 mg/kg/day in 3-4 divided doses; reduce other anticonvulsants (valproic acid, phenytoin, carbamazepine, and derivatives) by 20% to control plasma concentrations; may increase felbamate 15 mg/kg/day qwk up to 45 mg/day

Available forms: Tab 400, 600 mg; susp 600 mg/5 ml

Side effects/adverse reactions

CNS: Dizziness, fatigue, *headache, insomnia,* anxiety, tremor, unsteady gait, depression, paresthesia
CV: Chest pain
EENT: Dry mouth, blurred vision, diplopia, otitis media
GI: *Nausea, constipation, diarrhea, anorexia, vomiting,* abdominal pain, increased liver enzymes, hiccups, *dyspepsia*
GU: Urinary incontinence, intramenstrual bleeding, *UTI*
HEMA: Purpura, ***leukopenia***
INTEG: Rash, acne
RESP: Upper respiratory tract infection, rhinitis, sinusitis, pharyngitis, coughing

Contraindications: Hypersensitivity to this drug, other carbamates

Precautions: Hepatic disease, renal disease, cardiac disease,
P psychosis, pregnancy **C**, lacta-
G tion, child <6 yr, elderly

Pharmacokinetics

Absorption	Well absorbed (PO)
Distribution	Crosses placenta, plamsa protein binding (22%-25% to albumin)
Metabolism	Liver
Excretion	Kidneys—unchanged (40%-50%)
Half-life	20-23 hr

Pharmacodynamics

	PO
Onset	Unknown
Peak	Unknown
Duration	Unknown

Interactions

Drug/drug:

Individual drugs

Carbenazine: ↓ levels of carbenazine
Phenytoin: ↑ levels of phenytoin
Valproic acid: ↑ levels of phenytoin

NURSING CONSIDERATIONS

Assessment

- Assess mental status: mood, sensorium, affect, memory (long, short), especially in
G elderly
- Assess for blood dyscrasias: fever, sore throat, bruising, rash, jaundice, epistaxis (long-term treatment only)
- Assess seizure activity including type, location, duration, and character; provide seizure precaution

Associated nursing diagnoses

✓ Injury, risk for (side effects)
✓ Knowledge deficit (teaching)

Implementation

PO route

- Give on empty stomach for best absorption

Patient/family education

- Teach patient to carry Medic Alert ID stating name, drugs taken, condition, prescriber's name, phone number
- Advise patient to avoid driving, other activities that require alertness
- Teach patient not to discontinue medication abruptly after long-term use

Evaluation

Positive therapeutic outcome

- Decreased seizure activity

Treatment of overdose: Lavage, vital signs

felodipine

(fell-oh'di-peen)

Plendil

Func. class.: Calcium-channel blocker, antihypertensive

Chem. class.: Dihydropyridine

Pregnancy category C

Action: Inhibits calcium ion influx across cell membrane, resulting in dilation of peripheral arteries

Therapeutic Outcome: Decreased B/P in hypertension

Uses: Essential hypertension, alone or with other antihypertensives

Dosage and routes

Adult: PO 5 mg qd initially, usual range 5-10 mg qd; do not exceed 20 mg qd; do not adjust dosage at intervals of <2 wk

Available forms: Ext rel tab 5, 10 mg

Side effects/adverse reactions

CNS: Headache, fatigue, drowsiness, dizziness, anxiety, depression, nervousness, insomnia, light-headedness, paresthesia, tinnitus, psychosis, somnolence

CV: Dysrhythmias, edema, CHF, hypotension, palpitations, ***MI, pulmonary edema,*** tachycardia, syncope, AV block, angina

GI: Nausea, vomiting, diarrhea, gastric upset, constipation, increased liver function studies, dry mouth

HEMA: Anemia

INTEG: Rash, pruritus

MISC: Flushing, sexual difficulties, cough, nasal congestion, shortness of breath, wheezing, epistaxis, respiratory infection, chest pain

Contraindications: Hypersensitivity, sick sinus syndrome, 2nd- or 3rd-degree heart block

Precautions: CHF, hypotension <90 mm Hg systolic, hepatic injury, pregnancy **C**, P lactation, children, renal dis- G ease, elderly

Pharmacokinetics

Absorption	Well absorbed
Distribution	Unknown; protein binding >99%
Metabolism	Liver, extensively
Excretion	Kidneys
Half-life	11-16 hr

Pharmacodynamics

	PO
Onset	2-3 hr
Peak	2½-5 hr
Duration	<24 hr

Interactions

Drug/drug:

Individual drugs

Alcohol: ↑ hypotension
Carbamazepine: ↑ toxicity
Digoxin: ↑ digoxin levels, ↑ bradycardia, CHF
Phenobarbital: ↓ effectiveness
Phenytoin: ↓ effectiveness
Propranolol: ↑ toxicity

Drug classifications

Antihypertensives: ↑ hypotension
Beta-adrenergic blockers: ↑ bradycardia, CHF
Nitrates: ↑ nitrates

NURSING CONSIDERATIONS

Assessment

- Assess fluid volume status: I&O ratio and record; weight; skin turgor; adequacy of pulses; moist mucous membranes; bilateral lung sounds; peripheral pitting edema—dehydration symptoms of decreasing output, thirst, hypotension, dry mouth, and mucous membranes should be reported
- Monitor ALT (SGPT), AST (SGOT), bilirubin daily; if these are elevated
- Monitor cardiac status: B/P, pulse, respiration, ECG

Associated nursing diagnoses

✓ Cardiac output, decreased (uses)
✓ Knowledge deficit (teaching)

Implementation

PO route

- Give once a day, with food for GI symptoms

Patient/family education

- Caution patient to avoid hazardous activities until stabilized on drug, and dizziness is no longer a problem
- Instruct patient to limit caffeine consumption; to avoid alcohol and OTC drugs unless directed by prescriber
- Urge patient to comply in all areas of medical regimen: diet, exercise, stress reduction, drug therapy; to notify prescriber of irregular heart beat, shortness of breath, swelling of feet and hands, pronounced dizziness, constipation, nausea, hypotension
- Teach patient to use as directed even if feeling better; may be taken with other cardiovascular drugs (nitrates, beta blockers)

Evaluation

Positive therapeutic outcome

- Decreased B/P

F

fenofibrate

(fen-oh-fee′ brate)

Lipidil

Func. class.: Antilipemic

Chem. class.: Aryloxisobutyric acid derivative

Pregnancy category **C**

Action: Inhibits biosynthesis of low-density and very low-density lipoproteins, which are responsible for triglyceride development; mobilizes triglycerides from tissue; increases excretion of neutral sterols

Therapeutic Outcome: Decreasing cholesterol levels and low-density lipoproteins, decreased pruritus

Uses: Types IV, V; hyperlipidemia

Dosage and routes

Adult: PO 100 mg/day

Available forms: Cap 100 mg

Side effects/adverse reactions

CNS: Fatigue, weakness, drowsiness, dizziness
CV: Angina, dysrhythmias, thrombophlebitis, ***pulmonary emboli***
GI: Nausea, vomiting, dyspepsia, increased liver enzymes, stomatitis, flatulence, hepatomegaly, gastritis, increased cholethiasis, weight gain
GU: Decreased libido, impotence, dysuria, proteinuria, oliguria, ***hematuria***
HEMA: ***Leukopenia,*** anemia, ***eosinophilia,*** bleeding
INTEG: *Rash,* urticaria, pruritus, dry hair and skin, alopecia
MISC: Polyphagia, weight gain
MS: Myalgias, arthralgias

Contraindications: Severe hepatic disease, severe renal disease, primary biliary cirrhosis

Precautions: Peptic ulcer, pregnancy **C**, lactation

Pharmacokinetics

Absorption	Unknown
Distribution	Unknown
Metabolism	Unknown
Excretion	Unknown
Half-life	Unknown

Pharmacodynamics

	PO
Onset	Unknown
Peak	Unknown
Duration	Unknown

Interactions

Drug/drug:

Drug classifications

Anticoagulants, oral: ↑ effect of anticoagulants
Diuretics, thiazide: ↓ action of fenofibrate
Estrogens: ↓ action of fenofibrate

Lab test interferences

Increase: Liver function studies, CPK, BSP, thymol turbidity, glucose
Decrease: Hgb, Hct, WBC

NURSING CONSIDERATIONS

Assessment

- Assess nutrition: fat, protein, carbohydrates, nutritional analysis should be completed by dietician
- Assess skin integrity after patient has been receiving drug; itching, pruritus often occur from bile deposits on skin
- Monitor cardiac glycoside level if both drugs are being administered—cardiac glycoside levels will be decreased
- Monitor for signs of Vit A, D, K deficiency; serum cholesterol, triglyceride levels, electrolytes if on extended therapy
- Monitor bowel pattern daily; increase bulk, water in diet if constipation develops

Associated nursing diagnoses

✓ Knowledge deficit (teaching)
✓ Noncompliance (teaching)

Implementation

PO route

- Give with evening meal; if dose is increased, take with breakfast and evening meal
- Store in cool environment in tight, light-resistant container

Patient/family education

- Inform patient that compliance is needed because toxicity may result if doses are missed
- Teach patient that risk factors—high-fat diet, smoking, alcohol consumption, absence of exercise—should be decreased
- Caution patient to practice birth control while on this drug
- Teach patient to notify prescriber if the GI symptoms of diarrhea, abdominal or epigastric pain, nausea, or vomiting occur
- Instruct patient to report GU symptoms: dysuria, proteinuria, oliguria, decreased libido, impotence

Evaluation

Positive therapeutic outcome

- Decrease in cholesterol to desired level after 8 wk

fenoprofen

(fen-oh-proe'fen)

fenoprofen, Nalfon

Func. class.: Nonsteroidal antiinflammatory, nonnargotic analgesic

Chem. class.: Propionic acid derivative

Pregnancy category **B**

Action: Inhibits prostaglandin synthesis by decreasing enzyme needed for biosynthesis; analgesic, antiinflammatory, antipyretic

➔ Therapeutic Outcome: Decreased pain, inflammation

Uses: Mild to moderate pain, osteoarthritis, rheumatoid arthritis, acute gout, arthritis, ankylosing spondylitis, inflammation, dysmenorrhea

Dosage and routes

Pain

Adult: PO 200 mg q4-6h as needed

Arthritis

Adult: PO 300-600 mg qid, not to exceed 3.2 g/day

Available forms: Cap 200, 300 mg; tab 600 mg

Side effects/adverse reactions

CNS: Dizziness, headache, drowsiness, fatigue, tremors, confusion, insomnia, anxiety, depression
CV: Tachycardia, peripheral edema, palpitations, dysrhythmias
EENT: Tinnitus, hearing loss, blurred vision
GI: Nausea, anorexia, vomiting, diarrhea, jaundice, ***cholestatic hepatitis,*** constipation, flatulence, cramps, dry mouth, peptic ulcer
GU: ***Nephrotoxicity: dysuria, hematuria, oliguria, azotemia***
HEMA: ***Blood dyscrasias***
INTEG: Purpura, rash, pruritus, sweating

Contraindications: Hypersensitivity, asthma, severe renal disease, severe hepatic disease

Precautions: Pregnancy, **B** 1st and 2nd trimester, lactation, P children, bleeding disorders, GI disorders, cardiac disorders, hypersensitivity to other antiinflammatory agents

Pharmacokinetics

Absorption	Well absorbed (PO)
Distribution	Does not cross placenta
Metabolism	Extensively—liver
Excretion	Unchanged—kidneys
Half-life	3½ hr

Pharmacodynamics

	PO
Onset	15-30 min
Peak	2 hr
Duration	4-6 hr

Interactions

Drug/drug:

Individual drugs

Cefamandole: ↑ bleeding
Furosemide: ↑ toxic effects
Heparin: ↑ bleeding
Insulin: ↑ effects
Methotrexate: ↑ effects
Phenytoin: ↑ effects
Plicamycin: ↑ bleeding
Probenecid: ↓ effects
Spironolactone: ↓ effects
Sulfinpyrazone: ↓ effects
Valproic acid: ↑ effects, ↑ bleeding
Vancomycin: ↑ ototoxicity

Drug classifications

Antacids: ↓ effects of fenoprofen
Anticoagulants: ↑ effects
Carbonic anhydrase inhibitors: ↑ toxic effects
Nonsteroidal antiinflammatories: ↑ gastric ulcers
Salicylates: ↓ blood sugar levels
Steroids: ↓ effects of fenoprofen, ↑ gastric ulcers
Sulfonylamides: ↓ effects

NURSING CONSIDERATIONS

Assessment

- Monitor liver function; renal function, other blood studies: AST (SGOT), ALT (SGPT), bilirubin, creatinine, BUN, CBC, Hct, Hgb, pro-time if patient is on long-term therapy
- Check I&O ratio; decreasing

output may indicate renal failure (long-term therapy)
• Assess for allergic reactions: rash, urticaria; if these occur, drug may have to be discontinued
• Assess for ototoxicity: tinnitus, ringing, roaring in ears; audiometric testing needed before, after long-term therapy
• Assess for visual changes: blurring, halos; corneal, retinal damage
• Check edema in feet, ankles, legs
• Identify prior drug history; there are many drug interactions
• Monitor pain: location, duration, type, intensity, prior to dose and 1 hr after; ROM prior to dose and after

Associated nursing diagnoses

✓ Pain (uses)
✓ Mobility, impaired (uses)
✓ Knowledge deficit (teaching)
✓ Injury, risk for (adverse reactions)

Implementation

PO route
• Administer to patient crushed or whole; chewable tab may be chewed (do not crush enteric product)
• Give with food or milk to decrease gastric symptoms; absorption may be slowed; give 30 min ac or 2 hr pc

Patient/family education

• Teach patient to report any symptoms of renal toxicity, visual changes, ototoxicity, allergic reactions, bleeding (long-term therapy)
• Advise patient to take with 8 oz of water and sit upright for ½ hr after dose to prevent ulceration
• Caution patient not to exceed recommended dosage—acute poisoning may result—and to take as prescribed, do not double dose
• Instruct patient to read label on other OTC drugs; many contain other antiinflammatories
• Inform patient that the therapeutic response takes 2 wk (arthritis)
• Teach patient to report tinnitus, confusion, diarrhea, sweating, hyperventilation, blurred vision, fever, joint aches
• Caution patient to avoid alcohol ingestion; GI bleeding may occur

Evaluation

Positive therapeutic outcome
• Decreased pain
• Decreased inflammation
• Increased mobility

fentanyl

(fen'ta-nill)
fentanyl, Sublimaze
Func. class.: Narcotic analgesic
Chem. class.: Opiate, synthetic phenylpiperidine derivative

Pregnancy category **C**
Controlled substance schedule **II**

Action: Inhibits ascending pain pathways in CNS, increases pain threshold, alters pain perception by binding to opiate receptors

Therapeutic Outcome: Relief of pain, supplement to anesthesia

Uses: Preoperatively, postoperatively; adjunct to general anesthetic, when combined with droperidol

Dosage and routes

Anesthetic

Adult: **IV** 0.05-0.1 mg q2-3 min prn

Preoperatively

Adult: IM 0.05-0.1 mg q30-60 min before surgery

Postoperatively

Adult: IM 0.05-0.1 mg q1-2hr prn

P *Child:* IM 0.02-0.03 mg/9 kg

Available forms: Inj 0.05 mg/ml

Side effects/adverse reactions

CNS: Dizziness, delirium, euphoria, light-headedness, sedation, dysphoria, agitation, anxiety
CV: ***Bradycardia, cardiac arrest,*** hypotension or hypertension, facial flushing, chills
EENT: Blurred vision, miosis
GI: Nausea, vomiting, diarrhea, cramps
MS: Muscle rigidity
RESP: ***Respiratory depression, arrest, laryngospasm***

Contraindications: Hypersensitivity to opiates, myasthenia gravis

G **Precautions:** Elderly, respiratory depression, increased intracranial pressure, seizure disorders, severe respiratory disorders, cardiac dysrhythmias, pregnancy **C**

Pharmacokinetics

Absorption	Well absorbed (IM), completely absorbed (IV)
Distribution	Unknown, crosses placenta
Metabolism	Extensively—liver, 80% bound to plasma proteins
Excretion	Kidneys—up to 25% unchanged, breast milk
Half-life	2½-4 hr

Pharmacodynamics

	IM	IV
Onset	7-15 min	Rapid
Peak	30 min	3-5 min
Duration	1-2 hr	½-1 hr

Interactions

Drug/drug:

Individual drugs

Alcohol: ↑ respiratory depression, hypotension, ↑ sedation
Cimetidine: ↑ recovery
Erythromycin: ↑ recovery
Nalbuphine: ↓ analgesia
Pentazocine: ↓ analgesia

Drug classifications

Antihistamines: ↑ respiratory depression, hypotension
CNS depressants: ↑ respiratory depression, hypotension
MAOI: Do not use 2 wk before fentanyl
Phenothiazines: ↑ respiratory depression, hypotension
Sedative/hypnotics: ↑ respiratory depression, hypotension

Lab test interferences

Increase: Amylase, lipase

NURSING CONSIDERATIONS

Assessment

- Monitor vital signs after parenteral route (B/P, pulse, respiration); note muscle rigidity; take drug history before administering drug; check liver, kidney function tests; assess for respiratory dysfunction: respiratory depression, character, rate, rhythm; notify prescriber if respirations are <10/min
- Monitor CNS changes: dizziness, drowsiness, hallucinations, euphoria, LOC, pupil reaction
- Monitor allergic reactions: rash, urticaria; drug should be discontinued
- Assess for pain: intensity, location, duration, type, before and 15 min after IM route or 3-5 min after **IV** route

Associated nursing diagnoses

- ✓ Pain (uses)
- ✓ Sensory-perceptual alteration: visual, auditory (adverse reactions)
- ✓ Breathing pattern, ineffective (adverse reactions)
- ✓ Knowledge deficit (teaching)

Implementation

- Give by inj (IM, **IV**), only with resuscitative equipment available; give slowly to prevent rigidity
- Give **IV** undiluted by anesthesiologist or diluted with 5 ml or more sterile water or 0.9% NcCl given through Y-tube or 3-way stopcock given at 0.1 mg or less/1.2 min
- Store in light-resistant area at room temp

Syringe compatibilities:

Atropine, butorphanol, chlorpromazine, cimetidine, dimenhydrinate, diphenhydramine, droperidol, heparin, hydromorphone, hydroxyzine, meperidine, metoclopramide, midazolam, morphine, pentazocine, perphenazine, prochlorperazine edisylate, promazine, promethazine, ranitidine, scopolamine

Syringe incompatibility:

Pentobarbital

Y-site compatibilities:

Atracurium, enalaprilat, esmool, heparin, hydrocortisone sodium succinate, labetalol, nafcillin, pancuronium, potassium chloride, vecuronium

Additive compatibility:

Bupivacaine

Additive incompatibilities:

Methohexital, pentobarbital, thiopental

Solution compatibilities:

D_5W, 0.9% NaCl

Patient/family education

- Advise patient to report any symptoms of CNS changes, allergic reactions
- Instruct patient to avoid CNS depressants: alcohol, sedative/hypnotics for at least 24 hr after taking this drug
- Teach with patient that dizziness, drowsiness, confu-

F

sion are common, and to avoid getting up without assistance
- Discuss in detail with patient all aspects of the drug

Evaluation

Positive therapeutic outcome
- Maintenance of anesthesia
- Decreased pain

Treatment of overdose: Narcan 0.2-0.8 **IV**, O_2, **IV** fluids, vasopressors

fentanyl transdermal

(fen'ta-nill)

Duragesic-25, Duragesic-50, Duragesic-75, Duragesic-100

Func. class.: Narcotic, analgesic

Chem. class.: Opiate, synthetic phenylpiperidine

Pregnancy category **C**

Controlled substance schedule **II**

Action: Inhibits ascending pain pathways in CNS, increases pain threshold, alters pain perception by binding to opiate receptors

Therapeutic Outcome: Relief of chronic pain

Uses: Management of chronic pain for those requiring opioid analgesia

Dosage and routes

Adult: 25 μg/hr; may increase until pain relief occurs; apply patch to flat surface on upper torso and wear for 72 hr; apply new patch on different site for continued relief

Available forms: Patch 2.5, 5, 7.5, 10 mg

Side effects/adverse reactions

CNS: Dizziness, delirium, euphoria, light-headedness, sedation, dysphoria, agitation, anxiety
CV: Bradycardia, ***cardiac arrest***, hypotension or hypertension, facial flushing, chills
EENT: Blurred vision, miosis
GI: Nausea, vomiting, diarrhea, cramps
RESP: ***Respiratory depression, laryngospasm, bronchospasm;*** depresses cough; hypoventilation

Contraindications: Hypersensitivity to opiates, myasthenia gravis

G **Precautions:** Elderly, respiratory depression, increased intracranial pressure, seizure disorders, severe respiratory disorders, cardiac dysrhythmias, pregnancy **C**, fever

Pharmacokinetics

Absorption	92% (skin), continuously for 72 hr
Distribution	Crosses placenta
Metabolism	Extensively—liver
Excretion	Up to 25%—kidneys unchanged
Half-life	17 hr after removal of patch

Pharmacodynamics

	TD
Onset	6 hr
Peak	12-24 hr
Duration	72 hr

Interactions

Drug/drug:

Individual drugs

Alcohol: ↑ respiratory depression, hypotension, ↑ sedation
Cimetidine: ↑ recovery
Erythromycin: ↑ recovery
Nalbuphine: ↓ analgesia
Pentazocine: ↓ analgesia

Drug classifications

Antihistamines: ↑ respiratory depression, hypotension
CNS depressants: ↑ respiratory depression, hypotension
MAOI: Do not use 2 wk before fentanyl
Phenothiazines: ↑ respiratory depression, hypotension
Sedative/hypnotics: ↑ respiratory depression, hypotension

Lab test interferences

Increase: Amylase, lipase

NURSING CONSIDERATIONS

Assessment

- Assess for respiratory dysfunction: respiratory depression, character, rate, rhythm; notify prescriber if respirations are <10/min
- Monitor CNS changes: dizziness, drowsiness, hallucinations, euphoria, LOC, pupil reaction
- Monitor allergic reactions: rash, urticaria; drug should be discontinued
- Assess for pain: intensity, location, duration, type—before and after administration

Associated nursing diagnoses

- ✓ Pain (uses)
- ✓ Sensory-perceptual alteration: visual, auditory (adverse reactions)
- ✓ Breathing pattern, ineffective (adverse reactions)
- ✓ Knowledge deficit (teaching)

F

Implementation

Trans route

- Narcotic analgesics should be used to control pain until relief is obtained with transdermal patch. Patients may continue to require other narcotics for breakthrough pain. If >100 μg/hr is required, use multiple systems
- Apply patch to chest on a flat area with skin intact. For skin preparation, use clear water with no soap; clip hair, skin should be dry before applying patch. Apply immediately after removing from package and press firmly in place with palm of hand. Flush old patch down toilet immediately upon removal.

Use pain dosing

- Dosage is titrated based on patient's report of pain; dosage is determined by calculating the previous 24-hr requirement and converting to equianalgesic morphone dose
- To convert to another narcotic analgesic, remove transdermal patch and begin treatment with half the equal pain controlling dose of the new analgesic in 12-18 hr
- Medication should be tapered gradually after long-term use to prevent withdrawal symptoms

Patient/family education

- Advise patient to report any symptoms of CNS changes, allergic reactions
- Instruct patients to avoid CNS depressants: alcohol, sedative/hypnotics for at least 24 hr after this drug
- Discuss with patient that dizziness, drowsiness, and confusion are common and to avoid getting up without assistance
- Discuss all aspects of the drug in detail

Evaluation

Positive therapeutic outcome

- Decreased pain

Treatment of overdose:

Narcan 0.2-0.8 **IV**, O2, **IV** fluids, vasopressors

ferrous fumarate/ ferrous gluconate/ ferrous sulfate

(fer'us)

Femiron, Feostat, Ferrets, Ferrous Fumarate, Fumasorb, Fumerin, Hemocyte, Ircon, Nephro-Fer, Span-FF, Fergon, Ferralet, Ferralet S.R., ferrous gluconate, Simron, Feosol, Feratab, Fer-In-Sol, Fer-Iron, Fero-Gradumet, Ferospace, Ferralyn, Ferra-TD, ferrous sulfate, Mol-Iron, Slow-Fe

Func. class.: Hematinic

Chem. class.: Iron preparation

Pregnancy category A

Action: Replaces iron stores needed for red blood cell development, energy and O_2 transport, utilization; fumarate contains 33% elemental iron; gluconate, 12%; sulfate, 20%; iron, 30%; ferrous sulfate exsiccated

➡ **Therapeutic Outcome:** Prevention and correction of iron deficiency

Uses: Iron deficiency anemia, prophylaxis for iron deficiency in pregnancy

Dosage and routes

Fumarate

Adult: PO 200 mg tid-qid

P ***Child 2-12 yr:*** PO 3 mg/kg/day (elemental iron) tid-qid

P *Child 6 mo-2 yr:* PO up to 6 mg/kg/day (elemental iron) tid-qid

P *Child 6 mo-2 yr:* PO 6 mg/kg/day in 3-4 divided doses

P *Infants:* PO 10-25 mg/day (elemental iron) in 3-4 divided doses

Gluconate

Adult: PO 200-600 mg tid

P *Child 6-12 yr:* PO 300-900 mg qd

P *Child <6 yr:* PO 100-300 mg-qd

Sulfate

Adult: PO 0.750-1.5 g/day in divided doses tid

P *Child 6-12 yr:* 600 mg/day in divided doses

Pregnancy

Adult: PO 300-600 mg/day in divided doses

Available forms:

Fumarate:

Tab 63, 195, 200, 324, 325 mg; tab chewable 100 mg; tab controlled-release 300 mg; oral susp 100 mg/5 ml, 45 mg/0.6 ml

Gluconate:

Tab 300, 320, 325, mg; cap 86, 325, 435 mg; tab film-coated 300 mg; elix 300 mg/5 ml

Sulfate:

Tab 195, 300, 325, mg; tab enteric-coated 325 mg; tab extended-release, time-release cap 525 mg

Side effects/adverse reactions

GI: *Nausea, constipation, epigastric pain, black and red tarry stools,* vomiting, diarrhea

INTEG: Temporarily discolored tooth enamel and eyes

Contraindications: Hypersensitivity, ulcerative colitis/regional enteritis, hemosiderosis/hemochromatosis, peptic ulcer disease, hemolytic anemia, cirrhosis

Precautions: Anemia (long-term), pregnancy **A**

Pharmacokinetics

Absorption	Up to 30%
Distribution	Bound to transferrin, crosses placenta
Metabolism	Recycled
Excretion	Feces, urine, skin, breast milk
Half-life	Unknown

Pharmacodynamics

	PO
Onset	Unknown
Peak	Unknown
Duration	Unknown

Interactions

Drug/drug:

Individual drugs

Chloramphenicol: ↑ absorption of iron products

Levodopa: ↓ absorption of levodopa

Methyldopa: ↓ absorption of methyldopa

Penicillamine: ↓ absorption of penicillamine

Quinolone: ↓ absorption of quinolone

Tetracycline: ↓ absorption of iron products
Vitamin C: ↑ absorption of iron products

Lab test interferences

False-positive: Occult blood

NURSING CONSIDERATIONS

Assessment

- Monitor blood studies: Hct, Hgb, reticulocytes, bilirubin before treatment, at least monthly
- Assess for toxicity: nausea, vomiting, diarrhea (green, then tarry stools,) hematemesis, pallor, cyanosis, shock, coma
- Assess bowel elimination; if constipation occurs, increase water, bulk, activity before laxatives are required
- Assess nutrition: amount of iron in diet (meat, dark green leafy vegetables, dried beans, dried fruits, eggs); provide referral to dietician if indicated
- Identify cause of iron loss or anemia, including salicylates, sulfonamides, antimalarials, quinidine

Associated nursing diagnoses

✓ Nutrition, less than body requirements (uses)
✓ Fatigue (uses)
✓ Knowledge deficit (teaching)

Implementation

PO route

- Give only with Vit E supplements to infants or hemolytic anemia may occur [P]
- Give between meals for best absorption; may give with juice; do not give with antacids or milk, delay at least 1 hr; if GI symptoms occur, give PC even if absorption is decreased; eggs, milk products, chocolate, caffeine interfere with absorption
- Give liq preparations through plastic straw to avoid discoloration of tooth enamel; dilute thoroughly
- Give at least 1 hr before bedtime because corrosion may occur in stomach
- Give for <6 mo for anemia
- Store in air-tight, light-resistant container

Patient/family education

- Advise patient that iron will make stools black or dark green; that iron poisoning may occur if increased beyond recommended level
- Tell patient not to crush; swallow tab whole; to keep out of reach of children [P]
- Caution patient not to substitute one iron salt for another; elemental iron content differs (e.g., 300 mg ferrous fumarate contains about 100 mg elemental iron, whereas 300 mg ferrous gluconate contains only about 30 mg elemental iron)
- Caution patient to avoid reclining position for 15-30 min after taking drug to avoid esophageal corrosion; to follow diet high in iron

Evaluation

Positive therapeutic outcome

- Decreased fatigue, weakness
- Improvement in Hct, Hgb, reticulocytes

Treatment of overdose:

Induce vomiting; give eggs, milk until lavage can be done

fibrinolysin/ desoxyribonuclease

(fye-brin-oe-lye'sin/dez-ox-ee-rye-boe-nuke'lee-ase)

Elase

Func. class.: Enzyme

Chem. class.: Proteolytic-bovine

Pregnancy category **C**

Action: Dissolves fibrin in clots and fibrinous exudates, attacks DNA in areas of disintegrating cells

Therapeutic Outcome: A clean wound

Uses: Debridement of wounds, vaginitis, cervicitis, ulcerative colitis, 2nd-, 3rd-degree burns; irrigating wounds, topically

Dosage and routes

Debridement/intravaginally

Adult: Oint 5 g × 5 applications

Irrigating

Adult: IRRIG dilution depends on type of wound

Available forms: Fibrinolysin with desoxyribonuclease 666.6 U/g; powder for reconstitution fibrinolysin 25 U/desoxyribonuclease 15,000 U

Side effects/adverse reactions

INTEG: Hyperemia

Contraindications: Hypersensitivity to bovine or mercury products, hematoma

Precautions: Pregnancy **C**

Pharmacokinetics

Absorption	Not absorbed
Distribution	Unknown
Metabolism	Unknown
Excretion	Unknown
Half-life	Unknown

Pharmacodynamics

	TOP
Onset	Unknown
Peak	Unknown
Duration	Unknown

Interactions: None

NURSING CONSIDERATIONS

Assessment

- Assess for signs of irritation and inflammation around wound; drug should be discontinued
- Assess wound for drainage, color, odor, size, depth before and during therapy

Associated nursing diagnoses

- ✓ Skin integrity, altered (uses)
- ✓ Knowledge deficit (teaching)

Implementation

Top route

- Apply after reconstituting top sol with 10-50 ml sterile NaCl sol; use only fresh sol; reconstituted sol is stable for 24 hr; remove necrotic debris, dry eschar
- Saturate gauze with sol; pack area; remove in 6-8 hr and clean; repeat tid-qid
- Apply top oint after flushing wound with saline, water or hydrogen peroxide, let dry or pat dry, then apply a small

amount of oint to area and cover with a nonadhesive dressing; change qd or bid

Vag route

• Place 5 ml in applicator, apply with patient recumbent

Patient/family education

• Teach patient reason for treatment and expected results

Evaluation

Positive therapeutic outcome

• Decrease in wound scarring, tissue necrosis

filgrastim

(fill-gras'stim)

Neupogen

Func. class.: Biologic modifier

Chem. class.: Granulocyte colony-stimulating factor

Pregnancy category **C**

Action: Stimulates proliferation and differentiation of neutrophils; a glycoprotein

Therapeutic Outcome: Absence of infection

Uses: To decrease infection in patients receiving antineoplastics that are myelosuppressive; to increase WBC in patients with drug-induced neutropenia

Dosage and routes

Adult: **IV**/SC 5 μg/kg/day in a single dose; may increase by 5 μg/kg in each chemotherapy cycle; give qd for up to 2 wk until the absolute neutrophil count (ANC) has reached 10,000/mm^3; response to G-CSF is much greater with SC than **IV** therapy

Available forms: Inj 300 μg/ml

Side effects/adverse reactions

CNS: Fever

GI: Nausea, vomiting, diarrhea, mucositis, anorexia

HEMA: ***Thrombocytopenia***

INTEG: Alopecia, exacerbation of skin conditions

MS: Osteoporosis, skeletal pain

RESP: ***Respiratory distress syndrome***

Contraindications: Hypersensitivity to proteins of *E. coli*

Precautions: Pregnancy **C**, lactation, cardiac conditions, P children, myeloid malignancies

Pharmacokinetics

Absorption	Well absorbed (SC), completely absorbed (IV)
Distribution	Unknown
Metabolism	Unknown
Excretion	Unknown
Half-life	Unknown

Pharmacodynamics

	IV/SC
Onset	Unknown
Peak	Unknown
Duration	Unknown

Interactions

Drug/drug:

Drug classifications

Antineoplastics: ↑ neutrophils, do not use together 24

hr before or after antineoplastics

Lab test interferences

Increase: Uric acid, lactate dehydrogenase, alk phosphatase

NURSING CONSIDERATIONS

Assessment

- Monitor blood studies: CBC, platelet count before treatment and twice weekly; neutrophil counts (ANC) may be increased for 2 days after therapy, but treatment should continue until ANC >10,000/mm^3
- Assess for bone pain: frequency, intensity, duration; analgesics may be given; opiates should not be used
- Check B/P, heart rate, respiration, baseline and during treatment

Associated nursing diagnoses

✓ Infection, risk for (uses)
✓ Pain, acute (adverse reaction)
✓ Knowledge deficit (teaching)

Implementation

IV **IV route**

- Give 300 µg/ml or 480 µg/1.6 ml; allow to warm to room temp; give single dose over 1 min or less through Y-tube or medport
- Use single-use vials; after dose is withdrawn, do not reenter vial
- Give for 2 wk or until ANC is 10,000/mm^3 after the expected chemotherapy neutrophil nadir
- Store in refrigerator; do not freeze; may store at room temp for up to 6 hr; avoid shaking

Patient/family education

- Teach patient technique for self-administration: dose, side effects, disposal of containers and needles; provide instruction sheet

Evaluation

Positive therapeutic outcome
- Absence of infection

F

finasteride

(fin-ass'te-ride)

Proscar

Func. class.: Androgen hormone inhibitor

Chem. class.: 5-α-reductase inhibitor

Pregnancy category X

Action: Inhibits 5-α-reductase and reduction in DHT; DHT induces androgenic effects by binding to androgen receptors in the cell nuclei of the prostate gland, liver, skin; produces lower levels of 5-α-reductase, which prevents development of benign prostatic hypertrophy (BPH)

➔ Therapeutic Outcome: Reduced prostate size

Uses: Symptomatic benign prostatic hyperplasia

Dosage and routes

Adult: PO 5 mg qd × 6-12 mo

Available forms: Tab 5 mg

Side effects/adverse reactions

GU: Impotence, decreased libido, decreased volume of ejaculate

Contraindications: Hypersensitivity, pregnancy **X**, P children, women

Precautions: Large residual urinary volume, severely diminished urinary flow, liver function abnormalities

Pharmacokinetics

Absorption	PO (63%)
Distribution	Plasma protein binding, crosses blood-brain barrier
Metabolism	Liver
Excretion	Kidneys—metabolites (39%), feces (57%)
Half-life	6-15 hr

Pharmacodynamics

	PO
Onset	Immediate
Peak	8 hr
Duration	14 days

Interactions

Drug/drug:

Anticholinergics: ↓ effect of finasteride
Bronchodilators, adrenergic: ↓ effect of finasteride
Theophylline: ↓ effect of finasteride

NURSING CONSIDERATIONS

Assessment

- Assess urinary patterns, residual urinary volume, severely diminished urinary flow; PSA levels and digital rectal exam before initiating therapy and periodically thereafter
- Monitor liver function studies before initiating treatment; extensively metabolized in liver

Associated nursing diagnoses

✓ Urinary elimination, altered (uses)
✓ Knowledge deficit (teaching)

Implementation

PO route

- Administer without regard to meals
- Store at temp <86° F (30° C); protect from light; keep container tightly closed

Patient/family education

- Advise patient that pregnant women should not touch crushed tab or come into contact with semen of a patient taking this drug; may adversely affect development of male fetus
- Inform patient that volume of ejaculate may be decreased during treatment; impotence and decreased libido may also occur

Evaluation

Positive therapeutic outcome

- Decreased postvoiding dribbling, frequency, nocturia
- Increased urinary flow

flecainide

(flek'a-nide)

Tambocor

Func. class.: Antidysrhythmic (Class IC)

Pregnancy category **C**

Action: Decreases conduction in all parts of the heart, with greatest effect on the His-Purkinje system, which stabilizes the cardiac membrane

Therapeutic Outcome: Absence of dysrhythmias

Uses: Life-threatening ventricular dysrhythmias, sustained ventricular tachycardia; supraventricular tachydysrhythmias

Dosage and routes

Adult: PO 50-100 mg q12h; may increase every 4 days by 50 mg q12h to desired response, not to exceed 400 mg/day

Available forms: Tab 50, 100, 150 mg

Side effects/adverse reactions

CNS: Headache, dizziness, involuntary movement, confusion, psychosis, restlessness, irritability, paresthesias, ataxia, flushing, somnolence, depression, anxiety, malaise

CV: Hypotension, bradycardia, angina, PVCs, ***heart block, cardiovascular collapse, arrest,*** *dysrhythmias,* ***CHF, fatal ventricular tachycardia***

EENT: Tinnitus, *blurred vision,* hearing loss

GI: Nausea, vomiting, anorexia, constipation, abdominal pain, flatulence, change in taste

GU: Impotence, decreased libido, polyuria, urinary retention

HEMA: Leukopenia, thrombocytopenia

INTEG: Rash, urticaria, edema, swelling

RESP: Dyspnea, ***respiratory depression***

Contraindications: Hypersensitivity, severe heart block, cardiogenic shock, nonsustained ventricular dysrhythmias, frequent PVCs, non–life-threatening dysrhythmias

Precautions: Pregnancy **C**, lactation, children, renal disease, liver disease, CHF, respiratory depression, myasthenia gravis

Pharmacokinetics

Absorption	Well absorbed (PO)
Distribution	Widely distributed
Metabolism	Liver
Excretion	30% kidneys, unchanged
Half-life	14 hr

Pharmacodynamics

	PO
Onset	Unknown
Peak	3 hr
Duration	Unknown

Interactions

Drug/drug:

Individual drugs

Amiodarone: ↑ blood levels, ↑ toxicity

Digoxin: ↑ blood levels, ↑ toxicity
Disopyramide: ↑ levels, ↑ toxicity
Flecainide: ↑ levels, ↑ toxicity
Lidocaine: Bradycardia, arrest
Mexiletine: ↑ levels, ↑ toxicity
Phenytoin: ↑ blood levels
Procainamide: ↑ levels, ↑ toxicity
Quinidine: ↑ levels, ↑ toxicity
Warfarin: ↑ level, ↑ bleeding

Drug classifications
Beta blockers: ↑ dysrhythmias, arrest
Calcium channel blockers: ↑ dysrhythmias, arrest

NURSING CONSIDERATIONS

Assessment

- Monitor ECG continuously to determine drug effectiveness; measure PR, QRS, QT intervals; check for PVCs, other dysrhythmias; monitor B/P continuously for hypotension, hypertension and rebound hypertension (after 1-2 hr); check for dehydration or hypovolemia
- Monitor I&O ratio; electrolytes: [K (potassium), Na (sodium)], Cl (chloride); check weight daily and for signs of CHG or pulmonary toxicity: dyspnea, fatigue, cough, fever, chest pain; if these occur, drug should be discontinued
- Monitor liver function studies: AST (SGOT), ALT (SGPT), bilirubin, alk phosphatase
- Assess patient for CNS symptoms: confusion, psychosis, numbness, depression, involuntary movements; if these occur, drug should be discontinued
- Assess patient for hyperthyroidism: lethargy, dizziness, constipation, enlarged thyroid gland, edema of extremities, cool, pale skin; assess patient for hyperthyroidism: restlessness; tachycardia; eyelid puffiness; weight loss; frequent urination; menstrual irregularities; dyspnea; warm, moist skin
- Monitor cardiac rate, respiration: rate, rhythm, character, chest pain; watch for ventricular tachycardia, supraventricular tachycardia, or fibrillation

Associated nursing diagnoses

✓ Cardiac output, decreased (uses)
✓ Knowledge deficit (teaching)

Implementation

PO route

- Give reduced dosage slowly with ECG monitoring; do not increase dose fewer than 4 days apart
- Give with meals if GI upset occurs

Patient/family education

- Instruct patient to report side effects immediately to health care provider
- Instruct patient to complete follow-up appointment with health care provider including pulmonary function studies, chest x-ray

Evaluation

Positive therapeutic outcome

- Absence of dysrythmias

floxuridine

(flox-yoor′i-deen)

floxuridine, FUDR

Func. class.: Antineoplastic, antimetabolite

Chem. class.: Pyrimidine antagonist

Pregnancy category **D**

Action: Inhibits DNA synthesis; interferes with cell replication by competitively inhibiting thymidylate synthesis S phase of cell cycle

➔ Therapeutic Outcome: Prevention of rapidly growing malignant cells

Uses: GI adenocarcinoma metastatic to liver; cancer of breast, head, neck, liver, brain, gallbladder, bile duct

Dosage and routes

Adult: INTRAARTERIAL by continuous inf 0.1-0.6 mg/kg/day × 1-6 wk; HEPATIC ARTERY INJ 0.4-0.6 mg/kg/day × 1-6 wk

Available forms: Powder for inj 500 mg/5 ml vial

Side effects/adverse reactions

CNS: Lethargy, malaise, weakness

EENT: Epistaxis

GI: *Anorexia*, diarrhea, nausea, vomiting, ***hemorrhage***, stomatitis

GU: ***Renal failure***

HEMA: ***Thrombocytopenia, leukopenia, myelosuppression, anemia***

INTEG: *Rash*, fever, alopecia

Contraindications: Hypersensitivity, myelosuppression, pregnancy **D**, poor nutritional status, serious infections

Precautions: Renal disease, hepatic disease, bone marrow depression

Pharmacokinetics

Absorption	Direct to tumor
Distribution	To tumor, crosses blood-brain barrier
Metabolism	Liver
Excretion	60%-80% lungs, kidneys (small)
Half-life	Initial 10-20 min, 20 hr terminal

Pharmacodynamics

	IA
Onset	1 wk
Peak	1-3 wk
Duration	4 wk

Interactions

Drug/drug:

Individual drugs

Radiation: ↑ toxicity, bone marrow suppression

Drug classifications

Antineoplastics: ↑ toxicity bone marrow suppression

Live virus vaccine: ↑ adverse reactions

Lab test interferences

Increase: Liver function studies

NURSING CONSIDERATIONS

Assessment

- Assess buccal cavity q8h for dryness, sores or ulceration,

white patches, oral pain, bleeding, dysphagia; obtain prescription for viscous lidocaine (Xylocaine)
- Monitor CBC, differential, platelet count weekly; withhold drug if WBC count is <4000/mm^3 or platelet count is <100,000/mm^3; notify prescriber of results if WBC <20,000/mm^3, platelets <50,000/mm^3
- Monitor renal function studies: BUN, creatinine, serum uric acid, urine CrCl before and during therapy; I&O ratio; report fall in urine output to <30 ml/hr
- Monitor temp q4h (may indicate beginning of infection)
- Monitor liver function tests before and during therapy (bilirubin, AST (SGOT), ALT (SGPT), LDH) as needed or monthly
- Assess for bleeding: hematuria, stool guaiac, bruising or petechiae, mucosa or orifices q8h; inflammation of mucosa, breaks in skin
- Identify effects of alopecia on body image; discuss feelings about body changes

Associated nursing diagnoses

- ✓ Injury, risk for (adverse reactions)
- ✓ Body image disturbance (adverse reactions)
- ✓ Infection, risk for (adverse reactions)
- ✓ Knowledge deficit (teaching)

Implementation

- Avoid contact with skin, very irritating, wash completely to remove
- Give fluids **IV** or PO before chemotherapy to hydrate patient
- Give antiemetic 30-60 min before giving drug to prevent vomiting, and prn; administer antibiotics for prophylaxis of infection
- Give top or syst analgesics for pain
- Give in AM so drug can be eliminated before hs
- Provide liq diet: carbonated beverages; gelatin may be added if patient is not nauseated or vomiting
- Recommend that patient rinse mouth tid-qid with water, club soda; brushing of teeth bid-qid with soft brush or cotton-tipped applicators for stomatitis; use unwaxed dental floss

IA route

- Give by intraarterial inf pump after diluting 5 ml drug/5 ml sterile H_2O for inj; dilute further with D_5W or normal saline to required dilution; stable if refrigerated for 14 days.

Additive compatibilites:

Carboplatin, cisplatin, cisplatin with etoposide, cisplatin with leucovorin, etoposide, fluorouracil, fluorouracil with leucovorin, leucovorin

Y-site compatibilities:

Fludarabine, melphalan, ondansetron, sargramostim, paclitaxel, vinorelbine

Patient/family education

- Tell patient that contraceptive measures are recommended during therapy

• Teach patient to avoid use of products containing aspirin or ibuprofen, razors, commercial mouthwash because bleeding may occur; to report symptoms of bleeding (hematuria, tarry stools), irritability, faintness, shortness of breath
• Caution patient that hair loss may occur during treatment; a wig or hairpiece may make patient feel better; new hair may be different in color, texture
• Instruct patient not to have any vaccinations without the advice of the prescriber—serious reactions can occur

Evaluation

Positive therapeutic outcome
• Prevention of rapid division of malignant cells

fluconazole

(floo-kon′a-zole)
Diflucan
Func. class.: Antifungal
Pregnancy category **B**

Action: Inhibits ergosterol biosynthesis, causes direct damage to membrane phospholipids in the cell wall of fungi

Therapeutic Outcome: Fungistatic fungicidal against the following susceptible organisms: ***Candida, Crytococcus neoforms***

Uses: Oropharyngeal esophageal candidiasis in AIDS patients, chronic mucocutaneous candidiasis, urinary candidiasis, cryptococcal meningitis, peritonitis

Dosage and routes

Vaginal candidiasis
Adult: PO 150 mg as a single dose

Serious fungal infections
Adult: PO/**IV** 50-400 mg initially, then 200 mg once daily for 4 wk

Oropharyngeal candidiasis in AIDS patients
Adult: PO 200 mg initially, then 100 mg daily for at least 2 wk

Available forms: Tab 50, 100, 200 mg, inj 200, 400 mg

Side effects/adverse reactions

CNS: Headache
GI: Nausea, vomiting, diarrhea, cramping, flatus, increased AST (SGOT), ALT (SGPT), ***hepatotoxicity***
INTEG: Stevens-Johnson syndrome

Contraindications: Hypersensitivity

Precautions: Renal disease, pregnancy **B**

Pharmacokinetics

Absorption	Well absorbed (PO)
Distribution	Widely distributed (peritoneum, cerebrospinal fluid)
Metabolism	<10%—liver
Excretion	>90% kidneys (unchanged)
Half-life	30 hr, increased in renal disease

Pharmacodynamics

	PO	IV
Onset	Unknown	Immediate
Peak	1-2 hr	Infusion's end
Duration	Unknown	Unknown

Interactions

Drug/drug:

Individual drugs

Warfarin: ↑ anticoagulation

Drug classification

Cyclosporines: ↑ renal dysfunction

NURSING CONSIDERATIONS

Assessment

- Assess for signs and symptoms of infection
- Obtain cultures for C&S before beginning treatment; therapy may be started after culture is taken
- Monitor for renal toxicity: increasing BUN, serum creatinine; if BUN is >40 mg/dl or if serum creatinine is >3 mg/dl, drug may be discontinued or dosage reduced
- Monitor for hepatotoxicity: increased AST (SGOT), ALT (SGPT), alk phosphatase, bilirubin; drug will be discontinued if hepatotoxicity occurs

Associated nursing diagnoses

✓ Infection, risk for (uses)
✓ Injury, risk for (adverse reactions)
✓ Knowledge deficit (teaching)

Implementation

IV route

- Give after diluting according to package directions; run at 200 mg/hr or less; do not use plastic containers in connections
- Do not admix
- Administer **IV** using an in-line filter, using distal veins; check for extravasation and necrosis q2h
- Give drug only after C&S confirms organism, drug needed to treat condition
- Store protected from moisture and light, diluted sol is stable for 24 hr

Y-*site compatibilities:*

Acyclovir, amikacin, aminophylline, ampicillin/sulbactam, aztreonam, benztropine, cefazolin, cefotetan, cefoxitin, chlorpromazine, cimetidine, dexamethasone sodium phosphate, diphenhydramine, droperidol, famotidine, fludarabine, foscarnet, ganciclovir, gentamicin, heparin, hydrocortisone, immune globulin, leucovorin, meperidine, metoclopramide, metronidazole, midazolam, morphine, nafcillin, ondansetron, oxacillin, penicillin G, potassium, phenytoin, prochlorperazine, promethazine, sargramostim, ticarcillin/clavulanate, tobramycin, vancomycin, zidovudine

Y-*site incompatibilities:*

Amphotericin B, ampicillin, calcium gluconate, cefotaxime, ceftriaxone, ceftazidime, cefuroxime, chloramphenicol, clindamycin, diazepam, digoxin, erythromycin lactobionate, furosemide, haloperidol, hydroxyzine, imipenem/cilastatin, pentamidine, ticarcillin, trimethoprim/sulfamethoxazole

Patient/family education

- Caution patient that long-term therapy may be needed to clear infection; to take entire course of medication; take in equal intervals (PO)
- Teach patient the signs and symptoms of hepatotoxicity: nausea, vomiting, clay-colored stools, dark urine, anorexia, fatigue, jaundice—health care prescriber should be notified immediately

Evaluation

Positive therapeutic outcome

- Decreasing oral candidiasis, fever, malaise, rash
- Negative C&S for infecting organism

flucytosine

(floo-sye'toe-seen)

Ancobon, Ancotil ✦, 5-FC

Func. class.: Antifungal

Chem. class.: Pyrimidine (fluorinated)

Pregnancy category **C**

Action: Converted to fluorouracil after entering fungi; inhibits RNA, DNA synthesis; synergism action when used with amphotericin B in some infections

➡ **Therapeutic Outcome:** Fungicidal against the following susceptible organisms: ***Candida, cryptococcus***

Uses: ***Candida*** infections (septicemia, endocarditis, pulmonary, urinary tract infections), *Cryptococcus* (meningitis, pulmonary, urinary tract infections)

Dosage and routes

P *Adult and child >50 kg:* PO 50-150 mg/kg/day q6h

P *Adult and child <50 kg:* PO 1.5-4.5 g/m^2/day in 4 divided doses

Available forms: Cap 250, 500 mg

Side effects/adverse reactions

CNS: Headache, confusion, dizziness, sedation, vertigo

GI: *Nausea, vomiting, anorexia,* diarrhea, abdominal distention, cramps, enterocolitis, increased AST (SGOT), ALT (SGPT), alk phosphatase, ***bowel perforation*** (rare)

GU: Increased BUN, creatinine

HEMA: ***Thrombocytopenia, agranulocytosis, anemia, leukopenia, pancytopenia***

INTEG: Rash

Contraindications: Hypersensitivity

Precautions: Renal disease, impaired hepatic function, bone marrow depression, blood dyscrasias, radiation/chemotherapy, pregnancy **C**

Pharmacokinetics

Absorption	Well absorbed (PO)
Distribution	Widely distributed, crosses blood-brain barrier, crosses placenta
Metabolism	Unknown
Excretion	90% kidneys—unchanged
Half-life	3-6 hr, increased in renal disease

Pharmacodynamics

	PO
Onset	Rapid
Peak	2½-6 hr
Duration	6 hr

Interactions

Drug/drug:

Individual drugs

Amphotericin B: ↑ toxicity

Cytarabine: ↓ antifungal action

Drug classifications

Antineoplastics: ↑ bone marrow depression

Radiation: ↑ bone marrow depression

Lab test interferences

False increase: Creatinine

NURSING CONSIDERATIONS

Assessment

• Assess patient for signs and symptoms of infection before beginning treatment and during therapy

• Obtain cultures for C&S before initiating treatment; therapy may be started after culture is taken

• Monitor renal toxicity: increasing BUN, serum creatinine; if BUN is >40 mg/dl or if serum creatinine is >3 mg/dl, drug may be discontinued or dosage reduced

• Monitor for hepatotoxicity: increased AST (SGOT), ALT (SGPT), alk phosphatase, bilirubin; drug will be discontinued if hepatotoxicity occurs

Associated nursing diagnoses

✓ Infection, risk for (uses)
✓ Diarrhea (adverse reactions)
✓ Knowledge deficit (teaching)

Implementation

PO route

• Give a few cap at a time to decrease nausea, vomiting over 15 min; store in tight, light-resistant containers at room temp

• Use symptomatic treatment as ordered for adverse reactions: aspirin, antihistamines, antiemetics, antispasmodics

Patient/family education

• Advise patient that medication may cause dizziness, drowsiness, and confusion; to avoid hazardous activities until side effects are determined

• Instruct patient to notify prescriber if rash, fever, sore throat, fatigue, muscle weakness, diarrhea, bruising, bleeding occur

• Caution patient to take medication exactly as prescribed; not to double doses—missed doses should be taken when remembered within 1 hr of next dose

Evaluation

Positive therapeutic outcome

• Decreasing oral candidiasis, fever, malaise, rash

• Negative C&S for infection organism

fludarabine
(floo-dar'a-been)
Fludara
Func. class.: Antineoplastic, antimetabolite
Chem. class.: Vidarabine derivative
Pregnancy category **D**

Action: Competes with physiologic substrate that inhibits DNA synthesis

Therapeutic Outcome: Prevention of rapid growth of malignant cells

Uses: Chronic lymphocytic leukemia; non-Hodgkins lymphoma

Dosage and routes
Adult: **IV** 25 mg/m_2 over 30 min qd × 5 days, may repeat q28 days; reconstitute with 2 ml of sterile water for inj; dissolution should occur in <15 sec

Available forms: Lyophilized powder for reconstitution 50 mg/vial

Side effects/adverse reactions
CNS: Weakness, confusion, headache, depression, sleep disorder, impaired mentation, ***coma,*** peripheral neuropathy
CV: Edema
EENT: Visual disturbances, sinusitis
GI: *Nausea, vomiting, anorexia,* diarrhea, ***hepatotoxicity,*** abdominal pain, hematemesis, ***hemorrhage***
GU: Dysuria, infection
HEMA: Thrombocytopenia, bleeding, ***thrombocytopenia, leukopenia, myelosuppression, anemia***
INTEG: Rash
META: Hyperuricemia, hyperphosphatemia, hypocalcemia, metabolic acidosis, hyperkalemia
RESP: ***Pneumonia,*** dyspnea, cough, interstitial pulmonary infiltrate
SYST: *Fever, chills, malaise, fatigue*

Contraindications: Hypersensitivity, pregnancy **D**

Precautions: Renal disease, hepatic disease, infants

Pharmacokinetics

Absorption	Complete (IV)
Distribution	Unknown
Metabolism	To active metabolite
Excretion	23% kidneys—unchanged
Half-life	Of metabolite 10 hr

Pharmacodynamics

	IV
Onset	Unknown
Peak	Unknown
Duration	Unknown

Interactions
Drug/drug:
Individual drugs
Radiation: ↑ toxicity, bone marrow suppression
Drug classifications
Antineoplastics: ↑ toxicity, bone marrow suppression

Live virus vaccines: ↑ adverse reactions

Lab test interferences

Increase: Liver function studies

NURSING CONSIDERATIONS

Assessment

- Assess buccal cavity q8h for dryness, sores or ulcers, white patches, oral pain, bleeding, dysphagia; obtain prescription for viscous lidocaine (Xylocaine)
- Monitor CBC, differential, platelet count weekly; withhold drug if WBC count is <4000/mm^3 or platelet count is <100,000/mm^3, notify prescriber of results
- Monitor renal function studies: BUN, creatinine, serum uric acid, urine CrCl before and during therapy; I&O ratio; report fall in urine output to <30 ml/hr
- Monitor temp q4h (may indicate beginning of infection)
- Monitor liver function tests before and during therapy [bilirubin, AST (SGOT), ALT (SGPT), LDH] as needed or monthly; yellowing of skin, sclera, dark urine, clay-colored stools, itchy skin, abdominal pain, fever, diarrhea
- Assess for bleeding: hematuria, stool guaiac, bruising or petechiae, mucosa or orifices q8h; inflammation of mucosa, breaks in skin
- Identify patient's food preferences; list likes, dislikes
- Identify effects of alopecia on body image; discuss feelings about body changes
- Identify edema in feet, joint pain, stomach pain, tremors
- Identify inflammation of mucosa, breaks in skin

Associated nursing diagnoses

- ✓ Injury, risk for (adverse reactions)
- ✓ Body image disturbance (adverse reactions)
- ✓ Infection, risk for (adverse reactions)
- ✓ Knowledge deficit (teaching)

Implementation

- Administer fluids **IV** or PO before chemotherapy to hydrate patient
- Give antacid before oral agent, give drug after evening meal, before bedtime; antiemetic 30-60 min before giving drug to prevent vomiting, and prn; antibiotics for prophylaxis of infection
- Give top or syst analgesics for pain
- Give in AM so drug is eliminated before hs
- Put patient on liq diet: carbonated beverages; gelatin may be added if patient is not nauseated or vomiting
- Recommend that patient rinse mouth tid-qid with water, club soda; brush teeth bid-qid with soft brush or cotton-tipped applicators for stomatitis; use unwaxed dental floss

IV **IV route**

- Reconstitute with 2 ml of sterile water for injection; dissolve lyophilized powder; sol is stable for 8 hr
- Give by intermittent inf; dilute further in 100-125 ml of 0.9% NaCl or D_5W give over ½ hr

Y-*site incompatibilities:*

Acyclovir, amphotericin B chlorpromazine, daunorubicin, ganciclovir, hydroxyzine, melphalan, miconazole, prochloperazine, vinorelbine

Patient/family education

- Caution patient that contraceptive measures are recommended during therapy
- Teach patient to avoid aspirin- or ibuprofen-containing products, razors, commercial mouthwash (bleeding may occur); to report symptoms of bleeding (hematuria, tarry stools)
- Instruct patient to report signs of anemia (fatigue, headache, faintness, shortness of breath)
- Caution patient that hair loss may occur during treatment; a wig or hairpiece may make patient feel better; new hair may be different in color, texture

Evaluation

Positive therapeutic outcome

- Prevention of rapid division of malignant cells

fludrocortisone

(floo-droe-kor′ti-sone)

Florinef Acetate

Func. class.: Corticosteroid

Chem. class.: Mineralocorticoid

Pregnancy category C

Action: Promotes increased reabsorption of sodium and loss of potassium, water, hydrogen from the distal renal tubules

Therapeutic Outcome: Treatment of adrenal insufficiency symptoms

Uses: Adrenal insufficiency, salt-losing adrenogenital syndrome

Dosage and routes

Adult: PO 0.1-0.2 mg qd

Available forms: Tab 0.1 mg

Side effects/adverse reactions

CNS: Flushing, sweating, headache

CV: Hypertension, ***circulatory collapse, thrombophlebitis, embolism,*** tachycardia

MS: Fractures, osteoporosis, weakness

Contraindications: Hypersensitivity, acute glomerulonephritis, amebiasis

Precautions: Pregnancy **C**, osteoporosis, CHF

Pharmacokinetics

Absorption	Well absorbed (PO)
Distribution	Widely
Metabolism	Liver
Excretion	Kidneys, breast milk
Half-life	3½ hr

Pharmacodynamics

	PO
Onset	Unknown
Peak	Unknown
Duration	Unknown

Interactions

Drug/drug:

Amphotericin B: ↑ hypokalemia
Mezlocillin: ↑ hypokalemia
Phenobarbital: ↓ effect of fludrocortisone
Piperacillin: ↑ hypokalemia
Rifampin: ↓ effect of fludrocortisone

Drug classifications

Diuretics: ↑ hypokalemia
Nondepolarizing neuromuscular blocking agents: ↑ neuromuscular blockade

Drug/food:

↑ salt/sodium ingestion: ↑ hypokalemia, ↑ hypernatremia

Lab test interferences

Increase: potassium, chloride
Decrease: Hematocrit

NURSING CONSIDERATIONS

Assessment

- Monitor patient for fluid retention: weigh daily, notify prescriber of weekly gain >5 lb; B/P q4h, pulse; notify prescriber if chest pain occurs: I&O ratio; be alert for decreasing urinary output and increasing edema
- Check for potassium depletion: paresthesias, fatigue, nausea, vomiting, depression, polyuria, dysrhythmias, weakness

Associated nursing diagnoses

- ✓ Fluid volume deficit (uses)
- ✓ Fluid volume excess (adverse reactions)
- ✓ Knowledge deficit (teaching)

Implementation

PO route

- Administer titrated dose; use lowest effective dose; scored tab may be broken if lower dose is necessary
- Give with food or milk to decrease GI symptoms

Patient/family education

- Advise patient to carry ID as steroid user at all times during diagnosis and treatment
- Caution patient not to discontinue this medication abruptly—Addisonian crisis may occur
- Counsel patient to follow dietary regimen recommended by prescriber—should include high potassium and, possibly, low sodium
- Advise patient to report weight gain >5 lbs; edema in legs, hands; abdominal cramping; nausea; vomiting, anorexia; dizziness or weakness

Evaluation

Positive therapeutic outcome

- Correction of adrenal insufficiency
- Electrolytes and fluids in normal range

flumazenil
(flu-maz'e-nil)
Mazicon, Ronazicon
Func. class.: Benzodiazepine receptor antagonist
Chem. class.: Imidazobenzodiazepine derivative
Pregnancy category C

Action: Antagonizes the actions of benzodiazepines on the CNS, competitively inhibits the activity at the benzodiazepine receptor complex

➡ **Therapeutic Outcome:** Reversed benzodiazepine toxic effects

Uses: Reversal of the sedative effects of benzodiazepines

Dosage and routes

Reversal of conscious sedation or in general anesthesia

Adult: **IV** 0.2 mg (2 ml) given over 15 sec; wait 45 sec, then give 0.2 mg (2 ml) if consciousness does not occur; may be repeated at 60-sec intervals as needed, up to 4 additional times (max total dose 1 mg); dose is to be individualized

Management of suspected benzodiazepine overdose

Adult: **IV** 0.2 mg (2 ml) given over 30 sec; wait 30 sec, then give 0.3 mg (3 ml) over 30 sec if consciousness does not occur; further doses of 0.5 mg (5 ml) can be given over 30 sec at intervals of 1 min up to cumulative dose of 3 mg

Available forms: Inj 0.1 mg/ml

Side effects/adverse reactions

CNS: Dizziness, agitation, emotional lability, confusion, ***convulsions,*** somnolence
CV: Hypertension, palpitations, cutaneous vasodilation, dysrhythmias, bradycardia, tachycardia, chest pain
EENT: Abnormal vision, blurred vision, tinnitus
GI: Nausea, vomiting, hiccups
SYST: Headache, injection site pain, increased sweating, fatigue, rigors

Contraindications: Hypersensitivity to this drug or benzodiazepines, serous tricyclic antidepressant overdose, patients given benzodiazepine for control of life-threatening condition

Precautions: Pregnancy **C**, P lactation, children, elderly, G renal disease, seizures, head injury, labor and delivery, hepatic disease, hypoventilation, panic disorder, drug and alcohol dependency, ambulatory patients

Pharmacokinetics

Absorption	Complete (IV)
Distribution	Unknown
Metabolism	Liver
Excretion	Unknown
Half-life	41-79 min

F

Pharmacodynamics

	IV
Onset	1 min
Peak	10 min
Duration	Unknown

Interactions: None

NURSING CONSIDERATIONS

Assessment

- Assess cardiac status using continuous monitoring
- Assess for seizures; protect patient from injury
- Assess for GI symptoms: nausea, vomiting; place in side-lying position to prevent aspiration
- Assess for allergic reactions: flushing, rash, urticaria, pruritus

Associated nursing diagnoses

✓ Injury, risk for (uses)
✓ Poisoning (uses)

Implementation

IV **IV route**

- Give directly undiluted or diluted in 0.9% NaCl, D_5W, or LR; give over 15 sec
- Check airway and **IV** access before administration

Patient/family education

- Caution patient that amnesia may continue
- Instruct patient to avoid any hazardous activities for 18-24 hr after discharge
- Inform patient not to take any alcohol or nonprescription drugs for 18-24 hr—serious reactions may occur

Evaluation

Positive therapeutic outcome

- Decreased sedation, respiratory depression
- Absence of toxicity

flunisolide

(floo-nis'oh-lide)
AeroBid, Aero-Bib-M, Nasalide, Rhinalar ✦
Func. class.: Steroid, intranasal
Chem. class.: Glucocorticoid (long-acting)
Pregnancy category **C**

Action: Long-acting synthetic adrenocorticoid with antiinflammatory activity, minimal mineralocorticoid properties, immune-modifying properties

➔ **Therapeutic Outcome:** Absence of running nose and tearing eyes

Uses: Rhinitis (seasonal or perennial), nasal polyps; chronic steroid dependent asthma (Inh)

Dosage and routes

Adult: Instill 2 sprays in each nostril bid, then increase to tid if needed, not to exceed 8 sprays/day in each nostril

P *Child 6-14 yr:* Instill 1 spray in each nostril tid or 2 sprays bid, not to exceed 4 sprays/day in each nostril

P *Adult and child >6 yr:* Spray 2 puffs bid, not to exceed 4 puffs bid

Available forms: Aerosol 25 µg/spray; nasal sol 25 µg/metered dose (Nasalide), 250 µg/metered dose (Aerobid)

Side effects/adverse reactions

CNS: Headache, dizziness
EENT: Nasal irritation, dryness, rebound congestion, epistaxis, sneezing
INTEG: Urticaria
SYST: ***CHF, convulsions,*** increased Na, hypertension

Contraindications: Hypersensitivity, child <12 yr; fungal, bacterial infection of nose

Precautions: Lactation, pregnancy **C**

Pharmacokinetics

Absorption	Nasal (readily absorbed), INH (local absorbed)
Distribution	Unknown
Metabolism	Liver
Excretion	Kidneys
Half-life	6 min, 1.8 hr

Pharmacodynamics

	INH	AERO
Onset	Unknown	2-3 days
Peak	Unknown	2-3 days
Duration	Unknown	Unknown

Interactions: None

NURSING CONSIDERATIONS

Assessment

- Assess patient for infection: increased temp, WBC, even after withdrawal of medication—drug masks symptoms of infection; redness, swelling, pain in nasal passages
- Check nasal passages during long-term treatment for changes in mucus; check for burning, stinging
- Assess patient for glucocorticoid withdrawal: dizziness, hypotension, fatigue, muscle/joint pain—notify prescriber immediately
- Assess patient's respiratory status: rate, rhythm, characteristics; ausculate lungs bilaterally before and during treatment

Associated nursing diagnoses

- ✓ Airway clearance, ineffective (uses)
- ✓ Oral mucous membranes, altered (adverse reactions)
- ✓ Knowledge deficit (teaching)
- ✓ Noncompliance (teaching)

Implementaion

- Use after cleaning aerosol top daily with warm water, dry thoroughly
- Store in cool environment; do not puncture or incinerate container

Patient/family education

- Instruct patient to continue using product even if mild nasal bleeding occurs; this is usually transient
- Teach patient method of installation after providing written instructions from manufacturer
- Teach patient to clear nasal passages before administration; use decongestant if needed; shake inhaler, invert, tilt head backward, insert nozzle into nostril, away from septum; hold other nostril closed and depress activator, inhale

through nose, exhale through mouth

Evaluation

Positive therapeutic outcome
- Decreased congestion, runny nose

fluoride

ACT, Checkmate, Fluor-A-Day ✤, Fluorigard, Fluorinse, Fluoritab, Fluotic ✤, Flura, Flura-Drops, Flura-Loz, Gel II, Gel-Kam, Gel-Tin, Karidium, Karigel, Karigel-N, Listermint with Fluoride, Loz-Tabs, Luride, Luride-SF, Luride Lozi-Tabs, Luride 0.25 Lozi-Tabs, Luride 0.5 Lozi-Tabs, Minute-Gel, Pediaflor, Pharmaflur, Pharmaflur 1.1, Pharmaflur df, Phos-Flur, Point-Two, Prevident, Sodium Fluoride, Stop, Thera-Flur, Thera-Flur-N

Func. class.: Trace elements

Chem. class.: Fluorideion

Pregnancy category D

Action: Needed for hard tooth enamel and for resistance to periodontal disease; reduces acid production by dental bacteria

➔ **Therapeutic Outcome:** Prevention of dental caries in
P children

Uses: Prevention of dental
P caries in children

Dosage and routes

P *Adult and child >12 yr:* Top 10 ml 0.2% sol qd after brushing teeth, rinse mouth for >1 min with sol

P *Child 6-12 yr:* Top 5 ml 0.2% sol

P *Child >3 yr:* PO 1 mg qd

P *Child <3 yr:* PO 0.5 mg

Available forms: Tab chewable 0.25 mg; tab 0.5, 1 mg; tab effervescent 10 mg; gtt 0.125, 0.25, 0.5 mg/ml; rinse supplements 0.2 mg/ml; rinse 0.01%, 0.02%, 0.09%; gel 0.1%, 0.5%, 1.23%

Side effects/adverse reactions

ACUTE OVERDOSE: ***Black tarry stools, bloody vomit, diarrhea, decreased respiration, increased salivation, watery eyes***

CHRONIC OVERDOSE: ***Hypocalcemia and tetany, respiratory arrest, sores in mouth, constipation, loss of appetite, nausea, vomiting, weight loss, discoloration of teeth*** (white, black, brown)

Contraindications: Hypersensitivity, pregnancy **D**

P **Precautions:** Child <6 yr

Pharmacokinetics

Absorption	Well absorbed (PO)
Distribution	To bone, teeth, crosses placenta
Metabolism	Unknown
Excretion	50% kidneys—unchanged
Half-life	Unknown

Pharmacodynamics

	PO
Onset	Unknown
Peak	½-1 hr
Duration	Unknown

Interactions

Drug/drug:

Individual drugs

Aluminum hydroxide: ↓ absorption of fluoride

Drug classification

Calcium products: ↓ absorption of fluoride

Drug/food:

Calcium foods or dairy products: Blocked absorption of fluoride

NURSING CONSIDERATIONS

Assessment

• Assess nutritional status: increased fluoride content of water, decreased carbohydrate snacks; increased fish, tea, mineral water

Associated nursing diagnoses

✓ Nutrition: less than body requirements (uses)
✓ Knowledge deficit (teaching)
✓ Noncompliance (teaching)

Implementation

PO route

• Give drops pc with fluids or mixed with soda or tab; may be chewed; do not swallow whole; may be given with water or juice; avoid milk

Patient/family education

• Advise patient to monitor P children—gel or rinse should not be swallowed
• Advise patient not to drink, eat, or rinse mouth for at least ½ hr; to apply after brushing and flossing hs
• Caution patient not to use during pregnancy—this drug crosses placenta
• Instruct patient to store drug P out of children's reach

Evaluation

Positive therapeutic outcome

• Absence of dental caries in children

F

fluorometholone

(flure-oh-meth′oh-lone)

Flarex, Fluor-Op, FML, FML Forte, FML Liquifilm

Func. class.: Ophthalmic antiinflammatory

Pregnancy category C

Action: Decreases inflammation, resulting in decreased pain, photophobia, hyperemia, cellular infiltration

➔ **Therapeutic Outcome:** Absence of eye inflammation

Uses: Inflammation of eye, eyelids, conjunctiva, cornea;

uveitis, iridocyclitis, allergic conditions, burns, foreign bodies, postoperatively in cataract

Dosage and routes

P *Adult and child:* Instill 1-2 gtt into conjunctival sac qh × 2 days, if needed, then bid-qid or a thin strip of ointment q3-4h

Available forms: Oint 0.1%; ophth susp 0.1%, 0.25%

Side effects/adverse reactions

EENT: Increased intraocular pressure, poor corneal wound healing, increased possibility of corneal infections, glaucoma exacerbation, ***optic nerve damage,*** decreased acuity, visual field, cataracts

Contraindications: Hypersensitivity, acute superficial herpes simplex, fungal/viral diseases of the eye or conjunctiva, active diabetes mellitus, ocular TB, infections of the eye

Precautions: Corneal abrasions, glaucoma, pregnancy **C**, P lactation, children

Pharmacokinetics

Absorption	Unknown
Distribution	Unknown
Metabolism	Unknown
Excretion	Unknown
Half-life	Unknown

Pharmacodynamics

	OPHTHALMIC
Onset	Immediate
Peak	Unknown
Duration	Unknown

Interactions

Drug/drug:

Acetylcholine: ↓ effect of acetylcholine
Carbachol: ↓ effect of carbachol

NURSING CONSIDERATIONS

Assessment

- Assess patient for inflammation, redness before and during treatment; check for changes in vision; notify prescriber if vision changes occur

Associated nursing diagnoses

✓ Knowledge deficit (teaching)

Implementation

Ophth route
- Administer after shaking susp
- Store in airtight, light-resistant container

Patient/family education

- Teach patient instillation method: apply pressure on lacrimal duct for 1 min when using sol
- Caution patient not to share eye medications with others; not to touch applicator to eye
- Advise patient not to use if purulent drainage or other signs of infection are present

Evaluation

Positive therapeutic outcome
- Absence of swelling, redness, exudate

fluorouracil (5-fluorouracil)

(flure-oh-yoor'a-sil)

Adrucil, 5-FU

Func. class.: Antineoplastic, antimetabolite

Chem. class.: Pyrimidine antagonist

Pregnancy category **D**

Action: Inhibits DNA synthesis; interferes with cell replication by competitively inhibiting thymidylate synthesis, S phase of cell cycle-specific vesicant

Therapeutic Outcome: Prevention of rapidly growing malignant cells

Uses: Cancer of breast, colon, rectum, stomach, pancreas; multiple active keratoses; basal cell carcinoma (TOP)

Dosage and routes

Adult: **IV** 12 mg/kg/day × 4 days, not to exceed 800 mg/day; may repeat with 6 mg/kg on day 6, 8, 10, 12; maintenance is 10-15 mg/kg/wk as a single dose, not to exceed 1 g/wk

Adult: Top 1, 2% sol apply to lesion on head, neck or on other areas 5% bid

Available forms: Inj 50 mg/ml; cream 1, 5%; sol 1, 2, 5%

Side effects/adverse reactions

CNS: Lethargy, malaise, weakness

CV: Myocardial ischemia, angina

EENT: Epistaxsis

GI: Anorexia, stomatitis, diarrhea, nausea, vomiting, ***hemorrhage, enteritis glossitis***

GU: ***Renal failure***

HEMA: ***Thrombocytopenia, leukopenia, myelosuppression, anemia, agranulocytosis***

INTEG: Rash, fever

Contraindications: Hypersensitivity, myelosuppression, pregnancy **D**, poor nutritional status, serious infections

Precautions: Renal disease, hepatic disease, bone marrow depression, angina, lactation, children

Pharmacokinetics

Absorption	Completely bioavailable (**IV**), minimal (Top)
Distribution	Widely distributed, concentration in tumor
Metabolism	Liver—converted to active metabolite
Excretion	Lungs (60%-80%), kidneys (up to 15%)
Half-life	20 hr terminal

Pharmacodynamics

	IV/TOP
Onset	Unknown
Peak	Unknown
Duration	Unknown

Interactions

Drug/drug:

Individual drugs

Radiation: ↑ toxicity, bone marrow suppression

Drug classifications

Antineoplastics: ↑ toxicity bone marrow suppression

Lab test interferences

Increase: Liver function studies, 6-HIAA
Decrease: Albumin

NURSING CONSIDERATIONS

Assessment

- Monitor ECG; watch for ST-T wave changes, low QRS and T, possible dysrhythmias (sinus tachycardia, heart block, PVCs)
- Assess buccal cavity q8h for dryness, sores or ulceration, white patches, oral pain, bleeding, dysphagia; obtain prescription for viscous lidocaine (Xylocaine)
- Assess symptoms indicating severe allergic reaction: rash, pruritus, urticaria, purpuric skin lesions, itching, flushing
- Assess tachypnea, ECG changes, dyspnea, edema, fatigue; identify dyspnea, rales, unproductive cough, chest pain, tachypnea
- Monitor CBC, differential, platelet count weekly; withhold drug if WBC count is <4000/mm^3 or platelet count is <100,000/mm^3; notify prescriber of results if WBC <20,000/mm^3, platelets <50,000/mm^3
- Monitor renal function studies: BUN, creatinine, serum uric acid, urine CrCl before and during therapy; I&O ratio; report fall in urine output to <30 ml/hr
- Monitor temp q4h (may indicate beginning of infection)
- Monitor liver function tests before and during therapy (bilirubin, AST [SGOT], ALT [SGPT], LDH) as needed or monthly; yellowing of skin, sclera, dark urine, clay-colored stools, itchy skin, abdominal pain, fever, diarrhea
- Assess for bleeding: hematuria, stool guaiac, bruising or petechiae, mucosa or orifices q8h; inflammation of mucosa, breaks in skin

Associated nursing diagnoses

- ✓ Injury, risk for (adverse reactions)
- ✓ Body image disturbance (adverse reactions)
- ✓ Infection, risk for (adverse reactions)
- ✓ Knowledge deficit (teaching)

Implementation

- Avoid contact with skin (very irritating); wash completely to remove
- Give fluids **IV** or PO before chemotherapy to hydrate patient
- Give antiemetic 30-60 min before giving drug to prevent vomiting, and prn; antibiotics for prophylaxis of infection
- Provide liq diet: carbonated beverages; gelatin may be added if patient is not nauseated or vomiting
- Provide rinsing of mouth tid-qid with water, club soda; brushing of teeth bid-qid with soft brush or cotton-tipped applicators for stomatitis; use unwaxed dental floss

IV **IV route**

- **IV** undiluted; may inject through Y-tube or 3-way stopcock; give over 1-3 min

• May be diluted in NS, D_5W, given over 2-8 hr as an **IV** inf

Top route

• Wear gloves when applying; may use with a loose dressing

Syringe incompatibility: Droperidol

Syringe compatibilities: Bleomycin, cisplatin, cyclophosphamide, doxorubicin, furosemide, heparin, leucovorin, methotrexate, metoclopramide, mitomycin, vinblastine, vincristine

Y-site incompatibilities: Droperidol, vinorelbine

Y-site compatibilities: Bleomycin, cisplatin, cyclophosphamide, doxorubicin, furosemide, heparin, leucovorin, mannitol, melphalan, methotrexate, metoclopramide, mitomycin, paclitaxel, vinblastine, vincristine, sargramstim

Additive incompatibilities: Carboplatin, cisplatin, cytarabine, diazepam, doxorubicin

Additive compatibilities: Bleomycin, cephalothin, etoposides, floxuridine, ifosfamide, leucovorin, methotrexate, prednisolone, vincristine, cyclophosphamide, cyclophosphamide mitoxantrone

Solution compatibilities: Amino acids 4.25%/D_{25}, D_5/LR, $D_{3.3}$/0.3 NaCl, D_5W, 0.9% NaCl, TPN #23

Patient/family education

• Caution patient that contraceptive measures are recommended during therapy

• Teach patient to avoid using aspirin- or ibuprofen-containing products, razors, commercial mouthwash because bleeding may occur; to report symptoms of bleeding (hematuria, tarry stools)

• Instruct patient to report signs of anemia, (fatigue, headache, irritability, faintness, shortness of breath)

Evaluation

Positive therapeutic outcome

• Prevention of rapid division of malignant cells

fluoxetine

(floo-ox'e-teen)

Prozac

Func. class.: Bicyclic antidepressant

Pregnancy category **B**

Action: Inhibits CNS neuron uptake of serotonin, but not of norepinephrine

Therapeutic Outcome: Decreased symptoms of depression after 2-3 wk

Uses: Major depressive disorder

Investigational uses: Obsessive-compulsive disorder

Dosage and routes

Adult: PO 20 mg qd AM; after 4 wk if no clinical improve-

F

ment is noted, dose may be increased to 20 mg bid in AM, afternoon, not to exceed 80 mg/day

Available forms: Pulvules 20 mg, cap 10 mg, liq 20 mg/5 ml

Side effects/adverse reactions

CNS: Headache, nervousness, insomnia, drowsiness, anxiety, tremor, dizziness, fatigue, sedation, poor concentration, abnormal dreams, agitation, ***convulsions***
CV: Hot flashes, palpitations, angina pectoris, ***hemorrhage,*** hypertension, first-degree tachycardia
EENT: Visual changes, ear/eye pain, photophobia, tinnitus
GI: Nausea, diarrhea, dry mouth, anorexia, dyspepsia, constipation, cramps, vomiting, taste changes, flatulence, decreased appetite
GU: Dysmenorrhea, decreased libido, urinary frequency, urinary tract infection, amenorrhea, cystitis, impotence
INTEG: Sweating, rash, pruritus, acne, alopecia, urticaria
MS: Pain, arthritis, twitching
RESP: Infection, pharyngitis, nasal congestion, sinus headache, sinusitis, cough dyspnea, bronchitis, asthma, hyperventilation, pneumonia
SYST: Asthenia, viral infection, fever, allergy, chills

Contraindications: Hypersensitivity

P G **Precautions:** Pregnancy **B**, lactation, children, elderly

Pharmacokinetics

Absorption	Well absorbed (PO)
Distribution	Crosses blood-brain barrier
Metabolism	Liver, extensively to norfluoxetine
Excretion	Kidneys, unchanged (12%), metabolite (7%)
Half-life	2-7 days, metabolite up to 1 wk

Pharmacodynamics

	PO
Onset	Unknown
Peak	6-8 hr
Duration	Unknown

Interactions

Drug/drug:

Individual drugs
Alcohol: ↑ CNS depression
Drug classifications
Barbiturates: ↑ CNS depression
Benzodiazepines: ↑ CNS depression
CNS depressants: ↑ CNS depression
MAOI: Hypertensive crisis, convulsions
Oral anticoagulants: ↑ effects, toxicity
Sedative/hypnotics: ↑ CNS depression

Lab test interferences

Increase: Serum bilirubin, blood glucose, alk phosphatase
Decrease: VMA, 5-HIAA, blood glucose
False increase: Urinary catecholamines

NURSING CONSIDERATIONS

Assessment

• Monitor B/P (lying, standing), pulse q4h; if systolic B/P drops 20 mm hg, hold drug and notify prescriber; take vital signs q4h in patients with cardiovascular disease
• Monitor blood studies: CBC, leukocytes, differential, cardiac enzymes if patient is receiving long-term therapy
• Monitor hepatic studies: AST (SGOT), ALT (SGPT), bilirubin
• Check weight qwk; appetite may increase with drug
• Assess ECG for flattening of T wave, bundle branch block, AV block, dysrhythmias in cardiac patients
• Assess for EPS primarily in elderly: rigidity, dystonia, akathisia
• Assess mental status: mood, sensorium, affect, suicidal tendencies; increase in psychiatric symptoms: depression, panic
• Monitor urinary retention, constipation; constipation is [P] more likely to occur in children [G] or elderly
• Assess for withdrawal symptoms: headache, nausea, vomiting, muscle pain, weakness; do not usually occur unless drug is discontinued abruptly
• Identify patient's alcohol consumption; if alcohol is consumed, hold dose until AM

Associated nursing diagnoses

✓ Coping, ineffective individual (uses)
✓ Injury, risk for (side effects)
✓ Knowledge deficit (teaching)
✓ Noncompliance (teaching)

Implementation

PO route

• Give with food or milk for GI symptoms
• Give dosage hs if oversedation occurs during day; may [G] take entire dose hs; elderly may not tolerate once/day dosing
• Store at room temp; do not freeze

Patient/family education

• Teach patient that therapeutic effects may take 2-3 wk
• Instruct patient to use caution in driving or other activities requiring alertness because of drowsiness, dizziness, blurred vision; to avoid rising quickly from sitting to standing, [G] especially elderly
• Caution patient to avoid alcohol ingestion, other CNS depressants
• Advise patient not to discontinue medication quickly after long-term use: may cause nausea, headache, malaise
• Instruct patient to increase fluids, bulk in diet if constipation, urinary retention occur, [G] especially elderly
• Advise patient to take gum, hard sugarless candy, or frequent sips of water for dry mouth

Evaluation

Positive therapeutic outcome

• Decrease in depression
• Absence of suicidal thoughts

fluphenazine

(floo-fen'a-zeen)

Apo-Fluphenazine ♣, Permitil, Prolixin, fluphenazine decanoate, Prolixin Decanoate, Prolixin Enanthate, fluphenazine HCl

Func. class.: Antipsychotic/neuroleptic

Chem. class.: Phenothiazine, piperazine

Pregnancy category C

Action: Depresses cerebral cortex, hypothalamus, limbic system, which control activity and aggression; blocks neurotransmission produced by dopamine at synapse; exhibits strong α-adrenergic and anticholinergic blocking action; mechanism for antipsychotic effects is unclear

➡ **Therapeutic Outcome:** Decreased signs and symptoms of psychosis

Uses: Psychotic disorders, schizophrenia

Dosage and routes

Enanthate, decanoate

P ***Adult and child >12 yr:*** IM 12.5-25 mg q1-3 wk

HCl

Adult: PO 2.5-10 mg, in divided doses q6-8h, not to exceed 20 mg qd; IM initially 1.25 mg then 2.5-10 mg in divided doses q6-8h

P ***Child:*** PO 0.25-3.5 mg qd in divided doses q4-6h, max 10 mg/qd

Available forms: HCl tabs 1, 2.5, 5, 10 mg; elix 2.5 mg/5 ml; conc 5 mg/ml; inj IM 10 mg/ml, enanthate, decanoate, inj SC, IM 25 mg/ml

Side effects/adverse reactions

CNS: Extrapyramidal symptoms: pseudoparkinsonism, akathisia, dystonia, tardive dyskinesia, drowsiness, headache, ***seizures, neuroleptic malignant syndrome***

CV: Orthostatic hypotension, hypertension, ***cardiac arrest,*** ECG changes, ***tachycardia***

EENT: Blurred vision, glaucoma, dry eyes

GI: Dry mouth, nausea, vomiting, anorexia, constipation, diarrhea, jaundice, weight gain, ***paralytic ileus, hepatitis***

GU: Urinary retention, urinary frequency, enuresis, impotence, amenorrhea, gynecomastia

HEMA: Anemia, ***leukopenia, leukocytosis, agranulocytosis***

INTEG: Rash, photosensitivity, dermatitis

RESP: ***Laryngospasm,*** dyspnea, ***respiratory depression***

Contraindications: Hypersensitivity, circulatory collapse, liver damage, cerebral arteriosclerosis, coronary disease, severe hypertension/hypotension, blood dyscrasias,
P coma, child <12 yr, brain damage, bone marrow depression, alcohol and barbiturate withdrawal

Precautions: Pregnancy **C**, lactation, seizure disorders, hypertension, hepatic disease, cardiac disease

Pharmacokinetics

Absorption	Well absorbed (PO, IM)
Distribution	Widely absorbed, crosses blood-brain barrier, placenta
Metabolism	Liver, extensively
Excretion	Kidneys (metabolites)
Half-life	HCl-4.7-15.3 hr, enanthate 3½-4 days, decanoate 6.8-14.3 days

Pharmacodynamics

	PO/IM	IM	IM
	HCl	Enanthate	Decanoate
Onset	1 hr	1-2 days	1-3 days
Peak	1½-2 hr	2-3 days	1-2 days
Duration	6-8 hr	1-3 wk	>4 wk

Interactions

Drug/drug:

Individual drugs

Alcohol: ↑ effects of both drugs, oversedation
Aluminum hydroxide: ↓ absorption of fluphenazine
Bromocriptine: ↓ antiparkinson activity
Disopyramide: ↑ anticholinergic effects
Epinephrine: ↑ toxicity
Guanethidine: ↓ antihypertensive response
Levodopa: ↓ antiparkinson activity
Lithium: ↓ fluphenazine levels, ↑ extrapyramidal symptoms, masking of lithium toxicity
Magnesium hydroxide: ↓ absorption of fluphenazine
Norepinephrine: ↓ vasoresponse, ↑ toxicity
Phenobarbital: ↓ effectiveness, ↑ metabolism

Drug classifications

Antacids: ↓ absorption of fluphenazine
Anticholinergics: ↑ anticholinergic effects
Antidepressants: ↑ CNS depression
Antidiarrheals, adsorbent: ↓ absorption
Antihistamines: ↑ CNS depression
Antihypertensives: ↑ hypotension
Antithyroid agents: ↑ agranulocytosis
Barbiturate anesthetics: ↑ CNS depression
Beta adrenergics: ↑ effects of both drugs
General anesthetics: ↑ CNS depression
MAOI: ↑ CNS depression
Narcotics: ↑ CNS depression
Sedative/hypnotics: ↑ CNS depression

Lab test interferences

Increase: Liver function tests, cardiac enzymes, cholesterol, blood glucose, prolactin, bilirubin, PBI, cholinesterase I, alk phosphatase, leukocytes, granulocytes, platelets
Decrease: Hormones (blood and urine)
False positive: Pregnancy tests, PKU, urine bilirubin
False negative: Urinary steroids, 17-OHCS

NURSING CONSIDERATIONS

Assessment

- Assess mental status: orientation, mood, behavior, presence of hallucinations, and type before initial administration

and monthly; this drug should significantly reduce psychotic behavior
- Check for swallowing of PO medication; check for hoarding or giving of medication to other patients
- Monitor I&O ratio, palpate bladder if low urinary output G occurs, especially in elderly; urinalysis recommended before, during prolonged therapy
- Monitor bilirubin, CBC, liver function studies monthly
- Assess affect, orientation, LOC, reflexes, gait, coordination, sleep pattern disturbances
- Monitor B/P with patient sitting, standing, and lying down; take pulse and respirations q4h during initial treatment; establish baseline before starting treatment; report drops of 30 mm Hg; obtain baseline ECG, Q-wave and T-wave changes
- Check for dizziness, faintness, palpitations, tachycardia on rising; severe orthostatic hypotension is common
- Identify for neuroleptic malignant syndrome: hyperpyrexia, muscle rigidity, increased CPK, altered mental status; drug should be discontinued
- Assess for extrapyramidal symptoms including akathisia (inability to sit still, no pattern to movements), tardive dyskinesia (bizarre movements of the jaw, mouth, tongue, extremities), pseudoparkinsonism (ragged, tremors, pill rolling, shuffling gate), an antiparkinson drug should be prescribed
- Assess for constipation, urinary retention daily; if these occur, increase bulk, water in diet

Associated nursing diagnoses

- ✓ Thought processes, altered (uses)
- ✓ Coping, ineffective individual (uses)
- ✓ Knowledge deficit (teaching)
- ✓ Noncompliance (teaching)

Implementation

PO route

- Give drug in liq form mixed in glass of juice or cola if hoarding is suspected; do not mix in caffeine drinks, tannics, or pectinates; decrease dose in G elderly
- Give PO with full glass of water, milk; or give with food to decrease GI upset
- Store in tight, light-resistant container, oral sol in amber bottle

SC route

- May be given by this route; however, it is painful

IM route

- Inject in deep muscle mass, use a 21-G needle into dorsal gluteal site, keep patient recumbent for ½ hr—prevents orthostatic hypotension

Patient/family education

- Teach patient to use good oral hygiene; frequent rinsing of mouth, sugarless gum for dry mouth
- Caution patient to avoid hazardous activities until drug response is determined; dizziness, blurred vision may occur
- Inform patient that orthostatic hypotension occurs often and to rise from sitting or lying position gradually, to remain lying down after IM inj for at least 30 min; tell patient to avoid hot tubs, hot showers,

tub baths because hypotension may occur; tell patient that in hot weather, heat stroke may occur—extra precautions are necessary to stay cool

- Instruct patient to avoid abrupt withdrawal of this drug, or extrapyramidal symptoms may result; drug should be withdrawn slowly
- Teach patient to avoid OTC preparations (cough, hayfever, cold) unless approved by physician because serious drug interactions may occur; avoid use with alcohol, CNS depressants; increased drowsiness may occur
- Instruct patient to use a sunscreen and sunglasses to prevent burns
- Teach patient about extrapyramidal symptoms and necessity of meticulous oral hygiene beause oral candidiasis may occur
- Instruct patient to take antacids 2 hr before or after this drug
- Advise patient to report sore throat, malaise, fever, bleeding, mouth sores; if these occur, CBC should be drawn and drug discontinued

Evaluation

Positive therapeutic outcome

- Decrease in emotional excitement, hallucinations, delusions, paranoia
- Reorganization of patterns of thought, speech

Treatment of overdose:

Lavage if orally ingested; provide airway; *do not induce vomiting or use epinephrine*

flurandrenolide

(flure-an-dren'oh-lide)

Cordran, Cordran SP, Cordran Tape, Drenison ¼ ✤, Drenison Tape ✤

Func. class.: Topical corticosteroid

Chem. class.: Synthetic fluorinated agent

Pregnancy category **C**

F

Action: Antipruritic, anti-inflammatory

Therapeutic Outcome: Absence of severe itching, patches on skin, flaking

Uses: Psoriasis, eczema, contact dermatitis, pruritus; usually reserved for severe dermatoses that have not responded to less potent formulation

Dosage and routes

Adult and child: Top apply to affected area tid-qid; apply tape q12-24h

Available forms: Oint 0.025%, 0.05%; cream 0.025%, 0.05%; lotion 0.05%; tape 4 μg/cm²

Side effects/adverse reactions

INTEG: Burning, dryness, itching, irritation, acne, folliculitis, hypertrichosis, perioral dermatitis, hypopigmentation, atrophy, striae, miliaria, allergic contact dermatitis, secondary infection

Contraindications: Hypersensitivity to corticosteroids,

fungal infections, viral infections

Precautions: Pregnancy **C**, lactation, viral infections, bacterial infections

Pharmacokinetics

Absorption	Minimally absorbed; systemically absorbed on large areas
Distribution	Site only
Metabolism	Not metabolized
Excretion	Not excreted
Half-life	Unknown

Pharmacodynamics

	TOP
Onset	Up to 1 hr
Peak	Up to several days
Duration	Up to several days

Interactions: None

NURSING CONSIDERATIONS

Assessment

• Monitor patient for fever or rash: if fever develops drug should be discontinued
• Monitor patient for signs of systemic absorption: increased temp, inflammation, irritation

Associated nursing diagnoses

✓ Infection, risk for (advise reactions)
✓ Knowledge deficit (teaching)
✓ Noncompliance (noncompliance)

Implementation

Top route

• Apply only to affected areas; do not get in eyes
• Leave site uncovered or lightly covered; occlusive dressing is not recommended—systemic absorption may occur
• Use only on dermatoses; do not use on weeping, denuded, or infected area
• Cleanse before application of drug
• Continue treatment for a few days after area has cleared
• Store at room temp

Patient/family education

• Caution patient to avoid sunlight on affected area; burns may occur
• Advise patient to limit treatment to 14 days

Evaluation

Positive therapeutic outcome

• Absence of severe itching, patches on skin, flaking

flurazepam

(flure-az'e-pam)

Apo-flurazepam ✤, Dalmane, Durapam, flurazepam, Novoflupam ✤, Somnol ✤, Som-Pam ✤

Func. class.: Sedative-hypnotic

Chem. class.: Benzodiazepine derivative

Pregnancy category **D**

Controlled substance schedule **IV** (USA), schedule **F** (Canada)

Action: Produces CNS depression at the limbic, thalamic, hypothalamic levels of CNS; may be mediated by neurotransmitter γ-aminobutyric acid (GABA); results are sedation, hypnosis, skeletal muscle relaxation, anticonvulsant activity, anxiolytic action

Therapeutic Outcome: Ability to sleep, relaxation

Uses: Insomnia

Dosage and routes

Adult: PO 15-30 mg hs; may repeat dose once if needed

G ***Geriatric:*** PO 15 mg hs; may increase if needed

Available forms: Cap 15, 30 mg

Side effects/adverse reactions

CNS: Lethargy, drowsiness, daytime sedation, dizziness, confusion, light-headedness, headache, anxiety, irritability

CV: Chest pain, pulse changes

GI: Nausea, vomiting, diarrhea, heartburn, abdominal pain, constipation

HEMA: Leukopenia, granulocytopenia (rare)

Contraindications: Hypersensitivity to benzodiazepines, pregnancy **D**, lactation, intermittent porphyria, uncontrolled pain

Precautions: Anemia, hepatic disease, renal disease, suicidal G individuals, drug abuse, elderly, P psychosis, child <15 yr

Pharmacokinetics

Absorption	Well absorbed (PO)
Distribution	Widely absorbed, crosses blood-brain barrier, crosses placenta
Metabolism	Liver to active, inactive metabolites
Excretion	Kidneys, breast milk
Half-life	2½ hr, 30-200 hr active metabolites

Pharmacodynamics

	PO
Onset	15-30 min
Peak	½-1 hr
Duration	7-8 hr

Interactions

Drug/drug:

Individual drugs

Alcohol: ↑ CNS depression

Cimetidine: ↑ action of flurazepam

Disulfiram: ↑ action of flurazepam

Fluoxetine: ↑ action of flurazepam

Isoniazid: ↑ action of flurazepam

Ketoconazole: ↑ action of flurazepam

Levodopa: ↓ action of levodopa

Metoprolol: ↑ action of flurazepam

Propoxyphene: ↑ action of flurazepam

Propranolol: ↑ action of flurazepam

Rifampin: ↓ action of flurazepam

Theophylline: ↓ sedative effects

Valproic acid: ↑ action of flurazepam

F

Drug classifications

Analgesics, opioid: ↑ CNS depression
Antidepressants: ↑ CNS depression
Antihistamines: ↑ CNS depression
Barbiturates: ↓ effect of flurazepam
Contraceptives: ↑ effect

Lab test interferences

Increase: AST(SGOT)/ ALT(SGPT), serum bilirubin
False increase: Urinary 17-OHCS
Decrease: RAI uptake

NURSING CONSIDERATIONS

Assessment

- Assess anxiety reaction: inability to sleep, apprehension, dread, foreboding, or uneasiness related to unidentified source of danger
- Assess for previous drug dependence or tolerance; if drug dependent or tolerant, amount of medication should be restricted
- Monitor B/P (lying, standing), pulse; if systolic B/P drops 20 mm Hg, hold drug, notify prescriber; I&O; may indicate renal dysfunction
- Monitor blood studies: CBC during long-term therapy; blood dyscrasias have occurred rarely
- Monitor hepatic studies: AST (SGOT), ALT (SGPT), bilirubin, creatinine, LDH, alk phosphatase
- Monitor patient's mental status: mood, sensorium, affect, sleeping patterns, drowsiness, dizziness, suicidal tendencies

Associated nursing diagnoses

✓ Sleep pattern disturbance (uses)
✓ Knowledge deficit (teaching)
✓ Noncompliance (teaching)

Implementation

PO route

- Give ½-1 hr before hs for sleeplessness; give on empty stomach with full glass of water or juice for best absorption and to decrease corrosion (do not chew); give pc to decrease GI symptoms if used for sedation

Patient/family education

- Caution patient that drug may be taken with food; if dose is missed take as soon as remembered; do not double doses
- Advise patient to avoid OTC preparations unless approved by a physician, to avoid alcohol ingestion or other psychotropic medications unless prescribed by a health care provider, that 1-2 wk of therapy may be required before therapeutic effects occur
- Caution patient to avoid driving, activities requiring alertness—drowsiness may occur; until medication response is known, tell patient that drowsiness may worsen at beginning of treatment
- Instruct patient not to discontinue medication abruptly after long-term use
- Caution patient to rise slowly or fainting may occur, especially in elderly [G]

Evaluation

Positive therapeutic outcome

- Increased well-being

• Decreased anxiety, restlessness, sleeplessness, dread

Treatment of overdose: Lavage, activated charcoal; monitor electrolytes, vital signs

flurbiprofen

(flure-bi'proe-fen)

Ansaid, Froben ✦, Ocufen

Func. class.: Nonsteroidal antiinflammatory

Chem. class.: Phenylalkanoic acid

Pregnancy category C

Action: Inhibits prostaglandin synthesis by decreasing enzyme needed for biosynthesis; analgesic, antiinflammatory, antipyretic; inhibits enzyme system necessary for biosynthesis of prostaglandins; inhibits miosis

Therapeutic Outcome: Decreased pain, inflammation

Uses: Mild-to-moderate pain, osteoarthritis, rheumatoid arthritis, acute gout, arthritis, ankylosing spondylitis, inflammation, dysmenorrhea; inhibition of intraoperative miosis, corneal edema

Dosage and routes

Adult: PO 200-300 mg qd in 2-4 divided doses, max 300 mg/day or 100 mg/dose; ophth 1 gtt q½-2h before surgery (4 gtt total)

Available forms: Sol 0.03%; tabs 50, 100 mg

Side effects/adverse reactions

CNS: Depression, flushing, sweating, headache, mood changes

CV: Hypertension, ***circulatory collapse,*** thrombophlebitis, embolism, tachycardia, edema

EENT: Burning, stinging in the eye, irritation, bleeding or redness; fungal infections, increased intraocular pressure, blurred vision

GI: Diarrhea, nausea, abdominal distention, ***GI hemmorrhage,*** increased appetite, pancreatitis

INTEG: Acne, poor wound healing, ecchymosis, petechiae

MS: Fractures, osteoporosis, weakness

Contraindications: Hypersensitivity, epithelial herpes simplex keratitis

Precautions: Pregnancy **C**, lactation, child, aspirin or NSAID hypersensitivity, allergy, bleeding disorder

Pharmacokinetics

Absorption	Well absorbed (PO)
Distribution	Widely distributed (PO)
Metabolism	Liver—extensively
Excretion	Kidneys
Half-life	3-6 hr

Pharmacodynamics

	PO/OPHTH
Onset	Unknown
Peak	Unknown
Duration	Unknown

Interactions

Drug/drug:

Individual drugs

Alcohol: ↑ GI upset
Aspirin: ↓ effect of flurbiprofen
Carbachol: ↓ effect when used with other ophthalmics
Epinephrine: ↓ effect of epinephrine
Heparin: ↑ bleeding
Radiation: ↑ effects

Drug classifications

Antihypertensives: ↓ antihypertensive effect
Cephalosporins: ↑ bleeding
Hypoglycemics, oral: ↑ hypoglycemic effect
Nonsteroidal antiinflammatory agents: ↑ GI upset

NURSING CONSIDERATIONS

Assessment

- Assess for pain: joint pain (duration, intensity, ROM); baseline and during treatment

Implementation

Ophth route

- Excess sol must be wiped away promptly to prevent its flow into lacrimal system, producing systemic symptoms
- Protect sol from sun

PO route

- Give ½ hr ac or 2 hr pc

Patient/family education

- Advise patient to report change in vision, blurring, or loss of sight during miosis; rash, tinnitus, black stools, headache, chills, fever (systemic)
- Caution patient not to use for any other condition than prescribed
- Inform patient to avoid use with OTC medications for pain or with alcohol unless approved by prescriber
- Advise patient to avoid hazardous activities because dizziness or drowsiness occurs

Evaluation

Positive therapeutic outcome

- Absence of corneal edema, intraoperative miosis (ophth)
- Decreased pain, inflammation

flutamide

(floo'ta-mide)

Eulexin

Func. class.: Antineoplastic hormone

Chem. class.: Antiandrogen

Pregnancy category **D**

Action: Interferes with testosterone uptake in the nucleus or testosterone activity in target tissues; arrests tumor growth in androgen-sensitive tumors

Therapeutic Outcome: Prevention of rapidly growing malignant cells

Uses: Metastatic prostatic carcinoma, stage D2 in combination with LHRH agonistic analogs (leuprolide)

Dosage and routes

Adult: PO 250 mg q8h tid, for a daily dosage of 750 mg

Available forms: Cap 125 mg

Side effects/adverse reactions

CNS: Hot flashes, drowsiness, confusion, depression, anxiety
GI: Diarrhea, nausea, vomiting, increased liver function studies, ***hepatitis,*** anorexia
GU: Decreased libido, impotence, gynecomastia
INTEG: Irritation at site, rash photosensitivity
MISC: Edema, hematopoietic symptoms, neuromuscular and pulmonary symptoms, hypertension

Contraindications: Hypersensitivity, pregnancy **D**

Pharmacokinetics

Absorption	Well absorbed
Distribution	Unknown
Metabolism	Liver
Excretion	Unknown
Half-life	6 hr

Pharmacodynamics

	PO
Onset	Unknown
Peak	Unknown
Duration	Unknown

Interactions

Drug/drug:

Individual drugs
Leuprolide: ↑ synergistic effect

NURSING CONSIDERATIONS

Assessment

- Monitor bilirubin, creatinine, AST (SGOT), ALT (SGPT), alk phosphatase, which may be elevated
- Identify CNS symptoms: drowsiness, confusion, depression, anxiety

Associated nursing diagnoses

- ✓ Injury, risk for (adverse reactions)
- ✓ Sexual dysfunction (adverse reactions)
- ✓ Body image disturbance (adverse reactions)
- ✓ Infection, risk for (adverse reactions)
- ✓ Knowledge deficit (teaching)

Implementation

- Used in combination with LHRH agonist (leuprolide)
- May be given with food or fluids

Patient/family education

- Tell the patient to report side effects: decreased libido, impotence, breast enlargement, hot flashes, diarrhea, which occur when the two drugs are given together
- Inform patient that this drug is taken with leuprolide

Evaluation

Positive therapeutic outcome
- Prevention of rapid division of malignant cells

Treatment of overdose:

Induce vomiting, provide supportive care

F

folic acid (vitamin B_9)
(foe-lik a'sid)
Apo-Folic ♣, Folate, Folvite, Novofolacid ♣, Vitamin B/q
Func. class.: Vitamin B-complex group
Chem. class.: Supplement
Pregnancy category **A**

Action: Needed for erythropoiesis; increases RBC, WBC, and platelet formation in megaloblastic anemias

➔ **Therapeutic Outcome:** Absence of macrocytic, megaloblastic anemias

Uses: Megaloblastic or macrocytic anemia caused by folic acid deficiency; liver disease; alcoholism; hemolysis; intestinal obstruction; pregnancy

Dosage and routes

Supplement

Adult: PO/IM/SC/**IV** 0.1 mg qd

P *Child:* PO/IM/SC/**IV** 0.05 mg qd

Megaloblastic/macrocytic anemia

P *Adult and child >4 yr:* PO/SC/IM/**IV** 1 mg qd × 4-5 days

P *Child <4 yr:* PO/SC/IM/**IV** 0.3 mg or less qd

Pregnancy/lactation: PO/SC/IM/**IV** 0.8 mg qd

Prevention of megaloblastic/macrocytic anemia

Pregnancy: PO/SC/IM/**IV** 1 mg qd

Available forms: Tab 0.1, 0.4, 0.8, 1 mg; inj 5, 10 mg/ml

Side effects/adverse reactions

INTEG: Flushing
RESP: ***Bronchospasm***

Contraindications: Hypersensitivity, anemias other than megaloblastic/macrocytic anemia, Vit B_{12} deficiency anemia, uncorrected pernicious anemia

Precautions: Pregnancy **A**

Pharmacokinetics

Absorption	Well absorbed
Distribution	Liver, crosses placenta
Metabolism	Liver (converted to active metabolite)
Excretion	Kidneys (unchanged)
Half-life	Unknown

Pharmacodynamics

Onset	Unknown
Peak	½-1 hr
Duration	Unknown

Interactions

Drug/drug:

Individual drugs

Methotrexate: ↓ action of folic acid
Phenytoin: ↑ need for folic acid
Sulfasalazine: ↓ action of folic acid
Triamterene: ↓ action of folic acid

Drug classifications

Estrogens: ↑ need for folic acid
Glucocorticoids: ↑ need for folic acid
Sulfonamides: ↓ action of folic acid

NURSING CONSIDERATIONS

Assessment

- Assess patient for fatigue, dyspnea, weakness, shortness of breath, activity intolerance (signs of megaloblastic anemia)
- Monitor Hgb, Hct, and reticulocyte count; folate levels: 6-15 µg/ml baseline and throughout treatment
- Assess nutritional status: bran, yeast, dried beans, nuts, fruits, fresh vegetables, asparagus; if high folic acid foods are missing from the diet, a referral to a dietician may be indicated
- Identify drugs currently taken: alcohol, oral contraceptives, hydantoins, trimethoprim; these drugs may cause increased folic acid use by the body and contribute to deficiency

Associated nursing diagnoses

- ✓ Nutrition, less than body requirements (uses)
- ✓ Fatigue (uses)
- ✓ Activity intolerance (uses)
- ✓ Knowledge deficit (teaching)

Implementation

IV **IV route**

- Give **IV** directly, undiluted 5 mg or less/min—or may be added to most **IV** sol or TPN
- Store in light-resistant container

Syringe incompatibility:

Doxapram

Y-site compatibility:

Famotidine

Solution compatibility:

$D_{20}W$

Solution incompatibilities:

$D_{40}W$, $D_{50}W$, calcium gluconate

Patient/family education

- Advise patient to take drug exactly as prescribed; not to double doses, toxicity may occur
- Instruct patient to notify prescriber of side effects—rash or fever may indicate hypersensitivity
- Advise patient that urine may become more yellow
- Instruct patient to increase intake of foods rich in folic acid in diet as recommended by dietician or health care provider

Evaluation

Positive therapeutic outcome

- Absence of fatigue, weakness, dyspnea
- Absence of symptoms of megaloblastic anemia

F

foscarnet sodium

(foss-kar'net)
Foscavir
Func. class.: Antiviral
Chem. class.: Inorganic pyrophosphate organic analog
Pregnancy category **C**

Action: Antiviral activity is produced by selective inhibition at the pyrophosphate binding site on virus-specific DNA polymerases and reverse transcriptases at concentrations that do not affect cellular DNA polymerases

Therapeutic Outcome: Virostatic agents against CMV retinitis

Uses: Treatment of CMV (cytomegalovirus), retinitis

Dosage and routes

Adult: **IV** inf 60 mg/kg given over at least 1 hr, q8h × 2-3 wk initially, then 90-120 mg/kg/day over 2 hr, usually give with at least 750-1000 ml 0.9% NaCl qd

In renal abnormalities

Adult: **IV** male:

$$\frac{140\text{–age} = \text{creatinine clearance}}{\text{serum creatinine} \times 72}$$

Female: 0.85 x above value

Dose based on table provided in package insert

Available forms: Inj 24 mg/ml

Side effects/adverse reactions

CNS: Fever, dizziness, headache, ***seizures,*** fatigue, neuropathy, tremor, ataxia, dementia, stupor, EEG abnormalities, vertigo, ***coma,*** abnormal gait, hypertonia, extrapyramidal disorders, hemiparesis, ***paralysis,*** hyperreflexia, paraplegia, ***tetany,*** hyporeflexia, neuralgia, neuritis, celebral edema, paresthesia, depression, confusion, anxiety, insomnia, somnolence, amnesia, hallucinations, agitation
CV: Hypertension, palpitations, ECG abnormalities, 1st degree AV block, nonspecific ST-T segment changes, hypotension, cerebrovascular disorder, cardiomyopathy, ***cardiac arrest,*** bradycardia, dysrhythmias
EENT: Visual field defects, vocal cord paralysis, speech disorders, taste perversion, eye pain, conjunctivitis, tinnitus, otitis
GI: *Nausea, vomiting,* anorexia, abdominal pain, constipation, dysphagia, rectal hemorrhage, dry mouth, melena, flatulence, ulcerative stomatitis, pancreatitis, enteritis, enterocolitis, glossitis, proctitis, stomatitis, increased amylases, gastroenteritis, ***pseudomembranous colitis,*** duodenal ulcer, ***paralytic ileus, esophageal ulceration,*** abnormal A-G ratio, increased AST (SGPT), ALT (SGOT), cholecystitis, ***hepatitis,*** dyspepsia, tenesmus, hepatosplenomegaly, jaundice
GU: ***Acute renal failure,*** decreased Ccr and increased

serum creatinine, ***glomerulonephritis, toxic nephropathy, nephrosis, renal tubular disorders, pyelonephritis, uremia, hematuria, albuminuria,*** dysuria, polyuria
HEMA: Anemia, ***granulocytopenia, leukopenia, thrombocytopenia,*** platelet abnormalities, ***thrombosis, pulmonary embolism, coagulation disorders, decreased prothrombin, hypochromic anemia, pancytopenia, hemolysis, leukocytosis,*** lymphadenopathy, epistaxis, lymphopenia
INTEG: Rash, sweating, pruritus, skin ulceration, seborrhea, skin discoloration, alopecia, acne, dermatitis, pain/inflammation at injection site, facial edema, dry skin, urticaria
MS: Arthralgia, myalgia
RESP: Coughing, dyspnea, pneumonia, sinusitis, pharyngitis, ***pulmonary infiltration,*** stridor, ***pneumothorax, hemoptysis, bronchospasm,*** bronchitis, ***respiratory depression, pleural effusion, pulmonary hemorrhage,*** rhinitis
SYST: Hypokalemia, hypocalcemia, hypomagnesemia, increased alk phosphatase, LDH, BUN, acidosis, hypophosphatemia, hyperphosphatemia, dehydration, glycosuria, increased creatine phosphokinase, hypervolemia, infection, ***sepsis, death, ascites,*** hyponatremia, hypochlormia, hypercalcemia

Contraindications: Hypersensitivity

Precautions: Pregnancy **C**, P lactation, children, elderly, G renal disease, seizure disorders, electrolyte/mineral imbalances, severe anemia

Pharmacokinetics

Absorption	Complete (IV)
Distribution	14%-17% plasma protein binding
Metabolism	Not metabolized
Excretion	Kidneys (90%) unchanged, breast milk
Half-life	2-8 hr; ↑ in renal disease

Pharmacodynamics

	PO
Onset	48 hr
Peak	2 wk
Duration	Unknown

Interactions

Drug/drug:

Individual drugs

Amphotericin B: ↑ nephrotoxicity
Pentamide: ↑ nephrotoxicity
Zidovudine: ↑ anemia

Drug classification

Aminoglycosides: ↑ nephrotoxicity

NURSING CONSIDERATIONS

Assessment

- Culture should be done before treatment with foscarnet is begun. Cultures of blood, urine, and throat may all be taken; CMV is not confirmed by this method. The diagnosis is made by an ophth exam.
- Assess kidney and liver function. Increased hemopoietic studies: BUN, serum creatinine, creatitinine clearance AST (SGOT), ALT (SGPT),

A-G ratio, baseline and during treatment. Blood counts should be done q2wk; watch for decreasing granulocytes, Hgb; if low, therapy may have to be discontinued and restarted after hematologic recovery; blood transfusions may be required
• Assess for GI symptoms: severe nausea, vomiting, diarrhea; severe symptoms may necessitate discontinuing drug
• Monitor electrolytes and minerals: calcium, phosphorous, magnesium, sodium, potassium; watch closely for tetany during first administration
• Assess for symptoms of blood dyscrasias (anemia, granulocytopenia); bruising, fatigue, bleeding, poor healing
• Assess for symptoms of allergic reactions: flushing, rash, urticaria, pruritus

Associated nursing diagnoses

✓ Infection, risk for (uses)
✓ Injury, risk for (adverse reactions)
✓ Knowledge deficit (teaching)

Implementation

IV **IV route**
• Administer increased fluids before and during drug administration to induce diuresis and minimize renal toxicity
• Administer via inf pump, at no more than 1 mg/kg/min; do not give by rapid or bolus **IV**; give by central venous line or peripheral vein; standard 24 mg/ml sol may be used without dilution if using by central line; dilute the 24 mg/ml sol to 12 mg/ml with D_5W or 0.9% NaCl if using peripheral vein
• Monitor patient closely during therapy; if tingling, numbness, paresthesias occur, stop inf and obtain lab sample for electrolytes

Y-*site incompatibilities:*

Acyclovir, amphotericin B, calcium, co-trimoxazole, diazepam, digoxin, gancyclovir, haloperidol, leucovorin, midazolam, pentamidine, phenytoin, prochlorperazine, vancomycin

Y-*site compatibilities:*

Aminophylline, amikacin, ampicillin, aztreonam, benzquinamide, cephalorsporins, dexamethasone, dopamine, erythromycin lactobionate, fluconazole, flucytosine, furosemide, gentamicin, heparin, hydromorphone, hydroxyzine, metronidazole, miconazole, morphine, nafcillin, oxacillin, penicillin G potassium, phenytoin, piperacillin, rantidine, tobramycin

Patient/family education

• Advise patient to notify prescriber if sore throat, swollen lymph nodes, malaise, fever occur—may indicate presence of other infections
• Advise patient to report perioral tingling, numbness in extremities, and paresthesias; inf should be stopped and electrolytes should be requested
• Caution patient that serious drug interactions may occur if OTC products are ingested; check first with prescriber

• Inform patient that drug is not a cure, but will control symptoms
• Advise patient that ophth exams must be continued

Evaluation

Positive therapeutic outcome
• Improvement in CMV retinitis

fosinopril
(foss-in-o′pril)
Monopril
Func. class.: Antihypertensive
Chem. class.: Angiotensin-converting enzyme (ACE) inhibitor
Pregnancy category **D**

Action: Selectively suppresses renin-angiotensin-aldosterone system; inhibits ACE; prevents conversion of angiotensin I to angiotensin II; results in dilation of arterial, venous vessels

Therapeutic Outcome: Decreased B/P in hypertension

Uses: Hypertension, alone or in combination with thiazide diuretics

Dosage and routes

Adult: PO 10 mg qd initially, then 20-40 mg/day divided bid or qd

Available forms: Tab 10, 20 mg

Side effects/adverse reactions

CNS: *Insomnia, paresthesia, headache, dizziness,* fatigue, memory disturbance, tremor, mood change
CV: *Hypotension,* chest pain, palpitations, angina, orthostatic hypotension
GI: *Nausea,* constipation, vomiting, diarrhea
GU: ***Proteinuria,*** increased BUN, creatinine, decreased libido
HEMA: Decreased Hct, Hgb, ***eosinophilia, leukopenia, neutropenia***
INTEG: ***Angioedema,*** rash, flushing, sweating, photosensitivity, pruritus
META: Hyperkalemia
MS: Arthralgia, myalgia
RESP: Cough, sinusitis, dyspnea, ***bronchospasm***

Contraindications: Hypersensitivity to ACE inhibitors, pregnancy **D**, lactation, P children

Precautions: Impaired liver function, hypovolemia, blood dyscrasias, CHF, COPD, asthma, G elderly

Pharmacokinetics

Absorption	30% (PO)
Distribution	Crosses placenta
Metabolism	Liver—converted to fosinoprilate
Excretion	50% kidneys (metabolities), 50% feces
Half-life	12 hr—fosinoprilat

Pharmacodynamics

	PO
Onset	1 hr
Peak	2-6 hr
Duration	24 hr

Interactions

Drug/drug:

Individual drugs

Alcohol: ↑ hypotension (large amounts)
Allopurinol: ↑ hypersensitivity
Digoxin: ↑ serum levels
Hydralazine: ↑ toxicity
Indomethacin: ↓ antihypertensive effect
Lithium: ↑ serum levels
Prazosin: ↑ toxicity

Drug classifications

Adrenergic blockers: ↑ hypotension
Antacids: ↓ absorption
Antihypertensives: ↑ hypotension
Diuretics: ↑ hypotension
Diuretics, potassium sparing: ↑ toxicity
Ganglionic blockers: ↑ hypotension
Potassium supplements: ↑ toxicity
Sympathomimetics: ↑ toxicity

Lab test interferences

False positive: Urine acetone

NURSING CONSIDERATIONS

Assessment

- Monitor blood studies: neutrophils, decreased platelets
- Monitor B/P, check for orthostatic hypotension, syncope; if changes occur, dosage change may be required
- Monitor renal studies: protein, BUN, creatinine; watch for increased levels that may indicate nephrotic syndrome and renal failure; monitor renal symptoms: polyuria, oliguria, frequency, dysuria
- Establish baselines in renal, liver function tests before therapy begins
- Check potassium levels throughout treatment although hyperkalemia rarely occurs
- Check for edema in feet, legs daily, monitor weight daily
- Assess for allergic reactions: rash, fever, pruritus, urticaria; drug should be discontinued if antihistamines fail to help

Associated nursing diagnoses

✓ Cardiac output, decreased (uses)
✓ Injury, risk for (side effects)
✓ Knowledge deficit (teaching)
✓ Noncompliance (teaching)

Implementation

PO route

- Store in air-tight container at 86° F (30° C) or less
- Severe hypotension may occur after 1st dose of this medication; ↓ hypotension may be prevented by reducing or discontinuing diuretic therapy 3 days before beginning benzapril therapy

Patient/family education

- Advise patient not to discontinue drug abruptly—warn patient to tell all persons associated with his care
- Teach patient not to use OTC products (cough, cold, allergy) unless directed by prescriber because serious side effects can occur; xanthines such as coffee, tea, chocolate, cola can prevent action of drug
- Teach patient the importance of complying with dosage schedule, even if feeling better; to continue with medical regimen to decrease B/P: exercise,

smoking cessation, decreasing stress, diet modifications

- Emphasize the need to rise slowly to sitting or standing position to minimize orthostatic hypotension; not to exercise in hot weather or increased hypotension can occur
- Teach patient to notify prescriber of mouth sores, sore throat, fever, swelling of hands or feet, irregular heartbeat, chest pain, coughing, shortness of breath
- Instruct patient to report excessive perspiration, dehydration, vomiting, diarrhea; may lead to fall in B/P
- Caution patient that drug may cause dizziness, fainting, light-headedness; may occur during 1st few days of therapy; to avoid activities that may be hazardous
- Teach patient how to take B/P, and normal readings for age group

Evaluation

Positive therapeutic outcome

- Decreased B/P in hypertension

Treatment of overdose:

0.9% NaCl **IV** inf, hemodialysis

furosemide 🗝

(fur-oh'se-mide)

Apo-Furosemide ✦, Fumide, Furomide M.D., Furosemide, Furoside, Lasix, Lasix Special ✦, Luramide, Myrosemide, Novosemide ✦, Uritol ✦

Func. class.: Loop diuretic
Chem. class.: Sulfonamide derivative

Pregnancy category **C**

Action: Acts on the ascending loop of Henle in the kidney, inhibiting the reabsorption of the electrolytes sodium and chloride, causing excretion of sodium, calcium, magnesium, chloride, water, and some potassium; decreases reabsorption of sodium and chloride and increases the excretion of potassium in the distal tubule of the kidney; responsible for slight antihypertensive effect and peripheral vasodilation.

➔ **Therapeutic Outcome:** Decreased edema in lung tissue, peripherally; decreased B/P

Uses: Edema in congestive heart failure, nephrotic syndrome, ascites, caused by hepatic disease, hepatic cirrhosis; may be used alone or as adjunct with antihypertensives such as spironolatone, triamterene; should not be used with ethacrynic acid

Investigational uses: Hypercalcemia in malignancy

Dosage and routes

Adult: PO 20-80 mg/day in AM, may give another dose in 6 hrs, up to 600 mg/day; IM/**IV** 20-40 mg, increased by 20 mg q2h until desired response

P *Child:* PO/IM/**IV** 2 mg/kg, may increase by 1-2 mg/kg/ q6-8h up to 6 mg/kg

Pulmonary edema

Adult: **IV** 40 mg given over several min, repeated in 1 hr; increase to 80 mg if needed

Available forms: Tab 20, 40, 80 mg; oral sol 10 mg/ml; inj IM, **IV** 10 mg/ml

Side effects/adverse reactions

CNS: Headache, fatigue, weakness, vertigo, paresthesias

CV: Orthostatic hypotension, chest pain, ECG changes, ***circulatory collapse***

ELECT: Hypokalemia, hypochloremic alkalosis, hypomagnesemia, hyperuricania, hypocalcemia, hyponatremia, metabolic alkalosis

EENT: ***Loss of hearing,*** ear pain, tinnitus, blurred vision

GI: Nausea, diarrhea, dry mouth, vomiting, anorexia, cramps, oral or gastric irritations, pancreatitis

GU: Polyuria, ***renal failure,*** *glycosuria*

HEMA: ***Thrombocytopenia, agranulocytosis, leukopenia neutropenia, anemia***

INTEG: Rash, pruritus, prurpura, ***Stevens-Johnsons syndrome,*** sweating, photosensitivity, uticaria

MS: Cramps, stiffness

Contraindications: Hypersensitivity to sulfonamides, anuria, P hypovolemia, infants, lactation, electrolyte depletion

Precautions: Diabetes mellitus, dehydration, severe renal disease, pregnancy **C**

Pharmacokinetics

	PO
Absorption	GI tract (60%-70%)
	PO/IM/IV
Distribution	Crosses placenta
Metabolism	Liver (30%-40%)
Excretion	Breast milk, urine, feces
Half-life	½-1 hr

Pharmacodynamics

	PO	IM	IV
Onset	1 hr	½ hr	5 mins
Peak	1-2 hrs	Unknown	½ hr
Duration	6-8 hrs	4-8 hrs	2 hrs

Interactions

Drug/drug:

Individual drugs

Alcohol: ↑ orthostatic hypotension

Cisplatin: ↑ risk of ototoxicity

Ethacrynic acid: Combination with furosemide may cause ↑ chance of dysrhythmias (do not use together)

Indomethacin: ↑ diuretic and antihypertives of furosemide

Lithium: ↓ renal clearance, causing increased toxicity

Phenytoin: ↓ diuretic effect caused by ↓ absorption

Succinylcholine: Action of succinylcholine is ↑ by low doses and ↓ by high doses of furosemide

Theophylline: May ↑ or ↓ the effect of theophylline

Vancomycin: ↑ risk of ototoxicity

Drug classifications

Adrenergic blockers: ↑ effects
Aminoglycosides: ↑ ototoxicity, nephrotoxicity
Anticoagulants: ↑ anticoagulant effect caused by ↓ plasma protein binding
Antidiabetics: ↓ hypoglycemic effect
Antihypertensives: ↑ antihypertensive effect
Barbiturates: ↑ orthostatic hypotension
Cephalosporins: ↑ nephrotoxicity
Chloral hydrate: ↑ sweating, flushing when given with **IV** furosemide
Clofibrate: ↑ furosemide effects
Corticosteroids: ↑ potassium loss caused by potassium depletion effects of both drugs
Digitalis glycosides: ↑ potassium and magnesium loss with relating dysrhythmias
Ganglionic blockers: ↑ effect
Narcotics: ↑ orthostatic hypotension
Salicylates: ↑ risk of salicylate toxicity caused by ↓ renal excretion

Drug/food:

Food: ↓ diuresis

NURSING CONSIDERATIONS

Assessment

- Assess patient for tinnitus, hearing loss, ear pain. Periodic testing of hearing is needed when high doses of this drug are given by **IV** route
- Monitor for renal, cardiac, neurologic, GI, pulmonary manifestations of hypokalemia: acidic urine, reduced urine osmolality, nocturia, polyuria and polydipsia; hypotension, broad T-wave, U-wave, ectopy, tachycardia, weak pulse; muscle weakness, altered LOC, drowsiness, apathy, lethargy, confusion, depression; anorexia, nausea, cramps, constipation, distension, paralyticileus; hypoventilation, respiratory muscle weakness
- Monitor for CNS, GI, cardiovascular, integumentary, neurologic manifestations of hypocalcemia: personality changes, anxiety, disturbances, depression and psychosis; nausea, vomiting, constipation, abdominal pain from muscle spasm; decreased contractility, decreased cardiac output, hypotension, lengthened ST segment, prolonged QT interval; scaling eczema, alopecia, hyperpigmentation; tetany, muscle twitching, cramping grimacing, seizure, altered deep tendon reflexes, spasm
- Monitor for CNS, neuromuscular, GI, cardiac manifestations of hypomagnesemia, agitation; muscle twitching, paresthesias, hyperactive reflexes, positive Babinski reflex, dysphagia, nystagmus seizures, tetnany; nausea, vomiting, diarrhea, anorexia, abdominal distention; ectopy, tachycardia, broad, flat or inverted T-waves, depressed ST segment, prolonged OT, decreased cardiac output, hypotension
- Monitor for CV, GI, neurologic manifestations of hyponatremia: ↑ B/P, cold, clammy skin, hypovolemia or hypervolemia; anorexia, nausea, vomiting, diarrhea, abdominal cramps; lethargy,

F

increased ICP, confusion headache, seizures, coma, fatigue, tremors, hyperreflexia
- Monitor for neurologic, respiratory manifestations of hyperchloremia: weakness, lethargy, coma; deep rapid breathing
- Assess fluid volume status: I&O ratios and record, count or weigh diapers as appropriate, weight, distended red veins, crackles in lung, color, quality and sp. gr. of urine, skin turgor, adequacy of pulses, moist mucous membranes, bilateral lung sounds, peripheral pitting edema. Dehydration symptoms of decreasing output, thirst, hypotension, dry mouth and mucous membranes should be reported
- Monitor electrolytes: potassium, sodium, calcium, magnesium; also include BUN, blood pH, ABGs, uric acid, CBC, blood sugar
- Assess B/P before and during therapy lying, standing and sitting as appropriate; orthostatic hypotension can occur rapidly

Associated nursing diagnoses

✓ Fluid volume deficit (side effects)
✓ Fluid volume excess (uses)
✓ Knowledge deficit (teaching)

Implementation

- Give in AM to avoid interference with sleep
- Potassium replacement if potassium level is <3.0 whole, or use oral sol slightly, drug may be crushed if patient is unable to swallow

PO route
- With food, if nausea occurs, absorption may be reduced

IV **IV route**
- Do not use sol that is yellow, or has a precipitate, or crystals

Implementation

IV **Direct IV**
- Give undiluted through y-tube on 3-way stopcock; give 20 mg or less/min.

Int Inf
- May be added to NS, D_5W, $D_{10}W$, $D_{20}W$. Invert sugar 10% in electrolyte #1, LR, Sodium lactate y_6m, use within 24 hr to assure compatibility; give through y-tube or 3 way stopcock; give at 4 mg/min or less, use inf pump

Syringe incompatibilities:

Doxapram, doxorubicin, droperidol, metaclopramide, milrinone

Y-site incompatibilities:

Amsacrine, bleomycin, doxorubicin, droperidol, esmolol HCl, fluconazole, gentamicin, idarubicin, metoclopramide, milrinone, netilmicin, ondansetron, quinidine, vinblastine, vincristine

Additive incompatibilities:

Bleomycin, dobutamine, gentamicin, chlorpromazine, diazepam, erythromycin lactobionate, isoproterenol, meperidine, metoclopramide, netilmicin, opium alkaloids prochlorperazine, tetracycline

Y-site compatibilities:

Amikacin sulfate, cisplatin, cyclophosphamide, dobuternine, fumotidine, fludarabine, fluorouracil, foscarnet, heparin, hydrocortisone dintrate, sodium succinate, kanamycin, leucovorin, methotrexate, mitomycin, potassium chloride, sargramostim, tobramycin, tolazoline, vitamin B complex with C

Additive compatibilities:

Amikacin, aminophylline, amiodarone, ampicillin, atropine, flumetanide, calcium gluconate, cefumandole, cefuroxime, cimetidine, cloxacillin, digoxin, epinephrine, heparin, isosorbide, kanamycin, lidocaine, morphine, nitroglycerin, tobramycin, verapamil, ranitidine, sodium bicarbonate

Patient/family education

General

- Teach patient to take the medication early in the day to prevent nocturia
- Instruct the patient to take with food or milk if GI symptoms of nausea and anorexia occur
- Teach patient to maintain a record of weight on a weekly basis and notify physician of weight loss of >5 lbs.
- Caution the patient that this drug causes a loss of potassium, that food rich in potassium should be added to the diet; refer to a dietician for assistance in planning
- Caution the patient not to exercise in hot weather or stand for prolonged periods of time because orthostatic hypotension will be enhanced
- Advise patient to wear protective clothing and sunscreen to prevent photosensitivity
- Teach patient not to use alcohol or any over-the-counter medications without physician's approval, serious drug reactions may occur
- Emphasize the need to contact physician immediately if muscle cramps, weakness, nausea, dizziness or numbness occurs
- Teach patient to take and record their own B/P and pulse
- Caution the patient that orthostatic hypotension may occur and patient should rise slowly from sitting or reclining positions and lie down if dizziness occurs
- Teach patient to continue taking medication even if feeling better, this drug controls symptoms but does not cure the condition
- Advise the patient with hypertension to continue other medical treatment (exercise, weight loss, relaxation techniques, cessation of smoking)

Evaluation

Positive therapeutic outcome

- Decreased edema
- Decreased B/P
- Lowered calcium level in malignancy
- Increased diuresis

F

gallamine
(gal'a-meen)
Flaxedil
Func. class.: Neuromuscular blocker (nondepolarizing)
Pregnancy category **C**

Action: Inhibits transmission of nerve impulses by binding with cholinergic receptor sites, antagonizing action of acetylcholine; no analgesic response

Therapeutic Outcome: Paralysis of all skeletal muscles

Uses: Facilitation of endotracheal intubation, skeletal muscle relaxation during mechanical ventilation, surgery, or general anesthesia

Dosage and routes

P *Adult and child >1 mo:* **IV** 1 mg/kg, not to exceed 100 mg, then 0.5-1 mg/kg q30-40 min

P *Child <1 mo, >5 kg:* **IV** 0.25-0.75 mg/kg, then 0.01-0.05 mg/kg q30-40 min

Available forms: Inj 20 mg/ml

Side effects/adverse reactions

CNS: Malignant hyperthermia
CV: Bradycardia, tachycardia, increased, decreased B/P
EENT: Increased secretions
GI: Decreased motility
INTEG: Rash, flushing, pruritus, urticaria
RESP: Prolonged apnea, bronchospasm, cyanosis, respiratory depression

Contraindications: Hypersensitivity to iodides

Precautions: Pregnancy **C**, thyroid disease, collagen disease, cardiac disease, lactation, P children <2 yr, electrolyte imbalances, dehydration, neuromuscular disease (myasthenia gravis), respiratory disease, renal disease

Pharmacokinetics

Absorption	Complete bioavailability (IV)
Distribution	Extracellular space, crosses placenta
Metabolism	Plasma
Excretion	Kidneys—unchanged
Half-life	2½ hr

Pharmacodynamics

	IV
Onset	2 min
Peak	5 min
Duration	30 min

Interactions

Drug/drug:

Individual drugs
Clindamycin: ↑ paralysis, length, and intensity
Colistin: ↑ paralysis, length, and intensity
Lidocaine: ↑ paralysis, length, and intensity
Lithium: ↑ paralysis, length, and intensity
Magnesium: ↑ paralysis, length, and intensity
Polymyxin B: ↑ paralysis, length, and intensity
Procainamide: ↑ paralysis, length, and intensity
Quinidine: ↑ paralysis, length, and intensity
Succinylcholine: ↑ paralysis, length, and intensity

Drug classifications

Aminoglycosides: ↑ paralysis, length, and intensity

Beta blockers: ↑ paralysis, length, and intensity

Diuretics, potassium-losing: ↑ paralysis, length, and intensity

General anesthetics: ↑ paralysis, length, and intensity

NURSING CONSIDERATIONS

Assessment

- Monitor for electrolyte imbalances (potassium, magnesium), before drug is used; electrolyte imbalances may lead to increased action of this drug
- Monitor vital signs (B/P, pulse, respirations, airway) until fully recovered; rate, depth, pattern of respirations, strength of hand grip; patient should be intubated before use
- Monitor recovery: decreased paralysis of face, diaphragm, leg, arm, rest of body; residual weakness and respiratory problems may occur during recovery period
- Monitor allergic reactions: rash, fever, respiratory distress, pruritus; if present, drug should be discontinued

Associated nursing diagnoses

✓ Breathing pattern, ineffective (uses)

✓ Communication, impaired verbal (adverse reactions)

✓ Fear (adverse reactions)

✓ Knowledge deficit (teaching)

Implementation

IV route

- Use peripheral nerve stimulator by anesthesiologist to determine neuromuscular blockade; deep tendon reflexes should be monitored during extended use
- Give **IV** undiluted by direct **IV** over 1 min, or diluted in 10-50 ml of D_5W, ½ NaCl or NS and give as an infusion at prescribed rate (only by qualified person, usually an anesthesiologist); do not administer IM
- Further dilute in D_5W, 0.9% NaCl, D_5/0.9% NaCl q15-25 min (intermittent infusion)
- Maintenance dose is given q20-45 min after 1st dose (continuous infusion); titrate to patient response
- Store in light-resistant area

Patient/family education

- Provide reassurance if communication is difficult during recovery from neuromuscular blockade
- Provide explanation regarding all procedures or treatments; patient will remain conscious if anesthetic is not given also

Evaluation

Positive therapeutic outcome

- Paralysis of jaw, eyelid, head, neck, rest of body as evaluated by peripheral nerve stimulator

Treatment of overdose:

Administer edrophonium or neostigmine, atropine—monitor VS; may require mechanical ventilation

gallium nitrate
(gal'ee-yum nye-trate)
Ganite
Func. class.: Electrolyte modifier
Chem. class.: Hypocalcemic drug
Pregnancy category **C**

Action: Lowers serum calcium levels by inhibiting calcium resorption from bone

➔ **Therapeutic Outcome:** Decrease calcium level to 5-9 mg/dl

Uses: Cancer-related hypercalcemia

Dosage and routes
Adult: IV 100-200 mg/m^2 qd × 5 days; inf over 24 hr

Available forms: 25 mg/ml inj

Side effects/adverse reactions
CV: Tachycardia
EENT: Blurred vision, optic neuritis, hearing loss
GU: ***Nephrotoxicity,*** increased BUN, creatinine
HEMA: ***Anemia, leukopenia***
META: *Hypophosphatemia,* hypocalcemia, decreased serum bicarbonate

Contraindications: Hypersensitivity, severe renal disease

Precautions: Pregnancy **C**, P lactation, children, mild renal disease

Pharmacokinetics

Absorption	Completely absorbed (IV)
Distribution	Unknown
Metabolism	Unknown
Excretion	Kidneys (unchanged)
Half-life	Unknown

Pharmacodynamics

	IV
Onset	12-24 hr
Peak	Unknown
Duration	Unknown

Interactions
Drug/drug:
Amphotericin B: ↑ nephrotoxicity
Drug classifications
Aminoglycosides: ↑ nephrotoxicity

NURSING CONSIDERATIONS
Assessment
- Renal status: BUN, creatinine, urine output; if creatinine level is 2.5 mg/dl or more, drug should be discontinued
- Monitor calcium, phosphate, bicarbonate—all levels may be decreased and supplements of phosphate may be needed; calcium daily, phosphate 2-3 ×/wk
- Assess for hypercalcemia: nausea, vomiting, fatigue, weakness, thirst, dehydration, dysrhythmias, headache, confusion, coma, decreased reflexes
- For hypocalcemia: dysrhythmias, hypotension, paresthesia; twitching, colic, laryngospasm; hypercalcemia: poor coordination, myalgia, hypotonia, shortened ST segment and QT interval, prolonged PR inter-

val, cone-shaped T wave, sinus bradycardia; Trousseau's, Chvostek's sign: tremors, tetany, cramping, grimacing, seizures, altered deep tendon reflexes and spasms, personality changes including irritability, depression, psychosis
• Monitor for indications of hypophosphatemia: weakness, malaise, tremors, memory loss, inattention, confusion, decreased reflexes, aching bone pain, joint stiffness, rapid, shallow respiration, decreased tidal volume, nausea, vomiting, anorexia, portal hypertension

Associated nursing diagnoses

✓ Injury, risk for (uses)
✓ Knowledge deficit (teaching)

Implementation

IV route
• Provide adequate hydration with **IV** saline, 2 L/day during treatment; saline increases the extracellular calcium
• Give by continuous **IV** inf after dilution of dose/1 L 0.9% NaCl or D_5W, run over 24 hr, use inf pump
• Store solution for 48 hr at room temp or 1 wk in refrigerator

Patient/family education

• Instruct patient to follow dietary guidelines given by prescriber, including adequate calcium (dietary products, broccoli) and Vit D (fortified milk, grain products, fish oil)
• Explain purpose of drug and expected results

Evaluation

Positive therapeutic outcome
• Decreased serum calcium levels to 5-9 mg/dl

ganciclovir (DHPG)

(gan-sye'kloe-vir)
Cytovene
Func. class.: Antiviral
Chem. class.: Synthetic nucleoside analog
Pregnancy category **C**

Action: Inhibits replication of herpes viruses in vitro, in vivo by selective inhibition of the human CMV DNA polymerase and by direct incorporation into viral DNA

Therapeutic Outcome: Decreased proliferation of virus responsible for CMV retinitis

Uses: Cytomegalovirus (CMV) retinitis in immunocompromised persons, including those with AIDS, after indirect ophthalmoscopy confirms diagnosis

Dosage and routes

Induction treatment
Adult: **IV** 5 mg/kg given over 1 hr q12h × 2-3 wk

Maintenance treatment
Adult: **IV** inf 5 mg/kg given over 1 hr, qd × 7 days/wk; or 6 mg/kg qd × 5 days/wk; dosage must be reduced in renal impairment; Intravenous **IV** 200 μg every week

Prevention of CMV

Adult: **IV** 5 mg/kg q12h × 1-2 wks, then 5 mg/kg/day or 6 mg/kg × 5 day of each week

Available forms: Powder 500 mg/vial ganciclovir

Side effects/adverse reactions

CNS: *Fever,* chills, ***coma,*** confusion, abnormal thoughts, dizziness, bizarre dreams, headache, psychosis, tremors, somnolence, paresthesia

CV: Dysrhythmia, hypertension/hypotension

EENT: Retinal detachment in CMV retinitis

GI: *Abnormal LFTs,* nausea, vomiting, anorexia, diarrhea, abdominal pain, ***hemorrhage***

GU: ***Hematuria,*** increased creatinine, BUN

HEMA: ***Granulocytopenia, thrombocytopenia, irreversible neutropenia, anemia, eosinophilia***

INTEG: Rash, alopecia, pruritus, urticaria, pain at site, phlebitis

RESP: Dyspnea

Contraindications: Hypersensitivity to acyclovir or ganciclovir

Precautions: Preexisting cytopenias, renal function impairment pregnancy **C**, lactation, children <6 mo, elderly, platelet count <25,000/mm

Pharmacokinetics

Absorption	Completely absorbed (IV)
Distribution	Crosses blood-brain barrier, CSF
Metabolism	Not metabolized
Excretion	Kidneys (90%) unchanged, breast milk
Half-life	3 hr

Pharmacodynamics

	IV
Onset	Unknown
Peak	Unknown
Duration	Unknown

Interactions

Drug/drug:

Individual drugs

Imipemen with cilastin: ↑ chance of seizures

Probenecid: ↑ toxicity

Zidovudine: ↑ bone marrow depression

Radiation: ↑ bone marrow depression

Drug classifications

Antineoplastics: ↑ bone marrow depression

NURSING CONSIDERATIONS

Assessment

- Culture should be done before treatment with ganciclovir is initiated. Cultures of blood, urine, and throat may all be taken; CMV is not confirmed by this method. The diagnosis is made by an ophth exam
- Assess kidney, liver function; increased hemopoietic studies: BUN, serum creatinine, AST creatinine clearance (SGOT), ALT (SGPT), A-G ratio, baseline, and drip treatment. Blood counts should be done q2wk;

watch for decreasing granulocytes, Hgb; if low, therapy may have to be discontinued and restarted after hematologic recovery; blood transfusions may be required
• Assess for GI symptoms: severe nausea, vomiting, diarrhea; severe symptoms may necessitate discontinuing drug
• Monitor electrolytes and minerals: calcium, phosphorous, magnesium, sodium, potassium; watch closely for tetany during 1st administration
• Assess for symptoms of blood dyscrasias (anemia, granulocytopenia); brusing, fatigue, bleeding, poor healing
• Assess for symptoms of allergic reactions: flushing, rash, urticaria, pruritus
• Monitor for leukopenia/neutropenia/thrombocytopenia: WBCs, platelets q2day during 2 ×/day dosing and q1wk thereafter; check for leukopenia with qd WBC count in patients with prior leukopenia with other nucleoside analogs or for whom leukopenia counts are <1000 cells/mm^3 at start of treatment
• Monitor serum creatinine or creatine clearance at least q2wk

Associated nursing diagnoses

- ✓ Infection, risk for (uses)
- ✓ Injury, risk for (uses, adverse reactions)
- ✓ Knowledge deficit (teaching)

Implementation

IV route
• Medicine should be mixed under strict aseptic conditions using gloves, gown, and mask, and using precautions for antineoplastics
• Administer **IV** after diluting 500 mg/10 ml sterile water for inj (50 mg/ml); shake; further dilute in 100 ml D_5W, 0.9% NaCl, LR and run over 1 hr; use inf pump
• Give slowly; do not give by bolus **IV**, IM, SC inj
• Use diluted sol within 12 hr, do not refrigerate or freeze; do not use sol with particulate matter or discoloration, fludarabine, sargramostin

Y-site incompatibilities:

Amsacrine, fludarabine, foscarnet, ondansetron, sargramostin, vinorelbine

Y-site compatibilities:

Enalaprilat, fluconazole, melphalan, paclitaxel

Patient/family education

• Advise patient to notify prescriber if sore throat, swollen lymph nodes, malaise, fever occur—may indicate other infections
• Advise patient to report perioral tingling, numbness in extremities, and paresthesias
• Caution patient that serious drug interactions may occur if OTC products are ingested; check first with prescriber
• Inform patient that drug is not a cure, but will control symptoms
• Advise patient that regular ophth exams must be continued
• Inform patient that major toxicities may necessitate discontinuing drug
• Instruct patient to use contraception during treatment

G

and that infertility may occur; men should use barrier contraception for 90 days after treatment

Evaluation

Positive therapeutic outcome
- Decreased symptoms of CMV

Treatment of overdose:
Discontinue drug, use hemodialysis, and increase hydration

gemfibrozil
(gem-fye'broe-zil)
Lopid
Func. class.: Antilipemic
Chem. class.: Aryloxisobutyric acid derivative
Pregnancy category B

Action: Inhibits biosynthesis of VLDL, LDL, which are responsible for cholesterol development

➡ Therapeutic Outcome: Decreased cholesterol levels and low-density lipoproteins, decreased pruritus

Uses: Type III, IV, V hyperlipidemia as adjunct with diet therapy

Dosage and routes
Adult: PO 1200 mg in divided doses bid 30 min ac

Available forms: Cap 300, 600 mg

Side effects/adverse reactions
CNS: Dizziness, blurred vision
GI: Nausea, vomiting, dyspepsia, diarrhea, abdominal pain
HEMA: Leukopenia, anemia, eosinophilia
INTEG: Rash, urticaria, pruritus

Contraindications: Severe hepatic disease, preexisting gallbladder disease, severe renal disease, primary biliary cirrhosis, hypersensitivity

Precautions: Monitor hematologic and hepatic function, pregnancy **B**, lactation

Pharmacokinetics

Absorption	Well absorbed (PO)
Distribution	Unknown, plasma protein binding >90%
Metabolism	Liver—minimal
Excretion	Kidney—unchanged (70%), feces (6%)
Half-life	1½ hr

Pharmacodynamics

	PO
Onset	1-2 hr
Peak	1-2 hr
Duration	2-4 months

Interactions
Drug/drug:

Drug classifications
Anticoagulants, oral: ↑ effect of anticoagulants
Diuretics, thiazide: ↓ action of gemfibrozil
Estrogens: ↓ action of gemifibrozil

Lab test interferences

Increase: Liver function studies, CPK, BSP, thymol turbidity, glucose
Decrease: Hgb, Hct, WBC

NURSING CONSIDERATIONS

Assessment

- Assess nutrition: fat, protein, carbohydrates—nutritional analysis should be performed by dietitian before treatment is initiated
- Monitor bowel pattern daily; diarrhea may be a problem
- Monitor triglycerides, cholesterol baseline and throughout treatment. LDL and VLDL should be watched closely if increased drug should be discontinued

Associated nursing diagnoses

✓ Diarrhea (adverse reactions)
✓ Knowledge deficit (teaching)
✓ Noncompliance (teaching)

Implementation

PO route

- Give 30 min before AM and PM meals

Patient/family education

- Inform patient that compliance is needed for positive results to occur; not to double doses
- Caution patient to decrease risk factors: high-fat diet, smoking, alcohol consumption, lack of exercise
- Advise patient to notify health care prescriber if the GI symptoms of diarrhea, abdominal or epigastric pain, nausea, vomiting occur; or if chills, fever, sore throat, occur

Evaluation

Positive therapeutic outcome

- Decreased cholesterol levels, serum triglyceride and improved ratio with high-density lipoproteins (HDLs)

gentamicin

(jen-ta-mye'sin)

Alcomicin ♣, Apogen, Cidomycin ♣, Garamycin, Garamycin Intrathecal, Garamycin IV Piggyback, Garamycin Pediatric, Gentamicin Sulfate, gentamicin sulfate IV Piggyback, Jenamicin, Pediatric Gentamicin Sulfate

Func. class.: Antibiotic
Chem. class.: Aminoglycoside

Pregnancy category **C**

Action: Interferes with protein synthesis in bacterial cell by binding to ribosomal subunit, causing misreading of genetic code; inaccurate peptide sequence forms in protein chain, causing bacterial death

➡ **Therapeutic Outcome:** Bactericidal effects for the following organisms *P. aeruginosa, Proteus, Klebsiella, Serratia, E. coli, Enterobacter, Citrobacter, Staphylococcus, Shigella, Salmonella*

Uses: Severe systemic infections of CNS; respiratory, GI, and urinary tracts; bone; skin; soft tissues caused by susceptible strains

Dosage and routes

Severe systemic infections

Adult: **IV** inf 3-5 mg/kg/day in 3 divided doses q8h; dilute in 50-200 ml NS or D_5W given over 30 min-2 hr; IM 3 mg/kg/day in divided doses q8h

Adult: Intrathec 4-8 mg qd

P *Child:* **IV**/IM 2-2.5 mg/kg q8h

P *Neonates and infants:* **IV**/IM 2.5 mg/kg q8h

P *Neonates <1 wk:* 2.5 mg/kg q12h

P *Infants and child >3 mo:* Intrathec 1-2 mg qd

Dental/respiratory procedures/GI/GU surgery (prophylaxis endocarditis)

Adult: IM 1.5 mg/kg 1/2-1 hr before procedure with ampicillin

Top

P *Adult, child:* Apply to cleansed area 3-4 times daily

Ophth

P *Adult, child:* 1-2 drops of ophth sol q2-4h or ophth oint 2-3 times daily

P *Child:* IM 2.5 mg/kg ½-1 hr before procedure with ampicillin

Available forms: Inj 10, 40, 60, 80, 100 mg; intrathec 2 mg/ml; ophth sol 0.3%, ophth oint 0.3%, top oint 0.1%, top cream 0.1%

Side effects/adverse reactions

CNS: Confusion, depression, numbness, tremors, ***convulsions,*** muscle twitching, ***neurotoxicity,*** dizziness, vertigo

CV: Hypotension, hypertension, palpitations

EENT: Ototoxicity, deafness, visual disturbances, tinnitus

GI: Nausea, vomiting, anorexia, increased ALT (SGPT), AST (SGOT), bilirubin, hepatomegaly, ***hepatic necrosis,*** splenomegaly

GU: Oliguria, hematuria, renal damage, azotemia, renal failure, nephrotoxicity

HEMA: Agranulocytosis, thrombocytopenia, leukopenia, eosinophilia, anemia

INTEG: Rash, burning, urticaria, dermatitis, alopecia

Contraindications: Severe renal disease, hypersensitivity

P **Precautions:** Neonates, mild renal disease, pregnancy **C**, hearing deficits, myasthenia G gravis, lactation, elderly, Parkinson's disease

Pharmacokinetics

Absorption	Well absorbed (IM)
Distribution	Distributed in extracellular fluids, poorly distributed in CSF; crosses placenta
Metabolism	Liver, minimal
Excretion	Mostly unchanged (79%) kidneys
Half-life	1-3 hr, increased in renal disease

Pharmacodynamics

	IM	IV
Onset	Rapid	Rapid
Peak	½-1½ hr	Infusion's end

Interactions

Drug/drug:

Individual drugs

Amphotericin B: ↑ ototoxicity, neurotoxicity, nephrotoxicity
Cisplatin: ↑ ototoxicity, neurotoxicity, nephrotoxicity
Ethacrynic acid: ↑ ototoxicity, neurotoxicity, nephrotoxicity
Furosemide: ↑ ototoxicity, neurotoxicity, nephrotoxicity
Mannitol: ↑ ototoxicity, neurotoxicity, nephrotoxicity
Methoxyflurane: ↑ ototoxicity, neurotoxicity, nephrotoxicity
Polymyxin: ↑ ototoxicity, neurotoxicity, nephrotoxicity
Succinylcholine: ↑ neuromuscular blockade, respiratory depression
Vancomycin: ↑ ototoxicity, neurotoxicity, nephrotoxicity

Drug classifications

Anesthetics: ↑ neuromuscular blockade, respiratory depression
Aminoglycosides: ↑ otoxicity, neurotoxicity
Nondepolarizing neuromuscular blockers: ↑ neuromuscular blockade, respiratory depression

NURSING CONSIDERATIONS

Assessment

- Assess patient for previous sensitivity reaction
- Assess patient for signs and symptoms of infection including characteristics of wounds, sputum, urine, stool, WBC >10,000, fever. Obtain baseline information and during treatment.
- Complete culture and sensitivity before beginning drug therapy. This will ensure that correct treatment has been initiated.
- Assess for allergic reactions: rash, urticaria, pruritus, chills, fever, joint pain may occur a few days after therapy begins.
- Identify urine output; if decreasing, notify prescriber (may indicate nephrotoxicity). Also, increase BUN, creatinine, urine CrCl <80 ml/min
- Monitor blood studies: AST (SGOT), ALT (SGPT), CBC, Hct, bilirubin, LDH, alk phosphatase, Coombs' test monthly if patient is on long-term therapy
- Monitor electrolytes: potassium, sodium, chloride monthly if patient is on long-term therapy
- Monitor for bleeding: ecchymosis, bleeding gums, hematuria; assess stool guaiac daily if on long-term therapy
- Assess for overgrowth of infection: perineal itching, fever, malaise, redness, pain, swelling, drainage, rash, diarrhea, change in cough, sputum
- Obtain weight before treatment; calculation of dosage is usually based on ideal body weight, but may be calculated on actual body weight
- Monitor I&O ratio; urinalysis daily for proteinuria, cells, casts; report sudden change in urine output
- Monitor VS during inf, watch for hypotension, change in pulse

G

• Assess **IV** site for thrombophlebitis including pain, redness, swelling q30 min, change site if needed; apply warm compresses to discontinued site
• Obtain serum peak, drawn at 30-60 min after **IV** inf or 60 min after IM inj, trough level drawn just before next dose; blood level should be 2-4 times bacteriostatic level
• Assess urine pH if drug is used for UTI; urine should be kept alkaline
• Assess for deafness by audiometric testing, ringing, roaring in ears, vertigo; assess hearing before, during, after treatment
• Assess for dehydration: high sp gr, decrease in skin turgor, dry mucous membranes, dark urine

Associated nursing diagnoses

✓ Infection, Risk for (uses)
✓ Diarrhea (side effects)
✓ Knowledge deficit (teaching)
✓ Noncompliance (teaching)
✓ Injury, risk for (side effects)

Implementation

IM route
• Give deeply in large muscle mass; rotate sites
Top route
• Wash hands, wear gloves, clean skin before applying
IV **IV route**
• Give in even doses around the clock. Drug must be given for 10-14 days to ensure organism death and prevent superimposed infection.
• Store in tight container

Y-site incompatibilities:

Idarubicin, indomethacin, zidovudine

Y-site compatibilities:

Acyclovir, aldesleukin, atracurium, cyclophosphamide, enalaprilat, esmolol, famotidine, fluconazole, fludarabine, foscarnet, hydromorphone, insulin, labetalol, hydromorphone, magnesium sulfate, meperidine, morphine, multivitamins, ondansetron, pancuronium, vecuronium, vitamin B with C, zidovudine

Additive compatibility:

Ciprofloxacin

Patient/family education

• Teach patient to report sore throat, bruising, bleeding, joint pain—may indicate blood dyscrasias (rare)
• Advise patient to contact prescriber if vaginal itching, loose, foul-smelling stools, furry tongue occur—may indicate superimposed infection

Evaluation

Positive therapeutic outcome
• Absence of signs/symptoms of infection (WBC <10,000, temp WNL, absence of red, draining wounds)
• Reported improvement in symptoms of infection

Treatment of overdose:

Withdraw drug, hemodialysis

glutethimide

(gloo-teth'i-mide)

glutethimide, Doriglute

Func. class.: Sedative-hypnotic

Chem. class.: Piperidine derivative

Pregnancy category **C**

Controlled substance schedule **II** (USA), schedule **F** (Canada)

Action: Depresses activity in brain cells primarily in reticular activating system in brainstem; also selectively depresses neurons in posterior hypothalamus, limbic structures; pronounced anticholinergic activity; suppresses REM sleep

➔ **Therapeutic Outcome:** Ability to sleep, relaxation

Uses: Insomnia

Dosage and routes

Adult: PO 250-500 mg hs; may repeat dose >4 hr before usual awakening, not to exceed 1 g

Available forms: Tab 500 mg

Side effects/adverse reactions

CNS: Residual sedation, dizziness, ataxia, stimulation, headache, hangover

EENT: Dry mouth, blurred vision

GI: Nausea, vomiting, hiccups, diarrhea, jaundice

GU: Porphyria

HEMA: ***Thrombocytopenia, aplastic anemia, leukopenia, megaloblastic anemia***

INTEG: Rash, urticaria, purpura, ***exfoliative dermatitis (rare)***

Contraindications: Hypersensitivity to this drug or piperidine derivatives, severe pain, severe renal disease, porphyria

Precautions: Depression, suicidal individuals, drug abuse, cardiac dysrhythmias, narrow-angle glaucoma, prostatic hypertrophy, stenosed peptic ulcer, pyloroduodenal/bladder neck obstruction, pregnancy **C**

Pharmacokinetics

Absorption	Erratically absorbed (PO)
Distribution	Crosses placenta to fatty tissue
Metabolism	Liver (95%)
Excretion	Kidneys, breast milk
Half-life	10-12 hr

Pharmacodynamics

	PO
Onset	½ hr
Peak	1-2 hr
Duration	4-8 hr

Interactions

Drug/drug:

Individual drugs

Alcohol: ↑ CNS depression

Fluoxetine: ↑ action

Propoxyphene: ↑ action

Drug classifications

Analgesics, opioid: ↑ CNS depression

Anticoagulants, oral: ↓ action of anticoagulants

Antidepressants, tricyclic: ↑ CNS depression
Antihistamines: ↑ CNS depression
Sedative/hypnotics: ↑ CNS depression

Lab test interferences

Interferences: Urinary 17-OHCS

NURSING CONSIDERATIONS

Assessment

- Assess patient's sleep pattern and note physical (sleep apnea, obstructed airway, pain/discomfort, urinary frequency) and psychologic (fear, anxiety) circumstances that interrupt sleep
- Assess patient's bedtime routine, pre-sleep cues/props
- Assess potential for abuse; this drug may lend to physical and psychologic dependency; amount of drug should be limited
- Monitor blood studies: Hct, Hgb, RBCs, serum folate (if on long-term therapy) protime in patients receiving anticoagulants because action of anticoagulant may be increased
- Assess for blood dyscrasias: fever, sore throat, bruising, rash, jaundice, epistaxis (rare)
- Assess previous history of substance abuse, cardiac disease or gastritis

Associated nursing diagnoses

✓ Sleep pattern disturbance (uses)
✓ Knowledge deficit (teaching)
✓ Noncompliance (teaching)

Implementation

General

- Regulate environmental stimuli (light, noise, temp, remove foods and fluids that interfere with sleep
- Place side rails up after giving medication for hypnotic; remove cigarettes/matches from patient's environment to prevent fires

PO route

- Give ½-1 hr before hs for sleeplessness; several hr before patient is to rise (to avoid hangover)
- Store in tight container in cool environment

Patient/family education

- Caution patient to avoid driving or other activities requiring alertness; to avoid alcohol ingestion or CNS depressants—serious CNS depression may result plus tachycardia, flushing, headache, hypotension
- Inform patient not to discontinue medication quickly after long-term use; drug should be tapered over 1-2 wk; that effects may take 2 nights for benefits to be noticed; withdrawal symptoms include tremors, anxiety, hallucinations, delirium
- Inform patient of alternate measures to improve sleep (reading, exercise several hr before hs, warm bath, warm milk, TV, self-hypnosis, deep breathing)
- Teach patient that hangover G is common in elderly but less common than with barbiturates
- Caution patient to watch for blood dyscrasias: fever, sore

throat, bruising rash, jaundice (rare)
- Teach patient to watch for allergic reaction: rash; discontinue drug if rash occurs

Evaluation

Positive therapeutic outcome
- Ability to sleep at night
- Decreased amount of early morning awakenings

Treatment of overdose: Lavage, activated charcoal; monitor electrolytes, vital signs

glycerin

(gli'ser-in)

Fleet Babylax, glycerin USP, Glycerol, Ophthalgan, Osmoglyn, Sani-Supp

Func. class.: Laxative, hyperosmotic, antiglaucoma agent

Chem. class.: Trihydric alcohol

Pregnancy category **C**

Action: Increases osmotic pressure by drawing fluid into colon lumen from extravascular spaces to intravascular

➡ **Therapeutic Outcome:** Absence of constipation, intraocular pressure, intracranial pressure, absence of edema in the cornea

Uses: Constipation, intraocular pressure in glaucoma; intracranial pressure, edema in the superficial layers of the cornea

Dosage and routes

P *Adult and child >6 yr:* Rec supp 3 g; enema 5-15 ml

P *Child <6 yr:* Rec supp 1-1.5 g; enema 2-5 ml

Corneal edema

Adult Ophth: 1-2 gtt q3-4 h

Intraocular pressure reduction

Adult: PO 1-1.5 g/kg once, then 500 mg/kg q6h

P *Child:* PO 1-1.5 g/kg qd once, then 500 mg/kg 4-8 hr after first dose

Available forms: Rec sol 4 ml/applicator; supp; oral sol 0.6/ml; opth sol 7.5 ml/container

Side effects/adverse reactions

CNS: Headache, confusion, ***convulsions***

GI: Nausea, vomiting, diarrhea

META: Dehydration

Contraindications: Hypersensitivity

Precautions: Pregnancy **C**

Pharmacokinetics

Absorption	Well absorbed (PO), not absorbed (rectal)
Distribution	To intravascular space
Metabolism	Liver—80%, kidneys—20%
Excretion	Kidneys
Half-life	30 min

Pharmacodynamics

	PO	RECT	OPHTH
Onset	10-30 min	Unknown	Unknown
Peak	30-120 min	30 min	Unknown
Duration	6-8 hr	Unknown	Up to 4 hr

Interactions

Drug/drug:

Drug classifications

Diuretics: ↓ effect of glycerin (ophth)

NURSING CONSIDERATIONS

Assessment

- Assess patient for cause of constipation; identify whether fluids, bulk, or exercise is missing form life-style; check for distention, bowel sounds
- After administration, check for cramping, rec bleeding, nausea, vomiting; if these symptoms occur, drug should be discontinued
- Identify stool characteristics: consistency, color, amount, shape, volume

Associated nursing diagnoses

✓ Constipation (uses)
✓ Knowledge deficit (teaching)

Implementation

Rec route

- Insert glycerin supp after removing wrapper; may cause evacuation in ½ hr
- For evening use 4-ml applications of fluid, have patient in side-lying position, have patient retain for a few min

Ophth route

- Instill 1-2 gtt in one or both eyes by pulling down on conjunctival sac
- Do not use ophth sol that is discolored, has a precipate, or is cloudy

PO route

- Pour over cracked ice and sip through a straw
- To prevent severe cerebral dehydration headache have patient recumbent during and after administration
- Give by mixing 50% glycerine sol with 0.9% NaCl with flavoring, or use oral sol that is already flavored—flavoring improves taste and prevents GI symptoms
- Storage in cool environment; do not freeze

Patient/family education

- Caution patient not to use laxatives for long-term therapy; normal bowel tone will be lost; that normal bowel movements do not always occur daily
- Advise patient not to use in presence of abdominal pain, nausea, vomiting
- Instruct patient to notify prescriber if constipation is unrelieved or if weakness, dizziness, excessive thirst occur

Evaluation

Positive therapeutic outcome

- Decreased constipation
- Decreased intraocular pressure

glycopyrrolate

(glye-koe-pye'roe-late)

glycopyrrolate, Robinul, Robinul Forte

Func. class.: Cholinergic blocker

Chem. class.: Quaternary ammonium compound

Pregnancy category **C**

Action: Inhibits action of acetylcholine at receptor sites in autonomic nervous system, which controls secretions, free acids in stomach

Therapeutic Outcome: Decreased secretions in the respiratory tract, GI system

Uses: Decreased secretions before surgery, reversal of neuromuscular blockade, peptic ulcer disease, irritable bowel syndrome

Dosage and routes

Preoperatively

Adult: IM 0.002 mg/lb ½-1 hr before surgery

P *Child 2-12 yr:* IM 0.002-0.004 mg/lb

P *Child <2 yr:* IM 0.004 mg/lb

Reversal of neuromuscular blockage

Adult: **IV** 0.2 mg for each mg of neostigmine or 5 mg **IV** of pyridostigmine simultaneously

GI disorders

Adult: PO 1-2 mg bid-tid; IM/**IV** 0.1-0.2 mg tid-qid, titrated to patient response

Available forms: Tab 1, 2 mg; inj 0.2 mg/ml

Side effects/adverse reactions

CNS: Confusion, anxiety, restlessness, irritability, delusions, hallucinations, headache, sedation, depression, incoherence, dizziness, lethargy, flushing, weakness

CV: Palpitations, tachycardia, postural hypotension, paradoxical bradycardia

EENT: Blurred vision, photophobia, dilated pupils, difficulty swallowing, increased intraocular pressure, mydriasis, cycloplegia

GI: *Dryness of mouth, constipation,* nausea, vomiting, abdominal distress, paralytic ileus, altered taste perception

GU: Hesitancy, retention, impotence

INTEG: Urticaria, allergic reactions

MISC: Suppression of lactation, nasal congestion, decreased sweating

Contraindications: Hypersensitivity, narrow-angle glaucoma, myasthenia gravis, GI/GU obstruction, P child <3 yr, tachycardia, myocardial ischemia, hepatic disease, ulcerative colitis, toxic megacolon

Precautions: Pregnancy **C**, G elderly, lactation, prostatic hypertrophy, renal disease, CHF, pulmonary disease, hyperthyroidism

Pharmacokinetics

Absorption	Well absorbed (PO, SC, IM)
Distribution	Unknown
Metabolism	Not metabolized
Excretion	Unchanged feces
Half-life	2 hr

Pharmacodynamics

	PO	IM	IV
Onset	Unknown	15-30 min	Immediate
Peak	1 hr	30-45 min	10-15 min
Duration	8-12 hr	2-7 hr	2-7 hr

Interactions
Drug/drug:
Individual drugs
Amantadine: ↑ anticholinergic effect
Disopyramide: ↑ anticholinergic effect
Potassium chloride, oral: ↑ GI lesions
Quinidine: ↑ anticholinergic effect
Drug classifications
Antacids: ↓ absorption of glycopyrrolate
Antidiarrheals: ↓ absorption of glycopyrrolate
Anticholinergics: ↑ anticholinergic effect
Antidepressants, tricyclic: ↑ anticholinergic effect
Antihistamines: ↑ anticholinegic effect

NURSING CONSIDERATIONS
Assessment
- Monitor I&O ratio; retention commonly causes decreased urinary output; check for urinary hesitation; palpate bladder if retention occurs
- Monitor ECG for ectopic ventricular beats, PVC, tachycardia
- Monitor for bowel sounds; check for constipation; increase fluids, bulk, exercise if constipation occurs
- Assess for tolerance over long-term therapy; dose may have to be increased or changed
- Assess mental status: affect, mood, CNS depression, worsening of psychiatric symptoms during early therapy

Associated nursing diagnoses
✓ Knowledge deficit (teaching)

Implementation
IV route
- Administer **IV** undiluted, give at a rate of 0.2 mg or less over 1-2 min through Y-tube or 3-way stopcock; do not add to **IV** sol
- Administer parenteral dose with patient recumbent to prevent postural hypotension

Syringe compatibilities:
Atropine, benzquinamide, butorphanol, chlorpromazine, cimetidine, codeine, dimenhydrinate, diphenhydramine, droperidol, fentanyl, glycopyrrolate, heparin, hydromorphone, hydroxyzine, levorphanol, lidocaine, meperidine, midazolam, morphine, nalbuphine, pentazocine, prochlorperazine, promazine, promethazine, propionmazine, ranitidine, scopolamine

PO route
- Give PO with or after meals to prevent GI upset; may give with fluids other than water

IM route
- Give IM deeply in large muscle mass

Patient/family education
- Caution patient not to operate machinery or engage in hazardous activities if drowsiness occurs
- Advise patient not to take OTC products, cough, cold preparations with alcohol, antihistamines without approval of prescriber
- Caution patient not to discontinue this drug abruptly—tapering should be done over 1 wk

Evaluation
Positive therapeutic outcome
- Decreased secretions, bronchial, GI

gonadorelin acetate
(goe-nad-oh-rell'in)
(ass'e-tate)
Lutrepulse
Func. class.: Gonadotropin hormone
Chem. class.: Synthetic endogenous gonadotropin-releasing hormone (GnRH)
Pregnancy category B

Action: Induces ovulation in women by release of LH in the anterior pituitary gland

Therapeutic Outcome: Ovulation

Uses: Primary hypothalamic amenorrhea to produce ovulation

Dosage and routes
Adult: **IV** pump: 5 μg q1½ hr × 21 days; after three treatment intervals, it may be necessary to increase the dose in a stepwise program

Available forms: Powder for inj, 0.8, 3.2 mg vial to use with Lutrepulse pump

Side effects/adverse reactions
INTEG: Inflammation at inj site, phlebitis, hematoma at catheter site
REPRO: Ovarian hyperstimulation, multiple pregnancy
SYST: ***Anaphylaxis (bronchospasm, tachycardia, flushing, urticaria, induration of inj site)***

Contraindications: Hypersensitivity, patients with ovarian cysts or hormonally dependent tumors, anovulation other than that of hypothalamic origin

Precautions: Pregnancy **B**

Pharmacokinetics

Absorption	Completely absorbed (IV)
Distribution	Unknown
Metabolism	Liver—to inactive compounds
Excretion	Kidneys
Half-life	Up to 40 min

Pharmacodynamics

	INTRANASAL
Onset	Unknown
Peak	3 wk
Duration	Unknown

Interactions
Drug/drug:
Drug classifications
Ovarian stimulators: ↑ effect, avoid using together

NURSING CONSIDERATIONS
Assessment
- Assess by ultrasound before and during treatment to determine ovarian function (usually baseline), after 1 wk, after 2 wk; also monitor midluteal-phase serum progesterone
- Assess for hyperstimulation syndrome of the ovaries: pleural effusion, edema, ascites, ovarian growth—treatment should be discontinued immediately

Associated nursing diagnoses
✓ Sexual dysfunction (uses)
✓ Knowledge deficit (teaching)

Implementation
IV pump route
- Give by Lutrepulse pump only; detailed instructions are given with the pump
- Administer after reconstituting 8 ml of diluent provided and transferring to plastic reservoir; withdraw 8 ml of diluent and inject into lyophile drug cake, shake well, fill reservoir bag with reconstituted sol and administer **IV** using pump provided (8 ml = 1 wk supply). Set pump to 25-50 µl of sol/min and pulse frequency of 1½ hr
- Do not use sol if discolored or particulate is present
- Store at room temp: use prepared sol within 24 hr

Patient/family education
- Advise patient to report changes at **IV** site: redness, inflammation, pain
- Instruct patient on proper use of drug and pump; provide demonstration, request return demonstration

Evaluation
Positive therapeutic outcome
- Ovulation

gonadorelin hydrochloride
(goe-nad-oh-rell′in) (hye-droe-klor′ide)
Factrel
Func. class.: Gonadotropin hormone
Chem. class.: Synthetic luteinizing–hormone-releasing hormone
Pregnancy category **B**

Action: Combination luteinizing–hormone-releasing hormone that acts on anterior pituitary

Therapeutic Outcome: Elevated luteinizing hormone (LH) levels released by the anterior pituitary

Uses: Evaluation of response of gonadotropic hormone

Dosage and routes

Women: SC/**IV** 100 μg usually given between day 1-7 of menstrual cycle

Available forms: Powder for inj 100, 500 μg/vial

Side effects/adverse reactions

CNS: Dizziness, headache, flushing
GI: *Nausea*
INTEG: Inflammation at injection site
SYST: ***Anaphylaxis,*** antibody formation (large doses, extended time period)

Contraindications: Hypersensitivity

Precautions: Pregnancy **B**

Pharmacokinetics

Absorption	Completely absorbed (**IV**)
Distribution	Unknown
Metabolism	Liver—inactive compound
Excretion	Kidneys
Half-life	Up to 40 min

Pharmacodynamics

	FEMALES **(SC/IV)**	MALES **(SC)**	MALES **(IV)**
Onset	5 min	5 min	5 min
Peak	½ hr	1 hr	15 min
Duration	2-4 hr	2-4 hr	2-4 hr

Interactions

Drug/drug:

Individual drugs

Digoxin: ↓ level of gonadorelin
Levodopa: ↑ level of gonadorelin
Spironolactone: ↑ level of gonadorelin

Drug classifications

Dopamine antagonists: ↓ level of gonadorelin
Oral contraceptives: ↓ level of gonadorelin
Phenothiazines: ↓ level of gonadorelin

Lab test interferences

False test results: Androgus, glucocorticoids, estrogens, progestins

NURSING CONSIDERATIONS

Assessment

- Assess test results: pituitary/hypothalamus dysfunction (decreased LH); postmenopausal (increased LH)
- Assess menstrual cycle in females. Test should be done during the first wk of menstrual cycle
- Monitor levels by having lab personnel draw blood samples at intervals. Baseline levels are drawn 15 min before and just before administration

Associated nursing diagnoses

✓ Knowledge deficit (teaching)

Implementation

IV route

- Administer rapidly by direct **IV** after diluting 100 μg/1 ml or 500 μg/2 ml of provided diluent
- Repeated doses may be necessary to elevate pituitary gonadotropin reserve
- Discard unused portions

Patient/family education

- Teach patient purpose for medication and expected results
- Advise patient to report rash, hives, difficulty breathing, flushing; these should be reported immediately

Evaluation

Positive therapeutic outcome
- Completed test results for gonadotropin-releasing hormone

goserelin
(goe′se-rel-lin)

Zoladex

Func. class.: Gonadotropin-releasing hormone, antineoplastic

Chem. class.: Synthetic decapeptide analog of LHRH

Pregnancy category **X**

Action: Inhibitor of pituitary gonadotropin secretion. Initially increases LH and FSH, with increases in testosterone, reduction in sex steroid levels

Therapeutic Outcome: Decrease in tumor size and spread of malignant cells

Uses: Advanced prostate cancer

Dosage and routes

Adult: SC 3.6 mg q28 days (implant)

Available forms: Depot inj 3.6 mg

Side effects/adverse reactions

CNS: Headaches, ***spinal cord compression,*** anxiety, depression
CV: ***Dysrhythmia, cerebrovascular accident,*** hypertension, ***MI,*** chest pain
ENDO: Gynecomastia, breast tenderness, hot flashes
GI: Nausea, vomiting, constipation, diarrhea, ulcer
GU: *Spotting, breakthrough bleeding, decreased libido,* renal insufficiency, urinary obstruction, urinary tract infection
INTEG: Rash, pain on inj
MS: Osteoneuralgia

Contraindications: Hypersensitivity, pregnancy **X**

P **Precautions:** Children, lactation

Pharmacokinetics

Absorption	Well absorbed (SC)
Distribution	Unknown
Metabolism	Unknown
Excretion	Unknown
Half-life	4½ hr

Pharmacodynamics

	SC
Onset	Unknown
Peak	14-28 days
Duration	Treatment length

Interactions: None

Lab test interferences

Increased: Alk phosphatase, estradiol, FSH, LH, testosterone levels
Decreased: Testosterone levels, progesterone

NURSING CONSIDERATIONS

Assessment

- Assess for relief of bone pain (back pain)
- Monitor I&O ratios, palpate bladder for distention (urinary obstruction) at beginning of treatment—renal insufficiency and obstruction may occur

Associated nursing diagnoses

✓ Sexual dysfunction (uses)
✓ Knowledge deficit (teaching)

Implementation

SC route
- Administer via implant inserted by qualified persons into upper subcutaneous tissue in abdominal wall q28 days

Patient/family education

- Caution patient that gynecomastia and postmenopausal symptoms may occur but will decrease after treatment is discontinued
- Teach patient to contact prescriber if difficulty urinating occurs during treatment

Evaluation

Positive therapeutic outcome
- More normal levels of prostate-specific antigen, acid phosphatase, alk phosphatase; testosterone level of <25 mg/dl

granisetron

(grane-iss′e-tron)
Kytril
Func. class.: Antiemetic
Chem. class.: 5-HT_3 receptor antagonist
Pregnancy category **C**

Action: Prevents nausea, vomiting by blocking serotinin peripherally, centrally, and in the small intestine

➔ **Therapeutic Outcome:** Absence of nausea and vomiting

Uses: Prevention of nausea, vomiting associated with cancer chemotherapy including high-dose cisplatin

Dosage and routes

Adult: **IV** 10 μg/kg over 5 min, 30 min before the start of cancer chemotherapy

Available forms: Inj

Side effects/adverse reactions

CNS: Headache
GI: Diarrhea, constipation, increased AST (SGOT), ALT (SGPT)
MISC: Rash, ***bronchospasm***

Contraindications: Hypersensitivity

P G **Precautions:** Pregnancy **C**, lactation, children, elderly

G

Pharmacokinetics

Absorption	Unknown
Distribution	Unknown
Metabolism	Unknown
Excretion	Unknown
Half-life	Unknown

Pharmacodynamics

	IV
Onset	Unknown
Peak	Unknown
Duration	Unknown

Interactions: None

NURSING CONSIDERATIONS

Assessment

- Assess patient for absence of nausea, vomiting during chemotherapy
- Assess patient for hypersensitive reaction: rash, bronchospasm

Associated nursing diagnoses

✓ Fluid deficit (uses)
✓ Knowledge deficit (teaching)

Implementation

IV **IV route**

- Administer **IV** directly over 5 min
- Store at room temp for 48-hr dilution

Patient/family education

- Advise patient to report diarrhea, constipation, rash, or changes in respirations

Evaluation

Positive therapeutic outcome

- Absence of nausea, vomiting during cancer chemotherapy

griseofulvin microsize/ griseofulvin ultramicrosize

(gris-ee-oh-ful'vin)

Fulvicin P/G, Fulvicin-U/F, Grifulvin V, Grisactin, Grisactin 500, Grisactin-Ultra, Grisoven-FP ✤, Gris-PEG

Func. class.: Antifungal
Chem. class.: Penicillium griseofulvum derivative

Pregnancy category C

Action: Arrests fungal cell division at metaphase (mitosis); binds to human keratin, making it resistant to disease

➡ **Therapeutic Outcome:** Absence of fungicidal infection

Uses: Mycotic infections: *Tinea corporis, Tinea pedis, Tinea cruris, Tinea barbae, Tinea capitis, Tinea unguium* if caused by *Epidermophyton, Microsporum, Trichophyton*

Dosage and routes

Adult: PO 500-1000 mg qd in single or divided doses (microsize), 125-165 mg bid (ultramicrosize) or 250-330 mg qd; may need 500-660 mg in divided doses for severe infections

P *Child:* PO 10 mg/kg/day or 30 mg/m^2/day (microsize) or 5 mg/kg/day (ultramicrosize)

Available forms: Microcaps 125, 250 mg; tab 250, 500 mg; oral susp 125 mg/5 ml; ultratabs 125, 165, 250, 330 mg

Side effects/adverse reactions

CNS: *Headache,* peripheral neuritis, paresthesias, confusion, dizziness, fatigue
EENT: Transient hearing loss
GU: Proteinuria, cylinduria, precipitate porphyria, increased thirst
GI: *Nausea, vomiting, anorexia,* diarrhea, cramps, dry mouth, flatulence
HEMA: ***Leukopenia, granulocytopenia, neutropenia, monocytosis***
INTEG: *Rash, urticaria,* photosensitivity, lichen planus

Contraindications: Hypersensitivity, porphyria, hepatic disease, lupus erythematosus

Precautions: Penicillin sensitivity, pregnancy **C**

Pharmacokinetics

Absorption	Ultra products (completely absorbed), others (variably absorbed)
Distribution	Keratin in skin; liver, muscle, fat
Metabolism	Liver
Excretion	Feces
Half-life	10-24 hr

Pharmacodynamics

Onset	4 hr
Peak	1 day
Duration	2 day

Interactions

Drug/drug:

Individual drugs
Alcohol: ↑ CNS depression, tachycardia
Phenobarbital: ↓ action of griseofulvin
Drug classifications
Anticoagulants, oral: ↓ action of anticoagulant
Contraceptives, oral: ↓ effect of contraceptive

Drug/food:

Fat, (meat, dairy products): ↑ absorption

NURSING CONSIDERATIONS

G

Assessment

- Assess patient's skin for fungal infections: peeling, dryness, itching before and throughout treatment
- Monitor blood studies: leukocytes, CBC, platelets although blood dyscrasias are rare
- Monitor for renal toxicity: increased BUN, serum creatinine—if serum creatinine >1.7 mg/100 dl, dosage may be reduced (rare)
- Monitor for hepatotoxicity: increasing AST (SGOT), ALT (SGPT), alk phosphatase
- Monitor for allergic reaction: dermatitis, rash; drug should be discontinued, give antihistamines for mild reaction or epinephrine for severe reaction; if patient is allergic to penicillin a cross-sensitivity may exist with this medication

Associated nursing diagnoses

- ✓ Skin integrity, impaired (uses)
- ✓ Infection, risk for (uses)
- ✓ Knowledge deficit (teaching)

Implementation

PO route
- Give with meals (fatty) to prevent GI upset

• Administer drug carefully, making sure there is no confusion with dosage form (microsize vs ultrasize); with meals to decrease GI symptoms; store in tight, light-resistant container at room temp
• Administer drug until three separate cultures are negative for infective organism

Patient/family education

• Teach patient that long-term therapy may be needed to clear infection (2 wk-6 mo depending on organism); compliance is needed even after feeling better
• Instruct patient in proper hygiene: hand-washing technique, nail care, use of concomitant top agents if prescribed to clear infection
• Advise patient to avoid alcohol because nausea, vomiting, hypertension may occur
• Advise patient to use sunscreen or avoid direct sunlight to prevent photosensitivity
• Caution patient to notify prescriber of sore throat, fever, skin rash, which may indicate overgrowth of organisms
• Advise patient to use a nonhormonal form of contraception during treatment and to notify prescriber if pregnancy is anticipated

Evaluation

Positive therapeutic outcome
• Decrease in itching, peeling, dryness

guaifenesin

(gwye-fen'e-sin)
Amonidrin, Anti-tuss, Balminil ♣, Breonesin, Fenesin, Gee-Gee, Genatuss, GG-Cen, Glyate, Glycotuss, Glytuss, Guaifenesin, Guiatuss, Halotussin, Humibid, Humibid L.A., Hytuss, Hytuss 2X, Malotuss, Mytussin, Naldecon Senior EX, Resyl ♣, Robitussin, Scot-Tussin Expectorant, Sinumist-SR, Uni-Tussin
Func. class.: Expectorant
Pregnancy category C

Action: Acts as an expectorant by stimulating a gastric mucosal reflex to increase the production of lung mucus

Therapeutic Outcome: Decreased cough

Uses: Dry, nonproductive cough

Dosage and routes

Adult: PO 100-400 mg q4-6h, or 600-1200 mg q12h (sus-rel) not to exceed 2.4 g/day
P ***Child 6-12 yr:*** PO 100-200 mg q4h or 600 mg q12h (sus-rel); not to exceed 1.2 g/day
P ***Child 2-6 yr:*** PO: 50-100 mg q4h; not to exceed 600 mg/day

Available forms: Tab 100, 200 mg; cap 200 mg; syr 100

mg/5 ml; liq 200 mg/5 ml; sus-rel cap 300 mg; sus-rel tab 600 mg

Side effects/adverse reactions

CNS: Drowsiness
GI: Nausea, anorexia, vomiting

Contraindications: Hypersensitivity, persistent cough

Precautions: Pregnancy **C**

Pharmacokinetics

Absorption	Well absorbed (PO)
Distribution	Unknown
Metabolism	Unknown
Excretion	Unknown
Half-life	Unknown

Pharmacodynamics

	PO	PO SR
Onset	½ hr	Unknown
Peak	Unknown	Unknown
Duration	4-6 hr	12 hr

Interactions: None

NURSING CONSIDERATIONS

Assessment

- Assess cough: type, frequency, character, including characteristics of sputum; lung sounds bilaterally; fluids should be increased to 2 L/day to decrease secretion viscosity (thickness)

Associated nursing diagnoses

- ✓ Airway clearance, ineffective (uses)
- ✓ Knowledge deficit (teaching)

Implementation

PO route

- Store at room temp; provide room humidification to assist with liquefying secretions
- Avoid fluids for ½ hr after administration

Patient/family education

- Caution patient to avoid driving, other hazardous activities if drowsiness occurs (rare)
- Advise patient to avoid smoking, smoke-filled rooms, perfumes, dust, environmental pollutants, cleansers
- Instruct patient to notify prescriber if dry, nonproductive cough lasts over 7 days

Evaluation

Positive therapeutic outcome

- Absence of dry cough
- Thinner, more productive cough that raises secretions

guanabenz

(gwan'a-benz)
Wytensin
Func. class.: Antihypertensive
Chem. class.: Central α_2-adrenergic agonist
Pregnancy category **C**

Action: Stimulates central α_2-adrenergic receptors in the CNS, resulting in decreased sympathetic outflow from brain with decreased peripheral resistance

➔ Therapeutic Outcome: Decreased B/P in hypertension

G

Uses: Hypertension

Dosage and routes

Adult: PO 4 mg bid, increasing in increments of 4-8 mg/day q1-2 wk, not to exceed 32 mg bid

Available forms: Tab 4, 8 mg

Side effects/adverse reactions

CNS: *Drowsiness, dizziness, sedation, headache, depression, weakness*
CV: ***Severe rebound hypertension,*** chest pain, dysrhythmias, palpitations, hypotension
EENT: Nasal congestion, blurred vision, miosis
GI: Nausea, diarrhea, constipation, dry mouth, anorexia, abnormal taste
GU: Impotence, frequency, gynecomastia
MS: Backache, extremity pain
RESP: Dyspnea

Contraindications: Hypersensitivity to guanabenz

Precautions: Pregnancy **C**, P lactation, children <12 yr, severe coronary insufficiency, recent MI, cerebrovascular disease, severe hepatic or renal failure

Pharmacokinetics

Absorption	70%-80% (PO)
Distribution	Widely distributed
Metabolism	Liver, extensively
Excretion	Kidneys
Half-life	6 hr

Pharmacodynamics

	PO
Onset	1 hr
Peak	2-4 hr
Duration	12 hr

Interactions

Individual drugs

Alcohol: ↑ hypotension, ↑ sedation

Drug classifications

Analgesics, narcotic: ↑ sedation
Antihypertensives: ↑ hypotension
Beta-adrenergic blockers: ↑ bradycardia, CHF
MAOI: ↓ effectiveness of guanabenz
Nitrates: ↑ nitrates
Sedatives/hypnotics: ↑ sedation

NURSING CONSIDERATIONS

Assessment

- Monitor blood studies: neutrophils, decreased platelets
- Monitor renal studies: protein, BUN, creatinine; watch for increased levels that may indicate nephrotic syndrome; polyuria, oliguria, frequency
- Obtain baselines in renal, liver function tests before therapy begins; potassium levels, although hyperkalemia rarely occurs
- Monitor B/P, pulse if the drug is being used for hypertension; notify prescriber of change
- Watch for allergic reaction: rash, fever, pruritus, urticaria; drug should be discontinued if antihistamines fail to help

• Watch for symptoms of CHF: edema, dyspnea, wet rales, B/P, weight gain

Associated nursing diagnoses

✓ Cardiac output, decreased (uses)
✓ Injury, risk for (side effects)
✓ Knowledge deficit (teaching)
✓ Noncompliance (teaching)

Implementation

PO route
• Give in AM and at bedtime
• Store in air-tight container at room temp

Patient/family education

• Instruct patient not to discontinue drug abruptly—withdrawal symptoms may occur: anxiety, increased B/P, headache, insomnia, increased pulse, tremors, nausea, sweating
• Advise patient not to use OTC cough, cold, or allergy products unless directed by prescriber
• Teach patient to comply with dosage schedule even if feeling better; drug controls symptoms, does not cure
• Caution patient to rise slowly to sitting or standing position to minimize orthostatic hypotension, especially in the G elderly
• Teach patient that excessive perspiration, dehydration, vomiting may occur; diarrhea may lead to fall in blood pressure; consult prescriber if these occur
• Inform patient that drug may cause dizziness, fainting; light-headedness may occur during first few days of therapy; drug may cause dry mouth—use hard candy, saliva product, or frequent rinsing of mouth; that compliance is necessary; not to skip or stop drug unless directed by prescriber; that drug may cause skin rash or impaired perspiration
• Teach patient to avoid hazardous activities because drug may cause drowsiness, dizziness

Evaluation

Positive therapeutic outcome
• Decreased B/P

Treatment of overdose:
Vasopressor for hypotension, discontinue drug

guanadrel
(gwahn'a-drel)
Hylorel
Func. class.: Antihypertensive
Chem. class.: Adrenergic blocker, (peripheral guanethidine derivative)
Pregnancy category **B**

Action: Inhibits sympathetic vasoconstriction by inhibiting release of norepinephrine; depletes norepinephrine stores in adrenergic nerve endings and the adrenal medulla

➡ Therapeutic Outcome: Decreased B/P in hypertension

Uses: Hypertension (moderate to severe) as an adjunct

Dosage and routes

Adult: PO 5 mg bid, adjusted to desired response weekly or monthly; may need 20-75 mg/day in divided doses, higher doses are given tid or qid

Available forms: Tab 10, 25 mg

Side effects/adverse reactions

CNS: *Drowsiness, fatigue, weakness, feeling of faintness, insomnia, dizziness, mental changes,* memory loss, hallucinations, *depression,* anxiety, *confusion, paresthesia, headache*
CV: *Orthostatic hypotension, bradycardia,* ***CHF,*** palpitations, chest pain, tachycardia, dysrhythmias
EENT: *Nasal stuffiness, tinnitus, visual changes,* sore throat, double vision, dry burning eyes
GI: *Nausea, cramps, diarrhea, constipation, dry mouth, anorexia, indigestion*
GU: *Ejaculation failure, impotence,* dysuria, nocturia, urinary frequency
INTEG: Rash, purpura, alopecia
MS: *Leg cramps, aching,* pain, inflammation
RESP: *Bronchospasm,* dyspnea, cough, rales, SOB

Contraindications: Hypersensitivity, pregnancy **B**, pheochromocytoma, lactation, P CHF, child <18 yr

G **Precautions:** Elderly, bronchial asthma, peptic ulcer, electrolyte imbalances, vascular disease

Pharmacokinetics

Absorption	Well absorbed (PO)
Distribution	Widely distributed, minimally distributed in the CNS
Metabolism	Liver (50%)
Excretion	Kidneys, unchanged (50%)
Half-life	10-12 hr

Pharmacodynamics

	PO
Onset	½-2 hr
Peak	4-6 hr
Duration	4-14 hr

Interactions

Drug/drug:

Individual drugs
Alcohol: ↑ hypotension
Ephedrine: Block antihypertensive effect
Levodopa: ↑ hypotension
Norepinephrine: ↑ pressor, mydriatic effects
Phenylephrine: ↑ pressor, mydriatic effects

Drug classifications
Antidepressants, tricyclic: Blocked effect of guanadrel
Antihypertensive: ↑ hypotension
Amphetamines: ↑ pressor, mydriatic effect
MAOI: Block antihypertensive effect
Nitrates: ↑ hypotension

Lab test interferences

False positive: Urine acetone

NURSING CONSIDERATIONS

Assessment

- Monitor blood studies: neutrophils, decreased platelets
- Monitor renal studies: protein, BUN, creatinine; watch

for increased levels that may indicate nephrotic syndrome; polyuria, oliguria, urinary frequency
• Obtain baselines in renal, liver function tests before therapy begins; potassium levels, although hyperkalemia rarely occurs
• Monitor B/P, pulse if the drug is being used for hypertension; notify prescriber of changes
• Assess for allergic reaction: rash, fever, pruritus, urticaria; drug should be discontinued if antihistamines fail to help
• Symptoms of CHF: edema, dyspnea, wet rales, increased B/P, weight gain

Associated nursing diagnoses

✓ Cardiac output, decreased (uses)
✓ Injury, risk physical (side effects)
✓ Knowledge deficit (teaching)
✓ Noncompliance (teaching)

Implementation

• Usually given as adjunct with other cardiovascular drugs (diuretics) to decrease edema

PO route

• Store in air-tight container at 86° F (30° C) or less

Patient/family education

• Instruct patient not to discontinue drug abruptly, or withdrawal symptoms may occur: anxiety, increased B/P, headache, insomnia, increased pulse, tremors, nausea, sweating
• Advise patient not to use OTC (cough, cold, or allergy) products unless directed by prescriber
• Teach patient to comply with dosage schedule even if feeling better; drug controls symptoms, does not cure
• Caution patient to change position slowly, to rise slowly to sitting or standing position to minimize orthostatic hypotension, especially in the G elderly
• Caution patient that drug may cause dizziness, fainting; light-headedness may occur during first few days of therapy; that drug may cause dry mouth—use hard candy, saliva product, or frequent rinsing of mouth
• Instruct patient that compliance is necessary; not to skip or stop drug unless directed by prescriber
• Inform patient that drug may cause skin rash
• Teach patient to avoid hazardous activities because drug may cause drowsiness, dizziness

Evaluation

Positive therapeutic outcome

• Decreased B/P

guanethidine

(gwahn-eth-i'deen)

Apo-Guanethidine ♣, guanethidine sulfate, Ismelin

Func. class.: Antihypertensive

Chem. class.: Adrenergic blocker, (peripheral guanethidine derivative)

Pregnancy category **B**

Action: Inhibits sympathetic vasoconstriction by inhibiting release of norepinephrine, depletes norepinephrine stores in adrenergic nerve endings and the adrenal medulla

Therapeutic Outcome: Decreased B/P

Uses: Moderate to severe hypertension

Dosage and routes

Adult: PO 10 mg qd, increase by 10-12.5 mg qwk; may require 25-50 mg qd

Adult: (hospitalized) 25-50 mg; may increase by 25-50 mg/day or qod

P *Child:* PO 0.2 mg/kg/day (6 mg/m^2/day); increase q 7-10 day 0.2 mg/kg or 6 mg/m^2/day

Available forms: Tab 10, 25 mg

Side effects/adverse reactions

CNS: Depression, anxiety, drowsiness, fatigue, confusion, headache, sleeping problems

CV: *Orthostatic hypotension, dizziness, chest pain, weakness, edema*

EENT: *Nasal congestion,* ptosis, blurred vision

GI: Nausea, vomiting, *diarrhea, constipation, dry mouth,* weight gain, *anorexia,* abdominal pain

GU: *Ejaculation failure, impotence, nocturia,* edema, *retention,* increased BUN, *frequency*

INTEG: Dermatitis, loss of scalp hair

MS: Aches, leg cramps

RESP: Dyspnea, cough, shortness of breath

Contraindications: Hypersensitivity, pheochromocytoma, recent MI, CHF, cardiac failure, sinus bradycardia

Precautions: Pregnancy **B**, lactation, peptic ulcer, asthma

Pharmacokinetics

Absorption	Incompletely absorbed (up to 50%)
Distribution	Widely distributed, does not cross blood-brain barrier
Metabolism	Liver—partially
Excretion	Kidneys, breast milk (minimal)
Half-life	5 days

Pharmacodynamics

	PO
Onset	4 wk
Peak	4 wk
Duration	4 wk

Interactions

Drug/drug:

Individual drugs

Alcohol: ↑ hypotension

Ephedrine: Blocks antihypertensive effect
Levodopa: ↑ hypotension
Metharaminol: ↑ pressor, mydriatic effects
Norepinephrine: ↑ pressor, mydriatic effects
Phenylephrine: ↑ pressor, mydriatic effects

Drug classifications
Antidepressants, tricyclics: ↑ hypotension
Antihypertensive: ↑ hypotension
Amphetamines: ↑ pressor, mydriatic effect
Contraceptives, oral: Blocks antihypertensive effect, ↑ hypertension
MAOI: ↑ hypertension
Nitrates: ↑ hypotension
Phenothiazines: Blocks antihypertensive effect, ↑ hypertension

Lab test interferences

Increase: BUN
Decrease: Blood glucose, VMA excretion, urinary norepinephrine

NURSING CONSIDERATIONS

Assessment

- Monitor blood studies: neutrophils, decreased platelets
- Monitor B/P, orthostatic hypotension, syncope
- Monitor renal studies: protein, BUN, creatinine; watch for increased levels that may indicate nephrotic syndrome; polyuria, oliguria, urinary frequency
- Obtain baselines of renal, liver function tests before therapy begins
- Obtain potassium levels, although hyperkalemia rarely occurs
- Check for edema in feet, legs daily; monitor I&O; check for decreasing output
- Assess for allergic reaction: rash, fever, pruritus, urticaria; drug should be discontinued if antihistamines fail to help
- Assess for symptoms of CHF: edema, dyspnea, wet rales, B/P, weight gain

G

Associated nursing diagnoses

✓ Cardiac output, decreased (uses)
✓ Injury, risk for (adverse reactions)
✓ Knowledge deficit (teaching)

Implementation

PO route

- Usually given as adjunct with other cardiovascular drugs (diuretics) to decrease edema
- Store in air-tight container at 86° F (30° C) or less

Patient/family education

- Instruct patient not to discontinue drug abruptly because withdrawal symptoms may occur: anxiety, increased B/P, headache, insomnia, increased pulse, tremors, nausea, sweating
- Teach patient to comply with dosage schedule even if feeling better; drug controls symptoms, does not cure
- Caution patient to rise slowly to sitting or standing position to minimize orthostatic hypotension, especially in the G elderly

• Instruct patient to notify prescriber of sore throat, fever, swelling of hands or feet, irregular heartbeat, chest pain
• Caution patient that drug may cause dizziness, fainting, light-headedness may occur during first few days of therapy; that drug may cause dry mouth—use hard candy, saliva product, or frequent rinsing of mouth; that compliance is necessary—not to skip or stop drug unless directed by physician; that drug may cause skin rash or impaired perspiration
• Teach patient to avoid hazardous activities—drug may cause drowsiness, dizziness

Evaluation

Positive therapeutic outcome
• Decreased B/P in hypertension

Treatment of overdose: Administer vasopressors; discontinue drug

guanfacine
(gwahn'fa-seen)
Tenex
Func. class.: Antihypertensive
Chem. class.: Central α_2-adrenergic agonist
Pregnancy category B

Action: Stimulates central α_2-adrenergic receptors in the CNS resulting in decreased sympathetic outflow from brain with decreased peripheral resistance

➔ Therapeutic Outcome: Decreased B/P in hypertension

Uses: Hypertension in individual using a thaizide diuretic

Dosage and routes
Adult: PO 1 mg/day hs; may increase dose in 2-3 wk to 2-3 mg/day

Available forms: Tab 1 mg

Side effects/adverse reactions
CNS: Somnolence, dizziness, headache, fatigue
CV: Bradycardia, chest pain
EENT: Taste change, tinnitus, vision change, rhinitis, nasal congestion
GI: Dry mouth, constipation, cramps, nausea, diarrhea
GU: Impotence, urinary incontinence
INTEG: Dermatitis, pruritus, purpura
MS: Leg cramps
RESP: Dyspnea

Contraindications: Hypersensitivity

Precautions: Pregnancy **B**, P lactation, children <12 yr, severe coronary insufficiency, recent MI, renal or hepatic disease, CVA

Pharmacokinetics

Absorption	Well absorbed (80%)
Distribution	Widely distributed
Metabolism	Liver (50%)
Excretion	Kidneys—unchanged (50%)
Half-life	17 hr

Pharmacodynamics

	PO
Onset	Unknown
Peak	1-4 hr
Duration	Unknown

Interactions

Drug/drug:

Individual drugs

Alcohol: ↑ hypotension, ↑ sedation

Drug classifications

Analgesics, narcotic: ↑ sedation

Antidepressants, tricyclic: ↓ effectiveness of guanabenz

Antihypertensives: ↑ hypotension

Beta-adrenergic blockers: ↑ bradycardia, CHF

MAOI: ↓ effectiveness of guanabenz

Nitrates: ↑ nitrates

Sedatives/hypnotics: ↑ sedation

NURSING CONSIDERATIONS

Assessment

- Monitor blood studies: neutrophils, decreased platelets
- Monitor renal studies: Protein, BUN, creatinine; watch for increased levels that may indicate nephrotic syndrome; polyuria, oliguria, frequency
- Obtain baselines in renal, liver function tests before therapy begins; potassium levels, although hyperkalemia rarely occurs
- Monitor B/P, pulse if the drug is being used for hypertension; notify prescriber of changes
- Assess for edema in feet, legs daily; monitor I&O; check weight for decreasing output
- Assess for allergic reaction: rash, fever, pruritus, urticaria; drug should be discontinued if antihistamines fail to help
- Assess for symptoms of CHF: edema, dyspnea, wet rales, BP, weight gain

Associated nursing diagnoses

- ✓ Cardiac output, decreased (uses)
- ✓ Injury, risk for (adverse reactions)
- ✓ Knowledge deficit (teaching)
- ✓ Noncompliance (teaching)

Implementation

PO route

- Give hs
- Store in air-tight container at room temp

Patient/family education

- Instruct patient not to discontinue drug abruptly, or withdrawal symptoms may occur: anxiety, increased B/P, headache, insomnia, increased pulse, tremors, nausea, sweating
- Caution patient not to use OTC (cough, cold, or allergy) products unless directed by prescriber
- Teach patient to comply with dosage schedule even if feeling better; drug controls symptoms, does not cure
- Caution patient (especially G the elderly) to change position slowly, to rise slowly to sitting or standing position to minimize orthostatic hypotension
- Instruct patient to notify prescriber of sore throat, fever, swelling of hands or feet, irregular heartbeat, chest pain, increased weight

G

• Inform patient that drug may cause dizziness, fainting; light-headedness may occur during 1st few days of therapy; drug may cause dry mouth—use hard candy or saliva product, or rinse mouth frequently
• Teach patient that compliance is necessary; not to skip or stop drug unless directed by prescriber
• Caution patient that drug may cause skin rash
• Teach patient to avoid hazardous activities—drug may cause drowsiness; dizziness

Evaluation

Positive therapeutic outcome
• Decreased B/P

halazepam
(hal-az'e-pam)
Paxipam
Func. class.: Sedative/hypnotic
Chem. class.: Benzodiazepine
Pregnancy category **D**
Controlled substance schedule **IV**

Action: Depresses subcortical levels of CNS, including limbic system, reticular formation; potentiates GABA

Therapeutic Outcome: Decreased anxiety

Uses: Adjunct in anxiety

Dosage and routes

Adult: PO 20-40 mg tid-qid
G *Geriatric:* PO 20 mg qd-bid

Available forms: Tab 20, 40 mg

Side effects/adverse reactions

CNS: Dizziness, drowsiness, confusion, headache, anxiety, tremors, stimulation, fatigue, depression, insomnia, hallucinations
CV: Orthostatic hypotension, ***ECG changes, tachycardia,*** hypotension
EENT: Blurred vision, tinnitus, mydriasis
GI: Constipation, dry mouth, nausea, vomiting, anorexia, diarrhea
INTEG: Rash, dermatitis, itching

Contraindications: Hypersensitivity to benzodiazepines, narrow angle glaucoma, psychosis, pregnancy **D**, P child <18 yr

G **Precautions:** Elderly, debilitated, hepatic disease, renal disease

Pharmacokinetics

Absorption	Well absorbed (PO)
Distribution	Widely distributed; crosses placenta
Metabolism	Liver, extensively
Excretion	Kidneys, breast milk
Half-life	2 hr, 30-100 hr active metabolite

Pharmacodynamics

	PO
Onset	Unknown
Peak	1-3 hr
Duration	3-6 hr

Interactions

Drug/drug:

Individual drugs

Alcohol: ↑ CNS depression
Cimetidine: ↑ action
Digoxin: ↑ risk of digoxin toxicity
Disulfiram: ↑ action
Fluoxetine: ↑ action
Isoniazid: ↑ action
Ketoconazole: ↑ action
Levodopa: ↓ action of levodopa
Metoprolol: ↑ action
Propoxyphene: ↑ action
Propranolol: ↑ action
Rifampin: ↓ action of halazepam
Theophylline: ↓ sedative effects
Valproic acid: ↑ action

Drug classifications

Analgesics, opioid: ↑ CNS depression
Antidepressants: ↑ CNS depression
Antihistamines: ↑ CNS depression
Barbiturates: ↓ effect of halazepam
Contraceptives: ↑ effect

Lab test interferences

Increase: AST (SGOT)/ALT (SGPT), serum bilirubin
False increase: 17-OHCS
Decrease: RAIU

NURSING CONSIDERATIONS

Assessment

- Assess mental status: mood, sensorium, anxiety, affect, sleeping pattern, drowsiness, G dizziness, especially elderly; physical dependency, withdrawal symptoms: anxiety, panic attacks, agitation, convulsions, headache, nausea, vomiting, muscle pain, weakness; suicidal tendencies; for indications of increasing tolerance and abuse
- Monitor B/P (with patient lying, standing), pulse; if systolic B/P drops 20 mm Hg, hold drug, notify prescriber
- Monitor hepatic studies: AST (SGOT), ALT (SGPT), bilirubin, creatinine LDH, alkaline phosphatase

Associated nursing diagnoses

- ✓ Anxiety (uses)
- ✓ Injury, risk for (adverse reactions)
- ✓ Knowledge deficit (teaching)

Implementation

PO route

- Give with food or milk for GI symptoms; tab may be crushed, if patient is unable to swallow medication whole, and mixed with foods or fluids
- Give sugarless gum, hard candy, frequent sips of water for dry mouth

Patient/family education

- Advise patient that drug may be taken with food, or fluids and tab may be crushed or swallowed whole
- Caution patient not to use for everyday stress or longer than 3 mo unless directed by prescriber; not to take more than prescribed amount; may be habit forming; not to double doses or skip doses
- Advise patient to avoid OTC preparations unless approved by prescriber
- Instruct patient to avoid driving and activities that require alertness, since drowsi-

ness may occur; to avoid alcohol and psychotropic medications; to rise slowly to prevent fainting, especially G elderly; that drowsiness may worsen at beginning of treatment
• Instruct patient not to discontinue medication abruptly after long-term use; withdrawal symptoms include vomiting, cramping, tremors, seizures

Evaluation

Positive therapeutic outcome
• Decreased anxiety, restlessness, sleeplessness (short-term treatment only)

Treatment of overdose: Lavage, VS, supportive care, give flumazenil

halcinonide
(hal-sin′oh-nide)
Halog, Halog-E
Func. class.: Corticosteroid, synthetic
Chem. class.: Fluorinated corticosteroid
Pregnancy category C

Action: Antipruritic, antiinflammatory

Therapeutic Outcome: Decreased inflammation

Uses: Psoriasis, eczema, contact dermatitis, pruritus; usually reserved for severe dermatoses that have not responded to less potent formulation

Dosage and routes

Adult: Top apply to affected area bid-tid

Available forms: Cream 0.025%, 0.1%; oint 0.1%; sol 0.1%

Side effects/adverse reactions

INTEG: *Acne, atrophy, epidermal thinning, purpura, striae*

Contraindications: Hypersensitivity, viral infections, fungal infections

Precautions: Pregnancy **C**

Pharmacokinetics

Absorption	Minimal; systemic absorption on large areas
Distribution	Site only
Metabolism	Not metabolized
Excretion	Not excreted
Half-life	Unknown

Pharmacodynamics

	TOP
Onset	Up to 1 hr
Peak	Up to several days
Duration	Up to several days

Interactions: None

NURSING CONSIDERATIONS

Assessment

• Monitor temp; if fever develops, drug should be discontinued
• Check for systemic absorption: increased temp, inflammation, irritation

Associated nursing diagnoses

- ✓ Infection, risk for (adverse reactions)
- ✓ Knowledge deficit (teaching)
- ✓ Noncompliance (teaching)

Implementation

Top route
- Apply only to affected areas; do not get in eyes
- Leave area uncovered or lightly covered; occlusive dressing is not recommended; systemic absorption may occur
- Apply only to dermatoses; do not use on weeping, denuded, or infected area
- Cleanse area before application of drug
- Treat for a few days after area has cleared
- Store at room temp

Patient/family education

- Instruct patient to avoid sunlight on affected area; burns may occur
- Instruct patient to limit treatment to 14 days using <50 g/wk

Evaluation

Positive therapeutic outcome
- Absence of severe itching, inflammation, patches on skin, flaking

haloperidol

(ha-loe-per'i-dole)

Apo-Haloperidol ♣, Haldol, Haloperidol, Haloperidol Decanoate 50, Haloperidol 100, Haldol L.A. ♣, Novoperidol ♣, Peridol ♣

Func. class.: Antipsychotic/neuroleptic

Chem. class.: Butyrophenone

Pregnancy category **C**

H

Action: Depresses cerebral cortex, hypothalamus, limbic system, which control activity and aggression; blocks neurotransmission produced by dopamine at synapse; exhibits strong α-adrenergic, anticholinergic blocking action; mechanism for antipsychotic effects unclear

Therapeutic Outcome: Decreased signs and symptoms of psychosis

Uses: Psychotic disorders, control of tics, vocal utterances in Gilles de la Tourette syndrome, short-term treatment of hyperactive children showing excessive motor activity, prolonged parenteral therapy in chronic schizophrenia

Dosage and routes

Psychosis

Adult: PO 0.5-5 mg bid or tid initially depending on severity of condition; increase to desired dosage, max 100 mg/day; IM 2-5 mg q1-8h

P *Child 3-12 yr:* PO/IM 0.05-0.15 mg/kg/day

Decanoate: Initial dosage IM is 10-15 times daily oral dosage at 4-wk intervals; do not administer IV; not to exceed 100 mg

Chronic schizophrenia

Adult: IM 10-15 times the PO dosage q4 wk (decanoate)
P *Child 3-12 yr:* PO/IM 0.05-0.15 mg/kg/day

Tics/vocal utterances

Adult: PO 0.5-5 mg bid or tid, increased until desired response occurs
P *Child 3-12 yr:* PO 0.05-0.075 mg/kg/day

Hyperactive children

P *Child 3-12 yr:* PO 0.05-0.075 mg/kg/day

Available forms: Tab 0.5, 1, 2, 5, 10, 20 mg; conc 2 mg/ml; inj IM 5 mg/ml

Side effects/adverse reactions

CNS: *Extrapyramidal symptoms: pseudoparkinsonism, akathisia, dystonia, tardive dyskinesia, drowsiness, headache,* ***seizures neuroleptic malignant syndrome,*** confusion
CV: *Orthostatic hypotension,* hypertension, ***cardiac arrest,*** ECG changes, ***tachycardia***
EENT: Blurred vision, glaucoma, dry eyes
GI: *Dry mouth, nausea, vomiting, anorexia, constipation,* diarrhea, jaundice, weight gain, ***ileus, hepatitis***
GU: Urinary retention, urinary frequency, enuresis, impotence, amenorrhea, gynecomastia
INTEG: *Rash,* photosensitivity, dermatitis
RESP: ***Laryngospasm,*** dyspnea, ***respiratory depression***

Contraindications: Hypersensitivity, blood dyscrasias, P coma, child <3 yr, brain damage, bone marrow depression, alcohol and barbiturate withdrawal states, Parkinson's disease, angina, epilepsy, urinary retention, narrow angle glaucoma

Precautions: Pregnancy **C**, lactation, seizure disorders, hypertension, hepatic disease, cardiac disease

Pharmacokinetics

Absorption	Well absorbed (PO, IM); decanoate (IM) absorbed slowly
Distribution	High concentrations in liver, crosses placenta
Metabolism	Liver, extensively
Excretion	Kidneys, breast milk
Half-life	21-24 hr

Pharmacodynamics

	PO	IM	IM **(decanoate)**
Onset	Erratic	½ hr	3-9 days
Peak	2-6 hr	30-45 min	4-11 days
Duration	8-12 hr	4-8 hr	3 wk

Interactions

Drug/drug:

Individual drugs

Alcohol: ↑ effects of both drugs, oversedation
Aluminum hydroxide: ↓ absorption
Bromocriptine: ↓ antiparkinson activity
Disopyramide: ↑ anticholinergic effects
Epinephrine: ↑ toxicity
Guanethidine: ↓ antihypertensive response
Levodopa: ↓ antiparkinsonian activity
Lithium: ↓ haloperidol levels, ↑ extrapyramidal symptoms, masking of lithium toxicity
Magnesium hydroxide: ↓ absorption
Norepinephrine: ↓ vasoresponse, ↑ toxicity
Phenobarbital: ↓ effectiveness, ↑ metabolism

Drug classifications

Antacids: ↓ absorption
Anticholinergics: ↑ anticholinergic effects
Antidepressants: ↑ CNS depression
Antidiarrheals, adsorbent: ↓ absorption
Antihistamines: ↑ CNS depression
Antihypertensives: ↑ hypotension
Antithyroid agents: ↑ agranulocytosis
Barbiturate anesthetics: ↑ CNS depression
β-Adrenergics: ↑ effects of both drugs
General anesthetics: ↑ CNS depression
MAOI: ↑ CNS depression
Narcotics: ↑ CNS depression
Sedative/hypnotics: ↑ CNS depression

Lab test interferences

Increase: Liver function tests, cardiac enzymes, cholesterol, blood glucose, prolactin, bilirubin, PBI, cholinesterase
Decrease: Hormones (blood and urine)
False positive: Pregnancy tests, PKU, urine bilirubin
False negative: Urinary steroids, 17-OHCS

NURSING CONSIDERATIONS

Assessment

- Assess mental status: orientation, mood, behavior, presence and type of hallucinations before initial administration and monthly; this drug should significantly reduce psychotic behavior
- Check for swallowing of PO medication; check for hoarding or giving of medication to other patients
- Monitor I&O ratio; palpate bladder if low urinary output occurs, especially in elderly; urinalysis is recommended before, during prolonged therapy
- Monitor bilirubin, CBC, liver function studies monthly
- Assess affect, orientation, LOC, reflexes, gait, coordination, sleep pattern disturbances
- Monitor B/P with patient sitting, standing, and lying; take pulse and respirations q4h during initial treatment; establish baseline before starting treatment; report drops of 30 mm Hg; obtain baseline ECG, Q wave and T wave changes
- Check for dizziness, faintness, palpitations, tachycardia on rising; severe orthostatic hypotension is common

• Identify for neuroleptic malignant syndrome: hyperpyrexia, muscle rigidity, increased CPK, altered mental status; drug should be discontinued immediately
• Assess for extrapyramidal symptoms including akathisia (inability to sit still, no pattern to movements), tardive dyskinesia (bizarre movements of the jaw, mouth, tongue, extremities), pseudoparkinsonism (ragged tremors, pill rolling, shuffling gate); an antiparkinsonian drug should be prescribed
• Assess for constipation and urinary retention daily; if these occur, increase bulk, water in diet

Associated nursing diagnoses

✓ Thought processes, altered (uses)
✓ Coping, ineffective individual (uses)
✓ Knowledge deficit (teaching)
✓ Noncompliance (teaching)

Implementation

PO route
• Give drug in liquid form mixed in glass of juice or cola if hoarding is suspected; do not mix in caffeine drinks, tannics, pectins
• Give decreased dosage in elderly because of slower G metabolism
• Give PO with full glass of water, milk; or give with food to decrease GI upset
• Store in tight, light-resistant container, oral sol in amber bottle

IM route
• Inject in deep muscle mass, do not give SC; use 21 G 2-inch needle; do not administer sol with a precipitate; give <3 ml per inj site; give slowly, may be painful

Syringe incompatibility:

Heparin

Y-site compatibilities:

Cimetidine, dobustamine, dopamine, famotidine, fludarabine, lidocaine, melphalan, nitroglycerin, norepinephrine, ondansetron, paclitaxel, phenylephrine, theophylline, vinorelbine

Y-site incompatibilities:

Fluconazole, foscarnet, heparin, sargramostim

Patient/family education

• Teach patient to use good oral hygiene; use frequent rinsing of mouth, sugarless gum for dry mouth
• Advise patient to avoid hazardous activities until drug response is determined; dizziness, blurred vision are common
• Inform patient that orthostatic hypotension occurs often and to rise from sitting or lying position gradually to remain lying down after IM inj for at least 30 min; tell patient to avoid hot tubs, hot showers, tub baths, since hypotension may occur; tell patient that in hot weather heat stroke may occur; take extra precautions to stay cool
• Instruct patient to avoid abrupt withdrawal of this drug,

or extrapyramidal symptoms may result; drug should be withdrawn slowly
• Caution patient to avoid OTC preparations (cough, hay fever, cold) unless approved by prescriber, since serious drug interactions may occur; avoid use with alcohol, CNS depressants since increased drowsiness may occur
• Advise patient to use a sunscreen and sunglasses to prevent burns
• Teach patient about extrapyramidal symptoms and necessity of meticulous oral hygiene, since oral candidiasis may occur
• Instruct patient to take antacids 2 hr before or after this drug
• Tell patient to report sore throat, malaise, fever, bleeding, mouth sores; if these occur, CBC should be completed and drug discontinued

Evaluation

Positive therapeutic outcome
• Decrease in emotional excitement, hallucinations, delusions, paranoia
• Reorganization of patterns of thought, speech

Treatment of overdose:

Lavage if orally ingested; provide airway; *do not induce vomiting*

haloprogin (topical)

(ha-loe-proe'jin)
Halotex
Func. class.: Local antiinfective, antifungal
Chem. class.: Iodinated phenolic ester
Pregnancy category **B**

Action: Interferes with fungal cell membrane, which increases permeability, causing leakage of cell nutrients

H

Uses: Tinea pedis, tinea cruris, tinea corporis, tinea manus, tinea versicolor

Therapeutic Outcome: Fungistatic/fungicidal against susceptible organisms: tinea pedis, tinea cruris, tinea corporis, tinea versicolor

Dosage and routes

P *Adult and child:* Top apply to affected area bid × 14-28 days

Available forms: Cream 1%, sol 1%

Side effects/adverse reactions

INTEG: Rash, urticaria, stinging, burning, vesiculation, pruritus, erythema, scaling, folliculitis sensitization

Contraindications: Hypersensitivity

Precautions: Pregnancy **B**, P lactation, children

Pharmacokinetics

Absorption	Minimal
Distribution	Unknown
Metabolism	None
Excretion	None
Half-life	Unknown

Pharmacodynamics

Onset	Unknown
Peak	Unknown
Duration	Unknown

Interactions: None

NURSING CONSIDERATIONS

Assessment

- Assess skin for fungal infections: peeling, dryness, itching before and throughout treatment
- Monitor for allergic reaction: burning, stinging, swelling, redness, dermatitis, rash; drug should be discontinued, antihistamines (mild reaction) or epinephrine (severe reaction) administered; if patient is allergic to penicillin a cross-sensitivity may exist

Associated nursing diagnoses

- ✓ Skin integrity, impaired (uses)
- ✓ Infection, risk for (uses)
- ✓ Knowledge deficit (teaching)

Implementation

Top route

- Administer enough medication to cover lesions completely after cleansing with soap, water before each application: dry well
- Store at room temp in dry place

Patient/family education

- Teach patient to apply with glove to prevent further infection; do not cover with occlusive dressings
- Teach patient that long-term therapy may be needed to clear infection (2 wk-6 mo depending on organism); compliance is needed even after feeling better
- Teach patient proper hygiene: hand-washing technique, nail care, use of concomitant top agents if prescribed
- Advise patient to avoid use of OTC creams, ointments, lotions unless directed by prescriber
- Teach patient to wash hands before, after each application
- Advise patient to change socks and shoes once a day during treatment of tinea pedis
- Advise patient to report to prescriber if infection persists or returns; if blisters, burning, oozing, swelling occur

Evaluation

Positive therapeutic outcome

- Decrease in size, number of lesions

heparin calcium/ heparin sodium

(hep'a-rin)

Calcilean ✤, Calciparine, Hepalean ✤, Heparin Sodium and 0.45% Sodium Chloride, Heparin Sodium and 0.9% Sodium Chloride, Heparin Leo ✤, Heparin Lock Flush, Heparin Sodium, Hep-Lock, Hep-Lock U/P, Liquaemin Sodium

Func. class.: Anticoagulant

Pregnancy category **C**

Action: Prevents conversion of fibrinogen to fibrin and prothrombin to thrombin by enhancing inhibitory effects of antithrombin III

Therapeutic Outcome: Prevention of thrombi

Uses: Deep vein thrombosis and pulmonary emboli (treatment and prevention), MI, open heart surgery, disseminated intravascular clotting syndrome, atrial fibrillation with embolization, as an anticoagulant in transfusion and dialysis procedures

Dosage and routes

Deep vein thrombosis/MI

Adult: **IV** push 5000-7000 U q4h then titrated to PTT or ACT level; **IV** bol 5000-7500 U, then **IV** inf; **IV** inf after bolus dose, then 1000 U/hr titrated to PTT or ACT level

P *Child:* **IV** inf 50 U/kg, maintenance 100 U/kg q4h or 20,000 U/m^2 qd

Pulmonary embolism

Adult: **IV** push 7500-10,000 q4h then titrated to PTT or ACT level; **IV** bol 7500-10,000, then **IV** inf; **IV** inf after bol dose, then 1000 U/hr titrated to PTT or ACT level

P *Child:* **IV** inf 50 U/kg; maintenance 100 U/kg q4h or 20,000 U/m^2 qd

Open heart surgery

Adult: **IV** inf 150-300 U/kg, prophylaxis for DVT/PE; SC 5,000 U q8-12h

Heparin flush

P *Adult/child:* **IV** 10-100 U

Available forms: Heparin sodium inj 10, 1000, 5000, 10,000, 20,000, 40,000 U/ml; heparin calcium inj 5000, 12,500, 20,000 U/dose, 5000 U/0.2 ml

Side effects/adverse reactions

CNS: *Fever,* chills
GI: *Diarrhea,* nausea, vomiting, anorexia, stomatitis, abdominal cramps, ***hepatitis***
GU: Hematuria
HEMA: Hemorrhage, thrombocytopenia
INTEG: *Rash,* dermatitis, urticaria, alopecia, pruritus

Contraindications: Hypersensitivity, hemophilia, leukemia with bleeding, peptic ulcer disease, thrombocytopenic purpura, hepatic disease (severe), renal disease (severe), blood dyscrasias, severe hypertension, subacute bacterial endocarditis, acute nephritis

Precautions: Alcoholism, G elderly, pregnancy **C**

Pharmacokinetics

Absorption	Well absorbed (SC)
Distribution	Unknown
Metabolism	Unknown
Excretions	Lymph, spleen
Half-life	1½ hr

Pharmacodynamics

	SC	IV
Onset	½-1 hr	5 min
Peak	2 hr	10 min
Duration	8-12 hr	2-6 hr

Lab test interferences

False increase: T_3 uptake, serum thyroxine, BSP
Decrease: Uric acid
False negative: ^{125}I fibrinogen uptake

NURSING CONSIDERATIONS

Assessment

- Assess for blood studies (Hct, occult blood in stools) q3 mo if patient is on long-term therapy
- Monitor PPT, which should be 1½-2 times control, PTT; often done qd, APTT, ACT
- Monitor platelet count q2-3 days; thrombocytopenia may occur on 4th day of treatment and resolve, or continued thrombocytopenia on 8th day
- Assess for bleeding gums, petechiae, ecchymosis, black tarry stools, hematuria, epistaxis, decrease in Hct, B/P; may indicate bleeding and possible hemorrhage; notify prescriber immediately
- Monitor for hypersensitivity: fever, skin rash, urticaria; notify prescriber immediately

Associated nursing diagnoses

- ✓ Injury, risk for (uses, adverse reactions)
- ✓ Tissue perfusion, altered (uses)
- ✓ Knowledge deficit (teaching)

Implementation

IV **IV route**

- Give directly; **IV** loading dose over 1 min
- Give **IV** diluted in 0.9% NaCl, dextrose, Ringer's sol and by intermittent or cont inf; inf may run from 4-24 hr; use inf pump

Y-site compatibilities:

Acyclovir, aminophylline, ampicillin, atracurium, atropine, betamethasone, bleomycin, calcium gluconate, cephalothin, cephapirin, chlordiazepoxide, chlorpromazine, cimetidine, cisplatin, conjugated estrogens, cyancobalamin, cyclophosphamide, dexamethasone, digoxin, diphenhydramine, dopamine, edrophonium, enalaprilat, epinephrine, esmolol, ethacrynate, famotidine, fentanyl, fluconazole, fludarabine, fluorouracil, foscarnet, furosemide, hydralazine, insulin, isoproterenol, kanamycin, labetalol, leucovorin, lidocaine, magnesium sulfate, melphalan, menadiol sodium, meperidine, methicillin, methotrexate, methoxamine, methylergonovine, metoclopramide, minocycline, mitomycin, morphine, neostigmine, norepinephrine, ondansetron, oxacillin, oxytocin, paclitaxel, pancuronium, penicillin G potassium, pentazocine, phytonadione, prednisolone, procainamide, prochlorperazine, propranolol, pyridostigmine, ranitidine, sargramostim, scopolamine, sodium bicarbonate, streptokinase, succinylcholine, trimethophan camsylate, trimethobenzamide, vecuronium, vinblastine, vincristine, vinorelbine, zidovudine

Y-site incompatibilities:

Alteplase, ciprofloxacin, dacarbazine, diazepam, dobutamine, doxorubicin, ergotamine tartrate, gentamicin, haloperidol, idarubicin, methotrimeprazine, phenytoin, promethazine, tobramycin, triflupromazine

Additive compatibilities:

Amphotericin, calcium gluconate, cephalothin, cephapirin, chloramphenicol, clindamycin, colistimethate, dimenhydrinate, erythromycin gluceptate, furosemide, methyldopate methylprednisolone, nafcillin, octreotide, potassium chloride, prednisolone, promazine, ranitidine, sodium bicarbonate, verapamil, vitamin B complex, vitamin B complex with C

Additive incompatibilities:

Amikacin, erythromycin lactobionate, gentamicin, kanamycin, meperidine, methadone, morphine, polymyxin B, streptomycin

Heparin lock route
- Inject 10-100 U/0.5-1 ml after each inf or q8-12h

SC route
- Give SC with at least 25 G ⅜-in needle; do not massage area or aspirate fluid when giving SC inj; give in abdomen between pelvic bones, rotate sites; do not pull back on plunger, leave in for 10 sec; apply gentle pressure for 1 min
- Give at same time each day to maintain steady blood levels
- Changing needles is not recommended

Patient/family education

- Advise patient to avoid OTC preparations that may cause serious drug interactions unless directed by prescriber; may contain aspirin or other anticoagulants
- Tell patient that drug may be held during active bleeding (menstruation), depending on condition
- Caution patient to use soft-bristle toothbrush to avoid bleeding gums; avoid contact sports; use electric razor; avoid IM inj
- Instruct patient to carry a Medic Alert ID or other identification identifying drug taken and condition treated
- Advise patient to report any signs of bleeding: gums, under skin, urine, stools; or unusual bruising

H

Evaluation

Positive therapeutic outcome
- Decrease of deep vein thrombosis
- PTT of 1.5-2.5 times control
- Free-flowing IV

Treatment of overdose:

Withdraw drug, give frotamine sulfate

hepatitis B vaccine
(hep-a-tite'iss)
H-BIG, Hep-B-Gammagee, Hyper Hep
Func. class.: Vaccine
Pregnancy category **C**

Action: Provides active immunity to hepatitis B

Therapeutic Outcome: Passive immunity to hepatitis B

Uses: Prevention of hepatitis B virus in exposed patients, including passive immunity in neonates born to HBsAg-positive mother

Dosage and routes
P *Adult and child >10 yr:* IM 1 ml, then 1 ml after 1 mo, then 1 ml 6 mo after initial dose
P *Child 3 mo-10 yr:* IM 0.5 ml, then 0.5 ml after 1 mo, then 0.5 ml 6 mo after initial dose

Patients with decreased immunity: IM 2 ml, then 2 ml after 1 mo, then 2 ml 6 mo after initial dose

Available forms: Inj 10 mg/0.5 ml, 20 μg/ml

Side effects/adverse reactions
CNS: Headache, dizziness, fever, faintness, weakness
INTEG: Soreness at inj site, urticaria, erythema, swelling, pruritus
MS: Joint pain
SYST: ***Anaphylaxis, angioedema***

Contraindications: Hypersensitivity to immune globulins, thimerosal, glycine

Precautions: Pregnancy, G elderly, lactation, children, P active infection, IgA deficiency

Pharmacokinetics

Absorption	Slowly absorbed (IM)
Distribution	Unknown
Metabolism	Unknown
Excretion	Unknown
Half-life	3 wk

Pharmacodynamics

	IM
Onset	1-7 days
Peak	3-10 days
Duration	2-6 mo

Interactions
Drug/drug:
Live vaccines: ↓ or ↑ immune response

NURSING CONSIDERATIONS
Assessment
- Assess for history of allergies, skin conditions (eczema, psoriasis, dermatitis), reactions to vaccinations
- Assess for skin reactions: rash, induration, urticaria
- Assess for sneezing, pruritus, angioedema, dysphagia, vomiting, abdominal pain
- Assess for anaphylaxis: inability to breathe, bronchospasm, hypotension, wheezing, diaphoresis, fever, flushing; epinephrine and emergency equipment should be available

Associated nursing diagnoses

- ✓ Infection, risk for (uses)
- ✓ Knowledge deficit (teaching)

Implementation

IM route

- Give after rotating vial; do not shake
- Give in deltoid or anterolateral thigh for better protection; give 2-ml dose in two different sites; do not give **IV**
- Refrigerate unused portion; sol should be clear, light amber, and thick

Patient/family education

- Teach patient purpose of medication and expected results
- Give patient a list of adverse reactions that need to be reported immediately: wheezing, vomiting, sneezing, abdominal pain, sweating, tightness in chest
- Advise patient that pain, rash, swelling at inj site can be expected
- Give patient written record of immunization

Evaluation

Positive therapeutic outcome

- Prevention of hepatitis B

hetastarch

(het'a-starch)

Hespan

Func. class.: Plasma expander

Chem. class.: Synthetic polymer

Pregnancy category **C**

Action: Similar to human albumin, which expands plasma volume by colloidal osmotic pressure

➔ **Therapeutic Outcome:** Increased plasma volume

Uses: Plasma volume expander for sepsis, trauma, burns, leukophresis

Dosage and routes

Adult: **IV** inf 500-1000 ml (30-60 g); total dose not to exceed 1500 ml/day, not to exceed 20 ml/kg/hr (hemorrhagic shock)

Leukapheresis

Adult: **IV** inf 250-700 ml infused at 1 : 8 ratio with whole blood; may be repeated twice weekly up to 10 treatments

Available forms: 6% hetastarch/0.9% NaCl (6 g/100 ml)

Side effects/adverse reactions

CNS: Headache
GI: Nausea, vomiting
HEMA: Decreased hematocrit, platelet function, increased bleeding/coagulation

times, increased erythrosedintation rate
INTEG: Rash, urticaria, pruritus, angioedema, chills, fever, flushing, peripheral edema
RESP: Wheezing, dyspnea, ***bronchospasm, pulmonary edema***
SYST: ***Anaphylaxis***

Contraindications: Hypersensitivity, severe bleeding disorders, renal failure, CHF (severe)

Precautions: Pregnancy **C**, liver disease, pulmonary edema

Pharmacokinetics

Absorption	Completely absorbed (**IV**)
Distribution	Unknown
Metabolism	Degraded
Excretion	Kidneys, unchanged
Half-life	17 days (90%); 48 days (10%)

Pharmacodynamics

	IV
Onset	Immediate
Peak	Infusion's end
Duration	Over 24 hr

Interactions: None

Lab test interferences

False increase: Bilirubin

NURSING CONSIDERATIONS

Assessment

- Monitor VS q5 min for 30 min; CVP during inf (5-10 cm H_2O normal range); PCWP; urine output q1h: watch for increase which is common; if output does not increase, inf should be decreased or discontinued
- Monitor CBC with differential, Hgb, Hct, Pro-time, PTT, platelet count, clotting time during treatment; treatment may increase clotting time, PTT, pro-time, sedimentary rates, Hct may drop due to increase volume and hemodilution; do not allow Hct to be <30% by volume
- Monitor I&O ratio and sp gr, urine osmolarity; if sp gr is very low, renal clearance is low; drug should be discontinued
- Assess for allergy: rash, urticaria, pruritus, wheezing, dyspnea, bronchospasm; drug should be discontinued immediately
- Assess for circulatory overload: increased pulse, respirations, SOB, wheezing, chest tightness, chest pain, increased CVP, jugular vein distention
- Assess for dehydration after inf; decreased output, increased temp, poor skin turgor, increased sp gr, dry skin

Associated nursing diagnoses

- ✓ Fluid volume deficit (uses)
- ✓ Tissue perfusion, altered (uses)
- ✓ Fluid volume excess (adverse reactions)
- ✓ Knowledge deficit (teaching)

Implementation

IV route

- Give by IV cont inf, undiluted, run at 20 ml/kg/hr; reduced rate in septic shock, burns; rate is calculated by blood volume and response of patient

- Give up to 20 ml kg (1.2 g/kg)/hr
- Store at room temp; discard unused portions; do not freeze; do not use if turbid or deep brown or precipitate forms

Y-site incompatibilities:

Amikacin, cefamandole, cefoperazone, cefotaxime, cefoxitin, gentamicin, theophylline, tobramycin

Y-site compatibilities:

Cimetidine, doxycycline, enalaprilat

Additive compatibility:

Cloxacillin

Patient/family education

- Teach patient the reason for administration and expected results
- Advise patient to notify prescriber if flulike symptoms or allergic symptoms occur

Evaluation

Positive therapeutic outcome

- Increased plasma volume as evidenced by higher B/P, blood volume, output

hydralazine

(hye-dral'a-zeen)

Alazine, Apresoline, Dralzine, Novo-Hylazin*, hydralazine HCl, Rolzine

Func. class.: Antihypertensive, direct-acting peripheral vasodilator

Chem. class.: Phthalazine

Pregnancy category **C**

Action: Vasodilates arterioles in smooth muscle by direct relaxation; reduces B/P with reflex increases in cardiac function

Therapeutic Outcome: Decreased B/P in hypertension, decreased afterload in CHF

Uses: Essential hypertension; *parenteral:* severe essential hypertension, CHF

Dosage and routes

Adult: PO 10 mg qid 2-4 days, then 25 mg for rest of 1st wk, then 50 mg qid individualized to desired response, not to exceed 300 mg qd; **IV**/IM bol 20-40 mg q4-6h; administer PO as soon as possible; IM 20-40 mg q4-6h

Child: PO 0.75-3 mg/kg/day in 4 divided doses; max 7.5 mg/kg/24 hr; **IV** bol 0.1-0.2 mg/kg q4-6h; IM 0.1-0.2 mg/kg q4-6h

Available forms: Inj 20 mg/ml; tab 10, 25, 50, 100 mg

Side effects/adverse reactions

CNS: Headache, tremors, dizziness, anxiety, peripheral neuritis, depression
CV: Palpitations, reflex tachycardia, angina, ***shock,*** edema, rebound hypertension
GI: Nausea, vomiting, anorexia, diarrhea, constipation
GU: Impotence, urinary retention, Na^+, H_2O retention
HEMA: ***Leukopenia, agranulocytosis,*** anemia
INTEG: Rash, pruritus
MISC: Nasal congestion, muscle cramps, *lupuslike symptoms*

Contraindications: Hypersensitivity to hydralazines, coronary artery disease, mitral valvular rheumatic heart disease, rheumatic heart disease

Precautions: Pregnancy **C**, CVA, advanced renal disease

Pharmacokinetics

Absorption	Rapidly absorbed (PO); well absorbed (IM); completely absorbed (**IV**)
Distribution	Widely distributed; crosses placenta
Metabolism	GI mucosa, liver extensively
Excretion	Kidneys
Half-life	2-8 hr

Pharmacodynamics

	PO	IM	IV
Onset	½ hr	10-30 min	5-20 min
Peak	1 hr	1 hr	10-80 min
Duration	2-4 hr	4-6 hr	4-6 hr

Interactions

Drug/drug:

Individual drugs

Alcohol: ↑ hypotension

Drug classifications

Antihypertensives: ↑ hypotension
β-Adrenergic blockers: ↑ bradycardia, CHF
MAOI: ↑ hypotension
Nitrates: ↑ action of nitrates
NSAIDs: ↓ antihypertensive effect

NURSING CONSIDERATIONS

Assessment

- Assess B/P q5 min for 2 hr, then q1h for 2 hr, then q4h; pulse, jugular venous distention q4h
- Monitor electrolytes, blood studies: potassium, sodium, chloride, carbon dioxide, CBC, serum glucose
- Monitor weight daily, I&O; edema in feet, legs daily; check skin turgor, dryness of mucous membranes for hydration status
- Assess for rales, dyspnea, orthopnea; peripheral edema, fatigue, weight gain, jugular vein distention (CHF)

Associated nursing diagnoses

✓ Cardiac output, decreased (adverse reactions)
✓ Injury, risk for physical (side effects)
✓ Knowledge deficit (teaching)

Implementation

PO route

- Give with meals to enhance absorption
- Store protected from light and heat

IV **IV route**

• Give by **IV** undiluted through Y-tube or 3-way stopcock each 10 mg or less/min
• Administer with patient in recumbent position; keep in that position for 1 hr after administration

Y-site incompatibilities:

Aminophylline, ampicillin, diazoxide, furosemide, paclitaxel

Y-site compatibilities:

Heparin, hydrocortisone, potassium chloride, verapamil, vitamin B with C

Additive incompatibilities:

Aminophylline, ampicillin, chlorothiazide, edetate calcium disodium, ethacrynate, hydrocortisone, melphalan, mephenteramine, methohexital, nitroglycerin, phenobarbital, verapamil, vinorelbine

Additive compatibility:

Dobutamine

Patient/family education

• Teach patient to take with food to increase bioavailability
• Teach patient to avoid OTC preparations unless directed by prescriber
• Advise patient to notify prescriber if chest pain, severe fatigue, fever, muscle or joint pain occur

Evaluation

Positive therapeutic outcome

• Decreased B/P in hypertension

Treatment of overdose:

Administer vasopressors, volume expanders for shock; if PO, lavage or give activated charcoal, digitalization

hydrochlorothiazide

(hye-droe-klor-oh-thye′a-zide)

Diaqua, Diachlor H ✦, Esidrix, Hydro-Chlor, hydrochlorothiazide, HydroDiuril, Hydromal, Hydro-T, Hydrozide ✦, Neo-Codema ✦, Novohydrazide ✦, Oretic, Thiuretic, Urozide ✦

Func. class: Diuretic, antihypertensive

Chem. class: Thiazide, sulfonamide derivative

Pregnancy category **D**

Action: Acts on the distal tubule in the kidney, increasing excretion of sodium, water, chloride, magnesium, potassium, and bicarbonate

Therapeutic Outcome: Decreased B/P, decreased edema in lung tissues peripherally

Uses: Edema in CHF, nephrotic syndrome; may be used alone or as adjunct with antihypertensives

Dosage and routes

Adult: PO 25-100 mg/day

P *Child >6 mo:* PO 2.2 mg/kg/day

H

P *Child <6 mo:* PO up to 3.3 mg/kg/day in divided doses

Available forms: Tab 25, 50, 100 mg; sol 50 mg/5 ml, 100 mg/ml

Side effects/adverse reactions

CNS: Drowsiness, paresthesia, anxiety, depression, headache, *dizziness, fatigue, weakness*
CV: Irregular pulse, orthostatic hypotension, palpitations, volume depletion
EENT: Blurred vision
ELECT: Hypokalemia, hypercalcemia, hyponatremia, hypochloremia, hypomagnesemia
GI: Nausea, vomiting, anorexia, constipation, diarrhea, cramps, pancreatitis, GI irritation, ***hepatitis***
GU: Frequency, polyuria, ***uremia,*** glucosuria
HEMA: Aplastic anemia, hemolytic anemia, leukopenia, agranulocytosis, thrombocytopenia, neutropenia
INTEG: Rash, urticaria, purpura, photosensitivity, fever
META: Hyperglycemia, hyperuricemia, increased creatinine, BUN

Contraindications: Hypersensitivity to thiazides or sulfonamides, anuria, renal decompensation, pregnancy **D,** lactation

Precautions: Hypokalemia, renal disease, hepatic disease, gout, COPD, lupus erythematosus, diabetes mellitus, G elderly

Pharmacokinetics

	PO
Absorption	Variable
	PO/IV
Distribution	Extracellular spaces; crosses placenta
Metabolism	Excreted unchanged in urine
Excretion	Breast milk
Half-life	6-15 hr

Pharmacodynamics

	PO
Onset	2 hr
Peak	4 hr
Duration	6-12 hr

Interactions

Drug/drug:

Individual drugs
Cholestyramine:↓ absorption of hydrochlorothiazide
Colestipol:↓ absorption of hydrochlorothiazide
Diazoxide: ↓ hyperglycemia, hyperuricemia, hypotension
Digitalis:↑ toxicity
Indomethacin: ↓ hypotensive response
Lithium: ↑ toxicity
Mezlocillin: ↑ hypokalemia
Piperacillin: ↑ hypokalemia
Ticarcillin: ↑ hypokalemia

Drug classifications
Antidiabetics: ↓ effect of antidiabetic agent
Antihypertensives: ↑ antihypertensive effect
Nondepolarizing skeletal muscle relaxants: ↑ toxicity
Glucocorticoids: ↑ hypokalemia
Sulfonylureas: ↓ effect of sulfonylurea

Drug/food:

Food: ↑ absorption

Lab test interferences

Increase: BSP retention, calcium, amylase, parathyroid test
Decrease: PBI, PSP

NURSING CONSIDERATIONS

Assessment

- Monitor glucose in urine if patient is diabetic
- Assess improvement in CVP q8h
- Check for rashes, temp elevation qd
- G Assess for confusion, especially in elderly; take safety precautions if needed
- Monitor manifestations of hypokalemia: acidic urine, reduced urine, osmolality, nocturia; hypotension, broad T wave, U wave, ectopy, tachycardia, weak pulse; muscle weakness, altered LOC, drowsiness, apathy, lethargy, confusion, depression; anorexia, nausea, cramps, constipation, distention, paralytic ileus; hypoventilation, respiratory muscle weakness
- Monitor for manifestations of hypomagnesemia: agitation, muscle twitching, paresthesias, hyperactive reflexes, positive Babinski reflex, dysphagia, nystagmus seizures, tetany; nausea, vomiting, diarrhea, anorexia, abdominal distention; ectopy, tachycardia, broad, flat, or inverted T waves, depressed ST segment, prolonged QT, decreased cardiac output, hypotension
- Monitor for manifestations of hyponatremia: increased B/P, cold, clammy skin, hypovolemia or hypervolemia; anorexia, nausea, vomiting, diarrhea, abdominal cramps; lethargy, increased ICP, confusion, headache, seizures, coma, fatigue, tremors, hyperreflexia
- Monitor for manifestations of hyperchloremia: weakness, lethargy, coma, deep rapid breathing
- Assess fluid volume status: I&O ratios, record, count, or weigh diapers as appropriate, weight, distended red veins, crackles in lungs, color, quality and sp gr of urine, skin turgor, adequacy of pulses, moist mucous membranes, bilateral lung sounds, peripheral pitting edema; assess for dehydration symptoms of decreasing output, thirst, hypotension; dry mouth and mucous membranes should be reported
- Monitor electrolytes: potassium, sodium, calcium, magnesium; also include BUN, blood pH, ABGs, uric acid, CBC, blood sugar
- Assess B/P before and during therapy with patient lying, standing and sitting as appropriate; orthostatic hypotension can occur rapidly

Associated nursing diagnosis

- ✓ Altered urinary elimination (side effect)
- ✓ Fluid volume deficit (side effects)
- ✓ Fluid volume excess (uses)
- ✓ Knowledge deficit (teaching)

Implementation

- Give in AM to avoid interference with sleep
- Provide potassium replacement if potassium level is 3.0;

give whole tab or use oral sol lightly; drug may be crushed if patient is unable to swallow
- Administer with food; if nausea occurs, absorption may be increased

Patient/family education

- Teach patient to take the medication early in the day to prevent nocturia
- Instruct the patient to take with food or milk if GI symptoms of nausea and anorexia occur
- Teach patient to maintain a weekly record of weight and notify prescriber of weight loss >5 lb
- Caution the patient that this drug causes a loss of potassium and that food rich in potassium should be added to the diet; refer to a dietitian for assistance in planning
- Caution the patient not to exercise in hot weather or stand for prolonged periods since orthostatic hypotension will be enhanced
- Teach patient not to use alcohol or any OTC medications without prescriber's approval; serious drug reactions may occur
- Emphasize the need to contact prescriber immediately if muscle cramps, weakness, nausea, dizziness or numbness occurs
- Teach patient to take own B/P and pulse and record findings
- Caution the patient that orthostatic hypotension may occur; patient should rise slowly from sitting or reclining positions and lie down if dizziness occurs
- Teach patient to continue taking medication even if feeling better; this drug controls symptoms but does not cure the condition
- Advise the patient with hypertension to continue other medical treatment (exercise, weight loss, relaxation techniques, cessation of smoking)

Evaluation

Positive therapeutic outcome
- Decreased edema
- Decreased B/P
- Increased diuresis

Treatment of overdose: Lavage if taken orally, monitor electrolytes, administer dextrose in saline, monitor hydration, CV, renal status

hydrocodone

(hye-droe-koe'done)
Hycodan ✤, Robidone ✤
Func. class.: Narcotic analgesic
Chem. class.: Opiate
Pregnancy category C
Controlled substance schedule III

Action: Depresses pain impulse transmission at the spinal cord level by interacting with opioid receptors

Therapeutic Outcome: Pain relief, decreased cough, decreased diarrhea

Uses: Hyperactive and nonproductive cough, mild pain

Dosages and routes

Adult: PO 5 mg q4h prn or 10 mg q12h (long acting)

P *Child:* PO 2-12 mg 1.25-5 mg q4h prn

Available forms: Cap 5 mg, susp 5 mg/ml, tab 5 mg, 10 mg (long acting)

Side effects/adverse reactions

CNS: Drowsiness, dizziness, lightheadedness, confusion, headache, sedation, euphoria, dysphoria, weakness, hallucinations, disorientation, mood changes, dependence, ***convulsions***

CV: Palpitations, tachycardia, bradycardia, change in B/P, ***circulatory depression,*** syncope

EENT: Tinnitus, blurred vision, miosis, diplopia

GI: Nausea, vomiting, anorexia, constipation, cramps, dry mouth

GU: Increased urinary output, dysuria, urinary retention

INTEG: Rash, urticaria, flushing, pruritus

RESP: Respiratory depression

Contraindications: Hypersensitivity, addiction (narcotic)

Precautions: Addictive personality, pregnancy **C**, lactation, increased intracranial pressure, MI (acute), severe heart disease, respiratory depression, hepatic disease, renal

P disease, child <18 yr

Pharmacokinetics

Absorption	Well absorbed
Distribution	Unknown; crosses placenta
Metabolism	Liver, extensively
Excretion	Kidneys
Half-life	3-4 hr

Pharmacodynamics

	PO (analgesic)	PO (antitussive)
Onset	10-20 min	Unknown
Peak	30-60 min	Unknown
Duration	3-6 hr	4-6 hr

H

Interactions

Drug/drug:

Individual drugs

Alcohol: ↑ respiratory depression, hypotension, sedation
Cimetidine: ↑ recovery
Erythromycin: ↑ recovery
Nalbuphine: ↓ analgesia
Pentazocine: ↓ analgesia

Drug classifications

Antihistamines: ↑ respiratory depression, hypotension
CNS depressants: ↑ respiratory depression, hypotension
MAOI: Do not use for 2 wk before taking hydrocodone
Phenothiazines: ↑ respiratory depression, hypotension
Sedative/hypnotics: ↑ respiratory depression, hypotension

Lab test interferences

Increase: Amylase, lipase

NURSING CONSIDERATIONS

Assessment

- Monitor VS after parenteral route; note muscle rigidity, drug history, liver, kidney function tests, respiratory dysfunction: respiratory de-

pression, character, rate, rhythm; notify prescriber if respirations are <10/min
- Monitor CNS changes: dizziness, drowsiness, hallucinations, euphoria, LOC, pupil reaction
- Monitor allergic reactions: rash, urticaria

Associated nursing diagnoses

- ✓ Pain (uses)
- ✓ Sensory-perceptual alteration: visual, auditory (adverse reactions)
- ✓ Breathing pattern, ineffective (adverse reactions)
- ✓ Knowledge deficit (teaching)

Implementation

- Give with antiemetic if nausea, vomiting occur
- Give when pain is beginning to return; determine dosage interval by patient response; continuous dosing of medication is more effective given prn
- Medication should be slowly withdrawn after long-term use to prevent withdrawal symptoms
- Store in light-resistant container at room temp
- May be given with food or milk to lessen GI upset

Patient/family education

- Instruct patient to report any symptoms of CNS changes, allergic reactions; to avoid CNS depressants: alcohol, sedative/hypnotics for at least 24 hr after taking this drug
- Teach patient that dizziness, drowsiness, and confusion are common and to avoid getting up without assistance
- Discuss in detail all aspects of the drug

Evaluation

Positive therapeutic outcome

- Decreased pain
- Decreased cough

Treatment of overdose:

Naloxone HCl (Narcan) 0.2-0.8 IV, O_2, IV fluids, vasopressors

hydrocortisone/ hydrocortisone acetate/hydrocortisone valerate
(hye-droe-kor'ti-sone)
Aeroseb-HC, A-Hydrocort, Ala-Cort, Ala-Scalp, Alphaderm, Bactine Hydrocortisone, Caldecort Anti-Itch, Cetacort, Cortaid, Cortaid Maximum Strength, Cort-Dome, Cortef, Cortef Acetate, Cortef Feminine Itch, Cortenema Acticort 100, Cortizone-5, Cortizone-10, Cortril, Delacort, Delcort, Dermacort, Dermicort, Dermolate Anti-Itch, Dermtex HC, HI-COR-1.0, HI-COR-2.5, Hycort, Hydrocortone, Hydrocortone Acetate, Hydrocortone Phosphate, HydroTex, Hytone, Lacticare-HC, Nutracort, Penecort 1% HC, Solu-Cortef, S-T Cort, Synacort, Tega-Cort, Tega-Cort Forte, Texacort, Westcort
Func. class.: Short-acting glucocorticoid
Chem. class.: Natural nonfluorinated, group IV potency (valerate), group VI potency (acetate and plain)
Pregnancy category C

Action: Decreases inflammation by suppressing migration of polymorphonuclear leukocytes and fibroblasts and reversing increased capillary permeability and lysosomal stabilization (systemic); antipruritic, antiinflammatory (top)

➔ Therapeutic Outcome: Decreased inflammation

Uses: Severe inflammation, septic shock, adrenal insufficiency, ulcerative colitis, collagen disorders (systemic), psoriasis, eczema, contact dermatitis, pruritus (top)

Dosage and routes

Adrenal insufficiency/ inflammation

Adult: PO 5-30 mg bid-qid; IM/**IV** 100-250 mg (succinate), then 50-100 mg IM as needed; IM/**IV** 15-240 mg q12h (phosphate)

Shock

Adult: 500 mg-2 g q2-6h (succinate)

P ***Child:*** IM/**IV** 0.16-1 mg/kg bid-tid (succinate)

Colitis

Adult: Enema 100 mg nightly for 21 days

Top

P ***Adult and child >2 yr:*** Apply to affected area qd-qid

Available forms: Oint 0.5%, 1%, 2.5%; cream 0.25%, 0.5%, 1%, 2.5%; lotion 0.25%, 0.5%, 1%, 2%, 2.5%; gel 1%; sol 1%; aerosol/pump spray 0.5%; *acetate:* oint 0.5%, 1%, 2.5%; cream 0.5%; lotion 0.05%; aerosol 1%; *valerate:*

H

oint 0.2%; cream 0.2% (many others)

Side effects/adverse reactions

CNS: Depression, flushing, sweating, headache, mood changes
CV: Hypertension, circulatory collapse, thrombophlebitis, embolism, tachycardia, edema
EENT: Fungal infections, increased intraocular pressure, blurred vision
GI: Diarrhea, nausea, abdominal distention, *GI hemorrhage,* increased appetite, pancreatitis
HEMA: Thrombocytopenia
INTEG: Acne, poor wound healing, ecchymosis, petechiae (top) Burning, dryness, itching, irritation, acne, folliculitis, hypertrichosis, perioral dermatitis, hypopigmentation, atrophy, striae, miliaria, allergic contact dermatitis, secondary infection
MS: Fractures, osteoporosis, weakness

Contraindications: Psychosis, hypersensitivity, idiopathic thrombocytopenia, acute glomerulonephritis, amebiasis, fungal infections, nonasthmatic bronchial disease, P child <2 yr, AIDS, TB, fungal infections (top)

Precautions: Pregnancy **C**, diabetes mellitus, glaucoma, osteoporosis, seizure disorders, ulcerative colitis, CHF, myasthenia gravis, renal disease, esophagitis, peptic ulcer, lactation, (top) viral infections, bacterial infections

Pharmacokinetics

Absorption	Well absorbed (PO); systemic (top)
Distribution	Crosses placenta
Metabolism	Liver, extensively
Excretion	Kidney
Half-life	3-5 hr, adrenal suppression 3-4 days

Pharmacodynamics

	PO	IM	IV	TOP
Onset	1-2 hr	20 min	Rapid	Min to hr
Peak	1 hr	4-8 hr	Unkn	Hr to days
Duration	1½ days	1½ days	1½ days	Hr to days

Interactions

Drug/drug:

Individual drugs
Amphotericin B: ↑ hypokalemia
Cholestyramine: ↓ action of hydrocortisone
Colestripol: ↓ action of hydrocortisone
Ephedrine: ↓ action of hydrocortisone
Insulin: ↑ need for insulin
Mezlocillin: ↑ hypokalemia
Phenytoin: ↓ action, ↑ metabolism
Rifampin: ↓ action, ↑ metabolism
Ticarcillin: ↑ hypokalemia
Theophylline: ↓ action of hydrocortisone

Drug classifications
Anticoagulants: ↓ action of anticoagulant
Barbiturates: ↓ action, ↑ metabolism
Diuretics: ↑ hypokalemia

Hypoglycemia agents: ↑ need for hypoglycemic agents

Lab test interferences

Increase: Cholesterol, sodium, blood glucose, uric acid, calcium, urine glucose
Decrease: Calcium, potassium, T_4, T_3, thyroid ^{131}I uptake test, urine 17-OHCS, 17-KS, PBI
False negative: Skin allergy tests

NURSING CONSIDERATIONS

Assessment

- Monitor potassium, blood sugar, urine glucose while patient on long-term therapy; hypokalemia and hyperglycemia may occur
- Monitor I&O ratio; be alert for decreasing urinary output and increasing edema; weigh daily; notify prescriber of weekly gain >5 lb or edema, hypertension, cardiac symptoms
- Monitor plasma cortisol levels during long-term therapy (normal level is 138-635 nmol/L when drawn at 8 AM); check adrenal function periodically for HPA axis suppression
- Assess for infection: increased temp, WBC even after withdrawal of medication; drug masks infection symptoms; if fever develops, drug should be discontinued
- Check for potassium depletion: paresthesias, fatigue, nausea, vomiting, depression, polyuria, dysrhythmias, weakness
- Assess mental status: affect, mood, behavioral changes, aggression
- Check nasal passages during long-term treatment for changes in mucus (nasal)
- Assess for systemic absorption: increased temp, inflammation, irritation (top)

Associated nursing diagnoses

✓ Infection, risk for (adverse reactions)
✓ Knowledge deficit (teaching)
✓ Noncompliance (teaching) (top/nasal preparation)

Implementation

PO route
- Give with food or milk to decrease GI symptoms

IV **IV route**
- Give only sodium phosphate product **IV**; reconstitute with sol provided; give 100 mg over >1 min
- May be given by intermittent inf in compatible sol
- Give titrated dose; use lowest effective dosage

Sodium phosphate preparations

Syringe compatibilities:

Fluconazole, fludarabine, metoclopramide

Additive compatibilities:

Amphotericin B, bleomycin, dacarbazine

Sodium succinate preparations

Syringe compatibilities:

Metoclopramide, thiopental

Y-site compatibilities:

Acyclovir, aminophylline, ampicillin, amrinone, atracurium, atropine, betamethasone,

H

calcium gluconate, cephalothin, cephapirin, chlordiazepoxide, chlorpromazine, cyanocobalamin, dexamethasone, digoxin, diphenhydramine, dopamine, droperidol, edrophonium, enalaprilat, epinephrine, esmolol, conjugated estrogens, ethacrynate, famotidine, fentanyl, fentanyl/droperidol, fludarabine, fluorouracil, foscarnet, furosemide, hydralazine, insulin, isoproterenol, kanamycin, lidocaine, magnesium sulfate, melphalan, menadiol, methicillin, methoxamine, methylergonovine, minocycline, morphine, neostigmine, norepinephrine, ondansetron, oxacillin, oxytocin, paclitaxel, pancuronium, penicillin G potassium, pentazocine, phytonadione, prednisolone, procainamide, prochlorperazine, propranolol, pyridostigmine, scopolamine, sodium bicarbonate, succinylcholine, trimethobenzamide, trimethaphan camsylate, vecuronium, vinrelobine

Y-site incompatibilities:

Diazepam, ergotamine tartrate, idarubicin, phenytoin, sargramostim

Additive compatibilities:

Aminophylline, amphotericin, daunorubicin, mitoxantrone, potassium chloride

Additive incompatibilities:

Bleomycin, doxorubicin

Rec route

- Use applicator provided
- Clean applicator after each use

Top route

- Apply only to affected areas; do not get in eyes
- Cleanse and dry area before applying medication, then cover with occlusive dressing (only if prescribed); seal to normal skin; change q12h; syst absorption may occur; use only on dermatoses; do not use on weeping, denuded, or infected area
- Use for a few days after area has cleared
- Store at room temp

Nasal route

- Patient should clear nasal passages before administration; use decongestant if needed; shake inhaler, invert, tilt head backward, insert nozzle into nostril, away from septum; hold other nostril closed and depress activator, inhale through nose, exhale through mouth

Patient/family education

- Teach patient all aspects of drug usage, including cushingoid symptoms
- Advise patient that ID as steroid user should be carried; not to discontinue abruptly; adrenal crisis can result
- Instruct patient to notify prescriber if therapeutic response decreases; dosage adjustment may be needed
- Caution patient to avoid OTC products unless directed by perscriber: salicylates, alcohol in cough products, cold preparations
- Teach patient symptoms of adrenal insufficiency: nausea, anorexia, fatigue, dizziness, dyspnea, weakness, joint pain, and when to notify prescriber

- Advise patient that long-term therapy may be needed to clear infection (1-2 mo depending on type of infection)

Nasal route

- Instruct patient to clear nasal passages if sneezing attack occurs, then repeat dose; to continue using product even if mild nasal bleeding occurs; bleeding is usually transient
- Teach method of instillation after providing written instruction from manufacturer on instillation

Evaluation

Positive therapeutic outcome

- Decrease in runny nose (nasal)
- Ease of respirations, decreased inflammation
- Absence of severe itching, patches on skin, flaking (top)

hydromorphone

(hye-droe-mor'fone)

Dihydromorphinone, Dilaudid, Dilaudid-HP, Dilaudid Cough Syrup (combination with guaifenesin/alcohol)

Func. class.: Antitussive, narcotic; opioid analgesic agonist

Chem. class.: Phenanthrene derivative, guaifenesin

Pregnancy category **C**

Controlled substance schedule **II**

Action: Depresses pain impulse transmission at the spinal cord level by interacting with opioid receptors; increases respiratory tract fluid by decreasing surface tension and adhesiveness, which increases removal of mucus; analgesic, antitussive

Therapeutic Outcome: Decreased cough, decreased pain

Uses: As an antitussive to suppress cough; moderate to severe pain

Dosage and routes

Antitussive

Adult: PO 1 mg q3-4h prn

Child 6-12 yr: PO 0.5 mg q3-4h prn

Analgesic

Adult: PO 2 mg q3-6h prn; may increase to 4 mg q4-6h; SC/IM 1-2 mg q3-6h prn; may increase to 3-4 mg q4-6h; **IV** 0.5-1 mg q3h prn; rect 3 mg q4-8h prn

Available forms: Syr 1 mg/5 ml; tab 1, 2, 3, 4 mg; inj 2, 3, 4, 10 mg/ml; supp 3 mg

Side effects/adverse reactions

CNS: Dizziness, drowsiness, *sedation, confusion,* headache, euphoria, dreaming, hallucinations

CV: Hypotension, bradycardia

EENT: Miosis, diplopia, blurred vision

GI: Nausea, constipation, vomiting, anorexia

GU: Retention

INTEG: Urticaria, rash, sweating, flushing

RESP: ***Respiratory depression***

Contraindications:
Hypersensitivity, increased intracranial pressure, status asthmaticus

Precautions:
Hypothyroidism, Addison's disease, CNS depression, brain tumor, asthma, hepatic disease, renal disease, COPD, psychosis, alcoholism, convulsive disorders, pregnancy **C**

Pharmacokinetics

Absorption	Well absorbed (PO), complete (IV)
Distribution	Unknown; crosses placenta
Metabolism	Liver, extensively
Excretion	Kidneys
Half-life	4 hr

Pharmacodynamics

	PO	IM	SC	IV	REC
Onset	15-30 min	15-30 min	15-30 min	10-15 min	15-30 min
Peak	30-90 min	30-90 min	30-90 min	15-30 min	30-90 min
Duration	4-5 hr	4-5 hr	4-5 hr	2-3 hr	4-5 hr

Interactions
Drug/drug:
Individual drugs
Alcohol: ↑ respiratory depression, hypotension, sedation
Nalbuphine: ↓ analgesia
Pentazocine: ↓ analgesia

Drug classifications
Antihistamines: ↑ respiratory depression, hypotension
Antidepressants: ↑ respiratory depression, hypotension
CNS depressants: ↑ respiratory depression, hypotension
MAOI: Serious reactions; dosage should be reduced
Phenothiazines: ↑ respiratory depression, hypotension
Sedative/hypnotics: ↑ respiratory depression, hypotension

Lab test interferences
Increase: Amylase, lipase

NURSING CONSIDERATIONS
Assessment
- Monitor VS after parenteral route; note muscle rigidity, drug history, liver, kidney function tests, respiratory dysfunction: respiratory depression, character, rate, rhythm; notify prescriber if respirations are <10/min
- Monitor CNS changes: dizziness, drowsiness, hallucinations, euphoria, LOC, pupil reaction
- Monitor allergic reactions: rash, urticaria

Associated nursing diagnoses
- ✓ Pain (uses)
- ✓ Sensory-perceptual alteration: visual, auditory (adverse reactions)
- ✓ Breathing pattern, ineffective (adverse reactions)
- ✓ Knowledge deficit (teaching)

Implementation
- Give with antiemetic if nausea, vomiting occur
- Give when pain is beginning to return; determine dosage interval by patient response; continuous dosing of medication is more effective given prn; explain analgesic effect

- Withdraw medication slowly after long-term use to prevent withdrawal symptoms
- Store in light-resistant container at room temp

PO route

- May be given with food or milk to lessen GI upset

IM/SC route

- Do not give if sol is cloudy or a precipitate has formed

IV **IV route**

- Give by direct **IV** after diluting with 5 ml or more sterile water or 0.9% NaCl for inj
- Give slowly at 2 mg over 3-5 min or less

Syringe compatibilities:

Atropine, chlorpromazine, cimetidine, diphenhydramine, fentanyl, glycopyrrolate, hydroxyzine, midazolam, pentazocine, pentobarbital, promethazine, ranitidine, scopolamine, tetracaine, thiethylperazine, trimethobenzamide

Y-site compatibilities:

Acyclovir, amikacin, ampicillin, cefamandole, cefazolin, cefoperazone, ceforanide, cefotaxime, ceftazidine, cefoxitin, ceftizoxime, cefuroxime, cephalothin, cephapirin, chloramphenicol, clindamycin, doxycycline, erythromycin lactobionate, fludarabine, foscarnet, gentamicin, kanamycin, magnesium sulfate, melphalan, metronidazole, mezlocillin, moxalactam, nafcillin, ondansetron, oxacillin, paclitaxel, penicillin G potassium, piperacillin, ticarcillin, tobramycin, trimethoprim/sulfamethoxazole, vancomycin, vinorelbine

Y-site incompatibilities:

Ampicillin, diazepam, minocycline, phenobarbital, phenytoin, sargramostim

Solution compatibilities:

D_5W, D_5/0.45% NaCl, D_5/0.9% NaCl, D_5/LR, D_5/Ringer's sol, 0.45% NaCl, 0.9% NaCl, Ringer's and lactated Ringer's sol

Additive incompatibilities:

Sodium bicarbonate, thiopental

Patient/family education

- Instruct patient to report any symptoms of CNS changes, allergic reactions; to avoid CNS depressants: alcohol, sedative/hypnotics for at least 24 hr after taking this drug
- Advise patient that dizziness, drowsiness, and confusion are common and to avoid getting up without assistance
- Discuss in detail all aspects of the drug

Evaluation

Positive therapeutic outcome

- Decreased pain
- Decreased cough

Treatment of overdose:

Naloxone HCl (Narcan) 0.2-0.8 IV, O_2, **IV** fluids, vasopressors

H

hydroxychloroquine
(hye-drox-ee-klor'oh-kwin)
Plaquenil
Func. class.: Antimalarial, antiarthritic
Chem. class.: 4-Aminoquinoline derivative
Pregnancy category C

Action: Inhibits parasite replications, transcription of DNA to RNA by forming complexes with DNA in the parasite

➔ Therapeutic Outcome: Absence of malaria, absence of inflammation in arthritis

Uses: Malaria caused by *Plasmodium vivax, P. malariae, P. ovale, P. falciparum* (some strains); SLE, rheumatoid arthritis

Dosage and routes

Malaria

P ***Adult and child:*** PO 5 mg/kg/wk on same day of week, not to exceed 400 mg; treatment should begin 2 wk before entering endemic area; continue 8 wk after leaving; if treatment begins after exposure, 800 mg for adult, 10 mg/kg for children in 2 divided doses 6 hr apart

Lupus erythematosus

Adult: PO 400 mg qd-bid; length depends on patient response; maintenance 200-400 mg qd

Rheumatoid arthritis

Adult: PO 400-600 mg qd, then 200-300 mg qd after good response

Available forms: Tab 200 mg (base 155 mg)

Side effects/adverse reactions

CNS: Headache, stimulation, fatigue, irritability, ***convulsions,*** bad dreams, dizziness, confusion, psychosis, decreased reflexes
CV: Hypotension, heart block, ***asystole with syncope***
EENT: Blurred vision, corneal changes, retinal changes, difficulty focusing, tinnitus, vertigo, deafness, photophobia, corneal edema
GI: Nausea, vomiting, anorexia, diarrhea, cramps
HEMA: Thrombocytopenia, agranulocytosis, hemolytic anemia, leukopenia
INTEG: Pruritus, pigmentation changes, skin eruptions, lichen planus–like eruptions, eczema, ***exfoliative dermatitis,*** alopecia

Contraindications: Hypersensitivity, retinal field changes, P porphyria, children (long-term)

Precautions: Blood dyscrasias, severe GI disease, neurologic disease, alcoholism, hepatic disease, G6PD deficiency, psoriasis, eczema, pregnancy **C**

Pharmacokinetics

Absorption	Well absorbed (PO)
Distribution	Widely distributed; high concentration in liver
Metabolism	Partially metabolized
Excretion	Kidneys, partially unchanged
Half-life	3-5 days

Pharmacodynamics

	PO
Onset	Rapid
Peak	1-2 hr
Duration	Unknown

Interactions

Drug/drug:

Individual drugs

Digoxin: ↑ levels of digoxin
Penicillamine: ↑ toxicity
Rabies vaccine: ↑ rabies antibody titer

Drug classifications

Magnesium compounds: ↓ action of hydroxchloroquine
Aluminum compounds: ↓ action of hydoxchloroquine
Urine acidifiers: ↑ renal excretion

NURSING CONSIDERATIONS

Assessment

- Monitor CBC, platelets before and throughout treatment; platelets, WBC, RBC may be decreased
- Monitor liver studies weekly: ALT (SGPT), AST (SGOT), bilirubin before and throughout treatment
- Monitor renal status before treatment and monthly BUN, creatinine, output, sp gr, urinalysis
- Assess mental status often: affect, mood, behavioral changes; psychosis may occur
- Assess hepatic status: decreased appetite, jaundice, dark urine, fatigue related to density of parasites in the blood
- Assess for pain in rheumatoid arthritis: type of pain, duration, intensity, aggravation, ameliorating factors; check for swelling around joints and range of motion
- Assess for improvement in malaria: decreasing shaking chills, sweating, headache, aching, orthostatic hypotension, anemia; lupus erythematosus: decreased fever, malar rash, alopecia, photosensitivity, facial rash, low-grade fever

Associated nursing diagnoses

✓ Infection, risk for (uses)
✓ Injury, risk for (adverse reactions)
✓ Knowledge deficit (teaching)

Implementation

PO route

- Give with meals or milk to decrease GI symptoms; crush tab and mix with food for swallowing difficulty
- Give an antiemetic if vomiting occurs
- Give after C&S completed and every mo to detect resistance

Patient/family education

- Advise patient that compliance with dosage schedule, duration is necessary; if dose is missed take as soon as remembered; do not double dose

• Caution patient that scheduled appointments must be kept or relapse may occur; to report if improvement does not occur
• Advise patient to use sunglasses, protective clothing, sunscreen to prevent retinopathy, visual damage, and dermatoses
• Caution patient if dizziness occurs to avoid hazardous activities and driving until drug response is determined
• Instruct patient to keep out of reach of children; deaths have occurred with minimal doses

Evaluation

Positive therapeutic outcome
• Decreased symptoms of malaria
• Decreased symptoms of rheumatoid arthritis
• Decreased symptoms of SLE

hydroxyprogesterone

(hye-drox-ee-pro-jess'te-rone)
Delalatin, Duralutin, Gesterol L.A. 250, Hylutin, Hyprogest 250, Hyproval PA, Pro-Depo, Prodrox
Func. class.: Progestin, hormone
Chem. class.:
Pregnancy category X

Action: Inhibits secretion of pituitary gonadotropins, which prevents follicular maturation and ovulation and stimulates growth of mammary tissue; antineoplastic action against endometrial cancer

Therapeutic Outcome: Regular menstrual periods in menstrual disorders; decreased size and spread of malignant cells

Uses: Uterine carcinoma, menstrual disorders (abnormal uterine bleeding, amenorrhea)

Dosage and routes

Menstrual disorders
Adult: IM 125-375 mg q4 wk; discontinue after 4 cycles

Uterine cancer
Adult: IM 1 g 5-7 times/wk

Available forms: Inj 125, 250 mg/ml

Side effects/adverse reactions

CNS: Dizziness, headache, migraines, depression, fatigue
CV: Hypotension, thrombophlebitis, edema, ***thromboembolism, stroke, pulmonary embolism, MI***
EENT: Diplopia
GI: *Nausea,* vomiting, anorexia, cramps, increased weight, ***cholestatic jaundice***
GU: Amenorrhea, cervical erosion, breakthrough bleeding, dysmenorrhea, vaginal candidiasis, breast changes, *gynecomastia,* endometriosis, ***spontaneous abortion***
INTEG: Rash, urticaria, acne, hirsutism, alopecia, oily skin, seborrhea, purpura, melasma, photosensitivity
META: Hyperglycemia

Contraindications: Breast cancer, hypersensitivity, thromboembolic disorders, reproductive cancer, genital bleeding (abnormal, undiagnosed), pregnancy **X**

Precautions: Lactation, hypertension, asthma, blood dyscrasias, gallbladder disease, diabetes mellitus, bone disease, depression, migraine headache, convulsive disorders, hepatic disease, renal disease, family history of breast or reproductive tract cancer

Pharmacokinetics

Absorption	Unknown
Distribution	Unknown
Metabolism	Unknown
Excretion	Breast milk
Half-life	Unknown

Pharmacodynamics

	IM
Onset	Unknown
Peak	Unknown
Duration	24 hr

Interactions

Drug/drug:

Individual drugs

Bromocriptine: ↓ effectiveness of bromocriptine

Lab test interferences

Increase: Alkaline phosphatase, nitrogen (urine), pregnanediol, amino acids, factors VII, VIII, IX, X

Decrease: GTT, HDL

Interfere: Thyroid hormone assays

NURSING CONSIDERATIONS

Assessment

- Monitor weight daily; notify prescriber of weekly weight gain >5 lb
- Monitor B/P at beginning of treatment and periodically thereafter
- Monitor I&O ratio: be alert for decreasing urinary output, increasing edema and report to prescriber; do complete pad count daily to determine amount of vaginal bleeding
- Assess liver function studies: ALT (SGPT), AST (SGOT), bilirubin periodically during long-term therapy
- Assess mental status: affect, mood, behavioral changes, depression; if depression occurs, drug may need to be discontinued

Associated nursing diagnoses

- ✓ Sexual dysfunction (uses)
- ✓ Tissue perfusion, altered (adverse reactions)
- ✓ Injury, risk for (adverse reactions)
- ✓ Knowledge deficit (teaching)

Implementation

IM route

- Give deep in large muscle mass

Patient/family education

- Caution patient to avoid sunlight or use sunscreen; photosensitivity can occur
- Teach patient to report breast lumps, vaginal bleeding, edema, jaundice, dark urine, clay-colored stools, dyspnea, headache, blurred vision, abdominal pain, numbness or stiffness in legs, chest pain

• Advise patient to report suspected pregnancy to prescriber; drug is tetatogenic to fetus

Evaluation

Positive therapeutic outcome
• Absence of amenorrhea
• Decreased abnormal uterine bleeding
• Decreased growth of malignant cells in uterine carcinoma

hydroxyurea

(hye-drox-ee-yoo-ree′ah)
Hydrea
Func. class.: Antineoplastic, antimetabolite
Chem. class.: Synthetic urea analog
Pregnancy category **D**

Action: Acts by inhibiting DNA synthesis without interfering with RNA or protein synthesis; incorporates thymidine into DNA, causing direct damage to DNA strands; S phase specific of cell cycle

➡ Therapeutic Outcome: Prevention of rapidly growing malignant cells

Uses: Melanoma, chronic myelocytic leukemia, recurrent or metastatic ovarian cancer, squamous cell carcinoma of the head and neck

Dosage and routes

Solid tumors

Adult: PO 80 mg/kg as a single dose q 3 days or 20-30 mg/kg as a single dose qd

In combination with radiation

Adult: PO 80 mg/kg as a single dose q 3 days; should be started 7 days before irradiation

Resistant chronic myelocytic leukemia

Adult: PO 20-30 mg/kg/day as a single daily dose

Available forms: Cap 500 mg

Side effects/adverse reactions

CNS: Headache, confusion, hallucinations, dizziness, ***convulsions***
CV: Angina, ischemia
GI: Nausea, vomiting, anorexia, diarrhea, stomatitis, constipation
GU: Increased BUN, uric acid, creatinine, temporary renal function impairment
HEMA: Leukopenia, anemia, thrombocytopenia
INTEG: Rash, urticaria, pruritus, dry skin

Contraindications: Hypersensitivity, leukopenia (<2500/mm^3), thrombocytopenia (<100,000/mm^3), anemia (severe), pregnancy **D**

Precautions: Renal disease (severe)

Pharmacokinetics

Absorption	Well absorbed (PO)
Distribution	Crosses blood-brain barrier
Metabolism	Liver (50%)
Excretion	Kidneys, unchanged (50%)
Half-life	4 hr

Pharmacodynamics

	PO
Onset	Unknown
Peak	2 hr
Duration	Unknown

Interactions

Drug/drug:

Individual drugs

Cyclophosphamide: ↑ cardiotoxicity, CHF

Radiation: ↑ toxicity, bone marrow suppression

Drug classifications

Antineoplastics: ↑ toxicity, bone marrow suppression

Lab test interferences

Increase: Renal function studies

NURSING CONSIDERATIONS

Assessment

- Assess buccal cavity q8h for dryness, sores or ulceration, white patches, oral pain, bleeding, dysphagia; obtain prescription for viscous lidocaine (Xylocaine)
- Assess symptoms indicating severe allergic reaction: rash, pruritus, urticaria, purpuric skin lesions, itching, flushing
- Monitor CBC, differential, platelet count weekly; withhold drug if WBC count is <4000/mm^3 or platelet count is <100,000/mm^3; notify prescriber of results if WBC <20,000/mm^3, platelets <150,000/mm^3
- Assess for increased uric acid levels, swelling, joint pain primarily in extremities; patient should be well hydrated to prevent urate deposits
- Monitor renal function studies: BUN, creatinine, serum uric acid, urine CrCl before and during therapy; I&O ratio; report fall in urine output to <30 ml/hr
- Monitor temp q4h (may indicate beginning of infection)
- Monitor liver function tests before and during therapy (bilirubin, AST [SGOT], ALT [SGPT], LDH) as needed or monthly
- Assess for bleeding: hematuria, stool guaiac, bruising or petechiae, mucosa or orifices q8h; check for inflammation of mucosa, breaks in skin

Associated nursing diagnoses

- ☑ Injury, risk for (adverse reactions)
- ☑ Body image disturbance (adverse reactions)
- ☑ Infection, risk for (adverse reactions)
- ☑ Knowledge deficit (teaching)

Implementation

- Avoid contact with skin, very irritating; wash completely to remove
- Give fluids **IV** or PO before chemotherapy to hydrate patient
- Give antiemetic 30-60 min before giving drug and prn to prevent vomiting; antibiotics for prophylaxis of infection
- Provide liq diet: carbonated beverages; gelatin may be added if patient is not nauseated or vomiting
- Provide rinsing of mouth tid-qid with water, club soda; brushing of teeth bid-qid with soft brush or cotton-tipped

applicators for stomatitis; use unwaxed dental floss

PO route

- For difficulty swallowing, cap contents may be mixed with water

Patient/family education

- Advise patient that contraceptive measures are recommended during therapy
- Teach patient to avoid use of products containing aspirin or ibuprofen, razors, commercial mouthwash, since bleeding may occur; instruct patient to report symptoms of bleeding (hematuria, tarry stools)
- Instruct patient to report signs of anemia (fatigue, headache, irritability, faintness, shortness of breath)
- Advise patient to report any changes in breathing or coughing even several mo after treatment; to avoid crowds and persons with respiratory tract or other infections
- Caution patient not to have any vaccinations without the advice of the prescriber, serious reactions can occur

Evaluation

Positive therapeutic outcome

- Prevention of rapid division of malignant cells

hydroxyzine

(hye-drox'i-zeen)

Anxanil, Apo-hydroxyzine ♣, Atarax, Atarax 100, Durrex, E-Vista, Hydroxacen, Hydroxyzine HCl, hydroxyzine pamoate, Hyzine-50, Multipax ♣, Novohydroxyzine ♣, Quiess, Vistaject-25, Vistaject-50, Vistaquel 50, Vistaril, Vistazine 50

Func. class.: Sedative/hypnotic, antihistamine

Chem. class.: Piperazine derivative

Pregnancy category C

Action: Depresses subcortical levels of CNS, including limbic system, reticular formation; anticholinergic, antiemetic, antihistaminic responses

➔ Therapeutic Outcome: Absence of allergy symptoms, rhinitis, pruritus, absence of nausea/vomiting, sedation, absence of anxiety

Uses: Anxiety preoperatively, postoperatively to prevent nausea, vomiting; to potentiate narcotic analgesics; sedation; pruritus; prevention of alcohol, drug withdrawal

Dosage and routes

Adult: PO 25-100 mg tid-qid

P *Child >6 yr:* 50-100 mg/day in divided doses

P *Child <6 yr:* 50 mg/day in divided doses

Preoperatively/postoperatively

Adult: IM 25-100 mg q4-6h

P *Child:* IM 1.1 mg/kg q4-6h

Available forms: Tab 10, 25, 50, 100 mg; cap 25, 50, 100 mg; syrup 100 mg/5 ml; oral susp 25 mg/5 ml; IM inj 25, 50 mg/ml

Side effects/adverse reactions

CNS: Dizziness, drowsiness, confusion, headache, tremors, fatigue, depression, ***convulsions***

GI: Dry mouth

Contraindications: Hypersensitivity, pregnancy **C**

G **Precautions:** Elderly, debilitated patients, hepatic disease, renal disease

Pharmacokinetics

Absorption	Well absorbed
Distribution	Not known
Metabolism	Liver, completely
Excretion	Feces, bile
Half-life	3 hr

Pharmacodynamics

	PO/IM
Onset	15-30 min
Peak	2-4 hr
Duration	4-6 hr

Interactions

Drug/drug:

Individual drugs

Alcohol: ↑ CNS depression
Atropine: ↑ anticholinergic reactions
Disopyramide: ↑ anticholinergic reactions
Haloperidol: ↑ anticholinergic reactions
Quinidine: ↑ anticholinergic reactions

Drug classifications

Antidepressants: ↑ anticholinergic reactions
Antihistamines: ↑ anticholinergic reactions
CNS depressants: ↑ CNS depression
Narcotics: ↑ CNS depression
Phenothiazines: ↑ anticholinergic reactions
Sedative/hypnotics: ↑ CNS depression

Lab test interferences

False increase: 17-OHCS

NURSING CONSIDERATIONS

Assessment

- Assess respiratory status: rate, rhythm, increase in bronchial secretions, wheezing, chest tightness; provide fluids to 2 L/day to decrease secretion thickness
- Monitor I&O ratio: be alert for urinary retention, frequency, dysuria, especially in G the elderly; drug should be discontinued if these occur
- Observe for drowsiness, dizziness
- Assess cough characteristics including type, frequency, thickness of secretions; evaluate response to this medication if using for cough

Associated nursing diagnoses

✓ Injury, risk for (side effects)
✓ Anxiety (uses)
✓ Knowledge deficit (teaching)

H

Implementation

PO route

- Give with meals if GI symptoms occur; absorption may be slightly decreased; cap may be opened and drug mixed with food/fluids for patients with swallowing difficulties

IM route

- Give IM inj in large muscle mass; aspirate to avoid **IV** administration; use Z-track method; severe necrosis can result with improper technique

Y-site compatibilities:

Melphan, vinorelbine

Y-site incompatibility:

Paclitaxel

Syringe incompatibilities:

Aminophylline, chloramphenicol, dimenhydrinate, heparin, penicillin G potassium, pentobarbital, phenobarbital, phenytoin

Syringe compatibilities:

Atropine, benzquinamide, butorphanol, chlorpromazine, cimetidine, codeine, diphenhydramine, doxapram, droperidol, fentanyl, glycopyrrolate, hydromorphone, lidocaine, meperidine, metoclopromide, morphine, nalbuphine, oxymorphone, pentazocine, procaine, prochlorperazine, promazine, ranitidine, scopolamine

Patient/family education

- Caution patient to avoid hazardous activities and activities requiring alertness, since dizziness may occur; instruct patient to request assistance with ambulation
- Advise patient to avoid alcohol, other CNS depressants including cough, cold preparations; CNS depression may occur
- Teach all aspects of drug use; to notify prescriber if confusion, sedation, hypotension occur; to avoid driving and other hazardous activity if drowsiness occurs; to avoid alcohol and other CNS depressants that may potentiate effect
- Instruct patient to take 1 hr pc or 2 hr ac to facilitate absorption
- Caution patient not to exceed recommended dosage; dysrhythmias may occur
- Tell patient hard candy, gum, frequent rinsing of mouth may be used for dryness

Evaluation

Positive therapeutic outcome

- Absence of nausea, vomiting
- Decreased anxiety

Treatment of overdose:

Lavage if orally ingested, VS, supportive care, **IV** norepinephrine for hypotension

ibuprofen 🔑
(eye-byoo-proe'fen)
Aches-N-Pain, Actiprofen ✤, Advil, Amersol ✤, Apo-Ibuprofen ✤, Children's Advil, Excedrin IB, Genpril, Haltran, Ibuprin, ibuprofen, Ibuprohm, I-Tab, Medipren, Menadol, Midol-200, Motrin, Motrin IB, Novoprosen ✤, Nuprin, Pamprin-IB, Rufen, Saleto-200, Saleto-400, Saleto-600, Saleto-800, Trendar

Func. class.: Nonsteroidal antiinflammatory; nonnarcotic analgesic
Chem. class.: Propionic acid derivative

Pregnancy category B

Action: Inhibits prostaglandin synthesis by decreasing enzyme needed for biosynthesis; analgesic, antiinflammatory, antipyretic

Therapeutic Outcome: Decreased pain, inflammation, fever

Uses: Rheumatoid arthritis, osteoarthritis, primary dysmenorrhea, gout, dental pain, musculoskeletal disorders, fever

Dosage and routes

Analgesia

Adult: PO 200-400 mg q4-6h, not to exceed 3.2 g/day

Antipyretic

P *Child 6 mo-12yr:* PO 5 mg/kg (temp <102.5° F), 10 mg/kg (temp >102.5° F), may repeat q4-6h; max 40 mg/kg/day

Anti-inflammatory

Adult: PO 300-800 mg tid-qid; max 3.2 g/day

P *Child:* PO 30-40 mg/kg/day in 3-4 divided doses; max 50 mg/kg/day

Available forms: Tab 200, 300, 400, 600, 800 mg; oral susp 100 mg/5 ml

Side effects/adverse reactions

CNS: Dizziness, drowsiness, fatigue, tremors, confusion, insomnia, anxiety, depression
CV: Tachycardia, peripheral edema, palpitations, dysrhythmias, hypertension
EENT: Tinnitus, hearing loss, blurred vision
GI: Nausea, anorexia, vomiting, diarrhea, jaundice, ***cholestatic hepatitis,*** constipation, flatulence, cramps, dry mouth, peptic ulcer
GU: ***Nephrotoxicity;*** dysuria, hematuria, oliguria, azotemia
HEMA: ***Blood dyscrasias***
INTEG: Purpura, rash, pruritus, sweating

Contraindications: Hypersensitivity, asthma, severe renal disease, severe hepatic disease

Precautions: Pregnancy **B** 1st and 2nd trimester, lactation, P children, bleeding disorders, GI disorders, cardiac disorders, hypersensitivity to other antiinflammatory agents

Pharmacokinetics

Absorption	Well absorbed
Distribution	Not known; crosses placenta
Metabolism	Liver, extensively
Excretion	Kidneys, unchanged (10%)
Half-life	3½ hr

Pharmacodynamics

	PO
Onset	½ hr
Peak	1-2 hr
Duration	4-6 hr

Interactions

Drug/drug:

Individual drugs

Acetaminophen (long-term use): ↑ renal reactions
Alcohol: ↑ adverse reactions
Aspirin: ↓ effectiveness, ↑ adverse reactions
Coumarin: ↑ anticoagulant effects
Digoxin: ↑ toxicity, levels
Insulin: ↓ insulin effect
Lithium: ↑ toxicity
Methotrexate: ↑ toxicity
Phenytoin: ↑ toxicity
Probenecid: ↑ toxicity
Sulfonylurea: ↑ toxicity

Drug classifications

Anticoagulants: ↑ risk of bleeding
Antihypertensives: ↓ effect of antihypertensives
Antineoplastics: ↑ risk of hematologic toxicity
β-Blockers: ↑ antihypertension
Cephalosporins: ↑ risk of bleeding
Diuretics: ↓ effectiveness of diuretics
Glucocorticoids: ↑ adverse reactions
Hypoglycemics: ↓ hypoglycemic effect
NSAIDs: ↑ adverse reactions
Potassium supplements: ↑ adverse reactions
Radiation: ↑ risk of hematologic toxicity
Sulfonamides: ↑ toxicity

Lab test interferences

Increase: Bleeding time

NURSING CONSIDERATIONS

Assessment

- Monitor liver function studies: AST (SGOT), ALT (SGPT), bilirubin, creatinine if patient is on long-term therapy
- Monitor renal function studies: BUN, urine creatinine if patient is on long-term therapy
- Monitor blood studies: CBC, Hct, Hgb, pro-time if patient is on long-term therapy
- Check I&O ratio; decreasing output may indicate renal failure if patient is on long-term therapy
- Assess hepatotoxicity: dark urine, clay-colored stools, yellowing of skin and sclera, itching, abdominal pain, fever, diarrhea if patient is on long-term therapy
- Assess for allergic reactions: rash, urticaria; if these occur, drug may have to be discontinued
- Assess for ototoxicity: tinnitus, ringing, roaring in ears; audiometric testing needed before, after long-term therapy
- Assess for visual changes: blurring, halos; may indicate corneal, retinal damage
- Identify prior drug history; there are many drug interactions

• Monitor pain: location, duration, type, intensity before dose and 1 hr after
• Monitor musculoskeletal status: ROM before dose and 1 hr after
• Identify fever: length of time in evidence and related symptoms

Associated nursing diagnoses

✓ Pain (uses)
✓ Mobility, impaired (uses)
✓ Injury, risk for (side effects)
✓ Knowledge deficit (teaching)

Implementation

PO route
• Administer to patient crushed or whole; 800-mg tab may be dissolved in water
• Give with food or milk to decrease gastric symptoms; give 30 min pc or 2 hr ac; absorption may be slowed

Patient/family education

• Teach patient to report any symptoms of hepatotoxicity, renal toxicity, visual changes, ototoxicity, allergic reactions, bleeding if patient is on long-term therapy
• Caution patient not to exceed recommended dosage; acute poisoning may result
• Advise patient to read label on other OTC drugs
• Inform patient that the therapeutic response takes 1 mo (arthritis)
• Caution patient to avoid alcohol ingestion; GI bleeding may occur
• Advise patient with allergies that allergic reactions may develop

Evaluation

Positive therapeutic outcome
• Decreased pain
• Decreased inflammation
• Decreased fever
• Increased mobility

idarubicin

(eye-da-roo'bi-sin)
Idamycin
Func. class.: Antineoplastic, antibiotic
Chem. class.: Anthracycline glycoside
Pregnancy category **D**

Action: Inhibits DNS synthesis derived from daunorubicin by binding to DNA, which causes strand splitting; cell cycle specific (S phase); a vesicant

Therapeutic Outcome: Prevention of rapidly growing malignant cells

Uses: Used in combination with other antineoplastics for acute myelocytic leukemia in adults

Dosage and routes

Adult: **IV** 12 mg/m²/day × 3 days in combination with cytosine arabinoside, or 25 mg/m² **IV** bolus followed by 200 mg/m²/day × 5 days by cont inf

Available forms: Inj 5, 10 mg vials

Side effects/adverse reactions

CNS: Fever, chills, headache
CV: ***Dysrhythmias, CHF, pericarditis, myocarditis,*** peripheral edema
GI: Nausea, vomiting, abdominal pain, mucositis, diarrhea, ***hepatotoxicity***
HEMA: ***Thrombocytopenia, leukopenia, anemia***
INTEG: Rash, extravasation, dermatitis, reversible alopecia, urticaria, thrombophlebitis at inj site

Contraindications:
Hypersensitivity, pregnancy **D**

Precautions:
Renal and hepatic disease, gout, bone marrow depression, children

Pharmacokinetics

Absorption	Complete bioavailability
Distribution	Rapidly distributed; high tissue binding
Metabolism	Liver, extensively
Excretion	Bile
Half-life	22 hr

Pharmacodynamics

Onset	Unknown
Peak	Unknown
Duration	Unknown

Interactions
Drug/drug:
Individual drugs
Radiation: ↑ toxicity, bone marrow suppression
Drug classifications
Antineoplastics: ↑ toxicity, bone marrow suppression

Lab test interferences
Increase: Uric acid

NURSING CONSIDERATIONS
Assessment

- Assess symptoms indicating severe allergic reaction: rash, pruritus, urticaria, purpuric skin lesions, itching, flushing; drug should be discontinued
- Assess for tachypnea, ECG changes, dyspnea, edema, fatigue
- Monitor CBC, differential, platelet count weekly; withhold drug if WBC count is <4000/mm^3 or platelet count is <100,000/mm^3; notify prescriber of results if WBC <20,000/mm^3, platelets <150,000/mm^3
- Monitor temp q4h (may indicate beginning of infection)
- Monitor liver function tests before and during therapy (bilirubin, AST [SGOT], ALT [SGPT], LDH) as needed or monthly; note yellowing of skin and sclera, dark urine, clay-colored stools, itchy skin, abdominal pain, fever, diarrhea; hepatoxicity can be severe
- Assess for bleeding: hematuria, stool guaiac, bruising or petechiae, mucosa or orifices q8h; assess for inflammation of mucosa, breaks in skin
- Identify effects of alopecia on body image; discuss feelings about body changes

Associated nursing diagnoses

- ✓ Injury, risk for (adverse reactions)
- ✓ Cardiac output, decreased (adverse reactions)

✓ Body image disturbance (adverse reactions)
✓ Infection, risk for (adverse reactions)
✓ Knowledge deficit (teaching)

Implementation

- Avoid contact with skin; very irritating; wash completely to remove
- Give fluids **IV** or PO before chemotherapy to hydrate patient
- Administer antiemetic 30-60 min before giving drug and prn to prevent vomiting; administer antibiotics for prophylaxis of infection
- Give a liq diet: carbonated beverages; gelatin may be added if patient is not nauseated or vomiting
- Provide rinsing of mouth tid-qid with water, club soda; brushing of teeth bid-qid with soft brush or cotton-tipped applicators for stomatitis; use unwaxed dental floss

IV **IV route**

- Drug should be prepared by experienced personnel using proper precautions (biologic cabinet, wearing gown, gloves, mask)
- Give after reconstituting 5-mg vial with 5 ml 0.9% NaCl (1 mg/1 ml); give over 10-15 min through Y-tube or 3-way stopcock of inf of D_5 or normal saline; discard unused portion
- Inject hydrocortisone for extravasation; apply ice compress after stopping inf
- Store at room temp for 3 days after reconstituting or 7 days refrigerated

Y-*site compatibilities:*

Amikacin, cimetidine, cyclophosphamide, cytarabine, diphenhydramine, droperidol, erythromycin, lactobionate, heparin, magnesium sulfate, mannitol, melphalan, metoclopromide, potassium chloride, ranitidine, vinorelbine

Y-*site incompatibilities:*

Acyclovir, ampicillin/sulbactam, cefazolin, ceftazidine, clindamycin, dexamethasone sodium phosphate, etoposide, furosemide, gentamicin, heparin, hydrocortisone sodium succinate, lorazepam, meperidine, methotrexate, mezlocillin, sargramostim, sodium bicarbonate, vancomycin, vincristine

Solution compatibilities:

$D_{3.3}$/0.3% NaCl, D_5/0.9% NaCl, D_5W, Ringer's, 0.9% NaCl

Patient/family education

- Teach patient to avoid use of products containing aspirin or ibuprofen, razors, commercial mouthwash, since bleeding may occur; to report symptoms of bleeding (hematuria, tarry stools)
- Instruct patient to report signs of anemia (fatigue, headache, irritability, faintness, shortness of breath)
- Advise patient that hair may be lost during treatment; a wig or hair piece may make patient feel better; new hair may be different in color, texture
- Tell patient not to have any vaccinations without the advice of the prescriber; serious reactions can occur

• Advise patient contraception is needed during treatment and for several mo after the completion of therapy

Evaluation

Positive therapeutic outcome
• Prevention of rapid division of malignant cells

idoxuridine-IDU
(eye-dox-yoor'i-deen)
Herplex, Stoxil
Func. class.: Antiviral
Chem. class.: Pyrimidine nucleoside
Pregnancy category **C**

Action: Inhibits viral replication by interfering with DNA synthesis

Therapeutic Outcome: Decreased symptoms of infection in the eye

Uses: Herpes simplex keratitis, CMV, varicella zoster (alone or with corticosteroids)

Dosage and routes

Adult and child: Instill 1 gtt q1h during day and q2h during night

Available forms: Sol 0.1%; ointment 0.5%

Side effects/adverse reactions

EENT: Poor corneal wound healing, temporary visual haze, overgrowth of nonsusceptible organisms

Contraindications: Hypersensitivity

Precautions: Antibiotic hypersensitivity, pregnancy **C**

Pharmacokinetics	
Absorption	Minimally absorbed
Distribution	Not distributed
Metabolism	Not metabolized
Excretion	Not excreted
Half-life	Unknown

Pharmacodynamics	
Onset	Rapid
Peak	Unknown
Duration	Unknown

Interactions
Drug/drug:

Individual drugs
Boric acid: Do not use together

NURSING CONSIDERATIONS
Assessment

• Assess for allergy: itching, lacrimation, redness, swelling
• Assess for infection: pain, inflammation, redness, crusts, drainage; report to prescriber

Associated nursing diagnoses

✓ Infection, risk for (uses)
✓ Knowledge deficit (teaching)

Implementation

• Administer after washing hands; cleanse crusts or discharge from eye before application
• Store in refrigerator in light-resistant container until used

Patient/family education

- Advise patient to use drug exactly as prescribed; to avoid use of eye makeup, towels, washcloths, eye medication of others; reinfection may occur
- Instruct patient to report itching, increased redness, burning, stinging, swelling; drug should be discontinued
- Caution patient that drug may cause blurred vision when ointment is applied; to wait until vision is clear to drive or operate machinery

Evaluation

Positive therapeutic outcome

- Absence of redness, inflammation, tearing, photophobia

ifosfamide

(i-foss′fa-mide)

Ifex

Func. class.: Antineoplastic alkylating agent

Chem. class.: Nitrogen mustard

Pregnancy category **D**

Action: Alkylates DNA, RNA; inhibits enzymes that allow synthesis of amino acids in proteins; also responsible for cross-linking DNA strands; activity is not cell cycle stage specific

Therapeutic Outcome: Prevention of rapidly growing malignant cells

Uses: Testicular cancer

Dosage and routes

Adult: **IV** 1.2 g/m^2/day × 5 days; repeat course q3 wk; give with mesna

Available forms: Inj 1, 3 g

Side effects/adverse reactions

CNS: Facial paresthesia, fever, malaise, somnolence, confusion, depression, hallucinations, dizziness, disorientation, ***seizures, coma***

GI: Nausea, vomiting, anorexia, ***hepatotoxicity***, stomatitis, constipation

GU: ***Hematuria, nephrotoxicity, hemorrhagic cystitis,*** dysuria, urinary frequency

HEMA: ***Thrombocytopenia, leukopenia, anemia***

INTEG: Dermatitis, alopecia, pain at inj site

Contraindications: Hypersensitivity, bone marrow suppression, pregnancy **D**

Precautions: Renal disease, P lactation, children

Pharmacokinetics

Absorption	Complete bioavailability
Distribution	Saturation at high dosages
Metabolism	Liver
Excretion	Breast milk
Half-life	15 hr

Pharmacodynamics

Onset	Unknown
Peak	Unknown
Duration	Unknown

Interactions

Drug/drug:

Individual drugs

Radiation: ↑ toxicity, bone marrow suppression

Drug classifications

Antineoplastics: ↑ toxicity, bone marrow suppression

NURSING CONSIDERATIONS

Assessment

- Monitor CBC, differential, platelet count weekly; withhold drug if WBC is <4000 or platelet count is <75,000; notify prescriber of results if WBC <20,000/mm^3, platelets <150,000/mm^3
- Monitor renal function studies: BUN, serum uric acid, urine CrCl before, during therapy; I&O ratio; report fall in urine output of 30 ml/hr
- Monitor for cold, fever, sore throat (may indicate beginning infection); identify edema in feet and joints, stomach pain, shaking; prescriber should be notified
- Assess for bleeding: hematuria, guaiac, bruising or petechiae, mucosa or orifices q8h; no rec temp

Associated nursing diagnoses

- ✓ Injury, risk for (adverse reactions)
- ✓ Body image disturbance (adverse reactions)
- ✓ Infection, risk for (adverse reactions)
- ✓ Knowledge deficit (teaching)

Implementation

- Give fluids **IV** or PO before chemotherapy to hydrate patient
- Give antiemetic 30-60 min before giving drug and prn to prevent vomiting
- Provide liq diet: carbonated beverages; gelatin may be added if patient is not nauseated or vomiting

IV IV route

- Give **IV** after diluting 1 g/20 ml sterile or bacteriostatic water for inj with parabens or benzyl only; shake
- Give by intermittent inf after further diluting with D_5W, LR, 0.9% NaCl, sterile water for inj (1 g/20 ml = 50 mg/ml); (1 g/50 ml = 20 mg/ml; 1 g/200 ml = 5 mg/ml); give over 30 min
- Store powder at room temp; always give with mesna to prevent ifosfamide-induced hemorrhagic cystitis

Syringe compatibility:

Mesna

Y-site compatibilities:

Fludarabine, melphalan, paclitaxel, ondansetron, sargramostim, vinorelbine

Additive compatibilities:

Carboplatin, cisplatin, epirubicin, etoposide, fluorouracil, mesna

Patient/family education

- Teach patient to avoid use of products containing aspirin or ibuprofen, razors, commercial mouthwash, since bleeding may occur; to report symptoms of bleeding (hematuria, tarry stools)
- Instruct patient to report signs of anemia (fatigue, head-

ache, irritability, faintness, shortness of breath)

- Advise patient to report any changes in breathing or coughing even several mo after treatment; to avoid crowds and persons with respiratory tract or other infections
- Teach patient that hair loss is common; discuss the use of wigs or hair pieces
- Caution patient not to have any vaccinations without the advice of the prescriber; serious reactions can occur
- Advise patient contraception is needed during treatment and for several mo after the completion of therapy

Evaluation

Positive therapeutic outcome

- Prevention of rapid division of malignant cells
- Absence of swelling at night
- Increased appetite, increased weight

imipenem/cilastatin

(i-me-pen'em sye-la-stat'in)

Primaxin IM, Primaxin IV

Func. class.: Antiinfective; miscellaneous penicillin

Pregnancy category **C**

Action: Interferes with cell wall replication of susceptible organisms; osmotically unstable cell wall swells and bursts from osmotic pressure; addition of cilastatin prevents renal inactivation that occurs with high urinary concentrations of imipenem

Therapeutic Outcome: Bactericidal action against the following: *Streptococcus pneumoniae,* group A β-hemolytic streptococci, *Staphylococcus aureus,* enterococcus; gram-negative organisms: *Klebsiella, Proteus, Escherichia coli, Acinetobacter, Serratia, Pseudomonas aeruginosa; Salmonella, Shigella*

Uses: Serious infections caused by gram-positive or gram-negative organisms

Dosage and routes

Adult: **IV** 250-500 mg q6h; severe infections may require 1 g q6h; may give IM q12h (total daily IM dose >1500 mg not recommended)

Available forms: **IV** inj 250, 500; IM inj 500, 750 mg

Side effects/adverse reactions

CNS: Fever, somnolence, ***seizures,*** dizziness, weakness

CV: Hypotension, palpitations

GI: Diarrhea, nausea, vomiting, ***pseudomembranous colitis, hepatitis,*** glossitis

HEMA: ***Eosinophilia, neutropenia,*** decreased HGb, Hct

INTEG: Rash, urticaria, pruritus, pain at inj site, phlebitis, erythema at inj site

RESP: Chest discomfort, dyspnea, hyperventilation

SYST: ***Anaphylaxis***

Contraindications: Hypersensitivity, IM hypersensitivity to local anesthetics of the amide type

Precautions: Pregnancy **C**, G lactation, elderly, hypersensitivity to penicillins, seizure disorders, P renal disease, children

Pharmacokinetics

Absorption	Complete bioavailability (IV)
Distribution	Widely distributed; crosses placenta
Metabolism	Liver
Excretion	Kidneys, unchanged (70%); breast milk
Half-life	1 hr; increased in renal disease

Pharmacodynamics

	IV	IM
Onset	Rapid	Unknown
Peak	½-1 hr	Unknown

Interactions

Drug/drug:

Individual drugs

Ganciclovir: ↑ seizures
Probenecid: ↓ renal excretion, ↑ blood level

Drug classifications

Cephalosporins: ↓ action
Penicillins: ↓ action

Lab test interferences

False increase: Creatinine (serum urine), urinary 17-KS
False positive: Urinary protein, direct Coombs' test, urine glucose
Interference: Cross-matching

NURSING CONSIDERATIONS

Assessment

- Assess patient for previous sensitivity reaction
- Assess patient for signs and symptoms of infection, including characteristics of wounds, sputum, urine, stool, WBC >10,000, fever; obtain baseline information before and during treatment
- Complete C&S tests before beginning drug therapy to identify if correct treatment has been initiated
- Assess for allergic reactions: rash, urticaria, pruritus, chills, fever, joint pain; angioedema may occur a few days after therapy begins; epinephrine, resuscitation equipment should be available for anaphylactic reaction
- Identify urine output; if decreasing, notify prescriber (may indicate nephrotoxicity); also check for increased BUN, creatinine
- Monitor blood studies: AST (SGOT), ALT (SGPT), CBC, Hct, bilirubin, LDH, alkaline phosphatase, Coombs' test monthly if patient is on long-term therapy
- Monitor electrolytes: potassium, sodium, chloride monthly if patient is on long-term therapy
- Assess bowel pattern qd; if severe diarrhea occurs, drug should be discontinued; may indicate pseudomembranous colitis
- Monitor for bleeding: ecchymosis, bleeding gums, hematuria, stool guaiac daily if on long-term therapy
- Assess for overgrowth of infection: perineal itching, fever, malaise, redness, pain, swelling, drainage, rash, diarrhea, change in cough, sputum

Associated nursing diagnoses

✓ Infection, risk for (uses)
✓ Diarrhea (adverse reactions)

✓ Injury, risk for (adverse reactions)
✓ Knowledge deficit (teaching)
✓ Noncompliance (teaching)

Implementation

IM route
- Reconstitute 500 mg/2 ml or 750 mg/3 ml lidocaine without epinephrine; shake well, withdraw and administer entire vial; give deep in large muscle mass, massage

IV **IV route**
- Reconstitute each 250 or 500 mg/10 ml of compatible diluent; shake well; transfer the resulting susp to not less than 100 ml of compatible diluent; add 10 ml to each previously reconstituted vial and shake to ensure all medication is used; transfer the remaining contents of the vial to the inf container; do not administer susp by direct inj; reconstitute 120-ml inf bottles/100 ml of a compatible diluent; shake until clear; may use 0.9% NaCl, D_5W, $D_{10}W$, D_5/0.2% sodium bicarbonate, D_5/0.9% NaCl, D_5/0.45% NaCl, D_5/0.225% NaCl, mannitol 2.5%, 5%, or 10%
- Give by intermittent inf: each 250- or 500-mg dose over 20-30 min, and each 1-g dose over 40-60 min; administer over 15-20 min for P pediatric patients; do not administer direct **IV**; do not admix with other antibiotics

Y-site compatibilities:

Acyclovir, famotidine, fludarabine, foscarnet, idarubicin, regular insulin, melphalan, ondansetron, vinorelbine, zidovudine

Y-site incompatibilities:

Fluconazole, meperidine, sargramostim

Additive incompatibilities:

Fluconazole, meperidine, sargramostim

Patient/family education

- Teach patient to report sore throat, bruising, bleeding, joint pain; may indicate blood dyscrasias (rare)
- Advise patient to contact prescriber if vaginal itching, loose, foul-smelling stools, furry tongue occur; may indicate superinfection
- Advise patient to notify prescriber of diarrhea with blood or pus, which may indicate pseudomembranous colitis

Evaluation

Positive therapeutic outcome
- Absence of signs/symptoms of infection (WBC <10,000, temp WNL, absence of red, draining wounds)
- Reported improvement in symptoms of infection

Treatment of anaphylaxis:

Epinephrine, antihistamines, resuscitate if needed

imipramine

(im-ip'ra-meen)
Apo-Imipramine ♣, Imipramine HCl, Impril ♣, Janimine, Novo-Pramine ♣, SK-Pramine, Tipramine, Tofranil, Tofranil PM

Func. class.: Antidepressant, tricyclic
Chem. class.: Dibenzazepine, tertiary amine

Pregnancy category C

Action: Blocks reuptake of norepinephrine and serotonin into nerve endings, increasing action of norepinephrine and serotonin in nerve cells; has anticholinergic effects

Therapeutic Outcome: Decreased symptoms of depression after 2-3 wk; decreased bedwetting in children

Uses: Depression, enuresis in children

Investigational uses: Chronic pain, migraine headaches, cluster headaches as adjunct

Dosage and routes

Adult: PO/IM 75-100 mg/day in divided doses; may increase by 25-50 mg up to 200 mg, not to exceed 300 mg/day; may give daily dose hs

Child: PO 25-75 mg/day

Available forms: Tab 10, 25, 50 mg; inj 25 mg/2 ml; cap 75, 100, 125, 150 mg

Side effects/adverse reactions

CV: Orthostatic hypotension, ECG changes, tachycardia, ***hypertension,*** palpitations

CNS: Dizziness, drowsiness, confusion, headache, anxiety, tremors, stimulation, weakness, insomnia, nightmares, extrapyramidal symptoms (elderly), increased psychiatric symptoms, paresthesia

EENT: Blurred vision, tinnitus, mydriasis

GI: Diarrhea, dry mouth, nausea, vomiting, ***paralytic ileus,*** increased appetite, cramps, epigastric distress, jaundice, ***hepatitis,*** stomatitis

GU: Retention, ***acute renal failure***

HEMA: ***Agranulocytosis, thrombocytopenia, eosinophilia, leukopenia***

INTEG: Rash, urticaria, sweating, pruritus, photosensitivity

Contraindications: Hypersensitivity to tricyclic antidepressants, recovery phase of MI, convulsive disorders, prostatic hypertrophy

Precautions: Suicidal patients, severe depression, increased intraocular pressure, narrow angle glaucoma, urinary retention, cardiac disease, hepatic disease, hyperthyroidism, electroshock therapy, elective surgery, elderly, pregnancy **C**

Pharmacokinetics

Absorption	Well absorbed
Distribution	Widely distributed; crosses placenta
Metabolism	Liver, extensively
Excretion	Kidneys, breast milk
Half-life	6-20 hr

Pharmacodynamics

	PO	IM
Onset	1 hr	1 hr
Peak	Unknown	Unknown
Duration	Unknown	Unknown

Interactions

Drug/drug:

Individual drugs

Alcohol: ↑ CNS depression
Cimetidine: ↑ levels, toxicity
Clonidine: Severe hypotension; avoid use
Disulfiram: Organic brain syndrome
Fluoxetine: ↑ levels, toxicity
Guanethidine: ↓ effects

Drug classifications

Analgesics: ↑ CNS depression
Anticholinergics: ↑ side effects
Antihistamines: ↑ CNS depression
Antihypertensives: May block antihypertensive effect
Barbiturates: ↑ effects
Benzodiazepines: ↑ effects
CNS depressants: ↑ effects
MAOI: Hypertensive crisis, convulsions
Oral contraceptives: ↑ effects, toxicity
Phenothiazines: ↑ toxicity
Sedative/hypnotics: ↑ CNS depression
Sympathomimetics, indirect acting: ↓ effects

Drug/smoking:

↑ metabolism, ↓ effects

Lab test interferences

Increase: Serum bilirubin, blood glucose, alkaline phosphatase
Decrease: VMA, 5-HIAA, blood glucose
False increase: Urinary catecholamines

NURSING CONSIDERATIONS

Assessment

- Monitor B/P (with patient lying, standing), pulse q4h; if systolic B/P drops 20 mm Hg, hold drug, notify prescriber; take vital signs q4h in patients with cardiovascular disease
- Monitor blood studies: CBC, leukocytes, differential, cardiac enzymes if patient is receiving long-term therapy
- Monitor hepatic studies: AST (SGOT), ALT (SGPT), bilirubin
- Check weight weekly; appetite may increase with drug
- Assess ECG for flattening of T wave, bundle branch block, AV block, dysrhythmias in cardiac patients
- Assess for extrapyramidal G symptoms primarily in elderly: rigidity, dystonia, akathisia
- Assess mental status: mood, sensorium, affect, suicidal tendencies; increase in psychiatric symptoms: depression, panic
- Monitor urinary retention, constipation; constipation is P more likely to occur in children G or elderly
- Assess for withdrawal symptoms: headache, nausea, vomiting, muscle pain, weak-

I

ness; do not usually occur unless drug was discontinued abruptly
• Identify alcohol consumption; if alcohol is consumed, hold dose until AM

Associated nursing diagnoses

✓ Coping, ineffective individual (uses)
✓ Injury, risk for physical (side effects)
✓ Knowledge deficit (teaching)
✓ Noncompliance (teaching)

Implementation

PO route
• Give with food or milk
• Store at room temp; do not freeze

IM route
• Put ampule under warm running water for 1 min to dissolve crystals; sol may be yellow or red

Patient/family education

• Teach patient that therapeutic effects may take 2-3 wk
• Teach patient to use caution in driving and other activities requiring alertness because of drowsiness, dizziness, blurred vision; to avoid rising quickly from sitting position, especially G elderly
• Teach patient to avoid alcohol ingestion, other CNS depressants
• Teach patient not to discontinue medication quickly after long-term use: may cause nausea, headache, malaise
• Teach patient to wear sunscreen or large hat, since photosensitivity occurs
• Teach patient to increase fluids, bulk in diet if constipation, urinary retention occur, G especially elderly
• Teach patient to take gum, hard sugarless candy, or frequent sips of water for dry mouth

Evaluation

Positive therapeutic outcome
• Decreased depression
• Absence of suicidal thoughts
• Decreased enuresis in children

Treatment of overdose: ECG monitoring, induce emesis, lavage, activated charcoal, administer anticonvulsant

immune globulin

Gamma Globulin, IG, IGIV ISG, Gamimune N, Gammagard, Gammar, Gamastan, Gammar-IV, Iveegam, Sandoglobulin, Venoglobulin-I, immune serum globulin

Func. class.: Immune serum

Chem. class.: IgG

Pregnancy category **C**

Action: Provides passive immunity to hepatitis A, measles, varicella, rubella, immune globulin deficiency; contains γ-globulin antibodies (IgG)

➔ **Therapeutic Outcome:** Absence of infection

Uses: Agammaglobulinemia, hepatitis A exposure, measles exposure, measles vaccine complications, purpura, rubella exposure, chickenpox exposure

Dosage and routes

Adult: IM 30-50 ml q mo; **IV** 100 mg/kg q mo, 0.01-0.02 ml/kg/min over 30 min (Gamimune); **IV** 200 mg/kg qmo, 0.05-1 ml/min over 15-30 min, then increase to 1.5-2.5 ml/min (Sandoglobulin)

P *Child:* IM 20-40 ml q mo

Hepatitis A exposure

P *Adult and child:* IM 0.02-0.04 ml/kg or 0.1 mg/kg if treatment is delayed

Hepatitis B exposure

P *Adult and child:* IM 0.06 ml/kg within 1 wk, q mo

Measles (postexposure)

P *Child:* IM 0.25 ml/kg within 6 days

Immunoglobulin deficiency

P *Adult and child:* IM 1.3 ml/kg, then 0.66 ml/kg after 2-4 wk and q2-4 wk thereafter

Idiopathic thrombocytopenic purpura

P *Adult and child:* **IV** 0.4 g/kg/day × 5 days or 1g/kg/day × 1-2 days

Available forms: IM inj 2, 10 ml/vial; **IV** inj 5% sol, 0.5, 1, 2.5, 3, 6, 10 g vials

Side effects/adverse reactions

CNS: Headache, fatigue, malaise
GI: Abdominal pain
INTEG: Pain at inj site, rash, pruritus, chills, chest pain
MS: Arthralgia
SYST: Lymphadenopathy, ***anaphylaxis***

Contraindications: Hypersensitivity

Precautions: Pregnancy **C**

Pharmacokinetics

Absorption	Well absorbed (IM); completely absorbed (IV)
Distribution	Rapidly
Metabolism	Liver, catabolism
Excretion	Kidneys
Half-life	3-4 wk

Pharmacodynamics

	IM	IV
Onset	Unknown	Rapid
Peak	Unknown	Unknown
Duration	Unknown	Unknown

Interactions

Drug/drug:

Live virus vaccines: Do not give within 3 mo

NURSING CONSIDERATIONS

Assessment

- Assess for exposure date: this drug should be given within 6 days of measles, 1 wk of hepatitis B, 14 days of hepatitis A; if the date of exposure is outside these limits, immune globulin will not be effective
- Monitor blood studies in leukemia, idiopathic thrombocytopenic purpura: WBCs (leukemia), platelets

• Identify the number of inj of this drug the patient has received; multiple inj may lead to sensitization (diaphoresis, fever, chills, malaise)
• Assess for anaphylaxis in patient receiving **IV** immune globulin: diaphoresis, flushing, nausea, vomiting, wheezing, difficulty breathing, hypotension, chest tightness, fever, weakness, sneezing, abdominal pain; VS should be monitored during inf and 1 hr after beginning inf; emergency equipment should be available with epinephrine and antihistamines to treat anaphylaxis

Associated nursing diagnoses

✓ Infection, risk for (uses)
✓ Knowledge deficit (teaching)

Implementation

IM route

• Give IM (IGIM) in deltoid or anterolateral thigh in adults or anterolateral thigh in young P children; if large amounts are given, several inj may be needed
• Do not give the IM preparation **IV**, SC, or intradermally
• Sol should be transparent and clear or slightly colored

IV **IV route**

• Warm to room temp before administration (diluent, powder for inj)
• A transfer device is provided by manufacturer; this drug should not be agitated or shaken
• Do not give the **IV** preparation SC, IM, or intradermally
• Check for adverse reaction during inf; stop inf if adverse reactions are present

Gamimune N: Dilute **IV** with D_5; give 0.01 ml/kg/min; may increase to 0.02-0.04 ml/kg/min if no adverse reactions are present; may increase to 0.08 ml/kg/hr; sol should be refrigerated; do not freeze

Gammagard: Reconstitute with sterile water for inj (50 mg protein/ml); give within 2 hr of reconstitution; give 0.5 ml/kg/hr; may increase to 4 ml/kg/hr if no adverse reactions occur; use inf set provided

Gammar-IV: Give 0.01 ml/kg/min (50 mg/ml sol) over 15-30 min; may increase to 0.02 ml/kg/min; if adverse reactions are not present, may increase to 0.03-0.06 ml/kg/min; do not freeze; store at room temp

Iveegam (5%): Give 1-2 ml/min; refrigerate, do not freeze

Sandoglobulin: **IV** diluted with provided diluent; give 0.5-1 ml/min over 15-30 min; may increase to 1.5-2.5 ml/min; other inf may be given 2-2.5 ml/min; store at room temp

Venoglobulin-I: Give 50 mg/ml sol 0.01-0.02 ml/kg/min over 30 min if no adverse reactions; increase 0.04 ml/kg/min; store at room temp

Patient/family education

• Advise patient that passive immunity is temporary; explain reason for and expected results of this drug

• Advise patient that pain and tenderness may occur at inj site

Evaluation

Positive therapeutic outcome

• Prevention of infection
• Increased platelets

Treatment of anaphylaxis: Epinephrine, diphenhydramine, O_2, vasopressors, corticosteroids

indapamide

(in-dap'a-mide)

Lozol, Lozide

Func. class.: Diuretic, antihypertensive

Chem. class.: Thiazide-like sulfonamide derivative

Pregnancy category B

Action: Acts on the distal tubule in the kidney, increasing excretion of sodium, water, chloride, magnesium, potassium, and bicarbonate

Therapeutic Outcome: Decreased B/P, decreased edema in lung tissues, peripherally

Uses: May be used alone or as adjunct with antihypertensives (mild to moderate)

Investigational uses: May be used alone or in combination with other antihypertensives for edema in CHF

Dosage and routes

Adult: PO 2.5 mg qd in AM, may be increased to 5 mg qd if needed

Available forms: Tab 2.5 mg

Side effects/adverse reactions

CNS: Depression, *headache, dizziness, fatigue, weakness*
CV: Orthostatic hypotension, palpitations, volume depletion
EENT: Blurred vision, loss of hearing, tinnitus, nasal congestion, increased intraocular pressure
ELECT: Hypokalemia, hypercalcemia, hyponatremia, hypochloremia, hypomagnesemia
GI: Nausea, vomiting, anorexia, constipation, diarrhea, cramps, pancreatitis, GI irritation, ***hepatitis,*** abdominal pain
GU: Frequency, polyuria, dysuria
HEMA: Anemia, leukopenia, agranulocytosis, thrombocytopenia, neutropenia
INTEG: Rash, urticaria, *pruritus,* photosensitivity
META: Hyperglycemia, *hyperuricemia,* increased creatinine, BUN
MS: Cramps

Contraindications: Hypersensitivity to thiazides or sulfonamides, anuria, lactation

Precautions: Hypokalemia, renal disease, hepatic disease, gout, diabetes mellitus, elderly, ascites, dehydration, pregnancy **B**

Pharmacokinetics

Absorption	Well absorbed
Distribution	Widely distributed
Metabolism	Liver; 7% excreted unchanged (urine)
Half-life	14-18 hr

Pharmacodynamics

Onset	1-2 hr
Peak	2 hr
Duration	Up to 36 hr

Interactions

Drug/drug:

Individual drugs

Alcohol: ↑ hypotension
Lithium: ↑ toxicity
Mezlocillin: ↑ hypokalemia
Piperacillin: ↑ hypokalemia
Ticarcillin: ↑ hypokalemia

Drug classifications

Antihypertensives: ↑ antihypertensive effect
Cardiac glycosides: ↑ hypokalemia
Glucocorticoids: ↑ hypokalemia

Lab test interferences

Increase: Calcium, parathyroid test

NURSING CONSIDERATIONS

Assessment

- Check for rashes, temp elevation qd
- Monitor patients that receive cardiac glycosides for increased hypokalemia, toxicity
- Monitor manifestations of hypokalemia: acidic or reduced urine, osmolality, nocturia; hypotension, broad T wave, U wave, ectopy, tachycardia, weak pulse; muscle weakness, altered LOC, drowsiness, apathy, lethargy, confusion, depression; anorexia, nausea, cramps, constipation, distention, paralytic ileus; hypoventilation, respiratory muscle weakness
- Monitor for manifestations of hypomagnesemia: agitation, muscle twitching, paresthesias, hyperactive reflexes, positive Babinski reflex, dysphagia, nystagmus seizures, tetany; nausea, vomiting, diarrhea, anorexia, abdominal distention; ectopy, tachycardia, broad, flat or inverted T waves, depressed ST segment, prolonged QT, decreased cardiac output, hypotension
- Monitor for manifestations of hyponatremia: increased B/P, cold, clammy skin, hypovolemia or hypervolemia; anorexia, nausea, vomiting, diarrhea, abdominal cramps; lethargy, increased ICP, confusion, headache, seizures, coma, fatigue, tremors, hyperreflexia
- Monitor for manifestations of hyperchloremia: weakness, lethargy, coma, deep rapid breathing
- Assess fluid volume status: I&O ratios and record, weight, distended red veins, crackles in lung, color, quality and sp gr of urine, skin turgor, adequacy of pulses, moist mucous membranes, bilateral lung sounds, peripheral pitting edema; dehydration symptoms of decreasing output, thirst, hypotension, dry mouth and mucous membranes should be reported
- Monitor electrolytes: potassium, sodium, calcium, magnesium; also include BUN, blood pH, ABGs, uric acid, CBC, blood sugar

• Assess B/P before and during therapy with patient lying, standing and sitting as appropriate; orthostatic hypotension can occur rapidly

Associated nursing diagnoses

✓ Altered urinary elimination (side effect)
✓ Fluid volume deficit (side effects)
✓ Fluid volume excess (uses)
✓ Knowledge deficit (teaching)

Implementation

• Give in AM to avoid interference with sleep
• Provide potassium replacement if potassium level is <3.0; give whole

PO route

• Give with food; if nausea occurs, absorption may be increased

Patient/family education

• Teach patient to take the medication early in the day to prevent nocturia
• Instruct the patient to take with food or milk if GI symptoms of nausea and anorexia occur
• Teach patient to maintain weekly record of weight and notify prescriber of weight loss >5 lb
• Caution the patient that this drug causes a loss of potassium, so food rich in potassium should be added to the diet; refer to a dietitian for assistance in planning
• Caution the patient not to exercise in hot weather or stand for prolonged periods, since orthostatic hypotension will be enhanced
• Teach patient not to use alcohol or any OTC medications without prescriber's approval; serious drug reactions may occur
• Emphasize the need to contact prescriber immediately if muscle cramps, weakness, nausea, dizziness, or numbness occurs
• Teach patient to take own B/P and pulse and record findings
• Caution the patient that orthostatic hypotension may occur and to rise slowly from sitting or reclining positions and lie down if dizziness occurs
• Teach patient to continue taking medication even if feeling better; this drug controls symptoms but does not cure the condition
• Advise the patient with hypertension to continue other medical treatment (exercise, weight loss, relaxation techniques, cessation of smoking)

Evaluation

Positive therapeutic outcome

• Decreased edema
• Decreased B/P
• Increased diuresis

Treatment of overdose:

Lavage, monitor electrolytes, administer IV fluids, monitor hydration, CV, renal status

indomethacin

(in-doe-meth'a-sin)
Apo-Indomethacin ♣, Indameth ♣, Indocid ♣, Indocin PDA ♣, Novomethacin ♣, indomethacin, Indocin, Indocin SR, Indocin IV
Func. class.: NSAID
Chem. class.: Propionic acid derivative
Pregnancy category **B**

Action: Inhibits prostaglandin synthesis by decreasing enzyme needed for biosynthesis; analgesic, antiinflammatory, antipyretic

➡ **Therapeutic Outcome:** Decreased pain, inflammation; or closure of patent ductus arteriosus (premature infants)

Uses: Rheumatoid arthritis, ankylosing rheumatoid spondylitis, acute gouty arthritis, closure of patent ductus P arteriosus in premature infants

Dosage and routes

Arthritis/antiinflammatory

Adult: PO/rec 25 mg bid-tid; may increase by 25 mg/day q wk, not to exceed 200 mg/day; sus rel 75 mg qd; may increase to 75 mg bid

Acute arthritis

Adult: PO/rec 50 mg tid; use only for acute attack, then reduce dosage

Patent ductus arteriosus

P ***Infant <2 days:*** **IV** 0.2 mg/kg, then 0.1 mg/kg q12-24h

P ***Infant 2-7 days:*** **IV** 0.2 mg/kg, then 0.2 mg × 2 doses after 12, 24 hr

P ***Infant >7 days:*** **IV** 0.2 mg/kg, then 0.25 mg/kg × 2 doses after 12, 24 hr

Available forms: Cap 25, 50 mg; sus rel cap 75 mg; oral susp 25 mg/5 ml; rec supp 50 mg; inj 1 mg vials

Side effects/adverse reactions

CNS: Dizziness, drowsiness, fatigue, tremors, confusion, insomnia, anxiety, depression
CV: Tachycardia, peripheral edema, palpitations, dysrhythmias, hypertension
EENT: Tinnitus, hearing loss, blurred vision
GI: Nausea, anorexia, vomiting, diarrhea, jaundice, ***cholestatic hepatitis,*** constipation, flatulence, cramps, dry mouth, peptic ulcer
GU: ***Nephrotoxicity (dysuria, hematuria, oliguria, azotemia)***
HEMA: ***Blood dyscrasias***
INTEG: Purpura, rash, pruritus, sweating

Contraindications: Hypersensitivity, asthma, severe renal disease, severe hepatic disease, ulcer disease

Precautions: Pregnancy, P lactation, children, bleeding disorders, GI disorders, cardiac disorders, hypersensitivity to other antiinflammatory agents, pregnancy **B** 1st and 2nd trimesters, depression

Pharmacokinetics

Absorption	Well absorbed (PO); erratic (rec); complete (**IV**)
Distribution	Crosses blood-brain barrier; placenta, 99% plasma protein binding
Metabolism	Liver, extensively
Excretion	Breast milk
P **Half-life**	2.6-11 hr

Pharmacodynamics

	IV	PO	PO–EXT REL
Onset	2 day	1-2 hr	½ hr
Peak	Unknown	3 hr	Unknown
Duration	Unknown	4-6 hr	4-6 hr

Interactions

Drug/drug:

Individual drugs

Acetaminophen (long-term use): ↑ renal reactions
Alcohol: ↑ adverse reactions
Aspirin: ↓ effectiveness, ↑ adverse reactions
Coumarin: ↑ anticoagulant effects
Cyclosporine: ↑ nephrotoxicity
Digoxin: ↑ toxicity, levels
Insulin: ↓ insulin effect
Lithium: ↑ toxicity, levels
Methotrexate: ↑ toxicity
Phenytoin: ↑ toxicity
Probenecid: ↑ toxicity
Zidovudine: ↑ toxicity, levels

Drug classifications

Anticoagulants: ↑ risk of bleeding
Antihypertensives: ↓ effect of antihypertensives
Antineoplastics: ↑ risk of hematologic toxicity
β-Blockers: ↑ antihypertension
Cephalosporins: ↑ risk of bleeding
Glucocorticoids: ↑ adverse reactions
Hypoglycemics: ↓ hypoglycemic effect
Diuretics: ↓ effectiveness of diuretics
NSAIDs: ↑ adverse reactions
Potassium supplements: ↑ adverse reactions
Radiation: ↑ risk of hematologic toxicity
Sulfonamides: ↑ toxicity
Sulfonylureas: ↑ toxicity

NURSING CONSIDERATIONS

Assessment

- Assess for joint pain (duration, intensity, ROM), baseline and during treatment

Associated nursing diagnoses

- ✓ Pain (uses)
- ✓ Chronic pain (uses)
- ✓ Impaired mobility (uses)
- ✓ Knowledge deficit (teaching)

Implementation

PO route

- Administer to patient whole; do not crush, chew, or break sus rel cap
- Give with food or milk to decrease gastric symptoms

IV **IV route**

- Give after diluting 1 mg/ml or more normal saline or sterile water for inj without preservative; give over 5-10 sec; avoid extravasation

Rec route

- Have patient retain rec supp for 1 hr after insertion

Patient/family education

- Advise patient to report change in vision, blurring, rash, tinnitus, black stools

- Tell patient not to use for any other condition than prescribed
- Advise patient to avoid use with OTC medications for pain unless approved by prescriber
- Advise patient to avoid hazardous activities, since dizziness or drowsiness can occur

Evaluation

Positive therapeutic outcome

- Decreased stiffness
- Increased joint mobility
- Decreased pain

insulin, isophane suspension (NPH) 🔑

NPH Iletin II, Humulin N, Iletin NPH, Lentard Insulatard NPH, Novolin N, NPH Insulin, NPH Purified

Func. class.: Pancreatic hormone

Chem. class.: Exogenous unmodified insulin

Pregnancy category **B**

Action: Decreases blood sugar; by transport of insulin into cells and the conversion of glucose to glycogen indirectly increases blood pyruvate and lactate, decreases phosphate and potassium; insulin may be beef, pork, human (processed by recombinant DNA technologies)

➡ Therapeutic Outcome: Decreased blood glucose levels in diabetes mellitus

Uses: Adult-onset diabetes, juvenile diabetes, ketoacidosis types I and II, type II (non–insulin-dependent) diabetes mellitus, type I (insulin-dependent) diabetes mellitus

Dosage and routes

Adult: SC dosage individualized by blood, urine glucose; usual dose 7-26 U; may increase by 2-10 U/day if needed

Available forms: Inj 100 U/ml

Side effects/adverse reactions

EENT: Blurred vision, dry mouth

INTEG: Flushing, rash, urticaria, warmth, *lipodystrophy,* lipohypertrophy, swelling, redness

META: *Hypoglycemia,* rebond hyperglycemia (Somogyi effect 12-72 hr or longer)

SYST: ***Anaphylaxis***

Contraindications: Hypersensitivity to protamine

Precautions: Pregnancy **B**

Pharmacokinetics	
Absorption	Rapidly absorbed (SC)
Distribution	Widely distributed
Metabolism	Liver, muscle, kidney
Excretion	Kidneys
Half-life	10 min

Pharmacodynamics	
Onset	1-2 hr
Peak	4-12 hr
Duration	18-24 hr

Interactions

Drug/drug:

Individual drugs

Alcohol: ↑ hypoglycemia
Diltiazem: ↑ insulin need
Dobutamine: ↑ insulin need
Fenfluramine: ↓ insulin need
Guanethidine: ↓ insulin need
Phenylbutazone: ↓ insulin need
Rifampin: ↑ insulin need
Sulfinpyrazone: ↓ insulin need
Tetracycline: ↓ insulin need

Drug classifications

Anabolic steroids: ↓ insulin need
β-Blockers: Signs/symptoms of hypoglycemia may be masked
Glucocorticoid steroids: ↑ insulin need
Estrogens: ↑ insulin need
MAOI: ↓ insulin need
Oral anticoagulants: ↓ insulin need
Oral hypoglycemics: ↑ hypoglycemia
Thiazide diuretics: ↑ insulin need
Thyroid hormones: ↑ insulin need

Drug/smoking:

Tobacco: ↑ insulin need

Lab test interferences

Increase: VMA
Decrease: Potassium, magnesium, inorganic phosphate
Interference: Liver function studies, thyroid function studies

NURSING CONSIDERATIONS

Assessment

- Monitor fasting blood glucose, 2 hr PP (80-150 mg/dl, normal fasting level; 70-130 mg/dl, normal 2-hr level); also glycosylated Hgb may be drawn to identify treatment effectiveness
- Monitor urine ketones during illness; insulin requirements may increase during stress, illness, surgery
- Assess for hypoglycemic reaction that can occur during peak time (sweating, weakness, dizziness, chills, confusion, headache, nausea, rapid weak pulse, fatigue, tachycardia, memory lapses, slurred speech, staggering gait, anxiety, tremors, hunger)
- Assess for hyperglycemia: acetone breath, polyuria, fatigue, polydipsia, flushed, dry skin, lethargy

Associated nursing diagnoses

✓ Injury, risk for (adverse reactions)
✓ Knowledge deficit (teaching)
✓ Noncompliance (teaching)

Implementation

SC route

- Give after warming to room temp by rotating in palms to prevent injecting cold insulin; use only insulin syringes with markings or syringe matching U/ml; rotate inj sites within one area: abdomen, upper back, thighs, upper arm, buttocks; keep record of sites
- Give increased dosages if tolerance occurs; give human insulin to those allergic to beef or pork
- Store at room temp for <1 mo; keep away from heat and sunlight; refrigerate all other supply; do not use if discolored; do not freeze

Patient/family education

- Advise patient that blurred vision occurs; not to change corrective lenses until vision is stabilized after 1-2 mo of therapy
- Advise patient to keep insulin and equipment available at all times
- Advise patient to carry Medic Alert ID as diabetic
- Teach patient dosage, route, mixing instructions, disease process; tell patient to continue to use the same brand of insulin and to rotate inj sites
- Instruct patient to carry candy or lump of sugar to treat hypoglycemia; have glucagon emergency kit available; teach how to use these
- Teach patient symptoms of ketoacidosis: nausea, thirst, polyuria, dry mouth, decreased B/P, dry, flushed skin, acetone breath, drowsiness, Kussmaul respirations; to have insulin available at all times
- Advise patient that a plan is necessary for diet, exercise; all food on diet should be eaten, exercise routine should not vary
- Teach patient to avoid OTC drugs and alcohol unless approved by a prescriber
- Instruct patient to notify prescriber if pregnancy is planned
- Caution patient that treatment is lifelong; insulin does not cure condition

Evaluation

Positive therapeutic outcome

- Decrease in polyuria, polydipsia, polyphagia; clear sensorium, absence of dizziness, stable gait
- Blood glucose level under control

Treatment of overdose: Glucose 25 g **IV**, via dextrose 50% sol, 50 ml or 1 mg glucagon

insulin, isophane suspension and regular insulin

Humulin 70/30, Mixtard 70/30, Novolin 70/30

Func. class.: Pancreatic hormone

Chem. class.: Exogenous unmodified insulin

Pregnancy category **B**

Action: Decreases blood sugar; by transport of insulin into cells and the conversion of glucose to glycogen indirectly increases blood pyruvate and lactate, decreases phosphate and potassium; insulin may be beef, pork, human (processed by recombinant DNA technologies)

Therapeutic Outcome: Decreased blood glucose levels in diabetes mellitus

Uses: Ketoacidosis, type I (insulin-dependent) diabetes mellitus, type II (non–insulin dependent) diabetes mellitus

Dosage and routes

Adult: SC individualized dosage based on serum glucose levels

Available forms: 70 U/ml isophane insulin with 30 U/ml regular insulin = 100 U/ml

Side effects/adverse reactions

EENT: Blurred vision, dry mouth
INTEG: Flushing, rash, urticaria, warmth, *lipodystrophy*, lipohypertrophy, swelling, redness
META: *Hypoglycemia*, rebond hyperglycemia (Somogyi effect 12-72 hr or longer)
SYST: ***Anaphylaxis***

Contraindications: Hypersensitivity to protamine

Precautions: Pregnancy **B**

Pharmacokinetics

Absorption	Rapidly absorbed (SC)
Distribution	Widely distributed
Metabolism	Liver, muscle, kidney
Excretion	Kidneys
Half-life	10 min

Pharmacodynamics

Onset	½ hr
Peak	4-8 hr
Duration	12-24 hr

Interactions

Drug/drug:

Individual drugs
Alcohol: ↑ hypoglycemia
Diltiazem: ↑ insulin need
Dobutamine: ↑ insulin need
Fenfluramine: ↓ insulin need
Guanethidine: ↓ insulin need
Phenylbutazone: ↓ insulin need
Rifampin: ↑ insulin need
Sulfinpyrazone: ↓ insulin need
Tetracycline: ↓ insulin need

Drug classifications
Anabolic steroids: ↓ insulin need
β-Blockers: Signs/symptoms of hypoglycemia may be masked
Glucocorticoid steroids: ↑ insulin need
Estrogens: ↑ insulin need
MAOI: ↓ insulin need
Oral anticoagulants: ↓ insulin need
Oral hypoglycemics: ↑ hypoglycemia
Thiazide diuretics: ↑ insulin need
Thyroid hormones: ↑ insulin need

Drug/smoking:

Tobacco: ↑ insulin need

Lab test interferences

Increase: VMA
Decrease: Potassium, magnesium, inorganic phosphate
Interference: Liver function studies, thyroid function studies

NURSING CONSIDERATIONS

Assessment

- Monitor fasting blood glucose, 2 hr PP (80-150 mg/dl, normal fasting level; 70-130 mg/dl-normal 2-hr level); also glycosylated Hgb may be drawn to identify treatment effectiveness
- Monitor urine ketones during illness; insulin requirements may increase during stress, illness, surgery
- Assess for hypoglycemic reaction that can occur during peak time (sweating, weakness, dizziness, chills, confusion, headache, nausea, rapid weak

pulse, fatigue, tachycardia, memory lapses, slurred speech, staggering gait, anxiety, tremors, hunger)
• Assess for hyperglycemia: acetone breath, polyuria, fatigue, polydipsia, flushed, dry skin, lethargy

Associated nursing diagnoses

✓ Injury, risk for (adverse reactions)
✓ Knowledge deficit (teaching)
✓ Noncompliance (teaching)

Implementation

SC route
• Give after warming to room temp by rotating in palms to prevent injecting cold insulin; use only insulin syringes with markings or syringe matching U/ml; rotate inj sites within one area: abdomen, upper back, thighs, upper arm, buttocks; keep record of sites
• Give increased dosages if tolerance occurs; give human insulin to those allergic to beef or pork
• Store at room temp for <1 mo; keep away from heat and sunlight; refrigerate all other supply; do not use if discolored; do not freeze

Patient/family education

• Advise patient that blurred vision occurs; not to change corrective lenses until vision is stabilized after 1-2 mo of therapy
• Advise patient to keep insulin, equipment available at all times
• Advise patient to carry Medic Alert ID as diabetic
• Teach patient dosage, route, mixing instructions, disease process; tell patient to continue to use the same brand of insulin and to rotate inj sites
• Instruct patient to carry candy or lump of sugar to treat hypoglycemia; have glucagon emergency kit available; teach how to use these
• Teach patient symptoms of ketoacidosis: nausea, thirst, polyuria, dry mouth, decreased B/P, dry, flushed skin, acetone breath, drowsiness, Kussmaul respirations; to have insulin available at all times
• Advise patient that a plan is necessary for diet, exercise; all food on diet should be eaten, exercise routine should not vary
• Teach patient to avoid OTC drugs and alcohol unless approved by a prescriber
• Instruct patient to notify prescriber if pregnancy is planned
• Caution patient that treatment is lifelong; insulin does not cure condition

Evaluation

Positive therapeutic outcome
• Decrease in polyuria, polydipsia, polyphagia; clear sensorium, absence of dizziness, stable gait
• Blood glucose level under control

Treatment of overdose:

Glucose 25 g **IV**, via dextrose 50% sol, 50 ml or 1 mg glucagon

insulin, regular

Actrapid Iletin II, Humulin R, Iletin I, Novolin R, Novolin R Velosulin

Func. class.: Pancreatic hormone

Chem. class.: Exogenous unmodified insulin

Pregnancy category **B**

Action: Decreases blood sugar; by transport of insulin into cells and the conversion of glucose to glycogen indirectly increases blood pyruvate and lactate, decreases phosphate and potassium; insulin may be beef, pork, human (processed by recombinant DNA technologies)

Therapeutic Outcome: Decreased blood glucose levels in diabetes mellitus

Uses: Adult-onset diabetes, juvenile diabetes, ketoacidosis types I and II, type II (non–insulin-dependent) diabetes mellitus, type I (insulin-dependent) diabetes mellitus

Dosage and routes

Ketoacidosis

Adult: **IV** 5-10 U, then 5-10 U/hr until desired response, then switch to SC dose; **IV**/inf 2-12 U (50 U/500 ml of normal saline)

P ***Child:*** **IV** 0.1 U/kg

Replacement

P ***Adult and child:*** SC 0.5-1 U/kg/day qid given 30 min pc

Adolescents: SC 0.8-1.2 mg/kg/day; this dosage is used during rapid growth

Available forms: **IV**/IM/SC inj 40 U, 100 U/ml

Side effects/adverse reactions

EENT: Blurred vision, dry mouth

INTEG: Flushing, rash, urticaria, warmth, *lipodystrophy,* lipohypertrophy, swelling, redness

META: *Hypoglycemia,* rebond hyperglycemia (Somogyi effect 12-72 hr or longer)

SYST: ***Anaphylaxis***

Contraindications: Hypersensitivity

Precautions: Pregnancy **B**

Pharmacokinetics

Absorption	Rapidly absorbed (SC)
Distribution	Widely distributed
Metabolism	Liver, muscle, kidney
Excretion	Kidneys
Half-life	3-5 min; may be extended

Pharmacodynamics

	SC	IV
Onset	½-1 hr	10-30 min
Peak	2-4 hr	30-60 min
Duration	5-7 hr	½-1 hr

Interactions

Drug/drug:

Individual drugs

Alcohol: ↑ hypoglycemia
Diltiazem: ↑ insulin need
Dobutamine: ↑ insulin need
Fenfluramine: ↓ insulin need
Guanethidine: ↓ insulin need

Phenylbutazone: ↓ insulin need
Rifampin: ↑ insulin need
Sulfinpyrazone: ↓ insulin need
Tetracycline: ↓ insulin need

Drug classifications

Anabolic steroids: ↓ insulin need
β-Blockers: Signs/symptoms of hypoglycemia may be masked
Glucocorticoid steroids: ↑ insulin need
Estrogens: ↑ insulin need
MAOI: ↓ insulin need
Oral anticoagulants: ↓ insulin need
Oral hypoglycemics: ↑ hypoglycemia
Thiazide diuretics: ↑ insulin need
Thyroid hormones: ↑ insulin need

Drug/smoking:

Tobacco: ↑ insulin requirements

Lab test interferences

Increase: VMA
Decrease: Potassium, magnesium, inorganic phosphate
Interference: Liver function studies, thyroid function studies

NURSING CONSIDERATIONS

Assessment

- Monitor fasting blood glucose, 2 hr PP (80-150 mg/dl, normal fasting level; 70-130 mg/dl, normal 2-hr level); also, glycosylated Hgb may be drawn to identify treatment effectiveness
- Monitor urine ketones during illness; insulin requirements may increase during stress, illness, surgery
- Assess for hypoglycemic reaction that can occur during peak time (sweating, weakness, dizziness, chills, confusion, headache, nausea, rapid weak pulse, fatigue, tachycardia, memory lapses, slurred speech, staggering gait, anxiety, tremors, hunger)
- Assess for hyperglycemia: acetone breath, polyuria, fatigue, polydipsia, flushed, dry skin, lethargy

Associated nursing diagnoses

✓ Injury, risk for (adverse reactions)
✓ Knowledge deficit (teaching)
✓ Noncompliance (teaching)

Implementation

SC route

- Give after warming to room temp by rotating in palms to prevent injecting cold insulin; use only insulin syringes with markings or syringe matching U/ml; rotate inj sites within one area: abdomen, upper back, thighs, upper arm, buttocks; keep record of sites
- Give increased dosages if tolerance occurs; give human insulin to those allergic to beef or pork
- Store at room temp for <1 mo; keep away from heat and sunlight; refrigerate all other supply; do not use if discolored; do not freeze

IV **IV route**

- Do not use if cloudy, thick, or discolored
- Give **IV** direct, undiluted via vein, Y-site, 3-way stopcock; give at 50 U/min or less

• Give by cont inf after diluting with **IV** sol and run at prescribed rate; use **IV** inf pump for correct dosing; give reduced dose at serum glucose level of 250 mg/100 ml

Syringe compatibility:

Metoclopramide

Y-site incompatibility:

Nafcillin

Y-site compatibilities:

Dobutamine, famotidine, heparin, ampicillin, ampicillin/sulbactam, aztreonam, cefazolin, cefotetan, gentamicin, imipenen/cilastatin, magnesium sulfate, oxytocin, ritodrine, terbutalin, ticarcillin, ticarcillin/clavulanate, tobramycin, vancomycin, vitamin B with C, indomethacin sodium trihydrate, meperidine, morphine, pentobarbital, potassium chloride, regular insulin, sodium bicarbonate

Additive incompatibilities:

Aminophylline, amobarbital, chlorothiazide, cytarabine, dobutamine, pentobarbital, phenobarbital, phenytoin, secobarbital, sodium bicarbonate, thiopental

Additive compatibilities:

Bretylium, cimetidine, lidocaine, verapamil

Patient/family education

• Advise patient that blurred vision occurs; not to change corrective lenses until vision is stabilized after 1-2 mo of therapy
• Advise patient to keep insulin, equipment available at all times
• Advise patient to carry Medic Alert ID as diabetic
• Teach patient dosage, route, mixing instructions, disease process; tell patient to continue to use the same brand of insulin and to rotate inj sites
• Instruct patient to carry candy or lump of sugar to treat hypoglycemia; have glucagon emergency kit available; teach how to use these
• Teach patient symptoms of ketoacidosis: nausea, thirst, polyuria, dry mouth, decreased B/P, dry, flushed skin, acetone breath, drowsiness, Kussmaul respirations; to have insulin available at all times
• Advise patient that a plan is necessary for diet, exercise; all food on diet should be eaten, exercise routine should not vary
• Teach patient to avoid OTC drugs and alcohol unless approved by prescriber
• Instruct patient to notify prescriber if pregnancy is planned
• Caution patient that treatment is lifelong; insulin does not cure condition

Evaluation

Positive therapeutic outcome
• Decrease in polyuria, polydipsia, polyphagia, clear sensorium, absence of dizziness, stable gait
• Blood glucose level under control

Treatment of overdose:

Glucose 25 g **IV**, via dextrose 50% sol, 50 ml or 1 mg glucagon

insulin, regular concentrated

Iletin II U-500

Func. class.: Pancreatic hormone

Chem. class.: Exogenous unmodified insulin

Pregnancy category **B**

Action: Decreases blood sugar; by transport of insulin into cells and the conversion of glucose to glycogen indirectly increases blood pyruvate and lactate, decreases phosphate and potassium; insulin may be beef, pork, human (processed by recombinant DNA technologies)

➡ **Therapeutic Outcome:** Decreased blood glucose levels in diabetes mellitus

Uses: Treatment of diabetic patients with marked insulin resistance (>200 U/day)

Dosage and routes

Adult: SC dosage individualized by blood, urine glucose qd-tid

Available forms: Inj 500 U/ml

Side effects/adverse reactions

EENT: Blurred vision, dry mouth

INTEG: Flushing, rash, urticaria, warmth, *lipodystrophy,* lipohypertrophy, swelling, redness

META: Hypoglycemia, rebond hyperglycemia (Somogyi effect 12-72 hr or longer)

SYST: Anaphylaxis

Contraindications: Hypersensitivity

Precautions: Pregnancy **B**

Pharmacokinetics

Absorption	Rapidly absorbed (SC)
Distribution	Widely distributed
Metabolism	Liver, muscle, kidney
Excretion	Kidneys
Half-life	10 min

Pharmacodynamics

Onset	½-1 hr
Peak	2-5 hr
Duration	5-7 hr

Interactions

Drug/drug:

Individual drugs

Alcohol: ↑ hypoglycemia
Diltiazem: ↑ insulin need
Dobutamine: ↑ insulin need
Fenfluramine: ↓ insulin need
Guanethidine: ↓ insulin need
Phenylbutazone: ↓ insulin need
Rifampin: ↑ insulin need
Sulfinpyrazone: ↓ insulin need
Tetracycline: ↓ insulin need

Drug classifications

Anabolic steroids: ↓ insulin need
β-Blockers: Signs/symptoms of hypoglycemia may be masked
Glucocorticoid steroids: ↑ insulin need
Estrogens: ↑ insulin need
MAOI: ↓ insulin need

Oral anticoagulants: ↓ insulin need
Oral hypoglycemics: ↑ hypoglycemia
Thiazide diuretics: ↑ insulin need
Thyroid hormones: ↑ insulin need

Drug/smoking:

Tobacco: ↑ insulin requirements

Lab test interferences

Increase: VMA
Decrease: Potassium, magnesium, inorganic phosphate
Interference: Liver function studies, thyroid function studies

NURSING CONSIDERATIONS

Assessment

- Monitor fasting blood glucose, 2 hr PP (80-150 mg/dl, normal fasting level; 70-130 mg/dl, normal 2-hr level); also glycosylated Hgb may be drawn to identify treatment effectiveness
- Monitor urine ketones during illness; insulin requirements may increase during stress, illness, surgery
- Assess for hypoglycemic reaction that can occur during peak time (sweating, weakness, dizziness, chills, confusion, headache, nausea, rapid weak pulse, fatigue, tachycardia, memory lapses, slurred speech, staggering gait, anxiety, tremors, hunger)
- Assess for hyperglycemia: acetone breath, polyuria, fatigue, polydipsia, flushed, dry skin, lethargy

Associated nursing diagnoses

✓ Injury, risk for (adverse reactions)
✓ Knowledge deficit (teaching)
✓ Noncompliance (teaching)

Implementation

SC route

- Give after warming to room temp by rotating in palms to prevent injecting cold insulin; use only insulin syringes with markings or syringe matching U/ml
- Rotate inj sites within one area: abdomen, upper back, thighs, upper arm, buttocks; keep record of sites
- Give increased dosages if tolerance occurs; give human insulin to those allergic to beef or pork
- Store at room temp for <1 mo; keep away from heat and sunlight; refrigerate all other supply; do not use if discolored; do not freeze

Patient/family education

- Advise patient that blurred vision occurs; not to change corrective lenses until vision is stabilized after 1-2 mo of therapy
- Instruct patient to keep insulin, equipment available at all times
- Advise patient to carry Medic Alert ID as diabetic
- Teach patient dosage, route, mixing instructions, disease process; tell patient to continue to use the same brand of insulin and to rotate inj sites
- Advise patient to carry candy or lump of sugar to treat hypoglycemia; to have gluca-

gon emergency kit available; teach how to use these
• Teach patient symptoms of ketoacidosis: nausea, thirst, polyuria, dry mouth, decreased B/P, dry, flushed skin, acetone breath, drowsiness, Kussmaul respirations; to have insulin available at all times
• Advise patient that a plan is necessary for diet, exercise; all food on diet should be eaten, exercise routine should not vary
• Teach patient to avoid OTC drugs and alcohol unless approved by prescriber
• Instruct patient to notify prescriber if pregnancy is planned
• Caution patient that treatment is lifelong; insulin does not cure condition

Evaluation

Positive therapeutic outcome
• Decrease in polyuria, polydipsia, polyphagia, clear sensorium, absence of dizziness, stable gait
• Blood glucose level under control

Treatment of overdose:
Glucose 25 g **IV**, via dextrose 50% sol, 50 ml or 1 mg glucagon

insulin, zinc suspension (Lente)
Humulin L, Monotard, Lente Iletin, Lente Insulin, Novolin L
Func. class.: Pancreatic hormone
Chem. class.: Exogenous unmodified insulin
Pregnancy category **B**

Action: Decreases blood sugar; by transport of insulin into cells and the conversion of glucose to glycogen indirectly increases blood pyruvate and lactate, decreases phosphate and potassium; insulin may be beef, pork, human (processed by recombinant DNA technologies)

➔ Therapeutic Outcome: Decreased blood glucose levels in diabetes mellitus

Uses: Ketoacidosis, type I (insulin-dependent) diabetes mellitus, type II (non–insulin-dependent) diabetes mellitus

Dosage and routes
Adult: SC individualized

Available forms: 100 U/ml

Side effects/adverse reactions
EENT: **Blurred vision, dry mouth**
INTEG: **Flushing, rash, urticaria, warmth, *lipodystrophy*, lipohypertrophy, swelling, redness**
META: ***Hypoglycemia*, rebond hyperglycemia**

(Somogyi effect 12-72 hr or longer)
SYST: Anaphylaxis

Contraindications: Hypersensitivity to protamine

Precautions: Pregnancy **B**

Pharmacokinetics

Absorption	Rapidly absorbed (SC)
Distribution	Widely distributed
Metabolism	Liver, muscle, kidney
Excretion	Kidneys
Half-life	10 min

Pharmacodynamics

Onset	1-2½ hr
Peak	7-15 hr
Duration	12-24 hr

Interactions
Drug/drug:
Individual drugs
Alcohol: ↑ hypoglycemia
Diltiazem: ↑ insulin need
Dobutamine: ↑ insulin need
Fenfluramine: ↓ insulin need
Guanethidine: ↓ insulin need
Phenylbutazone: ↓ insulin need
Rifampin: ↑ insulin need
Sulfinpyrazone: ↓ insulin need
Tetracycline: ↓ insulin need
Drug classifications
Anabolic steroids: ↓ insulin need
β-Blockers: Signs/symptoms of hypoglycemia may be masked
Glucocorticoid steroids: ↑ insulin need
Estrogens: ↑ insulin need
MAOI: ↓ insulin need
Oral anticoagulants: ↓ insulin need
Oral hypoglycemics: ↑ hypoglycemia
Thiazide diuretics: ↑ insulin need
Thyroid hormones: ↑ insulin need

Drug/smoking:
↑ insulin requirements

Lab test interferences
Increase: VMA
Decrease: Potassium, magnesium, inorganic phosphate
Interference: Liver function studies, thyroid function studies

NURSING CONSIDERATIONS
Assessment

- Monitor fasting blood glucose, 2 hr PP (80-150 mg/dl, normal fasting level; 70-130 mg/dl, normal 2-hr level); also glycosylated Hgb may be drawn to identify treatment effectiveness
- Monitor urine ketones during illness; insulin requirements may increase during stress, illness, surgery
- Assess for hypoglycemic reaction that can occur during peak time (sweating, weakness, dizziness, chills, confusion, headache, nausea, rapid weak pulse, fatigue, tachycardia, memory lapses, slurred speech, staggering gait, anxiety, tremors, hunger)
- Assess for hyperglycemia: acetone breath, polyuria, fatigue, polydipsia, flushed, dry skin, lethargy

Associated nursing diagnoses

- ✓ Injury, risk for physical (adverse reactions)
- ✓ Knowledge deficit (teaching)
- ✓ Noncompliance (teaching)

Implementation

SC route

- Give after warming to room temp by rotating in palms to prevent injecting cold insulin; use only insulin syringes with markings or syringe matching U/ml; rotate inj sites within one area: abdomen, upper back, thighs, upper arm, buttocks; keep record of sites
- Give increased dosages if tolerance occurs; give human insulin to those allergic to beef or pork
- Store at room temp for <1 mo; keep away from heat and sunlight; refrigerate all other supply; do not use if discolored; do not freeze

Patient/family education

- Advise patient that blurred vision occurs; not to change corrective lenses until vision is stabilized after 1-2 mo of therapy
- Advise patient to keep insulin, equipment available at all times
- Advise patient to carry Medic Alert ID as diabetic
- Teach patient dosage, route, mixing instructions, disease process; tell patient to continue to use the same brand of insulin and to rotate inj sites
- Instruct patient to carry candy or lump of sugar to treat hypoglycemia; have glucagon emergency kit available; teach how to use these
- Teach patient symptoms of ketoacidosis: nausea, thirst, polyuria, dry mouth, decreased B/P, dry, flushed skin, acetone breath, drowsiness, Kussmaul respirations; to have insulin available at all times
- Advise patient that a plan is necessary for diet, exercise; all food on diet should be eaten, exercise routine should not vary
- Teach patient to avoid OTC drugs and alcohol unless approved by prescriber
- Instruct patient to notify prescriber if pregnancy is planned
- Caution patient that treatment is lifelong; insulin does not cure condition

Evaluation

Positive therapeutic outcome

- Decrease in polyuria, polydipsia, polyphagia, clear sensorium, absence of dizziness, stable gait
- Blood glucose level under control

Treatment of overdose:

Glucose 25 g **IV**, via dextrose 50% sol, 50 ml or 1 mg glucagon

insulin, zinc suspension extended (Ultralente)

Humulin U, Ultralente, Ultralente Iletin, Ultralente Insulin, Ultratard

Func. class.: Pancreatic hormone

Chem. class.: Exogenous unmodified insulin

Pregnancy category **B**

Action: Decreases blood sugar; by transport of insulin into cells and the conversion of glucose to glycogen indirectly increases blood pyruvate and lactate, decreases phosphate and potassium; insulin may be beef, pork, human (processed by recombinant DNA technologies)

Therapeutic Outcome: Decreased blood glucose levels in diabetes mellitus

Uses: Adult-onset diabetes, juvenile diabetes, ketoacidosis types I and II, type II (non–insulin-dependent) diabetes mellitus, type I (insulin-dependent) diabetes mellitus

Dosage and routes

Adult: SC individualized

Available forms: Inj 40, 100 U/ml

Side effects/adverse reactions

EENT: Blurred vision, dry mouth

INTEG: Flushing, rash, urticaria, warmth, ***lipodystrophy***, lipohypertrophy, swelling, redness

META: ***Hypoglycemia***, rebond hyperglycemia (Somogyi effect 12-72 hr or longer)

SYST: ***Anaphylaxis***

Contraindications: Hypersensitivity to protamine

Precautions: Pregnancy **B**

Pharmacokinetics

Absorption	Rapidly absorbed (SC)
Distribution	Widely distributed
Metabolism	Liver, muscle, kidney
Excretion	Kidneys
Half-life	10 min

Pharmacodynamics

Onset	4-8 hr
Peak	10-30 hr
Duration	7-36 hr

Interactions

Drug/drug:

Individual drugs

Alcohol: ↑ hypoglycemia
Diltiazem: ↑ insulin need
Dobutamine: ↑ insulin need
Fenfluramine: ↓ insulin need
Guanethidine: ↓ insulin need
Phenylbutazone: ↓ insulin need
Rifampin: ↑ insulin need
Sulfinpyrazone: ↓ insulin need
Tetracycline: ↓ insulin need

Drug classifications

Anabolic steroids: ↓ insulin need
β-Blockers: Signs/symptoms of hypoglycemia may be masked

Glucocorticoid steroids: ↑ insulin need
Estrogens: ↑ insulin need
MAOI: ↓ insulin need
Oral anticoagulants: ↓ insulin need
Oral hypoglycemics: ↑ hypoglycemia
Thiazide diuretics: ↑ insulin need
Thyroid hormones: ↑ insulin need

Drug/smoking:

Tobacco: ↑ insulin requirements

Lab test interferences

Increase: VMA
Decrease: Potassium, magnesium, inorganic phosphate
Interference: Liver function studies, thyroid function studies

NURSING CONSIDERATIONS

Assessment

- Monitor fasting blood glucose, 2 hr PP (80-150 mg/dl, normal fasting level; 70-130 mg/dl, normal 2-hr level); also glycosylated Hgb may be drawn to identify treatment effectiveness
- Monitor urine ketones during illness; insulin requirements may increase during stress, illness, surgery
- Assess for hypoglycemic reaction that can occur during peak time (sweating, weakness, dizziness, chills, confusion, headache, nausea, rapid weak pulse, fatigue, tachycardia, memory lapses, slurred speech, staggering gait, anxiety, tremors, hunger)
- Assess for hyperglycemia: acetone breath, polyuria, fatigue, polydipsia, flushed, dry skin, lethargy

Associated nursing diagnoses

- ✓ Injury, risk for (adverse reactions)
- ✓ Knowledge deficit (teaching)
- ✓ Noncompliance (teaching)

Implementation

SC route

- Give after warming to room temp by rotating in palms to prevent injecting cold insulin; use only insulin syringes with markings or syringe matching U/ml; rotate inj sites within one area: abdomen, upper back, thighs, upper arm, buttocks; keep record of sites
- Give increased dosages if tolerance occurs; give human insulin to those allergic to beef or pork
- Store at room temp for <1 mo; keep away from heat and sunlight; refrigerate all other supply; do not use if discolored; do not freeze

Patient/family education

- Advise patient that blurred vision occurs; not to change corrective lenses until vision is stabilized after 1-2 mo of therapy
- Advise patient to keep insulin, equipment available at all times
- Advise patient to carry Medic Alert ID as diabetic
- Teach patient dosage, route, mixing instructions, disease process; tell patient to continue to use the same brand of insulin and to rotate inj sites

- Instruct patient to carry candy or lump of sugar to treat hypoglycemia; have glucagon emergency kit available; teach how to use these
- Teach patient symptoms of ketoacidosis: nausea, thirst, polyuria, dry mouth, decreased B/P, dry, flushed skin, acetone breath, drowsiness, Kussmaul respirations; to have insulin available at all times
- Advise patient that a plan is necessary for diet, exercise; all food on diet should be eaten, exercise routine should not vary
- Teach patient to avoid OTC drugs and alcohol unless approved by prescriber
- Instruct patient to notify prescriber if pregnancy is planned
- Caution patient that treatment is lifelong; insulin does not cure condition

Evaluation

Positive therapeutic outcome
- Decrease in polyuria, polydipsia, polyphagia, clear sensorium, absence of dizziness, stable gait
- Blood glucose level under control

Treatment of overdose:
Glucose 25 g **IV**, via dextrose 50% sol, 50 ml or 1 mg glucagon

insulin, zinc suspension, prompt (Semilente)

Semilente Iletin I, Semilente Insulin, Semitard

Func. class.: Pancreatic hormone

Chem. class.: Exogenous unmodified insulin

Pregnancy category **B**

Action: Decreases blood sugar; by transport of insulin into cells and the conversion of glucose to glycogen indirectly increases blood pyruvate and lactate, decreases phosphate and potassium; insulin may be beef, pork, human (processed by recombinant DNA technologies)

Therapeutic Outcome: Decreased blood glucose levels in diabetes mellitus

Uses: Adult-onset diabetes, juvenile diabetes, ketoacidosis types I and II, type II (non–insulin-dependent) diabetes mellitus, type I (insulin-dependent) diabetes mellitus

Dosage and routes

Adult: SC dosage individualized by blood, urine glucose qd-tid

Available forms: 100 U/ml

Side effects/adverse reactions

EENT: Blurred vision, dry mouth

INTEG: Flushing, rash, urticaria, warmth, *lipodystrophy,* lipohypertrophy, swelling, redness
META: *Hypoglycemia,* rebound hyperglycemia (Somogyi effect 12-72 hr or longer)
SYST: ***Anaphylaxis***

Contraindications: Hypersensitivity

Precautions: Pregnancy **B**

Pharmacokinetics

Absorption	Rapidly absorbed (SC)
Distribution	Widely distributed
Metabolism	Liver, muscle, kidney
Excretion	Kidneys
Half-life	10 min

Pharmacodynamics

	SC
Onset	1-1½ hr
Peak	5-10 hr
Duration	12-16 hr

Interactions

Drug/drug:

Individual drugs
Alcohol: ↑ hypoglycemia
Diltiazem: ↑ insulin need
Dobutamine: ↑ insulin need
Fenfluramine: ↓ insulin need
Guanethidine: ↓ insulin need
Phenylbutazone: ↓ insulin need
Rifampin: ↑ insulin need
Sulfinpyrazone: ↓ insulin need
Tetracycline: ↓ insulin need
Drug classifications
Anabolic steroids: ↓ insulin need
β-blockers: Signs/symptoms of hypoglycemia may be masked
Glucocorticoid steroids: ↑ insulin need
Estrogens: ↑ insulin need
MAOI: ↓ insulin need
Oral anticoagulants: ↓ insulin need
Oral hypoglycemics: ↑ hypoglycemia
Thiazide diuretics: ↑ insulin need
Thyroid hormones: ↑ insulin need

Drug/smoking:

Tobacco: ↑ insulin requirements

Lab test interferences

Increase: VMA
Decrease: Potassium, magnesium, inorganic phosphate
Interference: Liver function studies, thyroid function studies

NURSING CONSIDERATIONS

Assessment

- Monitor fasting blood glucose, 2 hr PP (80-150 mg/dl, normal fasting level; 70-130 mg/dl, normal 2-hr level); also glycosylated Hgb may be drawn to identify treatment effectiveness
- Monitor urine ketones during illness; insulin requirements may increase during stress, illness, surgery
- Assess for hypoglycemic reaction that can occur during peak time (sweating, weakness, dizziness, chills, confusion, headache, nausea, rapid weak pulse, fatigue, tachycardia, memory lapses, slurred speech, staggering gait, anxiety, tremors, hunger)

- Assess for hyperglycemia: acetone breath, polyuria, fatigue, polydipsia, flushed, dry skin, lethargy

Associated nursing diagnoses

✓ Injury, risk for (adverse reactions)
✓ Knowledge deficit (teaching)
✓ Noncompliance (teaching)

Implementation

SC route

- Give after warming to room temp by rotating in palms to prevent injecting cold insulin; use only insulin syringes with markings or syringe matching U/ml; rotate inj sites within one area; abdomen, upper back, thighs, upper arm, buttocks; keep record of sites
- Give increased dosages if tolerance occurs; give human insulin to those allergic to beef or pork
- Store at room temp for <1 mo; keep away from heat and sunlight; refrigerate all other supply; do not use if discolored; do not freeze

Patient/family education

- Advise patient that blurred vision occurs; not to change corrective lenses until vision is stabilized after 1-2 mo of therapy
- Advise patient to keep insulin, equipment available at all times
- Advise patient to carry Medic Alert ID as diabetic
- Teach patient dosage, route, mixing instructions, disease process; tell patient to continue to use the same brand of insulin and to rotate inj sites
- Instruct patient to carry candy or lump of sugar to treat hypoglycemia; have glucagon emergency kit available; teach how to use these
- Teach patient symptoms of ketoacidosis: nausea, thirst, polyuria, dry mouth, decreased B/P, dry, flushed skin, acetone breath, drowsiness, Kussmaul respirations; to have insulin available at all times
- Advise patient that a plan is necessary for diet, exercise; all food on diet should be eaten, exercise routine should not vary
- Teach patient to avoid OTC drugs and alcohol unless approved by prescriber
- Instruct patient to notify prescriber if pregnancy is planned
- Caution patient that treatment is lifelong; insulin does not cure condition

Evaluation

Positive therapeutic outcome

- Decrease in polyuria, polydipsia, polyphagia, clear sensorium, absence of dizziness, stable gait
- Blood glucose level under control

Treatment of overdose:

Glucose 25 g **IV**, via dextrose 50% sol, 50 ml or 1 mg glucagon

I

interferon alfa-2a/ interferon alfa 2b

(in-ter-feer'on)

Roferon-A/Intron-A, a-2-Interferon

Func. class.: Miscellaneous antineoplastic

Chem. class.: Protein product

Pregnancy category **C**

Action: Antiviral action inhibits viral replication by reprogramming virus; antitumor action suppresses cell proliferation; immunomodulating action phagocytizes target cells

➡ Therapeutic Outcome: Prevention of rapid growth of malignant cells; treatment of hepatitis non-A, non-B (liver function improvement)

Uses: Hairy cell leukemia in persons >18 yr, condylomata acuminata (alfa 2b), metastatic melanoma, AIDS-related Kaposi's sarcoma, chronic hepatitis non-A, non-B (alfa 2b), chronic hepatitis B (alfa 2b)

Dosage and routes

Hairy cell leukemia (2a)

Adult: SC/IM 3 million IU/day × 16-24 wk, then 3 million IU 3 times a wk maintenance

Hairy cell leukemia (2b)

2 million IU/m^2 3 times a wk; if severe adverse reactions occur, dose should be skipped or reduced by one half

Kaposi's sarcoma (2a)

Adult: SC/IM 36 million IU/day × 10-12 wk or 3 million IU/day × 3 days, then 9 million IU/day × 3 days, then 18 million IU/day × 3 days, then 36 million IU/day for the rest of the course; if severe reaction occurs reduce dose by one half

Condylomata acuminata (2b)

1 million IU/lesion 3 times a wk × 3 wk

Chronic hepatitis B (2b)

Adult: SC/IM 5 million IU/day or 10 million IU 3 times a wk

Chronic hepatitis

Non-A, Non-B (2b)

Adult: SC/IM 36 million IU 3 times a wk

Available forms: Alfa-2a inj 3, 6, 36 million IU/ml; alfa-2b inj 3, 5, 10, 18, 25, 50 million U/vial

Side effects/adverse reactions

CNS: Dizziness, confusion, numbness, paresthesias, hallucinations, ***convulsions, coma,*** amnesia, anxiety, mood changes

CV: Edema, hypotension, hypertension, chest pain, palpitations, dysrhythmias, **CHF, MI, CVA**

GI: Weight loss, taste changes

GU: Impotence

INTEG: Rash, dry skin, itching, alopecia, flushing

MISC: Flulike syndrome: fever, fatigue, myalgias, headache, chills

Contraindications: Hypersensitivity

Precautions: Severe hypotension, dysrhythmia, tachycardia, P pregnancy C, lactation, children, severe renal or hepatic disease, convulsion disorder

Pharmacokinetics

Absorption	80%-90% (SC/IM)
Distribution	Unknown
Metabolism	Renal tubular (degraded)
Excretion	Kidneys
Half-life	3.7-8.5 hr (2a); 2-7 hr (2b)

Pharmacodynamics

Onset	Unknown
Peak	3-8 hr
Duration	Unknown

Interactions

Drug/drug:

Individual drugs

Aminophylline: ↑ toxicity, blood levels
Radiation: ↑ toxicity, bone marrow suppression
Zidovudine: ↑ neutropenia

Drug classifications

Antineoplastics: ↑ toxicity, bone marrow suppression

Lab test interferences

Interference: AST (SGOT), ALT (SGPT), LDH, alkaline phosphatase, WBC, platelets, granulocytes, creatinine

NURSING CONSIDERATIONS

Assessment

- Assess for symptoms of infection; may be masked by drug fever; fever, chills, headache, sore throat may occur 6 hr after dose; give acetaminophen for symptoms
- In AIDS patients with Kaposi's sarcoma, assess characteristics of lesions during therapy; symptoms should decrease
- Assess for bleeding: hematuria, stool guaiac, bruising or petechiae, mucosa or orifices q8h; check for inflammation of mucosa, breaks in skin; avoid IM injection, rectal temp, or any other procedures that break the skin
- Assess for CNS reaction: LOC, mental status, dizziness, confusion, poor coordination, difficulty speaking, behavior changes; notify prescriber

Associated nursing diagnoses

- ✓ Injury, risk for (adverse reactions)
- ✓ Body image disturbance (adverse reactions)
- ✓ Infection, risk for (adverse reactions)
- ✓ Knowledge deficit (teaching)

Implementation

- Sol should be prepared by qualified personnel only under controlled conditions in biologic cabinet using gown, gloves, and mask
- Use Luer-Lok tubing to prevent leakage; do not let sol come in contact with skin; if contact occurs, wash well with soap and water
- Give at hs to minimize side effects

• Give acetaminophen as ordered to alleviate fever and headache

IM/SC route

• Give by IM/SC after reconstituting 3-5 million IU/1 ml, 10 million IU/2 ml, 25 million IU/5 ml, of diluent provided; mix gently

• Store reconstituted sol for 1 mo in refrigerator

Intralesional route (2b)

• Give by intralesional route after reconstituting 10 million IU/1 ml bacteriostatic water for inj; no more than 5 lesions can safely be treated at a time; using a 25 G needle inject 0.1 ml into base at center

Patient/family education

• Caution patient to avoid hazardous tasks, since confusion, dizziness may occur; fatigue is common; activity may have to be altered

• Advise patient that brands of this drug should not be changed; each form is different, with different dosages

• Caution patient not to become pregnant while taking drug; possible mutagenic effects; impotence may occur during treatment but is temporary

• Advise patient to report signs of infection: sore throat, fever, diarrhea, vomiting

• Advise patient that emotional lability is common; notify prescriber if severe or incapacitating

Evaluation

Positive therapeutic outcome

• Leukocytes, Hgb, platelets, WNL

• Decreased amount of lesions in AIDS patients with Kaposi's sarcoma

• Decreased amount of genital warts

interferon β-1b

(in-ter-feer′on)

Betaseron

Func. class.: Multiple sclerosis agent, immune modifier

Chem. class.: Escherichia coli derivative

Pregnancy category C

Action: Antiviral, immunoregulatory; action not clearly understood; biologic response-modifying properties mediated through specific receptors on cells, inducing expression of interferon-induced gene products

➔ Therapeutic Outcome: Correcting symptoms of multiple sclerosis

Uses: Ambulatory patients with relapsing or remitting multiple sclerosis

Investigational uses: May be useful in treatment of AIDS, AIDS-related Kaposi's sarcoma, malignant melanoma, metastatic renal cell carcinoma, cutaneous T cell lymphoma, acute non-A, non-B hepatitis

Dosage and routes

Relapsing/remitting multiple sclerosis

Adult: SC 0.25 mg (8 IU) qod

Available forms: Powder for inj lyophilized 0.3 mg (9.6 mIU)

Side effects/adverse reactions

CNS: *Headache, fever, pain, chills, mental changes,* hypertonia, ***suicide attempts,*** gait disturbances, depression
CV: *Migraine, palpitations, hypertension,* tachycardia, peripheral vascular disorders
EENT: Conjunctivitis, blurred vision, laryngitis
GI: *Diarrhea, constipation, vomiting, abdominal pain*
GU: *Dysmenorrhea, irregular menses, metrorrhagia,* cystitis, breast pain, spontaneous abortion
HEMA: ***Decreased lymphocytes, WBC;*** *lymphadenopathy*
INTEG: *Sweating, inj site reaction,* necrosis
MS: *Myalgia,* ***myasthenia,*** back pain
RESP: *Sinusitis,* dyspnea

Contraindications: Hypersensitivity to natural or recombinant interferon-β or human albumin

Precautions: Pregnancy **C**, P lactation, child <18 yr, chronic progressive MS, depression, mental disorders

Pharmacokinetics

Absorption	50% is absorbed (SC)
Distribution	Unknown
Metabolism	Unknown
Excretion	Unknown
Half-life	8 min-4½ hr

Pharmacodynamics

	SC
Onset	Rapid
Peak	Up to 8 hr
Duration	Unknown

Interactions: None

NURSING CONSIDERATIONS

Assessment

- Monitor blood, renal, hepatic studies: CBC, differential, platelet counts, BUN, creatinine, ALT (SGPT), urinalysis; if neutrophil count is <750/mm^3, or if AST (SGOT), ALT (SGPT), is 10 times greater than upper normal limit, or if bilirubin is 5 times greater than upper normal limit; when neutrophil count exceeds 750/mm^3 and liver function or renal studies return to normal, treatment may resume at 50% original dosage
- Assess for CNS symptoms: headache, fatigue, depression; if depression occurs and is severe, drug should be discontinued
- Monitor GI status: diarrhea or constipation, vomiting, abdominal pain
- Monitor cardiac status: increased B/P, tachycardia

Associated nursing diagnoses

✓ Physical mobility, impaired (uses)
✓ Knowledge deficit (teaching)

Implementation

SC route

- Reconstitute 0.3 mg (9.6 million IU)/1.2 ml of supplied diluent (0.2 mg or 8 million

IU concentration); rotate vial gently, do not shake; withdraw 1 ml using a syringe with 27 G needle; administer SC into hip, thigh, arm; discard unused portion
- Give acetaminophen for fever, headache; use SC route only; do not give IM or **IV**
- Store reconstituted sol in refrigerator; do not freeze; do not use sol that contains precipitate or is discolored

Patient/family education

- Provide patient or family member with written, detailed instructions about the drug; provide initial and return demonstrations on inj procedure; give information on use and disposal of drug
- Inform patient that blurred vision, sweating may occur
- Advise women patients that irregular menses, dysmenorrhea, or metrorrhagia as well as breast pain may occur; use contraception during treatment; drug may cause spontaneous abortion

Evaluation

Positive therapeutic outcome
- Decreased symptoms of multiple sclerosis

interferon gamma-1b

(in-ter-feer'on)
Actimmune
Func. class.: Biologic response modifier
Chem. class.: Lymphokine, interleukin type
Pregnancy category C

Action: Species-specific protein synthesized in response to viruses; potent phagocyte-activating effects; capable of mediating the killing of *Staphylococcus aureus, Toxoplasma gondii, Leishmania donovani, Listeria monocytogenes, Mycobacterium avium-intracellulare;* enhances oxidative metabolism of macrophages; enhances antibody-dependent cellular cytotoxicity

Therapeutic Outcome: Decreased signs/symptoms of infection (serious) in chronic granulomatous disease

Uses: Serious infections associated with chronic granulomatous disease

Dosage and routes

Adult: SC 50 μg/m^2 (1.5 million U/m^2) for patients with a surface area of >0.5 m^2; 1.5 μg/kg/dose for patient with a surface area of <0.5/m^2; give on Monday, Wednesday, Friday for 3 times a wk dosing

Available forms: Inj 100 μg (3 million U)/single-dose vial

Side effects/adverse reactions

CNS: *Headache, fatigue,* depression, fever, chills
GI: *Nausea, anorexia,* abdominal pain, weight loss, diarrhea, vomiting
INTEG: Rash, pain at inj site
MS: Myalgia, arthralgia

Contraindications: Hypersensitivity to interferon gamma, *E. coli*–derived products

Precautions: Pregnancy **C**, cardiac disease, seizure disorders, CNS disorders, myelosuppression, lactation, P children

Pharmacokinetics

Absorption	Slowly absorbed (SC); 89%
Distribution	Unknown
Metabolism	Unknown
Excretion	Unknown
Half-life	5.9 hr

Pharmacodynamics

Onset	Unknown
Peak	7 hr
Duration	Unknown

Interactions

Drug/drug:

Individual drugs
Radiation: ↑ toxicity, bone marrow suppression

Drug classifications
Antineoplastics: ↑ toxicity, bone marrow suppression

NURSING CONSIDERATIONS

Assessment

- Monitor blood, renal, hepatic studies: CBC with differential, platelet count, BUN, creatinine, ALT (SGPT), urinalysis before and q3 mo during treatment
- Assess for infection: headache, fever, chills, fatigue; these are common adverse reactions
- Monitor CNS symptoms: headache, fatigue, depression

Associated nursing diagnoses

✓ Infection, risk for (uses)
✓ Knowledge deficit (teaching)

Implementation

- Give at hs to minimize adverse reactions; administer acetaminophen for fever, headache; use 50% of the dosage prescribed if severe reactions occur or discontinue treatment until reactions subside

SC route

- Administer using sterilized glass or plastic disposable syringes; give in right or left deltoid and anterior thigh; warm to room temp before use; do not leave at room temp over 12 hr (unopened vial); does not contain preservatives
- Store in refrigerator upon receipt; do not freeze; do not shake

Patient/family education

- Provide patient or family member with written, detailed instructions about the drug; provide initial and return demonstrations on inj procedure; give information on use and disposal of drug
- Caution patient to use contraception during treatment

Evaluation

Positive therapeutic outcome
- Decrease serious infections
- Improvement in existing infections and inflammatory conditions

ipecac syrup

(ip'e-kak)
Func. class.: Emetic
Chem. class.: Cephaelis ipecacuanha derivative
Pregnancy category **C**

Action: Acts on chemoreceptor trigger zone to induce vomiting; irritates gastric mucosa

➡ **Therapeutic Outcome:** Emesis

Uses: In poisoning from noncaustic substances to induce vomiting

Dosage and routes

Adult: PO 15-30 ml, then 200-300 ml water; may repeat in 30 min
P *Child >1 yr:* PO 15 ml, then 200-300 ml water; may repeat in 30 min
P *Child <1 yr:* PO 5-10 ml, then 100-200 ml water; may repeat dose if needed

Available forms: Liq

Side effects/adverse reactions

CNS: ***Depression, convulsions, coma***
CV: ***Circulatory failure, atrial fibrillation, fatal myocarditis, dysrhythmias***
GI: Nausea, vomiting, bloody diarrhea

Contraindications: Hypersensitivity, unconscious/semiconscious, depressed gag reflex, poisoning with petroleum products or caustic substances, convulsions, shock, alcohol intolerance

Precautions: Lactation, pregnancy **C**, P child <6 mo

Pharmacokinetics

Absorption	Not absorbed
Distribution	Unknown
Metabolism	Unknown
Excretion	Unknown
Half-life	Unknown

Pharmacodynamics

Onset	15-30 min
Peak	Unknown
Duration	½ hr

Interactions

Drug/drug:

Individual drugs
Activated charcoal: ↓ effect; do not use together
Drug classifications
Antiemetics: ↓ effect, do not use together

Drug/food:

Milk: ↓ effect
Carbonated drinks: ↑ abdominal distention

NURSING CONSIDERATIONS

Assessment

• Assess type of poisoning; do not administer if petroleum products or caustic substances have been ingested: kerosene, gasoline, lye, Drano
• Assess respiratory status before, during, after administration of emetic; check rate, rhythm, character; respiratory depression can occur rapidly G with elderly or debilitated patients
• Monitor LOC; do not give to patients who are semiconscious or unconscious or if gag reflex is not present

Associated nursing diagnoses

✓ Injury, risk for (uses)
✓ Poisoning (uses)
✓ Knowledge deficit (teaching)

Implementation

PO route
• Give **ipecac *syrup*, not ipecac,** which is 14 times stronger or death may occur
• Give activated charcoal after the patient has finished vomiting; may begin lavage after 10-15 min after 2 doses of ipecac syrup without results
• Give with the patient upright; give water immediately after the ipecac syrup (200-300 ml for adults; 100- P 200 ml child <1 yr; 200-300 ml for a child >1 yr)

Patient family education

• Give patient phone number for poison control
• Give patient written guidelines on poisoning and when to induce vomiting; suggest patient keep ipecac syrup in P house if young children are present

Evaluation

Positive therapeutic outcome
• Vomiting within 30 min

ipratropium

(i-pra-troe'pee-um)
Atrovent
Func. class.: Anticholinergic, bronchodilator
Chem. class.: Synthetic quaternary ammonium compound
Pregnancy category **B**

Action: Inhibits interaction of acetylcholine at receptor sites on the bronchial smooth muscle, resulting in decreased cyclic guanosine monophosphate (cGMP) and bronchodilatation

➔ **Therapeutic Outcome:** Bronchodilatation

Uses: Bronchodilatation during bronchospasm for patients with COPD

Dosage and routes

Adult: 2 inh qid, not to exceed 12 inh/24 hr

Available forms: Aerosol 18 µg/actuation

Side effects/adverse reactions

CNS: *Anxiety, dizziness, headache,* nervousness
CV: Palpitations

I

EENT: Dry mouth, blurred vision
GI: *Nausea, vomiting, cramps*
INTEG: Rash
RESP: *Cough, worsening of symptoms, **bronchospasms***

Contraindications: Hypersensitivity to this drug, atropine, soya lecithin

Precautions: Pregnancy **B**, P lactation, children <12 yr, narrow angle glaucoma, prostatic hypertrophy, bladder neck obstruction

Pharmacokinetics

Absorption	Minimal
Distribution	Does not cross blood-brain barrier
Metabolism	Liver, minimal
Excretion	Unknown
Half-life	2 hr

Pharmacodynamics

Onset	5-15 min
Peak	1-1½ hr
Duration	3-6 hr

Interactions

Drug/drug:

Drug classifications

Bronchodilators, aerosol: ↑ action of bronchodilator

NURSING CONSIDERATIONS

Assessment

- Monitor respiratory function: vital capacity, FEV, ABGs, lung sounds, heart rate, rhythm (baseline and during treatment); if severe bronchospasm is present, a more rapid medication is required
- Monitor for evidence of allergic reactions, paradoxic bronchospasm; withhold dose and notify prescriber; identify if patient is allergic to belladonna products or atropine; allergy to this drug may occur

Associated nursing diagnoses

- ✓ Airway clearance, ineffective (uses)
- ✓ Gas exchange, impaired (uses)
- ✓ Knowledge deficit (teaching)

Implementation

Aerosol route

- Give after shaking container; have patient exhale, place mouthpiece in mouth, inhale slowly, hold breath, remove, exhale slowly; allow at least 1 min between inhalations
- Store in light-resistant container; do not expose to temp over 86° F (30° C)

Patient/family education

- Advise patient not to use OTC medications unless approved by prescriber; extra stimulation may occur; to use this medication before other medications and allow at least 5 min between each to prevent overstimulation
- Teach patient the proper use of the inhaler; review package insert with patient; to avoid getting aerosol in eyes; blurring may result; to wash inhaler in warm water qd and dry; to avoid smoking, smoke-filled rooms, persons with respiratory tract infections
- Teach patient if paradoxic bronchospasm occurs to stop drug immediately and notify prescriber; to limit caffeine

products such as chocolate, coffee, tea, and colas

- Instruct patient on administration of dose, not to use more than prescribed; serious side effects may occur; if dose is missed, take when remembered; space other doses on new time schedule; do not double doses

Evaluation

Positive therapeutic outcome

- Absence of dyspnea, wheezing after 1 hr
- Improved airway exchange
- Improved ABGs

iron dextran

Imferon ✦, InFed

Func. class.: Hematinic

Chem. class.: Ferric hydroxide complex with dextran

Pregnancy category **C**

Action: Iron is carried by transferrin to the bone marrow, where it is incorporated into hemoglobin

Therapeutic Outcome: Prevention and resolution of iron-deficiency anemia

Uses: Iron-deficiency anemia in patients who cannot take oral preparations

Dosage and routes

P *Adult and child:* IM 0.5 ml as a test dose by Z-track, then no more than the following per day:

Adult <50 kg: IM 100 mg

Adult >50 kg: IM 250 mg

P *Infant <5 kg:* IM 25 mg

P *Child <9 kg:* IM 50 mg

Adult: **IV** 0.5 ml test dose, then 100 mg qd after 2-3 days; **IV** 250/1000 ml of NaCl; give 25 mg test dose, wait 5 min, then inf over 6-12 hr or follow equation:

$$\frac{0.3 \times \text{weight (lb)} \times 100\text{-Hgb (g/dl)} \times 100}{14.8}$$

Patients <30 lb (66 kg) should be given 80% of above formula dose

Available forms: Inj IM/**IV** 50 mg/ml; inj IM only 50 mg/ml

Side effects/adverse reactions

CNS: Headache, paresthesia, dizziness, shivering, weakness, ***seizures***

CV: Chest pain, ***shock,*** hypotension, tachycardia

GI: *Nausea,* vomiting, metallic taste, abdominal pain

HEMA: ***Leukocytosis***

INTEG: Rash, pruritus, urticaria, fever, sweating, chills, brown skin discoloration, pain at inj site, necrosis, sterile abscesses, phlebitis

MISC: ***Anaphylaxis***

RESP: Dyspnea

Contraindications: Hypersensitivity, all anemias excluding iron-deficiency anemia, hepatic disease

Precautions: Acute renal P disease, children, asthma, lactation, rheumatoid arthritis

(**IV**), infants <4 mo, pregnancy **C**

Pharmacokinetics

Absorption	Well absorbed; lymphatics over wk or mo
Distribution	Crosses placenta
Metabolism	Slow; blood loss, desquamation
Excretion	Breast milk, feces, urine, bile
Half-life	6 hr

Pharmacodynamics

	IM/IV
Onset	Unknown
Peak	Unknown
Duration	Unknown

Interactions

Drug/drug:

Individual drugs

Chloramphenicol: ↓ reticulocyte response
Oral iron: Do not use together
Vitamin E: ↓ reticulocyte response

Lab test interferences

False increase: Serum bilirubin
False decrease: Serum calcium
False positive: ^{99m}Tc diphosphate bone scan, iron test (large doses >2 ml)

NURSING CONSIDERATIONS

Assessment

- Monitor blood studies: Hct, Hgb, reticulocytes, bilirubin before treatment, at least monthly
- Assess for allergic reaction and ***anaphylaxis;*** rash, pruritus, fever, chills, wheezing, notify prescriber immediately
- Assess cardiac status: anginal pain, hypotension, tachycardia
- Assess for nutrition: amount of iron in diet (meat, dark green leafy vegetables, dried fruits, eggs); cause of iron loss or anemia, including salicylates, sulfonamides
- Monitor pulse, B/P during **IV** administration

Associated nursing diagnoses

- ✓ Fatigue (uses)
- ✓ Activity intolerance (uses)
- ✓ Knowledge deficit (teaching)

Implementation

IM route

- D/C oral iron before parenteral; give only after test dose of 25 mg by preferred route; wait at least 1 hr before giving remaining portion
- Give IM deep in large muscle mass; use Z-track method and 19-20 G 2-, 3-inch needle; ensure needle is long enough to place drug deep in muscle; change needles after withdrawing medication and injecting to prevent skin and tissue staining

IV **IV route**

- Give **IV** after flushing tubing with 10 ml of 0.9% NaCl; give undiluted; give 1 ml (50 mg) or less over 1 min or more; flush line after use with 10 ml of 0.9% NaCl; patient should remain recumbent for 30-60 min to prevent orthostatic hypotension
- **IV** inj requires single-dose vial without preservative; verify on label **IV** use is approved
- Give by cont inf after diluting in 50-250 normal saline for inf; administer over 4-5 hr

• Give only with epinephrine available in case of anaphylactic reaction during dose
• Store at room temp in cool environment

Patient/family education

• Caution patient that iron poisoning may occur if increased beyond recommended level; to not take oral iron preparation unless approved by prescriber
• Advise patient that delayed reaction may occur 1-2 days after administration and last 3-4 days (**IV**) or 3-7 days (IM); report fever, chills, malaise, muscle, joint aches, nausea, vomiting, backache

Evaluation

Positive therapeutic outcome
• Increased serum iron levels, Hct, Hb

Treatment of overdose:

• Discontinue drug, treat allergic reaction, give diphenhydramine or epinephrine as needed for anaphylaxis; give iron-chelating drug in acute poisoning

isoniazid

(eye-soe-nye'a-zid)
INH, isoniazid, Isotamine ✦, Laniazid, Laniazid C.T., Nydrazid, PMS-Isoniazid ✦, Tubizid
Func. class.: Antitubercular
Chem. class.: Isonicotinic acid hydrazide
Pregnancy category **C**

Action: Inhibits RNA synthesis, decreases tubercle bacilli replication

Therapeutic Outcome: Resolution of TB infection

Uses: Pulmonary TB as an adjunct; other infections caused by mycobacteria

Dosage and routes

Treatment

Adult: PO/IM 5 mg/kg qd as single dose for 9-24 mo, not to exceed 300 mg/day

P ***Child and infant:*** PO/IM 10-20 mg/kg qd as single dose for 18-24 mo, not to exceed 300 mg/day

Prevention

Adult: PO 300 mg qd as single dose × 12 mo

P ***Child and infant:*** PO/IM 10 mg/kg qd as single dose for 12 mo, not to exceed 300 mg/day

Available forms: Tab 100, 300 mg; inj 100 mg/ml; powder 50 mg/5 ml; syrup 50 mg/5 ml

Side effects/adverse reactions

Hypersensitivity: fever, skin eruptions, lymphadenopathy, vasculitis
CNS: *Peripheral neuropathy*, memory impairment, ***toxic encephalopathy, convulsions***, psychosis
EENT: Blurred vision, optic neuritis, visual disturbance
GI: Nausea, vomiting, epigastric distress, ***jaundice, fatal hepatitis***
HEMA: ***Agranulocytosis, hemolytic anemia, aplastic anemia, thrombocytopenia, eosinophilia, methemoglobinemia***
MISC: Dyspnea, vitamin B_6 deficiency, pellagra, hyperglycemia, metabolic acidosis, gynecomastia, rheumatic syndrome, SLE-like syndrome

Contraindications: Hypersensitivity, optic neuritis

Precautions: Pregnancy **C**, renal disease, diabetic retinopathy, cataracts, ocular defects, hepatic disease, P child <13 yr

Pharmacokinetics

Absorption	Well
Distribution	Widely
Metabolism	Liver
Excretion	Kidneys
Half-life	1-4 hr

Pharmacodynamics

	PO	IM
Onset	Rapid	Rapid
Peak	1-2 hr	45-60 min
Duration	6-8 hr	6-8 hr

Interactions

Drug/drug:

Individual drugs
Alcohol: ↑ toxicity
BCG vaccine: ↓ effectiveness of BCG vaccine
Carbamazepine: ↑ toxicity
Cycloserine: ↑ toxicity
Ethionamide: ↑ toxicity
Phenytoin: ↓ metabolism of phenytoin
Rifampin: ↑ toxicity
Drug classifications
Antacids, aluminum: ↓ absorption

Drug/food:

Tyramine foods: ↑ toxicity

NURSING CONSIDERATIONS

Assessment

- Obtain C&S tests, including sputum tests, before treatment; monitor every mo to detect resistance
- Monitor liver studies weekly: ALT (SGPT), AST (SGOT), bilirubin; renal studies treatment and monthly before: BUN, creatinine, output, sp gr, urinalysis, uric acid
- Assess mental status often: affect, mood, behavioral changes; psychosis may occur with hallucinations, confusion
- Assess hepatic status: decreased appetite, jaundice, dark urine, fatigue
- Assess for visual disturbance that may indicate optic neuritis: blurred vision, change in color perception; may lend to blindness

Associated nursing diagnoses

✓ Infection, risk for (uses)
✓ Diarrhea (adverse reactions)

✓ Injury, risk for (adverse reactions)
✓ Knowledge deficit (teaching)
✓ Noncompliance (teaching)

Implementation

- Give antiemetic for vomiting

PO route

- Give with meals to decrease GI symptoms; it is better to take on empty stomach for better absorption, 1 hr ac or 2 hr pc

IM route

- Give deep in large muscle mass, massage; rotate inj sites

Patient/family education

- Instruct patient that compliance with dosage schedule for duration is necessary; not to skip or double doses; that scheduled appointments must be kept or relapse may occur
- Caution patient to avoid alcohol while taking drug or hepatoxicity may result; to avoid ingestion of aged cheeses, fish or hypertensive crisis may result; give patient written directions or which foods to avoid while taking this medication
- Tell patient to report peripheral neuritis: weakness, tingling/numbness of hands/feet, fatigue, hepatoxicity: loss of appetite, nausea, vomiting, yellowing of skin or eyes

Evaluation

Positive therapeutic outcome

- Decreased symptoms of TB
- Culture negative for TB

isoproterenol

(eye-soe-proe-ter'e-nole)

Aerolone, Dispos-a-Med, Isoproterenol HCl, Isuprel, Isuprel Glossets, Isuprel Mistometer, Medihaler-Iso, Vapo-Iso

Func. class.: β-Adrenergic-agonist, antidysrhythmic, inotropic

Chem. class.: Catecholamine

Pregnancy category **C**

I

Action: Has β_1- and β_2-adrenergic action; relaxes bronchial smooth muscle and dilates the trachea and main bronchi by increasing levels of cAMP, which relaxes smooth muscles; causes increased contractility and heart rate by acting on β-receptors in heart

➔ **Therapeutic Outcome:** Bronchodilatation, increased heart rate and cardiac output from action on β-receptors in the heart

Uses: Bronchospasm, asthma, heart block, ventricular dysrhythmias, shock

Dosage and routes

Asthma, bronchospasm

Adult: SL tab 10-20 mg q6-8h; inh 1 puff; may repeat in 2-5 min; maintenance 1-2 puffs 4-6 times/day; **IV** 10-20 mg during anesthesia

P *Child:* SL tab 5-10 mg q6-8h; inh 1 puff; may repeat in 2-5 min; maintenance 1-2 puffs 4-6 times/day

Heart block/ventricular dysrhythmias

Adult: **IV** 0.02-0.06 mg, then 0.01-0.2 mg or 5 μg/min HCl; 0.2 mg, then 0.02-1 mg as needed

P *Child:* **IV** ½ of beginning adult dosage

Shock

Adult: **IV** inf 0.5-5 μg/min (1 mg/500 ml D_5W) titrate to B/P, CVP, hourly urine output

Available forms: Sol for nebulization 1:400 (0.25%), 1:200 (0.5%), 1:100 (1%); aerosol 0.25%, 0.2%; powder for inh 0.1 mg/cartridge; inj 1:5000 (0.2 mg/ml) **IV**; glossets (SL) 10, 15 mg

Side effects/adverse reactions

CNS: Tremors, anxiety, insomnia, headache, dizziness, stimulation
CV: Palpitations, tachycardia, hypertension, ***cardiac arrest***
GI: Nausea, vomiting
META: Hyperglycemia
RESP: Bronchial irritation, edema, dryness of oropharynx, ***bronchospasms*** (overuse)

Contraindications: Hypersensitivity to sympathomimetics, narrow angle glaucoma

Precautions: Pregnancy **C**, cardiac disorders, hyperthyroidism, diabetes mellitus, prostatic hypertrophy

Pharmacokinetics

Absorption	Erratic (SL, rec), rapid (inh, IV)
Distribution	Unknown
Metabolism	Lungs, liver, GI tract
Excretion	Kidneys, unchanged (50%)
Half-life	Unknown

Pharmacodynamics

	SL	INH	IV	REC
Onset	1-2 hr	Rapid	Rapid	2-4 hr
Peak	Unknown	Unknown	Unknown	Unknown
Duration	2 hr	1 hr	10 min	3-4 hr

Interactions

Drug/drug:

Drug classifications

β-Adrenergic blockers: Block therapeutic effect
Bronchodilators, aerosol: ↑ action of bronchodilator
MAOI: ↑ chance of hypertensive crisis
Sympathomimetics: ↑ adrenergic side effects

NURSING CONSIDERATIONS

Assessment

- Assess respiratory function: vital capacity, FEV, ABGs, lung sounds, heart rate, rhythm (baseline and during therapy)
- Monitor for evidence of allergic reactions, paradoxic bronchospasm; withhold dose; notify prescriber

Associated nursing diagnoses

✓ Airway clearance, ineffective (uses)
✓ Impaired gas exchange (uses)
✓ Knowledge deficit (teaching)

Implementation

Inh

- Give after diluting dose in sterile water or 0.9% NaCl, 0.45% NaCl; give over 15-20 min
- Store in light-resistant container; do not expose to temp over 86° F (30° C)

IV **IV route**

- Give by direct **IV** after diluting 0.2 mg or 1 ml (1:5000 sol)/10 ml 0.9% NaCl for inj or D_5W (1:50,000 sol); give 1:50,000 sol over 1 min
- Give by cont inf by diluting 2 mg or 10 ml (1:5000 sol)/500 ml 0.9% NaCl, D_5W, $D_{10}W$, 0.45% NaCl, Ringer's, LR (1:250,000 sol); give at a rate of 1 ml/min by inf pump; ratio is adjusted according to patient response

Y-site compatibilities:

Amiodarone, amrinone, atracurium, bretyllium, famotidine, heparin, hydrocortisone sodium succinate, pancuronium, potassium chloride, vecuronium, vitamin B with C

Syringe compatibility:

Ranitidine

Additive compatibilities:

Calcium chloride, calcium gluceptate, cephalothin, cimetidine, dobutamine, floxacillin, heparin, magnesium sulfate, multivitamins, netilmicin, potassium chloride, succinylchloride, tetracycline, verapamil, vitamin B with C

Patient/family education

- Caution patient not to use OTC medications before consulting prescriber; extra stimulation may occur
- Instruct patient to use this medication before other medications and allow at least 5 min between each; to prevent overstimulation by limiting caffeine products such as chocolate, coffee, tea, and colas
- Teach patient use of inhaler; review package insert with patient; to avoid getting aerosol in eyes; blurring may result; to wash inhaler in warm water qd and dry; rinse mouth after using; to avoid smoking, smoke-filled rooms, persons with respiratory tract infections
- Instruct patient if paradoxic bronchospasm occurs to stop drug immediately and notify prescriber; to limit caffeine products such as chocolate, coffee, tea, and colas
- Instruct patient on administration of dose; not to use more than prescribed; serious side effects may occur; if taking PO regularly and dose is missed, take when remembered; space other doses on new time schedule; do not double doses

Evaluation

Positive therapeutic outcome

- Absence of dyspnea, wheezing
- Improved airway exchange
- Improved ABGs

Treatment of overdose: Administer a β_2-adrenergic blocker

I

isosorbide

(eye-soe-sor'bide)

Apo-ISDN ✤, Cedocard-SR ✤, Coronex ✤, Dilatrate-SR, Imdur, ISDN, Iso-Bid, Isonate, Isorbid, Isordil, Isordil Tembids, Isordil Titradose, Isosorbide Dinitrate, Isotrate Timecelles, Monoket, Novasorbide ✤, Sorbitrate, Sorbitrate SA, Sorbitrate/ISMO

Func. class.: Antianginal, Vasodilator

Chem. class.: Nitrate

Pregnancy category **C**

Action: Decreases preload, afterload, thus decreasing LVEDP, systemic vascular resistance, and reducing cardiac O_2 demand

Therapeutic Outcome: Relief and prevention of angina pectoris

Uses: Chronic stable angina pectoris, prophylaxis of angina pain

Dosage and routes

Adult: PO 5-40 mg qid; SL tab 2.5-10 mg; may repeat q2-3h; chew tab 5-10 mg prn or q2-3h as prophylaxis; sus rel cap 40-80 mg q8-12h

Available forms: Sus rel cap 40 mg; tab 5, 10, 20, 30, 40 mg; chew tab 5, 10 mg; SL tab 2.5, 5, 10 mg

Side effects/adverse reactions

CNS: Vascular headache, flushing, dizziness, weakness, faintness

CV: Postural hypotension, tachycardia, ***collapse,*** syncope

GI: Nausea, vomiting

INTEG: Pallor, sweating, rash

MISC: Twitching, hemolytic anemia, ***methemoglobinemia***

Contraindications: Hypersensitivity to this drug or nitrates, severe anemia, increased intracranial pressure, cerebral hemorrhage, acute MI

Precautions: Postural hypotension, pregnancy **C**, lactation, P children

Pharmacokinetics

Absorption	Well
Distribution	Unknown
Metabolism	Liver
Excretion	Urine, metabolites
Half-life	Dinitrate 1 hr, mononitrate 5 hr

Pharmacodynamics

	SUS REL	SL	PO
Onset	20-45 min	2-5 min	15-30 min
Peak	Unknown	Unknown	Unknown
Duration	8-12 hr	1-4 hr	4-6 hr

Interactions

Drug/drug:

Individual drugs

Alcohol: ↑ hypotension

Drug classifications

Antihypertensives: ↑ hypotension

β-Blockers: ↑ hypotension
Calcium channel blockers: ↑ hypotension
Phenothiazines: ↑ hypotension

NURSING CONSIDERATIONS

Assessment

- Monitor for orthostatic B/P, pulse at baseline and during treatment
- Assess for pain: duration, time started, activity being performed, character, intensity

Associated nursing diagnoses

- ✓ Cardiac output, decreased (uses)
- ✓ Tissue perfusion, decreased (uses)
- ✓ Knowledge deficit (teaching)

Implementation

SL route

- Hold SL tab under tongue until dissolved (a few min); do not take anything PO when SL tab is in place

PO route

- Give 1 hr ac or 2 hr pc with 8 oz of water
- Sus rel tab should not be chewed, broken, or crushed; chew tab should be chewed thoroughly

Patient/family education

- Instruct patient to swallow sus rel tab whole, do not chew; SL tab should be dissolved under tongue, do not swallow; chew tab should be chewed thoroughly; do not skip or double doses; if dose is missed take when remembered if 2 hr before next dose (dinitrate), 6 hr before next dose (sus rel), or 8 hr before next dose (mononitrate)
- Caution patient to avoid alcohol and OTC medications unless approved by prescriber
- Inform patient that drug may be taken before stressful activity: exercise, sexual activity
- Advise patient that SL tab may sting mucous membranes
- Caution patient to avoid driving and hazardous activities if dizziness occurs
- Advise patient to comply with complete medical regimen
- Caution patient to make position changes slowly to prevent orthostatic hypotension

Evaluation

Positive therapeutic outcome

- Decrease in, prevention of anginal pain

isotretinoin

(eye-soe-tret'i-noyn)

Accutane, Accutane Roche ✱

Func. class.: Dermatologic antiacne agent

Chem. class.: Retinoic acid isomer, vitamin A derivative

Pregnancy category **X**

Action: Decreases sebum secretion; improves cystic acne

➡ **Therapeutic Outcome:** Decreased size and amount of severe recalcitrant cystic acne

Uses: Severe recalcitrant cystic acne

Dosage and routes

Adult: PO 0.5-2 mg/kg/day in 2 divided doses × 15-20 wk; if relapse occurs repeat after 8 wk off drug

Available forms: Cap 10, 20, 40 mg

Side effects/adverse reactions

CNS: Lethargy, fatigue, headache, depression, ***pseudotumor cerebri***
CV: Chest pain, palpitations, tachycardia
EENT: *Eye irritation, conjunctivitis, epistaxis, dry nose, mouth,* contact lens intolerance, optic neuritis, photophobia
GI: *Nausea, vomiting, anorexia, increased liver enzymes,* regional ileus, abdominal pain, weight loss
GU: ***Hematuria, proteinuria,*** hypouricemia, white cells in urine
HEMA: ***Thrombocytopenia,*** decreased Hgb and Hct, WBC, reticulocyte count
INTEG: *Dry skin, pruritus, cheilosis, joint pain, hair loss, photosensitivity,* urticaria, bruising, hirsutism, petechiae, hypopigmentation, hyperpigmentation, nail brittleness
MS: Hyperostosis, arthralgia, bone, joint, muscle pain

Contraindications: Hypersensitivity, inflamed skin, pregnancy **X**

Precautions: Lactation, diabetes, photosensitivity, hepatic disease, inflammatory bowel disease, obesity

Pharmacokinetics

Absorption	25% (PO)
Distribution	Widely distributed; crosses placenta
Metabolism	Liver
Excretion	Kidney
Half-life	10-20 hr

Pharmacodynamics

	PO
Onset	Unknown
Peak	2.9-3.2 hr
Duration	Unknown

Interactions

Drug/drug:

Individual drugs
Alcohol: ↑ triglyceride levels
Benzoyl peroxide: ↑ drying of skin
Minocycline: Pseudotumor cerebri
Sulfine: ↑ drying of skin
Tetracycline: ↑ chance of pseudotumor cerebri
Tretinoin: ↑ drying of skin
Vitamin A: ↑ toxic effects

Drug/food:

Vitamin A foods: ↑ toxicity

Lab test interferences

Increase: ESR, triglyceride, liver function studies
Decrease: RBC/WBC count

NURSING CONSIDERATIONS

Assessment

- Monitor triglyceride levels, cholesterol, HDLs, AST (SGOT), ALT (SGPT), alkaline phosphatase before, during treatment
- Perform urinalysis weekly for protein; blood studies: CBC, SMA, blood glucose, CPK

• Assess area of body involved, including time involved, what helps or aggravates condition; after beginning treatment acne may worsen
• Assess for pseudotumor cerebri: headache, vomiting, nausea, visual disturbance; discontinue drug

Associated nursing diagnoses

✓ Skin integrity, impaired (uses)
✓ Body image disturbances (uses)
✓ Knowledge deficit (teaching)

Implementation

PO route
• Give whole; do not crush; give with meals
• Give second course of treatment if needed after waiting 2 mo
• Store in tight, light-resistant container

Patient/family education

• Caution patient to avoid sunlight or wear sunscreen and protective clothing, since photosensitivity may occur
• Advise patient that an increase in acne may occur during initial treatment and decrease in 4-6 wk
• Instruct patient not to become pregnant while taking drug; to use contraceptives 1 mo before, during, and 6-8 wk after treatment; patient should stop medication if pregnancy is suspected; birth defects, fetal death can result
• Caution patient not to take vitamin A supplements; to take drug with meals, not to crush; give written list of food to avoid
• Advise patient to minimize or eliminate alcohol consumption; triglyceride levels may increase
• Instruct patient to repeat side effects: abdominal pain, diarrhea, nausea, vomiting, visual difficulty, rash, headache; drug should be discontinued; may indicate pseudotumor cerebri
• Teach patient that dry skin, lips, mouth, eyes will occur and to use rinses, gum, hard candy for dry mouth, lubricants for dry lips, eye lubricant for dry eyes; some patients may have to wear glasses instead of contact lenses during treatment

Evaluation

Positive therapeutic outcome
• Decrease in size and number of lesions

isradipine
(is-ra′di-peen)
DynaCirc
Func. class.: Calcium channel blocker, antihypertensive
Chem. class.: Dihydropyridine
Pregnancy category **C**

Action: Inhibits calcium ion influx across cell membrane during cardiac depolarization; produces relaxation of coronary vascular smooth muscle and peripheral vascular smooth muscle; dilates coronary vascular arteries; increases myocardial oxygen delivery in patients with vasospastic angina

Therapeutic Outcome: Decreased B/P

Uses: Hypertension

Dosage and routes

Adult: PO 2.5 mg bid; increase at 3-4 wk intervals up to 10 mg bid

Available forms: Cap 2.5, 5 mg

Side effects/adverse reactions

CNS: Headache, fatigue, dizziness, fainting, sleep disturbances
CV: Peripheral edema, tachycardia, hypotension, chest pain
GI: Nausea, vomiting, diarrhea, gastric upset, constipation, hepatitis
GU: Nocturia, polyuria, ***acute renal failure***
HEMA: ***Thrombocytopenia, leukopenia, anemia***
INTEG: Rash, pruritus, urticaria, photosensitivity, hair loss
MISC: Flushing

Contraindications: Sick sinus syndrome, 2nd- or 3rd-degree heart block, hypotension less than 90 mm Hg systolic, hypersensitivity

Precautions: CHF, hypotension, hepatic disease, pregnancy **C**, lactation, P children, G renal disease, elderly

Pharmacokinetics	
Absorption	Well absorbed
Distribution	High plasma protein binding (95%)
Metabolism	Liver, extensively and rapidly
Excretion	Kidney
Half-life	8 hr

Pharmacodynamics	
Onset	1-2 hr
Peak	2-3 hr
Duration	12 hr

Interactions

Drug/drug:

Individual drugs

Alcohol: ↑ hypotension
Fentanyl: ↑ hypotension

Drug classifications

Antihypertensives: ↑ hypotension
Nitrates: ↑ hypotension

NURSING CONSIDERATIONS

Assessment

- Assess fluid volume status: I&O ratio and record, weight, distended red veins, crackles in lung, color, quality and sp gr of urine, skin turgor, adequacy of pulses, moist mucous membranes, bilateral lung sounds, peripheral pitting edema; dehydration symptoms of decreasing output, thirst, hypotension, dry mouth and mucous membranes should be reported
- Monitor ALT (SGPT), AST (SGOT), bilirubin; if these are elevated, hepatotoxicity is suspected
- Monitor cardiac status: B/P, pulse, respiration, ECG

Associated nursing diagnoses

- ✓ Cardiac output, decreased (uses)
- ✓ Knowledge deficit (teaching)

Implementation

PO route

• Give once a day, with food for GI symptoms

Patient/family education

• Instruct patient to avoid hazardous activities until stabilized on drug and dizziness is no longer a problem
• Instruct patient to limit caffeine consumption; to avoid alcohol and OTC drugs unless directed by prescriber
• Advise patient to comply in all areas of medical regimen: diet, exercise, stress reduction, drug therapy; to notify prescriber of irregular heart beat, shortness of breath, swelling of feet and hands, pronounced dizziness, constipation, nausea, hypotension
• Teach patient to use as directed even if feeling better
• Teach patient to take with a full glass of water

Evaluation

Positive therapeutic outcome

• Decreased B/P

Treatment of overdose:

Defibrillation, atropine for AV block, vasopressor for hypotension

itraconazole

(it-tra-kon'a-zol)
Sporanox
Func. class.: Antifungal (systemic)
Chem. class.: Triazole derivative
Pregnancy category **C**

Action: Increases cell membrane permeability in susceptible organisms by binding sterols in fungal cell membrane; decreases potassium, sodium, and nutrients in cell

➔ **Therapeutic Outcome:** Fungistatic against *Histoplasma capsulatum, Blastomyces dermatitis, Cryptococcus neoformans, Aspergillus fumigatus, Candida*

Uses: Systemic candidiasis, chronic mucocandidiasis, oral thrush, candiduria, coccidioidomycosis, histoplasmosis, chromomycosis, paracoccidioidomycosis, blastomycosis (pulmonary and extrapulmonary)

Dosage and routes

Adult: PO 200 mg tid × 3 days with food; may increase to 400 mg qd if needed; divide doses over 200 mg in 2 doses/day

Available forms: Cap 100 mg

Side effects/adverse reactions

CNS: Headache, dizziness, insomnia, somnolence, depression

I

GI: Nausea, vomiting, anorexia, diarrhea, cramps, abdominal pain, flatulence, ***GI bleeding, hepatotoxicity***
GU: Gynecomastia, impotence, decreased libido
INTEG: Pruritus, fever, rash
MISC: Edema, fatigue, malaise, hypertension, hypokalemia, tinnitus

Contraindications: Hypersensitivity, lactation, fungal meningitis, coadministration with terfenadine

Precautions: Hepatic disease, achlorhydria or hypochlorhydria (drug-induced), P children, pregnancy **C**

Pharmacokinetics

Absorption	Variable (PO)
Distribution	Tissue, plasma, CSF
Metabolism	Liver, extensively
Excretion	Feces, breast milk
Half-life	20-21 hr

Pharmacodynamics

Onset	Unknown
Peak	4 hr
Duration	Unknown

Interactions

Drug/drug:

Individual drugs

Astemizole: ↑ dysrhythmias
Carbamazepine: ↑ metabolism, ↓ effect of itraconazole
Cyclosporine: ↑ effects of cyclosporine
Digoxin: ↑ effects of digoxin
Isoniazid: ↑ metabolism, ↓ effect of itraconazole
Phenytoin: ↑ metabolism, ↓ effect of itraconazole
Phenobarbital: ↑ metabolism, ↓ effect of itraconazole
Rifampin: ↑ metabolism, ↓ effect of itraconazole
Terfenadine: ↑ dysrhythmias
Warfarin: ↑ effects of warfarin

Drug classifications

Cardiac glycosides: ↑ effects of cardiac glycosides
Oral hypoglycemics: ↑ effects of oral hypoglycemics

Drug/food:

↑ absorption

NURSING CONSIDERATIONS

Assessment

- Monitor for hepatotoxicity: increasing AST (SGOT), ALT (SGPT), alkaline phosphatase, bilirubin
- Monitor for allergic reaction: dermatitis, rash; drug should be discontinued, antihistamines (mild reaction) or epinephrine (severe reaction) administered; check inj site for thrombophlebitis
- Monitor for hypokalemia: anorexia, drowsiness, weakness, decreased reflexes, dizziness, increased urinary output, increased thirst, paresthesias; if these occur, drug should be decreased or discontinued and potassium administered

Associated nursing diagnoses

- ✓ Infection, risk for (uses)
- ✓ Injury, risk for physical (adverse reaction)
- ✓ Knowledge deficit (teaching)

Implementation

PO route

- Give with food or milk to prevent nausea and vomiting

• Store in tight container at room temp

Patient/family education

• Advise patient that long-term therapy may be needed to clear infection (2 wk-3 mo depending on type of infection)
• Teach patient side effects and when to notify prescriber

Evaluation

Positive therapeutic outcome
• Decreased fever, malaise, rash
• Negative C&S for infectious organism

kanamycin

(kan-a-mye'sin)
kanamycin sulfate, Kantrex
Func. class.: Antiinfective
Chem. class.: Aminoglycoside
Pregnancy category **D**

Action: Interferes with protein synthesis in bacterial cell by binding to the 30s ribosomal subunit, causing inaccurate peptide sequence to form in protein chain, resulting in bacterial death

Therapeutic Outcome: Bactericidal effects for *Escherichia coli, Acinetobacter, Proteus, Serratia, Pseudomonas aeruginosa*

Uses: Severe systemic infections of CNS, respiratory tract, GI tract, urinary tract, bone, skin, soft tissues; also used as adjunct in hepatic coma, peritonitis, preoperatively to sterilize bowel; decreases ammonia-producing bacteria in bowel and intraperitoneally after fecal spill during surgery

Dosage and routes

Severe systemic infections

P *Adult and child:* **IV** inf 15 mg/kg/day in divided doses q8-12h; diluted 500 mg/200 ml of NS or D_5W given over 30-60 min, not to exceed 1.5 g/day; IM 15 mg/kg/day in divided doses q8-12h, not to exceed 1.5 g/day; irrigation not to exceed 1.5 g/day

Hepatic coma

Adult: PO 8-12 g/day in divided doses

Preoperative bowel sterilization

Adult: PO 1 g qh × 4 doses, then q6h × 36-72 hr

Available forms: Inj 75, 500 mg/2 ml, 1 g/3 ml; cap 500 mg

Side effects/adverse reactions

CNS: Confusion, depression, numbness, tremors, ***convulsions,*** muscle twitching, ***neurotoxicity***
CV: Hypotension
EENT: ***Ototoxicity,*** deafness, visual disturbances, dizziness, vertigo, tinnitus
GI: Nausea, vomiting, anorexia, increased ALT (SGPT), AST (SGOT), bilirubin, hepatomegaly, ***hepatic necrosis,*** splenomegaly

GU: Oliguria, hematuria, renal damage, azotemia, renal failure, nephrotoxicity
HEMA: Agranulocytosis, thrombocytopenia, leukopenia, eosinophilia, anemia
INTEG: *Rash,* burning, urticaria, dermatitis, alopecia
RESP: Respiratory depression

Contraindications: Bowel obstruction, severe renal disease, hypersensitivity, pregnancy **D**

P **Precautions:** Neonates, myasthenia gravis, hearing deficits, mild renal disease, lactation, Parkinson's disease

Pharmacokinetics

Absorption	Well absorbed (IM)
Distribution	Widely distributed in extracellular fluids; crosses placenta
Metabolism	Liver, minimally
Excretion	Kidneys, mostly unchanged (79%)
Half-life	2-3 hr; increased in renal disease

Pharmacodynamics

	IM	IV
Onset	Rapid	Rapid
Peak	1-2 hr	1-2 hr

Interactions
Drug/drug:
Individual drugs
Amphotericin B: ↑ ototoxicity, neurotoxicity, nephrotoxicity
Cisplatin: ↑ ototoxicity, neurotoxicity, nephrotoxicity
Ethacrynic acid: ↑ ototoxicity, neurotoxicity, nephrotoxicity
Furosemide: ↑ ototoxicity, neurotoxicity, nephrotoxicity
Mannitol: ↑ ototoxicity, neurotoxicity, nephrotoxicity
Methoxyflurane: ↑ ototoxicity, neurotoxicity, nephrotoxicity
Polymyxin: ↑ ototoxicity, neurotoxicity, nephrotoxicity
Succinylcholine: ↑ neuromuscular blockade, respiratory depression
Vancomycin: ↑ ototoxicity, neurotoxicity, nephrotoxicity
Drug classifications
Anesthetics: ↑ neuromuscular blockade, respiratory depression
Aminoglycosides: ↑ otoxicity, neurotoxicity, neurotoxicity
Nondepolarizing neuromuscular blockers: ↑ neuromuscular blockade, respiratory depression

NURSING CONSIDERATIONS
Assessment
- Assess patient for previous sensitivity reaction
- Assess patient for signs and symptoms of infection including characteristics of wounds, sputum, urine, stool, WBC >10,000, fever; obtain baseline information and during treatment
- Obtain C&S tests before beginning drug therapy to identify if correct treatment has been initiated
- Assess for allergic reactions: rash, urticaria, pruritus, chills, fever, joint pain; angioedema may occur a few days after therapy begins
- Identify urine output; if decreasing, notify prescriber (may indicate nephrotoxicity); also check for increased BUN,

creatinine, urine CrCl <80 ml/min
- Monitor blood studies: AST (SGOT), ALT (SGPT), CBC, Hct, bilirubin, LDH, alkaline phosphatase, Coombs' test monthly if patient is on long-term therapy
- Monitor electrolytes: potassium, sodium, chloride, calcium, magnesium monthly if patient is on long-term therapy
- Assess bowel pattern qd; if severe diarrhea occurs, drug should be discontinued; may indicate pseudomembranous colitis
- Monitor for bleeding: ecchymosis, bleeding gums, hematuria, stool guaiac daily if on long-term therapy
- Assess for overgrowth of infection: perineal itching, fever, malaise, redness, pain, swelling, drainage, rash, diarrhea, change in cough, sputum
- Obtain weight before treatment; calculation of dosage is usually based on ideal body weight, but may be calculated on actual body weight
- Monitor I&O ratio; perform urinalysis daily for proteinuria, cells, casts; report sudden change in urine output
- Monitor VS during inf; watch for hypotension, change in pulse
- Assess **IV** site for thrombophlebitis including pain, redness, swelling q30 min; change site if needed; apply warm compresses to discontinued site
- Obtain serum peak, drawn at 30-60 min after **IV** inf or 60 min after IM inj; draw trough level just before next dose; blood level should be 2-4 times bacteriostatic level
- Assess hearing by audiometric testing, ringing, roaring in ears, vertigo before, during, after treatment
- Assess for dehydration: high sp gr, decrease in skin turgor, dry mucous membranes, dark urine
- Assess vestibular dysfunction: nausea, vomiting, dizziness, headache; drug should be discontinued if severe

Associated nursing diagnoses

- ✓ Infection, risk for (uses)
- ✓ Diarrhea (adverse reactions)
- ✓ Injury, risk for (adverse reactions)
- ✓ Knowledge deficit (teaching)

K

Implementation

PO route
- Give in even doses around the clock; if GI upset occurs, give with food; drug must be given for 10-14 days to ensure organism death and prevent superinfection; store in tight container.

IM route
- Inject deep in large muscle mass

IV **IV route**
- Dilute 500 mg/100-200 ml; or 1 g/200-400 ml D_5W, $D_{10}W$, D_5/0.9% NaCl, 0.9% NaCl, LR
- Do not admix; give aminoglycosides and penicillin at least 1 hr apart
- Give by intermittent inf over 30-60 min; flush with 0.9% NaCl or D_5W after inf is complete

Syringe incompatibilities: Ampicillin, culbercillin, heparin

Additive incompatibilities: Amphotericin B, cephalothin, cephapirin, chlorpheniramine, colistimethate, heparin, methohexital

Additive compatibilities: Ascorbic acid, cefoxitin, chloramphenicol, clindamycin, dopamine, furosemide, polymyxin B, sodium bicarbonate, tetracycline; admixing is not recommended

Y-site compatibilities: Cyclophosphamide, furosemide, heparin with hydrocortisone, sodium succinate, hydromorphone, magnesium sulfate, meperidine, morphine, perphenazine, potassium chloride

Patient/family education

• Teach patient to report sore throat, bruising, bleeding, joint pain, may indicate blood dyscrasias (rare)
• Advise patient to contact prescriber if vaginal itching, loose, foul-smelling stools, furry tongue occur; may indicate superinfection

Evaluation

Positive therapeutic outcome
• Absence of signs/symptoms of infection (WBC <10,000, temp WNL, absence of red, draining wounds)
• Reported improvement in symptoms of infection

Treatment of overdose: Withdraw drug, hemodialysis, monitor serum levels of drug

kaolin/pectin

(kay'-oh-lin pek'tin)
Func. class.: Antidiarrheal
Chem. class.: Hydrous magnesium aluminum silicate
Pregnancy category **C**

Action: Decreases gastric motility, water content of stool; adsorbent, demulcent

➔ **Therapeutic Outcome:** Absence of diarrhea

Uses: Diarrhea (cause undetermined)

Dosage and routes

Adult: PO 60-120 ml (45-90 ml conc) after each loose bowel movement

P ***Child >12 yrs:*** PO 60 ml after each loose bowel movement

P ***Child 6-12 yrs:*** PO 30-60 ml (15 ml conc) after each loose bowel movement

P ***Child 3-6 yrs:*** PO 15-30 ml (7.5 ml conc) after each loose bowel movement

Available forms: Susp kaolin 0.87 g/5 ml, pectin 43 mg/5 ml; kaolin 0.98 g/5 ml, pectin 21.7 mg/5 ml

Side effects/adverse reactions

GI: Constipation (chronic use)

Contraindications: Child <3 yr, severe abdominal pain

Precautions: Pregnancy **C**

Pharmacokinetics

Absorption	Not absorbed
Distribution	Unknown
Metabolism	Unknown
Excretion	Unknown
Half-life	Unknown

Pharmacodynamics

Onset	½ hr
Peak	Unknown
Duration	6 hr

Interactions

All drugs: ↓ action of all other drugs

NURSING CONSIDERATIONS

Assessment

- Assess bowel pattern before, during treatment; for rebound constipation after termination of medication; check bowel sounds
- Check response after 48 hr; if no response, drug should be discontinued and other treatment initiated

Associated nursing diagnoses

☑ Diarrhea (uses)
☑ Constipation (adverse reactions)
☑ Knowledge deficit (teaching)
☑ Noncompliance (teaching)

Implementation

PO route

- Shake susp before use
- Administer for 48 hr only

Patient/family education

- Advise patient not to exceed recommended dosage

Evaluation

Positive therapeutic outcome

- Decreased diarrhea

ketamine

(ket'a-meen)

Ketalar

Func. class.: General anesthetic

Chem. class.: Phencyclidine derivative

Pregnancy category C

Action: Acts on limbic system, cortex by blocking pain impulses to provide anesthesia

Uses: Short anesthesia for diagnostic/surgical procedures; as an adjunct with other anesthetics

Dosage and routes

P *Adult and child:* **IV** 1-4.5 mg/kg over 1 min

P *Adult and child:* IM 6.5-13 mg/kg

Available forms: Inj IM, **IV** 10, 50, 100 mg/ml vial

Side effects/adverse reactions

CNS: Hallucinations, confusion, delirium, tremors, polyneuropathy, fasciculations, pseudoconvulsions

CV: Increased B/P, hypotension, bradycardia

EENT: Diplopia, salivation, small increase in intraocular pressure

INTEG: Rash, pain at inj site

K

Contraindications: Hypersensitivity, CVA, increased intracranial pressure, severe hypertension, cardiac decompensation, P child <2 yr

Precautions: Pregnancy **C**, seizure disorders, G elderly, psychiatric disorders

Pharmacokinetics

Absorption	Rapidly absorbed (IM); completely absorbed (IV)
Distribution	Rapidly distributed; crosses placenta
Metabolism	Liver
Excretion	Kidneys
Half-life	2½ hr

Pharmacodynamics

	IV	IM
Onset	Unknown	Unknown
Peak	40 sec	3-8 min
Duration	10 min	25 min

Interactions

Drug/drug:

Individual drugs

Atropine: ↑ action of ketamine
Tubocurarine: ↑ action of tubocurarine

Drug classifications

Antihypertensive with CNS depressant effect: ↑ respiratory depression
Barbiturates: ↑ recovery time
Narcotics: ↑ action of ketamine
Thyroid hormone: ↑ tachycardia, hypertension

NURSING CONSIDERATIONS

Assessment

- Monitor VS q10 min during **IV** administration, q30 min after IM dose
- Assess for hallucinations, delusions, separation from environment
- Assess for extrapyramidal reactions: dystonia, akathisia
- Monitor for increasing heart rate or decreasing B/P; notify prescriber at once

Associated nursing diagnoses

- ✓ Sensory-perceptual alterations (adverse reactions)
- ✓ Knowledge deficit (teaching)

Implementation

IV route

- Administer **IV** after diluting 100 mg/ml with equal parts of D_5W, 0.9% NaCl, sterile water for inj; give over 1 min; may be diluted 10 ml (50 mg/ml)/ 500 ml of normal saline or D_5W = 1 mg/ml; run at 1-2 mg/min; titrate to patient response
- Administer anticholinergic preoperatively to decrease secretions
- Give only with resuscitative equipment nearby
- Give narcotic or diazepam to control recovery symptoms

Syringe incompatibilities: Barbiturates, diazepam, doxapram

Syringe compatibility: Benzequinamide

Patient/family education

Teach patient reason for medication and expected results

Evaluation

Positive therapeutic outcome

- Maintenance of anesthesia

ketoconazole

(kee-toe-koe'na-zole)

Nizoral

Func. class.: Antifungal

Chem. class.: Imidazole derivative

Pregnancy category **C**

Action: Alters cell membrane and inhibits several fungal enzymes; prevents production of adrenal sterols; prevents fungal metabolism

Therapeutic Outcome: Fungistatic/fungicidal against susceptible organisms: *Blastomycoses, Candida, Coccidioides, Cryptococcus, Histoplasma;* Top route: *tinea cruris, tinea corporis, tinea versicolor, pityrosporum ovale*

Uses: Systemic candidiasis, chronic mucocandidiasis, oral thrush, candiduria, coccidioidomycosis, histoplasmosis, chromomycosis, paracoccidioidomycosis, blastomycosis

Investigational uses: Cushing's syndrome, advanced prostatic cancer

Dosage and routes

Adult: PO 200-400 mg once daily

P ***Children >2 yr:*** 3.3-6.6 mg/kg/day as single daily dose; <2 yr daily dose not established

P ***Adult and child >2 yr:*** Top 2% cream applied qd or bid

Adult: Massage shampoo into scalp 1 min, reapply × 3 min, rinse; continue treatment twice/wk × 1 mo, no more than once q3 days

Available forms: Tab 200 mg; cream 2%; shampoo 2%

Side effects/adverse reactions

CNS: Headache, dizziness, somnolence

GI: Nausea, vomiting, anorexia, diarrhea, abdominal pain, ***hepatotoxicity***

GU: Gynecomastia, impotence

HEMA: ***Thrombocytopenia, leukopenia, hemolytic anemia***

INTEG: Pruritus, fever, chills, photophobia, rash, dermatitis, purpura, urticaria

SYST: ***Anaphylaxis***

Contraindications: Hypersensitivity, lactation, fungal meningitis; coadministration with terfenadine

Precautions: Renal disease, hepatic disease, achlorhydria (drug induced), pregnancy **C**, P children <2 yr, other hepatotoxic agents including terfenadine

Pharmacokinetics

Absorption	pH dependent; ↓ pH ↑ absorption
Distribution	Widely distributed; crosses placenta
Metabolism	Liver, partially
Excretion	Feces, bile, breast milk
Half-life	Biphasic: 2 hr, 8 hr

Pharmacodynamics

Onset	Unknown
Peak	1-3 hr
Duration	Unknown

K

Interactions

Drug/drug:

Individual drugs

Alcohol: ↑ hepatotoxicity
Astemizole: ↑ dysrhythmias
Carbamazepine: ↑ metabolism, ↓ effect of itraconazole
Cimetidine: ↓ absorption
Cyclosporine: ↑ effects of cyclosporine
Digoxin: ↑ effects of digoxin
Famotidine: ↓ absorption
Isoniazid: ↑ metabolism, ↓ effect of itraconazole
Nizatidine: ↓ absorption
Omeprazole: ↓ absorption
Phenobarbital: ↑ metabolism, ↓ effect of itraconazole
Phenytoin: ↑ metabolism, ↓ effect of itraconazole
Ranitidine: ↓ absorption
Rifampin: ↑ metabolism, ↓ effect of itraconazole
Terfenadine: ↑ dysrhythmias
Theophylline: ↓ effectiveness
Warfarin: ↑ effects of warfarin

Drug classifications

Cardiac glycosides: ↑ effects of cardiac glycosides
Oral anticoagulants: ↑ effects of oral anticoagulants
Oral hypoglycemics: ↑ effects of oral hypoglycemics

Drug/food: ↑ absorption

NURSING CONSIDERATIONS

Assessment

- Assess for signs and symptoms of infection: drainage, sore throat, urinary pain, hematuria, fever
- Obtain cultures for C&S before beginning treatment; therapy may be started after culture is taken
- Monitor for hepatotoxicity: increased AST (SGOT), ALT (SGPT), alkaline phosphatase, bilirubin; drug is discontinued if hepatotoxicity occurs

Associated nursing diagnoses

- ✓ Infection, risk for (uses)
- ✓ Injury, risk for (adverse reactions)
- ✓ Knowledge deficit (teaching)

Implementation

PO route

- Give in the presence of acid products only; do not use alkaline products or antacids within 2 hr of drug; may give coffee, tea, acidic fruit juices; give with food to decrease GI symptoms
- Give with hydrochloric acid if achlorhydria is present
- Store in tight container at room temp

Top route

- Use enough medication to cover fungally infected area and surrounding area; rub in; do not use occlusive dressing; do not get in eyes

Shampoo

- Hair should be wet; apply shampoo, lather, rub gently into scalp and hair for 1 min; rinse; reapply × 3 min; continue treatment 2 times/wk for 1 mo, no more than once q3 days

Patient/family education

- Advise patient that long-term therapy may be needed to clear infection (1 wk-6 mo depending on infection)
- Advise patient to avoid hazardous activities if dizziness occurs
- Instruct patient to take 2 hr before administration of other

drugs that increase gastric pH (antacids, H_2-blockers, anticholinergics)
• Stress the importance of compliance with drug regimen
• Advise patient to notify prescriber of GI symptoms, signs of liver dysfunction (fatigue, nausea, anorexia, vomiting, dark urine, pale stools)
• Teach patient proper hygiene: hand washing, nail care, use of concomitant top agents if prescribed
• Caution patient to avoid alcohol, since nausea, vomiting, hypertension may occur
• Advise patient to use sunscreen or avoid direct sunlight to prevent photosensitivity
• Advise patient to notify prescriber of sore throat, fever, skin rash, which may indicate superinfection

Evaluation

Positive therapeutic outcome
• Decreased oral candidiasis, fever, malaise, rash
• Negative C&S for infectious organism
• Absence of dandruff, scaling

ketoprofen
(ke-to-proe'fen)
Ketoprofen, Orudis, Orudis-E ✤, Oruvail
Func. class.: NSAID; nonnarcotic analgesic
Chem. class.: Propionic acid derivative
Pregnancy category **B**

Action: Inhibits prostaglandin synthesis by decreasing enzyme needed for biosynthesis; analgesic, antiinflammatory

Therapeutic Outcome: Decreased pain, inflammation

Uses: Mild to moderate pain, osteoarthritis, rheumatoid arthritis, dysmenorrhea

Dosage and routes
Antiinflammatory
Adult: PO 150-300 mg in divided doses tid-qid, not to exceed 300 mg/day

Analgesic
Adult: PO 25-50 mg q6-8h

Available forms: Cap 25, 50, 75 mg

K

Side effects/adverse reactions
CNS: Dizziness, drowsiness, fatigue, tremors, confusion, insomnia, anxiety, depression
CV: Tachycardia, peripheral edema, palpitations, dysrhythmias, hypertension
EENT: Tinnitus, hearing loss, blurred vision
GI: Nausea, anorexia, vomiting, diarrhea, jaundice, ***cholestatic hepatitis,*** constipation, flatulence, cramps, dry mouth, peptic ulcer
GU: ***Nephrotoxicity: dysuria, hematuria, oliguria, azotemia***
HEMA: ***Blood dyscrasias***
INTEG: Purpura, rash, pruritus, sweating

Contraindications: Hypersensitivity, asthma, severe renal disease, severe hepatic disease, ulcer disease

Precautions: Pregnancy **B**, P lactation, children, bleeding disorders, GI disorders, cardiac disorders, hypersensitivity to other antiinflammatory agents, G elderly

Pharmacokinetics

Absorption	Well absorbed
Distribution	Not known
Metabolism	Liver
Excretion	Kidneys
Half-life	3-3½ hr

Pharmacodynamics

	PO
Onset	Unknown
Peak	2 hr
Duration	Unknown

Interactions

Drug/drug:

Individual drugs

Acetaminophen (long-term use): ↑ renal reactions
Alcohol: ↑ adverse reactions
Aspirin: ↓ effectiveness, ↑ adverse reactions
Coumarin: ↑ anticoagulant effects
Digoxin: ↑ toxicity, levels
Insulin: ↓ insulin effect
Lithium: ↑ toxicity
Methotrexate: ↑ toxicity
Phenytoin: ↑ toxicity
Probenecid: ↑ toxicity
Sulfonylurea: ↑ toxicity

Drug classifications

Anticoagulants: ↑ risk of bleeding
Antihypertensives: ↓ effect of antihypertensives
Antineoplastics: ↑ risk of hematologic toxicity
β-Blockers: ↑ antihypertension
Cephalosporins: ↑ risk of bleeding
Diuretics: ↓ effectiveness of diuretics
Glucocorticoids: ↑ adverse reactions
Hypoglycemics: ↓ hypoglycemic effect
NSAIDs: ↑ adverse reactions
Potassium supplements: ↑ adverse reactions
Radiation: ↑ risk of hematologic toxicity
Sulfonamides: ↑ toxicity

Lab test interferences

Increase: Bleeding time, liver function studies, serum uric acid, amylase, CO_2, urinary protein
Decrease: Serum potassium, PBI, cholesterol
Interfere: Urine catecholamines, pregnancy test, urine glucose tests (Clinistix, Tes-Tape)

NURSING CONSIDERATIONS

Assessment

- Monitor liver function, renal function, studies: AST (SGOT), ALT (SGPT), bilirubin, creatinine BUN, urine creatinine, CBC Hct, Hgb, pro-time if patient is on long-term therapy
- Check I&O ratio; decreasing output may indicate renal failure (long-term therapy)
- Assess hepatotoxicity: dark urine, clay-colored stools, yellowing of skin and sclera, itching, abdominal pain, fever, diarrhea if patient is on long-term therapy
- Assess for allergic reactions: rash, urticaria; if these occur, drug may have to be discontinued
- Assess for ototoxicity: tinnitus, ringing, roaring in ears;

audiometric testing needed before, after long-term therapy
- Assess for visual changes: blurring, halos; may indicate corneal, retinal damage
- Check edema in feet, ankles, legs
- Identify prior drug history; there are many drug interactions
- Monitor pain: location, duration, type, intensity, before dose and 1 hr after; ROM before dose and after

Associated nursing diagnoses

- ✓ Pain (uses)
- ✓ Mobility, impaired physical (uses)
- ✓ Injury, risk for (adverse reactions)
- ✓ Knowledge deficit (teaching)

Implementation

PO route
- Administer to patient whole; do not crush, break, or open cap
- Give with food or milk to decrease gastric symptoms; give 30 min ac or 2 hr pc; absorption may be slowed

Patient/family education

- Teach patient to report any symptoms of hepatotoxicity, renal toxicity, visual changes, ototoxicity, allergic reactions, bleeding (long-term therapy)
- Advise patient to take with 8 oz of water and sit upright for 30 min after dose to prevent ulceration
- Caution patient not to exceed recommended dosage; acute poisoning may result; to take as prescribed; do not double dose
- Advise patient to read label on other OTC drugs; many contain other antiinflammatories
- Inform patient that the therapeutic response takes 2 wk (arthritis)
- Teach patient to report tinnitus, confusion, diarrhea, sweating, hyperventilation, blurred vision, fever, joint aches
- Caution patient to avoid alcohol ingestion; GI bleeding may occur

Evaluation

Positive therapeutic outcome
- Decreased pain
- Decreased inflammation
- Increased mobility

ketorolac
(kee'toe-role-ak)
Toradol
Func. class.: NSAID, nonnarcotic analgesic
Chem. class.: Pyrrolopyrrole
Pregnancy category **C**

Action: Inhibits prostaglandin synthesis by decreasing an enzyme needed for biosynthesis; analgesic, needed for biosynthesis; analgesic, antiinflammatory, antipyretic effects

➡ **Therapeutic Outcome:** Decreased pain, inflammation, ocular itching

K

Uses: Mild to moderate pain (short term); decreased ocular itching in seasonal allergic conjunctivitis

Dosage and routes

Adult: IM 30-60 mg loading dose, then 15-30 mg q6h; PO prn; max 40 mg/day

Ophth

Adult: 1 gtt (0.25 mg) qid × 7 days

Available forms: Inj 15, 30 mg/ml (prefilled syringes); ophth 0.5% sol; tab 10 mg

Side effects/adverse reactions

CV: Hypertension, flushing, syncope, pallor
CNS: Dizziness, drowsiness, tremors
EENT: Tinnitus, hearing loss, blurred vision
GI: Nausea, anorexia, vomiting, diarrhea, constipation, flatulence, cramps, dry mouth, peptic ulcer
GU: Nephrotoxicity: dysuria, hematuria, oliguria, azotemia
HEMA: Blood dyscrasias
INTEG: Purpura, rash, pruritus, sweating

Contraindications: Hypersensitivity, asthma, severe renal disease, severe hepatic disease, peptic ulcer disease

Precautions: Pregnancy **C**, P lactation, children, bleeding disorders, GI disorders, cardiac disorders, hypersensitivity to other antiinflammatory agents

Pharmacokinetics

Absorption	Rapidly, completely absorbed
Distribution	Bound to plasma proteins (99%)
Metabolism	Liver (<50%)
Excretion	Kidney, metabolites (92%); breast milk (6%); feces
Half-life	6 hr; increased in renal disease

Pharmacodynamics

	IM	OPHTH/PO
Onset	Up to 10 min	Unknown
Peak	50 min	Unknown
Duration	4-6 hr	Unknown

Interactions

Drug/drug:

Individual drugs
Heparin: ↑ bleeding
Methotrexate: ↑ effects
Phenytoin: ↑ effects
Sulfinpyrazone: ↓ effects

Drug classifications
Anticoagulants: ↑ effects
NSAIDs: ↑ gastric ulcers
Salicylates: ↓ blood sugar levels
Sulfonamides: ↓ effects

Lab test interferences

Increase: Coagulation studies, liver function studies, serum uric acid, amylase, CO_2, urinary protein
Decrease: Serum potassium, PBI, cholesterol
Interfere: Urine catecholamines, pregnancy test, urine glucose tests (Clinistix, Tes-Tape)

NURSING CONSIDERATIONS

Assessment

- Monitor blood counts during therapy; watch for decreas-

ing platelets; if low, therapy may need to be discontinued and restarted after hematologic recovery; assess for blood dyscrasia (thrombocytopenia): bruising, fatigue, bleeding, poor healing
• Assess patient's eyes: redness swelling, tearing, itching

Associated nursing diagnoses

✓ Pain (uses)
✓ Mobility, impaired physical (uses)
✓ Injury, risk for (adverse reactions)
✓ Knowledge deficit (teaching)

Implementation

PO route
• Administer to patient crushed or whole
• Give with food or milk to decrease gastric symptoms; give 30 min ac or 2 hr pc; absorption may be slowed

Patient/family education

• Teach patient that drug must be continued for prescribed time to be effective; to avoid aspirin, alcoholic beverages
• Caution patient to report bleeding, bruising, fatigue, malaise, since blood dyscrasias do occur
• Instruct patient to use caution when driving; drowsiness, dizziness may occur
• Teach patient to take with a full glass of water to enhance absorption; do not crush, break, or chew
• Caution patient that this drug may cause eye redness, burning if soft contact lenses are worn

Evaluation

Positive therapeutic outcome
• Decreased pain
• Decreased inflammatory response
• Increased mobility
• Decreased ocular itching

labetalol

(la-bet'a-lole)
Normodyne, Trandate
Func. class.: Antihypertensive
Chem. class.: Nonselective β-blocker
Pregnancy category C

Action: Competitively blocks stimulation of β-adrenergic receptor within vascular smooth muscle; produces chronotropic, inotropic activity (decreases rate of SA node discharge, increases recovery time), slows conduction of AV node, decreases heart rate, which decreases O_2 consumption in myocardium; also has α-andrenergic blocking activity

➜ **Therapeutic Outcome:** Decreased B/P

Uses: Mild to moderate hypertension; treatment of severe hypertension (**IV**)

Investigational uses: Angina pectoris (PO), hypotension during surgery (**IV**)

Dosage and routes

Hypertension
Adult: PO 100 mg bid; may be given with a diuretic; may

increase to 200 mg bid after 2 days; may continue to increase q1-3 days; max 400 mg bid

Hypertensive crisis

Adult: **IV** inf 200 mg/160 ml D_5W, run at 2 ml/min; stop inf after desired response obtained; repeat q6-8h as needed; **IV** bol 20 mg over 2 min; may repeat 40-80 mg q10 min, not to exceed 300 mg

Available forms: Tab 100, 200, 300 mg; inj 5 mg/ml in 20 ml ampules

Side effects/adverse reactions

CNS: Dizziness, mental changes, drowsiness, fatigue, headache, catatonia, depression, anxiety, nightmares, paresthesias, lethargy
CV: Orthostatic hypotension, bradycardia, ***CHF,*** chest pain, ***ventricular dysrhythmias,*** AV block
EENT: Tinnitus, visual changes, sore throat, double vision, dry burning eyes
GI: Nausea, vomiting, diarrhea
GU: Impotence, dysuria, ejaculatory failure
HEMA: ***Agranulocytosis, thrombocytopenia, purpura*** (rare)
INTEG: Rash, alopecia, urticaria, pruritus, fever
RESP: ***Bronchospasm,*** dyspnea, wheezing

Contraindications: Hypersensitivity to β-blockers, cardiogenic shock, heart block (2nd or 3rd degree), sinus bradycardia, CHF, bronchial asthma

Precautions: Major surgery, pregnancy **C**, lactation, diabetes mellitus, renal disease, thyroid disease, COPD, well-compensated heart failure, CAD, nonallergic bronchospasm

Pharmacokinetics

Absorption	Bioavailability 25% (PO); complete (IV)
Distribution	Crosses placenta, CNS
Metabolism	Liver, extensively
Excretion	Breast milk, kidneys, bile
Half-life	6-8 hr

Pharmacodynamics

	PO	IV
Onset	1-2 hr	5 min
Peak	2-4 hr	15 min
Duration	8-12 hr	2-4 hr

Interactions

Drug/drug:

Individual drugs
Alcohol: ↑ hypotension (large amounts)
Epinephrine: α-Adrenergic stimulation
Hydralazine: ↑ hypotension, bradycardia
Indomethacin: ↓ antihypertensive effect
Insulin: ↑ hypoglycemia
Methyldopa: ↑ hypotension, bradycardia
Phenytoin (IV): ↑ myocardial depression
Prazosin: ↑ hypotension, bradycardia
Reserpine: ↑ hypotension, bradycardia
Thyroid: ↓ effectiveness
Verapamil: ↑ myocardial depression

Drug classifications

Antihypertensives: ↑ hypertension
β_2-Agonists: ↓ bronchodilatation
Cardiac glycosides: ↑ bradycardia
MAOIs: Avoid use
Nitrates: ↑ hypotension
Theophyllines: ↓ bronchodilatation

Lab test interferences

False increase: Urinary catecholamines

NURSING CONSIDERATIONS

Assessment

- Monitor B/P at beginning of treatment, periodically thereafter; pulse q4h; note rate, rhythm, quality: apical/radial pulse before administration; notify prescriber of any significant changes (pulse <50 bpm)
- Check for baselines in renal, liver function tests before therapy begins
- Assess for edema in feet, legs daily, monitor I&O, daily weight; check for jugular vein distention, rales bilaterally, dyspnea (CHF)
- Monitor skin turgor, dryness of mucous membranes for hydration status, especially G elderly

Associated nursing diagnoses

- ✓ Cardiac output, decreased (uses)
- ✓ Injury, potential for physical (side effects)
- ✓ Knowledge deficit (teaching)
- ✓ Noncompliance (teaching)

Implementation

PO route

- Given ac, hs, tab may be crushed or swallowed whole; give with food to prevent GI upset; reduce dosage in renal dysfunction
- Store protected from light, moisture; place in cool environment

IV **IV route**

- Give **IV** undiluted 20 mg/2 min; may increase q10 min 40-80 mg until desired effect
- Give **IV** cont inf by diluting in LR, D_5W, D_5 in 0.2%, 0.9%, 0.33% NaCl or Ringer's inj; inf is titrated to patient response; 200 mg of drug/160 ml sol (1 mg/ml); 300 mg of drug/240 ml sol (1 mg/ml); 200 mg of drug/250 ml sol (2 mg/3ml); use inf pump
- Keep patient recumbent for 3 hr after inf

Y-*site incompatibilities:*

Cefoperazone, nafcillin

Y-*site compatibilities:*

Amikacin, aminophylline, ampicillin, butorphanol, calcium gluconate, cefazolin, ceftazidine, ceftizoxine, chloramphenicol, cimetidine, clindamycin, co-trimoxazole, dopamine, enalaprilat, erythromycin, lactobionate, famotidine, fentanyl, gentamicin, heparin, lidocaine, magnesium sulfate, meperidine, metronidazole, morphine, oxacillin, penicillin G potassium, piperacillin, potassium chloride, potassium phosphate, ranitidine, sodium acetate, tobramycin, vancomycin

Solution incompatibility:
Sodium bicarbonate 5%

Solution compatibilities:
D_5R, D_5LR, $D_{2½}/0.45\%$ NaCl, $D_5/0.2\%$ NaCl, $D_5/0.33\%$ NaCl, $D_5/0.9\%$ NaCl, D_5W, Ringer's, LR

Patient/family education
- Teach patient not to discontinue drug abruptly, or precipitate angina might occur; taper over 2 wk
- Teach patient not to use OTC products containing α-adrenergic stimulants (such as nasal decongestants, cold preparations); to avoid alcohol, smoking and to limit sodium intake as prescribed
- Teach patient how to take pulse and B/P at home; advise when to notify prescriber
- Instruct patient to comply with weight control, dietary adjustments, modified exercise program
- Advise patient to carry/wear Medic Alert ID to identify drug being taken, allergies; teach patient drug controls symptoms but does not cure
- Caution patient to avoid hazardous activities if dizziness, drowsiness are present
- Teach patient to report symptoms of CHF: difficult breathing, especially on exertion or when lying down, night cough, swelling of extremities, bradycardia, dizziness, confusion, depression, fever
- Teach patient to take drug as prescribed, not to double or skip doses; take any missed doses as soon as remembered if at least 4 hr until next dose

Evaluation

Positive therapeutic outcome
- Decreased B/P in hypertension (after 1-2 wk)
- Absence of dysrhythmias

Treatment of overdose:
Lavage, **IV** atropine for bradycardia, **IV** theophylline for bronchospasm, digitalis, O_2, diuretic for cardiac failure, hemodialysis, **IV** glucose for hyperglycemia, **IV** diazepam (or phenytoin) for seizures

lactulose
(lak'tyoo-lose)
Cephulac, Cholac, Chronulac, Constilac, Constulose, Duphalac Emulose, Enulose, Lactulax ✤
Func. class.: Laxative (Hyperosmotic/ ammonia detoxicant)
Chem. class.: Lactose synthetic derivative
Pregnancy category C

Action: Increases osmotic pressure; draws fluid into colon; prevents absorption of ammonia in colon; increases water in stool

➡ **Therapeutic Outcome:** Decreased constipation, decreased blood ammonia level

Uses: Chronic constipation, portal-systemic encephalopathy in patients with hepatic disease

Dosage and routes

Constipation

Adult: PO 15-60 ml qd

Encephalopathy

Adult: PO 20-30 g tid or qid until stools are soft; retention enema 30-45 ml in 100 ml of fluid

Available forms: Oral sol, rec sol 3.33 g/5 ml

Side effects/adverse reactions

GI: *Nausea, vomiting, anorexia, abdominal cramps, diarrhea,* flatulence, *distention, belching*

Contraindications: Hypersensitivity, low-galactose diet

Precautions: Pregnancy **C**, lactation, diabetes mellitus, G elderly and debilitated patient

Pharmacokinetics

Absorption	Poorly absorbed
Distribution	Not known
Metabolism	Colonic bacteria to acids
Excretion	Kidneys, unchanged
Half-life	Unknown

Pharmacodynamics

	PO
Onset	Unknown
Peak	Unknown
Duration	Unknown

Interactions

Drug/drug:

Individual drugs

Neomycin: ↓ effectiveness (portal-systemic encephalopathy)

Drug classifications

Laxatives: Do not use together (portal-systemic encephalopathy)

NURSING CONSIDERATIONS

Assessment

- Monitor glucose levels in diabetic (increases)
- Monitor blood, urine, electrolytes if used often by patient; may cause diarrhea, hypokalemia, hypernatremia; check I&O ratio to identify fluid loss
- Assess cramping, rec bleeding, nausea, vomiting; if these symptoms occur, drug should be discontinued; identify cause of constipation; identify whether fluids, bulk, or exercise is missing from lifestyle
- Monitor blood ammonia level (30-70 mg/100 ml); monitor for clearing of confusion, lethargy, restlessness, irritability (hepatic encephalopathy); may decrease ammonia level by 50%

Associated nursing diagnoses

- ✓ Constipation (uses)
- ✓ Diarrhea (adverse reactions)
- ✓ Knowledge deficit (teaching)
- ✓ Noncompliance (teaching)

Implementation

PO route

- Give with full glass fruit juice, water, milk to increase palatability of oral form; give increased fluids of 2 L/day; do not give with other laxatives; if diarrhea occurs, reduce dosage

Rec route

- Administer retention enema by diluting 300 ml lactulose/

L

700 ml of water or 0.9% NaCl; administer by rec balloon catheter; retain for 30-60 min; repeat if evacuated too quickly

Patient/family education

- Discuss with the patient that adequate fluid consumption is necessary
- Teach patient that normal bowel movements do not always occur daily
- Teach patient not to use in presence of abdominal pain, nausea, vomiting; tell patient to notify prescriber if constipation unrelieved or if symptoms of electrolyte imbalance occur: muscle cramps, pain, weakness, dizziness, excessive thirst
- Teach patient not to use laxatives for long-term therapy; bowel tone will be lost
- Do not give at hs as a laxative; may interfere with sleep
- Notify prescriber if diarrhea occurs; may indicate overdosage

Evaluation

Positive therapeutic outcome

- Decreased constipation
- Decreased blood ammonia level
- Clearing of mental state

lamotrigine

(lam-o-trye′geen)

Lamictal

Func. class.: Anticonvulsant

Chem. class.: Phenyltriazine

Pregnancy category **C**

Action: Unknown; may inhibit voltage-sensitive sodium channels

Therapeutic Outcome: Decrease in intensity and amount of seizures

Uses: Adjunct in the treatment of partial seizures

Dosage and routes

Without valproic acid

Adult: 50 mg/day for weeks 1 and 2, then increase to 100 mg divided bid for weeks 3 and 4; maintenance 300-500 mg/day

With valproic acid

Adult: 25 mg every other day, weeks 1 through 4, then 150 mg/day in divided doses

Available forms: Tab 25, 100, 150, 200 mg

Side effects/adverse reactions

CNS: Fever, insomnia, tremor, depression, anxiety, **dizziness,** ataxia, **headache**
EENT: Nystagmus, **diplopia, blurred vision**
GI: **Nausea, vomiting, anorexia,** abdominal pain
GU: **Dysmenorrhea**
INTEG: Rash, alopecia, photosensitivity
RESP: **Rhinitis,** pharyngitis, cough

Contraindications: Hypersensitivity

Precautions: Pregnancy **C**, lactation, children <16 yr, renal, hepatic disease

Pharmacokinetics

Absorption	Well absorbed (PO)
Distribution	Unknown
Metabolism	Unknown
Excretion	Unknown
Half-life	Varies, depending on dose

Pharmacodynamics

Onset	Unknown
Peak	Unknown
Duration	Unknown

Interactions

Drug/drug:

Individual drugs

Carphenazine: ↑ metabolic clearance of lamotrigine
Phenobarbital: ↑ metabolic clearance of lamotrigine
Phenytoin: ↑ metabolic clearance of lamotrigine
Valproic acid: ↓ metabolic clearance of lamotrigine

NURSING CONSIDERATIONS

Assessment

- Assess for seizure activity: duration, type, intensity, halo before seizure
- Assess for hypersensitive reactions

Associated nursing diagnoses

✓ Injury, risk for (uses)
✓ Knowledge deficit (teaching)

Implementation

PO route

- May be given with food or fluids

Patient/family education

- Teach patient to take PO doses divided with or after meals to decrease adverse effects
- Caution patient not to discontinue drug abruptly; seizures may occur
- Caution patient to avoid hazardous activities until stabilized on drug
- Advise patient to notify prescriber of skin rash or increased seizure activity
- Instruct patient to report to prescriber if pregnant or if patient intends to become pregnant
- Teach patient to use sunscreen and protective clothing, photosensitivity occurs
- Advise patient to carry Medic Alert ID stating drug use

Evaluation

Positive therapeutic outcome

- Decrease in severity of seizures

leucovorin

(loo-koe-vor'in)

Citrovorum Factor, 5-Formyl Tetrahydrofolate, Folinic Acid, leucovorin calcium, Wellcovorin

Func. class.: Vitamin/folic acid antagonist antidote

Chem. class.: Tetrahydrofolic acid derivative

Pregnancy category **C**

Action: Needed for normal growth patterns; prevents toxicity during antineoplastic therapy by protecting normal cells

Therapeutic Outcome: Reversal of severe toxic effects of folic acid antagonists

Uses: Megaloblastic or macrocytic anemia caused by folic acid deficiency, overdose of folic acid antagonist, methotrexate toxicity, toxicity caused by pyrimethamine or trimethoprim, pneumocystosis, toxoplasmosis

Dosage and routes

Megaloblastic anemia caused by enzyme deficiency

P *Adult and child:* PO, IM, **IV** up to 1 mg/day

Megaloblastic anemia caused by deficiency of folate

P *Adult and child:* IM 1 mg or less qd until adequate response

Methotrexate toxicity

P *Adult and child:* PO/IM/ **IV** given 6-36 hr after dose of methotrexate 10 mg/m^2, then 10 mg/m^2 q6h × 72 hr

Pyrimethamine toxicity

P *Adult and child:* PO/IM 5 mg qd

Trimethoprim toxicity

P *Adult and child:* PO IM 400 μg qd

Available forms: Tab 5, 10, 15, 25 mg; inj 3, 5 mg/ml; powder for inj 10 mg/ml

Side effects/adverse reactions

INTEG: Rash, pruritus, erythema, thrombocytosis, urticaria

RESP: Wheezing

Contraindications: Hypersensitivity, anemias other than megaloblastic not associated with vitamin B_{12} deficiency

Precautions: Pregnancy **C**

Pharmacokinetics

Absorption	Rapidly absorbed (PO); completely absorbed (IV)
Distribution	Widely distributed
Metabolism	Liver
Excretion	Kidney
Half-life	3½ hr

Pharmacodynamics

	PO/IM/IV
Onset	Up to 5 min
Peak	Unknown
Duration	4-6 hr

Interactions

Drug/drug:

Individual drugs

Chloramphenicol: ↓ folate levels

Phenobarbital: ↑ metabolism of phenobarbital, ↓ effect

Drug classifications

Hydantoins: ↑ metabolism of hydantoins, ↓ effect

NURSING CONSIDERATIONS

Assessment

- Obtain CrCl before leucovorin rescue and qd to detect nephrotoxicity
- Monitor I&O; watch for nausea and vomiting; if vomiting occurs IM or **IV** route may be necessary
- Assess diet for inclusion of bran, yeast, dried beans, nuts, fruits, fresh vegetables, aspara-

gus, which have high folic acid levels

- Assess drugs currently taken: alcohol, hydantoins, trimethoprim may cause increased folic acid use by body
- Assess for allergic reactions: rash, dyspnea, wheezing

Associated nursing diagnoses

- ✓ Injury, risk for (uses)
- ✓ Nutrition, altered: less than body requirements (uses)
- ✓ Knowledge deficit (teaching)

Implementation

PO route

- Use PO route only if patient is not vomiting

IM route

- Give within 1 hr of folic acid antagonist
- Give increased fluid intake if used to treat folic acid inhibitor overdose
- Provide protection from light and heat when storing ampules

IV **IV route**

- Reconstitute 50 mg/5 ml bacteriostatic water or sterile water for inj (10 mg/ml) or 100 mg/10 ml; use immediately if sterile water for inj is used to reconstitute
- Give by direct **IV** over 160 mg/min or less
- Give by intermittent inf after diluting in 100-500 ml of 0.9% NaCl, D_5W, $D_{10}W$, LR, Ringer's

Syringe/Y-site compatibilities:

Bleomycin, cisplatin, cyclophosphamide, doxorubicin, fluorouracil, furosemide, heparin, methotrexate, metoclopramide, mitomycin, vinblastine, vincristine

Syringe/Y-site incompatibility:

Droperidol

Additive compatibilities:

Cisplatin, floxuridine, fluorouracil

Patient/family education

- Advise patient to take drug exactly as prescribed; to notify prescriber of side effects immediately
- Advise patient to report signs of hyposensitivity reaction immediately
- Instruct patient about leucovorin rescue have patient drink 3 L of fluid each day of rescue
- Advise patient with folic acid deficiency to eat folic acid–rich foods: bran, yeast, dried beans, nuts, fruits, fresh green leafy vegetables, asparagus

Evaluation

Positive therapeutic outcome

- Increased weight
- Improved orientation, well-being
- Absence of fatigue

leuprolide

(loo-proe′lide)

Leupron Depo Ped, Lupron Depot, Lupron

Func. class.: Antineoplastic hormone

Chem. class.: Gonadotropin-releasing hormone

Pregnancy category (depot) X

L

Action: Causes initial increase in circulating levels of LH, FSH; continuous administration results in decreased LH, FSH; in men testosterone is reduced to castration levels; in premenopausal women estrogen is reduced to menopausal levels

Therapeutic Outcome: Prevention of rapidly growing malignant cells in prostate cancer, decreased pain in endometriosis, resolution of central precocious puberty (CPP)

Uses: Metastatic prostate cancer, management of endometriosis (depot), CPP

Dosage and routes

Prostate cancer

Adult: SC 1 mg/day; IM 7.5 mg/mo

Endometriosis

Adult: IM 7.5 mg once a month

Central precocious puberty

P ***Child:*** SC 50 μg/kg/day; increase as needed by 10 μg/kg/day

P ***Child:*** IM 0.3 mg/kg/mo; may increase by 3.75 mg/mo

Available forms: Inj (depot) 3.75 mg, 7.5 mg single-dose, multiple-dose vials (5 mg/ml); pediatric depot 7.5, 11.25, 15 mg

Side effects/adverse reactions

GU: Edema, hot flashes, impotence, decreased libido, amenorrhea, vaginal dryness, gynecomastia

Contraindications: Hypersensitivity to GnRH or analogs, thromboembolic disorders, pregnancy **X**, lactation, undiagnosed vaginal bleeding

Precautions: Edema, hepatic disease, CVA, MI, seizures, hypertension, diabetes mellitus

Pharmacokinetics

Absorption	Rapidly absorbed (SC); slowly absorbed (IM depot)
Distribution	Unknown
Metabolism	Unknown
Excretion	Unknown
Half-life	3-4 hr

Pharmacodynamics

	SC
Onset	Unknown
Peak	Unknown
Duration	Unknown

Interactions

Drug/drug:

Megestrol: ↑ antineoplastic action

Flutamide: ↑ antineoplastic action

NURSING CONSIDERATIONS

Assessment

- Assess for symptoms of endometriosis including lower abdominal pain if drug is given for the diagnosis of endometriosis
- If giving this drug for CPP, the diagnosis should have been confirmed by development of secondary sex characteristics in P child <9 yr; also included to

confirm the diagnosis of CPP is estradiol/testosterone, GnRH test, tomography of head, adrenal steroid, chorionic gonadotropin, wrist x-ray, height, weight; patients diagnosed with CPP display the signs of testicular growth, facial, body hair (males), breast development, menses (females)
• Monitor liver function tests before, during therapy (bilirubin, AST [SGOT], ALT [SGPT], LDH) as needed or monthly
• Monitor pituitary gonadotropic and gonadal function during therapy and 4-8 wk after therapy is decreased; check LH, FSH, acid phosphate at beginning of treatment
• Monitor worsening of signs and symptoms (normal during beginning therapy): fatigue, increased pulse, pallor, lethargy, edema in feet, joints, stomach pain, shaking
• Monitor renal status: I&O ratio, check for bladder distention daily during beginning therapy (renal obstruction)

Associated nursing diagnoses

✓ Sexual dysfunction (adverse reactions)
✓ Injury, risk for (adverse reactions)
✓ Knowledge deficit (teaching)

Implementation

IM/SC route
• Use syringe and drug packaged together; give deep in large muscle mass; rotate sites
• Use depot only IM; never give SC
• Reconstitute vial (single dose)/1 ml of diluent; shake (appearance should be white); withdraw and use immediately
• Unused vials may be stored at room temp

Patient/family education

• Advise patient to notify prescriber if menstruation continues; menstruation should stop; to use a nonhormonal method of contraception during therapy
• Instruct patient to report any complaints, side effects to nurse or prescriber; hot flashes are common
• Teach patient how to prepare, administer; to rotate sites for SC inj; to keep accurate records of dosing (prostate cancer)
• Instruct patient that tumor flare may occur: increase in size of tumor, increased bone pain; tell patient that bone pain disappears after 1 wk; may take analgesics for pain; premenopausal women must use mechanical birth control; ovulation may be induced

Evaluation

Positive therapeutic outcome
• Decreased size, spread of malignancy
• Decreased pain in endometriosis
• Decreased signs of CPP

levamisole

(lee-vam′i-sol)
Ergamisol
Func. class.: Antineoplastic, immunomodulator
Pregnancy category C

Action: May increase the action of macrophages, monocytes, and T cells, which restore immune function; complete action is unknown; cholinergic properties

Therapeutic Outcome: Prevention of rapid growth of malignant cells when used with fluorouracil

Uses: Treatment of Dukes' stage C colon cancer when given with fluorouracil after surgical resection

Investigational uses: Malignant melanoma (advanced)

Dosage and routes

Adult: PO 50 mg q8h × 3 days; begin treatment at least 1 wk but no more than 4 wk after resection; give with fluorouracil 450 mg/m^2/day

Available forms: Tab 50 mg (base)

Side effects/adverse reactions

CNS: Dizziness, headache, paresthesia, somnolence, depression, anxiety, *fatigue*, fever, mental changes, ataxia, insomnia

CV: Chest pain, edema

EENT: Blurred vision, conjunctivitis

GI: ***Nausea, vomiting, anorexia, diarrhea, stomatitis,*** constipation, flatulence, dyspepsia, abdominal pain

HEMA: ***Granulocytopenia, leukopenia, thrombocytopenia***

INTEG: Rash, pruritus, ***alopecia, dermatitis,*** urticaria

META: Hyperbilirubinemia

MISC: Rigors, infection, altered sense of smell, arthralgia, myalgia

Contraindications: Hypersensitivity

Precautions: Pregnancy **C**, P lactation, children, blood dyscrasias

Pharmacokinetics

Absorption	Rapidly absorbed (PO)
Distribution	Unknown
Metabolism	Liver, extensively
Excretion	Unknown
Half-life	3-4 hr

Pharmacodynamics

	PO
Onset	Unknown
Peak	1½-2 hr
Duration	Unknown

Interactions

Drug/drug:

Individual drugs

Alcohol: ↑ disulfiram reaction

Phenytoin: ↑ plasma levels

Radiation: ↑ bone marrow depression

Drug classifications

Antineoplastics: ↑ bone marrow depression

NURSING CONSIDERATIONS

Assessment

- Monitor CBC, differential, platelet count weekly; withhold

drug if WBC is <4000 or platelet count is <100,000; notify prescriber of results; drug should be discontinued and restarted after recovery
- Monitor renal function studies: BUN, serum uric acid, urine CrCl before, during therapy; I&O ratio; report fall in urine output of 30 ml/hr; check for decreased hyperuricemia
- Monitor for cold, fever, sore throat (may indicate beginning infection)
- Assess for bleeding: hematuria, guaiac, bruising or petechiae, mucosa or orifices q8h; no rec temp
- Identify inflammation of mucosa, breaks in skin; use viscous lidocaine (Xylocaine) for oral pain

Associated nursing diagnoses

✓ Injury, risk for (adverse reactions)
✓ Body image disturbance (adverse reactions)
✓ Infection, risk for (adverse reactions)
✓ Knowledge deficit (teaching)

Implementation

PO route
- Give 7-20 days after surgery; start fluorouracil with 2nd course of levamisole; begin no sooner than 21 days and no later than 35 days after surgery; if levamisole therapy begins 21-30 days after resection, fluorouracil should be given with 1st course; apply pressure to venipuncture sites for 10 min, especially if platelets are low

Patient/family education

- Advise patient to call prescriber if sore throat, swollen lymph nodes, malaise, fever occur, since other infections may develop
- Advise patient that contraceptive measures are recommended during therapy and 4 mo after; teratogenic effects are possible
- Caution patient to avoid ingestion of alcohol, since disulfiram reaction may occur with flushing, severe nausea, vomiting, pounding headache; death can result; advise patient that tyramine-containing foods and cold, hay fever, weight-reducing products may cause hypertensive crisis
- Caution patient to avoid use of products containing aspirin or ibuprofen, razors, commercial mouthwash, since bleeding may occur; to report symptoms of bleeding (hematuria, tarry stools)
- Advise patient to report signs of anemia (fatigue, headache, irritability, faintness, shortness of breath) and CNS reactions including confusion, psychosis, nightmares, seizures, severe headaches
- Inform patient that hair may be lost during treatment; a wig or hair piece may make patient feel better; new hair may be different in color, texture
- Teach patient the reason for medication use and expected results

Evaluation

Positive therapeutic outcome
- Decreased spread of malignant cells when used with fluorouracil

levodopa

(lee'voe-doe-pa)

Dopar, Larodopa, L-Dopa

Func. class.: Antiparkinsonian agent

Chem. class.: Catecholamine, dopamine agonist

Pregnancy category **C**

Action: Decarboxylation to dopamine, which increases dopamine levels in brain

Therapeutic Outcome: Decreased symptoms of Parkinson's disease (involuntary movements)

Uses: Parkinsonism

Dosage and routes

Adult: PO 0.5-1 g qd divided bid-qid with meals; may increase by up to 0.75 g q3-7 days, not to exceed 8 g/day unless closely supervised

Available forms: Cap 100, 250, 500 mg; tab 100, 250, 500 mg

Side effects/adverse reactions

CNS: *Involuntary choreiform movements, hand tremors, fatigue, headache, anxiety, twitching, numbness, weakness, confusion, agitation, insomnia, nightmares,* psychosis, hallucinations, hypomania, severe depression, dizziness

CV: *Orthostatic hypotension,* tachycardia, hypertension, palpitations

EENT: Blurred vision, diplopia, dilated pupils

GI: *Nausea, vomiting, anorexia, abdominal distress, dry mouth, flatulence, dysphagia,* bitter taste, diarrhea, constipation

HEMA: Hemolytic anemia, leukopenia, agranulocytosis

INTEG: Rash, sweating, alopecia

MISC: Urinary retention, incontinence, weight change, dark urine

Contraindications: Hypersensitivity, narrow angle glaucoma, undiagnosed skin lesions

Precautions: Renal disease, cardiac disease, hepatic disease, respiratory disease, MI with dysrhythmias, convulsions, peptic ulcer, pregnancy **C**, asthma, endocrine disease, affective disorders, psychosis, lactation, P children <12 yr peptic ulcer

Pharmacokinetics

Absorption	Well absorbed (PO)
Distribution	Widely distributed
Metabolism	Liver, GI tract, extensively
Excretion	Kidneys to metabolites; breast milk
Half-life	1 hr

Pharmacodynamics

Onset	10-15 min
Peak	1-3 hr
Duration	Up to 24 hr

Interactions

Drug/drug:

Individual drugs

Haloperidol: ↓ effect of levodopa

Methyldopa: ↑ CNS toxicity
Papaverine: ↓ effects of levodopa
Phenytoin: ↓ effect of levodopa
Pyridoxine: ↓ effects of levodopa
Reserpine: ↓ effect of levodopa
Selegiline: ↑ adverse reaction

Drug classifications

Anticholinergics: ↓ effects of levodopa
Antihypertensives: ↑ hypotension
Hydantoins: ↓ effects of levodopa
MAOI: Hypertensive crisis

Drug/food:

↓ effect of levodopa from pyridoxine foods

Lab test interferences

False positive: Urine ketones, urine glucose, Coombs' test, urine, norepinephrine
False negative: Urine glucose (glucose oxidase)
False increase: Uric acid, urine protein
Decrease: VMA

NURSING CONSIDERATIONS

Assessment

- Monitor B/P, respiration during initial treatment; hypotension or hypertension should be reported
- Assess mental status: affect, mood, behavioral changes, depression; complete suicide assessment
- Monitor liver function enzymes: AST (SGOT), ALT (SGPT), alkaline phosphatase; also check LDH, bilirubin, CBC
- Assess for involuntary movements in parkinsonism: akinesia, tremors, staggering gait, muscle rigidity, drooling; these symptoms should improve with levodopa therapy
- Assess for levodopa toxicity: mental, personality changes, increased twitching, grimacing, tongue protrusion; these should be reported to prescriber

Associated nursing diagnoses

✓ Mobility, impaired (uses)
✓ Injury, risk for (uses)
✓ Knowledge deficit (teaching)
✓ Noncompliance (teaching)

Implementation

PO route

- Levodopa/carbidopa should not be started until this drug is withheld for 8 hr; toxicity may result if the two drugs are taken close together
- Give drug until NPO before surgery
- Adjust dosage to patient response
- Give with meals to decrease GI upset; limit protein taken with drug
- Give only after MAOIs have been discontinued for 2 wk

Patient/family education

- Advise patient that therapeutic effects may take several wk to a few mo
- Caution patient to change positions slowly to prevent orthostatic hypotension
- Instruct patient to report side effects: twitching, eye spasms; indicate overdose

L

• Instruct patient to use drug exactly as prescribed; if drug is discontinued abruptly, parkinsonian crisis may occur
• Inform patient that urine, sweat may darken
• Advise patient to avoid vitamin B_6 preparations, vitamin-fortified foods containing B_6; these foods can reverse effects of levodopa; also OTC preparations should be avoided unless approved by prescriber

Evaluation

Positive therapeutic outcome
• Decreased akathisia, other involuntary movements
• Increased mood

levorphanol

(lee-vor′ fan-ole)
Levo-Dromoran, Levorphan
Func. class.: Narcotic analgesic (opioid analgesic agonist)
Chem. class.: Opiate, synthetic morphine derivative

Pregnancy category B
Controlled substance schedule II

Action: Inhibits ascending pain pathways in limbic system, thalamus, midbrain, hypothalamus by binding to opiate receptor sites, altering pain perception and response

➡ **Therapeutic Outcome:** Relief of pain

Uses: Moderate to severe pain

Dosage and routes

Adult: PO/SC/**IV** 2-3 mg q4-5h prn

Available forms: Inj 2 mg/ml; tab 2 mg

Side effects/adverse reactions

CNS: ***Drowsiness, dizziness, confusion, headache, sedation, euphoria***
CV: Palpitations, bradycardia, change in B/P
EENT: Tinnitus, blurred vision, miosis, diplopia
GI: ***Nausea, vomiting, anorexia, constipation, cramps***
GU: Urinary retention, dysuria
INTEG: ***Rash,*** urticaria, diaphoresis, pruritus
RESP: ***Respiratory depression***

Contraindications: Hypersensitivity, addiction (narcotic)

Precautions: Addictive personality, pregnancy **B**, lactation, increased intracranial pressure, MI (acute), severe heart disease, respiratory depression, hepatic disease, renal disease, P child <18 yr

Pharmacokinetics	
Absorption	Well absorbed (SC, PO); completely absorbed (IV)
Distribution	Unknown
Metabolism	Liver, extensively
Excretion	Kidneys
Half-life	12-16 hr

Pharmacodynamics

	PO	SC	IV
Onset	Up to 60 min	Unknown	Unknown
Peak	1½-2 hr	1-1½ hr	20 min
Duration	6 hr	6 hr	6 hr

Interactions

Drug/drug:

Individual drugs

Alcohol: ↑ respiratory depression, hypotension, sedation
Nalbuphine: ↓ analgesia
Pentazocine: ↓ analgesia

Drug classifications

Antihistamines: ↑ respiratory depression, hypotension
Antidepressants: ↑ respiratory depression, hypotension
CNS depressants: ↑ respiratory depression, hypotension
MAOI: ↑ respiratory depression
Sedative/hypnotics: ↑ respiratory depression, hypotension

Lab test interferences

Increase: Amylase

NURSING CONSIDERATIONS

Assessment

- Monitor VS after parenteral route; note muscle rigidity, drug history, liver, kidney function tests, respiratory dysfunction: respiratory depression, character, rate, rhythm; notify prescriber if respirations are <10/min
- Monitor CNS changes: dizziness, drowsiness, hallucinations, euphoria, LOC, pupil reaction
- Monitor allergic reactions: rash, urticaria

Associated nursing diagnoses

- ✓ Pain (uses)
- ✓ Sensory-perceptual alteration: visual, auditory (adverse reactions)
- ✓ Breathing pattern, ineffective (adverse reactions)
- ✓ Injury, risk for (adverse reactions)
- ✓ Knowledge deficit (teaching)

Implementation

- Give with antiemetic if nausea, vomiting occur
- Administer when pain is beginning to return, determine dosage interval by patient response; continuous dosing of medication is more effective given prn; explain analgesic effect
- Medication should be slowly withdrawn after long-term use to prevent withdrawal symptoms
- Store in light-resistant container at room temp

PO route

- May be given with food or milk to lessen GI upset

IV **IV route**

- Give **IV** directly; give through Y-tube or 3-way stopcock over 5 min; do not administer rapidly or circulatory collapse may occur
- Store in light-resistant area at room temp

Syringe compatibility:

Glycopyrrolate

Additive incompatibilities:

Aminophylline, ammonium chloride, amobarbital, chlorothiazide, heparin, methicillin, pentobarbital, phenobarbital, phenytoin, secobarbital, so-

L

dium bicarbonate, sodium iodine, thiopental

Patient/family education

- Caution patients to avoid CNS depressants: alcohol, sedative/hypnotics for at least 24 hr after taking this drug
- Discuss with patient that dizziness, drowsiness, confusion are common; to avoid getting up without assistance
- Discuss in detail all aspects of the drug and what to expect after anesthesia
- Advise patient to make position changes carefully to lessen orthostatic hypotension

Evaluation

Positive therapeutic outcome

- Decreased pain

Treatment of overdose: Narcan 0.2-0.8 **IV**, O_2, **IV** fluids, vasopressors

levothyroxine 🔑

(lee-voe-thye-rox'een)

Eltroxin ✤, Levothroid, levothyroxine sodium, Levoxine, Synthroid, T_4

Func. class.: Thyroid hormone

Chem. class.: Levoisomer of thyroxine

Pregnancy category A

Action: Controls protein synthesis; increases metabolic rate, cardiac output, renal blood flow, O_2 consumption, body temp, blood volume, growth, development at cellular level

➔ Therapeutic Outcome: Correction of lack of thyroid hormone

Uses: Hypothyroidism, myxedema coma, thyroid hormone replacement, cretinism, thyrotoxicosis

Dosage and routes

Severe hypothyroidism

Adult: PO 12.5-50 μg qd, increased by 0.05-0.1 mg q1-4 wk until desired response; maintenance dosage 75-125 μg qd, IM/**IV** 50-100 μg/day as a single dose

P *Child >12 yr:* PO 2-3 μg/kg/day given as a single dose AM

P *Child 6-12 yr:* PO 4-5 μg/kg/day given as a single dose AM

P *Child 1-5 yr:* PO 5-6 μg/kg/day given as a single dose AM

P *Child 6-12 mo:* PO 6-8 μg/kg/day give as a single dose AM

P *Child to 6 mo:* PO 8-10 μg/kg/day given as a single dose AM

Myxedema coma

Adult: **IV** 200-500 μg; may increase by 100-300 μg after 24 hr; place on oral medication as soon as possible; maintenance 50-100 μg/day

Available forms: Inj 50, 200, 500 μg/vial; tab 0.025, 0.05, 0.075, 0.088, 0.1, 0.112, 0.125, 0.15, 0.175, 0.2, 0.3 mg

Side effects/adverse reactions

CNS: *Anxiety, insomnia, tremors,* headache, ***thyroid storm***

CV: Tachycardia, palpitations, angina, dysrhythmias, hypertension, ***cardiac arrest***
GI: Nausea, diarrhea, increased or decreased appetite, cramps
MISC: Menstrual irregularities, weight loss, sweating, heat intolerance, fever

Contraindications: Adrenal insufficiency, MI, thyrotoxicosis

G **Precautions:** Elderly, angina pectoris, hypertension, ischemia, cardiac disease, pregnancy **A**, lactation

Pharmacokinetics

Absorption	Erratic (PO); complete (IV)
Distribution	Widely distributed
Metabolism	Liver; enterohepatic recirculation
Excretion	Feces via bile; breast milk (small amounts)
Half-life	6-7 days

Pharmacodynamics

	PO	IV
Onset	Unknown	6-8 hr
Peak	12-48 hr	12-48 hr
Duration	Unknown	Unknown

Interactions

Drug/drug:

Individual drugs
Cholestyramine: ↓ absorption of thyroid hormone
Colestipol: ↓ absorption of levothyroxine
Digitalis: ↓ effect of digitalis
Insulin: ↑ requirement for insulin
Phenytoin (IV): ↑ release of thyroid hormone

Drug classifications
Amphetamines: ↑ CNS, cardiac stimulation
β-Adrenergic blockers: ↓ effect of β-blockers
Decongestants: ↑ CNS, cardiac stimulation
Oral anticoagulants: ↑ requirements for anticoagulants
Vasopressors: ↑ CNS, cardiac stimulation

Lab test interferences

Increase: CPK, LDH, AST (SGOT), PBI, blood glucose
Decrease: TSH, ^{131}I uptake test, uric acid, triglycerides

NURSING CONSIDERATIONS

Assessment

- Identify if the patient is taking anticoagulants, antidiabetic agents; document on chart
- Take B/P, pulse before each dose; monitor I&O ratio and weight every day in same clothing, using same scale, at same time of day
- Monitor height, weight, psychomotor development and growth rate if given to a child
- Monitor T_3, T_4, FTIs, which are decreased; radioimmunoassay of TSH, which is increased; radio uptake, which is increased if patient is on too low a dosage of medication
- Monitor pro-time (may require decreased anticoagulant); check for bleeding, bruising
- Assess for increased nervousness, excitability, irritability, which may indicate too high a dosage of medication, usually after 1-3 wk of treatment

- Assess cardiac status: angina, palpitations, chest pain, change in VS; the elderly patient may have undetected cardiac problems and baseline ECG should be completed before treatment

Associated nursing diagnoses

✓ Knowledge deficit (teaching)
✓ Noncompliance (teaching)

Implementation

PO route
- Give in AM if possible as a single dose to decrease sleeplessness; give at same time each day to maintain drug level
- Give only for hormone imbalances; not to be used for obesity, male infertility, menstrual conditions, lethargy; give lowest dosage that relieves symptoms; lower dosage for the elderly and in cardiac diseases
- Store in tight, light-resistant container
- Remove medication 4 wk before RAIU test

IV route
- Give **IV** after diluting with provided diluent (0.9% NaCl), 0.5 mg/5 ml; shake well; give through Y-tube or 3-way stopcock; give 0.1 mg or less over 1 min; do not add to IV inf; 0.1 mg = 1 ml; discard any unused portion

Patient/family education

- Teach patient that drug is not a cure but controls symptoms and treatment is long term
- Instruct patient to report excitability, irritability, anxiety, sweating, heat intolerance, chest pain, palpitations, which indicate overdose
- Advise patient not to switch brands unless approved by prescriber; bioavailability may differ; do not take with food; absorption will be decreased
- Teach patient that drug may be discontinued after giving birth; thyroid panel will be evaluated after 1-2 mo
- Teach patient or parent that hyperthyroid child will show almost immediate behavior/personality change; that hair loss will occur in child but is temporary
- Caution patient that drug is not to be taken to reduce weight
- Caution patient to avoid OTC preparations with iodine; read labels; other medications should not be used unless approved by prescriber
- Teach patient to avoid iodine-rich food: iodized salt, soybeans, tofu, turnips, some seafood, some bread

Evaluation

Positive therapeutic outcome
- Absence of depression
- Weight loss, increased diuresis, pulse, appetite
- Absence of constipation, peripheral edema, cold intolerance, pale, cool dry skin, brittle nails, alopecia, coarse hair, menorrhagia, night blindness, paresthesias, syncope, stupor, coma, rosy cheeks
- Improved levels of T_3, T_4 by laboratory tests

P • Child: age-appropriate weight, height and psychomotor development

Treatment of overdose: Withhold dose for up to 1 wk: acute overdose: gastric lavage or induced emesis, activated charcoal; provide supportive treatment to control symptoms

lidocaine

(lye'doe-kane)

Anestacon, Baylocaine, L-Caine, Lidocaine HCl IV for Cardiac Arrhythmias, Lidopen Auto-Injector, Xylocaine HCl IM for Cardiac Arrhythmias, Xylocaine HCl IV for Cardiac Arrhythmias

Func. class.: Antidysrhythmic (Class IB); local anesthetic

Chem. class.: Aminoacyl amide

Pregnancy category B

Action: Increases electrical stimulation threshold of ventricle and His-Purkinje system, which stabilizes cardiac membrane and decreases automaticity; locally produces anesthesia by preventing initiation and conduction of nerve impulses

Therapeutic Outcome: Decreased ventricular dysrhythmia; produces anesthesia locally

Uses: Ventricular tachycardia, ventricular dysrhythmias during cardiac surgery, MI, digitalis toxicity, cardiac catheterization; anesthesia locally

Dosage and routes

Adult: **IV** bol 50-100 mg (1 mg/kg) over 2-3 min; repeat q3-5 min, not to exceed 300 mg in 1 hr; begin **IV** inf 20-50 μg/kg/min; IM 200-300 mg (4.3 mg/kg) in deltoid muscle; may repeat in 1-1½ hr if needed

G *Elderly with CHF, reduced liver function:* **IV** bol give ½ adult dose

P *Child:* **IV** bol 1 mg/kg, then **IV** inf 30 μg/kg/min

P *Adult and child:* Top apply as needed to affected areas

Available forms: **IV** inf 0.2% (2 mg/ml), 0.4% (4 mg/ml), 0.8% (8 mg/ml); **IV** admixture 4% (40 mg/ml), 10% (100 mg/ml), 20% (200 mg/ml); **IV** dir 1% (10 mg/ml), 2% (20 mg/ml); IM 300 mg/3 ml; ointment (top) 2.5, 5%; cream (top) 0.5%; spray 10%; jelly 2%; viscous sol 2%; local infiltrative inj 0.5, 1%

Side effects/adverse reactions

CNS: Headache, dizziness, involuntary movement, confusion, tremor, *drowsiness,* euphoria, ***convulsions***

CV: Hypotension, bradycardia, ***heart block, cardiovascular collapse, arrest***

EENT: Tinnitus, blurred vision

GI: Nausea, vomiting, anorexia

INTEG: Rash, urticaria, edema, swelling, burning, stinging

MISC: Febrile response, phlebitis at inj site

Contraindications: Hypersensitivity to amides, severe heart block, supraventricular dysrhythmias, Adams-Stokes syndrome, Wolff-Parkinson-White syndrome

Precautions: Pregnancy **B**, P lactation, children, renal disease, liver disease, CHF, respiratory depression, malignant hyperthermia

Pharmacokinetics

Absorption	Complete bioavailability (IV)
Distribution	Erythrocytes, cardiovascular endothelium
Metabolism	Liver
Excretion	Kidneys
Half-life	Biphasic 8 min, 1-2 hr

Pharmacodynamics

	IV	IM	TOP
Onset	2 min	5-15 min	Unknown
Peak	Unknown	½ hr	5 min
Duration	20 min	1½ hr	½-1 hr

Interactions

Drug/drug:

Individual drugs

Cimetidine: ↓ metabolism, ↑ toxicity
Procainamide: ↑ toxicity
Propranolol: ↑ toxicity
Phenytoin: ↑ toxicity
Quinidine: ↑ toxicity

Drug classifications

β-Blockers: ↑ toxicity

Lab test interferences

Increase: Liver function tests

NURSING CONSIDERATIONS

Assessment

• Assess for oxygenation or perfusion deficit: decreased B/P, chest pain, dizziness, loss of consciousness
• Assess respiratory status: auscultate lung fields for bibasilar crackles in patients with advanced CHF
• Assess for urinary retention: check for pain, abdominal absorption, palpate bladder; check males with benign prostatic hypertrophy; anticholinergic reaction may cause retention
• Monitor I&O ratio, electrolytes (potassium, sodium, chloride); watch for decreasing urinary output, possible retention
• Monitor liver function studies: AST (SGOT), ALT (SGPT), bilirubin, alkaline phosphatase
• Monitor ECG continuously to determine drug effectiveness, measure PR, QRS, QT intervals, check for PVCs, other dysrhythmias; monitor B/P continuously for hypotension, hypertension; check for rebound hypertension after 1-2 hr, prolonged PR/QT intervals, QRS complex; if QT or QRS increases by 50% or more, withhold next dose, notify prescriber
• Monitor for CNS symptoms: confusion, numbness, depression, involuntary movements; if these occur, drug should be discontinued
• Monitor blood levels (therapeutic level 1.5-5 μg/ml),

notify prescriber of abnormal results

Associated nursing diagnoses

- ✓ Cardiac output, decreased (uses)
- ✓ Impaired gas exchange (adverse reactions)
- ✓ Knowledge deficit (teaching)

Implementation

IM route

- Administer in deltoid, aspirate to prevent **IV** administration
- Check site daily for extravasation

IV route

- Give **IV** bolus undiluted (1%, 2% only); give 6 mg or less over 1 min; if using an **IV** line, use port near insertion site, flush with normal saline (50 ml)
- Store at room temp; sol should be clear
- Give by cont inf after adding 1 g/250-1000 ml D_5W; give 1-4 mg/min; use inf pump for correct dosage; pediatric inf is 120 mg of lidocaine/100 ml of D_5W; 1-2.5 ml/kg/hr = 20-50 μg/kg/min; use only 1%, 2% sol

Solution compatibilities:

D_5W, D_5/0.9% NaCl, D_5/0.45% NaCl, D_5/LR, LR, 0.9% NaCl, 0.45% NaCl

Syringe compatibilities:

Carbenicillin, glycopyrrolate, heparin, hydroxyzine, methicillin, metoclopramide, milrinone, moxalactam, nalbuphine

Syringe incompatibility:

Cefazolin

Y-site compatibilities:

Altaplase, amiodarone, amrinone, cefazolin, diltiazem, dobutamine, enalaprilat, famotidine, haloperidol, heparin with hydrocortisone sodium succinate, labetalol, meperidine, morphine, nitroglycerin, nitroprusside, potassium chloride, streptokinase, vitamin B with C

Additive compatibilities:

Aminophylline, amiodarone, bretylium, calcium chloride, calcium gluceptate, calcium gluconate, chloramphenicol, chlorothiazide, cimetidine, dexamethasone, digoxin, diphenhydramine, dobutamine, dopamine, ephedrine, erythromycin lactobionate, floxacillin, furosemide, heparin, hydrocortisone sodium succinate, hydroxyzine, regular insulin, mephentermine, metaraminol, nitroglycerin, penicillin G potassium, oxytetracycline, pentobarbital, phenylephrine, potassium chloride, procainamide, prochlorperazine, promazine, ranitidine, sodium bicarbonate, tetracycline, verapamil, vitamin B with C

Additive incompatibilities:

Methohexital, phenytoin; do not admix with blood transfusions

Infiltration

Physician may order lidocaine with epinephrine to minimize

systemic absorption and prolong local anesthesia

Patient/family education

- Teach patient or family reason for use of medication and expected results
- Instruct patient in at-home use of Lidopen Auto-Injector; patient should call prescriber before use if heart attack is imminent

Evaluation

Positive therapeutic outcome

- Decreased B/P, dysrhythmias
- Decreased heart rate
- Normal sinus rhythm

Treatment of overdose: Oxygen, artificial ventilation, ECG, administer dopamine for circulatory depression, diazepam or thiopental for convulsions, decreased drug or discontinuation may be required

lindane

(lin-dane)

Bio-Well, GBH ✤, G-Well, Kwell, Kwellada ✤, Kwildane, lindane, Scabene, Thionex

Func. class.: Scabicide/pediculicide

Chem. class.: Chlorinated hydrocarbon (synthetic)

Pregnancy category B

Action: Stimulates nervous system of arthropods, resulting in seizures, death of organism

Therapeutic Outcome: Resolution of infestation

Uses: Scabies, lice (head/pubic/body), nits

Dosage and routes

Lice

P *Adult and child:* Cream/lotion: wash area with soap and water 8-12 hr after application; may reapply in 1 wk if needed; shampoo using 30 ml: work into lather, rub for 5 min, rinse, dry with towel; use fine-toothed comb to remove nits

Scabies

P *Adult and child:* Top apply 1% cream/lotion to skin from neck to bottom of feet, toes; repeat in 1 wk if necessary

Available forms: Lotion, shampoo, cream (1%)

Side effects/adverse reactions

CNS: Tremors, ***convulsions,*** stimulation, dizziness (chronic inhalation of vapors)
CV: ***Ventricular fibrillation*** (chronic inhalation of vapors)
GI: Nausea, vomiting, diarrhea, liver damage (inhalation of vapors)
HEMA: Aplastic anemia (chronic inhalation of vapors)
INTEG: Pruritus, rash, irritation, contact dermatitis

Contraindications: Hypersensitivity, P premature neonate, patients with known seizure disorders, inflammation of skin, abrasions, or breaks in skin

Precautions: Pregnancy **B**, P children <10 yr, infants, lactation; avoid contact with eyes

Pharmacokinetics

Absorption	20% (Top)
Distribution	Fat
Metabolism	Liver
Excretion	Kidneys
Half-life	18 hr

Pharmacodynamics

	TOP
Onset	Rapid
Peak	Rapid
Duration	3 hr

Interactions
Drug/drug:

Oil based hair dressing: ↑ absorption; wash, rinse, and dry hair before using lindane

NURSING CONSIDERATIONS
Assessment

- Assess head, hair for lice and nits before and after treatment; if scabies are present, check all skin surfaces
- Identify source of infection: school, family members, sexual contacts

Associated nursing diagnoses

✓ Skin integrity, impaired (uses)
✓ Knowledge deficit (teaching)

Implementation

Top route

- Apply to body areas, scalp only; do not apply to face, lips, mouth, eyes, any mucous membrane, anus, or meatus
- Give top corticosteroids as ordered to decrease contact dermatitis; provide antihistamines
- Apply menthol or phenol lotions to control itching
- Give top antibiotics for infection
- Provide isolation until areas on skin, scalp have cleared and treatment is completed
- Remove nits by using a fine-toothed comb rinsed in vinegar after treatment; use gloves

Patient/family education

- Advise patient to wash all inhabitants' clothing, using insecticide; preventive treatment may be required of all persons living in same house, using lotion or shampoo to decrease spread of infection; use rubber gloves when applying drug
- Instruct patient that itching may continue for 4-6 wk; that drug must be reapplied if accidently washed off, or treatment will be ineffective
- Advise patient not to apply to face; if accidental contact with eyes occurs, flush with water
- Advise patient that sexual contacts should be treated simultaneously

Evaluation

Positive therapeutic outcome

- Decreased crusts, nits, brownish trails on skin, itching papules in skinfolds
- Decreased itching after several wk

Treatment of ingestion:

Gastric lavage, saline laxatives,

L

IV diazepam (Valium) for convulsions (if taken orally)

liothyronine (T_3)
(lye-oh-thye'roe-neen)
Cytomel, L-Triiodothyronine, liothyronine sodium, Triostat, T_3
Func. class.: Thyroid hormone
Chem. class.: Synthetic T_3
Pregnancy category **A**

Action: Controls protein synthesis; increases metabolic rates, cardiac output, renal blood blow, O_2 consumption, body temp, blood volume, growth, development at cellular level

Therapeutic Outcome: Correction of lack of thyroid hormone

Uses: Hypothyroidism, myxedema coma, thyroid hormone replacement, cretinism, nontoxic goiter, T_3 suppression test

Dosage and routes

Adult: PO 25 μg qd, increased by 12.5-25 μg q1-2 wk until desired response, maintenance dosage 25-75 μg qd

Cretinism

P *Child >3 yr:* PO 50-100 μg qd

P *Child <3 yr:* PO 5 μg qd, increased by 5 μg q3-4 days titrated to response

Myxedema, severe hypothyroidism

Adult: PO 5 μg qd; may increase by 5-10 μg q1-2 wk; maintenance dosage 50-100 μg qd

Myxedema coma/precoma

Adult: **IV** 25-50 μg initially; G 5 μg in elderly; 10-20 μg in cardiac disease; give doses q4-12h

Nontoxic goiter

Adult: PO 5 μg qd, increased by 12.5-25 μg q1-2 wk; maintenance dosage 75 μg qd

Suppression test (T_3)

Adult: PO 75-100 μg qd × 1 wk; ^{131}I is given before and after 1st wk dose

Available forms: Tab 5, 25, 50 μg; inj 10 μg/ml

Side effects/adverse reactions

CNS: *Insomnia, tremors,* headache, ***thyroid storm***
CV: *Tachycardia, palpitations, angina, dysrhythmias,* hypertension, cardiac arrest
GI: Nausea, diarrhea, increased or decreased appetite, cramps
MISC: Menstrual irregularities, weight loss, sweating, heat intolerance, fever

Contraindications: Adrenal insufficiency, MI, thyrotoxicosis

G **Precautions:** Elderly, angina pectoris, hypertension, ischemia, cardiac disease, pregnancy **A**, lactation

Pharmacokinetics

Absorption	Well (PO); complete (IV)
Distribution	Widely distributed; does not cross placenta
Metabolism	Liver
Excretion	Feces via bile, breast milk
Half-life	6-7 days

Pharmacodynamics

	PO/IV
Onset	Unknown
Peak	12-24 hr
Duration	72 hr

Interactions

Drug/drug:

Individual drugs

Cholestyramine: ↓ absorption of thyroid hormone
Colestipol: ↓ absorption of thyroid hormone
Digitalis: ↓ effect of digitalis
Insulin: ↑ requirement for insulin
Phenytoin (IV): ↑ release of thyroid hormone

Drug classifications

Amphetamines: ↑ CNS, cardiac stimulation
β-Adrenergic blockers: ↓ effect of β-blockers
Decongestants: ↑ CNS, cardiac stimulation
Oral anticoagulants: ↑ requirements for anticoagulants
Vasopressors: ↑ CNS, cardiac stimulation

Lab test interferences

Increase: CPK, LDH, AST (SGOT), PBI, blood glucose
Decrease: TSH, RAIU, uric acid, triglycerides

NURSING CONSIDERATIONS

Assessment

• Identify if the patient is taking anticoagulants, antidiabetic agents; document on patient record
• Take B/P, pulse before each dose; monitor I&O ratio and weight every day in same clothing, using same scale, at same time of day
• Monitor height, weight, psychomotor development, and growth rate if given to a P child
• Monitor T_3, T_4, FTIs, which are decreased; radioimmunoassay of TSH, which is increased; RAIU, which is increased if patient is on too low a dosage of medication
• Monitor pro-time; may require decreased anticoagulant; check for bleeding, bruising
• Assess for increased nervousness, excitability, irritability, which may indicate too high a dosage, usually after 1-3 wk of treatment
• Assess cardiac status: angina, palpitations, chest pain, change G in VS; elderly patients may have undetected cardiac problems, and baseline ECG should be completed before treatment

Associated nursing diagnoses

✓ Knowledge deficit (teaching)
✓ Noncompliance (teaching)

Implementation

PO route

• Give in AM if possible as a single dose to decrease sleeplessness; give at same time each day to maintain drug level

L

• Give only for hormone imbalances; not to be used for obesity, male infertility, menstrual conditions, lethargy; give lowest dosage that relieves symptoms; give lower dosage **G** to the elderly and for cardiac diseases
• Store in air-tight, light-resistant container

IV **IV route**
• Administer **IV** for myxedema coma and precoma; do not give IM or SC; give q4-12h; use PO dose as soon as feasible

Patient/family education

• Teach patient that drug is not a cure but controls symptoms, and treatment is long term
• Instruct patient to report excitability, irritability, anxiety, sweating, heat intolerance, chest pain, palpitations, which indicate overdose
• Advise patient not to switch brands unless approved by prescriber; bioavailability may differ; do not take with food or absorption will be decreased
• Teach patient that drug may be discontinued after giving birth; thyroid panel will be evaluated after 1-2 mo
• Teach patient that hyperthy- **P** roid child will show almost immediate behavior/personality change; that hair loss will occur in child but is temporary
• Caution patient that drug is not to be taken to reduce weight
• Caution patient to avoid OTC preparations with iodine; read labels; other medications should not be used unless approved by prescriber
• Teach patient to avoid iodine-rich food: iodized salt, soybeans, tofu, turnips, some seafood, some bread

Evaluation

Positive therapeutic outcome
• Absence of depression
• Weight loss
• Increased diuresis, pulse, appetite
• Absence of constipation, peripheral edema, cold intolerance, pale, cool dry skin, brittle nails, alopecia, coarse hair, menorrhagia, night blindness, paresthesias, syncope, stupor, coma, rosy cheeks
• Improved levels of T_3, T_4 by laboratory tests
P • Child: age-appropriate weight, height, and psychomotor development

Treatment of overdose:

Withhold dose for up to 1 wk; for acute overdose: gastric lavage or induce emesis, then activated charcoal; provide supportive treatment to control symptoms

liotrix

(lye'oh-trix)
Euthroid, T_3/T_4, Thyrolar
Func. class.: Thyroid hormone
Chem. class.: Levothyroxine/liothyronine (synthetic T_4, T_3)
Pregnancy category **A**

Action: Controls protein synthesis; increases metabolic rates, cardiac output, renal blood blow, O_2 consumption, body temp, blood volume, growth, development at cellular level

Therapeutic Outcome: Correction of lack of thyroid hormone

Uses: Hypothyroidism, thyroid hormone replacement

Dosage and routes

P *Adult and child:* PO 15-30 mg qd, increased by 15-30 mg q1-2 wk until desired response; may increase by 15-30 mg q2 wk in child

G *Geriatric:* PO 15-30 mg; double dose q6-8 wk until desired response

Available forms: Euthroid ½, 1, 2, 3 gr; Thyrolar ¼, ½, 1, 2, 3, gr; ½ grain = 30 mg

Side effects/adverse reactions

CNS: *Insomnia, tremors,* headache, thyroid storm
CV: *Tachycardia, palpitations, angina, dysrhythmias,* hypertension, cardiac arrest
GI: Nausea, diarrhea, increased or decreased appetite, cramps
MISC: Menstrual irregularities, weight loss, sweating, heat intolerance, fever

Contraindications: Adrenal insufficiency, MI, thyrotoxicosis

G **Precautions:** Elderly, angina pectoris, hypertension, ischemia, cardiac disease, pregnancy **A**, lactation

Pharmacokinetics

Absorption	50%-80% (T_4); 95% (T_3)
Distribution	Widely distributed; does not cross placenta
Metabolism	Liver, tissues
Excretion	Feces via bile; breast milk
Half-life	6-7 days (T_4); 2 days (T_3)

Pharmacodynamics

	PO (T_4)	PO (T_3)
Onset	Unknown	Unknown
Peak	Unknown	24-72 hr
Duration	Unknown	72 hr

Interactions

Drug/drug:

Individual drugs

Cholestyramine: ↓ absorption of thyroid hormone
Colestipol: ↓ absorption of liotrix
Digitalis: ↓ effect of digitalis
Insulin: ↑ requirement for insulin
Phenytoin (IV): ↑ release of thyroid hormone

Drug classifications

Amphetamines: ↑ CNS, cardiac stimulation
β-Adrenergic blockers: ↓ effect of β-blockers
Decongestants: ↑ CNS, cardiac stimulation
Oral anticoagulants: ↑ requirements for anticoagulants
Vasopressors: ↑ CNS, cardiac stimulation

Lab test interferences

Increase: CPK, LDH, AST (SGOT), PBI, blood glucose
Decrease: TSH, RAIU, uric acid, triglycerides

NURSING CONSIDERATIONS

Assessment

- Identify if the patient is taking anticoagulants, antidiabetic agents; document on chart
- Take B/P, pulse before each dose; monitor I&O ratio and weight every day in same clothing, using same scale, at same time of day
- Monitor height, weight, psychomotor development, and growth rate if given to a P child
- Monitor T_3, T_4, FTIs, which are decreased; radioimmunoassay of TSH, which is increased; RAIU, which is increased if patient is on too low a dosage of medication
- Monitor pro-time; may require decreased anticoagulant; check for bleeding, bruising
- Assess for increased nervousness, excitability, irritability, which may indicate too high a dosage of medication, usually after 1-3 wk of treatment
- Assess cardiac status: angina, palpitations, chest pain, change G in VS; the elderly patient may have undetected cardiac problems, and baseline ECG should be completed before treatment

Associated nursing diagnoses

✓ Knowledge deficit (teaching)
✓ Noncompliance (teaching)

Implementation

PO route

- Give in AM if possible as a single dose to decrease sleeplessness; give at same time each day to maintain drug level
- Give only for hormone imbalances; not to be used for obesity, male infertility, menstrual conditions, lethargy; give lowest dosage that relieves symptoms; give lower dosage G to the elderly and for cardiac diseases
- Store in airtight, light-resistant container
- Remove medication 4 wk before RAIU test

Patient/family education

- Teach patient that drug is not a cure but controls symptoms, and treatment is long term
- Instruct patient to report excitability, irritability, anxiety, sweating, heat intolerance, chest pain, palpitations, which indicate overdose
- Advise patient not to switch brands unless approved by prescriber; bioavailability may differ; do not take with food or absorption will be decreased
- Teach patient that drug may be discontinued after giving birth; thyroid panel will be evaluated after 1-2 mo
- Teach patient that hyperthy- P roid child will show almost immediate behavior/personality change; that hair loss will occur in child but is temporary
- Caution patient that drug is not to be taken to reduce weight
- Caution patient to avoid OTC preparations with iodine; read labels; other medications should not be used unless approved by prescriber
- Teach patient to avoid iodine-rich food: iodized salt, soybeans, tofu, turnips, some seafood, some bread

Evaluation

Positive therapeutic outcome

- Absence of depression
- Weight loss
- Increased diuresis, pulse, appetite
- Absence of constipation, peripheral edema, cold intolerance, pale, cool dry skin, brittle nails, alopecia, coarse hair, menorrhagia, night blindness, paresthesias, syncope, stupor, coma, rosy cheeks
- Improved levels of T_3, T_4 by laboratory tests
- P Child: age-appropriate weight, height, and psychomotor development

Treatment of overdose:

Withhold dose for up to 1 wk; acute overdose: gastric lavage or induce emesis, then activated charcoal; provide supportive treatment to control symptoms

lisinopril

(lyse-in'oh-pril)

Prinivil, Zestril

Func. class.: Angiotensin converting enzyme (ACE) inhibitor

Chem. class.: Enalaprilat lysine analog

Pregnancy category **C**

Action: Selectively suppresses renin-angiotensin-aldosterone system; inhibits ACE; prevents conversion of angiotensin I to angiotensin II; results in dilatation of arterial, venous vessels

Therapeutic Outcome: Decreased B/P in hypertension, decreased preload, afterload in CHF

Uses: Mild to moderate hypertension, adjunctive therapy of CHF

Dosage and routes

Hypertension

Adult: PO 10-40 mg qd; may increase to 80 mg qd if required

CHF

Adult: PO 2.5-5 mg initially with diuretics/digitalis

Available forms: Tab 5, 10, 20, 40 mg

Side effects/adverse reactions

CNS: *Vertigo,* depression, stroke, insomnia, paresthesias, *headache,* fatigue, asthenia
EENT: Blurred vision, nasal congestion
GI: Nausea, vomiting, anorexia, constipation, flatulence, GI irritation
GU: ***Proteinuria, renal insufficiency,*** sexual dysfunction, impotence
INTEG: Rash, pruritus
RESP: Cough, dyspnea

Contraindications: Hypersensitivity

Precautions: Pregnancy **C**, lactation, renal disease, hyperkalemia

Pharmacokinetics

Absorption	Variable (PO)
Distribution	Unknown
Metabolism	Not metabolized
Excretion	Kidneys, unchanged
Half-life	12 hr

Pharmacodynamics

	PO
Onset	1 hr
Peak	6-8 hr
Duration	24 hr

Interactions

Drug/drug:

Individual drugs

Alcohol: ↑ hypotension (large amounts)
Allopurinol: ↑ hypersensitivity
Digoxin: ↑ serum levels
Hydralazine: ↑ toxicity
Indomethacin: ↓ antihypertensive effect
Lithium: ↑ levels of lithium
Prazosin: ↑ toxicity

Drug classifications

Adrenergic blockers: ↑ hypotension
Antacids: ↓ absorption
Antihypertensives: ↑ hypotension
Diuretics: ↑ hypotension
Diuretics, potassium-sparing: ↑ toxicity
Ganglionic blockers: ↑ hypotension
Potassium supplements: ↑ toxicity
Sympathomimetics: ↑ toxicity

Drug/food:

High-potassium diet (bananas, orange juice, avocados, broccoli, nuts, spinach) should be avoided; hyperucemia may occur

Lab test interferences

False positive: Urine acetone

NURSING CONSIDERATIONS

Assessment

- Monitor B/P, check for orthostatic hypotension, syncope; if changes occur, dosage change may be required
- Monitor renal studies: protein, BUN, creatinine; watch for increased levels that may indicate nephrotic syndrome and renal failure; monitor renal symptoms: polyuria, oliguria, frequency, dysuria
- Establish baselines in renal, liver function tests before therapy begins
- Check potassium levels throughout treatment, although hyperkalemia rarely occurs
- Check for edema in feet, legs daily
- Assess for allergic reactions: rash, fever, pruritus, urticaria; drug should be discontinued if antihistamines fail to help

Associated nursing diagnoses

- ✓ Cardiac output, decreased (uses)
- ✓ Injury, risk for (side effects)
- ✓ Knowledge deficit (teaching)
- ✓ Noncompliance (teaching)

Implementation

PO route

- Store in tight container at 86° F (30° C) or less
- Severe hypotension may occur after 1st dose of this medication; it may be prevented by reducing or discontinuing diuretic therapy 3 days before beginning lisinopril therapy

Patient/family education

- Caution patient not to discontinue drug abruptly; advise patient to inform all health

care providers about taking this drug
- Teach patient not to use OTC products (cough, cold, allergy) unless directed by prescriber; serious side effects can occur
- Teach patient the importance of complying with dosage schedule, even if feeling better; to continue with medical regimen to decrease B/P: exercise, cessation of smoking, decreasing stress, diet modifications
- Teach patient to notify prescriber of mouth sores, sore throat, fever, swelling of hands or feet, irregular heartbeat, chest pain, coughing, shortness of breath
- Caution patient to report excessive perspiration, dehydration, vomiting, diarrhea; may lead to fall in B/P
- Emphasize the need to rise slowly to sitting or standing position to minimize orthostatic hypotension; not to exercise in hot weather or increased hypotension can occur
- Caution patient that drug may cause dizziness, fainting, light-headedness; may occur during 1st few days of therapy; to avoid activities that may be hazardous
- Teach patient how to take B/P, and normal readings for age group; advise patient to take B/P regularly

Evaluation

Positive therapeutic outcome
- Decreased B/P in hypertension
- Decreased CHF symptoms

Treatment of overdose: 0.9% NaCl **IV** inf, hemodialysis

lithium

(li'thee-um)

Carbolith ♣, Cibalith-S, Duralith, Eskalith, Eskalith CR, Lithane, lithium carbonate, Lithizine ♣, Lithonate, Lithotabs

Func. class.: Antimanic

Chem. class.: Alkali metal ion salt

Pregnancy category D

Action: May alter sodium, potassium ion transport across cell membrane in nerve, muscle cells; may balance biogenic amines of norepinephrine, serotonin in CNS areas involved in emotional responses

➔ Therapeutic Outcome: Stable mood

Uses: Manic-depressive illness (manic phase), prevention of bipolar manic-depressive psychosis

Dosage and routes

Adult: PO 300-600 mg tid; maintenance 300 mg tid or qid; slow rel tab 300 mg bid; dosage should be individualized to maintain blood levels at 0.5-1.5 mEq/L

P ***Child:*** PO 15-20 mg (0.4-0.5 mEq)/kg/day in 2-3 divided doses

Available forms: Cap 300, 600 mg; tab 300 mg; controlled rel tab 450 mg; syrup 300 mg/5 ml (8 mEq/5 ml); slow rel cap 150, 300 mg ♣

Side effects/adverse reactions

CNS: *Headache, drowsiness, dizziness, tremors,* twitching, ataxia, ***seizure,*** slurred speech, restlessness, *confusion,* stupor, memory loss, clonic movements, *fatigue*
CV: *Hypotension,* ECG changes, dysrhythmias, ***circulatory collapse, edema***
EENT: Tinnitus, blurred vision, aphasia, dysarthria
ENDO: Hypothyroidism, goiter, hyperglycemia, hyperthyroidism
GI: *Dry mouth, anorexia, nausea, vomiting, diarrhea,* incontinence, abdominal pain, metallic taste
GU: Polyuria, glycosuria, proteinuria, albuminuria, urinary incontinence, polydipsia, edema, ***renal toxicity***
HEMA: Leukocytosis
INTEG: Drying of hair, alopecia, rash, pruritus, hyperkeratosis, *acneiform rash, folliculitis*
MS: *Muscle weakness,* rigidity
SYST: Hyponatremia

Contraindications: Hepatic disease, renal disease, brain trauma, OBS, pregnancy **D**, lactation, schizophrenia, severe cardiac disease, severe renal disease, severe dehydration

G **Precautions:** Elderly, thyroid disease, seizure disorders, diabetes mellitus, syst infection, urinary retention, P children <12 yr

Pharmacokinetics

Absorption	Completely absorbed (PO)
Distribution	Reabsorbed by renal tubules (80%); crosses blood-brain barrier; crosses placenta
Metabolism	Unknown
Excretion	Urine, unchanged
Half-life	18-36 hr depending on age

Pharmacodynamics

	PO
Onset	Rapid
Peak	½-4 hr
Duration	Unknown

Interactions

Drug/drug:

Individual drugs
Acetazolamide: ↑ renal clearance
Aminophylline: ↑ renal clearance
Calcium iodide: ↑ hypothyroid effect
Haloperidol: Brain damage
Iodinated glycerol: ↑ hypothyroid effect
Indomethacin: ↑ toxicity
Mannitol: ↑ renal clearance
Potassium: ↑ hypothyroid effect
Sodium bicarbonate: ↑ renal clearance
Thioridazine: Brain damage
Urea: ↑ toxicity
Drug classifications
Phenothiazines: ↑ effect of phenothiazines
Theophyllines: ↓ effect of lithium

Lab test interferences

Increase: Potassium excretion, urine glucose, blood glucose, protein, BUN

Decrease: VMA, T_3, T_4, PBI, ^{131}I

NURSING CONSIDERATIONS

Assessment

- Assess for minor lithium toxicity: vomiting, diarrhea, poor coordination, fine motor tremors, weakness, lassitude; major toxicity: course tremors, severe thirst, tinnitus, dilute urine
- Assess weight daily; check for edema in legs, ankles, wrists; report if present; check skin turgor at least daily
- Monitor sodium intake; decreased sodium intake with decreased fluid intake may lead to lithium retention; increased sodium and fluids may decrease lithium retention
- Monitor urine for albuminuria, glycosuria, uric acid during beginning treatment, q2 mo thereafter
- Assess neuro status: LOC, gait, motor reflexes, hand tremors
- Monitor serum lithium levels weekly initially, then q2 mo (therapeutic level: 0.5-1.5 mEq/L); toxicity and therapeutic levels are very close; toxicity may occur rapidly; blood levels are drawn before the AM dose

Associated nursing diagnoses

- ✓ Ineffective individual coping (uses)
- ✓ Thought processes, altered (uses)
- ✓ Knowledge deficit (teaching)
- ✓ Noncompliance (teaching)

Implementation

PO route

- Administer reduced dosage G to elderly; give with meals to avoid GI upset
- Provide adequate fluids (2-3 L/day) to prevent dehydration during initial treatment, 1-2 L/day during maintenance

Patient/family education

- Provide patient with written information on symptoms of minor toxicity: vomiting, diarrhea, poor coordination, fine motor tremors, weakness, lassitude; major toxicity: coarse tremors, severe thirst, tinnitus, dilute urine
- Advise patient to monitor urine sp gr; emphasize need for follow-up care to determine lithium effects
- Advise patient that contraception is necessary, since lithium may harm fetus
- Caution patient not to operate machinery until lithium levels are stable and response determined; that beneficial effects may take 1-3 wk
- Provide to the patient a list of drugs that interact with lithium and discuss need for adequate salt and fluid intake

Evaluation

Positive therapeutic outcome

- Decrease in excitement, poor judgment, insomnia (manic phase)
- Decreased mood swings and lability

Treatment of overdose:

Induce emesis or lavage, maintain airway, respiratory function; dialysis for severe intoxication

lomefloxacin

(lome-flocks'a-sin)

Maxaquin

Func. class.: Antiinfective

Chem. class.: Fluoroquinolone

Pregnancy category C

Action: Interferes with conversion of intermediate DNA fragments into high-molecular-weight DNA in bacteria; DNA gyrase inhibitor

Therapeutic Outcome: Bactericidal for gram-negative organisms *Aeromonas, Citrobacter, Enterobacter, Escherichia coli, Haemophilus influenzae, Klebsiella, Legionella, Moraxella catarrhalis, Morganella morganii, Proteus vulgaris, P. mirabilis, Providencia alcalifaciens, P. rettgeri, Pseudomonas aeruginosa, Serratia* gram-positive organisms *Staphylococcus aureus, S. epidermidis, S. saprophyticus* (methicillin-resistant strains also)

Uses: Treatment of lower respiratory tract infections (pneumonia, bronchitis), genitourinary tract infections (prostatitis, UTIs), preoperatively to reduce urinary tract infections in transurethral surgical procedures

Dosage and routes

Adult: PO 400 mg/day × 7-14 days depending on type of infection

In renal impairment

Adult: PO 200 mg/dose

Prophylaxis of UTI

Adult: PO 400 mg 2-6 hr before surgery

Available forms: Tab 400 mg

Side effects/adverse reactions

CNS: Dizziness, headache, somnolence, depression, insomnia, nervousness, confusion, agitation

EENT: Visual disturbances

GI: Diarrhea, nausea, vomiting, anorexia, flatulence, heartburn, dry mouth, increased AST (SGOT), ALT (SGPT), constipation, abdominal pain, oral thrush, glossitis, stomatitis

INTEG: Rash, pruritus, urticaria, photosensitivity

Contraindications: Hypersensitivity to quinolones

P G **Precautions:** Pregnancy **C**, lactation, children, elderly, renal disease, seizure disorders, excessive exposure to sunlight

Pharmacokinetics

Absorption	Well absorbed (PO)
Distribution	Widely distributed
Metabolism	Unknown
Excretion	Kidney, unchanged
Half-life	6-8 hr; increased in renal disease

Pharmacodynamics

	PO
Onset	Unknown
Peak	1-2 hr

Interactions

Drug/drug:

Individual drugs

Cimetidine: ↑ lomefloxacin levels
Probenicid: ↑ lomefloxacin levels
Warfarin: ↑ levels of warfarin
Cyclosporine: ↑ levels of cyclosporine
Nitrofurantoin: ↓ lomefloxacin levels
Sucralfate: ↓ lomefloxacin levels

Drug classifications

Antacids: ↓ levels of lomefloxacin
Iron sulfate: ↓ levels of lomefloxacin
Zinc sulfate: ↓ levels of lomefloxacin

NURSING CONSIDERATIONS

Assessment

- Assess patient for previous sensitivity reaction
- Assess patient for signs and symptoms of infection: characteristics of wounds, sputum, urine, stool, WBC >10,000, fever; obtain baseline information before and during treatment
- Obtain C & S before beginning drug therapy to identify if correct treatment has been initiated
- Assess for allergic reactions: rash, urticaria, pruritus
- Monitor blood studies: AST (SGOT), ALT (SGPT), CBC, Hct, bilirubin, LDH, alkaline phosphatase, Coombs' test monthly if patient is on long-term therapy
- Assess bowel pattern qd; if severe diarrhea occurs, drug should be discontinued
- Assess for overgrowth of infection: perineal itching, fever, malaise, redness, pain, swelling, drainage, rash, diarrhea, change in cough, sputum
- Assess for CNS symptoms: insomnia, vertigo, headaches, agitation, confusion

Associated nursing diagnoses

- ✓ Infection, risk for (uses)
- ✓ Diarrhea (adverse reactions)
- ✓ Injury, risk for (adverse reactions)
- ✓ Knowledge deficit (teaching)
- ✓ Noncompliance (teaching)

Implementation

PO route

- Give with food for GI symptoms; give with 8 oz of water
- Do not give with iron, calcium, magnesium products or antacids, which decrease absorption

Patient/family education

- Instruct patient to take all medication prescribed for the length of time ordered; drug must be taken around the clock to maintain blood levels; do not give medication to others
- Teach patient to use sunscreen when outdoors to decrease phototoxicity
- Advise patient to increase fluids to 2 L/day to prevent crystalluria
- Caution patient to avoid driving and other hazardous activities until response is known; dizziness, confusion, drowsiness may occur

L

Evaluation

Positive therapeutic outcome

- Absence of signs/symptoms of infection (WBC <10,000, temp WNL)
- Reported improvement in symptoms of infection

lomustine

(loe-mus'teen)

CCNU, CeeNU

Func. class.: Antineoplastic alkylating agent

Chem. class.: Nitrosourea

Pregnancy category **D**

Action: Changes essential cellular ions to covalent bonding with resultant alkylation; this interferes with normal biologic function of DNA; activity is not phase specific; action is due to myelosuppression

Therapeutic Outcome: Prevention of rapid growth of malignant cells in chronic myelocytic leukemia

Uses: Hodgkin's disease, lymphomas, multiple myeloma

Investigational uses: Brain, breast, renal, GI tract, bronchogenic carcinoma; melanomas

Dosage and routes

Adult: PO 100, 130 mg/m² as a single dose q6 wk; titrate dosage to WBC level; do not give repeat dose unless WBCs are >4000/mm³, platelet count >100,000/mm³

Available forms: Cap 10, 40, 100 mg

Side effects/adverse reactions

GI: Nausea, vomiting, anorexia, stomatitis, ***hepatotoxicity***

GU: Azotemia, renal failure

HEMA: Thrombocytopenia, leukopenia, myelosuppression, anemia

INTEG: Burning at inj site

RESP: Fibrosis, pulmonary infiltrate

Contraindications: Radiation, chemotherapy, lactation, pregnancy (3rd trimesters) **D,** "blastic" phase of chronic myelocytic leukemia, hypersensitivity

Precautions: Childbearing age men and women, leukopenia, thrombocytopenia, anemia, hepatotoxicity, renal toxicity

Pharmacokinetics

Absorption	Rapidly absorbed (PO)
Distribution	Widely
Metabolism	Liver
Excretion	Kidneys, breast milk
Half-life	16-48 hr

Pharmacodynamics

Onset	Unknown
Peak	Unknown
Duration	Unknown

Interactions

Drug/drug:

Individual drugs

Radiation: ↑ toxicity, bone marrow suppression

Drug classifications

Antineoplastics: ↑ toxicity, bone marrow suppression

Lab test interferences

False positive: Cytology tests for breast, bladder, cervix, lung

NURSING CONSIDERATIONS

Assessment

- Monitor CBC, differential, platelet count weekly; withhold drug if WBC is <4000 or platelet count is <75,000; notify prescriber of results if WBC <20,000 /mm^3, platelets <150,000/mm^3
- Monitor pulmonary function tests, chest x-ray films before, during therapy; chest film should be obtained q2 wk during treatment; assess for dyspnea, rales, unproductive cough, chest pain, tachypnea
- Monitor renal function studies: BUN, serum uric acid, urine CrCl before, during therapy; I&O ratio; report fall in urine output of 30 ml/hr; check for decreased hyperuricemia
- Monitor for cold, fever, sore throat (may indicate beginning infection); identify edema in feet, joint and stomach pain, shaking; prescriber should be notified
- Assess for bleeding: hematuria, guaiac, bruising or petechiae, mucosa or orifices q8h, no rec temp

Associated nursing diagnoses

✓ Injury, risk for (adverse reactions)
✓ Body image disturbance (adverse reactions)
✓ Infection, risk for (adverse reactions)
✓ Knowledge deficit (teaching)

Implementation

PO route

- Give drug after evening meal, before hs; administer antiemetic 30-60 min before giving drug to prevent vomiting
- Give antibiotics for prophylaxis of infection may be prescribed, since infection potential is high
- Store in tight container

Patient/family education

- Teach patient to avoid use of products containing aspirin or ibuprofen, razors, commercial mouthwash, since bleeding may occur; to report symptoms of bleeding (hematuria, tarry stools)
- Advise patient to report signs of anemia (fatigue, headache, irritability, faintness, shortness of breath)
- Caution patient to report any changes in breathing or coughing even several mo after treatment; to avoid crowds and persons with respiratory tract or other infections
- Caution patient not to have any vaccinations without the advice of prescriber; serious reactions can occur
- Tell patient contraception is needed during treatment and for several mo after the completion of therapy

Evaluation

Positive therapeutic outcome

- Decreased tumor sizes
- Decreased spread of malignancy

loperamide

(loe-per'a-mide)
loperamide solution, Imodium, Imodium A-D, Imodium A-D Caplet, Loperamide, A-D Kaopectate II Caplets, Maalox Antidiarrheal Caplets, Pepto Diarrhea Control
Func. class.: Antidiarrheal
Chem. class.: Piperidine derivative
Pregnancy category B

Action: Direct action on intestinal muscles to decrease GI peristalsis; reduces volume, increases bulk; electrolytes are not lost

Uses: Diarrhea (cause undetermined), chronic diarrhea, ileostomy discharge

Dosage and routes

Adult: PO 4 mg, then 2 mg after each loose stool, not to exceed 16 mg/day

P ***Child 2-5 yr:*** PO 1 mg on day 1, then 0.1 mg/kg after each loose stool

P ***Child 5-8 yr:*** PO 2 mg bid on day 1, then 0.1 mg/kg after each loose stool

P ***Child 8-12 yr:*** PO 2 mg tid on day 1, then 0.1 mg/kg after each loose stool

Available forms: Cap 2 mg; liq 1 mg/5 ml; tab 2 mg

Side effects/adverse reactions

CNS: Dizziness, drowsiness, fatigue, fever

GI: Nausea, dry mouth, vomiting, constipation, abdominal pain, anorexia, ***toxic megacolon***

INTEG: Rash

RESP: Respiratory depression

Contraindications: Hypersensitivity, severe ulcerative colitis, pseudomembranous colitis, acute diarrhea associated with *E. coli*

Precautions: Pregnancy **B**, P lactation, children <2 yr, liver disease, dehydration, bacterial disease

Pharmacokinetics

Absorption	Poor
Distribution	Unknown
Metabolism	Liver
Excretion	Feces, unchanged; small amount in urine
Half-life	7-14 hr

Pharmacodynamics

Onset	½-1 hr
Peak	Unknown
Duration	4-5 hr

Interaction

Drug/drug:

Solutions: Do not mix with other oral sol

NURSING CONSIDERATIONS

Assessment

• Monitor electrolytes (potassium, sodium, chloride) if patient is on long-term therapy; check fluid status, skin turgor

• Assess bowel pattern before, during treatment; check for rebound constipation after termination of medication; check bowel sounds
• Check response after 48 hr; if no response, drug should be discontinued and other treatment initiated
• Assess for abdominal distention, toxic megacolon, which may occur in ulcerative colitis

Associated nursing diagnoses

✓ Diarrhea (uses)
✓ Constipation (adverse reactions)
✓ Knowledge deficit (teaching)
✓ Noncompliance (teaching)

Implementation

PO route
• Store in airtight containers

Patient/family education

• Caution patient to avoid alcohol and OTC products unless directed by prescriber; may cause increased CNS depression
• Advise patient not to exceed recommended dosage; drug may be habit forming
• Advise patient that drug may cause drowsiness and to avoid hazardous activities until response to drug is determined
• Teach patient that dry mouth can be decreased by frequent sips of water, hard candy, sugarless gum

Evaluation

Positive therapeutic outcome
• Decreased diarrhea

loracarbef

(lor-a-kar′beff)
Lorabid
Func. class.: Antiinfective
Chem. class.: Cephalosporin (2nd generation)
Pregnancy category B

Action: Inhibits bacterial cell wall synthesis, which renders cell wall osmotically unstable

➔ Therapeutic Outcome: Bactericidal for the following organisms: *gram-negative Haemophilus influenzae, Escherichia coli, Proteus mirabilis, Klebsiella;* gram-positive *Streptococcus pneumoniae, S. pyogenes, Staphylococcus aureus*

Uses: Upper and lower respiratory tract, urinary tract, skin infections; otitis media, pharyngitis, tonsillitis

Dosage and routes

P *Adult and child >13 yr:* PO 200-400 mg q12h
P *Child to 12 yr:* PO 15-30 mg/kg/day in 2 divided doses given q12h

Available forms: Cap 200 mg; oral susp 100, 200 mg/5 ml

Side effects/adverse reactions

CNS: Dizziness, headache, fatigue, paresthesia, fever, chills, confusion
GI: Diarrhea, nausea, vomiting, anorexia, dysgeusia, glossitis, bleeding, increased AST (SGOT), ALT (SGPT),

bilirubin, LDH, alkaline phosphatase, abdominal pain, loose stools, flatulence, heartburn, stomach cramps, colitis, jaundice
GU: Vaginitis, pruritus, candidiasis, increased BUN, ***nephrotoxicity, renal failure,*** pyuria, dysuria, reversible interstitial nephritis
HEMA: Leukopenia, thrombocytopenia, agranulocytosis, anemia, ***neutropenia, lymphocytosis, eosinophilia, pancytopenia, hemolytic anemia, leukocytosis, granulocytopenia***
INTEG: Rash, urticaria, dermatitis
MISC: Anaphylaxis
RESP: Dyspnea

Contraindications: Hypersensitivity to cephalosporins or related antibiotics, seizures

Precautions: Pregnancy **B**, P lactation, children, renal disease

Pharmacokinetics

Absorption	Well absorbed (PO)
Distribution	Widely distributed; crosses placenta
Metabolism	Not metabolized
Excretion	Kidneys, unchanged; enters breast milk
Half-life	1 hr; increased in renal disease

Pharmacodynamics

Onset	Rapid
Peak	1 hr

Interactions: None

Lab test interferences

Increase (false): Creatinine (serum urine), urinary 17-KS
False positive: Urinary protein, direct Coombs' test, urine glucose testing (Clinitest)
Interfere: Cross-matching

NURSING CONSIDERATIONS

Assessment

- Assess patient for previous sensitivity reaction
- Assess patient for signs and symptoms of infection: characteristics of wounds, sputum, urine, stool, WBC >10,000, earache, fever; obtain baseline information and during treatment
- Obtain C & S before beginning drug therapy to identify if correct treatment has been initiated
- Assess for allergic reactions: rash, urticaria, pruritus, chills, fever, joint pain; angioedema may occur a few days after therapy begins; epinephrine, resuscitation equipment should be available for anaphylactic reaction
- Identify urine output; if decreasing, notify prescriber (may indicate nephrotoxicity); also check for increased BUN, creatinine
- Monitor blood studies: AST (SGOT), ALT (SGPT), CBC, Hct, bilirubin, LDH, alkaline phosphatase, Coombs' test monthly if patient is on long-term therapy
- Assess bowel pattern qd; if severe diarrhea occurs, drug should be discontinued; may indicate pseudomembranous colitis
- Assess for overgrowth of infection: perineal itching, fever, malaise, redness, pain, swelling, drainage, rash, diarrhea, change in cough, sputum

Associated nursing diagnoses

- ✓ Infection, risk for (uses)
- ✓ Diarrhea (adverse reactions)
- ✓ Injury, risk for (adverse reactions)
- ✓ Knowledge deficit (teaching)
- ✓ Noncompliance (teaching)

Implementation

PO route

- Give on an empty stomach, 1 hr ac or 2 hr pc
- Oral susp should be shaken before administration

Patient/family education

- Teach patient to report sore throat, bruising, bleeding, joint pain; may indicate blood dyscrasias (rare)
- Advise patient to contact prescriber if vaginal itching, loose, foul-smelling stools, furry tongue occur; may indicate superinfection
- Advise patient to notify prescriber of diarrhea with blood or pus, which may indicate pseudomembranous colitis

Evaluation

Positive therapeutic outcome

- Absence of signs/symptoms of infection (WBC <10,000, temp WNL, absence of red, draining wounds, earache)
- Reported improvement in symptoms of infection

Treatment of anaphylaxis:

Epinephrine, antihistamines, resuscitate if needed

loratidine

(lor-a'ti-deen)

Claritin

Func. class.: Antihistamine

Chem. class.: Selective histamine (H_1) receptor antagonist

Pregnancy category **B**

Action: Binds to peripheral histamine receptors, which provides antihistamine action without sedation

➔ **Therapeutic Outcome:** Decreased nasal stuffiness, itching, swollen eyes

Uses: Seasonal rhinitis

Dosage and routes

Adult: PO 10 mg qd

Available forms: Tab 10 mg

Side effects/adverse reactions

CNS: Sedation (more common with increased dosages)

Contraindications: Hypersensitivity, acute asthma attacks, lower respiratory tract disease

Precautions: Pregnancy **B**, increased intraocular pressure, bronchial asthma

Pharmacokinetics

Absorption	Well absorbed (PO)
Distribution	Unknown
Metabolism	Liver, extensively, to active metabolites
Excretion	Kidneys
Half-life	14½ hr

L

Pharmacodynamics

Onset	Unknown
Peak	1½ hr
Duration	Unknown

Interactions

Drug/drug:

Individual drugs
Alcohol: ↑ CNS depression
Drug classifications
CNS depressants: ↑ CNS depression
Narcotics: ↑ CNS depression
Sedative/hypnotics: ↑ CNS depression

Drug/food:

↑ absorption

Lab test interferences

False negative: Skin allergy tests (discontinue antihistamine 3 days before testing)

NURSING CONSIDERATIONS

Assessment

- Assess respiratory status: rate, rhythm, increase in bronchial secretions, wheezing, chest tightness; provide fluids to 2 L/day to decrease secretion thickness

Associated nursing diagnoses

- ✓ Airway clearance, ineffective (uses)
- ✓ Knowledge deficit (teaching)
- ✓ Noncompliance (teaching, overuse)

Implementation

PO route

- Give on an empty stomach, 1 hr ac or 2 hr pc to facilitate absorption
- Store in tight, light-resistant container

Patient/family education

- Teach all aspects of drug uses; to notify prescriber if confusion, sedation, hypotension occur; to avoid driving and other hazardous activity if drowsiness occurs; to avoid alcohol and other CNS depressants that may potentiate effect
- Teach patient to take 1 hr ac or 2 hr pc to facilitate absorption
- Caution patient not to exceed recommended dosage; dysrhythmias may occur
- Teach patient hard candy, gum, frequent rinsing of mouth may be used for dryness

Evaluation

Positive therapeutic outcome

- Absence of running or congested nose

lorazepam

(lor-az′e-pam)

Alzapam, Apo-Lorazepam ✤, Ativan, Loraz, lorazepam, Novolorazem ✤

Func. class.: Sedative/hypnotic, antianxiety agent

Chem. class.: Benzodiazepine

Pregnancy category **D**

Controlled substance schedule **IV**

Action: Potentiates the actions of GABA, an inhibitory neurotransmitter, especially in the limbic system and reticular formation, which depresses the CNS

Therapeutic Outcome: Decreased anxiety, relaxation

Uses: Anxiety, irritability in psychiatric or organic disorders, preoperatively, insomnia

Dosage and routes

Anxiety

Adult: PO 2-6 mg/day in divided doses, not to exceed 10 mg/day

G ***Elderly:*** PO 0.5-2 mg/day in divided doses

Insomnia

Adult: PO 2-4 mg hs; only minimally effective after 2 wk continuous therapy

G ***Elderly:*** PO 1-2 mg initially

Preoperatively

Adult: IM 50 μg/kg 2 hr before surgery; **IV** 44 μg/kg 15-20 min before surgery

Available forms: Tab 0.5, 1, 2 mg; inj 2, 4 mg/ml; conc sol 0.2 mg/ml

Side effects/adverse reactions

CNS: Dizziness, drowsiness, confusion, headache, anxiety, tremors, stimulation, fatigue, depression, insomnia, hallucinations, weakness, unsteadiness

CV: Orthostatic hypotension, ***ECG changes, tachycardia,*** hypotension

EENT: Blurred vision, tinnitus, mydriasis

GI: Constipation, dry mouth, nausea, vomiting, anorexia, diarrhea

INTEG: Rash, dermatitis, itching

Contraindications: Hypersensitivity to benzodiazepines, narrow angle glaucoma, psychosis, P pregnancy **D**, child <12 yr, history of drug abuse, COPD

G **Precautions:** Elderly, debilitated patients, hepatic disease, renal disease

Pharmacokinetics

Absorption	Well absorbed (PO); completely absorbed (IM)
Distribution	Widely distributed; crosses placenta, blood-brain barrier
Metabolism	Liver, extensively
Excretion	Kidneys, breast milk
Half-life	14 hr

Pharmacodynamics

	PO	IM	IV
Onset	½ hr	15-30 min	5-15 min
Peak	1-3 hr	1-1½ hr	Unknown
Duration	3-6 hr	3-6 hr	3-6 hr

Interactions

Drug/drug:

Individual drugs

Alcohol: ↑ CNS depression
Cimetidine: ↑ action
Disulfiram: ↑ action
Fluoxetine: ↑ action
Levodopa: ↓ action of levodopa

Drug classifications
Analgesics, opioid: ↑ CNS depression
Antidepressants: ↑ CNS depression
Antihistamines: ↑ CNS depression

Drug/smoking:
↑ metabolism, ↓ effect

Lab test interferences
Increase: AST (SGOT), ALT (SGPT), serum bilirubin
False increase: 17-OHCS
Decrease: RAIU

NURSING CONSIDERATIONS
Assessment
- Assess degree of anxiety; what precipitates anxiety and whether drug controls symptoms; other signs of anxiety: dilated pupils, inability to sleep, restlessness, inability to focus
- Assess for alcohol withdrawal symptoms, including hallucinations (visual, auditory), delirium, irritability, agitation, fine to coarse tremors
- Monitor B/P (with patient lying/standing), pulse, check respiratory rate; if systolic B/P drops 20 mm Hg, hold drug, notify prescriber; respirations q5-15 min if given **IV**
- Monitor CBC during long-term therapy; blood dyscrasias have occurred (rarely)
- Monitor for seizure control; type, duration, and intensity of convulsions; what precipitates seizures
- Monitor hepatic studies: AST (SGOT), ALT (SGPT), bilirubin, creatinine, LDH, alkaline phosphatase
- Assess mental status: mood, sensorium, affect, sleeping pattern, drowsiness, dizziness, suicidal tendencies, and ability of drug to control these symptoms; check for tolerance, withdrawal symptoms: headache, nausea, vomiting, muscle pain, weakness after long-term use

Associated nursing diagnoses
- ✓ Sleep pattern disturbance (uses)
- ✓ Coping, ineffective individual (uses)
- ✓ Knowledge deficit (teaching)
- ✓ Noncompliance (teaching)

Implementation
PO route
- Give with food or milk for GI symptoms; crush tab if patient is unable to swallow medication whole; provide sugarless gum, hard candy, frequent sips of water for dry mouth
- Use by SL route for rapid response (investigational use)

IM route
- Give deep in muscle mass; if using for preoperative sedation, give 2 hr or more before surgical procedure

IV **IV route**
- Dilute with sterile water for inj, 0.9% NaCl, or D_5W just before using; give by Y-site or 3-way stopcock at 2 mg/min
- Do not use sol that is discolored or contains a precipitate

Syringe compatibility:
Cimetidine

Y-site incompatibilities:
Idarubicin, ondansetron, sargramostim

Y-site compatibilities:
Acyclovir, atracurium, fludarabine, melphalan, paclitaxel, pancuronium, vecuronium, vinorelbine, zidovudine

Patient/family education

- Advise patient that drug may be taken with food; that drug is not to be used for everyday stress or used longer than 4 mo unless directed by a prescriber; to take no more than prescribed amount; may be habit forming
- Caution patient to avoid OTC preparations unless approved by prescriber; to avoid alcohol, other psychotropic medications unless prescribed by physician; not to discontinue medication abruptly after long-term use
- Inform patient to avoid driving and activities that require alertness; drowsiness may occur; to rise slowly or fainting G may occur, especially in elderly
- Inform patient that drowsiness may worsen at beginning of treatment

Evaluation

Positive therapeutic outcome

- Decreased anxiety, restlessness, insomnia

Treatment of overdose: Lavage, VS, supportive care

losartan
Cozaar
Func. class.: Antihypertensive
Chem. class.: Angiotensin II receptor (Type AT_1)
Pregnancy category N/A

Action: Blocks the vasoconstrictor and aldosterone-secreting effects of angiotensin II; selectively blocks the binding of angiotensin II to the AT_1 receptor found in tissues

Therapeutic Outcome: Decreased B/P

Uses: Hypertension, alone or in combination

Dosage and routes
Adult: PO mg qd alone or 25 mg qd when used in combination

Available forms: Tab 25, 50 mg

Side effects/adverse reactions
CNS: Dizziness, insomnia, anxiety, confusion, abnormal dreams, migraine, tremor, vertigo
CV: Angina pectoris, 2nd degree AV block, ***cerebrovascular accident,*** hypotension, *myocardial infarction, dysrhythmias*
EENT: Blurred vision, burning eyes, conjunctivitis, task perversion
GI: Diarrhea, dyspepsia, anorexia, constipation, dry mouth, flatulence, gastritis, vomiting
GU: Impotence, nocturia, urinary frequency, urinary tract infection
HEMA: Anemia
INTEG: Alopecia, dermatitis, dry skin, flushing, photosensitivity, rash, pruritus, sweating
META: Gout

MS: Cramps, myalgia, pain, stiffness
RESP: ***Cough, upper respiratory infection,*** congestion, dyspnea, bronchitis

Contraindications: Hypersensitivity

Precautions: Hypersensitivity to ACE inhibitors; Pregnancy category **C** 1st trimester, **D** 2nd, 3rd trimester; lactation, P children, G elderly

Pharmacokinetics

Absorption	Well (PO)
Distribution	Bound to plasma proteins
Metabolism	Extensive
Excretion	Feces, urine
Half-life	Biphasic, 2 hr, 6-9 hr

Pharmacodynamics

Onset	Unknown
Peak	Unknown
Duration	Unknown

Interactions: None significant

NURSING CONSIDERATIONS

Assessment

- Assess B/P, pulse q4h; note rate, rhythm, quality
- Monitor electrolytes: potassium, sodium, chloride
- Obtain baselines in renal, liver function tests before therapy begins
- Monitor for edema in feet, legs daily
- Assess for skin turgor, dryness of mucous membranes for hydration status

Associated nursing diagnoses

- ✓ Fluid volume deficit (side effects)
- ✓ Noncompliance (teaching)
- ✓ Knowledge deficit (teaching)

Implementation

- Administer without regard to meals

Patient/family education

- Teach patient to avoid sunlight or wear sunscreen if in sunlight; photosensitivity may occur
- Advise patient to comply with dosage schedule, even if feeling better
- Teach patient to notify prescriber of mouth sores, fever, swelling of hands or feet, irregular heartbeat, chest pain
- Advise patient excessive perspiration, dehydration, vomiting, diarrhea; may lead to fall in blood pressure—consult prescriber if these occur
- Inform patient that drug may cause dizziness, fainting; light-headedness may occur
- Caution patient to rise slowly to sitting or standing position to minimize orthostatic hypotension

Evaluation

Positive therapeutic outcome

- Decreased B/P

lovastatin

(loe'va-sta-tin)

Mevacor

Func. class.: Cholesterol-lowering agent

Chem. class.: Aspergillus terreus strain derivative

Pregnancy category X

Action: Inhibits biosynthesis of VLDL and LDL, which are responsible for cholesterol development

➔ **Therapeutic Outcome:** Decreased cholesterol levels and LDLs, increased HDLs

Uses: As an adjunct in primary hypercholesterolemia (types IIa, IIb), mixed hyperlipidemia

Dosage and routes

(Patient should first be placed on a cholesterol-lowering diet)

Adult: PO 20 mg qd with evening meal; may increase to 20-80 mg/day in single or divided doses; not to exceed 80 mg/day; dosage adjustments should be made monthly

Available forms: Tab 20, 40 mg

Side effects/adverse reactions

CNS: Dizziness, headache
EENT: Blurred vision, dysgeusia, lens opacities
GI: Nausea, constipation, diarrhea, dyspepsia, flatus, abdominal pain, heartburn, ***liver dysfunction***
INTEG: Rash, pruritus
MS: Muscle cramps, myalgia, ***myositis, rhabdomyolysis***

Contraindications: Hypersensitivity, pregnancy **X**, lactation, active liver disease

Precautions: Past liver disease, alcoholism, severe acute infections, trauma, hypotension, uncontrolled seizure disorders, severe metabolic disorders, electrolyte imbalances, visual condition, P children

Pharmacokinetics

Absorption	Poorly absorbed, erratic (PO)
Distribution	Crosses placenta, blood-brain barrier
Metabolism	Liver, extensively
Excretion	Bile, feces, kidneys
Half-life	Unknown

Pharmacodynamics

Onset	Unknown
Peak	2-4 hr
Duration	Unknown

Interactions

Drug/drug:

Individual drugs

Cholestyramine: ↑ action
Colestipol: ↑ action
Cyclosporine: ↑ risk of myopathy
Erythromycin: ↑ risk of myopathy
Gemfibrozil: ↑ risk of myopathy
Niacin: ↑ risk of myopathy

Drug/food:

↑ levels of lovastatin with food

Lab test interferences

Increased: CPK, liver function tests

NURSING CONSIDERATIONS

Assessment

- Assess nutrition: fat, protein, carbohydrates; nutritional

analysis should be completed by dietician before treatment
• Monitor bowel pattern daily; diarrhea may be a problem
• Monitor triglycerides, cholesterol at baseline and throughout treatment; LDL and VLDL should be watched closely; if increased, drug should be discontinued

Associated nursing diagnoses

✓ Diarrhea (adverse reactions)
✓ Knowledge deficit (teaching)
✓ Noncompliance (teaching)

Implementation

PO route
• Give with evening meal; if dosage is increased, take with breakfast and evening meal
• Store in cool environment in airtight, light-resistant container

Patient/family education

• Inform patient that compliance is needed for positive results to occur; not to double doses
• Teach patient that risk factors should be decreased: high-fat diet, smoking, alcohol consumption, absence of exercise
• Advise patient to notify prescriber if the GI symptoms of diarrhea, abdominal or epigastric pain, nausea, vomiting occur; or if chills, fever, sore throat occur

Evaluation

Positive therapeutic outcome
• Decreased cholesterol levels, serum triglyceride
• Improved ratio of HDLs

loxapine

(lox'a-peen)
Loxapac ✤, loxapine succinate, Loxitane IM, Loxitane, Loxitane-C
Func. class.: Antipsychotic/neuroleptic
Chem. class.: Dibenzoxazepine
Pregnancy category C

Action: Depresses cerebral cortex, hypothalamus, limbic system, which control activity and aggression; blocks neurotransmission produced by dopamine at synapse; exhibits strong α-adrenergic, anticholinergic blocking action; mechanism for antipsychotic effects is unclear

➡ **Therapeutic Outcome:** Decreased psychotic behavior

Uses: Psychotic disorders

Investigational uses: Depression, anxiety

Dosage and routes

Adult: PO 10 mg bid-qid initially; may be rapidly increased depending on severity of condition; maintenance 60-100 mg/day; IM 12.5-50 mg q4-6h or more until desired response, then start PO form

Available forms: Cap 5, 10, 25, 50 mg; conc 25 mg/ml; inj 50 mg/ml

Side effects/adverse reactions

CNS: Extrapyramidal symptoms: pseudoparkin-

sonism, akathisia, dystonia, tardive dyskinesia, drowsiness, headache, ***seizures,*** confusion, neuroleptic malignant syndrome
CV: Orthostatic hypotension, ***cardiac arrest,*** ECG changes, tachycardia
EENT: Blurred vision, glaucoma
GI: Dry mouth, nausea, vomiting, anorexia, constipation, diarrhea, jaundice, weight gain
GU: Urinary retention, urinary frequency, enuresis, impotence, amenorrhea, gynecomastia
HEMA: ***Anemia, leukopenia, leukocytosis, agranulocytosis***
INTEG: Rash, photosensitivity, dermatitis
RESP: ***Laryngospasm,*** dyspnea, ***respiratory depression***

Contraindications: Hypersensitivity, blood dyscrasias, coma, brain damage, bone marrow depression, alcohol and barbiturate withdrawal states

Precautions: Pregnancy **C**, lactation, seizure disorders, hepatic disease, cardiac disease, prostatic hypertrophy, cardiac conditions **P** child <16 yr, glaucoma, GI obstruction

Pharmacokinetics

Absorption	Well absorbed (PO)
Distribution	Unknown
Metabolism	Liver, extensively
Excretion	Kidneys
Half-life	Biphasic 5 hr, 19 hr

Pharmacodynamics

	PO	IM
Onset	½ hr	15-30 min
Peak	2-4 hr	15-20 min
Duration	12 hr	12 hr

Interactions

Drug/drug:

Individual drugs

Alcohol: ↑ effects of both drugs, oversedation
Aluminum hydroxide: ↓ absorption
Epinephrine: ↑ toxicity
Guanethidine: ↓ antihypertensive response
Guanadrel: ↓ antihypertensive response
Magnesium hydroxide: ↓ absorption

Drug classifications

Analgesics, narcotic: ↑ CNS depression
Anticholinergics: ↑ anticholinergic effects
Antidepressants: ↑ CNS depression
Antihistamines: ↑ CNS depression
Barbiturate anesthetics: ↑ CNS depression
MAOI: ↑ CNS depression
Sedatives/hypnotics: ↑ CNS depression

NURSING CONSIDERATIONS

Assessment

- Assess mental status: orientation, mood, behavior, presence and type of hallucinations before initial administration and monthly; this drug should significantly reduce psychotic behavior
- Check for swallowing of PO medication; check for hoarding

or giving of medication to other patients
- Monitor I&O ratio; palpate bladder if low urinary output G occurs, especially in elderly; urinalysis recommended before, during prolonged therapy
- Monitor bilirubin, CBC, liver function studies monthly
- Assess affect, orientation, LOC, reflexes, gait, coordination, sleep pattern disturbances
- Monitor B/P with patient sitting, standing, and lying; take pulse and respirations q4h during initial treatment; establish baseline before starting treatment; report drops of 30 mm Hg
- Check for dizziness, faintness, palpitations, tachycardia on rising; severe orthostatic hypotension is common
- Identify for neuroleptic malignant syndrome: hyperpyrexia, muscle rigidity, increased CPK, altered mental status; drug should be discontinued
- Assess for EPS including akathisia (inability to sit still, no pattern to movements), tardive dyskinesia (bizarre movements of the jaw, mouth, tongue, extremities), pseudoparkinsonism (ragged tremors, pill rolling, shuffling gate); an antiparkinsonian drug should be prescribed
- Assess for constipation, urinary retention daily; if these occur, increase bulk, water in diet

Associated nursing diagnoses

✓ Thought processes, altered (uses)
✓ Coping, ineffective individual (uses)
✓ Knowledge deficit (teaching)
✓ Noncompliance (teaching)

Implementation

PO route
- Administer drug in liq form mixed in glass of juice or cola if hoarding is suspected; do not mix in caffeine drinks, tannics, pectins
- Administer lowered dose in G elderly, since metabolism is slowed
- Administer with full glass of water or milk; or give with food to decrease GI upset
- Store in airtight, light-resistant container, oral sol in amber bottle

IM route
- Inject deep in muscle mass; do not give SC; do not administer sol with a precipitate; amber-colored sol can be used

Patient/family education

- Teach patient to use good oral hygiene; suggest frequent rinsing of mouth, sugarless gum for dry mouth
- Caution patient to avoid hazardous activities until drug response is determined; dizziness, blurred vision may occur
- Inform patient that orthostatic hypotension occurs often and to rise from sitting or lying position gradually; to remain lying down after IM inj for at least 30 min; caution patient to avoid hot tubs, hot showers, tub baths, since hypotension may occur; tell patient that in

hot weather heat stroke may occur; take extra precautions to stay cool

- Advise patient to avoid abrupt withdrawal of this drug, or EPS may result; drug should be withdrawn slowly
- Teach patient to avoid OTC preparations (cough, hay fever, cold) unless approved by prescriber, since serious drug interactions may occur; avoid use with alcohol, CNS depressants; increased drowsiness may occur
- Advise patient to use a sunscreen and sunglasses to prevent burns
- Teach patient about EPS and necessity of meticulous oral hygiene, since oral candidiasis may occur
- Suggest patient take antacids 2 hr before or after taking this drug
- Instruct patient to report sore throat, malaise, fever, bleeding, mouth sores; if these occur, CBC should be drawn and drug discontinued

Evaluation

Positive therapeutic outcome

- Decrease in emotional excitement, hallucinations, delusions, paranoia
- Reorganization of patterns of thought, speech

Treatment of overdose: Lavage if orally ingested; barbiturates; provide airway, **IV** fluids; do not use epinephrine, which may increase hypotension

magaldrate

(mag'al-drate)

Antiflux ♣, Lowsium, Riopan, Riopan Extra Strength

Func. class.: Antacid

Chem. class.: Aluminum/magnesium hydroxide

Pregnancy category **C**

Action: Neutralizes gastric acidity; drug is dissolved in gastric contents; this drug is a combination of aluminum and magnesium

➔ Therapeutic Outcome: Decreased pain of ulcers

Uses: Antacid, peptic ulcer disease (adjunct), indigestion/heartburn, duodenal and gastric ulcers, reflex esophagitis, hyperacidity

Dosage and routes

Adult: PO 1-2 tab (480-1080 mg) between meals, hs, not to exceed 20 tab/day; 1-2 chew tab (480-960 mg) between meals, hs, not to exceed 20 tab/day; susp 5-10 ml (400-800 mg) with water between meals, hs, not to exceed 100 ml/day

Available forms: Tab 480 mg; chew tab 480 mg; susp 540 mg/5 ml, 480 mg/5 ml, 1080 mg/5 ml

Side effects/adverse reactions

GI: Constipation, diarrhea
META: Hypermagnesemia, hypophosphatemia

M

Contraindications: Hypersensitivity to this drug or aluminum products

G **Precautions:** Elderly, fluid restriction, decreased GI motility, GI obstruction, dehydration, renal disease, sodium-restricted diets, pregnancy **C**

Pharmacokinetics

Absorption	Not absorbed
Distribution	Not distributed
Metabolism	Not metabolized
Excretion	Kidneys
Half-life	Unknown

Pharmacodynamics

Onset	Unknown
Peak	½ hrs
Duration	1 hr

Interactions

Drug/drug:

Individual drugs

Chlordiazepoxide:↓ absorption of chlordiazapoxide
Cimetidine: ↓ absorption of cimetidine
Ketoconazole: ↓ effect of ketoconazole
Phenytoin: ↓ absorption of phenytoin
Tetracycline: ↓ effect of tetracycline

Drug classifications

Anticholinergics: ↓ absorption of anticholinergics
Corticosteroids: ↓ absorption of corticosteroids
Iron salts: ↓ absorption of iron salts
Phenothiazines: ↓ absorption of phenothiazines
Salicylates: ↓ absorption of salicylates

NURSING CONSIDERATIONS

Assessment

- Assess GI status: location of pain, intensity, characteristics, what aggravates, ameliorates pain; heartburn/indigestion; hematemesis
- Monitor serum magnesium levels with impaired renal function
- Assess for constipation: increase bulk in diet if needed or obtain order for stool softener

Associated nursing diagnoses

✓ Pain (uses)
✓ Knowledge deficit (teaching)

Implementation

PO route

- Give laxatives or stool softeners if constipation occurs
- Give susp after shaking; give between meals and hs
- Give when stomach is empty pc and hs

Patient/family education

- Advise patient to separate ingestion of enteric-coated drugs and antacid by 1 hr
- Advise patient to use 2 wk or less; drug should not be used for long periods
- Teach patient to notify prescriber immediately if coffee-ground emesis, emesis with frank blood, or black tarry stools occur

Evaluation

Positive therapeutic outcome

- Absence of abdominal pain
- Decreased acidity

magnesium hydroxide

Concentrated Phillip's Milk of Magnesia, Milk of Magnesia, Phillip's Milk of Magnesia

Func. class.: Laxative, saline; antacid

Pregnancy category **B**

Action: Increases osmotic pressure; draws fluid into the lumen of the colon; neutralizes hydrochloric acid

➔ **Therapeutic Outcome:** Decreased constipation, decreased gastric acidity

Uses: Constipation, bowel preparation before surgery or examination; antacid

Dosage and routes

Laxative

Adult: PO 30-60 ml hs (milk of magnesia)

P ***Adult and child >6 yr:*** PO 15 g in 8 oz water; PO 10-20 ml (conc milk of magnesia)

Antacid

P ***Adult and child >12 yr:*** PO 5-15 ml (liq), 650-1300 mg (tab) qid

P ***Child 2-6 yr:*** 5-15 ml (milk of magnesia)

Available forms: Liq 395 mg/5 ml; chew tab 300, 600 mg; conc liq 1.2 gm/5 ml

Side effects/adverse reactions

CNS: Muscle weakness, flushing, sweating, confusion, sedation, depressed reflexes, ***flaccid paralysis,*** hypothermia

CV: Hypotension, heart block, ***circulatory collapse***

GI: Nausea, vomiting, anorexia, cramps

META: Electrolyte, fluid imbalances

Contraindications: Hypersensitivity, renal diseases, abdominal pain, nausea/vomiting, obstruction, acute surgical abdomen, rec bleeding

Precaution: Pregnancy **B**

Pharmacokinetics

Absorption	Up to 30% (PO)
Distribution	Widely distributed, crosses placenta
Metabolism	Not metabolized
Excretion	Kidneys, breast milk
Half-life	Unknown

M

Pharmacodynamics

Onset	Unknown
Peak	1-2 hr
Duration	Unknown

Interactions

Drug/drug:

Drug classifications

Neuromuscular blockers: ↑ action if absorbed systemically

Fluoroquinolones: ↓ absorption of fluoroquinolones

NURSING CONSIDERATIONS

Assessment

- Monitor blood, urine electrolytes if used often by patient; check I&O ratio to identify fluid loss
- Assess for cramping, rec bleeding, nausea, vomiting; if

these symptoms occur, drug should be discontinued; identify cause of constipation; identify whether fluids, bulk, or exercise is missing from lifestyle
• Assess stool for color, consistency, amount, presence of flatulence
• Assess for magnesium toxicity: thirst, confusion, decrease in reflexes

Associated nursing diagnoses

✓ Constipation (uses)
✓ Diarrhea (adverse reaction)
✓ Knowledge deficit (teaching)
✓ Noncompliance (teaching)

Implementation

PO route
• Chew tab well before swallowing; follow with 4 oz of water to prevent undissolved tab entering small intestine
• Susp should be shaken before use

Patient/family education

• Discuss with the patient that adequate fluid consumption is necessary
• Teach patient that normal bowel movements do not always occur daily
• Caution patient not to use in presence of abdominal pain, nausea, vomiting; tell patient to notify prescriber if constipation is unrelieved or if symptoms of electrolyte imbalance occur (muscle cramps, pain, weakness, dizziness, excessive thirst)
• Teach patient not to use laxatives for long-term therapy; bowel tone will be lost and will decrease
• Instruct patient to shake susp well before use
• Teach patient not to take at hs as a laxative; may interfere with sleep
• Teach patient not to use with food or vitamin preparations; delays digestion and absorption of fat-soluble vitamins

Evaluation

Positive therapeutic outcome
• Decreased constipation in 4-6 hr
• Absence of GI symptoms

magnesium sulfate

Func. class.: Anticonvulsant
Chem. class.: Magnesium product
Pregnancy category **C**

Action: Decreases acetylcholine in motor nerve terminals, which is responsible for anticonvulsant properties; osmotically retains fluid, which increases amount of water in feces when used as laxative; reduces SA node impulse formation, prolongs conduction time in myocardium

➔ **Therapeutic Outcome:** Absence of seizures

Uses: Hypomagnesemic seizures, control of seizures in pregnancy-induced hypertension, seizures in acute nephritis

Dosage and routes

Hypomagnesemic seizures
Adult: **IV** 1-2 g over 15 min,

then 1 g IM q4-6h, depending on response

Nephritis

P *Child:* IM 20-40 mg/kg in 20% sol; repeat as needed

Preeclampsia/eclampsia

Adult: **IV** 4 g/250 ml D_5W and 4 g IM, then 4 g IM q4h prn; or 4 g **IV** loading dose, then 1-4 g **IV** inf hourly, not to exceed 3 ml/min

Available forms: Inj 10%, 12.5%, 25%, 50%; granules

Side effects/adverse reactions

CNS: Sweating, depressed deep tendon reflexes, flushing, drowsiness, flaccid paralysis, hypothermia, weakness, sedation
CV: Hypotension, ***circulatory collapse, heart block,*** decreased cardiac function
RESP: Paralysis

Contraindications: Hypersensitivity, MI, renal disease

Precaution: Pregnancy **C**

Pharmacokinetics

Absorption	Well absorbed (IM); 15%-30% (PO)
Distribution	Widely distributed; crosses placenta
Metabolism	Unknown
Excretion	Kidneys, breast milk
Half-life	Unknown

Pharmacodynamics

	PO	IM	IV
Onset	3-6 hr	1 hr	1-5 min
Peak	Unknown	Unknown	Unknown
Duration	Unknown	3-4 hr	½ hr

Interactions

Drug/drug:

Drug classifications

Antipsychotics: ↑ CNS depression
Barbiturates: ↑ CNS depression
Fluoroquinolones: ↓ absorption of fluoroquinolones
Narcotics: ↑ CNS depression
Neuromuscular blockers: ↑ effect

NURSING CONSIDERATIONS

Assessment

- Monitor VS q15 min after **IV** dose; also check pulse, respirations
- Monitor cardiac function: magnesium levels
- Monitor timing of contractions; determine intensity; monitor fetal heart rate, reactivity; may decrease with this drug if using during labor
- Monitor I&O: should remain at 30 ml/hr or more; if less than this, notify prescriber; check urine output before each dose; output should be 100 ml/4 hr or more
- Assess mental status: mood, sensorium, affect, memory (long, short)
- Assess respiratory dysfunction: respiratory depression, character, rate, rhythm; hold drug if respirations are <16/min
- Assess for hypermagnesemia: depressed patellar reflex, flushing, polydipsia, confusion, weakness, flaccid paralysis, hypothermia, dyspnea begin to appear at blood levels of 4 mEQ/L

M

• Assess respiratory rate, rhythm of newborn if drug was given 24 hr before delivery or less; check reflexes of newborn whose mother received this drug before delivery
• Monitor reflexes: knee jerk, patellar; decreased signals in magnesium toxicity; mild depression will occur in therapeutic range

Associated nursing diagnoses

✓ Injury, risk for (uses)
✓ Knowledge deficit (teaching)

Implementation

IV route
• Give only when calcium gluconate available for magnesium toxicity
• Give **IV** undiluted 1.5 ml of 10% sol over 1 min; may dilute to 20% sol; inf over 3 hr; use inf pump to regulate rate accurately

Y-site compatibilities:
Acyclovir, amikacin, ampicillin, cefamandole, cefazolin, cefoperazone, ceforanide, cefotaxime, cefoxitin, cephalothin, cephapirin, chloramphenicol, clindamycin, dobutamine, doxycycline, enalaprilat, erythromycin lactobionate, esmolol, famotidine, fludarabine, gentamicin, heparin, hydrocortisone, hydromorphone, idarubicin, insulin, kanamycin, labetalol, meperidine, metronidazole, minocycline, morphine, nafcillin, ondansetron, oxacillin, paclitaxel, penicillin G potassium, piperacillin, potassium chloride, sargramostim, ticarcillin, tobramycin, trimethoprim/sulfamethoxazole, vancomycin, vitamin B complex with C

Additive compatibilities:
Calcium gluconate, cephalothin, chloramphenicol, cisplatin, hydrocortisone sodium succinate, methyldopate, penicillin G potassium, potassium phosphate, verapamil

Additive incompatibilities:
Calcium gluceptate, polymyxin, sodium bicarbonate, tobramycin

Patient/family education

• Teach patient symptoms of hypermagnesemia

Evaluation

Positive therapeutic outcome
• Absence of seizures

Treatment of overdose: Stop administration of drug; administer calcium gluconate, monitor reflexes, magnesium levels; ECG monitoring if calcium is administered

mannitol

(man′i-tole)
mannitol, Osmitrol, Resectisol
Func. class.: Osmotic diuretic
Chem. class.: Hexahydric alcohol
Pregnancy category **C**

Action: Increases osmolarity of glomerular filtrate, which raises osmotic pressure of fluid in renal tubules; there is a decrease in reabsorption of water, electrolytes; increases in urinary output, sodium, chloride, potassium, calcium, phosphorus, uric acid, urea, magnesium

Uses: Edema; promote systemic diuresis in cerebral edema, decrease intraocular pressure, improve renal function in acute renal failure, chemical poisoning

Dosage and routes

Oliguria, prevention

Adult: **IV** 50-100 g of a 5%-25% sol

Oliguria, treatment

Adult: **IV** 300-400 mg/kg of a 20%-25% sol up to 100 g of a 15%-20% sol over 30-60 min

P *Child:* **IV** 0.25-2 g/kg as a 15%-20% sol, run over 2-6 hr

Intraocular pressure/intracranial pressure

Adult: **IV** 1.5-2 g/kg of a 15%-25% sol over 30-60 min

P *Child:* **IV** 1-2 g/kg (30-60 g/m^2) as a 15%-20% sol run over 30-60 min

Renal failure

Adult: **IV** 50-200 g/24 hr, adjusting to maintain output of 30-50 mg/hr

Diuresis in drug intoxication

P *Adult and child >12 yr:* 5%-10% sol continuously up to 200 g **IV**, while maintaining 100-500 ml urine output/hr

Available forms: Inj **IV** 5%, 10%, 15%, 20%, 25%

Side effects/adverse reactions

CNS: Dizziness, headache, ***convulsions, rebound increased intracranial pressure,*** confusion
CV: Edema, hypotension, hypertension, tachycardia, ***CHF,*** thrombophlebitis
EENT: Loss of hearing, blurred vision, nasal congestion, decreased intraocular pressure
ELECT: Fluid, electrolyte imbalances, acidosis, electrolyte loss, dehydration
GI: Nausea, vomiting, dry mouth, diarrhea
GU: Marked diuresis, urinary retention, thirst
RESP: Pulmonary congestion

Contraindications: Active intracranial bleeding, hypersensitivity, anuria, severe pulmonary congestion, edema, severe dehydration, progressive heart, renal failure

M

Precautions: Dehydration, pregnancy **C**, severe renal disease, CHF, lactation

Pharmacokinetics

Absorption	Complete
Distribution	Extracellular spaces
Metabolism	Minimal
Excretion	Renal
Half-life	100 min

Pharmacodynamics

	IV
Onset	½-1 hr
Peak	1 hr
Duration	6-8 hr

Interactions

Drug/drug:

Individual drugs

EDTA: ↑ effects
Lithium: ↓ action, ↑ excretion

Drug/food:

Potassium foods: ↑ hyperkalemia

Lab test interferences

Interfere: Inorganic phosphorus, ethylene glycol

NURSING CONSIDERATIONS

Assessment

- Assess neurologic status: LOC, intracranial pressure reading, pupil size and reaction when drug is given for increased intracranial pressure
- Assess for visual changes or eye discomfort or pain
- Assess patient for tinnitus, hearing loss, ear pain; periodic testing of hearing is needed when high doses of this drug are given by **IV** route
- Monitor manifestations of hypokalemia: acidic urine, reduced urine osmolality, nocturia, polyuria, polydipsia; hypotension, broad T wave, U wave, ectopy, tachycardia, weak pulse; muscle weakness, altered LOC, drowsiness, apathy, lethargy, confusion, depression; anorexia, nausea, cramps, constipation, distention, paralytic ileus; hypoventilation, respiratory muscle weakness
- Monitor for manifestations of hyponatremia: increased B/P, cold, clammy skin, hypovolemia or hypervolemia; anorexia, nausea, vomiting, diarrhea, abdominal cramps; lethargy, increased intracranial pressure, confusion headache, seizures, coma, fatigue, tremors, hyperreflexia
- Assess fluid volume status: check I&O ratios and record hourly urine values, CVP, breath sounds, weight, distended red veins, crackles in lung, color, quality and sp gr of urine, skin turgor, adequacy of pulses, moist mucous membranes, bilateral lung sounds, peripheral pitting edema
- Assess for dehydration; symptoms of decreasing output, thirst, hypotension, dry mouth and mucous membranes should be reported.
- Monitor electrolytes: potassium, sodium, calcium, magnesium; also include BUN, ABGs, CBC; regularly monitor serum and urine levels of sodium and potassium
- Assess B/P before and during therapy with patient lying, standing, and sitting as appropriate; orthostatic hypotension can occur rapidly
- Monitor for rebound intracranial pressure: headache, confusion

Associated nursing diagnoses

- ✓ Urinary elimination, altered (adverse reactions)
- ✓ Fluid volume deficit (adverse reactions)
- ✓ Fluid volume excess (uses)
- ✓ Knowledge deficit (teaching)

Implementation

- Administer potassium replacement if potassium level is whole, or use oral sol lightly; drug may be crushed if patient is unable to swallow

IV route

- Use an in-line filter for 15%, 20%, 25% give with inf pump; check **IV** patency at inf site before and during administration; do not use sol that is yellow or has a precipitate or crystals; to redissolve, run bottle in hot water and shake vigorously; cool to body temp before giving
- Run at 30-50 ml/hr in oliguria
- Run over 30-60 min in increased intracranial pressure
- Run over 30 min for intraocular pressure; 60-90 min after surgery

Y-site incompatibilities: Amsacrine, bleomycin sulfate, doxorubicin HCl, fluconazole, gentamicin sulfate, quinidine gluconate, vinblastine sulfate, vincristine sulfate

Y-site compatibilities: Ondansetron, fluorouracil, idarubicin, melphalan, paclitaxel, vinorelbine sulfate

Additive compatibilities: Amikacin, bretylium, cefamandole, cefoxitin, cimetidine, cisplatin, dopamine, gentamicin, metoclopramide, netilmicin, nizatidine, tobramycin, verapamil

Additive incompatibilities: Blood, blood products, imipenem/cilastatin, potassium chloride, sodium chloride

Patient/family education

- Teach patient reason for and method of treatment

Evaluation

Positive therapeutic outcome

- Decreased intracranial pressure
- Decreased intraocular pressure
- Prevention of hypokalemia (diuretic use)
- Decreased edema
- Increased diuresis of >30 ml/hr
- Increased excretion of toxic substances

Treatment of overdose: Discontinue inf, correct fluid, electrolyte imbalances, hemodialysis, monitor hydration, CV, renal function

maprotiline

(ma-proe'ti-leen)

Ludiomil, maprotiline

Func. class.: Antidepressant

Chem. class.: Tetracyclic

Pregnancy category B

Action: Blocks reuptake of norepinephrine, serotonin into nerve endings, increasing action of norepinephrine, serotonin in nerve cells; has anticholinergic action

Therapeutic Outcome: Decreased symptoms of depression after 2-3 wk

Uses: Depression, dysthymic disorder, bipolar disorder: depression, agitated depression

Dosage and routes

Adult: PO 75 mg/day in moderate depression; may

increase to 150 mg/day; not to exceed 225 mg in hospitalized patients; severely depressed patients who are hospitalized may be given 300 mg/day

G *Elderly:* 50-75 mg/day

Available forms: Tab 25, 50, 75 mg

Side effects/adverse reactions

CNS: Dizziness, drowsiness, confusion, headache, anxiety, tremors, stimulation, weakness, insomnia, nightmares, G EPS (elderly), increased psychiatric symptoms, ***seizures***

CV: Orthostatic hypotension, ECG changes, tachycardia, ***hypertension,*** palpitations

EENT: Blurred vision, tinnitus, mydriasis

GI: Diarrhea, dry mouth, nausea, vomiting, ***paralytic ileus,*** increased appetite, cramps, epigastric distress, jaundice, ***hepatitis,*** stomatitis

GU: Retention, ***acute renal failure***

HEMA: ***Agranulocytosis, thrombocytopenia, eosinophilia, leukopenia***

INTEG: Rash, urticaria, sweating, pruritus, photosensitivity

Contraindications: Hypersensitivity to tricyclic antidepressants, recovery phase of MI, convulsive disorders, prostatic hypertrophy

Precautions: Suicidal patients, severe depression, increased intraocular pressure, narrow angle glaucoma, urinary retention, cardiac disease, hepatic disease, hypothyroidism, hyperthyroidism, electroshock therapy, elective G surgery, elderly, pregnancy **B**

Pharmacokinetics

Absorption	Slow, complete
Distribution	Widely distributed; crosses placenta
Metabolism	Liver, extensively
Excretion	Feces; breast milk
Half-life	21-25 hr

Pharmacodynamics

Onset	15-30 min
Peak	12 hr
Duration	3 wk

Interactions

Drug/drug:

Individual drugs

Alcohol: ↑ CNS depression
Cimetidine: ↑ levels, ↑ toxicity
Clonidine: Severe hypotension; avoid use
Disulfiram: Organic brain syndrome
Fluoxetine: ↑ levels, toxicity
Guanethidine: ↓ effects

Drug classifications

Analgesics: ↑ CNS depression
Anticholinergics: ↑ side effects
Antihistamines: ↑ CNS depression
Antihypertensives: May block antihypertensive effect
Barbiturates: ↑ effects
Benzodiazepines: ↑ effects
CNS depressants: ↑ effects
MAOI: Hypertensive crisis, convulsions
Oral contraceptives: ↑ effects, toxicity
Phenothiazines: ↑ toxicity
Sedative/hypnotics: ↑ CNS depression

Sympathomimetics, indirect acting: ↓ effects

Drug/smoking: ↑ metabolism, ↓ effects

Lab test interferences

Increase: Serum bilirubin, blood glucose, alkaline phosphatase
Decrease: VMA, 5-HIAA
False increase: Urinary catecholamines

NURSING CONSIDERATIONS

Assessment

- Monitor B/P (with patient lying, standing), pulse q4h during beginning treatment; if systolic B/P drops 20 mm Hg, hold drug, notify prescriber; take VS q4h in patients with cardiovascular disease
- Monitor blood studies: CBC, leukocytes, differential, cardiac enzymes if patient is receiving long-term therapy
- Monitor hepatic studies: AST (SGOT), ALT (SGPT), bilirubin
- Check weight weekly; drug may increase appetite
- Assess ECG for flattening of T wave, bundle branch block, AV block, dysrhythmias in cardiac patients
- Assess for EPS primarily in G elderly: rigidity, dystonia, akathisia
- Assess mental status: mood, sensorium, affect, suicidal tendencies; assess increase in psychiatric symptoms: depression, panic
- Monitor urinary retention, constipation; constipation is P more likely to occur in children G and elderly
- Assess for withdrawal symptoms: headache, nausea, vomiting, muscle pain, weakness; do not usually occur unless drug was discontinued abruptly
- Identify alcohol consumption; if alcohol is consumed, hold dose until AM

Associated nursing diagnoses

- ✓ Coping, ineffective individual (uses)
- ✓ Injury, risk for (side effects)
- ✓ Knowledge deficit (teaching)
- ✓ Noncompliance (teaching)

Implementation

PO route

- Give with food or milk for GI symptoms; crush if patient is unable to swallow medication whole
- Give dose hs if oversedation occurs during day; may take G entire dose hs; elderly may not tolerate once/day dosing
- Store at room temp; do not freeze

Patient/family education

- Inform patient that therapeutic effects may take 2-3 wk
- Advise patient to use caution in driving and other activities requiring alertness because of drowsiness, dizziness, blurred vision; to avoid rising quickly from sitting to standing, espe- G cially elderly
- Caution patient to avoid alcohol ingestion, other CNS depressants
- Caution patient not to discontinue medication quickly after long-term use: may cause nausea, headache, malaise

M

- Teach patient to wear sunscreen or large hat, since photosensitivity occurs
- Teach patient to increase fluids, bulk in diet if constipation, urinary retention occur, G especially elderly
- Teach patient to take gum, hard sugarless candy, or frequent sips of water for dry mouth

Evaluation

Positive therapeutic outcome
- Decrease in depression
- Absence of suicidal thoughts

Treatment of overdose: ECG monitoring, induce emesis, lavage, activated charcoal, administer anticonvulsant

mebendazole

(me-ben′da-zole)
Nemasole ✚, Vermox
Func. class.: Anthelmintic
Chem. class.: Carbamate
Pregnancy category **C**

Action: Inhibits glucose uptake, degeneration of cytoplasmic microtubules in the cell; interferes with absorption, secretory function

➡ **Therapeutic Outcome:** Parasite, cyst, egg death

Uses: Infestation with pinworms, roundworms, hookworms, whipworms, threadworms, pork tapeworms, dwarf tapeworms, beef tapeworms; hydatid cyst

Dosage and routes

P ***Adult and child >2 yr:*** PO 100 mg as a single dose or bid × 3 days, depending on type of infestation; course may be repeated in 3 wk if needed

Available forms: Chew tab 100 mg

Side effects/adverse reactions

CNS: Dizziness, fever
GI: Transient diarrhea, abdominal pain

Contraindication: Hypersensitivity

P **Precautions:** Child <2 yr, lactation, pregnancy (1st trimester) **C**

Pharmacokinetics	
Absorption	Minimal (PO)
Distribution	Highly bound to plasma proteins
Metabolism	Liver
Excretion	Feces in metabolites (>95%); urine, unchanged
Half-life	2½-9 hr; increased in hepatic disease

Pharmacodynamics	
Onset	Unknown
Peak	½-7 hr
Duration	Unknown

Interactions

Drug/drug:

Individual drugs

Carbamazepine: ↓ effect of mebendazole

Drug classifications

Hydantoins: ↓ effect of hydantoins

Drug/food:
High-fat foods ↑ absorption

NURSING CONSIDERATIONS
Assessment
- Assess stools during entire treatment; specimens must be sent to lab while still warm, also 1-3 wk after treatment is completed; monitor for diarrhea during expulsion of worms; avoid self-contamination with patient's feces
- Assess for allergic reaction: rash (rare)
- Identify infestation in other family members, since transmission from person to person is common
- If pinworms are suspected, a piece of cellophane tape should be placed over the anal area at night for 1 wk after treatment at night to identify ova; negative perianal swabs taken every AM for 3 days confirm that the patient is no longer infested
- Monitor blood studies: AST (SGOT), ALT (SGPT), alkaline phosphatase, BUN, CBC during treatment

Associated nursing diagnoses
✓ Infection, risk for (uses)
✓ Knowledge deficit (teaching)

Implementation
PO route
- Tabs may be chewed if patient is unable to swallow whole
- Give PO after meals to avoid GI symptoms, since absorption is not altered by food
- Give second course after 3 wk if needed; usually recommended (pinworms)
- Store in airtight container

Patient/family education
- Teach patient proper hygiene after BM, including handwashing technique; tell patient to avoid putting fingers in mouth; clean fingernails
- Advise patient that infested person should sleep alone; do not shake bed linen; wash bed linen daily in hot water; change and wash undergarments daily
- Advise patient to clean toilet daily with disinfectant (green soap sol)
- Inform patient that compliance is needed with dosage schedule, duration of treatment
- Tell patient to wear shoes, wash all fruits and vegetables well before eating, use commercial fruit and vegetable cleaner solution

Evaluation
Positive therapeutic outcome
- Expulsion of worms
- Three negative stool cultures after completion of treatment

mechlorethamine
(me-klor-eth'a-meen)
Mustargen, Nitrogen Mustard
Func. class.: Antineoplastic alkylating agent
Chem. class.: Nitrogen mustard
Pregnancy category **D**

Action: Alkylates DNA, RNA; inhibits enzymes that allow synthesis of amino acids in

M

proteins; activity is not cell cycle phase specific

Therapeutic Outcome: Prevention of rapidly growing malignant cells

Uses: Hodgkin's disease, lymphomas, leukemias, lymphosarcoma; ovarian, breast, lung carcinoma; neoplastic effusions

Dosage and routes

Adult: **IV** 0.4 mg/kg as 1 dose or 2-4 divided doses over 2-4 days; second course after 3 wk depending on blood cell count

Neoplastic effusions

Adult: Intracavity 10-20 mg (may be 200-400 μg/kg)

Available forms: Inj 10 mg/vial

Side effects/adverse reactions

CNS: Headache, dizziness, drowsiness, paresthesia, peripheral neuropathy, ***coma***
EENT: Tinnitus, hearing loss
GI: Nausea, vomiting, diarrhea, stomatitis, weight loss, colitis, ***hepatotoxicity***
HEMA: ***Thrombocytopenia, leukopenia, agranulocytosis,*** anemia
INTEG: Alopecia, pruritus, herpes zoster

Contraindications: Lactation, pregnancy (1st trimester) **D**, myelosuppression, acute herpes zoster

Precautions: Radiation therapy, chronic lymphocytic leukopenia

Pharmacokinetics

Absorption	Complete (IV)
Distribution	Unknown
Metabolism	Tissues/fluids
Excretion	Kidneys
Half-life	Unknown

Pharmacodynamics

	IV
Onset	1 day
Peak	1-2 wk
Duration	1-3 wk

Interactions

Drug/drug:

Individual drugs
Radiation: ↑ toxicity, bone marrow suppression
Drug classifications
Antineoplastics: ↑ toxicity, bone marrow suppression
Bone marrow–suppressing drugs: ↑ bone marrow suppression
Live vaccines: ↑ adverse reactions, ↓ antibody reaction

Lab test interferences

Increase: Uric acid

NURSING CONSIDERATIONS

Assessment

- Monitor CBC, differential, platelet count weekly; withhold drug if WBC is <4000 or platelet count is <75,000; notify prescriber of results if WBC <20,000/mm^3, platelets <150,000/mm^3
- Monitor pulmonary function tests, chest x-ray films before, during therapy; chest film should be obtained q2 wk during treatment; assess for dyspnea, rales, unproductive cough, chest pain, tachypnea

• Assess for increased uric acid levels, swelling, joint pain primarily in extremities; patient should be well hydrated to prevent urate deposits
• Monitor renal function studies: BUN, serum uric acid, urine CrCl before, during therapy; I&O ratio; report fall in urine output of 30 ml/hr; for decreased hyperuricemia
• Monitor for cold, fever, sore throat (may indicate beginning infection); identify edema in feet, joint and stomach pain, shaking; prescriber should be notified
• Assess for bleeding: hematuria, guaiac, bruising or petechiae, mucosa or orifices q8h; no rec temp

Associated nursing diagnoses

✓ Injury, risk for (adverse reactions)
✓ Body image disturbance (adverse reactions)
✓ Infection, risk for (adverse reactions)
✓ Knowledge deficit (teaching)

Implementation

• Give fluids **IV** or PO before chemotherapy to hydrate patient
• Give antacid before oral agent; give drug after evening meal, before hs; administer antiemetic 30-60 min before giving drug and prn to prevent vomiting; give antibiotics for prophylaxis of infection
• Give top or syst analgesics for pain
• Give in AM so drug can be eliminated before hs
• Use a liq diet: carbonated beverages; gelatin may be added if patient is not nauseated or vomiting

IV **IV route**
• Give **IV** after diluting 10 mg/10 ml sterile water or 0.9% NaCl; leave needle in vial, shake, withdraw dose, give through Y-tube or 3-way stopcock or directly over 3-5 min into running **IV** of 0.9% NaCl

Y-site compatibilities:

Fludarubine, melphalan, ondansetron, sargramostim, vinorelbine

Additive incompatibility:

Methohexital

Solution incompatibilities:

D_5W, 0.9% NaCl (**IV** only)

Intracavity route
• Further dilute in 100 ml 0.9% NaCl; administration is completed by presciber
• Watch for infiltration; if infiltration occurs, infiltrate area with isotonic sodium thiosulfate or 1% lidocaine; apply ice for 6-12 hr

Patient/family education

• Teach patient to avoid use of products containing aspirin or ibuprofen, razors, commercial mouthwash, since bleeding may occur; to report symptoms of bleeding (hematuria, tarry stools)
• Teach patient to report signs of anemia (fatigue, headache, irritability, faintness, shortness of breath)
• Advise patient to report any changes in breathing or coughing even several mo after treatment; to avoid crowds and

M

persons with respiratory tract or other infections
• Tell patient hair loss is common; discuss the use of wigs or hair pieces
• Caution patient not to have any vaccinations without the advice of the presciber, serious reactions can occur
• Advise patient contraception is needed during treatment and for several mo after the completion of therapy
• Have patient rinse mouth tid-qid with water, club soda; brush teeth bid-qid with soft brush or cotton-tipped applicators for stomatitis; use unwaxed dental floss

Evaluation

Positive therapeutic outcome
• Decreased size of tumor
• Decreased spread of malignancy
• Improved blood values
• Absence of sweating at night
• Increased appetite, increased weight

meclofenamate

(me-kloe-fen-am'ate)
meclofenamate,
Meclofen, Meclomen
Func. class.: Nonsteroidal antiinflammatory; analgesic (nonopioid)
Chem. class.: Anthranilic acid derivative
Pregnancy category **B**

Action: Inhibits prostaglandin synthesis by decreasing an enzyme needed for biosynthesis; analgesic, antiinflammatory

Therapeutic Outcome: Decreased pain, inflammation

Uses: Mild to moderate pain, osteoarthritis, rheumatoid arthritis, dysmenorrhea

Dosage and routes

Antiinflammatory
Adult: PO 200-400 mg/day in divided doses tid-qid

Analgesic
Adult: PO 50-100 mg q4-6h

Dysmenorrhea
Adult: PO 100 mg tid

Available forms: Cap 50, 100 mg

Side effects/adverse reactions

CNS: Dizziness, drowsiness, fatigue, tremors, confusion, insomnia, anxiety, depression
CV: Tachycardia, hypertension, peripheral edema, palpitations, dysrhythmias
EENT: Tinnitus, hearing loss, blurred vision
GI: Nausea, anorexia, vomiting, diarrhea, jaundice, ***cholestatic hepatitis,*** constipation, flatulence, cramps, dry mouth, peptic ulcer, ***ulceration, perforation***
GU: ***Nephrotoxicity: dysuria, hematuria, oliguria, azotemia***
HEMA: ***Blood dyscrasias***
INTEG: Purpura, rash, pruritus, sweating
SYST: Anaphylaxis, Stevens-Johnson syndrome

Contraindications: Hypersensitivity, asthma, severe renal disease, severe hepatic disease, ulcer disease

Precautions: Pregnancy **B**, P lactation, children, bleeding disorders, GI disorders, cardiac disorders, hypersensitivity to other antiinflammatory agents

Pharmacokinetics	
Absorption	Well absorbed (PO)
Distribution	Unknown
Metabolism	Liver, extensively
Half-life	½-2 hr

Pharmacodynamics	
Onset	Unknown
Peak	2 hr
Duration	Unknown

Interactions

Drug/drug:

Individual drugs

Acetaminophen (long-term use): ↑ renal reactions
Alcohol: ↑ adverse reactions
Aspirin: ↓ effectiveness, ↑ adverse reactions
Coumarin: ↑ anticoagulant effects
Digoxin: ↑ toxicity, levels
Insulin: ↓ insulin effect
Lithium: ↑ toxicity
Methotrexate: ↑ toxicity
Phenytoin: ↑ toxicity
Probenecid: ↑ toxicity
Sulfonylurea: ↑ toxicity

Drug classifications

Anticoagulants: ↑ risk of bleeding
Antihypertensives: ↓ effect of antihypertensives
Antineoplastics: ↑ risk of hematologic toxicity
β-Blockers: ↑ antihypertension
Cephalosporins: ↑ risk of bleeding
Glucocorticoids: ↑ adverse reactions
Gold preparations: ↑ renal toxicity
Hypoglycemics: ↓ hypoglycemic effect
Diuretics: ↓ effectiveness of diuretics
NSAIDs: ↑ adverse reactions
Potassium supplements: ↑ adverse reactions
Radiation: ↑ risk of hematologic toxicity
Sulfonamides: ↑ toxicity

NURSING CONSIDERATIONS

Assessment

- Monitor blood counts during therapy; watch for decreasing platelets; if low, therapy may need to be discontinued, restarted after hematologic recovery; assess for blood dyscrasia (thrombocytopenia): bruising, fatigue, bleeding, poor healing
- Assess pain: intensity, area involved
- Assess joint pain, range of motion, inflammation before and during treatment in arthritis

M

Associated nursing diagnoses

- ✓ Pain (uses)
- ✓ Pain, chronic (uses)
- ✓ Mobility, impaired physical (uses)
- ✓ Injury, risk for (adverse reaction)
- ✓ Knowledge deficit (teaching)

Implementation

PO route

- Administer to patient whole
- Give with food or milk to decrease gastric symptoms;

give 30 min ac or 2 hr pc; absorption may be slowed

Patient/family education

- Teach patient that drug must be continued for prescribed time to be effective; to avoid aspirin, alcoholic beverages, acetaminophen, ibuprofen
- Caution patient to report bleeding, bruising, fatigue, malaise, since blood dyscrasias do occur
- Instruct patient to use caution when driving; drowsiness, dizziness may occur
- Teach patient to take with a full glass of water to enhance absorption; do not crush, break or chew; patient should remain sitting up to prevent gastric irritation

Evaluation

Positive therapeutic outcome

- Decreased pain
- Decreased inflammation
- Increased mobility

medroxyprogesterone

(me-drox-ee-proe-jess'te-rone)

Amen, Curretab, Cycrin, Depo-Provera, medroxyprogesterone acetate, Provera

Func. class.: Hormone—progestogen; contraceptive; antineoplastic

Chem. class.: Progesterone derivative

Pregnancy category **X**

Action: Inhibits secretion of pituitary gonadotropins, which prevents follicular maturation and ovulation; stimulates growth of mammary tissue; antineoplastic action against endometrial cancer

➔ Therapeutic Outcome: Decreased abnormal uterine bleeding, absence of amenorrhea

Uses: Uterine bleeding (abnormal), secondary amenorrhea, endometrial cancer, renal cancer, contraceptive

Investigational uses: Pickwickian syndrome, sleep apnea

Dosage and routes

Secondary amenorrhea

Adult: PO 5-10 mg qd × 5-10 days

Endometrial/renal cancer

Adult: IM 400-1000 mg/wk

Uterine bleeding

Adult: PO 5-10 mg qd × 5-10 days starting on 16th day of menstrual cycle

Contraceptive

Adult: Inj q3 mo

Available forms: Tab 2.5, 5, 10 mg; inj susp 100, 150, 400 mg/ml; contraceptive injectable

Side effects/adverse reactions

CNS: Dizziness, headache, migraines, depression, fatigue
CV: Hypotension, thrombophlebitis, edema, ***thromboembolism, stroke, pulmo-***

nary embolism, myocardial infarction
EENT: Diplopia
GI: Nausea, vomiting, anorexia, cramps, increased weight, ***cholestatic jaundice***
GU: Amenorrhea, cervical erosion, breakthrough bleeding, dysmenorrhea, vaginal candidiasis, breast changes, *gynecomastia, testicular atrophy, impotence,* endometriosis, ***spontaneous abortion***
INTEG: Rash, urticaria, acne, hirsutism, alopecia, oily skin, seborrhea, purpura, melasma, photosensitivity
META: Hyperglycemia

Contraindications: Breast cancer, hypersensitivity, thromboembolic disorders, reproductive cancer, genital bleeding (abnormal, undiagnosed), pregnancy **X**

Precautions: Lactation, hypertension, asthma, blood dyscrasias, gallbladder disease, CHF, diabetes mellitus, bone disease, depression, migraine headache, convulsive disorders, hepatic disease, renal disease, family history of cancer of breast or reproductive tract

Pharmacokinetics

Absorption	Unknown
Distribution	Unknown
Metabolism	Unknown
Excretion	Unknown
Half-life	Unknown

Pharmacodynamics

	PO	IM
Onset	Unknown	Unknown
Peak	Unknown	Unknown
Duration	2-4 hr	Unknown

Interactions
Drug/drug:
Individual drugs
Aminoglutethimide: ↓ contraceptive effect
Bromocriptine: ↓ effectiveness

Lab test interferences
Increase: Alkaline phosphatase, pregnanediol, amino acids
Decrease: GTT, HDL

NURSING CONSIDERATIONS

Assessment

- Monitor B/P at beginning of treatment and periodically; check weight daily; notify prescriber of weekly weight gain >5 lb
- Monitor I&O ratio: be alert for decreasing urinary output, increasing edema, hypertension
- Assess liver function studies: ALT (SGPT), AST (SGOT), bilirubin, periodically during long-term therapy
- Assess for edema, hypertension, cardiac symptoms, jaundice
- Assess mental status: affect, mood, behavioral changes, depression

Associated nursing diagnoses

- ✓ Sexual dysfunction (uses)
- ✓ Tissue perfusion, altered (adverse reactions)
- ✓ Injury, risk for (adverse reactions)
- ✓ Knowledge deficit (teaching)

Implementation

PO route

- Give with food or milk to decrease GI symptoms; give in one dose in AM

IM route
- Store in dark area
- Give titrated dosage; use lowest effective dosage; give oil sol deep in large muscle mass (IM); rotate sites; use after warming to dissolve crystals

Patient/family education
- Advise patient to avoid sunlight or use sunscreen; photosensitivity and melasma (brown patches on the face) can occur
- Teach patient about cushingoid symptoms
- Teach patient to report breast lumps, vaginal bleeding, edema, jaundice, dark urine, clay-colored stools, dyspnea, headache, blurred vision, abdominal pain, numbness or stiffness in legs, chest pain; male to report impotence or gynecomastia
- Teach patient to report suspected pregnancy immediately

Evaluation
Positive therapeutic outcome
- Decreased abnormal uterine bleeding
- Absence of amenorrhea
- Prevented pregnancy
- Arrested spread of malignant cells

megestrol
(me-jess'trole)
Megace, megestrol acetate
Func. class.: Antineoplastic
Chem. class.: Hormone, progestin
Pregnancy category X

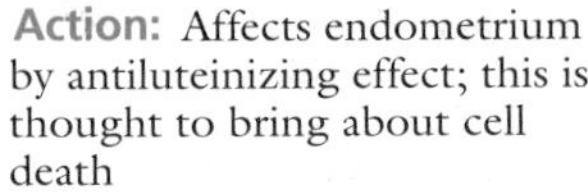

Action: Affects endometrium by antiluteinizing effect; this is thought to bring about cell death

Therapeutic Outcome: Prevention of rapidly growing malignant cells; weight gain, increased appetite in AIDS

Uses: Breast, endometrial, renal cell cancer; increase weight, decrease cachexia and anorexia associated with AIDS

Dosage and routes
Endometrial/ovarian carcinoma
Adult: PO 40-320 mg/day in divided doses

Breast carcinoma
Adult: PO 40 mg qid

Anorexia (AIDS)
Adult: PO 40 mg qid

Available forms: Tab 20, 40 mg; oral susp 40 mg/ml

Side effects/adverse reactions
CNS: Mood swings
CV: ***Thrombophlebitis***
GI: Nausea, vomiting, anorexia, diarrhea, abdominal cramps
GU: Gynecomastia, fluid retention, ***hypercalcemia***
INTEG: Alopecia, rash, pruritus, purpura, itching

Contraindications: Hypersensitivity, pregnancy **X**

Pharmacokinetics

Absorption	Well absorbed
Distribution	Unknown
Metabolism	Liver, completely
Excretion	Unknown
Half-life	1 hr

Pharmacodynamics

	PO
Onset	Several wk-mo
Peak	Unknown
Duration	1-3 days

Interactions: None

Lab test interferences

Increase: Alkaline phosphatase, urinary pregnanediol, plasma amino acids
False positive: Urine glucose
Decrease: HDL, glucose tolerance test

NURSING CONSIDERATIONS

Assessment

- Monitor effects of alopecia on body image; discuss feelings about body changes
- In AIDS patients monitor calorie counts, weight, appetite
- Assess for thrombophlebitis: pain, redness, swelling in legs; notify prescriber if these occur

Associated nursing diagnoses

✓ Knowledge deficit (teaching)

Implementation

PO route

- Administer with meals for GI symptoms
- Oral susp is usually used for AIDS patients

Patient/family education

- Teach patient to report any complaints or side effects to prescriber
- Advise patient that contraceptive measures must be used during and several mo after treatment; drug is teratogenic
- Explore need for wig or hair piece for hair loss
- Caution patient to report vaginal bleeding to prescriber
- Review with patient the need to comply with dosage schedule, not to miss or double doses; missed doses may be taken up to 1 hr before next dose

Evaluation

Positive therapeutic outcome

- Decreased spread of malignant cells
- Weight gain, increased appetite in AIDS patients

melphalan

(mel'fa-lan)

Alkeran, Alkeran IV, L-Pam, L-Sarcolysin

Func. class.: Antineoplastic alkylating agent

Chem. class.: Nitrogen mustard

Pregnancy category **D**

Action: Alkylates DNA, RNA; inhibits enzymes that allow synthesis of amino acids in proteins; activity is not cell cycle phase specific

Therapeutic Outcome: Prevention of rapidly growing malignant cells

Uses: Multiple myeloma, breast carcinoma, reticulum cell sarcoma, testicular seminoma, malignant melanoma, advanced ovarian cancer

Investigational uses: Breast, testicular, prostate carcinoma; osteogenic sarcoma, chronic myelogenous leukemia

Dosage and routes

Multiple myeloma

Adult: PO 6 mg qd × 2-3 wk; stop drug for 4 wk or until WBC level begins to rise; do not administer if WBC <3000/mm^3 or platelets <100,000/mm^3; may be given 0.15 mg/kg/day × 7 days; wait until platelets and WBCs rise, then 0.05 mg/kg/day

Ovarian carcinoma

Adult: **IV** inf 16 mg/m^2; reduce in renal insufficiency; give over 15-20 min; give at 2-wk intervals × 4 doses, then at 4-wk intervals

Available forms: Tab 2 mg, inj 50 mg

Side effects/adverse reactions

GI: Nausea, vomiting, stomatitis, diarrhea
GU: Amenorrhea, hyperuricemia, gonadal suppression
HEMA: Thrombocytopenia, neutropenia, leukopenia, anemia
INTEG: Rash, urticaria, alopecia, pruritus
RESP: Fibrosis, dysplasia
SYST: ***Anaphylaxis,*** allergic reaction

Contraindications: Lactation, pregnancy **D**, hypersensitivity to this drug or other nitrogen mustards

Precautions: Radiation therapy, bone marrow depression, infection, renal disease, P children

Pharmacokinetics

Absorption	Variable; incompletely absorbed
Distribution	Rapidly distributed
Metabolism	Bloodstream
Excretion	Kidneys, unchanged (10%)
Half-life	1½ hr

Pharmacodynamics

	PO/IV
Onset	Unknown
Peak	Unknown
Duration	Unknown

Interactions

Drug/drug:

Individual drugs
Radiation: ↑ toxicity, bone marrow suppression
Drug classifications
Antineoplastics: ↑ toxicity, bone marrow suppression
Bone marrow–suppressing drugs: ↑ bone marrow suppression
Live vaccines: ↑ adverse reactions, ↓ antibody reaction

Lab test interferences

Increase: Uric acid

NURSING CONSIDERATIONS

Assessment

- Monitor CBC, differential, platelet count weekly; withhold drug if WBC is <4000 or platelet count is <75,000; notify prescriber of results if WBC <20,000/mm^3, platelets <100,000/mm^3
- Monitor pulmonary function tests, chest x-ray films before, during therapy; chest film should be obtained q2 wk during treatment; check for dyspnea, rales, unproductive cough, chest pain, tachypnea
- Assess for increased uric acid levels, swelling, joint pain primarily in extremities; patient should be well hydrated to prevent urate deposits
- Monitor renal function studies: BUN, serum uric acid, urine CrCl before, during therapy; check I&O ratio; report fall in urine output of 30 ml/hr; check for decreased hyperuricemia; monitor AST (SGOT), ALT (SGPT)
- Monitor for cold, fever, sore throat (may indicate beginning infection); identify edema in feet, joint and stomach pain, shaking; prescriber should be notified
- Assess for bleeding: hematuria, guaiac, bruising or petechiae, mucosa or orifices q8h; no rec temp

Associated nursing diagnoses

- ✓ Injury, risk for (adverse reactions)
- ✓ Body image disturbance (adverse reactions)
- ✓ Infection, risk for (adverse reactions)
- ✓ Knowledge deficit (teaching)

Implementation

- Give fluids **IV** or PO before chemotherapy to hydrate patient
- Give antacid before oral agent; give drug after evening meal, before hs; provide antiemetic 30-60 min before giving drug and prn to prevent vomiting; give antibiotics for prophylaxis of infection
- Give top or syst analgesics for pain
- Give in AM so drug can be eliminated before hs
- Use a liq diet: carbonated beverages; gelatin may be added if patient is not nauseated or vomiting

PO route

- Give 1 hr ac or 2 hr pc to prevent nausea/vomiting

IV **IV route**

- Give as intermittent inf: reconstitute with provided diluent (10 ml) to 5 mg/ml; shake until clear; further dilute with 0.9% NaCl to <0.45 mg/ml; give over 15 min

Patient/family education

- Teach patient to avoid use of products containing aspirin or ibuprofen, razors, commercial mouthwash, since bleeding may occur; to report symptoms of bleeding (hematuria, tarry stools)
- Instruct patient to report signs of anemia (fatigue, headache, irritability, faintness, shortness of breath)
- Instruct patient to report any changes in breathing or coughing even several mo after treatment; to avoid crowds and persons with respiratory tract or other infections

- Tell patient hair loss is common; discuss the use of wigs or hair pieces
- Caution patient not to have any vaccinations without the advice of the prescriber, serious reactions can occur
- Advise patient contraception is needed during treatment and for several mo after the completion of therapy
- Teach patient to rinse mouth tid-qid with water, club soda; brush teeth bid-qid with soft brush or cotton-tipped applicators for stomatitis; use unwaxed dental floss

Evaluation

Positive therapeutic outcome

- Decreased size of tumor
- Decreased spread of malignancy

menotropins

(men-oh-troe'pinz)

HMG, Pergonal

Func. class.: Gonadotropin

Chem. class.: Exogenous gonadotropin

Pregnancy category **C**

Action: In women, increases follicular growth, maturation; in men, when given with HCG, stimulates spermatogenesis; contains FSH and LH

➔ Therapeutic Outcome: Pregnancy, ovulation

Uses: Infertility, anovulation in women; stimulates spermatogenesis in men; usually used with HCG

Dosage and routes

Infertility

Adult (men): IM 1 ampule 3 times a wk with HCG 2000 U 2 times a wk × 4 mo

Anovulation

Adult (women): IM 75 IU of FSH, LH qd × 9-12 days, then 10,000 U HCG 1 day after these drugs; repeat × 2 menstrual cycles, then increase to 150 IU of FSH, LH qd × 9-12 days, then 10,000 U HCG 1 day after these drugs × 2 menstrual cycles

Available forms: Powder for inj 17 IU/ampule

Side effects/adverse reactions

CNS: Fever

CV: ***Hypovolemia***, thrombophelibitis, ***pulmonary embolism, thromboembolism***

GI: *Nausea,* vomiting, diarrhea, anorexia, abdominal distention/pain

GU: *Ovarian enlargement,* multiple births, ovarian hyperstimulation, sudden ovarian enlargement, ascites with or without pain, pleural effusion, gynecomastia in men

HEMA: Hemoperitoneum, arterial thromboembolism

Contraindications: Primary ovarian failure, abnormal bleeding, thyroid/adrenal dysfunction, organic intracranial lesion, ovarian cysts, primary testicular failure

Precautions: Pregnancy **C**

Pharmacokinetics

Absorption	Well absorbed
Distribution	Unknown
Metabolism	Unknown
Excretion	Kidneys, unchanged (8%)
Half-life	70 hr (FSH); 4 hr (LH)

Pharmacodynamics

	IM FEMALE	IM MALE
Onset	Unknown	Unknown
Peak	Unknown	Unknown
Duration	Unknown	Unknown

Interactions: None

NURSING CONSIDERATIONS

Assessment

- Monitor weight qd; notify prescriber if weight gain increases rapidly
- Monitor estrogen excretion level; if >100 μg/24 hr, drug is withheld; hyperstimulation syndrome may occur
- Monitor I&O ratio; be alert for decreasing urinary output
- Assess for ovarian enlargement, abdominal distention/pain; report symptoms immediately

Associated nursing diagnoses

✓ Sexual dysfunction (uses)
✓ Knowledge deficit (teaching)

Implementation

IM route

- Give after reconstituting with 1-2 ml sterile saline inj; use immediately

Patient/family education

- Advise patient that multiple births are possible; if pregnancy occurs, it is usually 4-6 wk after start of treatment
- Instruct patient to keep daily appointment for 2 wk during treatment
- Tell patient that daily intercourse is necessary from day preceding administration of gonadotropin until ovulation occurs

Evaluation

Positive therapeutic outcome

- Pregnancy

meperidine

(me-per′i-deen)

Demerol, meperidine HCl, Pethandol, Pethidine

Func. class.: Narcotic analgesic

Chem. class.: Opiate, phenylpiperidine derivative

Pregnancy category **B**

Controlled substance schedule **II**

Action: Depresses pain impulse transmission at the spinal cord level by interacting with opioid receptors; produces CNS depression

Therapeutic Outcome: Relief of pain

Uses: Moderate to severe pain, preoperatively, during labor

Dosage and routes

Pain

Adult: PO/SC/IM 50-150 mg q3-4h prn; dosage should be decreased if given **IV**

P *Child:* PO/SC/IM 1 mg/kg q4-6h prn, not to exceed 100 mg q4h

Preoperatively

Adult: IM/SC 50-100 mg q30-90 min before surgery; dosage should be reduced if given **IV**

P *Child:* IM/SC 1-2.2 mg/kg 30-90 min before surgery

Labor analgesia

Adult: SC/IM 50-100 mg given when contractions are regulary spaced, repeat q1-3h prn

Available forms: Inj 10, 50, 75, 100 mg/ml; tab 50, 100 mg; syr 50 mg/5 ml

Side effects/adverse reactions

CNS: Drowsiness, dizziness, confusion, headache, sedation, euphoria, **increased intracranial pressure**

CV: Palpitations, bradycardia, change in B/P, tachycardia (**IV**)

EENT: Tinnitus, blurred vision, miosis, diplopia, depressed corneal reflex

GI: Nausea, vomiting, anorexia, constipation, cramps

GU: Urinary retention, dysuria

INTEG: Rash, urticaria, bruising, flushing, diaphoresis, pruritus

RESP: **Respiratory depression**

Contraindications: Hypersensitivity, addiction (narcotic)

Precautions: Addictive personality, pregnancy **B**, lactation, increased intracranial pressure, MI (acute), severe heart disease, respiratory depression, hepatic disease, renal disease, P child <18 yr

Pharmacokinetics

Absorption	Well absorbed (IM, SC); 50% (PO)
Distribution	Widely distributed; crosses placenta
Metabolism	Liver, extensively
Excretion	Kidneys; breast milk
Half-life	3-6 hr

Pharmacodynamics

	PO	IM	SC	IV
Onset	15 min	10 min	10 min	Rapid
Peak	1 hr	1 hr	1 hr	5-7 min
Duration	4-5 hr	4-5 hr	4-5 hr	2 hr

Interactions

Drug/drug:

Individual drugs

Alcohol: ↑ respiratory depression, hypotension, sedation
Cimetidine: ↑ recovery
Erythromycin: ↑ recovery
Nalbuphine: ↓ analgesia
Pentazocine: ↓ analgesia

Drug classifications

Antihistamines: ↑ respiratory depression, hypotension
Barbiturates: ↑ respiratory depression
CNS depressants: ↑ respiratory depression, hypotension
MAOI: Do not use for 2 wk before taking meperidine
Phenothiazines: ↑ respiratory depression, hypotension
Sedative/hypnotics: ↑ respiratory depression, hypotension

Lab test interferences

Increase: Amylase

NURSING CONSIDERATIONS

Assessment

- Assess pain: location, duration, intensity before and 1 hr after administration
- Monitor VS after parenteral route; note muscle rigidity, drug history, liver, kidney function tests, respiratory dysfunction: respiratory depression, character, rate, rhythm; notify prescriber if respirations are <10/min
- Monitor CNS changes: dizziness, drowsiness, hallucinations, euphoria, LOC, pupil reaction; these are due to metabolite produced
- Monitor allergic reactions: rash, urticaria

Associated nursing diagnoses

- ✓ Pain (uses)
- ✓ Sensory perceptual alteration: visual, auditory (adverse reactions)
- ✓ Breathing pattern, ineffective (adverse reactions)
- ✓ Injury, risk for (adverse reactions)
- ✓ Knowledge deficit (teaching)

Implementation

- Give with antiemetic if nausea, vomiting occur
- Administer when pain is beginning to return; determine dosage interval by patient response; continuous dosing of medication is more effective given prn
- Medication should be slowly withdrawn after long-term use to prevent withdrawal symptoms
- Store in light-resistant container at room temp

PO route

- May be given with food or milk to lessen GI upset
- Syrup should be mixed with 4 oz of water

IM/SC route

- Do not give if cloudy or a precipitate has formed
- Patient should remain recumbent for 1 hr after administration

IV **IV route**

- Give by direct **IV** after diluting to 10 mg/ml with sterile water, 0.9% NaCl for inj; give slowly at 25 mg/1 min; rapid administration may cause respiratory depression, hypotension, circulatory collapse
- Give cont inf after diluting to 1 mg/ml with D_5W, $D_{10}W$, dextrose/saline combinations, dextrose/Ringer's, inj combinations, 0.45% NaCl, 0.9% NaCl, Ringer's, LR; give by inf pump; titrate according to response

Syringe compatibilities: Atropine, benzquinamide, butorphanol, chlorpromazine, cimetidine, dimenhydrinate, diphenhydramine, droperidol fentanyl, glycopyrrolate, hydroxyzine, metochlopramide, midazolam, pentazocine, perphenazine, prochlorperazine, promazine, promethazine, ranitidine, scopolamine

Syringe incompatibilities: Heparin, morphine, pentobarbital

M

Additive compatibilities:
Scopolamine, triflupromazine

Y-site compatibilities:
Amikacin, ampicillin, bumetanide, cefamandole, cefazolin, ceforanide, cefotaxime, cefotetan, cefoxitin, ceftizoxime, ceftriaxone, cefuroxime, cephalothin, cephapirin, chloramphenicol, clindamycin, dexamethasone, diphenhydramine, dobutamine, dopamine, doxycycline, droperidol, erythromycin lactobionate, famotidine, fluconazole, fludarabine, gentamicin, heparin, hydrocortisone sodium succinate, insulin, kanamycin, labetalol, lidocaine, methyldopate, magnesium sulfate, melphalan methylprednisolone, metoclopramide, metoprolol, metronidazole, mezlocillin, minocycline, ondansetron, oxacillin, oxytocin, paclitaxel, penicillin G potassium, piperacillin, potassium chloride, propranolol, ranitidine, sargramostim, ticarcillin, ticarcillin/clavulanate, tobramycin, trimethoprim/sulfamethoxazole, vancomycin, verapamil, vinorelbine

Y-site incompatibilities:
Cefoperazone, idarubicin, imipenem/cilastatin, mezlocillin, minocycline

Patient/family education
- Advise patients to avoid CNS depressants (alcohol, sedative/hypnotics) for at least 24 hr after taking this drug
- Discuss with patient that dizziness, drowsiness, and confusion are common; to avoid getting up without assistance
- Discuss in detail all aspects of the drug, including its purpose and what to expect
- Caution patient to make position changes carefully to lessen orthostatic hypotension

Evaluation
Positive therapeutic outcome
- Decreased pain

Treatment of overdose:
Narcan 0.2-0.8 **IV**, O_2, **IV** fluids, vasopressors

meprobamate
(me-proe-ba'mate)
Apo-Meprobamate ✤, Equanil, Meditran ✤, meprobamate, Meprospan, Miltown, Miltown 600, Neuramate, Neo-Tran ✤, Novomepro ✤, Sedabamate, Trancot
Func. class.: Sedative/hypnotic; antianxiety
Chem. class.: Propanediol carbamate derivative
Pregnancy category D
Controlled substance schedule IV

Action: Produces widespread depression of the CNS

➡ **Therapeutic Outcome:** Decreased anxiety, sedation

Uses: Anxiety, sedation

Dosage and routes
Adult: PO 1.2-1.6 g/day in 2-3 divided doses, not to exceed 2.4 g/day or 800-1600

mg/day in 2 divided doses (sus rel); max 2.4 g/day

P *Child 6-12 yr:* PO 100-200 mg bid-tid or 200 mg (sus rel) bid

Available forms: Tab 200, 400, 600 mg; sust rel cap 200, 400 mg

Side effects/adverse reactions

CNS: Dizziness, drowsiness, headache, ***convulsions,*** ataxia
CV: Hypotension, tachycardia, palpitations, ***hyperthermia***
EENT: Blurred vision, tinnitus, mydriasis, slurred speech
GI: Nausea, vomiting, anorexia, diarrhea, stomatitis
HEMA: ***Thrombocytopenia, leukopenia, eosinophilia***
INTEG: Urticaria, pruritus, maculopapular rash

Contraindications: Hypersensitivity, renal failure, porphyria, pregnancy **D**, history of drug abuse or dependence

Precautions: Suicidal patients, severe depression, renal disease, hepatic disease, G elderly

Pharmacokinetics

Absorption	Well absorbed (PO)
Distribution	Widely distributed; crosses placenta
Metabolism	Liver
Excretion	Kidneys, feces, breast milk
Half-life	6-16 hr

Pharmacodynamics

	PO	PO–SUS REL
Onset	1 hr	Unknown
Peak	1-3 hr	Unknown
Duration	6-12 hr	Up to 12 hr

Interactions

Drug/drug:

Individual drugs
Alcohol: ↑ CNS depression
Fluoxetine: ↑ action
Propoxyphene: ↑ action
Drug classifications
Analgesics, opioid: ↑ CNS depression
Antidepressants: ↑ CNS depression
Antihistamines: ↑ CNS depression
Sedative/hypnotics: ↑ CNS depression

Lab test interferences

False increase: 17-OHCS
False positive: Phentolamine test

NURSING CONSIDERATIONS

Assessment

- Assess patient's sleep pattern and note physical (sleep apnea, obstructed airway, pain/discomfort, urinary frequency) and psychologic (fear, anxiety) circumstances that interrupt sleep
- Assess patient's bedtime routine, presleep cues, props
- Assess potential for abuse; this drug may lend to physical and psychologic dependency; amount of drug should be limited
- Monitor blood studies: Hct, Hgb, RBCs, serum folate (if on long-term therapy), protime in patients receiving anticoagulants, since action of anticoagulant may be increased
- Monitor mental status: mood, sensorium, affect, memory (long, short)

- Monitor physical dependency: more frequent requests for medication, shakes, anxiety, pinpoint pupils
- Monitor respiratory dysfunction: respiratory depression, character, rate, rhythm; hold drug if respirations are <10/min or if pupils are dilated (rare)
- Assess for blood dyscrasias: fever, sore throat, bruising, rash, jaundice, epistaxis (rare)
- Assess previous history of substance abuse, cardiac disease, or gastritis

Associated nursing diagnoses

✓ Anxiety (uses)
✓ Knowledge deficit (teaching)
✓ Noncompliance (teaching)

Implementation

PO route

- Give with food to minimize GI symptoms; do not break, crush, or chew sus rel cap
- Store in tight container in cool environment

Patient/family education

- Advise patient to avoid driving and other activities requiring alertness; to avoid alcohol and CNS depressants; serious CNS depression may result, as well as tachycardia, flushing, headache, hypotension
- Caution patient not to discontinue medication quickly after long-term use; drug should be tapered over 1-2 wk; effects may take 2 nights for benefits to be noticed; withdrawal symptoms include tremors, anxiety, hallucinations, delirium
- Teach patient alternate measures to improve sleep (reading, exercise several hr before hs, warm bath, warm milk, TV, self-hypnosis, deep breathing)
- Instruct patient that hangover is common in elderly but less common than with barbiturates [G]
- Teach patient symptoms of withdrawal: nausea, vomiting, anxiety, hallucinations, insomnia, tachycardia, fever, cramps, tremors, seizures
- Teach patient to watch for blood dyscrasias: fever, sore throat, bruising, rash, jaundice (rare)
- Teach patient to watch for allergic reaction (rash); discontinue drug if rash occurs

Evaluation

Positive therapeutic outcome

- Decreased anxiety, restlessness, insomnia

Treatment of overdose:

Lavage, VS, supportive care

mercaptopurine

(mer-kap-toe-pyoor'een)

6-MP, Purinethol

Func. class.: Antineoplastic, antimetabolite

Chem. class.: Purine analog

Pregnancy category **D**

Action: Inhibits purine metabolism at multiple sites, which inhibits DNA and RNA synthesis S phase of cell cycle

Therapeutic Outcome: Prevention of rapidly growing malignant cells

Uses: Chronic myelocytic leukemia, acute lymphoblastic leukemia in children, acute myelogenous leukemia

Investigational Uses: Polycythemia vera, psoriatic arthritis, colitis, lymphoma

Dosage and routes

Adult: PO 2.5 mg/kg/day, not to exceed 5 mg/kg/day; maintenance 1.5-2.5 mg/kg/day

Child: 75 mg/m^2/day (2.5 mg/kg/day)

Available forms: Tab 50 mg

Side effects/adverse reactions

CNS: Fever, headache, weakness

GI: Nausea, vomiting, anorexia, diarrhea, stomatitis, ***hepatotoxicity*** (with high doses), jaundice, gastritis

GU: ***Renal failure,*** hyperuricemia, ***oliguria,*** crystalluria, ***hematuria***

HEMA: ***Thrombocytopenia, leukopenia, myelosuppression, anemia***

INTEG: Rash, dry skin, urticaria

Contraindications: Patients with prior drug resistance, leukopenia (<2500/mm^3), thrombocytopenia (<100,000/mm^3), anemia, pregnancy **D**

Precautions: Renal disease

Pharmacokinetics

Absorption	Variable (PO)
Distribution	Widely-body water
Metabolism	Liver-extensively
Extensively	Kidneys unchanged (small amounts)
Half-life	Unknown

Pharmacodynamics

	PO
Onset	Unknown
Peak	Unknown
Duration	Unknown

Interactions

Drug/drug:

Individual drugs

Allopurinol: ↑ toxicity

Cyclophosphamide: ↑ cardiotoxicity, CHF

Radiation: ↑ toxicity, bone marrow suppression

Warfarin: ↑ or ↓ effect of warfarin

Drug classifications

Antineoplastics: ↑ toxicity, bone marrow suppression

Hepatotoxic agents: ↑ hepatotoxicity

Live virus vaccines: ↓ antibodies

Nondepolarizing muscle relaxants: Reversal of neuromuscular blockade

NURSING CONSIDERATIONS

Assessment

- Assess buccal cavity q8h for dryness, sores or ulceration, white patches, oral pain, bleeding, dysphagia; obtain prescription for viscous lidocaine (Xylocaine)
- Assess symptoms indicating severe allergic reaction: rash, pruritus, urticaria, purpuric

skin lesions, itching, flushing
• Monitor CBC, differential, platelet count weekly; withhold drug if WBC count is <4000/mm^3 or platelet count is <100,000/mm^3; notify prescriber of results if WBC <20,000/mm^3, platelets <150,000/mm^3
• Assess for increased uric acid levels, swelling, joint pain primarily in extremities; patient should be well hydrated to prevent urate deposits
• Monitor renal function studies: BUN, creatinine, serum uric acid, urine CrCl before and during therapy; check I&O ratio; report fall in urine output to <30 ml/hr
• Monitor temp q4h (may indicate beginning of infection)
• Monitor liver function tests before and during therapy (bilirubin, AST [SGOT], ALT [SGPT], LDH) as needed or monthly; check for yellowing of skin or sclera, dark urine, clay-colored stools, itchy skin, abdominal pain, fever, diarrhea
• Assess for bleeding: hematuria, stool guaiac, bruising or petechiae, mucosa or orifices q8h; check for inflammation of mucosa, breaks in skin
• Identify inflammation of mucosa, breaks in skin

Associated nursing diagnoses

✓ Injury, risk for (adverse reactions)
✓ Body image disturbance (adverse reactions)
✓ Infection, risk for (adverse reactions)
✓ Knowledge deficit (teaching)

Implementation

• Give fluids **IV** or PO before chemotherapy to hydrate patient
• Give antiemetic 30-60 min before giving drug and prn to prevent vomiting; give antibiotics for prophylaxis of infection
• Give top or syst analgesics for pain
• Give in AM so drug can be eliminated before hs
• Provide liq diet: carbonated beverages; gelatin may be added if patient is not nauseated or vomiting
• Encourage patient to rinse mouth tid-qid with water, club soda; brush teeth bid-qid with soft brush or cotton-tipped applicators for stomatitis; use unwaxed dental floss

PO route
• Tab may be crushed and added to fluids or food to facilitate swallowing

Patient/family education

• Advise patient that contraceptive measures are recommended during therapy; serious teratogenic effects may occur
• Teach patient to avoid use of products containing aspirin or ibuprofen, razors, commercial mouthwash, since bleeding may occur; to report symptoms of bleeding (hematuria, tarry stools)
• Instruct patient to report signs of anemia (fatigue, headache, irritability, faintness, shortness of breath)
• Instruct patient to report any changes in breathing or coughing even several mo after treatment; to avoid crowds and

persons with respiratory tract or other infections
• Caution patient not to have any vaccinations without the advice of the prescriber; serious reactions can occur

Evaluation

Positive therapeutic outcome
• Prevention of rapid division of malignant cells

mesalamine
(mez-al'a-meen)
Asacol, Pentusa, Rowasa, Salofulk 🍁
Func class.: GI antiinflammatory
Chem class.: 5-Aminosalicylic acid
Pregnancy category **B**

Action: May diminish inflammation by blocking cyclooxygenase, inhibiting prostaglandin production in colon, local action only

Therapeutic Outcome: Decreased cramping, pain in GI conditions

Uses: Mild to moderate active distal ulcerative colitis, proctosigmoiditis, proctitis

Dosage and routes

Adult: Rec 60 ml (4 g) hs, retained for 8 hr × 3-6 wk; PO 800 mg tid for 6 wk; supp 500 mg bid for 3-6 wk

Available forms: Rec susp 4 g/60 ml; supp 500 mg; delayed rel tab 400 mg

Side effects/adverse reactions

CNS: Headache, fever, dizziness, insomnia, asthenia, weakness, fatigue
CV: Pericarditis, myocarditis
EENT: Sore throat, cough, pharyngitis, rhinitis
GI: Cramps, gas, nausea, diarrhea, rec pain, constipation
INTEG: Rash, itching, acne
SYST: Flu, malaise, back pain, peripheral edema, leg and joint pain, arthralgia, dysmenorrhea

Contraindications: Hypersensitivity to this drug or salicylates

Precautions: Renal disease, pregnancy **B**, lactation, children, sulfite sensitivity

Pharmacokinetics

Absorption	20%-30% (PO), 10%-25% (rec)
Distribution	Unknown
Metabolism	Unknown
Excretion	Feces
Half-life	1 hr; metabolite 5-10 hr

Pharmacodynamics

	REC	PO
Onset	Unknown	Unknown
Peak	Unknown	Unknown
Duration	Unknown	Unknown

Interactions: None

NURSING CONSIDERATIONS

Assessment

• Assess for GI symptoms: cramping, gas, nausea, diarrhea, rec pain, abdominal pain;

if severe, the drug should be discontinued

Associated nursing diagnoses

- ✓ Pain (uses)
- ✓ Diarrhea (uses)
- ✓ Knowledge deficit (teaching)

Implementation

PO route

- May give orally; tab should be swallowed whole

Rec route (suppos)

- Give hs, retained until AM
- Store at room temp
- Usual course of therapy is 3-6 wk
- Give after shaking bottle well

Patient/family education

- Advise patient to notify prescriber if abdominal pain, cramping, diarrhea with blood, headache, fever, rash occur; drug should be discontinued
- Teach correct administration for PO, or enema

Evaluation

Positive therapeutic outcome

- Absence of pain, bleeding from GI tract

mesoridazine

(mez-oh-rid′a-zeen)

Serentil

Func. class.: Antipsychotic/neuroleptic

Chem. class.: Phenothiazine, piperidine

Pregnancy category C

Action: Depresses cerebral cortex, hypothalamus, limbic system, which control activity, aggression; blocks neurotransmission produced by dopamine at synapse; exhibits strong α-adrenergic, anticholinergic blocking action; mechanism for antipsychotic effects is unclear

➡ **Therapeutic Outcome:** Decreased signs and symptoms of psychosis, reorganization of thought patterns

Uses: Psychotic disorders, schizophrenia, anxiety, alcoholism, behavioral problems in mental deficiency, chronic brain syndrome

Dosage and routes

Schizophrenia

Adult: PO 50 mg tid; optimum dosage 100-400 mg/day; IM 25 mg; may repeat in 30-60 min; dosage range 25-200 mg/day

Behavior problems

Adult: PO 25 mg tid; optimum dosage 75-300 mg/day

Alcoholism

Adult: PO 25 mg bid; optimum dosage 50-200 mg/day

Schizoaffective disorders

Adult: PO 10 mg tid; optimum dosage 30-150 mg/day

Available forms: Tab 10, 25, 50, 100 mg; conc 25 mg/ml; inj 25 mg/ml

Side effects/adverse reactions

CNS: Extrapyramidal symptoms: pseudoparkinsonism, akathisia, dystonia,

tardive dyskinesia, drowsiness, headache, ***neuroleptic malignant syndrome***
CV: Orthostatic hypotension, hypertension, ***cardiac arrest,*** ECG changes, tachycardia
EENT: Blurred vision, glaucoma
GI: Dry mouth, nausea, vomiting, anorexia, constipation, diarrhea, jaundice, weight gain
GU: Urinary retention, urinary frequency, enuresis, impotence, amenorrhea, gynecomastia
HEMA: Anemia, leukopenia, leukocytosis, agranulocytosis
INTEG: Rash, photosensitivity, dermatitis
RESP: ***Laryngospasm,*** dyspnea, ***respiratory depression***

Contraindications: Hypersensitivity, circulatory collapse, liver damage, cerebral arteriosclerosis, coronary disease, severe hypertension/hypotension, blood dyscrasias, coma, brain damage, bone marrow depression, narrow angle glaucoma

Precautions: Pregnancy **C**, lactation, seizure disorders, hypertension, hepatic disease, cardiac disease, prostatic hypertrophy, intestinal obstruction, respiratory conditions

Pharmacokinetics

Absorption	Well absorbed (PO, IM)
Distribution	Widely distributed; crosses placenta, blood-brain barrier
Metabolism	Liver, extensively
Excretion	Kidneys, breast milk
Half-life	Unknown

Pharmacodynamics

	PO	IM
Onset	Erratic	15-30 min
Peak	2 hr	30 min
Duration	4-6 hr	6-8 hr

Interactions

Drug/drug:

Individual drugs

Alcohol: ↑ effects of both drugs, oversedation
Aluminum hydroxide: ↓ absorption
Bromocriptine: ↓ antiparkinsonian activity
Disopyramide: ↑ anticholinergic effects
Epinephrine: ↑ toxicity
Guanethidine: ↓ antihypertensive response
Levodopa: ↓ antiparkinsonian activity
Lithium: ↓ mesoridazine levels, ↑ extrapyramidal symptoms, masking of lithium toxicity
Magnesium hydroxide: ↓ absorption
Norepinephrine: ↓ vasoresponse, ↑ toxicity
Phenobarbital: ↓ effectiveness, ↑ metabolism

Drug classifications

Antacids: ↓ absorption
Anticholinergics: ↑ anticholinergic effects
Antidepressants: ↑ CNS depression
Antidiarrheals, adsorbent: ↓ absorption
Antihistamines: ↑ CNS depression
Antihypertensives: ↑ hypotension
Barbiturate anesthetics: ↑ CNS depression
β-Adrenergics: ↑ effects of both drugs

M

General anesthetics: ↑ CNS depression
MAOI: ↑ CNS depression
Narcotics: ↑ CNS depression
Sedative/hypnotics: ↑ CNS depression

Lab test interferences

Increase: Liver function tests, cardiac enzymes, cholesterol, blood glucose, prolactin, bilirubin, PBI, cholinesterase ^{131}I, alkaline phosphatase, leukocytes, granulocytes, platelets
Decrease: Hormones (blood and urine)
False positive: Pregnancy tests, PKU
False negative: Urinary steroids, 17-OHCS

NURSING CONSIDERATIONS

Assessment

- Assess mental status: orientation, mood, behavior, presence and type of hallucinations before initial administration and monthly; this drug should significantly reduce psychotic behavior
- Check for swallowing of PO medication; check for hoarding or giving of medication to other patients
- Monitor I&O ratio; palpate bladder if low urinary output G occurs, especially in elderly; urinalysis recommended before, during prolonged therapy
- Monitor bilirubin, CBC, liver function studies monthly
- Assess affect, orientation, LOC, reflexes, gait, coordination, sleep pattern disturbances
- Monitor B/P with patient sitting, standing, and lying; take pulse and respirations q4h during initial treatment; establish baseline before starting treatment; report drops of 30 mm Hg; obtain baseline ECG, Q wave and T wave changes
- Check for dizziness, faintness, palpitations, tachycardia on rising; severe orthostatic hypotension is common
- Identify for neuroleptic malignant syndrome: hyperpyrexia, muscle rigidity, increased CPK, altered mental status; drug should be discontinued
- Assess for EPS including akathisia (inability to sit still, no pattern to movements), tardive dyskinesia (bizarre movements of the jaw, mouth, tongue, extremities,) pseudoparkinsonism (ragged tremors, pill rolling, shuffling gate); an antiparkinsonism drug should be prescribed
- Assess for constipation, urinary retention daily; if these occur, increase bulk, water in diet

Associated nursing diagnoses

✓ Thought processes, altered (uses)
✓ Coping, ineffective individual (uses)
✓ Knowledge deficit (teaching)
✓ Noncompliance (teaching)

Implementation

PO route

- Administer drug in liq form mixed in glass of juice or cola if hoarding is suspected; do not mix in caffeine drinks or with tannics, pectins
- Administer decreased dosage G in elderly, since metabolism is slowed
- Administer PO with full glass of water, milk; or give with food to decrease GI upset

• Store in airtight, light-resistant container, oral sol in bottle

IM route

• Inject deeply in large muscle mass; do not give SC; do not administer sol with a precipitate

Patient/family education

• Teach patient to use good oral hygiene; frequent rinsing of mouth, sugarless gum for dry mouth
• Tell patient to avoid hazardous activities until drug response is determined; dizziness, blurred vision may occur
• Inform patient that orthostatic hypotension occurs often and to rise from sitting or lying position gradually; to remain lying down after IM inj for at least 30 min; tell patient to avoid hot tubs, hot showers, tub baths, since hypotension may occur; tell patient that in hot weather heat stroke may occur; take extra precautions to stay cool
• Caution patient to avoid abrupt withdrawal of this drug, or EPS may result; drug should be withdrawn slowly
• Teach patient to avoid OTC preparations (cough, hay fever, cold) unless approved by presciber, since serious drug interactions may occur; avoid use with alcohol, CNS depressants; increased drowsiness may occur
• Caution patient to use a sunscreen and sunglasses in case of photosensitivity
• Teach patient about EPS and necessity of meticulous oral hygiene, since oral candidiasis may occur
• Advise patient to take antacids 2 hr before or after taking this drug
• Instruct patient to report sore throat, malaise, fever, bleeding, mouth sores; if these occur, CBC should be drawn and drug discontinued
• Teach patient that urine may turn pink or red

Evaluation

Positive therapeutic outcome

• Decrease in emotional excitement, hallucinations, delusions, paranoia
• Reorganization of patterns of thought, speech

Treatment of overdose: Lavage if orally ingested; provide airway; *do not induce vomiting or use epinephrine*

metaproterenol

(met-a-proe-ter′e-nole)
Alupent, Arm-A-Med metaproterenol sulfate, Metaprel
Func. class.: Selective β_2-agonist, bronchodilator
Pregnancy category C

Action: Relaxes bronchial smooth muscle by direct action on β_2-adrenergic receptors, with increased levels of cAMP and increased bronchodilatation, diuresis, and cardiac and CNS stimulation

Therapeutic Outcome: Bronchodilatation with ease of breathing

M

Uses: Bronchial asthma, bronchospasm

Dosage and routes

P *Adult and child >12 yr:* Inh 2-3 puffs; may repeat q3-4h, not to exceed 12 puffs/day

Asthma/bronchospasm

Adult: PO 20 mg q6-8h

P *Child >9 yr or >27 kg:* PO 20 mg q6-8h or 0.4-0.9 mg/kg tid

P *Child 6-9 yr or <27 kg:* PO 10 mg q6-8h or 0.4-0.9 mg/kg tid

Available forms: Tab 10, 20 mg; aerosol 0.65 mg/dose; syr 10 mg/5 ml; sol nebulizer 0.4%, 0.6%, 5%

Side effects/adverse reactions

CNS: *Tremors,* anxiety, insomnia, headache, dizziness, stimulation
CV: Palpitations, tachycardia, hypertension, dysrhythmias, ***cardiac arrest***
GI: Nausea, vomiting

Contraindications: Hypersensitivity to sympathomimetics, narrow angle glaucoma

Precautions: Pregnancy **C**, cardiac disorders, hyperthyroidism, diabetes mellitus, prostatic hypertrophy

Pharmacokinetics

Absorption	Well absorbed (PO)
Distribution	Unknown
Metabolism	Liver, tissues
Excretion	Unknown
Half-life	2-4 hr

Pharmacodynamics

	PO	INH
Onset	15 min	5 min
Peak	1 hr	1 hr
Duration	4 hr	4 hr

Interactions

Drug/drug:

Drug classifications

β-Adrenergic blockers: Block therapeutic effect
Bronchodilators, aerosol: ↑ action of bronchodilator
MAOI: ↑ chance of hypertensive crisis
Sympathomimetics: ↑ adrenergic side effects

NURSING CONSIDERATIONS

Assessment

- Monitor respiratory function: vital capacity, FEV, ABGs, lung sounds, heart rate, rhythm (baseline)
- Determine that patient has not received theophylline therapy before giving dose; identify client's ability to self-medicate
- Monitor for evidence of allergic reactions; paradoxic bronchospasm; withhold dose; notify prescriber

Associated nursing diagnoses

✓ Airway clearance, ineffective (uses)
✓ Impaired gas exchange (uses)
✓ Knowledge deficit (teaching)

Implementation

Aerosol route

- Give after shaking, exhale, place mouthpiece in mouth, inhale slowly, hold breath,

remove, exhale slowly; allow at least 1 min between inh
• Store in light-resistant container, do not expose to temp over 86° F (30° C)

PO route
• Give PO with meals to decrease gastric irritation; syrup to children (no alcohol, sugar)

Patient/family education

• Advise patient not to use OTC medications; extra stimulation may occur; to use this medication before other medications and allow at least 5 min between each to prevent overstimulation
• Teach patient use of inhaler; review package insert with patient; teach patient to avoid getting aerosol in eyes, since blurring may result; to wash inhaler in warm water qd and dry; to avoid smoking, smoke-filled rooms, persons with respiratory tract infections
• Advise patient that paradoxic bronchospasm may occur and to stop drug immediately and notify prescriber; to limit caffeine products such as chocolate, coffee, tea, and colas
• Instruct patient on administration of dose; not to use more than prescribed; serious side effects may occur

Evaluation

Positive therapeutic outcome
• Absence of dyspnea, wheezing after 1 hr
• Improved airway exchange
• Improved ABGs

Treatment of overdose:

Administer a β_2-adrenergic blocker

methadone

(meth'a-done)
Dolophine HCl, methadone HCl, methadone HCl Diskets, methadone HCl Intensol, Methadose

Func. class.: Narcotic analgesic
Chem. class.: Opiate, synthetic diphenylheptane derivative

Pregnancy category **B**
Controlled substance schedule **II**

Action: Depresses pain impulse transmission at the spinal cord level by interacting with opioid receptors; produces CNS depression

Therapeutic Outcome: Relief of pain; successful narcotic withdrawal

Uses: Severe pain, narcotic withdrawal

Dosage and routes

Pain
Adult: PO/SC/IM 2.5-10 mg q4-12h prn

Narcotic withdrawal
Adult: PO 15-40 mg/day individualized initially, then 20-120 mg/day titrated to patient response

Available forms: Inj 10 mg/ml; tabs 5, 10 mg; oral sol 5, 10 mg/5 ml; dispersible tab 40 mg; oral cap 10 mg/ml

Side effects/adverse reactions

CNS: ***Drowsiness, dizziness, confusion, headache, sedation,*** euphoria
CV: Palpitations, bradycardia, change in B/P
EENT: Tinnitus, blurred vision, miosis, diplopia
GI: ***Nausea, vomiting, anorexia, constipation, cramps,*** biliary tract spasm
GU: Increased urinary output, dysuria, urinary retention
INTEG: ***Rash,*** urticaria, bruising, flushing, diaphoresis, pruritus
RESP: ***Respiratory depression***

Contraindications: Hypersensitivity to this drug, or hypersensitivity to chlorobutanol (inj route), addiction (narcotic)

Precautions: Addictive personality, pregnancy **B**, lactation, increased intracranial pressure, MI (acute), severe heart disease, respiratory depression, hepatic disease, renal disease, P child <18 yr

Pharmacokinetics

Absorption	Well absorbed (PO, SC, IM)
Distribution	Widely distributed; crosses placenta
Metabolism	Liver, extensively
Excretion	Kidneys, breast milk
Half-life	1-1½ days

Pharmacodynamics

	PO	IM	SC
Onset	½-1hr	20 min	20 min
Peak	1½-2 hr	1-2 hr	1-2 hr
Duration	4-12 hr	4-6 hr	4-6 hr

Interactions

Drug/drug:

Individual drugs
Alcohol: ↑ respiratory depression, hypotension, sedation
Cimetidine: ↑ recovery
Erythromycin: ↑ recovery
Nalbuphine: ↓ analgesia
Pentazocine: ↓ analgesia

Drug classifications
Antihistamines: ↑ respiratory depression, hypotension
CNS depressants: ↑ respiratory depression, hypotension
MAOI: Do not use for 2 wk before taking methadone
Phenothiazines: ↑ respiratory depression, hypotension
Sedative/hypnotics: ↑ respiratory depression, hypotension

Lab test interferences

Increase: Amylase, lipase

NURSING CONSIDERATIONS

Assessment

- Monitor VS after parenteral route; note muscle rigidity, drug history, liver, kidney function tests, respiratory dysfunction: respiratory depression, character, rate, rhythm; notify prescriber if respirations are <10/min
- Monitor CNS changes: dizziness, drowsiness, hallucinations, euphoria, LOC, pupil reaction
- Monitor allergic reactions: rash, urticaria

Associated nursing diagnoses

- ✓ Pain (uses)
- ✓ Sensory-perceptual alteration: visual, auditory (adverse reactions)

✓ Breathing pattern, ineffective (adverse reactions)
✓ Knowledge deficit (teaching)

Implementation

- Medication should be slowly withdrawn after long-term use to prevent withdrawal symptoms

PO route

- May be given with food or milk to lessen GI upset
- Store in light-resistant container at room temp

IM/SC route

- Do not give if cloudy or a precipitate has formed
- Give deeply in large muscle mass; rotate inj sites

Patient/family education

- Instruct patient to report any symptoms of CNS changes, allergic reactions; to avoid CNS depressants: alcohol, sedative/hypnotics for at least 24 hr after taking this drug
- Discuss with patient that dizziness, drowsiness, and confusion are common; to avoid getting up without assistance
- Discuss in detail all aspects of the drug
- Caution patient to make position changes slowly to prevent orthostatic hypotension

Evaluation

Positive therapeutic outcome

- Decreased pain
- Successful narcotic withdrawl

Treatment of overdose:

Naloxone (Narcan) 0.2-0.8 **IV**, O_2, **IV** fluids, vasopressors

methicillin

(meth-i-sill'in)
Staphcillin
Func. class.: Broad-spectrum antibiotic
Chem. class.: Penicillinase-resistant penicillin
Pregnancy category **B**

Action: Interferes with cell wall replication of susceptible organisms; osmotically unstable cell wall swells, bursts from osmotic pressure

Uses: Penicillinase-producing staphylococci, streptococci; infections of respiratory tract, skin, skin structures, urinary tract, bone, joint; sinusitis, endocarditis, septicemia, meningitis

Therapeutic Outcome: Bactericidal for the following gram-positive cocci: *Staphylococcus aureus, Streptococcus pyogenes, S. viridans, S. faecalis, S. bovis, S. pneumoniae;* improvement of infections caused by penicillinase-producing *staphylococci*

Dosage and routes

Adult: IM/**IV** 4-12 g/day in divided doses q4-6h

P *Child:* IM/**IV** 50-300 mg/kg/day in divided doses q4-12h

Available forms: Powder for inj 1, 4, 6, 10 g; **IV** inf only 1 g

Side effects/adverse reactions

CNS: Lethargy, hallucina-

M

tions, anxiety, depression, twitching, ***coma, convulsions***
GI: Nausea, vomiting, diarrhea, increased AST (SGOT), ALT (SGPT), abdominal pain, glossitis, colitis, interstitial nephritis
GU: Oliguria, ***proteinuria, hematuria, vaginitis, moniliasis, glomerulonephritis***
HEMA: Anemia, increased bleeding time, ***bone marrow depression, granulocytopenia***

Contraindications: Hypersensitivity to penicillins

Precautions: Pregnancy **B**, hypersensitivity to cephalosporins, P neonates

Pharmacokinetics

Absorption	Well absorbed
Distribution	Widely distributed; crosses placenta
Metabolism	Not metabolized
Excretion	Kidneys, unchanged; breast milk
Half-life	20-30 min; increased in renal disease

Pharmacodynamics

	IM	IV
Onset	Rapid	Rapid
Peak	½-1 hr	15 min
Duration	4 hr	4 hr

Interactions

Drug/drug:

Individual drugs
Probenecid: ↑ methicillin levels, ↓ renal excretion
Drug classifications
Erthromycins: ↓ antimicrobial effectiveness
Oral anticoagulants: ↑ anticoagulant effects
Oral contraceptives: ↓ contraceptive effectiveness
Tetracyclines: ↓ antimicrobial effectiveness

Lab test interferences

False positive: Urine glucose, urine protein

NURSING CONSIDERATIONS

Assessment

- Assess patient for previous sensitivity reaction to penicillins or other cephalosporins; cross-sensitivity between penicillins and cephalosporins is common
- Assess patient for signs and symptoms of infection including characteristics of wounds, sputum, urine, stool, WBC >10,000, fever; obtain baseline information and during treatment
- Obtain C & S before beginning drug therapy to identify if correct treatment has been initiated
- Assess for allergic reactions: rash, urticaria, pruritus, chills, fever, joint pain; angioedema may occur a few days after therapy begins; epinephrine, resuscitation equipment should be available for anaphylactic reaction
- Identify urine output; if decreasing, notify prescriber (may indicate nephrotoxicity); also check for increased BUN, creatinine
- Monitor blood studies: AST (SGOT), ALT (SGPT), CBC, Hct, bilirubin, LDH, alkaline phosphatase, Coombs' test monthly if patient is on long-term therapy
- Monitor electrolytes: potassium, sodium, chloride

monthly if patient is on long-term therapy
- Assess bowel pattern qd; if severe diarrhea occurs, drug should be discontinued
- Monitor for bleeding: ecchymosis, bleeding gums, hematuria, stool guaiac daily if on long-term therapy
- Assess for overgrowth of infection: perineal itching, fever, malaise, redness, pain, swelling, drainage, rash, diarrhea, change in cough, sputum

Associated nursing diagnoses

✓Infection, risk for (uses)
✓Diarrhea (adverse reactions)
✓Injury, risk for (adverse reactions)
✓Knowledge deficit (teaching)
✓Noncompliance (teaching)

Implementation

IM route
- Reconstitute 1 g/1.5 ml sterile water or 0.9% NaCl; 5 g/5.7 ml; 6 g/8.6 ml yielding conc of 500 mg/ml
- Give slowly in deep muscle mass; well tolerated by deep intragluteal inj; may be painful

IV **IV route**
- Reconstitute 1 g/1.5 ml sterile water or 0.9% NaCl; 5 g/5.7 ml; 6 g/8.6 ml yielding conc of 500 mg/ml
- Give by direct IV by further diluting in 20-25 ml of sterile water, 0.9% NaCl; give 10 ml/min
- Give by intermittent inf after diluting in D_5W, $D_{10}W$, 0.9% NaCl, D_5/0.9% NaCl, D_5/LR, LR, Ringer's, run over ½-8 hr; stable for 8 hr at room temp
- Do not admix with other drugs

Syringe incompatibilities:
Heparin, kanamycin, oxytetracycline, tetracycline

Syringe compatibilities:
Chloramphenicol, colistimethate, erythromycin, gentamicin, lidocaine, polymyxin B, procaine

Y-site compatibilities:
Heparin, hydrocortisone sodium succinate, potassium chloride, verapamil, vitamin B with C

Additive incompatibilities:
Amikacin, chlorpromazine, codeine, levorphanol, meperidine, metaraminol, methadone, methohexital, morphine, oxytetracycline, promethazine, tetracycline, vancomycin

Additive compatibilities:
Aminophylline, ascorbic acid, calcium chloride, gluconate, cephalothin, chloramphenicol, colistimethate, corticotropin, dimenhydrinate, diphenhydramine, erythromycin, gentamicin, penicillin G, polymyxin B, potassium chloride, prednisolone, procaine, verapamil

Patient/family education

- Teach patient to report sore throat, bruising, bleeding, joint pain; may indicate blood dyscrasias (rare)
- Advise patient to contact prescriber if vaginal itching, loose, foul-smelling stools, furry tongue occur; may indicate superinfection
- Advise patient to notify prescriber of diarrhea with

blood or pus, which may indicate pseudomembranous colitis

Evaluation

Positive therapeutic outcome
- Absence of signs/symptoms of infection (WBC <10,000, temp WNL, absence of red, draining wounds)
- Reported improvement in symptoms of infection

Treatment of anaphylaxis: Withdraw drug, maintain airway, administer epinephrine, aminophylline, O_2, **IV** corticosteroids

methimazole
(meth-im′a-zole)
Tapazole
Func. class.: Thyroid hormone antagonist (antithyroid)
Chem. class.: Thioamide
Pregnancy category **D**

Action: Inhibits synthesis of thyroid hormones by decreasing iodine use in the manufacture of thyroglobin and iodothyronine; does not affect already formed hormones

➔ **Therapeutic Outcome:** Decreased T_4 levels, hyperthyroid symptoms

Uses: Hyperthyroidism, preparation for thyroidectomy, thyrotoxic crisis, thyroid storm

Dosage and routes

Hyperthyroidism

Adult: PO 5-20 mg tid depending on severity of condition; continue until euthyroid; maintenance dosage 5-10 mg qd-tid; max dosage 150 mg qd

P *Child:* PO 0.4 mg/kg/day in divided doses q8h; continue until euthyroid; maintenance dosage 0.2 mg/kg/day in divided doses q8h

Preparation for thyroidectomy

P *Adult and child:* PO same as above; iodine may be added for 10 days before surgery

Thyrotoxic crisis

P *Adult and child:* PO same as hyperthyroidism with iodine and propranolol

Available forms: Tab 5, 10 mg

Side effects/adverse reactions

CNS: Drowsiness, headache, vertigo, fever, paresthesias, neuritis
ENDO: Enlarged thyroid
GI: Nausea, diarrhea, vomiting, ***jaundice, hepatitis,*** loss of taste
GU: Nephritis
HEMA: Agranulocytosis, leukopenia, thrombocytopenia, hypothrombinemia, lymphadenopathy, bleeding, vasculitis
INTEG: Rash, urticaria, pruritus, alopecia, hyperpigmentation, lupuslike syndrome
MS: Myalgia, arthralgia, nocturnal muscle cramps

Contraindications: Hypersensitivity, pregnancy (3rd trimester) **D**, lactation

Precautions: Infection, bone marrow depression, hepatic disease, pregnancy (1st, 2nd trimester), patient >40 yr

Pharmacokinetics

Absorption	Rapidly absorbed (PO)
Distribution	Crosses placenta
Metabolism	Liver, extensively
Excretion	Kidneys, unchanged; breast milk
Half-life	1-2 hr

Pharmacodynamics

Onset	½ hr
Peak	Unknown
Duration	2-4 hr

Interactions

Drug/drug:

Individual drugs

Lithium: ↑ antithyroid effect
Potassium iodide: ↑ antithyroid effect
Radiation: ↑ bone marrow depression

Drug classifications

Antineoplastics: ↑ bone marrow depression
Phenothiazines: ↑ granulocytosis

Lab test interferences

Increase: Pro-time, AST (SGOT), ALT (SGPT), alkaline phosphatase

NURSING CONSIDERATIONS

Assessment

- Monitor pulse, B/P, temp; check I&O ratio; check for edema (puffy hands, feet, periorbits); indicates hypothyroidism
- Check weight qd; same clothing, scale, time of day
- Monitor T_3, T_4, which are increased; serum TSH, which is decreased; free thyroxine index, which is increased if dosage is too low; discontinue drug 3-4 wk before RAIU
- Monitor blood work: CBC for blood dyscrasias (leukopenia, thrombocytopenia, agranulocytosis); liver function tests
- Assess for overdose (peripheral edema, heat intolerance, diaphoresis, palpitations, dysrhythmias, severe tachycardia, increased temp, delirium, CNS irritability); drug should be discontinued
- Assess for hypersensitivity (rash, enlarged cervical lymph nodes); drug may have to be discontinued
- Assess for hypoprothrombinemia (bleeding, petechiae, ecchymosis)
- Monitor clinical response: after 3 wk should include increased weight, pulse, decreased T_4
- Assess for bone marrow depression: sore throat, fever, fatigue

Associated nursing diagnoses

✓ Knowledge deficit (teaching)
✓ Noncompliance (teaching)

Implementation

PO route

- Give with meals to decrease GI upset; give at same time each day to maintain drug level
- Give lowest dosage that relieves symptoms
- Store in light-resistant container
- Increase fluids to 3-4 L/day, unless contraindicated

M

Patient/family education

- Advise patient to abstain from breastfeeding after delivery; drug appears in breast milk
- Instruct patient to take pulse daily; to keep graph of weight, pulse, mood
- Advise patient to report redness, swelling, sore throat, mouth lesions, which indicate blood dyscrasias
- Caution patient to avoid OTC products that contain iodine; that seafood and other iodine-containing products may be restricted by prescriber
- Caution patient not to discontinue this medication abruptly; thyroid crisis may occur; stress patient compliance
- Advise patient that response may take several mo if thyroid is large
- Teach patient symptoms/signs of overdose: periorbital edema, cold intolerance, mental depression; notify prescriber at once
- Teach patient symptoms of inadequate dosage: tachycardia, diarrhea, fever, irritability; prescriber should be notified to adjust
- Teach patient to take medication exactly as prescribed, not to skip or double doses; missed doses should be taken when remembered up to 1 hr before next dose
- Instruct patient to carry identification (Medic Alert) describing medication taken and condition being treated

Evaluation

Positive therapeutic outcome

- Decreased weight gain
- Decreased pulse
- Decreased T_4
- Decreased B/P

methocarbamol

(meth-oh-kar'ba-mole)

Delaxin, Marbaxin 750, methocarbamol, Robaxin, Robaxin-750, Robomol-500, Robomol-750, Tresortil ✤

Func. class.: Skeletal muscle relaxant, central acting

Chem. class.: Carbamate derivative

Pregnancy category **C**

Action: Depresses multisynaptic pathways in the spinal cord, causing skeletal muscle relaxation

➔ Therapeutic Outcome: Decreased pain, spasm

Uses: Adjunct for relief of spasm and pain in musculoskeletal conditions, tetanus management

Dosage and routes

Pain of muscle spasm

Adult: PO 1.5 g × 2-3 days, then 1 g qid; IM 500 mg in each gluteal region; may repeat q8h; **IV** bol 1-3 g/day at 3 ml/min; **IV** inf 1 g/250 ml D_5W or NS, not to exceed 3 g/day

Tetanus

Adult: **IV** inf 1-3 g/L of sol q6h; **IV** bol 1-2 g injected into running **IV**

P *Child:* **IV** 15 mg/kg q6h

Available forms: Tab 500, 750 mg; inj 100 mg/ml

Side effects/adverse reactions

CNS: ***Dizziness, weakness, drowsiness,*** headache, tremor, depression, insomnia, ***seizures***
CV: Postural hypotension, bradycardia
EENT: Diplopia, temporary loss of vision, blurred vision, nystagmus
GI: ***Nausea,*** vomiting, hiccups, anorexia, metallic taste
GU: Brown, black, green urine
HEMA: Hemolysis, increased hemoglobin (**IV** only)
INTEG: Rash, pruritus, fever, facial flushing, urticaria

Contraindications: Hypersensitivity, P child <12 yr, intermittent porphyria

Precautions: Renal disease, hepatic disease, addictive personalities, pregnancy **C**, myasthenia gravis, epilepsy

Pharmacokinetics

Absorption	Rapidly absorbed (PO)
Distribution	Widely distributed; crosses placenta
Metabolism	Liver, partially
Excretion	Kidney, unchanged
Half-life	1-2 hr

Pharmacodynamics

	PO	IM	IV
Onset	½ hr	Rapid	Rapid
Peak	1-2 hr	Unknown	Inf end
Duration	>8 hr	Unknown	Unknown

Interactions

Drug/drug:

Individual drugs
Alcohol: CNS depression
Drug classifications
Antidepressants, tricyclic: ↑ CNS depression
Barbiturates: ↑ CNS depression
Narcotics: ↑ CNS depression
Sedative/hypnotics: ↑ CNS depression

Lab test interferences

False increase: VMA, urinary 5 HIAA

NURSING CONSIDERATIONS

Assessment

- Assess for pain and spasm: location, duration, intensity, range of motion
- Monitor during and after inj: CNS effects, rash, conjunctivitis, and nasal congestion may occur
- Monitor ECG in epileptic patients; poor seizure control has occurred in patients taking this drug
- Assess allergic reactions: rash, fever, respiratory distress; check for severe weakness, numbness in extremities
- Assess for tolerance: increased need for medication, more frequent requests for medication, increased pain
- Assess for CNS depression: dizziness, drowsiness, psychiatric symptoms

Associated nursing diagnoses

- ✓ Physical mobility, impaired (uses)
- ✓ Injury, risk for (adverse reactions)

M

✓ Knowledge deficit (teaching)

Implementation

PO route
- Give with meals if GI symptoms occur
- Store in tight container at room temp

IV **IV route**
- Give **IV** undiluted over 1 min or more; give 300 mg or less/1 min or longer; may be diluted in 250 ml or less D_5 or isotonic NaCl sol
- Give by slow **IV** to prevent phlebitis; keep recumbent for 15 min to prevent orthostatic hypotension; check for extravasation

IM route
- Give deep in large muscle mass; rotate sites

Patient/family education

- Advise patient not to discontinue medication quickly; insomnia, nausea, headache, spasticity, tachycardia will occur; drug should be tapered off over 1-2 wk
- Inform patient that urine may turn green, black, or brown
- Caution patient not to take with alcohol, other CNS depressants; increased CNS depression can occur
- Advise patient to avoid altering activities while taking this drug
- Caution patient to avoid hazardous activities if drowsiness, dizziness occur; driving should be avoided until drug response is known
- Advise patient to avoid using OTC medications that are CNS depressants (cough preparations, antihistamines) unless directed by prescriber; CNS depression can occur

Evaluation

Positive therapeutic outcome
- Decreased pain, spasticity

Treatment of overdose:
Induce emesis in conscious patient; lavage, dialysis; have epinephrine, antihistamines, and corticosteroids available

methohexital
(meth-oh-hex′i-tal)
Brevital Sodium, Brietal Sodium ✤
Func. class.: General anesthetic
Chem. class.: Barbiturate
Pregnancy category **C**
Controlled substance schedule **IV**

Action: Acts in reticular activating system in the CNS to produce anesthesia; may be potentiated by GABA

➔ **Therapeutic Outcome:** Anesthesia

Uses: General anesthesia for electroshock therapy, reduction of fractures, adjunct with other anesthetics, balanced anesthesia

Dosage and routes
Induction
P ***Adult and child:*** **IV** 50-100 mg given 1 ml/5 sec

Maintenance
P ***Adult and child:*** **IV** 20-40 mg q4-7 min of a 0.1% sol

Available forms: Inj 500 mg, 2.5, 5g

Side effects/adverse reactions

CNS: Retrograde amnesia, prolonged somnolence, seizures
CV: Tachycardia, hypotension, ***myocardial depression, dysrhythmias***
EENT: Sneezing, coughing
GI: Nausea, vomiting, abdominal pain, hiccups
INTEG: Chills, *shivering*, necrosis, pain at inj site
MS: Muscle irritability
RESP: Respiratory depression, bronchospasm, **dyspnea**

Contraindications: Hypersensitivity, status asthmaticus, hepatic/intermittent porphyrias

Precautions: Severe cardiovascular disease, renal disease, pregnancy **C**, hypotension, liver disease, myxedema, myasthenia gravis, asthma, increased intracranial pressure

Pharmacokinetics

Absorption	Well absorbed (IM); completely absorbed (IV)
Distribution	Fatty tissues
Metabolism	Liver, kidneys, brain
Excretion	Kidneys, breast milk
Half-life	4 hr; increased in G elderly

Pharmacodynamics

	IM	IV
Onset	Unknown	30-40 sec
Peak	Unknown	Unknown
Duration	Unknown	6 min

Interactions

Drug/drug:

Individual drugs
Alcohol: ↑ action, CNS depression

Drug classifications
Analgesics, narcotics: ↑ action, CNS depression
Antihistamines: ↑ action, CNS depression
CNS depressants: ↑ action, CNS depression

NURSING CONSIDERATIONS

Assessment

- Monitor VS q10 min during **IV** administration, q30 min after IM dose
- Assess for hallucinations, delusions, separation from environment
- Assess for extrapyramidal reactions: dystonia, akathisia
- Check for increasing heart rate or decreasing B/P; notify prescriber at once

Associated nursing diagnoses

✓ Sensory-perceptural alterations (adverse reactions)
✓ Knowledge deficit (teaching)

Implementation

IV **IV route**

- Give by direct **IV** at 10 mg/5 sec or more
- Give by cont inf by reconstituting 2.5 g/15 ml or 5 g/30 ml sterile water, 0.9% NaCl, D_5W

Syringe incompatibility:
Glycopyrrolate

M

Additive incompatibilities:

Atropine, chlorpromazine, cimetidine, clindamycin, droperidol, fentanyl, hydralazine, kanamycin, lidocaine, mechlorethamine, metaraminol, methicillin, methyldopate, metocurine, oxytetracycline, pancuronium, penicillin G potassium, pentazocine, prochlorperazine, promazine, promethazine, propiomazine, scopolamine, succinylcholine, streptomycin, tetracycline, tubocurarine

Patient/family education

- Instruct patient to avoid CNS depressants for 24 hr after methohexital
- Teach patient reason for medication and expected results

Evaluation

Positive therapeutic outcome
- Maintenance of anesthesia

methotrexate

(meth-oh-trex'ate)

Amethopterin, Folex PFS, methotrexate, methotrexate LPF, Rheumatrex Dose Pack

Func. class.: Antineoplastic, antimetabolite

Chem. class.: Folic acid antagonist

Pregnancy category X

Action: Inhibits an enzyme that reduces folic acid, which is needed for nucleic acid synthesis in all cells; S phase of cell cycle specific; immunosuppressive

Therapeutic Outcome: Prevention of rapidly growing malignant cells; immunosuppression

Uses: Acute lymphocytic leukemia, in combination for breast, lung, head, neck carcinoma, lymphosarcoma, gestational choriocarcinoma, hydatidiform mole, psoriasis, rheumatoid arthritis, mycosis fungoides

Dosage and routes

Leukemia

P *Adult and child:* PO 3.3 mg/m^2/day given with prednisone IT 12 mg/m^2; maintenance 30 mg/m^2/day 2 times a wk; **IV** 2.5 mg/kg q2 wk

Choriocarcinoma

P *Adult and child:* PO 15-30 mg/ m^2 qd × 5 days, then off 1 wk; may repeat

Osteosarcoma

P *Adult and child:* **IV** 12 g/m^2 given over 4 hr, then leucovorin rescue is given

Mycosis fungoides

Adult: PO 2.5-10 mg/day until cleared (may be many mo); IM 50 mg q wk or 25 mg 2 times a wk

Psoriasis

Adult: PO/IM/**IV** 10 mg q wk; may increase to 25 mg q wk

Available forms: Tab 2.5 mg; inj 25 mg/ml; powder for inj 20, 25, 50, 100, 250

mg/g; sodium inj 2.5, 25 mg/ml

Side effects/adverse reactions

CNS: Dizziness, ***convulsions,*** headache, confusion, hemiparesis, malaise, fatigue, chills, fever
GI: Nausea, vomiting, anorexia, diarrhea, stomatitis, ***hepatotoxicity,*** cramps, ulcer, gastritis, ***GI hemorrhage,*** abdominal pain, hematemesis
GU: Urinary retention, ***renal failure,*** menstrual irregularities, defective spermatogenesis, ***hematuria, azotemia, uric acid nephropathy***
HEMA: ***Leukopenia, thrombocytopenia, myelosuppression, anemia***
INTEG: Rash, alopecia, dry skin, urticaria, photosensitivity, folliculitis, vasculitis, petechiae, ecchymosis, acne, alopecia

Contraindications: Hypersensitivity, leukopenia (<2500/mm^3), thrombocytopenia (<100,000/mm^3), anemia, psoriatic patients with severe renal/hepatic disease, pregnancy **X**

Precautions: Renal disease, lactation

Pharmacokinetics

Absorption	Well absorbed (GI)
Distribution	Widely distributed; crosses placenta
Metabolism	Not metabolized
Excretion	Kidneys, unchanged; breast milk (minimal)
Half-life	2-4 hr; increased in renal disease

Pharmacodynamics

	PO	IM/IV	IT
Onset	Unknown	Unknown	Unknown
Peak	1-4 hr	½-2 hr	Unknown
Duration	Unknown	Unknown	Unknown

Interactions

Drug/drug:

Individual drugs
Acyclovir: ↑ neurologic reactions (IT route)
Allopurinol: ↑ toxicity
Asparaginase: ↓ effects of methotrexate
Chloramphenicol: ↑ toxicity
Cyclophosphamide: ↑ cardiotoxicity, CHF
Phenylbutazone: ↑ toxicity
Phenytoin: ↑ toxicity
Probenecid: ↑ toxicity
Radiation: ↑ toxicity, bone marrow suppression
Warfarin: ↑ or ↓ effect of warfarin

Drug classifications
Antineoplastics: ↑ toxicity bone marrow suppression
Hepatotoxic agents: ↑ hepatotoxicity
Live virus vaccines: ↓ antibodies
Nephrotoxic drugs: ↑ toxicity
Nondepolarizing muscle relaxants: Reversal of neuromuscular blockade
NSAIDs: ↑ toxicity
Salicylates: ↑ toxicity
Sulfonylureas: ↑ toxicity
Tetracylines: ↑ toxicity

NURSING CONSIDERATIONS

Assessment

- Assess buccal cavity q8h for dryness, sores or ulceration,

M

white patches, oral pain, bleeding, dysphagia; obtain prescription for viscous lidocaine (Xylocaine)
• Assess symptoms indicating severe allergic reaction: rash, pruritus, urticaria, purpuric skin lesions, itching, flushing
• Assess tachypnea, ECG changes, dyspnea, edema, fatigue; identify dyspnea, rales, unproductive cough, chest pain, tachypnea
• Monitor CBC, differential, platelet count weekly; withhold drug if WBC count is <4000/mm^3 or platelet count is <100,000/mm^3; notify prescriber of results if WBC <20,000/mm^3, platelets <150,000/mm^3
• Assess for increased uric acid levels, swelling, joint pain primarily in extremities; patient should be well hydrated to prevent urate deposits
• Monitor renal function studies: BUN, creatinine, serum uric acid, urine CrCl before and during therapy; check I&O ratio; report fall in urine output to <30 ml/hr
• Monitor temp q4h (may indicate beginning of infection)
• Monitor liver function tests before and during therapy (bilirubin, AST [SGOT], ALT [SGPT], LDH) as needed or monthly; check for yellowing of skin and sclera, dark urine, clay-colored stools, itchy skin, abdominal pain, fever, diarrhea (hepatotoxicity)
• Assess for bleeding: hematuria, stool guaiac, bruising or petechiae, mucosa or orifices q8h; check for inflammation of mucosa, breaks in skin
• Identify effects of alopecia on body image; discuss feelings about body changes
• Identify edema in feet, joint and stomach pain, shaking; prescriber should be notified
• Identify inflammation of mucosa, breaks in skin

Associated nursing diagnoses

✓ Injury, risk for (adverse reactions)
✓ Body image disturbance (adverse reactions)
✓ Infection, risk for (adverse reactions)
✓ Knowledge deficit (teaching)

Implementation

• Avoid contact with skin, since drug is very irritating; wash completely to remove
• Administer leucovorin calcium within 12 hr of giving this drug to prevent tissue damage; check agency policy
• Give fluids **IV** or PO before chemotherapy to hydrate patient
• Give antacid before oral agent; give drug after evening meal, before hs; give antiemetic 30-60 min before giving drug and prn to prevent vomiting; administer antibiotics for prophylaxis of infection
• Give in AM so drug can be eliminated before hs
• Provide liq diet: carbonated beverages; gelatin may be added if patient is not nauseated or vomiting
• Encourage patient to rinse mouth tid-qid with water, club soda; brush teeth bid-qid with soft brush or cotton-tipped applicators for stomatitis; use unwaxed dental floss

PO route
- Give 1 hr ac or 2 hr pc to prevent vomiting

IM route
- Give deeply in large muscle mass

IV **IV route**
- Give **IV** after diluting 5 mg/2 ml of sterile water for inj; give through Y-tube or 3-way stopcock at 10 mg or less/min
- Give **IV** inf after diluting in 0.9% NaCl, D_5W, D_5/0.9% NaCl and give as prescribed

Syringe incompatibilities:
Droperidol, ranitidine

Syringe compatibilities:
Bleomycin, cisplatin, cyclophosphamide, doxapram, doxorubicin, fluorouracil, furosemide, leucovorin, mitomycin, vinblastine, vincristine

Y-site incompatibilities:
Droperidol, idarubicin

Y-site compatibilities:
Bleomycin, cisplatin, cyclophosphamide, doxorubicin, fludarabine, fluorouracil, furosemide, heparin, leucovorin, metoclopramide, melphalan, mitomycin, ondansetron, paclitaxel, sargramostim, vancomycin, vinblastine, vincristine, vinorelbine

Additive incompatibilities:
Bleomycin, prednisolone

Additive compatibilities:
Cephalothin, cyclophosphamide, cytarabine, fluorouracil, hydroxyzine, mercaptopurine, sodium bicarbonate, vincristine

Solution compatibilities:
Amino acids, 4.25%/D_{25}, D_5W, sodium bicarbonate 0.05 mol/L

Patient/family education

- Advise patient that contraceptive measures are recommended during therapy; drug is teratogenic; contraception should be used for 3 mo (male) and 4-6 wk (female)
- Teach patient to avoid use of products containing aspirin or ibuprofen, razors, commercial mouthwash, since bleeding may occur; to report symptoms of bleeding (hematuria, tarry stools)
- Caution patient to report signs of anemia (fatigue, headache, irritability, faintness, shortness of breath)
- Advise patient to report any changes in breathing or coughing even several mo after treatment; to avoid crowds and persons with respiratory tract or other infections
- Teach patient that hair may be lost during treatment; a wig or hair piece may make patient feel better; new hair may be different in color, texture
- Caution patient not to have any vaccinations without the advice of the prescriber; serious reactions can occur

Evaluation

Positive therapeutic outcome
- Prevention of rapid division of malignant cells

M

methotrimeprazine

(meth-oh-trye-mep′ra-zeen)
Levoprome, Nozinan ♣
Func. class.: Nonopioid analgesic
Chem. class.: Aliphatic (propylamine phenothiazine derivative)
Pregnancy category C

Action: Depresses cerebral cortex, hypothalamus, limbic system; blocks neurotransmission produced by dopamine at synapse; exhibits strong α-adrenergic, anticholinergic blocking action; antihistamine

Therapeutic Outcome: Decreased pain; analgesia

Uses: Sedation, analgesia, preoperative and postoperative analgesia, obstetric analgesia in nonambulatory patients

Dosage and routes

Analgesia/sedation

P *Adult and child >12 yr:* IM 10-20 mg q4-6h prn

G *Elderly:* IM 5-10 mg q4-6h

Preoperative medication

P *Adult and child >12 yr:* IM 2-20 mg 45 min to 3 hr before surgery

Postoperative medication

P *Adult and child >12 yr:* IM 2.5-7.5 mg q4-6h titrated to patient's needs

Obstetric analgesia

Adult: 15-20 mg; may be repeated

Available forms: Inj 20 mg/ml

Side effects/adverse reactions

CNS: ***Weakness, dizziness,*** drowsiness, confusion, delirium, euphoria, headache, sedation, EPS
CV: ***Orthostatic hypotension,*** palpitations, tachycardia, bradycardia
EENT: Nasal congestion, blurred vision, slurred speech
GI: ***Nausea, vomiting, abdominal pain, dry mouth,*** jaundice (long-term use)
GU: ***Hematuria,*** dysuria, hesitancy, retention, uterine inertia (rare)
HEMA: ***Thrombocytopenia, agranulocytosis, leukopenia, neutropenia, hemolytic anemia*** (long-term use, high dosage)
INTEG: Pain, edema at inj site, fever, chills

Contraindications: Hypersensitivity to this drug, phenothiazines, bisulfite; seizures, severe hepatic disease, severe renal disease, severe cardiac disease, coma

G **Precautions:** Elderly, pregnancy **C**

Pharmacokinetics

Absorption	Well absorbed (IM)
Distribution	CSF, placenta
Metabolism	Liver, extensively; to active metabolites
Excretion	Kidneys, unchanged (1%)
Half-life	15-30 hr

Pharmacodynamics

Onset	20-30 min
Peak	1-2 hr
Duration	4 hr

Interactions

Drug/drug:

Individual drugs

Alcohol: ↑ sedation, hypotension

Atropine: ↑ anticholinergic effect

Disopyramide: ↑ anticholinergic effect

Epinephrine: ↓ vasopressor effect

Meprobamate: ↑ sedation

Reserpine: ↑ sedation

Scopolamine: ↑ anticholinergic effect

Drug classifications

Antidepressants: ↑ CNS depression, anticholinergic effect

Antihistamines: ↑ CNS depression, anticholinergic effect

Antihypertensives: ↑ hypotension

MAOI: ↑ hypotension

Narcotic analgesics: ↑ CNS depression

Nitrates: ↑ hypotension

Phenothiazines: ↑ anticholinergic effect

Sedatives/hypnotics: ↑ CNS depression

NURSING CONSIDERATIONS

Assessment

- Assess pain: location, duration, intensity
- Monitor blood counts during therapy; watch for decreasing platelets; if low, therapy may need to be discontinued, restarted after hematologic recovery; check for blood dyscrasia (thrombocytopenia): bruising, fatigue, bleeding, poor healing
- Assess for effect on uterine contractions, fetal heart tones if drug is used for labor
- Assess patient for EPS (akathisia, dystonia), since drug is a phenothiazine derivative

Associated nursing diagnoses

- ✓ Pain (uses)
- ✓ Injury, risk for (adverse reactions)
- ✓ Knowledge deficit (teaching)

Implementation

- Give after removal of cigarettes to prevent fires
- Give lowest dosage, then gradually increase; lower dosages are required after general anesthesia
- Provide bed rest for several hours after inj if orthostatic hypotension occurs
- Provide safety measure: low side rails, night light, call bell within easy reach if drowsiness or dizziness occurs

IM route

- Give deeply in large muscle mass; rotate inj sites; do not give by **IV** or SC inj
- Do not allow to come in contact with skin, contact dermatitis may occur
- Store in darkness; product expires after 5 yr

Syringe compatibilities:

Atropine, hydroxyzine, metoclopramide, scopolamine

Syringe incompatibility:

Ranitidine

M

Patient/family education

- Teach patient that drug must be continued for prescribed time to be effective; to avoid aspirin, alcoholic beverages and other CNS depressants
- Caution patient to report bleeding, bruising, fatigue, malaise, since blood dyscrasias do occur
- Instruct patient to use caution when driving; drowsiness, dizziness may occur; to ask for assistance with ambulation for 6 hr after inj

Evaluation

Positive therapeutic outcome

- Decreased pain
- Increased sedation

Treatment of overdose: Monitor electrolytes, VS

methyldopa/ methyldopate

(meth-ill-doe′pa)

Aldomet, Amodopar, Apo-Methyldopa ✤, Dopamet ✤, Novamedopa ✤, methyldopa/ methyldopate HCl

Func. class.: Antihypertensive

Chem. class.: Centrally acting α-adrenergic inhibitor

Pregnancy category C

Action: Stimulates central α_2-adrenergic receptors in the CNS, resulting in decreased sympathetic outflow from the brain with decreased peripheral resistance

➔ **Therapeutic Outcome:** Decreased B/P in hypertension

Uses: Hypertension

Dosage and routes

Adult: PO 250-500 mg bid or tid, then adjusted q2 days prn, 0.5-3 g qd in 2-4 divided doses (maintenance), not to exceed 3 g/day; **IV** 250-500 mg in 100 ml D_5W q6h, run over 30-60 min, not to exceed 1 g q6h

P ***Child:*** PO 10 mg/kg/day in 2-4 divided doses, not to exceed 65 mg/kg or 3 g/day, whichever is less; **IV** 20-40 mg/kg/day in 4 divided doses, not to exceed 65 mg/kg

Available forms: Tab 125, 250, 500 mg; oral susp 250 mg/5 ml; inj 50 mg/ml (250 mg/5 ml)

Side effects/adverse reactions

CNS: Drowsiness, weakness, dizziness, sedation, headache, depression, psychosis

CV: Bradycardia, myocarditis, orthostatic hypotension, angina, edema, weight gain

EENT: Nasal congestion, eczema

GI: Nausea, vomiting, diarrhea, constipation, hepatic dysfunction

GU: Impotence, failure to ejaculate

HEMA: Leukopenia, thrombocytopenia, hemolytic anemia, positive Coombs' test

INTEG: Lupuslike syndrome

Contraindications: Active hepatic disease, hypersensitivity, blood dyscrasias

Precautions: Pregnancy **C**, liver disease, eclampsia, severe cardiac disease

Pharmacokinetics

Absorption	50% (PO)
Distribution	Crosses placenta, blood-brain barrier
Metabolism	Liver, moderately
Excretion	Kidneys, unchanged (partially)
Half-life	1½ hr

Pharmacodynamics

	PO	IV
Onset	Unknown	Unknown
Peak	2-4 hr	2 hr
Duration	12-24 hr	10-16 hr

Interactions

Drug/drug:

Individual drugs

Alcohol: ↑ hypotension
Levodopa: ↑ hypotension, toxicity
Lithium: ↑ lithium toxicity

Drug classifications

Amphetamines: ↓ antihypertensive effect
Antihypertensives: ↑ hypotension
Antidepressants, tricyclic: ↓ antihypertensive effect
NSAIDs: ↓ antihypertensive effect
Nitrates: ↑ hypotension
Phenothiazines: ↓ antihypertensive effect

NURSING CONSIDERATIONS

Assessment

- Monitor blood studies: neutrophils, decreased platelets
- Monitor renal studies: protein, BUN, creatinine; watch for increased levels that may indicate nephrotic syndrome: polyuria, oliguria, frequency
- Obtain baselines in renal, liver function tests before therapy begins; check potassium levels, although hyperkalemia rarely occurs
- Monitor B/P, pulse if the drug is being used for hypertension; notify prescriber of changes
- Monitor edema in feet, legs daily; monitor I&O; check weight for decreasing output
- Assess for allergic reaction: rash, fever, pruritus, urticaria; drug should be discontinued if antihistamines fail to help

Associated nursing diagnoses

- ✓ Cardiac output, decreased (uses)
- ✓ Injury, risk for (side effects)
- ✓ Knowledge deficit (teaching)
- ✓ Noncompliance (teaching)

Implementation

PO route

- Give ac
- Shake susp before using
- Store in tight container at room temp

IV **IV route**

- Give by intermittent inf after diluting in 100 ml 0.9% NaCl, D_5W, D_5/0.9% NaCl, 5% sodium bicarbonate, Ringer's sol; administer over 30-60 min

Y-site compatibilities:

Esmolol, meperidine, morphine

M

Additive incompatibilities:

Amphotericin B, barbiturates, methohexital, sulfonamides

Additive compatibilities:

Aminophylline, ascorbic acid, chloramphenicol, diphenhydramine, heparin, magnesium sulfate, multivitamins, netilmicin, potassium chloride, promazine, sodium bicarbonate, succinylcholine, verapamil, vitamin B with C

Solution compatibilities:

D_5W, D_5/0.9% NaCl, Ringer's, sodium bicarbonate 5%, 0.9% NaCl, amino acids 4.25%/D_{25}, $Dextran_6$/0.9% NaCl, Normosol R, Normosol M/D_5W

Patient/family education

- Instruct patient not to discontinue drug abruptly, or withdrawal symptoms may occur: anxiety, increased B/P, headache, insomnia, increased pulse, tremors, nausea, sweating
- Caution patient not to use OTC (cough, cold, or allergy) products unless directed by prescriber
- Teach patient to comply with dosage schedule even if feeling better; drug controls symptoms, does not cure
- Caution patient to change position slowly, to rise slowly to sitting or standing position to minimize orthostatic hypotension, especially elderly (G)
- Teach patient about excessive perspiration, dehydration, vomiting; diarrhea may lead to fall in B/P; consult prescriber if these occur
- Advise patient that drug may cause dizziness, fainting; lightheadedness may occur during 1st few days of therapy; that drug may cause dry mouth; use hard candy, saliva product, or frequent rinsing of mouth
- Caution patient that compliance is necessary; not to skip or stop drug unless directed by prescriber
- Teach patient that drug may cause skin rash
- Teach patient to avoid hazardous activities, since drug may cause drowsiness, dizziness
- Teach patient to take ac

Evaluation

Positive therapeutic outcome
- Decreased B/P

methylergonovine

(meth-ill-er-goe-noe'veen)
Methergine, Methylergobasine ✤, Methylergonovine
Func. class.: Oxytocic
Chem. class.: Ergot alkaloid
Pregnancy category C

Action: Stimulates uterine and vascular smooth muscle, causing contractions, decreased bleeding

➔ Therapeutic Outcome: Absence of hemorrhage

Uses: Treatment of hemorrhage post partum or after abortion

Dosage and routes

Adult: IM 0.2 mg q2-5h, not to exceed 5 doses; **IV** 0.2 mg given over 1 min; PO 0.2 mg given over 1 min; PO 0.2-0.4 mg q6-12h × 2-7 days after initial IM or **IV** dose

Available forms: Inj 0.2 mg/ml; tab 0.2 mg

Side effects/adverse reactions

CNS: *Headache, dizziness*
CV: Chest pain, palpitations, hypertension, *hypotension,* dysrhythmias
EENT: Tinnitus
GI: *Nausea, vomiting*
GU: Cramping
INTEG: Sweating, rash, allergic reactions
RESP: *Dyspnea*

Contraindications: Hypersensitivity to ergot preparations, indication of labor, before delivery of placenta, hypertension, pelvic inflammatory disease, respiratory disease, cardiac disease, peripheral vascular disease

Precautions: Pregnancy **C**, severe hepatic disease, severe renal disease, jaundice, diabetes mellitus, convulsive disorders

Pharmacokinetics

Absorption	Well absorbed (PO, IM)
Distribution	Unknown
Metabolism	Liver, possibly
Excretion	Unknown
Half-life	½-2 hr

Pharmacodynamics

	PO	IM	IV
Onset	5-15 min	5 min	Immediate
Peak	Unknown	Unknown	Unknown
Duration	3 hr	3 hr	Unknown

Interactions

Drug/drug:

Individual drugs

Cyclopropane anesthesia: ↑ hypotension

Drug classifications

Vasopressors: ↑ hypertension

Drug/smoking:

↑ vasoconstriction

NURSING CONSIDERATIONS

Assessment

- Monitor B/P, pulse; watch for change that may indicate hemorrhage; check respiratory rate, rhythm, depth; notify prescriber of abnormalities
- Assess fundal tone, nonphasic contractions; check for relaxation or severe cramping
- Assess for ergotism or overdose: nausea, vomiting, weakness, muscular pain, insensitivity to cold, paresthesia of extremities; drug should be decreased or inf discontinued
- Before administering ergonovine, calcium levels should be checked; if hypocalcemia is present, correction should be made to increase effectiveness of this drug
- Monitor prolactin levels and for decreased breast milk production

M

Associated nursing diagnoses

✓ Tissue perfusion, decreased (uses)
✓ Injury, risk for (adverse reactions)
✓ Knowledge deficit (teaching)

Implementation

PO route
- PO is the preferred route

IM route
- Give deeply in large muscle mass

IV **IV route**
- Give by this route for severe, life-threatening hemorrhage
- Give directly undiluted or diluted with 5 ml 0.9% NaCl given through Y-site or 3-way stopcock; give 0.2 mg/min; use clear, colorless sol
- Store up to 2 mo if unused

Y-site compatibilities:

Heparin, hydrocortisone sodium succinate, potassium chloride, vitamin B with C

Patient/family education

- Advise patient to stop smoking, since increased vasoconstriction will result
- Inform patient that abdominal cramps are a side effect of this medication
- Instruct patient to notify prescriber if chest pain, nausea, vomiting, headache, muscle pain, weakness or cold, numb extremities occur

Evaluation

Positive therapeutic outcome
- Prevention of hemorrhage

methylphenidate

(meth-ill-fen′i-date)
Methidate, Ritalin, Ritalin SR
Func. class.: Cerebral stimulant
Chem. class.: Piperidine derivative
Pregnancy category C
Controlled substance schedule II

Action: Increases release of norepinephrine and dopamine in cerebral cortex to reticular activating system; exact action not known

Therapeutic Outcome: Increased alertness, decreased fatigue, ability to stay awake (narcolepsy), increased attention span, decreased hyperactivity (ADHD)

Uses: Attention deficit disorder with hyperactivity, narcolepsy

Dosage and routes

ADHD

Adult: PO 5-20 bid-tid

P ***Child >6 yr:*** PO 5 mg before breakfast and lunch, increasing by 5-10 mg/wk, not to exceed 60 mg/day

Narcolepsy

Adult: PO 10 mg bid-tid, 30-45 min ac; may increase up to 40-60 mg/day

Available forms: Tab 5, 10, 20 mg; sus rel tab 20 mg

Side effects/adverse reactions

CNS: Hyperactivity, insomnia, restlessness, talkativeness, dizziness, headache, akathisia, dyskinesia, Gilles de la Tourette's syndrome
CV: Palpitations, tachycardia, B/P changes, angina, dysrhythmias, ***thrombocytopenic purpura***
ENDO: Growth retardation
GI: Nausea, anorexia, dry mouth, weight loss, abdominal pain
GU: Uremia
HEMA: Leukopenia, anemia
INTEG: Exfoliative dermatitis, urticaria, rash, erythema multiforme
MISC: Fever, arthralgia, scalp hair loss

Contraindications: Hypersensitivity, anxiety, history of Gilles de la Tourette's syndrome; P children <6 yr, glaucoma

Precautions: Hypertension, depression, pregnancy **C**, seizures, lactation, drug abuse

Pharmacokinetics

Absorption	Well absorbed (PO); delayed (sus rel)
Distribution	Widely distributed; crosses placenta
Metabolism	Liver
Excretion	Kidneys
Half-life	1-3 hr

Pharmacodynamics

	PO	PO–SUS REL
Onset	½-1 hr	2 hr
Peak	1-3 hr	4 hr
Duration	4-6 hr	6-8 hr

Interactions

Drug/drug:

Drug classifications
Anticonvulsants: ↑ effects
Antidepressants, tricyclics: ↑ effects
MAOI: Hypertensive crisis
Oral anticoagulants: ↑ effects
Sympathomimetics: ↑ effects
Vasopressors: Hypertensive crisis

NURSING CONSIDERATIONS

Assessment

- Monitor VS, B/P, since this drug may reverse antihypertensives; check patients with cardiac disease more often for increased B/P
- Perform CBC, urinalysis; for diabetic patients monitor blood sugar, urine sugar; insulin changes may be required, since eating will decrease
- Monitor height and weight q3 mo since growth rate in children may be decreased; appetite is suppressed, weight loss is common during the first few mo of treatment
- Monitor mental status: mood sensorium, affect, stimulation, insomnia; aggressiveness may occur; depression with crying spells may occur after drug has worn off
- Assess for tolerance; should not be used for extended time except in ADHD; dosage should be discontinued gradually to prevent withdrawal symptoms
- Assess for narcoleptic symptoms before medication and after; ability to stay awake should increase significantly
- In children or adults with ADHD, monitor for improved

M

organizational skills, attention span, attending to tasks, impulse control, socialization, and ability to get along better with others
- Assess for withdrawal symptoms: headache, nausea, vomiting, muscle pain, weakness; drug tolerance will develop after long-term use; dosage should not be increased if tolerance develops

Associated nursing diagnoses

- ✓ Thought processes, altered (uses, adverse reactions)
- ✓ Coping, ineffective individual (uses)
- ✓ Knowledge deficit (teaching)
- ✓ Family coping, impaired (uses)

Implementation

PO route
- Give at least 6 hr before hs to avoid sleeplessness; titrate to patient's response; lowest dosage should be used to control symptoms
- Give gum, hard candy, frequent sips of water for dry mouth at beginning of treatment; these symptoms tend to lessen with time

Patient/family education

- Teach patient to decrease caffeine consumption (coffee, tea, cola, chocolate), which may increase irritability and stimulation; to avoid OTC preparations unless approved by prescriber; to avoid alcohol ingestion; these may cause serious drug interactions
- Advise patient to taper off drug over several wk, or depression, increased sleeping, lethargy may occur
- Caution patient to avoid hazardous activities until stabilized on medication
- Instruct patient not to double doses if medication is missed; prescriber may suggest drug holidays (ADHD) during the school year to assess progress and determine continued drug necessity
- Instruct patient/family to notify presciber if significant side effects occur: tremors, insomnia, palpitations, restlessness; drug changes may be needed
- Inform patient that if dry mouth occurs to use frequent sips of water, sugarless gum, hard candy during beginning therapy; dry mouth lessens with continued treatment
- Encourage patient to get needed rest; patients will feel more tired at end of day; to take last dose at least 6 hr before hs to avoid insomnia

Evaluation

Positive therapeutic outcome
- Decreased activity in ADHD
- Improved attention span in ADHD
- Absence of sleeping during day in narcolepsy

Treatment of overdose:

Administer fluids, hemodialysis, peritoneal dialysis, antihypertensives for increased B/P

methylprednisolone/ methylprednisolone acetate/ methylprednisolone sodium succinate

(meth-ill-pred-niss'oh-lone)
Medrol/Depo-Medrol, Duralone, Medralone, Rep-Pred/A-Methapred, Solu-Medrol
Func. class.: Corticosteroid
Chem. class.: Glucocorticoid, immediate acting
Pregnancy category **C**

Action: Decreases inflammation by suppression of migration of polymorphonuclear leukocytes, fibroblasts; reverses increased capillary permeability and lysosomal stabilization; antipruritic, antiinflammatory (top)

Therapeutic Outcome: Decreased inflammation

Uses: Severe inflammation, shock, adrenal insufficiency, collagen disorders, psoriasis, eczema, contact dermatitis, pruritus (top)

Dosage and routes

Adrenal insufficiency/ inflammation

Adult: PO 2-60 mg if 4 divided doses; IM 40-80 mg (acetate); IM/**IV** 10-250 mg (succinate); intraarticular 4-30 mg (acetate)

P *Child:* **IV** 117 µg-1.66 mg/kg in 3-4 divided doses (succinate)

Shock

Adult: **IV** 100-250 mg q2-6h (succinate)

Pruritus

P *Adult and child:* Apply to affected area qd-qid

Available forms: Tab 2, 4, 6, 8, 16, 24, 32 mg; inj 20, 40, 80 mg/ml acetate; inj 40, 125, 500, 1000 mg/vial succinate; oint 0.25%, 1%

Side effects/adverse reactions

CNS: Depression, flushing, sweating, headache, mood changes
CV: Hypertension, ***circulatory collapse, thrombophlebitis, embolism,*** tachycardia
EENT: Fungal infections, increased intraocular pressure, blurred vision
GI: Diarrhea, nausea, abdominal distention, GI hemorrhage, increased appetite, pancreatitis
HEMA: Thrombocytopenia
INTEG: Burning, dryness, itching, irritation, acne, folliculitis, hypertrichosis, perioral dermatitis, hypopigmentation, atrophy, striae, miliaria, allergic contact dermatitis, secondary infection, poor wound healing, ecchymosis, petechiae
MS: Fractures, osteoporosis, weakness

Contraindications: Hypersensitivity to corticosteroids, fungal infections, psychosis, idiopathic thrombocytopenia, acute glomerulonephritis, amebiasis, nonasthmatic bron-

M

P chial disease, child <2 yr, AIDS, TB

Precautions: Pregnancy **C**, lactation, viral or bacterial infections, diabetes mellitus, glaucoma, osteoporosis

Pharmacokinetics

Absorption	Well absorbed (PO); systemic (top)
Distribution	Crosses placenta
Metabolism	Liver, extensively
Excretion	Kidney
Half-life	3-5 hr; adrenal suppression 3-4 days

Pharmacodynamics

	PO	IM	IV	TOP
Onset	Unknown	Unknown	Rapid	Min to hr
Peak	2 hr	4-8 days	Unknown	Hr to days
Duration	1½ days	1-4 wk	Unknown	Hr to days

Interactions

Drug/drug:

Individual drugs

Amphotericin B: ↑ hypokalemia
Insulin: ↑ need for insulin
Mezlocillin: ↑ hypokalemia
Phenytoin: ↓ action, ↑ metabolism
Rifampin: ↓ action, ↑ metabolism
Ticarcillin: ↑ hypokalemia

Drug classifications

Barbiturates: ↓ action, ↑ metabolism
Diuretics: ↑ hypokalemia
Hypoglycemic agents: ↑ need for hypoglycemic agents

Lab test interferences

Increase: Cholesterol, sodium, blood glucose, uric acid, calcium, urine glucose
Decrease: Calcium, potassium, T_4, T_3, thyroid RAIU test, urine 17-OHCS, 17-KS, PBI
False negative: Skin allergy tests

NURSING CONSIDERATIONS

Assessment

- Monitor potassium, blood sugar, urine glucose while patient is on long-term therapy; hypokalemia and hyperglycemia
- Monitor weight daily; notify prescriber of weekly gain >5 lb
- Monitor B/P q4h, pulse; notify prescriber if chest pain occurs
- Monitor I&O ratio; be alert for decreasing urinary output and increasing edema
- Monitor plasma cortisol levels during long-term therapy (normal level 138-635 nmol/L when drawn at 8 AM)
- Monitor adrenal function periodically for HPA axis suppression
- Assess for infection: increased temp, WBC even after withdrawal of medication; drug masks infection symptoms
- Assess for potassium depletion: paresthesias, fatigue, nausea, vomiting, depression, polyuria, dysrhythmias, weakness
- Assess for edema, hypertension, cardiac symptoms
- Assess mental status: affect, mood, behavioral changes, aggression
- Check temp; if fever develops, drug should be discontinued
- Assess for syst absorption: increased temp, inflammation, irritation (top)

Associated nursing diagnoses

✓Infection, risk for (adverse reactions)
✓Knowledge deficit (teaching)
✓Noncompliance (teaching)

Implementation

IV **IV route**
• Give IV, use only sodium phosphate product; give >1 min; may be given by IV inf in compatible sol
• Give after shaking susp (parenteral)
• Give titrated dosage; use lowest effective dosage

Y-site compatibilities:

Acyclovir, amrinone, enalaprilat, famotidine, fludarabine, melphalan, meperidine, morphine, vitamin B with C

Y-site incompatibilities:

Ondansetron, paclitaxel, sargramostina, vinorelbine

Syringe compatibility:

Metoclopramide

IM route
• Give IM inj deep in large mass; rotate sites; avoid deltoid; use 21 G needle
• Give in one dose in AM to prevent adrenal suppression; avoid SC administration; may damage tissue

PO route
• Give with food or milk to decrease GI symptoms

Inh route
• Give inh with water to decrease possibility of fungal infections
• Give titrated dosage; use lowest effective dosage
• Clean aerosol top daily with warm water; dry thoroughly
• Store in cool environment; do not puncture or incinerate container

Top route
• Cleanse area before applying drug
• Apply only to affected areas; do not get in eyes
• Apply medication, then cover with occlusive dressing (only if prescribed); seal to normal skin; change q12h; syst absorption may occur
• Apply only to dermatoses; do not use on weeping, denuded, or infected area
• Apply treatment for a few days after area has cleared
• Store at room temp

Patient/family education

• Teach patient that ID as steroid user should be carried
• Advise patient to notify prescriber if therapeutic response decreases; dosage adjustment may be needed
• Caution patient not to discontinue abruptly; adrenal crisis can result
• Caution patient to avoid OTC products: salicylates, alcohol in cough products, cold preparations unless directed by prescriber
• Teach patient all aspects of drug usage including cushingoid symptoms
• Teach patient symptoms of adrenal insufficiency: nausea, anorexia, fatigue, dizziness, dyspnea, weakness, joint pain
• Inform patient that long-term therapy may be needed to clear infection (1-2 mo depending on type of infection)

Nasal route
- Advise patient to clear nasal passages if sneezing attack occurs; repeat dose
- Advise patient to continue using product even if mild nasal bleeding occurs; is usually transient
- Teach patient method of instillation after providing written instructions from manufacturer

Top route
- Advise patient to avoid sunlight on affected area; burns may occur

Evaluation

Positive therapeutic outcome
- Ease of respirations, decreased inflammation
- Absence of severe itching, patches on skin, flaking (top)

methysergide
(meth-i-ser'jide)
Sansert
Func. class.: Serotonin antagonist
Chem. class.: Ergot derivative
Pregnancy category **C**

Action: Competitively blocks serotonin hydroxytryptamine receptors in CNS and periphery; potent vasoconstrictor

➡ **Therapeutic Outcome:** Absence of migraines and other vascular headaches

Uses: Prophylaxis for migraine and other vascular headaches

Dosage and routes
Adult: PO 2 mg bid with meals

Available forms: Tab 2 mg

Side effects/adverse reactions
CNS: Tremors, anxiety, insomnia, headache, dizziness, euphoria, confusion, depersonalization, hallucinations, paresthesias, drowsiness
CV: ***Retroperitoneal fibrosis,*** valvular thickening, palpitations, tachycardia, postural hypertension, angina, thrombophlebitis, ECG changes, ***cardiac fibrosis***
GI: Nausea, vomiting, weight gain
HEMA: ***Blood dyscrasias***
INTEG: Flushing, rash, alopecia
MS: Arthralgia, myalgia

Contraindications: Hypersensitivity to ergot, tartrazine, peripheral vascular occlusion, CAD, hepatic disease, renal disease, peptic ulcer, hypertension, connective tissue disease, fibrotic pulmonary disease

Precautions: Pregnancy **C**, P lactation, children

Pharmacokinetics

Absorption	Rapidly absorbed (PO)
Distribution	Widely distributed
Metabolism	Liver
Excretion	Kidneys, breast milk
Half-life	10 hr

Pharmacodynamics

Onset	Unknown
Peak	Unknown
Duration	Unknown

Interactions

Drug/drug:

Drug classifications

β-Blockers: ↑ vasoconstriction
Narcotic analgesics: ↓ effect of narcotics

Drug/smoking: ↑ vasoconstriction

NURSING CONSIDERATIONS

Assessment

- Monitor stress level, activity, reaction, coping mechanisms of patient
- Assess neurologic status: LOC, blurring vision, nausea, vomiting, tingling in extremities preceding headache
- Assess for ingestion of tyramine-containing foods (pickled products, beer, wine, aged cheese), food additives, preservatives, colorings, artificial sweeteners, chocolate, caffeine, which may precipitate these types of headaches

Associated nursing diagnoses

✓ Pain, chronic (uses)
✓ Injury, risk for (adverse reactions)
✓ Knowledge deficit (teaching)

Implementation

- Provide quiet, calm environment with decreased stimulation; no noise, bright lights, or excessive talking

PO route

- Give with or pc to avoid GI symptoms
- Store in dark area

Patient/family education

- Caution patient to avoid OTC medications and alcohol; serious drug interactions may occur
- Caution patient to maintain dosage at approved level; not to increase even if drug does not relieve headache
- Advise patient that an increase in headaches may occur when this drug is discontinued after long-term use
- Caution patient to keep drug out of the reach of children; death may occur
- Caution patient to use drug for less than 6 mo unless a 3-4 wk rest period has been taken

Evaluation

Positive therapeutic outcome

- Decreased in frequency, severity of headache

M

metipranolol

(met-ee-pran'oh-lole)
Optipranolol
Func. class.: β-Adrenergic blocker (ophth)
Chem. class.: I-isomer
Pregnancy category C

Action: Reduces production of aqueous humor by unknown mechanism

➔ **Therapeutic Outcome:** Decreased ocular hypertension

Uses: Ocular hypertension, chronic open angle glaucoma

Dosage and routes

Adult: Instill 1 gtt bid

Available forms: Sol 0.3%

Side effects/adverse reactions

CNS: Weakness, fatigue, depression, anxiety, headache, confusion
CV: ***Bradycardia***
EENT: Eye irritation, conjunctivitis, keratitis
GI: Nausea, anorexia, dyspepsia
INTEG: Rash, urticaria
RESP: ***Bronchospasm,*** dyspnea, bronchitis, coughing, rhinitis

Contraindications: Hypersensitivity, asthma, 2nd- or 3rd-degree heart block, right ventricular failure, congenital **P** glaucoma (infants)

Precautions: Pregnancy **C**

Pharmacokinetics

Absorption	Minimal
Distribution	Minimal
Metabolism	None
Excretion	Lacrimation
Half-life	Short

Pharmacodynamics

Onset	15-30 min
Peak	1-2 hr
Duration	24 hr

Interactions
Drug/drug:

Individual drugs
Metoprolol: ↑ effect
Propranolol: ↑ effect

NURSING CONSIDERATIONS
Assessment

- Monitor B/P, heart rate throughout treatment
- Assess for increased intraocular pressure during treatment
- Monitor for eye irritation, conjunctivitis

Associated nursing diagnoses

✓ Pain (uses)
✓ Sensory-perceptual alteration: visual (uses)
✓ Knowledge deficit (teaching)

Implementation

- Store at room temp for 21 days after reconstituting

Patient/family education

- Advise patient to report change in vision (blurring or loss of sight), trouble breathing, sweating, flushing
- Teach patient method of instillation, including pressure on lacrimal sac for 1 min, and not touching dropper to eye
- Advise patient that long-term therapy may be required
- Assure patient that blurred vision will decrease with continued use of drug

Evaluation

Positive therapeutic outcome
- Decreased intraocular pressure

metoclopramide
(met-oh-kloe-pra′mide)
Clopra, Emex ✤, Maxeran ✤, Maxolon, metoclopramide HCl, Octamide PFS, Reclomide, Reglan
Func. class.: Cholinergic, antiemetic
Chem. class.: Central dopamine receptor antagonist
Pregnancy category B

Action: Enhances response to acetylcholine of tissue in upper GI tract, which causes contraction of gastric muscle, relaxes pyloric, duodenal segments, increases peristalsis without stimulating secretions

➔ **Therapeutic Outcome:** Decreased symptoms of delayed gastric emptying, decreased nausea, vomiting

Uses: Prevention of nausea, vomiting induced by chemotherapy, radiation; delayed gastric emptying, gastroesophageal reflux

Dosage and routes

Nausea/vomiting

Adult: **IV** 2 mg/kg q2h × 5 doses 30 min before administration of chemotherapy

Delayed gastric emptying

Adult: PO 10 mg 30 min ac, hs × 2-8 wk

Gastroesophageal reflux

Adult: PO 10-15 mg qid 30 min ac

Available forms: Tab 5, 10 mg; syr 5 mg/5 ml; inj 5 mg/ml

Side effects/adverse reactions

CNS: Sedation, fatigue, restlessness, headache, sleeplessness, dystonia, dizziness, drowsiness

CV: Hypotension, supraventricular tachycardia

GI: Dry mouth, constipation, nausea, anorexia, vomiting

GU: Decreased libido, prolactin secretion, amenorrhea, galactorrhea

INTEG: Urticaria, rash

Contraindications: Hypersensitivity to this drug or procaine or procainamide, seizure disorder, pheochromocytoma, breast cancer (prolactin dependent), GI obstruction

Precautions: Pregnancy **B**, lactation, GI hemorrhage, CHF

Pharmacokinetics

Absorption	Well absorbed (PO)
Distribution	Widely distributed; crosses blood-brain barrier, placenta
Metabolism	Liver, minimally
Excretion	Kidneys, breast milk
Half-life	4 hr

Pharmacodynamics

	PO	IM	IV
Onset	½-1 hr	10-15 min	1-3 min
Peak	Unknown	Unknown	Unknown
Duration	1-2 hr	1-2 hr	1-2 hr

Interactions

Drug/drug:

Individual drugs

Alcohol: ↓ action of metoclopramide

Haloperidol: ↑ extrapyramidal reaction

Drug classifications

Anticholinergics: ↓ action of metoclopramide

Antidepressants: ↑ CNS depression

Antihistamines: ↑ CNS depression

M

CNS depressants: ↑ sedation
MAOI: ↑ catecholamine levels
Opiates: ↑ sedation
Phenothiazines: ↑ extrapyramidal reaction
Sedative/hypnotics: ↑ CNS depression

Lab test interferences

Increase: Prolactin, aldosterone, thyrotropin

NURSING CONSIDERATIONS

Assessment

- Assess GI complaints: nausea, vomiting, anorexia, constipation, abdominal distention before and after administration
- Assess for EPS and tardive dyskinesia: rigidity, grimacing, shuffling gait, tremors, rhythmic involuntary movements of tongue, mouth, jaw, feet, hands; these side effects should be reported to prescriber immediately; some effects may be irreversible
- Assess mental status: depression, anxiety, irritability during treatment

Associated nursing diagnoses

✓ Injury, risk for (adverse reactions)
✓ Knowledge deficit (teaching)

Implementation

IV IV route

- Give **IV** undiluted if dose is <10 mg; give over 2 min
- Dilute 10 mg or more in 50 ml or more D_5W, NaCl, Ringer's, LR and given over 15 min or more
- Discard open ampules

Syringe compatibilities:

Aminophylline, ascorbic acid, atropine, benztropine, bleomycin, chlorpromazine, cisplatin, cyclophosphamide, cytarabine, dexamethasone, dimenhydrinate, diphenhydramine, doxorubicin, droperidol, fentanyl, fluorouracil, heparin, hydrocortisone, hydroxyzine, regular insulin, leucovorin, lidocaine, magnesium sulfate, meperidine, methylprednisolone sodium succinate, midazolam, mitomycin, morphine, pentazocine, perphenazine, prochlorperazine, promazine, promethazine, ranitidine, scopolamine, vinblastine, vincristine

Syringe incompatibilities:

Ampicillin, calcium gluconate, cephalothin, chloramphenicol, furosemide, penicillin G potassium, sodium bicarbonate

Y-site incompatibility:

Furosemide

Additive compatibilities:

Clindamycin, multivitamins, potassium acetate, potassium chloride, potassium phosphate, verapamil

Additive incompatibilities:

Cisplatin, erythromycin lactobionate, tetracycline

PO route

- Give 30-60 min ac for better absorption and at hs
- Use gum, hard candy, frequent rinsing of mouth for dryness of oral cavity

Patient/family education

- Instruct patient to avoid driving, other hazardous activi-

ties until stabilized on this medication
• Advise patient to avoid alcohol and other CNS depressants that enhance sedating properties of this drug
• Advise patient to notify prescriber if involuntary movements occur

Evaluation

Positive therapeutic outcome
• Absence of nausea, vomiting, anorexia, fullness

metocurine
(me-toe-cure'een)
Metubine
Func. class.: Neuromuscular blocker (nondepolarizing)
Chem. class.: Methyl analog of tubocurarine
Pregnancy category **C**

Action: Inhibits transmission of nerve impulses by binding with cholinergic receptor sites, antagonizing action of acetylcholine; no analgesic response

Therapeutic Outcome: Paralysis of all skeletal muscles

Uses: Facilitation of endotracheal intubation, skeletal muscle relaxation during mechanical ventilation, surgery, or general anesthesia, reduction of fractures/dislocations

Dosage and routes

Surgery
Adult: **IV** 2-4 mg if given cyclopropane as an anesthetic; 1.5-3 mg if given ether as an anesthetic; 4-7 mg if given nitrous oxide

Electroconvulsive therapy adjunct
Adult: **IV** 2-3 mg

Available forms: Inj 2 mg/ml

Side effects/adverse reactions

CV: Bradycardia, tachycardia, increased, decreased B/P
EENT: Increased secretions, salivation
INTEG: Rash, flushing, pruritus, urticaria
RESP: ***Prolonged apnea, bronchospasm, cyanosis, respiratory depression***

Contraindications: Hypersensitivity to iodides

Precautions: Pregnancy **C**, cardiac disease, hepatic disease, renal disease, lactation, P children <2 yr, electrolyte imbalances, dehydration, neuromuscular disease (myasthenia gravis), respiratory disease, when histamine release is a definite hazard (e.g., asthma)

Pharmacokinetics	
Absorption	Completely absorbed (IV)
Distribution	Widely distributed; crosses placenta
Metabolism	Plasma
Excretion	Kidneys, unchanged (50%)
Half-life	3½ hr

Pharmacodynamics	
Onset	2-2½ min
Peak	5 min
Duration	½-1½ hr

M

Interactions

Drug/drug:

Individual drugs

Clindamycin: ↑ paralysis length and intensity
Colistin: ↑ paralysis length and intensity
Lidocaine: ↑ paralysis length and intensity
Lithium: ↑ paralysis length and intensity
Magnesium sulfate: ↑ paralysis length and intensity
Polymyxin B: ↑ paralysis length and intensity
Procainamide: ↑ paralysis length and intensity
Quinidine: ↑ paralysis length and intensity
Succinylcholine: ↑ paralysis length and intensity

Drug classifications

Aminoglycosides: ↑ paralysis length and intensity
β-Blockers: ↑ paralysis length and intensity
Diuretics, potassium-losing: ↑ paralysis length and intensity
General anesthesia: ↑ paralysis length and intensity

NURSING CONSIDERATIONS

Assessment

- Monitor VS (B/P, pulse, respirations, airway) until fully recovered; rate, depth, pattern of respirations, strength of hand grip; patient should be intubated before use
- Monitor for electrolyte imbalances (potassium, magnesium) before drug is used; electrolyte imbalances may lead to increased action of this drug
- Monitor for recovery: decreased paralysis of face, diaphragm, leg, arm, rest of body; residual weakness and respiratory problems may occur during recovery period
- Assess for hypersensitive reactions: rash, fever, respiratory distress, pruritus; drug should be discontinued

Associated nursing diagnoses

- ✓ Breathing pattern, ineffective (uses)
- ✓ Communication, impaired verbal (adverse reactions)
- ✓ Fear (adverse reactions)
- ✓ Knowledge deficit (teaching)

Implementation

IV **IV route**

- Use peripheral nerve stimulator (anesthesiologist) to determine neuromuscular blockade; deep tendon reflexes should be monitored during extended periods
- Give direct **IV** undiluted over 1 min; may give doses of 0.5-1 mg titrated to patient response; should be administered only by qualified person, usually an anesthesiologist; do not administer IM
- Store in light-resistant container
- Give anticholinesterase to reverse neuromuscular blockade

Patient/family education

- Provide reassurance if communication is difficult during recovery from neuromuscular blockade
- Provide explanation to patients regarding all procedures or treatments; patient will remain conscious if anesthesia is not given also

Evaluation

Positive therapeutic outcome
- Paralysis of jaw, eyelid, head, neck, rest of body as evaluated by peripheral nerve stimulator

Treatment of overdose:
Edrophonium or neostigmine, atropine, monitor VS; may require mechanical ventilation

metolazone
(me-tole'a-zone)
Diulo, MyKrox, Zaroxolyn
Func. class.: Diuretic, antihypertensive
Chem. class.: Thiazide-like quinazoline derivative
Pregnancy category **B**

Action: Acts on the distal tubule and cortical thick ascending limb of the loop of Henle in the kidney, increasing excretion of sodium, water, chloride, magnesium, potassium, and bicarbonate

➡ **Therapeutic Outcome:** Decreased BP, decreased edema in lung tissue and peripherally

Uses: Edema in CHF, nephrotic syndrome; may be used alone or as adjunct with antihypertensives for mild to moderate hypertension

Dosage and routes

Edema
Adult: PO 5-20 mg/day

Hypertension
Adult: PO 2.5-5 mg/day (Diulo, Zaroxolyn); PO 0.5 mg (MyKrox) qd in AM: may increase to 1 mg

Available forms: Mykrox Tab 0.5, Zaroxolyn 2.5, 5, 10 mg

Side effects/adverse reactions

CNS: Drowsiness, paresthesia, anxiety, depression, headache, *dizziness, fatigue, weakness*
CV: Irregular pulse, orthostatic hypotension, palpitations, volume depletion, chest pain
EENT: Blurred vision
ELECT: *Hypokalemia,* hypercalcemia, hyponatremia, hypochloremia, hypomagnesemia, hypophosphatemia
GI: *Nausea, vomiting, anorexia,* constipation, diarrhea, cramps, pancreatitis, GI irritation, ***hepatitis***
GU: *Frequency,* polyuria, ***uremia,*** glucosuria
HEMA: ***Aplastic anemia, hemolytic anemia, leukopenia, agranulocytosis, neutropenia***
INTEG: *Rash,* urticaria, purpura, photosensitivity, fever
META: *Hyperglycemia, hypomagnesemia, increased creatinine, BUN*

Contraindications: Hypersensitivity to thiazides or sulfonamides, anuria, renal decompensation

Precautions: Hypokalemia, renal disease, hepatic disease, gout, COPD, lupus erythema-

M

G tosus, diabetes mellitus, elderly, pregnancy **B**, lactation

Pharmacokinetics

Absorption	GI tract (10%-20%)
Distribution	Crosses placenta
Metabolism	Urine, unchanged
Excretion	Breast milk
Half-life	8 hr (extended); 14 hr (prompt)

Pharmacodynamics

Onset	1 hr
Peak	2 hr
Duration	12-24 hr

Interactions

Drug/drug:

Individual drugs

Cholestyramine: ↓ absorption of metolazone
Colestipol: ↓ absorption of metolazone
Diazoxide: ↓ hyperglycemia, hyperuricemia, hypotension
Digitalis: ↑ toxicity
Indomethacin: ↓ hypotensive response
Lithium: ↑ toxicity
Mezlocillin: ↑ hypokalemia
Piperacillin: ↑ hypokalemia
Ticarcillin: ↑ hypokalemia

Drug classifications

Antidiabetics: ↓ effect of antidiabetic agent
Antihypertensives: ↑ antihypertensive effect
Cardiac glycosides: ↑ hypokalemia
Glucocorticoids: ↑ hypokalemia
Sulfonylureas: ↓ effect of sulfonylurea
Nondepolarizing skeletal muscle relaxants: ↑ toxicity

Drug/food:

Food: ↑ absorption

Lab test interferences

Interfere: Urine steroid tests
Increase: BSP retention, calcium, amylase, parathyroid test
Decrease: PBI, PSP

NURSING CONSIDERATIONS

Assessment

- Monitor glucose in urine if patient is diabetic
- Check for rashes, temp elevation qd
- Monitor patients that receive cardiac glycosides for increased hypokalemia
- Monitor manifestations of hypokalemia; acidic urine, reduced urine, osmolality, nocturia; hypotension, broad T wave, U wave, ectopy, tachycardia, weak pulse; muscle weakness, altered LOC, drowsiness, apathy, lethargy, confusion, depression; anorexia, nausea, cramps, constipation, distention, paralytic ileus; hypoventilation, respiratory muscle weakness
- Monitor for manifestations of hypomagnesemia: agitation, muscle twitching, paresthesias, hyperactive reflexes, positive Babinski reflex, dysphagia, nystagmus seizures, tetany; nausea, vomiting, diarrhea, anorexia, abdominal distention; Ectopy, tachycardia, broad, flat, or inverted T waves, depressed ST segment, prolonged QT, decreased cardiac output, hypotension
- Monitor for manifestations of hyponatremia; increased B/P, cold, clammy skin, hypovolemia or hypervolemia; anorexia, nausea, vomiting, diarrhea, abdominal cramps; lethargy, increased ICP, confu-

sion, headache, seizures, coma, fatigue, tremors, hyperreflexia
- Monitor for manifestations of hyperchloremia: weakness, lethargy, coma, deep rapid breathing
- Assess and record fluid volume status: I&O ratios; monitor weight, distended red veins, crackles in lung, color, quality and sp gr of urine, skin turgor, adequacy of pulses, moist mucous membranes, bilateral lung sounds, peripheral pitting edema; dehydration symptoms of decreasing output, thirst, hypotension, dry mouth and mucous membranes should be reported
- Monitor electrolytes: potassium, sodium, calcium, magnesium; also include BUN, blood pH, ABGs, uric acid, CBC, blood sugar
- Assess B/P before and during therapy with patient lying, standing, and sitting as appropriate; orthostatic hypotension can occur rapidly

Associated nursing diagnoses

- ✓ Altered urinary elimination (adverse reactions)
- ✓ Fluid volume deficit (adverse reactions)
- ✓ Fluid volume excess (uses)
- ✓ Knowledge deficit (teaching)

Implementation

- Give in AM to avoid interference with sleep
- Provide potassium replacement if potassium level is 3.0; drug may be crushed if patient is unable to swallow
- Give with food; if nausea occurs, absorption may be increased; extended release products are Diulo, Zaroxolyn; prompt action product is MyKrox; the two formulations are not equivalent

Patient/family education

- Teach patient to take the medication early in the day to prevent nocturia
- Instruct the patient to take with food or milk if GI symptoms of nausea and anorexia occur
- Teach patient to maintain a weekly record of weight and notify prescriber of weight loss >5 lb
- Caution the patient that this drug causes a loss of potassium, so food rich in potassium should be added to the diet; refer to a dietician for assistance in planning
- Caution the patient not to exercise in hot weather or stand for prolonged periods, since orthostatic hypotension will be enhanced
- Teach patient not to use alcohol or any OTC medications without prescriber's approval; serious drug reactions may occur
- Emphasize the need to contact prescriber immediately if muscle cramps, weakness, nausea, dizziness or numbness occurs
- Teach patient to take own B/P and pulse and record
- Advise patient to use sunscreen to prevent burns
- Caution the patient that orthostatic hypotension may occur and to rise slowly from sitting or reclining positions, lie down if dizziness occurs
- Teach patient to continue

M

taking medication even if feeling better; this drug controls symptoms but does not cure the condition
• Advise the patient with hypertension to continue other medical treatment (exercise, weight loss, relaxation techniques, cessation of smoking)

Evaluation

Positive therapeutic outcome
• Decreased edema
• Decreased B/P

Treatment of overdose:

Lavage if taken orally, monitor electrolytes; administer dextrose in saline; monitor hydration, CV, renal status

metoprolol

(met-oh-proe'lole)
Apo-Metoprolol ✦, Betaloc ✦, Betaloc Durules ✦, Lopressor, Lopressor SR ✦, Novometoprol ✦, Toprol XL
Func. class.: Antihypertensive, antianginal
Chem. class.: β_1-Blocker
Pregnancy category **C**

Action: Competitively blocks stimulation of β_1-adrenergic receptor within vascular smooth muscle; produces chronotropic, inotropic activity (decreases rate of SA node discharge, increases recovery time), slows conduction of AV node, decreases heart rate, which decreases O_2 consumption in myocardium; also decreases renin-aldosterone-angiotensin system at high doses

➡ **Therapeutic Outcome:** Decreased B/P, heart rate, AV conduction

Uses: Mild to moderate hypertension, acute MI to reduce cardiovascular mortality, angina pectoris

Investigational uses: Dysrhythmias, hypertrophic cardiomyopathy, mitral valve prolapse, pheochromocytoma, tremors, prevention of vascular headaches, aggression

Dosage and routes

Hypertension

Adult: PO 50 mg bid, or 100 mg qd; may give 200-450 mg in divided doses; ext rel tabs give qd

MI

Adult: Early treatment, **IV** bol 5 mg q2 min × 3 doses, then 50 mg PO 15 min after last dose and q6h × 48 hr; late treatment, PO maintenance 100 mg bid for 3 mo

Available forms: Tab 50, 100 mg; inj 1 mg/ml; ext rel tab 50, 100, 200 mg

Side effects/adverse reactions

CNS: Insomnia, dizziness, mental changes, hallucinations, ***depression,*** anxiety, headaches, nightmares, confusion, fatigue

CV: Hypotension, *bradycardia, CHF: palpitations,* dysrhythmias, ***cardiac arrest, AV block***
EENT: Sore throat, dry burning eyes
GI: Nausea, vomiting, colitis, cramps, *diarrhea,* constipation, flatulence, dry mouth, *hiccups*
GU: Impotence
HEMA: Agranulocytosis, eosinophilia, thrombocytopenic purpura
INTEG: Rash, purpura, alopecia, dry skin, urticaria, pruritus
RESP: Bronchospasm, dyspnea, wheezing

Contraindications: Hypersensitivity to β-blockers, cardiogenic shock, heart block (2nd, 3rd degree), sinus bradycardia, CHF, bronchial asthma

Precautions: Major surgery, pregnancy **C**, lactation, diabetes mellitus, renal disease, thyroid disease, COPD, heart failure, CAD, nonallergic bronchospasm, hepatic disease

Pharmacokinetics

Absorption	Well absorbed (PO); completely absorbed (IV)
Distribution	Crosses blood-brain barrier, placenta
Metabolism	Liver, extensively
Excretion	Kidneys, breast milk
Half-life	3-4 hr

Pharmacodynamics

	PO	IV
Onset	15 min	Immediate
Peak	2-4 hr	20 min
Duration	6-19 hr	5-8 hr

Interactions
Drug/drug:
Individual drugs
Alcohol: ↑ hypotension (large amounts)
Epinephrine: α-Adrenergic stimulation
Hydralazine: ↑ hypotension, bradycardia
Indomethacin: ↓ antihypertensive effect
Insulin: ↑ hypoglycemia
Methyldopa: ↑ hypotension, bradycardia
Phenytoin (IV): ↑ myocardial depression
Prazosin: ↑ hypotension, bradycardia
Reserpine: ↑ hypotension, bradycardia
Thyroid: ↓ effectiveness
Verapamil: ↑ myocardial depression
Drug classifications
Amphetamines: ↑ hypertension, bradycardia
Antihypertensive: ↑ hypotension
β_2-Agonists: ↓ bronchodilatation
Cardiac glycosides: ↑ bradycardia
Nitrates: ↑ hypotension
Theophyllines: ↓ bronchodilatation

Lab test interferences
False increase: Urinary catecholamines

NURSING CONSIDERATIONS
Assessment
• Monitor B/P during beginning treatment, periodically thereafter; pulse q4h; note rate, rhythm, quality; check apical/radial pulse before administration; notify pre-

M

scriber of any significant changes (pulse <50 bpm)
- Check for baselines in renal, liver function tests before therapy begins and periodically thereafter
- Assess for edema in feet, legs daily; monitor I&O, daily weight; check for jugular vein distention, rales bilaterally, dyspnea (CHF)
- Monitor skin turgor, dryness of mucous membranes for hydration status, especially elderly

Associated nursing diagnoses

- ✓ Cardiac output, decreased (uses)
- ✓ Injury, risk for (adverse reactions)
- ✓ Knowledge deficit (teaching)
- ✓ Noncompliance (teaching)

Implementation

PO route
- Given ac, hs; tab may be crushed or swallowed whole; give with food to prevent GI upset; reduced dosage in renal dysfunction
- Do not crush or chew ext rel tab
- Store protected from light, moisture; place in cool environment

IV route
- Give by direct **IV** 5 mg/2 min or more; keep patient recumbent for 3 hr

Y-site compatibilities:

Alteplase, meperidine, morhpine

Patient/family education

- Teach patient not to discontinue drug abruptly; taper over 2 wk; may cause precipitate angina if stopped abruptly
- Teach patient not to use OTC products containing α-adrenergic stimulants (such as nasal decongestants, cold preparations); to avoid alcohol, smoking and to limit sodium intake as prescribed
- Teach patient how to take pulse and B/P at home; advise when to notify prescriber
- Instruct patient to comply with weight control, dietary adjustments, modified exercise program
- Tell patient to carry/wear Medic Alert ID to identify drug being taken, allergies; tell patient drug controls symptoms but does not cure
- Caution patient to avoid hazardous activities if dizziness, drowsiness is present, to avoid driving until drug response is known
- Teach patient to report symptoms of CHF; difficult breathing, especially on exertion or when lying down, night cough, swelling of extremities or bradycardia, dizziness, confusion, depression, fever
- Teach patient to take drug as prescribed, not to double doses or skip doses; take any missed doses as soon as remembered if at least 4 hr until next dose

Evaluation

Positive therapeutic outcome
- Decreased B/P in hypertension (after 1-2 wk)
- Absence of dysrhythmias

Treatment of overdose:

Lavage, **IV** atropine for bradycardia, **IV** theophylline for bronchospasm, digitalis, O_2, diuretic for cardiac failure, hemodialysis, **IV** glucose for hyperglycemia, **IV** diazepam (or phenytoin) for seizures

metronidazole

(me-troe-ni'da-zole)

Apo-Metronidazole ✤, Flagyl, Flagyl IV, Flagyl IV RTU, Metro IV, Metronidazole, Metronidazole Redi-Infusion, Metryl, Neo-Metric ✤, Novonidazole ✤, PMS-Metronidazole ✤, Protostat, Satric, Trikacide ✤

Func. class.: Trichomonacide, amebicide, anti-infective

Chem. class.: Nitroimidazole derivative

Pregnancy category **B**

Action: Direct-acting amebicide/trichomonacide; binds, degrades DNA in organism

➔ Therapeutic Outcome: Trichomonacidal, amebicidal, bactericidal for the following susceptible organism: *Bacteroides, Clostridium, Trichomonas vaginalis, Giardia lamblia, Entamoeba histolytica*

Uses: Intestinal amebiasis, amebic abscess, trichomoniasis, refractory trichomoniasis, bacterial anaerobic infections, giardiasis; septicemia, endocarditis, bone, joint, and lower respiratory tract infections

Dosage and routes

Trichomoniasis

Adult: PO 250 mg tid × 7 days or 2 g in single dose; do not repeat treatment for 4-6 wk

P *Child:* PO 15 mg/kg/day in divided doses × 7-10 days

Refractory trichomoniasis

Adult: PO 250 mg bid × 10 days

Amebic abscess

Adult: PO 500-750 mg tid × 5-10 days

P *Child:* PO 35-50 mg/kg/day in 3 divided doses × 10 days

Intestinal amebiasis

Adult: PO 750 mg tid × 5-10 days

P *Child:* PO 35-50 mg/kg/day in 3 divided doses × 10 days; then oral iodoquinol

Anaerobic bacterial infections

Adult: **IV** inf 15 mg/kg/over 1 hr, then 7.5 mg/kg **IV** or PO q6h, not to exceed 4 g/day; first maintenance dose should be administered 6 hr following loading dose

Giardiasis

Adult: PO 250 mg tid × 5 days

P *Child:* PO 5 mg/kg tid × 5 days

M

Available forms: Tab 250, 500 mg; film-coated tab 250, 1500 mg; inj 5 mg/vial; HCl inj 500 mg

Side effects/adverse reactions

CNS: Headache, dizziness, confusion, irritability, restlessness, ataxia, depression, fatigue, drowsiness, insomnia, paresthesia, peripheral neuropathy, ***convulsions,*** incoordination, depression
CV: Flat T waves
EENT: Blurred vision, sore throat, retinal edema, dry mouth, metallic taste, furry tongue, glossitis, stomatitis
GI: Nausea, vomiting, diarrhea, epigastric distress, *anorexia,* constipation, *abdominal cramps,* metallic taste, ***pseudomembranous colitis***
GU: Darkened urine, vaginal dryness, polyuria, ***albuminuria,*** dysuria, cystitis, decreased libido, ***nephrotoxicity,*** incontinence, dyspareunia
HEMA: Leukopenia, bone marrow depression, aplasia
INTEG: Rash, pruritus, urticaria, flushing
SYST: Superinfection

Contraindications: Hypersensitivity to this drug, renal disease, hepatic disease, contracted visual or color fields, blood dyscrasias, pregnancy (1st trimester), lactation, CNS disorders

Precautions: Candidal infections, pregnancy (2nd, 3rd trimesters) **B**

Pharmacokinetics

Absorption	80% (PO)
Distribution	Widely distributed, crosses placenta
Metabolism	Liver
Excretion	Urine, unchanged; feces
Half-life	6-11 hr

Pharmacodynamics

	PO	IV	TOP/VAG
Onset	Rapid	Immediate	Unknown
Peak	1-2 hr	Infusion's end	Unknown

Interactions

Drug/drug:

Individual drugs
Alcohol: ↑ disulfiram-like reaction
Azathioprine: ↑ leukopenia
Cimetidine: ↓ action of metronidazole
Phenobarbital: ↓ effect of metronidazole
Disulfiram: ↑ risk of psychosis
Fluorouracil: ↑ leukopenia
Drug classifications
Anticoagulants, oral: ↑ risk of bleeding

Lab test interferences

Decrease: AST (SGOT), ALT (SGPT)

NURSING CONSIDERATIONS

Assessment

- Assess patient for signs and symptoms of infection including characteristics of wounds, WBC >10,000, vaginal secretions, fever; obtain baseline information and during treatment
- Obtain C&S before begin-

ning drug therapy to identify if correct treatment has been initiated

- Assess for allergic reactions: rash, urticaria, pruritus
- Identify urine output; if decreasing, notify prescriber (may indicate nephrotoxicity); also check for increased BUN, creatinine
- Assess bowel pattern qd; if severe diarrhea occurs, drug should be discontinued
- Assess for overgrowth of infection: perineal itching, fever, malaise, redness, pain, swelling, drainage, rash, diarrhea, change in cough, sputum

Associated nursing diagnoses

- ✓ Infection, risk for (uses)
- ✓ Diarrhea (adverse reactions)
- ✓ Injury, risk for (adverse reactions)
- ✓ Knowledge deficit (teaching)
- ✓ Noncompliance (teaching)

Implementation

IV route

- Give intermittent **IV** prediluted; for Flagyl **IV** dilute with 4.4 ml sterile water or 0.9% NaCl; must be diluted further with 8 mg/ml or more 0.9% NaCl, D_5W, or LR; must neutralize with 5 mEq $NaHCO_3$/500 mg; CO_2 gas will be generated and may require venting; run over 1 hr; primary **IV** must be discontinued; may be given as cont inf; do not use aluminum products; **IV** may require venting

Top route

- A thin coating should be applied to affected area after cleaning with soap and water and patting dry

PO route

- Give with or pc to avoid GI symptoms, metallic taste; crush tab if needed
- Store in light-resistant container; do not refrigerate

Patient/family education

- Teach patient to report sore throat, bruising, bleeding, joint pain; may indicate blood dyscrasias (rare)
- Advise patient to contact prescriber if vaginal itching, loose, foul-smelling stools, furry tongue occur; may indicate superinfection
- Teach trichmoniasis patient that both partners need to be treated; condoms should be used during intercourse to prevent reinfection
- Advise patient of disulfiram-like reaction to alcohol ingestion; alcohol should not be used when taking this anti-infective
- Inform patient drug has a metallic taste and urine may turn dark
- If pregnancy is suspected, prescriber should be notified

Evaluation

Positive therapeutic outcome

- Decreased symptoms of infection

mexiletine

(mex-il'e-teen)

Mexitil

Func. class.: Antidysrhythmic (Class IB)

Chem. class.: Lidocaine analog

Pregnancy category **C**

Action: Increases electrical stimulation threshold of ventricle and His-Purkinje system, which stabilizes cardiac membrane and decreases automaticity

➡ **Therapeutic Outcome:** Decreased ventricular dysrhythmia

Uses: Ventricular tachycardia, ventricular dysrhythmias during cardiac surgery, MI

Dosage and routes

Adult: PO 400 mg (loading dose), then 200 mg q8h, then 200-400 mg q8h

Available forms: Cap 150, 200, 250 mg

Side effects/adverse reactions

CNS: Headache, dizziness, confusion, ***convulsions,*** tremors, psychosis, nervousness, paresthesias, weakness, fatigue, coordination difficulties, change in sleep habits

CV: Hypotension, bradycardia, angina, PVCs, ***heart block, cardiovascular collapse, arrest,*** sinus node slowing, ***left ventricular failure,*** syncope, ***cardiogenic shock***

EENT: Blurred vision, hearing loss, tinnitus

GI: Nausea, vomiting, anorexia, diarrhea, abdominal pain, ***hepatitis,*** dry mouth, peptic ulcer, altered taste, GI bleeding

GU: Urinary hesitancy, decreased libido

HEMA: ***Thrombocytopenia, leukopenia, agranulocytosis, hypoplastic anemia,*** SLE syndrome

INTEG: Rash, alopecia, dry skin

MISC: Edema, arthralgia, fever

RESP: Dyspnea, ***fibrosis, embolism,*** pneumonia

Contraindications: Hypersensitivity to amides, cardiogenic shock, blood dyscrasias, severe heart block

Precautions: Pregnancy **C**, P lactation, children, renal disease, liver disease, CHF, respiratory depression, myasthenia gravis

Pharmacokinetics

Absorption	Well absorbed (PO)
Distribution	Body tissues
Metabolism	Liver, extensively
Excretion	Kidneys, unchanged (10%)
Half-life	12 hr

Pharmacodynamics

Onset	½-2 hr
Peak	2-3 hr
Duration	8-12 hr

Interactions

Drug/drug:

Individual drugs

Cimetidine: ↑ toxicity
Digoxin: ↑ blood levels, toxicity
Disopyramide: ↑ levels, toxicity
Flecainide: ↑ levels, toxicity
Lidocaine: Bradycardia, arrest
Phenobarbital: ↓ effectiveness
Phenytoin: ↑ effectiveness
Procainamide: ↑ levels, toxicity

Quinidine: ↑ levels, toxicity
Rifampin: ↓ effectiveness
Warfarin: ↑ level, bleeding

Drug classifications
Antacids: ↓ absorption
Analgesics, opoid: ↓ absorption

Drug/smoking:
↓ effectiveness

Lab test interferences
Increase: CPK

NURSING CONSIDERATIONS
Assessment
- Assess for oxygenation or perfusion deficit: decreased B/P, chest pain, dizziness, loss of consciousness
- Assess respiratory status: auscultate lung fields for bibasilar crackles in patients with advanced CHF
- Assess for urinary retention: check for pain, abdominal absorption, palpate bladder; check males with benign prostatic hypertrophy; anticholinergic reaction may cause retention
- Monitor I&O ratio; electrolytes potassium, sodium, chloride; watch for decreasing urinary output, possible retention
- Monitor liver function studies: AST (SGOT), ALT (SGPT), bilirubin, alkaline phosphatase
- Monitor ECG periodically to determine drug effectiveness; measure PR, QRS, QT intervals; check for PVCs, other dysrhythmias; assess B/P for hypotension, hypertension, for rebound hypertension after 1-2 hr; for prolonged PR/QT intervals, QRS complex, if QT or QRS increase by 50% or more, withhold next dose, notify prescriber
- Monitor for dehydration and hypovolemia
- Monitor blood levels (therapeutic level 0.5-2 μg/ml), notify prescriber of abnormal results
- Assess pulmonary toxicity: dyspnea, fatigue, cough, fever, chest pain; drug should be discontinued
- Assess cardiac rate, respiration: rate, rhythm, character, chest pain, ventricular tachycardia, supraventricular tachycardia, fibrillation

Associated nursing diagnoses
- ✓ Cardiac output, decreased (uses)
- ✓ Impaired gas exchange (adverse reactions)
- ✓ Knowledge deficit (teaching)

Implementation
PO route
- Give with meals for GI upset

Patient/family education
- Teach patient to report side effects immediately to prescriber; to take exactly as prescribed; if dose is missed, take when remembered if within 3-4 hr of next dose; do not double doses
- Caution patient to avoid temp extremes; impairment of heat-regulating mechanism can occur
- Encourage patient to complete follow-up appointment with health care provider, including pulmonary function studies, chest-x-ray

M

- Instruct patient that dry mouth may be relieved by frequent sips of water, hard candy, sugarless gum
- Caution patient to make position changes from lying to standing slowly to prevent orthostatic hypotension

Evaluation

Positive therapeutic outcome

- Decreased B/P, dysrhythmias
- Decreased heart rate
- Normal sinus rhythm

Treatment of overdose:

O_2, artificial ventilation, ECG, administer dopamine for circulatory depression, administer diazepam or thiopental for convulsions, isoproterenol

mezlocillin

(mez-loe-sill'in)

Mezlin

Func. class.: Broad-spectrum antiinfective

Chem. class.: Extended-spectrum penicillin

Pregnancy category B

Action: Interferes with cell wall replication of susceptible organisms; osmotically unstable cell wall swells, bursts from osmotic pressure

Uses: Infection due to penicillinase-producing staphylococci, streptococci; respiratory tract, skin, skin structure, urinary tract, bone, joint infections; sinusitis, endocarditis, septicemia, meningitis; may be combined with an aminoglycoside for *Pseudomonas* infection

Therapeutic Outcome: Bactericidal effects on the following: gram-positive cocci *Staphylococcus aureus, Streptococcus viridans, S. faecalis, S. pneumoniae,* gram-negative coccus *Neisseria gonorrhoeae,* gram-positive bacilli *Clostridium perfringens, C. tetani,* gram-negative bacilli *Bacteroides, Escherichia coli, Haemophilus influenzae, Klebsiella, Proteus mirabilis, Peptococcus, Peptostreptococcus, Morganella morganii, Enterobacter, Serratia, Pseudomonas, Proteus vulgaris, P. rettgeri, Shigella, Citrobacter, Veillonella*

Dosage and routes

Adult: IM/**IV** 200-300 mg/kg/day in divided doses q4-6h; may give up to 24 g/day for severe infections

P *Child:* IM/**IV** 50 mg/kg q4-6h

P *Infants >8 days:* >2000 g, 75 mg/kg q6h; <2000 g, 75 mg/kg q8h

P *Infants <8 days:* 75 mg/kg q12h

Available forms: Powder for inj 1, 2, 3, 4 g; **IV** inf 2, 3, 4 g

Side effects/adverse reactions

CNS: Lethargy, hallucinations, anxiety, depression, twitching, ***coma, convulsions***

GI: Nausea, vomiting, diarrhea, increased AST (SGOT), ALT (SGPT), abdominal

pain, glossitis, colitis, abnormal taste
GU: Oliguria, proteinuria, hematuria vaginitis, moniliasis, ***glomerulonephritis,*** increased BUN, creatinine
HEMA: Anemia, increased bleeding time, ***bone marrow depression, granulocytopenia***
META: Hyperkalemia, hypokalemia, alkalosis, hypernatremia

Contraindications: Hypersensitivity to penicillins

Precautions: Pregnancy **B**, hypersensitivity to cephalosporins, P neonates

Pharmacokinetics

Absorption	Well absorbed
Distribution	Widely distributed; crosses placenta
Metabolism	Liver, small amounts
Excretion	Kidneys, unchanged (40%-70%); breast milk, bile (15%-30%)
Half-life	50-55 min; increased in renal disease

Pharmacodynamics

	IM	IV
Onset	Rapid	Rapid
Peak	5 min	Inf end

Interactions

Drug/drug:

Individual drugs

Aspirin: ↑ mezlocillin levels, ↓ renal excretion
Cholestyramine: ↓ effectiveness of mezlocillin
Chloramphenicol: ↑ half-life of chloramphenicol, ↓ effectiveness of mezlocillin
Colestipol: ↓ effectiveness of mezlocillin
Lithium: ↓ excretion, ↑ toxicity
Probenecid: ↑ mezlocillin levels, ↓ renal excretion

Drug classifications

Diuretics: ↑ hypokalemia
Erythromycins: ↓ antimicrobial effectiveness
Oral anticoagulants: ↑ anticoagulant effects
Oral contraceptives: ↓ contraceptive effectiveness
Tetracyclines: ↓ antimicrobial effectiveness

Drug/food:

Food, carbonated drinks, citrus fruit juices: ↓ absorption

Lab test interferences

False positive: Urine glucose, urine protein

M

NURSING CONSIDERATIONS

Assessment

- Assess patient for previous sensitivity reaction to penicillins or other cephalosporins; cross-sensitivity between penicillins and cephalosporins is common
- Assess patient for signs and symptoms of infection including characteristics of wounds, sputum, urine, stool, WBC >10,000, fever; obtain baseline information and during treatment
- Obtain C & S before beginning drug therapy to identify if correct treatment has been initiated
- Assess for allergic reactions: rash, urticaria, pruritus, chills, fever, joint pain; angioedema may occur a few days after therapy begins; epinephrine,

resuscitation equipment should be available for anaphylactic reaction
- Identify urine output; if decreasing, notify prescriber (may indicate nephrotoxicity); also check for increase BUN, creatinine
- Monitor blood studies: AST (SGOT), ALT (SGPT), CBC, Hct, bilirubin, LDH, alkaline phosphatase, Coombs' test monthly if patient is on long-term therapy
- Monitor electrolytes: potassium, sodium, chloride monthly if patient is on long-term therapy
- Assess bowel pattern qd; if severe diarrhea occurs, drug should be discontinued; may indicate pseudomembranous colitis
- Monitor for bleeding: ecchymosis, bleeding gums, hematuria, stool guaiac daily if on long-term therapy
- Assess for overgrowth of infection: perineal itching, fever, malaise, redness, pain, swelling, drainage, rash, diarrhea, change in cough, sputum

Associated nursing diagnoses

- ✓ Infection, risk for (uses)
- ✓ Diarrhea (adverse reactions)
- ✓ Injury, risk for (adverse reactions)
- ✓ Knowledge deficit (teaching)
- ✓ Noncompliance (teaching)

Implementation

IV **IV route**
- Dilute 1g or less/10 ml of sterile water, for inj; D_5, 0.9% NaCl, for inj; shake, dilute further with D_5W or 0.45 NaCl, give over 3-5 min

Patient/family education

- Teach patient to report sore throat, bruising, bleeding, joint pain; may indicate blood dyscrasias (rare)
- Advise patient to contact prescriber if vaginal itching, loose, foul-smelling stools, furry tongue occur; may indicate superinfection
- Advise patient to notify prescriber of diarrhea with blood or pus, which may indicate pseudomembranous colitis

Evaluation

Positive therapeutic outcome
- Absence of signs/symptoms of infection (WBC <10,000, temp WNL, absence of red, draining wounds)
- Reported improvement in symptoms of infection

Treatment of anaphylaxis: Withdraw drug, maintain airway, administer epinephrine, aminophylline, O_2, **IV** corticosteroids

miconazole

(mi-kon'a-zole)

Monistat, Monistat IV; topical: Micatin, Micatin Liquid, miconazole Nitrate, Monistat-Derm, Monistat 3, Monistat 7, Monistat Dual-Pak

Func. class.: Antifungal
Chem. class.: Imidazole

Pregnancy category **B**

Action: Alters cell membranes, inhibits fungal enzymes, inhibits sterols so intracellular contents are lost, prevents biosynthesis of phospholipids/triglycerides

Therapeutic Outcome: Fungistatic/fungicidal against: *Aspergillus, Coccidioides, Cryptococcus, Candida, Dermatophytes, Histoplasma*

Uses: Coccidioidomycosis, candidiasis, cryptococcosis, paracoccidioidomycosis, chronic mucocutaneous candidiasis, fungal meningitis; **IV** used for severe infections only; top tinea pedis, tinea cruris, tinea corporis, tinea versicolor, vaginal or vulva candidal infections

Dosage and routes

Adult: **IV** inf 200-3600 mg/day; may be divided in 3 inf at 200-1200 mg/inf; may have to repeat course; IT 20 mg given simultaneously with **IV** for fungal meningitis q3-7 days

P *Child:* **IV** 20-40 mg/kg/day, not to exceed 15 mg/kg/day

Top

P *Adult and child:* Top apply to affected area bid × 2-4 wk

Adult: Intravag give 1 applicator or suppository × 7 days hs

Available forms: Inj 10 mg/ml; aerosol 2%; cream 2%; lotion 2%; powder 2%; spray 2%; vag cream 2%; vag supp 100, 200 mg

Side effects/adverse reactions

CNS: Drowsiness, headache, laziness

CV: Tachycardia, dysrhythmias (rapid **IV**)

GI: Nausea, vomiting, anorexia, diarrhea, cramps

GU: Vulvovaginal burning, itching, hyponatremia, pelvic cramps (topical forms)

HEMA: Decreased Hct, thrombocytopenia, hyperlipidemia

INTEG: Pruritus, rash, fever, flushing, hives

SYST: Anaphylaxis

Contraindications: Hypersensitivity

Precautions: Renal disease, hepatic disease, pregnancy **B**

Pharmacokinetics

Absorption	Poorly absorbed (PO)
Distribution	Widely distributed (IV); bound to serum proteins (90%)
Metabolism	Liver, extensively
Excretion	Unknown
Half-life	Triphasic: 0.4, 2.1, 24 hr

Pharmacodynamics

	IV	TOP	VAG
Onset	Rapid	Unknown	Unknown
Peak	Infusion's end	Unknown	Unknown

Interactions

Drug/drug:

Individual drugs

Amphotericin B: ↓ effect of miconazole

Coumarin: ↑ anticoagulant effect

Isoniazid: ↓ effect of miconazole

Rifampin: ↓ effect of miconazole

Lab test interferences

False positive: Urine glucose, urine protein

NURSING CONSIDERATIONS

Assessment

- Assess for signs and symptoms of infection: drainage, sore throat, urinary pain, hematuria, fever
- Obtain cultures for C&S before beginning treatment; therapy may be started after culture is taken; monitor signs of infection before and throughout treatment
- Monitor bowel pattern before and during treatment; diarrhea may occur
- Monitor cardiac system: B/P, pulse; watch for increasing pulse, cardiac dysrhythmias; drug should be discontinued
- Monitor blood studies: WBC, RBC, Hgb, Hct, bleeding time; patients taking anticoagulants may need a decreased dosage; monitor liver and renal studies periodically for patients on long-term therapy
- Monitor I&O ratio; watch for decreasing urinary output, change in sp gr; discontinue drug to prevent renal damage; patients with renal disease may require lowered dose
- Monitor **IV** for thrombophlebitis; site should be changed q48-72h
- Monitor for allergies before initiation of treatment and reaction to each medication; highlight allergies on chart; check for allergic reaction: burning, stinging, swelling, redness (top); observe for skin eruptions after administration of drug to 1 wk after discontinuing drug

Associated nursing diagnoses

- ✓ Skin integrity, impaired (uses)
- ✓ Infection, risk (uses)
- ✓ Injury, risk for (adverse reactions)
- ✓ Knowledge deficit (teaching)

Implementation

- Have adrenalin, suction, tracheostomy set, endotracheal intubation equipment available

IV **IV route**

- Give 200 mg initially to prevent severe hypersensitive reaction
- Give by intermittent **IV** after diluting in 200 ml or more, D_5W or 0.9% NaCl; give over 30-60 min
- Store at room temp; reconstituted sol is stable for 24 hr refrigerated

Y-site incompatibility:

Fludarabine

Y-site compatibilities:

Foscarnet, ondansetron, sargramostim

Top route

- Apply after cleansing area with soap and water before each application; use enough medication to cover lesions completely; dry well
- Store at room temp in dry place

Vag route

- Administer 1 applicatorful every night high into the vagina
- Store at room temp in dry place

Patient/family education

- Inform patient that culture may be taken after completed course of medication
- Advise patient to notify nurse of diarrhea, symptoms of candidal vaginitis

Top route

- Teach patient to use medical asepsis (hand washing) before, after each application; to apply with glove to prevent further infection; to avoid contact with eyes; not to use occlusive dressings
- Caution patient to avoid use of OTC creams, ointments, lotions unless directed by prescriber
- Instruct patient to notify prescriber if no improvement in condition in 4 wk or if symptoms return in 2 mo; pregnancy or a serious medical condition may be the cause
- Teach patient to use for full prescribed treatment time, or reinfection may occur

Vag route

- Instruct patient in asepsis (hand washing) before, after each application
- Teach patient to apply with applicator only; to avoid use of any other vag product unless directed by prescriber; sanitary napkin may prevent soiling of undergarments; to abstain from sexual intercourse until treatment is completed; reinfection and irritation may occur
- Instruct patient to notify prescriber if symptoms persist

Evaluation

Positive therapeutic outcome

- Decreasing oral candidiasis, fever, malaise, rash
- Negative C&S for infectious organism
- Decrease in size, number of lesions
- Decrease in itching or white discharge (vaginal)

Treatment of overdose: Withdraw drug; maintain airway; administer epinephrine, aminophylline, O_2, **IV** corticosteroids for anaphylaxis

midazolam

(mid'ay-zoe-lam)

Versed

Func. class.: Sedative/hypnotic

Chem. class.: Benzodiazepine, short-acting

Pregnancy category D

Controlled substance schedule IV

M

Action: Depresses subcortical levels in CNS; may act on limbic system, reticular formation; may potentiate GABA by binding to specific benzodiazepine receptors

Therapeutic Outcome: Sedation for anesthesia induction and procedures

Uses: Preoperative sedation, general anesthesia induction, sedation for diagnostic endoscopic procedures, intubation

Dosage and routes

Preoperative sedation

Adult: IM 0.07-0.08 mg/kg

30-60 min before general anesthesia

Induction of general anesthesia

Adult: Unpremedicated patients, **IV** 0.3-0.35 mg/kg over 30 sec, wait 2 min, follow with 25% of initial dose if needed; premedicated patients, 0.15-0.35 mg/kg over 20-30 sec, allow 2 min for effect

Available forms: Inj 1, 5 mg/ml

Side effects/adverse reactions

CNS: Retrograde amnesia, euphoria, confusion, headache, anxiety, insomnia, slurred speech, paresthesia, tremors, weakness, chills
CV: Hypotension, PVCs, tachycardia, bigeminy, nodal rhythm
EENT: Blurred vision, nystagmus, diplopia, blocked ears, loss of balance
GI: Nausea, vomiting, increased salivation, hiccups
INTEG: Urticaria, pain, swelling at inj site, rash, pruritus
RESP: Coughing, ***apnea, bronchospasm, laryngospasm,*** dyspnea

Contraindications: Pregnancy **D**, hypersensitivity to benzodiazepines, shock, coma, alcohol intoxication, acute narrow angle glaucoma

Precautions: COPD, CHF, chronic renal failure, chills, G elderly, debilitated

Pharmacokinetics

Absorption	Well absorbed
Distribution	Crosses placenta, blood-brain barrier
Metabolism	Liver
Excretion	Kidneys, breast milk
Half-life	1-12 hr

Pharmacodynamics

	IM	IV
Onset	15 min	3-5 min
Peak	½-1 hr	Unknown
Duration	2-6 hr	2-6 hr

Interactions

Drug/drug:

Individual drugs
Alcohol: ↑ CNS depression
Drug classifications
Analgesics, opioid: ↑ CNS depression
Antihistamines: ↑ CNS depression
Antihypertensives: ↑ hypotension
Nitrates: ↑ hypotension
Sedative/hypnotics: ↑ CNS depression

NURSING CONSIDERATIONS

Assessment

- Monitor B/P, pulse, respiration during **IV**; O_2 and emergency equipment should be nearby
- Monitor inj site for redness, pain, swelling
- Assess degree of amnesia in G elderly; may be increased
- Assess anterograde amnesia
- Assess vital signs for recovery period in obese patient, since half-life may be extended

Associated nursing diagnoses

✓ Knowledge deficit (teaching)

Implementation

IV route

• Give **IV** undiluted or after diluting with D_5W or 0.9% NaCl to a conc of 0.25 mg/ml; give over 2 min (conscious sedation) or over 30 sec (anesthesia induction)

• Ensure immediate availability of resuscitation equipment, O_2 to support airway; do not give by rapid bol

Syringe compatibilities:
Atropine, benzquinamide, buprenorphine, butorphanol, chlorpromazine, cimetadine, diphenhydramine, droperidol, fentanyl, glycopyrrolate, hydromorphine, hydroxyzine, meperidine, metoclopramide, morphine, nalbuphine, promazine, promethazine, scopolamine, thiethylperazine, trimethobenzamide

Syringe incompatibilities:
Dimenhydrinate, pentobarbital, perphenazine, prochlorperazine, ranitidine

Y-site compatibilities:
Atracurium, famotidine, fluconazole, pancuronium, vecuronium

Y-site incompatibility:
Foscarnet

IM route

• Give IM deep in large muscle mass

• Store at room temp

Patient/family education

• Instruct patient to avoid hazardous activities until drowsiness, weakness subside

• Inform patient that amnesia occurs; events may not be remembered

• Caution patient to avoid CNS depressants including alcohol for 24 hr after taking this drug

Evaluation

Positive therapeutic outcome

• Induction of sedation, amnesia

Treatment of overdose:
O_2, vasopressors, physostigmine, resuscitation; flumazenil will reverse effects

milrinone

(mill-re′none)

Primacor

Func. class.: Inotropic/vasodilator agent with phosphodiesterase activity

Chem. class.: Bipyridine derivative

Pregnancy category **C**

Action: Positive inotropic agent with vasodilator properties; reduces preload and afterload by direct relaxation of vascular smooth muscle; increases myocardial contractility

Therapeutic Outcome: Increased inotropic effect resulting in increased cardiac output

Uses: Short-term management of CHF that has not responded to other medication; can be used with digitalis products

Dosage and routes

Adult: **IV** bol 50 μg/kg given over 10 min; start inf of 0.375-0.75 μg/kg/min; reduce dosage in renal impairment

Available forms: Inj 1 mg/ml

Side effects/adverse reactions

CV: Dysrhythmias, hypotension, chest pain
GI: Nausea, vomiting, anorexia, abdominal pain, ***hepatotoxicity,*** jaundice
HEMA: Thrombocytopenia
MISC: Headache, hypokalemia, tremor

Contraindications: Hypersensitivity to this drug, severe aortic disease, severe pulmonic valvular disease, acute MI

Precautions: Lactation, pregnancy **C**, **P** children, renal disease, hepatic disease, atrial flutter/fibrillation, **G** elderly

Pharmacokinetics

Absorption	Completely absorbed (IV)
Distribution	Unknown
Metabolism	Liver (50%)
Excretion	Kidney, unchanged and metabolites (60%-90%)
Half-life	3½-6 hr; increased in CHF

Pharmacodynamics

Onset	2-5 min
Peak	10 min
Duration	Variable

Interactions: None

NURSING CONSIDERATIONS

Assessment

- Monitor manifestations of hypokalemia: acidic urine, reduced urine, osmolality, nocturia; hypotension, broad T wave, U wave, ectopy, tachycardia, weak pulse; muscle weakness, altered LOC, drowsiness, apathy, lethargy, confusion, depression; anorexia, nausea, cramps, constipation, distention, paralytic ileus; hypoventilation, respiratory muscle weakness
- Assess fluid volume status: complete I&O ratio and record; note weight, distended red veins, crackles in lung, color, quality and sp gr of urine, skin turgor, adequacy of pulses, moist mucous membranes, bilateral lung sounds, peripheral pitting edema; dehydration symptoms of decreasing output, thirst, hypotension, dry mouth and mucous membranes should be reported
- Monitor electrolytes: potassium, sodium, calcium, magnesium; also include BUN, blood pH, ABGs
- Monitor B/P and pulse, PCWP, CVP, index, often during inf; if B/P drops 30 mm Hg, stop inf and call prescriber
- Monitor ALT (SGPT), AST (SGOT), bilirubin daily; if these are elevated, hepatoxicity is suspected
- Monitor platelets; if <150,000/mm^3, drug is usually discontinued and another drug started
- Assess for extravasation: change site q48h

Associated nursing diagnoses

- ✓ Cardiac output, decreased (uses)
- ✓ Fluid volume excess (uses)
- ✓ Knowledge deficit (teaching)

Implementation

IV route

- Do not mix directly with glucose sol; chemical reaction occurs over 24 hr; precipitate forms if milrinone and furosemide come in contact
- Administer by direct **IV** into inf through Y-connector or directly into tubing; may give undiluted over 2-3 min
- Give by cont inf diluted with normal saline to conc of 1-3 mg/ml, run at prescribed rate; give by inf pump for doses other than bol
- Administer potassium supplements if ordered for potassium levels <3.0

Y-site compatibility:

Furosemide

Patient/family education

- Teach patient reason for medication and expected results
- Instruct patient to make position changes slowly; orthostatic hypotension may occur
- Teach patient signs and symptoms of hypersensitivity reactions and hypokalemia

Evaluation

Positive therapeutic outcome

- Increased cardiac output
- Decreased PCWP, adequate CVP
- Decreased dyspnea, fatigue, edema, ECG

Treatment of overdose: Discontinue drug, support circulation

mineral oil

Agoral Plain, Fleet Mineral Oil Enema, Kondremul ♣, Kondremul Plain, Lansoyl ♣, Liqui-doss, Milkinol, Neo-Cultol, Nujol, Petrogalar Plain, Zymenol

Func. class.: Laxative, lubricant

Chem. class.: Petroleum hydrocarbon

Pregnancy category C

Action: Eases passage of stool by increasing water retention in feces; acts as a lubricant

Therapeutic Outcome: Decreased constipation, softening of impacted feces

Uses: Constipation, preparation for bowel surgery or examination

Dosage and routes

Adult: PO 15-30 ml hs; enema 4 oz

P ***Child 6-12 yr:*** PO 5-15 ml hs; enema 1-2 oz

P ***Child 2-11 yr:*** Enema 1-2 oz

Available forms: Oil; enema; jelly 55%; susp 1.4, 2.5, 2.75 mg/5 ml

M

Side effects/adverse reactions

CNS: Muscle weakness
GI: ***Nausea, vomiting, anorexia, diarrhea,*** pruritus ani, hepatic infiltration
META: Hypoprothrombinemia
RESP: Lipid pneumonia

Contraindications: Hypersensitivity, intestinal obstruction, abdominal pain, nausea/vomiting

Precautions: Pregnancy **C**

Pharmacokinetics

Absorption	Minimal (PO)
Distribution	Liver, spleen, lymph nodes, intestinal mucosa
Metabolism	Unknown
Excretion	Feces
Half-life	Unknown

Pharmacodynamics

	PO	REC
Onset	6 hr	15 min
Peak	Unknown	Unknown
Duration	Unknown	Unknown

Interactions

Drug/drug:

Individual drugs
Vitamins A, D, E, K: ↓ absorption of vitamins

Drug/food:

Foods containing fat-soluble vitamins: ↓ absorption of vitamins

NURSING CONSIDERATIONS

Assessment

• Monitor blood, urine electrolytes if preparation used often by patient; check I&O ratio to identify fluid loss
• Assess for cramping, rec bleeding, nausea, vomiting; if these symptoms occur, drug should be discontinued; identify cause of constipation; identify whether fluids, bulk, or exercise is missing from lifestyle
• Assess stool for color, consistency, amount, presence of flatulence

Associated nursing diagnoses

✓ Constipation (uses)
✓ Diarrhea (adverse reaction)
✓ Knowledge deficit (teaching)
✓ Noncompliance (teaching)

Implementation

PO route
• Administer hs; do not give within 2 hr of meals; absorption may be delayed; do not give within 2 hr of stool softener
G • Use cautiously in elderly to prevent aspiration (PO)
Rec route
• Moisten supp with mineral oil using slightly warm water for 30 sec before insertion
• Do not use lubricant before insertion; they interfere with absorption of mineral oil

Patient/family education

• Discuss with the patient that adequate fluid consumption is necessary
• Teach patient that normal bowel movements do not always occur daily
• Caution patient not to use in presence of abdominal pain, nausea, vomiting; tell patient to notify prescriber if constipa-

tion is unrelieved or if symptoms of electrolyte imbalance occur (muscle cramps, pain, weakness, dizziness, excessive thirst)
- Teach patient not to use laxatives for long-term therapy; bowel tone will be lost and will decrease
- Shake emulsion well before using
- Teach patient not to take at hs as a laxative; may interfere with sleep, or cause lipid pneumonia
- Teach patient not to use with food or vitamin preparations; delays digestion and absorption of fat-soluble vitamins

Evaluation

Positive therapeutic outcome
- Decreased constipation in 8-10 hr (PO); 15 min (rec)

minocycline

(min-oh-sye'kleen)
Minocin, Minocin IV
Func. class.: Antiinfective
Chem. class.: Tetracycline
Pregnancy category **D**

Action: Inhibits protein synthesis and phosphorylation in microorganisms by binding to 30S ribosomal subunits and reversibly binding to 50S ribosomal subunits; bacteriostatic

Therapeutic Outcome: Bactericidal action against susceptible organisms, including *Neisseria meningitidis, N. gonorrhoeae, Treponema pallidum, Chlamydia trachomatis, Ureaplasma urealyticum, Mycoplasma pneumoniae, Nocardia, Rickettsia*

Uses: Syphilis, chlamydial infection, gonorrhea, lymphogranuloma venereum, rickettsial infections, inflammatory acne, meningitis carriers

Dosage and routes

Adult: PO/**IV** 200 mg, then 100 mg q12h or 50 mg q6h, not to exceed 400 mg/24h **IV**
P *Child >8 yr:* PO/**IV** 4 mg/kg then 4 mg/kg/day PO in divided doses q12h

Gonorrhea
Adult: PO 200 mg, then 100 mg q12h × 4 days

Chlamydia trachomatis infection
Adult: PO 100 mg bid × 7 days

Syphilis
Adult: PO 200 mg, then 100 mg q12h × 10-15 days

Available forms: Tab 50, 100 mg; cap 50, 100 mg; oral susp 50 mg/5 ml; powder for inj 100 mg/vial

Side effects/adverse reactions

CNS: Dizziness, fever, lightheadedness, vertigo
CV: Pericarditis
EENT: Dysphagia, glossitis, decreased calcification, permanent discoloration of deciduous teeth, oral candidiasis
GI: Nausea, abdominal pain, *vomiting, diarrhea,* anorexia,

M

enterocolitis, ***hepatotoxicity,*** flatulence, abdominal cramps, epigastric burning, stomatitis
GU: Increased BUN, polyuria, polydipsia, ***renal failure, nephrotoxicity***
HEMA: Eosinophilia, neutropenia, thrombocytopenia, hemolytic anemia
INTEG: Rash, urticaria, photosensitivity, increased pigmentation, ***exfoliative dermatitis,*** pruritus, angioedema, blue-gray color of skin and mucous membranes

Contraindications: Hypersensitivity to tetracyclines, P children <8 yr, pregnancy **D**

Precautions: Hepatic disease, lactation

Pharmacokinetics

Absorption	Well absorbed (PO)
Distribution	Widely distributed (55%-88% protein bound); some distribution in CSF, crosses placenta
Metabolism	Liver, some
Excretion	Kidneys, unchanged (20%), bile, feces
Half-life	11-17 hr

Pharmacodynamics

	PO	IV
Onset	Rapid	Rapid
Peak	2-3 hr	Infusion's end

Interactions

Drug/drug:

Individual drugs

Calcium: Forms chelates, ↓ absorption
Carbamazepine: ↑ effect of carbamazepine
Iron: Forms chelates, ↓ absorption
Magnesium: Forms chelates, ↓ absorption

Drug classifications

Antidiarrheals, adsorbent: ↓ absorption
Anticoagulants, oral: ↑ effect of anticoagulants
Contraceptives, oral: ↓ effect of oral contraception

Lab test interferences

False negative: Urine glucose with Clinistix, Tes-Tape

NURSING CONSIDERATIONS

Assessment

- Assess patient for previous sensitivity reaction
- Assess patient for signs and symptoms of infection including characteristics of wounds, sputum, urine, stool, WBC >10,000, fever; obtain baseline information, before and during treatment
- Obtain C & S before beginning drug therapy to identify if correct treatment has been initiated
- Assess for allergic reactions: rash, urticaria, pruritus
- Monitor blood studies: AST (SGOT), ALT (SGPT), CBC, Hct, bilirubin, alkaline phosphatase, amylase monthly if patient is on long-term therapy
- Assess bowel pattern qd; if severe diarrhea occurs, drug should be discontinued
- Monitor for bleeding: ecchymosis, bleeding gums, hematuria, stool guaiac daily if on long-term therapy; blood dyscrasias may occur
- Assess for overgrowth of infection: perineal itching,

fever, malaise, redness, pain, swelling, drainage, rash, diarrhea, change in cough, sputum; black, furry tongue

Associated nursing diagnoses

- ✓ Infection, risk for (uses)
- ✓ Diarrhea (adverse reactions)
- ✓ Knowledge deficit (teaching)
- ✓ Noncompliance (teaching)

Implementation

PO route

- Give around the clock to maintain proper blood levels; give with food to increase absorption of drug; do not give within 3 hr of other agents; drug interactions may occur
- Give with 8 oz of water 1 hr before hs to prevent ulceration
- Shake liquid preparation well before giving; use calibrated device for proper dosing
- Do not give with iron, calcium, magnesium products or antacids, which decrease absorption and form insoluble chelate

IV **IV route**

- Check for irritation, extravasation, phlebitis daily; change site q72hr
- For intermittent inf, dilute each 100 mg/10 ml 0.9% NaCl, sterile water for inj; further dilute in 500-1000 ml 0.9% NaCl, D_5W, Ringer's, LR, D_5/LR; give over 6 hr

Y-site incompatibilities:

Hydromorphone, meperidine, morphine

Y-site compatibilities:

Cyclophosphamide, fludarabine, heparin, hydrocortisone, magnesium sulfate, melphalan, perphenazine, potassium chloride, sargramostim, sodium succinate, vinorelbine, vitamin B with C

Additive compatibilities:

Amikacin, cimetidine, clindamycin, gentamicin, kanamycin, multivitamins, rifampin, sodium bicarbonate, tobramycin, verapamil, vitamin B complex with C

Additive incompatibility:

Rifampin

Syringe compatibility:

Heparin

Syringe incompatibility:

Doxapram

Patient/family education

- Teach patient to use sunscreen when outdoors to decrease photosensitivity reaction
- Teach patient to report sore throat, bruising, bleeding, joint pain; may indicate blood dyscrasias (rare)
- Advise patient to contact prescriber if vaginal itching, loose, foul-smelling stools, furry tongue occur; may indicate superinfection; report itching, rash, pruritus, urticaria
- Instruct patient to take all medication prescribed for the length of time ordered; drug must be taken around the clock to maintain blood levels; do not give medication to others; take with a full glass of water; may take with food or milk
- Advise patient to use a form of contraception other than hormonal

M

Evaluation

Positive therapeutic outcome
- Absence of signs/symptoms of infection (WBC <10,000, temp WNL, absence of red, draining wounds)
- Reported improvement in symptoms of infection

minoxidil

(mi-nox'i-dill)

Loniten, Minodyl, minoxidil, Rogaine

Func. class.: Antihypertensive, hair growth stimulant

Chem. class.: Vasodilator, peripheral

Pregnancy category C

Action: Directly relaxes arteriolar smooth muscle, causing vasodilatation; increased cutaneous blood flow; stimulation of hair follicles

Therapeutic Outcome: Decreased B/P in hypertension; hair growth

Uses: Severe hypertension unresponsive to other therapy (use with diuretic); topically to treat alopecia

Dosage and routes

Adult: PO 5 mg/day not to exceed 100 mg daily; usual range 10-40 mg/day in single doses

P ***Child <12 yr:*** initial, 0.2 mg/kg/day; effective range, 0.25-1 mg/kg/day; max, 50 mg/day

Alopecia

Adult: Apply top, rub into scalp daily

Available forms: Tab 2.5, 10 mg; top 20 mg/ml

Side effects/adverse reactions

CNS: *Drowsiness, dizziness, sedation,* headache, depression, fatigue

CV: *Severe rebound hypertension,* tachycardia, angina, increased T wave, ***CHF, pulmonary edema, pericardial effusion,*** edema, sodium retention, water retention

GI: Nausea, vomiting

GU: Gynecomastia, breast tenderness

HEMA: Hct, Hgb, erythrocyte count may decrease initially

INTEG: Pruritus, ***Stevens-Johnson syndrome,*** rash, hirsutism

Contraindications: Acute MI, dissecting aortic aneurysm, hypersensitivity, pheochromocytoma

Precautions: Pregnancy **C**, P lactation, children, renal disease, CAD, CHF

Pharmacokinetics	
Absorption	Well absorbed (PO); minimally absorbed (top)
Distribution	Widely distributed
Metabolism	Liver
Excretion	Kidneys, breast milk
Half-life	4.2 hr

Pharmacodynamics

	PO	TOP
Onset	½ hr	4 mo
Peak	2-3 hr	Unknown
Duration	75 hr	4 mo

Interactions

Drug/drug:

Individual drugs

Alcohol: ↑ hypotension

Drug classifications

Antihypertensives: ↑ hypotension

Glucocorticoids (top route): ↑ absorption

Nitrates: ↑ nitrates

NSAIDs: ↓ antihypertensive effect

Retinoids (top route): ↑ absorption

NURSING CONSIDERATIONS

Assessment

- Monitor B/P, pulse, jugular venous distention periodically throughout treatment
- Monitor electrolytes, blood studies: potassium, sodium, chloride, carbon dioxide, CBC, serum glucose
- Monitor weight daily, I&O; assess edema in feet, legs daily; check skin turgor, dryness of mucous membranes for hydration status
- Assess for rales, dyspnea, orthopnea, peripheral edema, fatigue, weight gain, jugular vein distention (CHF)
- Assess for signs of hyperglycemia: acetone breath, increased urinary output, severe thirst, lethargy, dizziness

Associated nursing diagnoses

- ✓ Cardiac output, decreased (adverse reactions)
- ✓ Injury, risk for (side effects)
- ✓ Knowledge deficit (teaching)

Implementation

PO route

- Give with meals to decrease GI symptoms
- Give with β-blockers and/or diuretic for hypertension
- Store protected from light and heat

Top route

- Administer 1 ml dose no matter how much balding has occurred; increasing dose does not speed hair growth
- Treatment must continue long term or new hair will be lost again

M

Patient/family education

Top route

- Teach patient that new hair will be soft and hardly visible
- Caution patient not to use on other parts of the body; drug is to be used on the scalp only
- Instruct patient that hair should be clean before applying medication; do not get on clothing
- Caution patient not to get medication near mucus membranes (mouth, nose, eyes) and to contact prescriber if burning, stinging or rash occurs

Evaluation

Positive therapeutic outcome

- Decreased B/P in hypertension
- Hair growth (top)

misoprostol
(mye-soe-prost′ole)
Cytotec
Func. class.: Gastric mucosa protectant; antiulcer
Chem. class.: Prostaglandin E_1 analog
Pregnancy category **X**

Action: Inhibits gastric acid secretion; may protect gastric mucosa; can increase bicarbonate, mucus production

Therapeutic Outcome: Prevention of gastric ulcers

Uses: Prevention of NSAID-induced gastric ulcers

Dosage and routes
Adult: PO 200 μg qid with food for duration of NSAID therapy; if 200 μg is not tolerated, 100 μg may be given

Available forms: Tab 100, 200 μg

Side effects/adverse reactions
GI: ***Diarrhea,*** nausea, vomiting, flatulence, constipation, dyspepsia, abdominal pain
GU: Spotting, cramps, hypermenorrhea, menstrual disorders

Contraindications: Hypersensitivity, pregnancy **X**

P G **Precautions:** Lactation, children, elderly, renal disease

Pharmacokinetics
Absorption	Well absorbed (PO)
Distribution	Unknown
Metabolism	Liver
Excretion	Kidneys
Half-life	½-1 hr

Pharmacodynamics
Onset	½ hr
Peak	Unknown
Duration	3 hr

Interactions
Drug/drug:
Drug classifications
Antacids, magnesium: ↑ diarrhea

NURSING CONSIDERATIONS
Assessment
- Assess patient for GI symptoms: hematemesis, occult or frank blood in stools, also severe abdominal pain, cramping, severe diarrhea
- Obtain a negative pregnancy test in women if childbearing age before starting medication; miscarriages are common

Associated nursing diagnoses
✓ Pain (uses)
✓ Knowledge deficit (teaching)

Implementation
PO route
- Give with meals for prolonged drug effect; avoid use of magnesium antacids

Patient/family education
- Advise patient to avoid black pepper, caffeine, alcohol, harsh spices, extremes in temp of

food, which may aggravate condition
• Caution patient to avoid OTC preparations: aspirin, cough, cold preparations; condition may worsen
• Teach patient that drug must be continued for prescribed time to be effective and taken exactly as prescribed; doses are not to be doubled
• Instruct patient to report to prescriber diarrhea, black tarry stools, abdominal pain, cramping, menstrual disorders
• Caution patient to prevent pregnancy while taking this drug; spontaneous abortion may occur

Evaluation

Positive therapeutic outcome
• Prevention of ulcers

mitomycin
(mye-toe-mye'sin)
Mutamycin
Func. class.: Antineoplastic, antibiotic
Pregnancy category **D**

Action: Inhibits DNA synthesis, primarily; derived from *Streptomyces caespitosus*; appears to cause cross-linking of DNA, a vesicant

Therapeutic Outcome: Prevention of rapidly growing malignant cells

Uses: Pancreas, stomach, head and neck, breast cancer

Investigational uses: Palliative treatment of head, neck, colon, breast, biliary, cervical, lung malignancies

Dosage and routes

Adult: **IV** 20 mg/m^2/day × 5 days, stop drug for 2 days, then repeat cycle; or 10-20 mg/m^2 as a single dose; repeat cycle in 6-8 wk; stop drug if platelets are <75,000/mm^3 or WBC is <3000/mm^3

Available forms: Inj 5, 20, 40 mg/vial

Side effects/adverse reactions

CNS: Fever, headache, confusion, drowsiness, syncope, fatigue
EENT: Blurred vision, drowsiness, syncope
GI: Nausea, vomiting, anorexia, stomatitis, ***hepatotoxicity,*** diarrhea
GU: Urinary retention, ***renal failure,*** edema
HEMA: ***Thrombocytopenia, leukopenia, anemia***
INTEG: Rash, alopecia, ***extravasation***
RESP: ***Fibrosis, pulmonary infiltrate,*** dyspnea

Contraindications: Hypersensitivity, pregnancy (1st trimester) **D**, as a single agent, thrombocytopenia, coagulation disorders

Precautions: Renal disease, bone marrow depression

Pharmacokinetics

Absorption	Complete bioavailability (IV)
Distribution	Widely distributed; concentrates in tumor
Metabolism	Liver, extensively
Excretion	Kidneys, unchanged
Half-life	1 hr

Pharmacodynamics

Onset	Unknown
Peak	Unknown
Duration	Unknown

Interactions

Drug/drug:

Individual drugs

Radiation: ↑ toxicity, bone marrow suppression

Drug classifications

Antineoplastics: ↑ toxicity, bone marrow suppression

NURSING CONSIDERATIONS

Assessment

- Assess buccal cavity q8h for dryness, sores or ulceration, white patches, oral pain, bleeding, dysphagia; obtain prescription for viscous lidocaine (Xylocaine)
- Assess symptoms indicating severe allergic reaction: rash, pruritus, urticaria, purpuric skin lesions, itching, flushing
- Monitor CBC, differential, platelet count weekly; withhold drug if WBC count is <4000/mm^3 or platelet count is <100,000/mm^3, notify prescriber of results if WBC <20,000/mm^3, platelets <150,000/mm^3
- Monitor renal function studies: BUN, creatinine, serum uric acid, urine CrCl before and during therapy; check I&O ratio; report fall in urine output to <30 ml/hr
- Monitor temp q4h (may indicate beginning of infection)
- Monitor liver function tests before and during therapy (bilirubin, AST [SGOT], ALT [SGPT], LDH) as needed or monthly; check for yellowing of skin and sclera, dark urine, clay-colored stools, itchy skin, abdominal pain, fever, diarrhea
- Assess for bleeding: hematuria, stool guaiac, bruising or petechiae, mucosa or orifices q8h; inflammation of mucosa, breaks in skin
- Identify effects of alopecia on body image; discuss feelings about body changes
- Identify edema in feet, joint pain, stomach pain, shaking; check for inflammation of mucosa, breaks in skin

Associated nursing diagnoses

- ✓ Injury, risk for (adverse reactions)
- ✓ Body image disturbance (adverse reactions)
- ✓ Infection, risk for (adverse reactions)
- ✓ Knowledge deficit (teaching)

Implementation

- Avoid contact with skin, since medication is very irritating; wash completely to remove
- Give fluids **IV** or PO before chemotherapy to hydrate patient
- Provide antacid before oral agent; give drug after evening meal, before hs; administer antiemetic 30-60 min before

giving drug and prn to prevent vomiting; use antibiotics for prophylaxis of infection
• Give top or syst analgesics for pain
• Give in AM so drug can be eliminated before hs
• Provide a liq diet: carbonated beverages; gelatin may be added if patient is not nauseated or vomiting
• Encourage patient to rinse mouth tid-qid with water, club soda, brush teeth bid-qid with soft brush or cotton-tipped applicators for stomatitis, use unwaxed dental floss

IV **IV route**
• Drug should be prepared by experienced personnel using proper precautions in a biologic cabinet using gown, gloves, mask
• Give by direct **IV** after diluting 5 mg/10 sterile water for inj; shake, allow to stand, give through Y-tube or 3 way stopcock; give over 5-10 min through running D_5W, 0.9% NaCl **IV**
• Use sodium thiosulfate for extravasation; apply ice compress

Syringe compatibilities:
Bleomycin, cisplatin, cyclophosphamide, doxorubicin, droperidol, fluorouracil, furosemide, heparin, leucovorin, methotrexate, metoclopramide, vinblastine, vincristine

Y-site compatibilities:
Bleomycin, cisplatin, cyclophosphamide, doxorubicin, droperidol, fluorouracil, furosemide, heparin, leucovorin, melphalan, methotrexate, metoclopramide, ondansetron, vinblastine, vincristine

Y-site incompatibilities:
Sargramostim, vinorelbine

Additive incompatibility:
Bleomycin

Additive compatibility:
Sodium lactate

Solution compatibilities:
LR, 0.3% NaCl, 0.5% NaCl

Patient/family education
• Teach patient to avoid use of products containing aspirin or ibuprofen, razors, commercial mouthwash, since bleeding may occur; to report symptoms of bleeding (hematuria, tarry stools)
• Caution patient to report signs of anemia (fatigue, headache, irritability, faintness, shortness of breath)
• Advise patient to report any changes in breathing or coughing even several mo after treatment; to avoid crowds and persons with respiratory tract or other infections
• Inform patient that hair may be lost during treatment; a wig or hair piece may make patient feel better; new hair may be different in color, texture
• Advise patient not to have any vaccinations without the advice of the prescriber, serious reactions can occur
• Teach patient contraception is needed during treatment and for several mo after completion of therapy

Evaluation

Positive therapeutic outcome
- Prevention of rapid division of malignant cells

mitotane

(mye'toe-tane)
Lysodren, p'-DDD
Func. class.: Antineoplastic
Chem. class.: Hormone, adrenal cytotoxic agent
Pregnancy category **C**

Action: Cytotoxic and suppressive activity without cellular destruction in the adrenal cortex; related to DDT

Therapeutic Outcome: Prevention of rapid growth of malignant cells

Uses: Adrenocortical carcinoma

Investigational uses: Pituitary disorders with cushingoid symptoms

Dosage and routes

Adult: PO 9-10 g/day in divided doses tid or qid; may have to decrease dosage if severe reactions occur

Available forms: Tab 500 mg

Side effects/adverse reactions

CNS: Lightheadedness, flushing, sedation, vertigo
CV: Hypertension, orthostatic hypotension
EENT: Lethargy, blurring, retinopathy
GI: Nausea, vomiting, anorexia, diarrhea
GU: ***Proteinuria, hematuria***
INTEG: Rash
RESP: ***Fibrosis, pulmonary infiltrate***

Contraindications: Hypersensitivity

Precautions: Lactation, hepatic disease, pregnancy **C**

Pharmacokinetics

Absorption	40% (PO)
Distribution	Widely distributed
Metabolism	Liver, extensively
Excretion	Kidneys (10%), bile (15%)
Half-life	18 days-6 mo

Pharmacodynamics

Onset	Unknown
Peak	Unknown
Duration	Unknown

Interactions

Drug/drug:

Individual drugs
Alcohol: ↑ CNS depression
Phenytoin: ↓ effectiveness of phenytoin
Spironolactone: Blocked response in Cushing's disease
Warfarin: ↓ effectiveness of warfarin

Drug classifications
Antidepressants: ↑ CNS depression
Antihistamines: ↑ CNS depression
CNS depressants: ↑ CNS depression
Opioid analgesics: ↑ CNS depression

Sedative/hypnotics: ↑ CNS depression

Lab test interferences

Decrease: PBI, urinary 17-OHCS, uric acid

NURSING CONSIDERATIONS

Assessment

- Assess for adrenal insufficiency: fatigue, orthostatic hypotension, weight loss, weakness, nausea, vomiting, diarrhea
- Monitor renal function studies: BUN, serum uric acid, urine CrCl electrolytes before, during therapy; determine I&O ratio, urinary 17-OHCS, 8-hr plasma cortisol, before, during treatment
- Assess for dyspnea, chest pain, tachypnea, fatigue, increased pulse, pallor, lethargy, muscular weakness, fatigue, oliguria, hypoglycemia
- Assess for frequency of stools, and characteristics of stool: cramping, acidosis, signs of dehydration (rapid respirations, poor skin turgor, decreased urine output, dry skin, restlessness, weakness)
- Assess for symptoms indicating severe allergic reactions: rash, pruritus, itching, flushing
- Assess for signs of infection: increased temp, cough, fatigue, malaise

Associated nursing diagnoses

✓ Injury, risk for (adverse reactions)
✓ Body image disturbance (adverse reactions)
✓ Infection, risk for (adverse reactions)
✓ Knowledge deficit (teaching)

Implementation

PO route

- Give 1 hr ac or 2 hr pc to lessen nausea and vomiting or give antacid before oral agent; give drug after evening meal, before hs; administer antiemetic 30-60 min before giving drug to prevent vomiting
- Store in tight container

Patient/family education

- Instruct patient to report any complaints, side effects to the prescriber
- Instruct patient to report any changes in breathing, coughing; signs of wheezing
- Caution patient to avoid driving and other activities requiring alertness until response to drug is known
- Advise patient that a mechanical barrier method of contraception is needed to prevent pregnancy; drug is teratogenic
- Advise patient to use a Medic Alert bracelet or other form of identification to identify treatment and drug used
- Advise patient that if lethargy, somnolence, dizziness, tremors, or weakness occurs the prescriber should be contacted
- Caution patient not to use alcohol or OTC drugs unless approved by prescriber; serious adverse reactions may result

Evaluation

Positive therapeutic outcome

- Prevention of rapid division of malignant cells

M

mitoxantrone

(mye-toe-zan'trone)

Novantrone

Func. class.: Antineoplastic-antibiotic

Chem. class.: Synthetic anthraquinone

Pregnancy category **D**

Action: DNA reactive agent; cytocidal effect on both proliferating and nonproliferating cells, suggesting lack of cell cycle phase specificity; a vesicant

Therapeutic Outcome: Prevention of rapidly growing malignant cells

Uses: Acute nonlymphocytic leukemia (adult), relapsed leukemia, breast cancer

Investigational uses: Breast and liver malignancies, non-Hodgkin's lymphoma

Dosage and routes

Induction

Adult: **IV** inf 12 mg/m^2/day on days 1-3, and 100 mg/m^2 cytosine arabinoside × 7 days as a cont 24-hr inf; if complete remission occurs, 2nd inductor may be used

Consolidation

Adult: **IV** inf 12 mg/m^2/day × 2 days, given with cytosine arabinoside 100 mg/m^2/day × 5 days as cont inf usually 6 wk after induction

Available forms: Inj 2 mg/ml

Side effects/adverse reactions

CNS: Headache, seizures
CV: ***CHF, cardiomyopathy, dysrhythmias,*** ECG changes
EENT: Conjunctivitis, blue-green sclera
GI: *Nausea, vomiting, diarrhea, anorexia, mucositis,* ***hepatotoxicity***
HEMA: ***Thrombocytopenia, leukopenia, myelosuppression, anemia***
INTEG: *Rash, necrosis at inj site,* alopecia, dermatitis, thrombophlebitis at inj site
MISC: Fever, hypersensitivity, hyperuricemia
RESP: Cough, dyspnea

Contraindications: Hypersensitivity

Precautions: Myelosuppression, lactation, cardiac disease, P children, pregnancy **D**, renal, hepatic disease, gout

Pharmacokinetics

Absorption	Completely absorbed (IV)
Distribution	Widely distributed
Metabolism	Liver
Excretion	Bile; kidneys, unchanged (<10%)
Half-life	24-72 hr

Pharmacodynamics

Onset	Unknown
Peak	Unknown
Duration	Unknown

Interactions

Drug/drug:

Individual drugs

Radiation: ↑ toxicity, bone marrow suppression

Drug classifications
Antineoplastics: ↑ toxicity, bone marrow suppression
Live virus vaccines: ↑ adverse reactions

NURSING CONSIDERATIONS

Assessment

- Monitor ECG; watch for ST-T wave changes, low QRS and T, possible dysrhythmias (sinus tachycardia, heart block, PVCs)
- Assess buccal cavity q8h for dryness, sores or ulceration, white patches, oral pain, bleeding, dysphagia; obtain prescription for viscous lidocaine (Xylocaine)
- Assess symptoms indicating severe allergic reaction: rash, pruritus, urticaria, purpuric skin lesions, itching, flushing
- Assess tachypnea, ECG changes, dyspnea, edema, fatigue
- Monitor CBC, differential, platelet count weekly; withhold drug if WBC count is <4000/mm^3 or platelet count is <100,000/mm^3, notify prescriber of results if WBC <20,000/mm^3, platelets <150,000/mm^3
- Assess for increased uric acid levels, swelling, joint pain primarily in extremities; patient should be well hydrated to prevent urate deposits
- Monitor renal function studies: BUN, creatinine, urine CrCl before and during therapy; determine I&O ratio
- Monitor temp q4h (may indicate beginning of infection)
- Monitor liver function tests before and during therapy (bilirubin, AST [SGOT], ALT [SGPT], LDH) as needed or monthly; check for yellowing of skin and sclera, dark urine, clay-colored stools, itchy skin, abdominal pain, fever, diarrhea
- Assess for bleeding: hematuria, stool guaiac, bruising or petechiae, mucosa or orifices q8h; check for inflammation of mucosa, breaks in skin
- Identify effects of alopecia on body image; discuss feelings about body changes

Associated nursing diagnoses

- ✓ Injury, risk for (adverse reactions)
- ✓ Body image disturbance (adverse reactions)
- ✓ Infection, risk for (adverse reactions)
- ✓ Knowledge deficit (teaching)

Implementation

- Avoid contact with skin, since medication is very irritating; wash completely to remove
- Give fluids **IV** or PO before chemotherapy to hydrate patient
- Give antacid before oral agent; give drug after evening meal, before hs; provide antiemetic 30-60 min before giving drug and prn to prevent vomiting; administer antibiotics for prophylaxis of infection
- Give top or syst analgesics for pain
- Liq diet: carbonated beverages; gelatin may be added if patient is not nauseated or vomiting
- Encourage patient to rinse mouth tid-qid with water, club soda, brush teeth bid-qid with soft brush or cotton-tipped

M

applicators for stomatitis, use unwaxed dental floss

IV route

• Sol should be prepared by qualified personnel only under controlled conditions in a biologic cabinet using mask, gloves, gown

• Use Luer-Lok tubing to prevent leakage; do not let sol come in contact with skin; if contact occurs wash well with soap and water

• Give by direct **IV** after diluting with 50 ml or more normal saline or D_5W; give over 3-5 min, running **IV** of D_5W or 0.9% NaCl

• Intermittent inf may be diluted further in D_5W, 0.9% NaCl and run over 15-30 min; check for extravasation

Y-site compatibilities:
Ondansetron, fludarabine, melphalan, sargrasmostin, vinorelbine

Y-site incompatibility:
Paclitaxel

Additive incompatibility:
Heparin

Additive compatibilities:
Hydrocortisone sodium succinate, cyclophosphamide, cytarabine, fluorouracil, potassium chloride

Solution compatibilities:
D_5/0.9 NaCl, D_5W, 0.9% NaCl

Patient/family education

• Teach patient to avoid use of products containing aspirin or ibuprofen, razors, commercial mouthwash, since bleeding may occur; to report symptoms of bleeding (hematuria, tarry stools)

• Caution patient to report signs of anemia (fatigue, headache, irritability, faintness, shortness of breath)

• Inform patient that hair may be lost during treatment; a wig or hair piece may make patient feel better; new hair may be different in color, texture

• Caution patient not to have any vaccinations without the advice of the prescriber; serious reactions can occur

• Advise patient contraception is needed during treatment and for several mo after completion of therapy

Evaluation

Positive therapeutic outcome

• Prevention of rapid division of malignant cells

mivacurium

(mi-va-kure'ee-um)

Mivacron

Func. class.: Nondepolarizing neuromuscular blocker

Pregnancy category **C**

Action: Inhibits transmission of nerve impulses by binding with cholinergic receptor sites, antagonizing action of acetylcholine; no analgesic response

Therapeutic Outcome: Paralysis of all skeletal muscles

Uses: Facilitation of endotracheal intubation; skeletal muscle relaxation during mechanical ventilation, surgery, or general anesthesia; reduction of fractures/dislocations

Dosage and routes

Adult: **IV** 0.15 mg/kg; maintenance q15 min

P *Child:* 2-12 **IV** 0.2 mg/kg for a 10-min block

Available forms: 5, 10 ml single-use vial (2 mg/ml); premixed inf in D_5W 50 ml flex container

Side effects/adverse reactions

CV: Decreased B/P, bradycardia, tachycardia
EENT: Diplopia
INTEG: Rash, urticaria
MS: Weakness, prolonged skeletal muscle relaxation, ***paralysis***
RESP: ***Prolonged apnea, bronchospasm, wheezing, respiratory depression***

Contraindications: Hypersensitivity

Precautions: Pregnancy **C**, renal or hepatic disease, lactation, P children <3 mo, fluid and electrolyte imbalances, neuromuscular disease, respiratory G disease, obesity, elderly

Pharmacokinetics

Absorption	Completely absorbed (IV)
Distribution	Extracellular spaces; crosses placenta
Metabolism	Plasma
Excretion	Kidneys
Half-life	2 hr

Pharmacodynamics

Onset	2-2½ min
Peak	2-3 min
Duration	20-30 min

Interactions

Drug/drug:

Individual drugs

Clindamycin: ↑ paralysis length and intensity
Colistin: ↑ paralysis length and intensity
Lidocaine: ↑ paralysis length and intensity
Lithium: ↑ paralysis length and intensity
Magnesium: ↑ paralysis length and intensity
Polymyxin B: ↑ paralysis length and intensity
Procainamide: ↑ paralysis length and intensity
Quinidine: ↑ paralysis length and intensity
Succinylcholine: ↑ paralysis length and intensity

Drug classifications

Aminoglycosides: ↑ paralysis length and intensity
β-Blockers: ↑ paralysis length and intensity
Diuretics, potassium-losing: ↑ paralysis length and intensity
General anesthesia: ↑ paralysis length and intensity

NURSING CONSIDERATIONS

Assessment

- Monitor VS (B/P, pulse, respirations, airway) until fully recovered; rate, depth, pattern of respirations, strength of hand grip; patient should be intubated before use
- Monitor for electrolyte imbalances (potassium, magnesium) before drug is used;

M

electrolyte imbalances may lead to increased action of this drug
• Monitor for recovery: decreased paralysis of face, diaphragm, leg, arm, rest of body; residual weakness and respiratory problems may occur during recovery period
• Assess for hypersensitive reactions: rash, fever, respiratory distress, pruritus; drug should be discontinued

Associated nursing diagnoses

✓ Breathing pattern, ineffective (uses)
✓ Communication, impaired verbal (adverse reactions)
✓ Fear (adverse reactions)
✓ Knowledge deficit (teaching)

Implementation

IV **IV route**
• Use peripheral nerve stimulator (anesthesiologist) to determine neuromuscular blockade; deep tendon reflexes should be monitored during extended periods
• Give direct **IV** undiluted over 5-15 min
• Give cont **IV** diluted to 0.5 mg ml in D_5W, 0.9% NaCl, D_5/0.9% NaCl, LR, D_5/LR and give as an inf at prescribed rate (only by qualified person, usually an anesthesiologist); do not administer IM
• Store in light-resistant container
• Give anticholinesterase to reverse neuromuscular blockade

Y-site compatibilities: Alfentanil, droperidol, fentanyl, midazolam, sufentanil

Y-site incompatibility: Barbiturates

Patient/family education

• Provide reassurance if communication is difficult during recovery from neuromuscular blockade
• Provide explanation to patients regarding all procedures or treatments; patient will remain conscious if anesthesia is not given also

Evaluation

Positive therapeutic outcome
• Paralysis of jaw, eyelid, head, neck, rest of body as evaluated by peripheral nerve stimulator

Treatment of overdose: Edrophonium or neostigmine, atropine; monitor VS; may require mechanical ventilation

molindone
(moe-lin'done)
Moban
Func. class.: Antipsychotic/neuroleptic
Chem. class.: Dihydroindolone
Pregnancy category **C**

Action: Depresses cerebral cortex, hypothalamus, limbic system, which control activity, aggression; blocks neurotransmission produced by dopamine at synapse; exhibits strong α-adrenergic, anticholinergic blocking action; mechanism for antipsychotic effects is unclear

➡ Therapeutic Outcome: Decreased psychotic behavior

Uses: Psychotic disorders

Dosage and routes

Adult: PO 50-75 mg/day increasing to 225 mg/day if needed

Available forms: Tab 5, 10, 25, 50, 100 mg; conc 20 mg/ml

Side effects/adverse reactions

CNS: ESP: pseudoparkinsonism, akathisia, dystonia, tardive dyskinesia, drowsiness, headache, seizures, ***neuroleptic malignant syndrome***
CV: Orthostatic hypotension, hypertension, ***cardiac arrest,*** ECG changes, ***tachycardia***
EENT: Blurred vision, glaucoma
GI: Dry mouth, nausea, vomiting, anorexia, constipation, diarrhea, jaundice, weight gain
GU: Urinary retention, urinary frequency, enuresis, impotence, amenorrhea, gynecomastia
HEMA: ***Anemia, leukopenia, leukocytosis, agranulocytosis***
INTEG: Rash, photosensitivity, dermatitis
RESP: ***Laryngospasm,*** dyspnea, ***respiratory depression***

Contraindications: Hypersensitivity, coma, child

Precautions: Pregnancy **C**, lactation, hypertension, hepatic disease, cardiac disease, Parkinson's disease, brain tumor, glaucoma, urinary retention, diabetes mellitus, respiratory disease, prostatic hypertrophy

Pharmacokinetics

Absorption	Rapidly absorbed
Distribution	Widely distributed
Metabolism	Liver (>90%)
Excretion	Kidneys, unchanged
Half-life	1½ hr

Pharmacodynamics

Onset	Erratic
Peak	1½ hr
Duration	24-36 hr

Interactions

Drug/drug:

Individual drugs

Alcohol: ↑ effects of both drugs, oversedation
Disopyramide: ↑ anticholinergic effects
Guanethidine: ↓ antihypertensive response
Levodopa: ↓ antiparkinsonian activity
Lithium: ↓ molidone levels, ↑ EPS, masking of lithium toxicity
Norepinephrine: ↓ vasoresponse, ↑ toxicity
Phenobarbital: ↓ effectiveness, ↑ metabolism

Drug classifications

Antacids: ↓ absorption
Anticholinergics: ↑ anticholinergic effects
Antidepressants: ↑ CNS depression
Antihistamines: ↑ CNS depression

M

Antihypertensives: ↑ hypotension
Barbiturate anesthetics: ↑ CNS depression
General anesthetics: ↑ CNS depression
MAOI: ↑ anticholinergic effect
Narcotics: ↑ CNS depression
Sedative/hypnotics: ↑ CNS depression

Lab test interferences

Alterations in: BUN, RBC, serum glucose, WBC
Increase: Serum prolactin levels

NURSING CONSIDERATIONS

Assessment

- Assess mental status: orientation, mood, behavior, presence and type of hallucinations before initial administration and monthly; this drug should significantly reduce psychotic behavior
- Check for swallowing of PO medication; check for hoarding or giving of medication to other patients
- Monitor I&O ratio; palpate bladder if low urinary output [G] occurs, especially in elderly; urinalysis recommended before, during prolonged therapy
- Monitor bilirubin, CBC, liver function studies monthly
- Assess affect, orientation, LOC, reflexes, gait, coordination, sleep pattern disturbances
- Monitor B/P with patient sitting, standing, and lying; take pulse and respirations q4h during initial treatment; establish baseline before starting treatment; report drops of 30 mm Hg
- Check for dizziness, faintness, palpitations, tachycardia on rising; severe orthostatic hypotension is common
- Identify for neuroleptic malignant syndrome: hyperpyrexia, muscle rigidity, increased CPK, altered mental status; drug should be discontinued
- Assess for EPS including akathisia (inability to sit still, no pattern to movements), tardive dyskinesia (bizarre movements of the jaw, mouth, tongue, extremities), pseudoparkinsonism (ragged tremors, pill rolling, shuffling gate); an antiparkinsonism drug should be prescribed
- Assess for constipation, urinary retention daily; if these occur, increase bulk, water in diet

Associated nursing diagnoses

✓ Thought processes, altered (uses)
✓ Coping, ineffective individual (uses)
✓ Knowledge deficit (teaching)
✓ Noncompliance (teaching)

Implementation

PO route

- Administer decreased dosage [G] in elderly, since metabolism is slowed
- Administer PO with full glass of water, milk; or give with food to decrease GI upset
- Store in airtight, light-resistant container, oral sol in bottle

Patient/family education

- Teach patient to use good oral hygiene; frequent rinsing

of mouth, sugarless gum for dry mouth
• Caution patient to avoid hazardous activities until drug response is determined; dizziness, blurred vision may occur
• Inform patient that orthostatic hypotension occurs often and to rise from sitting or lying position gradually; to remain lying down after IM inj for at least 30 min; tell patient to avoid hot tubs, hot showers, tub baths, since hypotension may occur; teach patient that in hot weather heat stroke may occur; take extra precautions to stay cool
• Teach patient to avoid abrupt withdrawal of this drug, or EPS may result; drug should be withdrawn slowly
• Teach patient to avoid OTC preparations (cough, hay fever, cold) unless approved by prescriber, since serious drug interactions may occur; avoid use with alcohol, CNS depressants; increased drowsiness may occur
• Advise patient to use a sunscreen and sunglasses to prevent burns
• Teach patient about EPS and necessity of meticulous oral hygiene, since oral candidiasis may occur
• Advise patient to take antacids 2 hr before or after taking this drug
• Instruct patient to report sore throat, malaise, fever, bleeding, mouth sores; if these occur, CBC should be drawn and drug discontinued

Evaluation

Positive therapeutic outcome
• Decrease in emotional excitement, hallucinations, delusions, paranoia
• Reorganization of patterns of thought, speech

Treatment of overdose: Lavage if orally ingested; provide airway; *do not induce vomiting or use epinephrine*

moricizine
(more-i'siz-een)
Ethmozine
Func. class.: Antidysrhythmic, group I
Chem. class.: Phenothiazine
Pregnancy category **B**

Action: Decreased rate of rise of action potential, prolonging refractory peroid and shortening the action potential duration; depression of inward influx if sodium mediates the effects; may slow atrial and AV nodal conduction

Therapeutic Outcome: Resolution of ventricular and life-threatening dysrhythmias

Uses: Symptomatic ventricular and life-threatening dysrhythmias

Dosage and routes
Adult: PO 10-15 mg/kg/day in 2-3 divided doses or 600-900 mg/day given in 2-3 divided doses

Available forms: Film-coated tab 200, 250, 300 mg

M

Side effects/adverse reactions

CNS: Dizziness, headache, fatigue, perioral numbness, euphoria, nervousness, sleep disorders, depression, tinnitus, fatigue
CV: Palpitations, chest pain, CHF, hypertension, syncope, ***dysrythmias,*** bradycardia, ***MI,*** thrombophlebitis
GI: Nausea, abdominal pain, vomiting, diarrhea
GU: Sexual dysfunction, difficult urination, dysuria, incontinence
MISC: Sweating, musculoskeletal pain
RESP: Dyspnea, hyperventilation, ***apnea,*** asthma, pharyngitis, cough

Contraindications: 2nd- to 3rd-degree AV block, right bundle branch block, cardiogenic shock, hypersensitivity

Precautions: CHF, hypokalemia, hyperkalemia, sick sinus syndrome, pregnancy **B**, lactation, P children, impaired hepatic and renal function, cardiac dysfunction

Pharmacokinetics

Absorption	Well absorbed (PO)
Distribution	Plasma protein binding (95%)
Metabolism	Liver, extensively
Excretion	Kidneys, breast milk
Half-life	1½-3½ hr

Pharmacodynamics

Onset	Unknown
Peak	½-2 hr
Duration	8-12 hr

Interactions

Drug/drug:

Individual drugs
Cimetidine: ↑ effect of moricizine
Theophylline: ↓ effect of theophylline

NURSING CONSIDERATIONS

Assessment

- Monitor ECG at baseline and periodically to determine drug effectiveness; measure PR, QRS, QT intervals, check for PVCs, other dysrhythmias; check B/P for hypotension, hypertension and for rebound hypertension after 1-2 hr; check for dehydration or hypovolemia
- Monitor I&O ratio and electrolytes: potassium, sodium, chloride; check weight daily and for signs of CHF or pulmonary toxicity: dyspnea, fatigue, cough, fever, chest pain; drug should be discontinued
- Monitor liver function studies: AST (SGOT), ALT (SGPT), bilirubin, alkaline phosphatase
- Monitor cardiac rate; monitor respiration rate, rhythm, character, and chest pain; watch for ventricular tachycardia, supraventricular tachycardia, or fibrillation

Associated nursing diagnoses

✓ Cardiac output, decreased (uses)
✓ Impaired gas exchange (adverse reactions)
✓ Knowledge deficit (teaching)

Implementation

PO route

- Give with meals for GI upset; may be given in 2 divided doses if adverse reactions are minimal
- Make dosage adjustment q 3 days or more

Patient/family education

- Instruct patient to report side effects immediately to prescriber
- Instruct patient to complete follow-up appointment with health care provider including pulmonary function studies, chest-x-ray, ophth and otoscopic examinations
- Advise patient to carry identification (Medic-Alert) indicating condition and treatment
- Caution patient to avoid driving and other hazardous activities until drug response is determined
- Instruct patient to take medication as prescribed, not to double doses; missed doses may be taken up to 6 hr after previous dose

Treatment of overdose:

O_2, artificial ventilation, ECG, administer dopamine for circulatory depression, administer diazepam or thiopental for convulsions, isoproterenol

morphine

(mor'feen)

Astramorph PF, Duramorph, Epimorph ✤, Infumorph 200, Infumorph 500, Morphine H.P. ✤, morphine sulfate, Morphitec ✤, M.O.S. ✤, M.O.S.-S.R. ✤, MS Contin, MSIR, OMS Concentrate, Oramorph SR, RMS, Roxanol, Roxanol 100, Roxanol Rescudose, Roxanol SR

Func. class.: Opioid analgesic

Pregnancy category **B**

Controlled substance schedule **II**

M

Action: Depresses pain impulse transmission at the spinal cord level by interacting with opioid receptors, produces CNS depression

Therapeutic Outcome: Decreased pain

Uses: Severe pain; often given after or during an MI

Dosage and routes

Adult: SC/IM 4-15 mg q4h prn; PO 10-30 mg q4h prn; ext rel q8-12h; rec 10-20 mg q4h prn; **IV** 4-10 mg diluted in 4-5 ml water for inj, over 5 min; epidural 2-10 mg/day

Child: SC 0.1-0.2 mg/kg, not to exceed 15 mg; IM/**IV** 50-100 μg/kg, max 10 mg/dose initially

Pharmacodynamics

	PO	PO–EXT REL	IM	SC	REC	IV	IT
Onset	Variable	Unknown	10-30 min	20 min	Unknown	Rapid	Rapid
Peak	1 hr	Unknown	½-1 hr	1-1½ hr	½-1 hr	20 min	Unknown
Duration	4-5 hr	8-12 hr	4-5 hr	4-5 hr	4-5 hr	4-5 hr	Ext

Available forms: Inj 2, 4, 5, 8, 10, 15 mg/ml; sol tab 10, 15, 30 mg; oral sol 10, 20 mg/5 ml, 20 mg/10 ml, 20 mg/ml; oral tab 15, 30 mg; rec supp 5, 10, 20 mg; ext rel tab 300 mg

Side effects/adverse reactions

CNS: Drowsiness, dizziness, ***confusion***, headache, ***sedation***, euphoria hallucinations, dysphoria
CV: Palpitations, bradycardia, ***hypotension***
EENT: Tinnitus, blurred vision, miosis, diplopia
GI: Nausea, vomiting, anorexia, ***constipation***, cramps, biliary tract pressure
GU: Urinary retention
INTEG: Rash, urticaria, bruising, flushing, diaphoresis, pruritus
RESP: Respiratory depression

Contraindications: Hypersensitivity, addiction (narcotic), hemorrhage, bronchial asthma, increased intracranial pressure

Precautions: Addictive personality, pregnancy **B**, lactation, acute MI, severe heart disease, G elderly, respiratory depression, hepatic disease, renal disease, P child <18 yr

Pharmacokinetics

Absorption	Variably absorbed (PO); well absorbed (IM, SC, rec); completely absorbed (IV)
Distribution	Widely distributed; crosses placenta
Metabolism	Liver, extensively
Excretion	Kidneys
Half-life	2-3 hr

Interactions

Drug/drug:

Individual drugs

Alcohol: ↑ respiratory depression, hypotension, sedation
Nalbuphine: ↓ analgesia
Pentazocine: ↓ analgesia

Drug classifications

Antihistamines: ↑ respiratory depression, hypotension
CNS depressants: ↑ respiratory depression, hypotension
MAOI: Reduce dosage; unpredictable reaction may occur
Sedative/hypnotics: ↑ respiratory depression, hypotension

Lab test interferences

Increase: Amylase

NURSING CONSIDERATIONS

Assessment

- Assess pain: location, type, character, intensity; give dose before pain becomes extreme
- Monitor I&O ratio; check

for decreasing output; may indicate urinary retention; check for constipation; increase fluids, bulk in diet if needed or stool softeners may be prescribed
• Monitor CNS changes: dizziness, drowsiness, hallucinations, euphoria, LOC, pupil reactions
• Monitor allergic reactions: rash, urticaria
• Assess respiratory dysfunction: depression, character, rate, rhythm; notify prescriber if respirations are <10/min

Associated nursing diagnoses

✓ Pain (uses)
✓ Sensory-perceptual alteration: visual, auditory (adverse reactions)
✓ Breathing pattern, ineffective (adverse reactions)
✓ Knowledge deficit (teaching)

Implementation

• Give with antiemetic if nausea, vomiting occur
• Administer when pain is beginning to return; determine dosage interval by patient response; continuous dosing of medication is more effective than giving prn
• Medication should be slowly withdrawn after long-term use to prevent withdrawal symptoms
• Store in light-resistant container at room temp

PO route

• May be given with food or milk to lessen GI upset; may be crushed and mixed with food or fluids; ext rel tabs should be swallowed whole

IM/SC route

• Do not give if cloudy or a precipitate has formed

IV **IV route**

• Give direct **IV** by diluting with ≥5 ml of sterile water or 0.9% NaCl for inj; give 2.5-15 mg/4-5 min; rapid administration may lead to increased respiratory depression, death
• Give cont inf by adding to D_5W, $D_{10}W$, 0.9% NaCl, 0.45% NaCl, Ringer's, LR, any dextrose/saline sol, or any dextrose/Ringer's, 0.1-1 mg/ml
• Give by inf pump to deliver correct dosage; titrate to provide adequate pain relief without serious sedation, respiratory depression, hypotension
• May be given by patient-controlled analgesia (PCA) pump in terminal illnesses; patient is able to control amount of morphine

Syringe compatibilities:

Atropine, benzquinamide, butorphanol, chlorpromazine, cimetidine, dimenhydrinate, diphenhydramine, droperidol, fentanyl, glycopyrrolate, hydroxyzine, metoclopramide, midazolam, perphenazine, promazine, ranitidine, scopolamine

Syringe incompatibilities:

Meperidine, thiopental

Y-site compatibilities:

Acyclovir, aldesleukin, amikacin, aminophylline, ampicillin, ampicillin/sulbactam, atracurium, calcium chloride, cefamandole, cefazolin, cefopera-

M

zone, ceforanide, cefotaxime, cefotetan, cefoxitin, ceftizoxime, cefuroxime, cephalothin, cephapirin, chloramphenicol, clindamycin, co-trimoxazole, doxycycline, enalaprilat, erythromycin lactobionate, esmolol, famotidine, foscarnet, gentamicin, heparin, hydrocortisone sodium succinate, insulin, kanamycin, labetalol, magnesium sulfate, melphalan, metronidazole, mezlocillin, moxalactam, nafcillin, ondansetron, oxacillin, oxytocin, paclitaxel, pancuronium, penicillin G potassium, piperacillin, potassium chloride, ranitidine, sodium bicarbonate, ticarcillin, ticarcillin/clavulanate, tobramycin, vancomycin, vecuronium, vinorelbine, vitamin B with C, zidovadine

Y-site incompatibilities:
Furosemide, minocycline, tetracycline

Additive compatibilities:
Dobutamine, succinylcholine, verapamil

Additive incompatibility:
Aminophylline

Patient/family education

- Advise patient to report any symptoms of CNS changes, allergic reactions
- Caution patients to avoid CNS depressants (alcohol, sedative/hypnotics) for at least 24 hr after taking this drug
- Discuss with patient that dizziness, drowsiness, and confusion are common; to avoid getting up without assistance
- Discuss in detail all aspects of the drug and expected response

Evaluation

Positive therapeutic outcome
- Decreased pain

Treatment of overdose: Naloxone (Narcan) 0.2-0.8 **IV**, O_2, **IV** fluids, vasopressors

multivitamins

Adavite, Dayalets, LKV Drops, Multi-75, Multi-Day, One-A-Day, Optilets, Poly-Vi-Sol, Quintabs, Rulets, Sesame Street Vitamins, Tab-A-Vite, Therabid, Theragran, Unicaps, Vita-Bob, Vita-Kid, many other brands; Berocca Parenteral, M.V.C. 9+3, M.V.I. Pediatric

Func. class.: Vitamins, multiple

Pregnancy category **A**

Action: Needed for adequate metabolism

➔ **Therapeutic Outcome:** Prevention and treatment of vitamin deficiencies

Uses: Prevention and treatment of vitamin deficiencies

Dosage and routes

P *Adult and child:* PO depends on brand

Available forms: Many forms available

Side effects/adverse reactions

Rare at recommended dosage

Precautions: Pregnancy **A**

Pharmacokinetics	
Absorption	Well absorbed (PO)
Distribution	Widely distributed; crosses placenta
Metabolism	Widely metabolized
Excretion	Kidney, unchanged (water soluble)
Half-life	Unknown

Pharmacodynamics	PO/IV
Onset	Unknown
Peak	Unknown
Duration	Unknown

Interactions

Drug/drug:

Individual drugs

Levodopa: ↓ effect of levodopa (large amounts of B_6)

NURSING CONSIDERATIONS

Assessment

- Assess patient for vitamin deficiency; usually more than one vitamin is deficient

Associated nursing diagnoses

- ✓ Nutrition, less than body requirements (uses)
- ✓ Knowledge deficit (teaching)

Implementation

PO route

- Liq multivitamins can be diluted or dropped into patients' mouth using dropper provided with some brands
- Chew tab should be chewed and not swallowed whole

IV route

- Give by cont inf only after diluting 5-10 ml (multivitamins)/500-1000 ml of D_5W, $D_{10}W$, $D_{20}W$, LR, D_5/LR, D_5/0.9% NaCl, 0.9% NaCl, 3% NaCl
- Do not use sol with crystals, precipitate or color other than bright yellow

Y-site compatibilities:

Acyclovir, ampicillin, carbenicillin, cefazolin, cephalothin, cephapirin, erythromycin lactobionate, fludarabine, gentamicin, tetracycline

Additive compatibilities:

Cefoxitin, isoproterenol, methyldopate, metoclopramide, metronidazole, netilmicin, norepinephrine, sodium bicarbonate, verapamil

Additive incompatibilities:

Penicillin G, erythromycin, tetracycline, kanamycin, streptomycin, doxycycline, lincomycin should not be admixed

Patient/family education

- Advise patient that adequate nutrition must be maintained to prevent further deficiencies; to comply with treatment regimen
- Advise patient to avoid treating flavored multivitamins as candy; child may overdose
- Caution patient to store vitamins out of children's reach

Evaluation

Positive therapeutic outcome

- Check each individual vitamin for guidelines

• Absence of vitamin deficiencies

mupirocin

(myoo-peer'oh-sin)

Bactroban, Pseudomonic Acid A

Func. class.: Topical antiinfective

Chem. class.: Pseudomonic Acid A

Pregnancy category **B**

Action: Inhibits bacterial protein synthesis, shows no cross-resistance to most antibiotics

➡ **Therapeutic Outcome:** Decreased bacterial growth

Uses: Impetigo caused by *Staphylococcus aureus,* β-hemolytic *Streptococcus, S. pyogenes;* decreased carrier state of *S. aureus*

Dosage and routes

Adult: Top apply small amount to affected area tid; nasal up to qid

Available forms: Oint 2% (20 mg/g); nasal

Side effects/adverse reactions

INTEG: Burning, stinging, itching, rash, dry skin, swelling, contact dermatitis, erythema, tenderness, increased exudate

Contraindications: Hypersensitivity

Precautions: Pregnancy **B**, lactation

Pharmacokinetics	
Absorption	Minimal (top)
Distribution	Remains in skin layer
Metabolism	Skin
Excretion	Removed by desquamation
Half-life	Unknown

Pharmacodynamics	
Onset	Unknown
Peak	Unknown
Duration	Unknown

Interactions: None

NURSING CONSIDERATIONS

Assessment

• Assess affected area for continuing infection: increased size, number of lesions; or failure of medication to decrease size and number of lesions

Associated nursing diagnoses

✓ Skin integrity, impaired (uses)
✓ Infection, risk for (uses)
✓ Knowledge deficit (teaching)

Implementation

Top route

• Wash hands before use; apply a small amount to affected area; cover with 2 × 2 in gauze if needed
• Wash hands after applying oint
• Store at room temp

Patient/family education

• Teach patient to wash hands before and after applying oint;

to trim fingernails to prevent scratching
- Instruct patient to report irritation, worsening of condition, itching, or pain at site; if no improvement within 3-5 days, report to prescriber

Evaluation

Positive therapeutic outcome
- Reduction in size, number of lesions

muromonab-CD3
(mur-oe-mone'ab)
Orthoclone OKT3
Func. class.: Immunosuppressive
Chem. class.: Murine monoclonal antibody
Pregnancy category **C**

Action: Reverses graft rejection by blocking T cell function

Therapeutic Outcome: Prevention of graft rejection

Uses: Acute allograft rejection in renal, cardiac/hepatic transplant patients

Dosage and routes

Adult: **IV** bol 5 mg/day × 10-14 days; usually methylprednisolone sodium succinate, 1 mg/kg **IV**, is given before muromonab-CD3, 100 mg **IV** hydrocortisone sodium succinate is given 30 min after muromonab-CD3

P *Child:* **IV** 100 μg/kg/day × 10-14 day

Cardiac/hepatic allograft rejection, steroid resistant

Adult: **IV** bol 5 mg/day × 10-14 days; begin when it is known that rejection has not been reversed by steroids

Available forms: Inj 5 mg/5 ml

Side effects/adverse reactions

CNS: Pyrexia, chills, tremors
CV: Chest pain
GI: Vomiting, nausea, diarrhea
MISC: Infection
RESP: Dyspnea, wheezing, ***pulmonary edema***

Contraindications: Hypersensitivity to murine origin, fluid overload

Precautions: Pregnancy **C**, P child <2 yr, fever

Pharmacokinetics	
Absorption	Completely absorbed
Distribution	Unknown
Metabolism	Unknown
Excretion	Unknown
Half-life	Unknown

Pharmacodynamics	
Onset	Unknown
Peak	Unknown
Duration	Unknown

Interactions

Drug/drug:

Individual drugs

Allopurinol: ↑ toxicity
Cyclosporine: ↑ myelosuppression

Drug classifications

Antineoplastics: ↑ myelosuppression

NURSING CONSIDERATIONS

Assessment

- Assess for cytosine release syndrome (CRS): nausea, vomiting, chills, fever, joint pain, weakness, dizziness, diarrhea, tremors, abdominal pain; occurs 30-60 min after first dose; methylprednisolone sodium succinate may be prescribed to lessen this reaction
- Assess for hypersensitivity reaction: dyspnea, bronchospasm, urticaria, tachycardia, hypotension, angioedema; discontinue drug; all emergency equipment must be nearby
- Assess for headache, photophobia, fever, rigidity; indicate aseptic meningitis has developed
- Assess for sore throat, fever, chills, rash, dysuria which may indicate infection; therapy may be discontinued
- Assess for fluid overload: edema, pulmonary edema, increasing weight
- Monitor blood studies: CBC with differential, platelets, BUN, creatinine, alkaline phosphatase, bilirubin during treatment monthly
- Monitor AST (SGOT), ALT (SGPT), BUN, creatinine, alkaline phosphatase, bilirubin
- Obtain human-mouse antibody; if titer is over 1:1000, this drug should not be used
- Monitor T cell with CD_3 antigen qd; report should be CD_3 positive and T cells $<25/mm^3$

Associated nursing diagnoses

- ✓ Infection, risk for (uses)
- ✓ Knowledge deficit (teaching)

Implementation

IV IV route

- Give by direct **IV** undiluted; withdraw with a 0.2-0.22 low–protein binding μm filter; discard and use new needle for administration; give over 1 min
- Give for several days before transplant surgery

Patient/family education

- Instruct patient to report fever, chills, sore throat, fatigue, since serious infections may occur
- Advise patient to use contraceptive measures during treatment for 12 wk after ending therapy; drug is mutagenic
- Advise patient to avoid crowds and persons with known infections to reduce risk of infection

Evaluation

Positive therapeutic outcome

- Absence of graft rejection

nabumetone

(na-byoo′me-tone)

Relafen

Func. class.: Nonsteroidal antiinflammatory

Chem. class.: Acetic acid derivative

Pregnancy category C

Action: Inhibits prostaglandin synthesis by decreasing an enzyme needed for biosynthesis; analgesic, antiinflammatory

Therapeutic Outcome: Decreased pain, swelling of joints

Uses: Osteoarthritis, rheumatoid arthritis, acute or chronic treatment

Dosage and routes

Adult: PO 1 g as a single dose; may increase to 1.5-2 g/day if needed; may give qd or bid (as a divided dose)

Available forms: Tab 500, 750 mg

Side effects/adverse reactions

CNS: Dizziness, headache, drowsiness, fatigue, tremors, confusion, insomnia, anxiety, depression, nervousness
CV: Tachycardia, peripheral edema, palpitations, dysrhythmias, CHF
EENT: Tinnitus, hearing loss, blurred vision
GI: Nausea, anorexia, vomiting, diarrhea, jaundice, cholestatic hepatitis, constipation, flatulence, cramps, dry mouth, peptic ulcer, gastritis, ***ulceration, perforation***
GU: ***Nephrotoxicity, dysuria, hematuria, oliguria, azotemia,*** cystitis
HEMA: ***Blood dyscrasias***
INTEG: Purpura, rash, pruritus, sweating, photosensitivity
RESP: Dyspnea, pharyngitis, ***bronchospasm***

Contraindications: Hypersensitivity to this drug or aspirin, iodides, NSAIDs, asthma, severe renal disease

Precautions: Pregnancy **C** 1st and 2nd trimester, lactation, P children, bleeding disorders, GI disorders, cardiac disorders, renal disorders hepatic dys- G function, elderly

Pharmacokinetics

Absorption	Well absorbed (PO)
Distribution	Unknown
Metabolism	Liver, extensively, to inactive metabolite
Excretion	Unknown
Half-life	22-30 hr

Pharmacodynamics

Onset	Unknown
Peak	2½-4 hr
Duration	Unknown

Interactions

Drug/drug:

Individual drugs

Acetaminophen (long-term use): ↑ renal reactions
Alcohol: ↑ adverse reactions
Aspirin: ↓ effectiveness, ↑ adverse reactions
Cefamandole: ↑ bleeding
Cefoperazone: ↑ bleeding
Cefotetan: ↑ bleeding
Coumarin: ↑ anticoagulant effects
Digoxin: ↑ toxicity, levels
Insulin: ↓ insulin effect
Lithium: ↑ toxicity
Methotrexate: ↑ toxicity
Phenytoin: ↑ toxicity
Probenecid: ↑ toxicity
Sulfonylurea: ↑ toxicity
Valproic acid: ↑ bleeding

Drug classifications

Anticoagulants: ↑ risk of bleeding

N

Antihypertensives: ↓ effect of antihypertensives
Antineoplastics: ↑ risk of hematologic toxicity
Cephalosporins: ↑ risk of bleeding
Diuretics: ↓ effectiveness of diuretics
Glucocorticoids: ↑ adverse reactions
Hypoglycemics, oral: ↓ hypoglycemic effect
NSAIDs: ↑ adverse reactions
Potassium supplements: ↑ adverse reactions
Radiation: ↑ risk of hematologic toxicity
Sulfonamides: ↑ toxicity

NURSING CONSIDERATIONS

Assessment

- Assess for pain: location, duration, intensity; and for inflammation of joints ROM
- Monitor blood counts during therapy; watch for decreasing platelets; if low, therapy may need to be discontinued, restarted after hematologic recovery; check for blood dyscrasias (thrombocytopenia): brusing, fatigue, bleeding, poor healing; monitor liver function tests: AST (SGOT), ALT (SGPT), alkaline phosphatase

Associated nursing diagnoses

- ✓ Pain (uses)
- ✓ Mobility, impaired (uses)
- ✓ Injury, risk for (adverse reactions)
- ✓ Knowledge deficit (teaching)

Implementation

PO route

- Administer tab to patient crushed or whole
- Give with food or milk to decrease gastric symptoms

Patient/family education

- Tell patient that drug must be continued for prescribed time to be effective; to avoid aspirin, alcoholic beverages, ibuprofen, and OTC medications unless approved by prescriber
- Caution patient to report bleeding, bruising, fatigue, malaise, since blood dyscrasias do occur
- Instruct patient to use caution when driving; drowsiness, dizziness may occur
- Advise patient to use sunscreen, hat, and other protective clothing to prevent burning

Evaluation

Positive therapeutic outcome

- Decreased pain
- Decreased inflammation
- Increased mobility

nadolol

(nay-doe'lole)

Corgard

Func. class.: Antihypertensive, antianginal
Chem. class.: β-Adrenergic receptor blocker

Pregnancy category **C**

Action: Competitively blocks stimulation of β-adrenergic receptor within vascular smooth muscle; produces chronotropic, inotropic activity (decreases rate of SA node discharge, increases recovery time), slows conduction of AV node, decreases heart rate, which decreases O_2 consumption in myocardium; also decreases renin-aldosterone-angiotensin system at high doses, inhibits β_2-receptors in bronchial system

Therapeutic Outcome: Decreased B/P, heart rate

Uses: Chronic stable angina pectoris, mild to moderate hypertension, prophylaxis of migraine headaches

Investigational uses: Tachyarrhythmias, aggression, anxiety, tremors, esophageal varices (rebleeding only)

Dosage and routes

Adult: PO 40 mg qd; increase by 40-80 mg q3-7 days; maintenance 40-240 mg/day for angina, 40-320 mg/day for hypertension

Available forms: Tab 20, 40, 80, 120, 160 mg

Side effects/adverse reactions

CNS: Depression, hallucinations, dizziness, fatigue, lethargy, paresthesia, headache
CV: Bradycardia, hypotension, ***CHF,*** palpitations, AV block, chest pain, peripheral ischemia, flushing, edema, vasodilatation, conduction disturbances
EENT: Sore throat
GI: Nausea, vomiting, diarrhea, colitis, constipation, cramps, dry mouth, flatulence, hepatomegaly, pancreatitis, taste distortion
HEMA: Agranulocytosis, thrombocytopenia
INTEG: Rash, pruritus, fever
RESP: Dyspnea, respiratory dysfunction, ***bronchospasm,*** cough, wheezing, nasal stuffiness, pharyngitis, ***laryngospasm***

Contraindications: Hypersensitivity to this drug, cardiac failure, cardiogenic shock, 2nd- or 3rd-degree heart block, bronchospastic disease, sinus bradycardia, CHF, COPD

Precautions: Diabetes mellitus, pregnancy **C**, renal disease, lactation, hyperthyroidism, peripheral vascular disease, myasthenia gravis

Pharmacokinetics

Absorption	Variably absorbed (PO)
Distribution	Crosses placenta; minimal concentration in CNS
Excretion	Kidneys, unchanged
Half-life	10-24 hr; increased in renal disease

Pharmacodynamics

	PO
Onset	Variable
Peak	3-4 hr
Duration	17-24 hr

Interactions

Drug/drug:

Individual drugs
Alcohol: ↑ hypotension (large amounts)
Epinephrine: α-Adrenergic stimulation

N

Hydralazine: ↑ hypotension, bradycardia
Indomethacin: ↓ antihypertensive effect
Insulin: ↑ hypoglycemia
Methyldopa: ↑ hypotension, bradycardia
Phenytoin (IV): ↑ myocardial depression
Prazosin: ↑ hypotension, bradycardia
Reserpine: ↑ hypotension, bradycardia
Thyroid: ↓ effectiveness
Verapamil: ↑ myocardial depression

Drug classifications
Amphetamines: ↑ hypotension, bradycardia
Antihypertensives: ↑ hypertension
β_2-agonists: ↓ bronchodilatation
Cardiac glycosides: ↑ bradycardia
MAOI: ↑ hypertension
Nitrates: ↑ hypotension
NSAIDs: ↓ effect
Theophyllines: ↓ bronchodilatation

Lab test interferences

False increase: Urinary catecholamines

NURSING CONSIDERATIONS

Assessment

- Monitor B/P at beginning of treatment, periodically thereafter; note rate, rhythm, quality of apical/radial pulse before administration; notify prescriber of any significant changes (pulse <55 bpm)
- Check for baselines in renal, liver function tests before therapy begins
- Assess for edema in feet, legs daily; monitor I&O, daily weight; check for jugular vein distention and rales bilaterally, dyspnea (CHF)
- Monitor skin turgor, dryness of mucous membranes for hydration status, especially elderly [G]

Associated nursing diagnoses

- ✓ Cardiac output, decreased (uses)
- ✓ Injury, potential for (adverse reactions)
- ✓ Knowledge deficit (teaching)
- ✓ Noncompliance (teaching)

Implementation

PO route

- Given ac, hs, tab may be crushed or swallowed whole; give with food to prevent GI upset; give reduced dosage in renal dysfunction
- Store protected from light, moisture; placed in cool environment

Patient/family education

- Teach patient not to discontinue drug abruptly; taper over 2 wk; may cause precipitate angina if stopped abruptly
- Teach patient not to use OTC products containing α-adrenergic stimulants (such as nasal decongestants, cold preparations); to avoid alcohol, smoking and to limit sodium intake as prescribed
- Teach patient how to take pulse and B/P at home; advise when to notify prescriber
- Instruct patient to comply with weight control, dietary adjustments, modified exercise program

• Advise patient to carry/wear Medic Alert ID to identify drug being taken, allergies; teach patient drug controls symptoms but does not cure condition
• Caution patient to avoid hazardous activities if dizziness, drowsiness present
• Teach patient to report symptoms of CHF: difficult breathing, especially on exertion or when lying down, night cough, swelling of extremities or bradycardia, dizziness, confusion, depression, fever
• Teach patient to take drug as prescribed, not to double doses, skip doses; take any missed doses as soon as remembered if at least 4 hr until next dose

Evaluation

Positive therapeutic outcome
• Decreased B/P in hypertension

nafcillin

(naf-sill'in)

Nafcil, nafcillin sodium, Nallpen, Unipen

Func. class.: Broad-spectrum antiinfective

Chem. class.: Penicillinase-resistant penicillin

Pregnancy category **B**

Action: Interferes with cell wall replication of susceptible organisms; osmotically unstable cell wall swells, bursts from osmotic pressure

Uses: Infections caused by penicillinase-producing staphylococci, streptococci; respiratory tract, skin, skin structure, urinary tract, bone, joint infections, sinusitis, endocarditis, septicemia, meningitis

Therapeutic Outcome: Bactericidal effects for gram-positive cocci *Staphylococcus aureus, Streptococcus viridans, S. pneumoniae* and infections caused by penicillinase-producing *Staphylococcus*

Dosage and routes

Adult: IM/**IV** 2-6 g/day in divided doses q4-6h; PO 2-6 g/day in divided doses q4-6h

P *Child:* IM 25 mg/kg q12h; PO 25-50 mg/kg/day in divided doses q6h

P *Neonates:* IM 10 mg/kg bid

Available forms: Cap 250 mg; tab 500 mg; powder for oral susp 250 mg/5 ml; powder for inj 500 mg, 1, 2, 10 g; **IV** 1, 1.5, 2, 4 g

Side effects/adverse reactions

CNS: Lethargy, hallucinations, anxiety, depression, muscle twitching, ***coma, convulsions***

GI: Nausea, vomiting, diarrhea, increased AST (SGOT), ALT (SGPT), abdominal pain, glossitis, ***pseudomembranous colitis***

GU: Oliguria, ***proteinuria, hematuria, vaginitis, moniliasis, glomerulonephritis,*** interstitial nephritis

N

HEMA: Anemia, increased bleeding time, ***bone marrow depression, granulocytopenia***

Contraindications: Hypersensitivity to penicillins

Precautions: Pregnancy **B**, hypersensitivity to cephalosporins, **P** neonates

Pharmacokinetics

Absorption	Well absorbed (IM); erratic (PO)
Distribution	Widely distributed; crosses placenta
Metabolism	Not metabolized
Excretion	Kidneys, unchanged; breast milk
Half-life	1 hr; increased in renal disease

Pharmacodynamics

	PO	IM	IV
Onset	½ hr	½ hr	Immediate
Peak	1-2 hr	1-2 hr	Inf end

Interactions

Drug/drug:

Individual drugs

Aspirin: ↑ nafcillin levels, ↓ renal excretion

Probenecid: ↑ nafcillin levels, ↓ renal excretion

Drug classifications

Oral anticoagulants: ↑ anticoagulant effects

Oral contraceptives: ↓ contraceptive effectiveness

Drug/food:

Food, carbonated drinks, citrus fruit juices: ↓ absorption

Lab test interferences

False positive: Urine glucose, urine protein

NURSING CONSIDERATIONS

Assessment

- Assess patient for previous sensitivity reaction to penicillins or other cephalosporins; cross-sensitivity between penicillins and cephalosporins is common
- Assess patient for signs and symptoms of infection including characteristics of wounds, sputum, urine, stool, WBC >10,000, earache, fever; obtain baseline information and during treatment
- Obtain C & S before beginning drug therapy to identify if correct treatment has been initiated
- Assess for allergic reactions: rash, urticaria, pruritus, chills, fever, joint pain; angioedema may occur a few days after therapy begins; epinephrine, resuscitation equipment should be available for anaphylactic reaction
- Identify urine output; if decreasing, notify prescriber (may indicate nephrotoxicity); also check for increased BUN, creatinine
- Monitor blood studies: AST (SGOT), ALT (SGPT), CBC, Hct, bilirubin, LDH, alkaline phosphatase, Coombs' test monthly if patient is on long-term therapy
- Monitor electrolytes: potassium, sodium, chloride monthly if patient is on long-term therapy
- Assess bowel pattern qd; if severe diarrhea occurs, drug should be discontinued; may indicate pseudomembranous colitis
- Monitor for bleeding: ecchymosis, bleeding gums, hema-

turia, stool guaiac daily if on long-term therapy
• Assess for overgrowth of infection: perineal itching, fever, malaise, redness, pain, swelling, drainage, rash, diarrhea, change in cough, sputum

Associated nursing diagnoses

- ✓ Infection, risk for (uses)
- ✓ Diarrhea (adverse reactions)
- ✓ Injury, risk for (adverse reactions)
- ✓ Knowledge deficit (teaching)
- ✓ Noncompliance (teaching)

Implementation

PO route
• Give in even doses around the clock; if GI upset occurs, give with food; drug must be given for 10-14 days to ensure organism death and prevent superinfection; store in tight container.
• Shake susp; store in refrigerator for 2 wk, 1 wk at room temp

IM route
• Reconstitute 500 mg/1.7-1.8 ml; 1 g/3.4 ml; 2 g/6.6-6.8 ml with sterile water or bacteriostatic water for a conc of 250 mg/ml; store unused portion in refrigerator for up to 7 days
• Give deep in large muscle mass

IV **IV route**
• Reconstitute 500 mg/1.7 ml; 1 g/3.4 ml; 2 g/6.6-6.8 ml with sterile water or bacteriostatic water for a conc of 250 mg/ml; store unused portion in refrigerator for up to 7 days
• Give by direct **IV** by diluting reconstituted sol with 15-30 ml of sterile water or 0.9% NaCl; give over 5-10 min
• Give by intermittent inf by diluting to a conc of 2-40 mg/ml with 0.9% NaCl, D_5W, $D_{10}W$, D_5/0.9% NaCl, D_5/LR, LR, Ringer's; store in refrigerator for up to 96 hr or 24 hr room temp; run over 30-60 min

Syringe compatibilities:

Cimetidine, heparin

Y-site incompatibilities:

Droperidol, fentanyl/droperidol, labetalol, nalbuphine, pentazocine, regular insulin, verapamil

Y-site compatibilities:

Acyclovir, atropine, cyclophosphamide, diazepam, enalaprilat, esmolol, famotidine, fentanyl, fluconazole, foscarnet, hydromorphone, magnesium sulfate, morphine, perphenazine, zidovudine

Additive incompatibilities:

Ascorbic acid, aztreonam, bleomycin, cytarabine, gentamicin, hydrocortisone sodium succinate, methylprednisolone sodium succinate, promazine

Additive compatibilities:

Chloramphenicol, chlorothiazide, dexamethasone, diphenhydramine, ephedrine, heparin, hydroxyzine, potassium chloride, prochlorperazine, sodium bicarbonate, sodium lactate

Patient/family education

• Teach patient to report sore throat, bruising, bleeding,

joint pain; may indicate blood dyscrasias (rare)
• Advise patient to contact prescriber if vaginal itching, loose, foul-smelling stools, furry tongue occur; may indicate superinfection
• Instruct patient to take all medication prescribed for the length of time ordered
• Advise patient to notify prescriber of diarrhea with blood or pus, which may indicate pseudomembranous colitis

Evaluation

Positive therapeutic outcome
• Absence of signs/symptoms of infection (WBC <10,000, temp WNL, absence of red, draining wounds, earache)
• Reported improvement in symptoms of infection

Treatment of anaphylaxis: Withdraw drug, maintain airway, administer epinephrine, aminophylline, O_2, **IV** corticosteroids

naftifine

(naf'tih-feen)
Naftin
Func. class.: Topical antifungal
Chem. class.: Synthetic allylamine derivative
Pregnancy category **B**

Action: Interferes with cell membrane permeability and synthesis of sterols in fungi such as *Trichophyton rubrum, T. mentagrophytes, T. tonsurans, Epidermophyton floccosum, Microsporum canis, M. audouinii, M. gypseum, Candida;* broad-spectrum antifungal

Therapeutic Outcome: Fungistatic/fungicidal against tinea pedis, tinea cruris, tinea corporis, tinea versicolor

Uses: Tinea cruris, tinea corporis, tinea versicolor

Dosage and routes

Adult: Top, massage into affected area and surrounding area bid (gel), qd (cream); continue for 7-14 days

Available forms: Cream 1%, gel 1%

Side effects/adverse reactions

INTEG: Burning, stinging, dryness, itching, local irritation

Contraindications: Hypersensitivity

Precautions: Pregnancy **B** P lactation, children

Pharmacokinetics

Absorption	Minimal
Distribution	Unknown
Metabolism	Unknown
Excretion	Unknown
Half-life	Unknown

Pharmacodynamics

Onset	Unknown
Peak	Unknown
Duration	Unknown

Interactions: None

NURSING CONSIDERATIONS

Assessment

- Assess skin for fungal infections: peeling, dryness, itching before and throughout treatment
- Monitor for allergic reaction: dermatitis, rash; drug should be discontinued

Associated nursing diagnoses

- ✓ Skin integrity, impaired (uses)
- ✓ Infection, risk for (uses)
- ✓ Knowledge deficit (teaching)

Implementation

Top route
- Apply to affected area, surrounding area; do not cover with occlusive dressings
- Store below 30° C (86° F)

Patient/family education

- Teach patient proper hygiene: hand washing, nail care, use of concomitant top agents if prescribed
- Instruct patient to use sunscreen or avoid direct sunlight to prevent photosensitivity
- Teach patient to wear cotton clothing; to use clean towel, dry well; to avoid contact of medication with mucous membranes; to avoid covering areas unless directed to by prescriber
- Advise patient to report excessive itching, burning
- Teach patient how to apply; massage gel into affected area and surrounding skin in AM, PM; cream AM only; effects observed within 1 wk; continue 1-2 wk after symptoms decrease; wash hands after application

Evaluation

Positive therapeutic outcome
- Decrease in size, number of lesions

nalbuphine

(nal'byoo-feen)

Nubain, nalbuphine HCl

Func. class.: Opioid analgesic

Chem. class.: Synthetic opioid agonist/antagonist

Pregnancy category **C**

Controlled substance schedule **II**

Action: Inhibits ascending pain pathways in limbic system, thalamus, midbrain, hypothalamus by binding to opiate receptor sites, thus altering pain perception and response

➡ **Therapeutic Outcome:** Relief of pain

Uses: Moderate to severe pain, labor analgesia, balanced anesthesia (adjunct)

Dosage and routes

Analgesic

Adult: SC/IM/**IV** 10-20 mg q3-6h prn, not to exceed 160 mg/day

Balanced anesthesia supplement

Adult: **IV** 0.3-3 mg/kg given over 10-15 min; may give 0.25-0.5 mg/kg as needed (maintenance)

Available forms: Inj 10, 20 mg/ml

N

Side effects/adverse reactions

CNS: *Drowsiness, dizziness, confusion, headache, sedation, euphoria*, dysphoria (high doses), hallucinations, dreaming, tolerance, physical and psychologic dependency
CV: Palpitations, bradycardia, change in B/P, orthostatic hypotension
EENT: Tinnitus, blurred vision, miosis (high doses), diplopia
GI: *Nausea, vomiting, anorexia, constipation, cramps*
GU: Increased urinary output, dysuria, urinary retention, urgency
INTEG: *Rash*, urticaria, bruising, flushing, *diaphoresis*, pruritus
RESP: ***Respiratory depression***

Contraindications: Hypersensitivity, addiction (narcotic)

Precautions: Addictive personality, pregnancy **C**, lactation, increased intracranial pressure, MI (acute), severe heart disease, respiratory depression, hepatic disease, renal disease

Pharmacokinetics

Absorption	Well absorbed (SC, IM); completely absorbed (IV)
Distribution	Crosses placenta
Metabolism	Liver, extensively
Excretion	Feces, kidneys, unchanged (small amounts); breast milk
Half-life	5 hr

Pharmacodynamics

	IM	SC	IV
Onset	Up to 15 min	Up to 15 min	Rapid
Peak	1 hr	Unknown	½ hr
Duration	3-6 hr	3-6 hr	3-6 hr

Interactions

Drug/drug:

Individual drugs

Alcohol: ↑ respiratory depression, hypotension, sedation

Drug classifications

Antihistamines: ↑ respiratory depression, hypotension
CNS depressants: ↑ respiratory depression, hypotension
MAOI: Use cautiously, results are unpredictable
Phenothiazines: ↑ respiratory depression, hypotension
Opioid agonists: ↑ opioid withdrawals (dependency)
Sedative/hypnotics: ↑ respiratory depression, hypotension

Lab test interferences

Increase: Amylase, lipase

NURSING CONSIDERATIONS

Assessment

- Assess pain characteristics (location, intensity, type) before medication administration and following treatment
- Monitor VS after parenteral route; note muscle rigidity, drug history, liver, kidney function tests; respiratory dysfunction: respiratory depression, character, rate, rhythm; notify prescriber if respirations are <10/min
- Monitor CNS changes: dizziness, drowsiness, hallucina-

tions, euphoria, LOC, pupil reaction
• Monitor allergic reactions: rash, urticaria

Associated nursing diagnoses

✓ Pain (uses)
✓ Sensory-perceptual alteration: visual, auditory (adverse reactions)
✓ Breathing pattern, ineffective (adverse reactions)
✓ Knowledge deficit (teaching)

Implementation

• Give by inj (IM, **IV**), only with resuscitative equipment available; give slowly to prevent rigidity
• Store in light-resistant area at room temp

IM route
• Give deeply in large muscle mass; rotate inj sites

IV **IV route**
• Give direct **IV** undiluted 10 mg or less over 3-5 min or more

Syringe incompatibilities:
Diazepam, pentobarbital

Syringe compatibilities:
Atropine, cimetidine, droperidol, hydroxyzine, lidocaine, midazolam, prochlorperazine, promethazine, ranitidine, scopolamine, trimethobenzamide

Y-site incompatibilities:
Nafcillin, sargramostim

Y-site compatibilities:
Fludarabine, melphalan, paclitaxel, vinorelbine

Patient/family education

• Instruct patient to report any symptoms of CNS changes, allergic reactions
• Caution patients to avoid CNS depressants: alcohol, sedative/hypnotics for at least 24 hr after taking this drug
• Discuss with patient that dizziness, drowsiness, confusion are common; to avoid getting up without assistance
• Discuss in detail all aspects of the drug: reason for taking drug and expected results
• Instruct patient to change position slowly to prevent orthostatic hypotension
• Teach patient to turn, cough, deep breathe after surgery to prevent atelectasis

Evaluation

Positive therapeutic outcome
• Relief of pain

Treatment of overdose:
Naloxone (Narcan) 0.2-0.8 **IV**, O_2, **IV** fluids, vasopressors

naloxone
(nal-oks'one)
naloxone HCl, Narcan
Func. class.: Opioid antagonist
Chem. class.: Thebaine derivative
Pregnancy category **B**

Action: Competes with narcotics at narcotic receptor sites

➔ **Therapeutic Outcome:** Absence of opioid overdose

Uses: Respiratory depression induced by narcotics, pentazocine, propoxyphene; refractory circulatory shock

Dosage and routes

Opioid-induced respiratory depression, CNS depression

Adult: **IV**/SC/IM 0.4-2 mg; repeat q2-3 min if needed

Postoperative respiratory depression

Adult: **IV** 0.1-0.2 mg q2-3 min prn

P *Child:* **IV**/IM/SC 0.01 mg/kg q2-3 min prn

Asphyxia neonatorum

P *Neonates:* **IV** 0.01 mg/kg given into umbilical vein after delivery; may repeat in q2-3 min × 3 doses

Available forms: Inj 0.4, P 1 mg/ml; neonatal inj 0.02 mg/ml

Side effects/adverse reactions

CNS: Drowsiness, nervousness
CV: Ventricular tachycardia, fibrillation, increased systolic B/P (high doses)
GI: Nausea, vomiting
RESP: Hyperpnea

Contraindications: Hypersensitivity, respiratory depression

Precautions: Pregnancy **B**, P children, cardiovascular disease, opioid dependency, lactation

Pharmacokinetics

Absorption	Well absorbed (SC, IM); completely absorbed (IV)
Distribution	Rapidly distributed; crosses placenta
Metabolism	Liver
Excretion	Kidneys
P **Half-life**	1 hr; up to 3 hr (neonates)

Pharmacodynamics

	IV	IM/SC
Onset	1 min	2-5 min
Peak	Unknown	Unknown
Duration	45 min	45-60 min

Interactions

Drug/drug:

Drug classifications
Analgesics, opioids: ↑ withdrawal in those addicted to opioids

Lab test interferences

Interferences: Urine VMA, 5-HIAA, urine glucose

NURSING CONSIDERATIONS

Assessment

- Assess for opioid withdrawal: cramping, hypertension, anxiety, vomiting in drug-dependent individuals
- Monitor VS q3-5 min; ABGs including Po_2, Pco_2
- Assess cardiac status: tachycardia, hypertension; monitor ECG
- Assess for respiratory dysfunction: respiratory depression, character, rate, rhythm; if respirations are <10/min, administer naloxone; probably due to opioid overdose; monitor LOC

Associated nursing diagnoses

- ✓ Breathing pattern, ineffective (uses)
- ✓ Coping, ineffective individual (uses)
- ✓ Pain (adverse reactions)
- ✓ Knowledge deficit (teaching)

Implementation

IV **IV route**
- Give by direct **IV** undiluted; give 0.4 mg or less over 15 sec or titrate inf to response
- Give cont **IV** further diluted with 0.9% NaCl and D_5 and give as an inf
- Give only with resuscitative equipment, O_2 nearby
- Use only sol prepared within 24 hr
- Store at room temp in darkness

Patient/family education

- Explain reason for and expected results of medication when patient alert

Evaluation

Positive therapeutic outcome
- Reversal of respiratory depression
- LOC: alert

naphazoline

(naff-a-zoe'leen)
Privine
Func. class.: Nasal decongestant
Chem. class.: Sympathomimetic amine
Pregnancy category **C**

Action: Produces vasoconstriction (rapid, long acting) of arterioles, thereby decreasing fluid exudation and mucosal engorgement by stimulation of α-adrenergic receptors in vascular smooth muscle

➔ **Therapeutic Outcome:** Absence of nasal congestion

Uses: Nasal congestion

Dosage and routes

Adult: Instill 2 gtt or sprays to nasal mucosa q3-4h

P *Child 6-12 yr:* Instill 1-2 gtt or sprays; repeat q3-4h prn; not to exceed 5 days

Available forms: Nasal sol 0.05%

Side effects/adverse reactions

CNS: Anxiety, restlessness, tremors, weakness, insomnia, dizziness, fever, headache
EENT: Irritation, burning, sneezing, stinging, dryness, rebound congestion
GI: Nausea, vomiting, anorexia
INTEG: Contact dermatitis

Contraindications: Hypersensitivity to sympathomimetic amines

P G **Precautions:** Child <6 yr, elderly, diabetes, cardiovascular disease, hypertension, hyperthyroidism, increased ICP, prostatic hypertrophy, pregnancy **C**, glaucoma

N

Pharmacokinetics

Absorption	Minimal
Distribution	Site only
Metabolism	Not metabolized
Excretion	Not excreted
Half-life	Unknown

Pharmacodynamics

Onset	5-10 min
Peak	Unknown
Duration	Up to 6 hr

Interactions: None

NURSING CONSIDERATIONS

Assessment

- Assess for redness, swelling, pain in nasal passages before and during treatment
- Assess for systemic absorption: hypertension, tachycardia; notify prescriber; syst absorption occurs at high doses or after prolonged use

Associated nursing diagnoses

- ✓ Airway clearance, ineffective (uses)
- ✓ Knowledge deficit (teaching)
- ✓ Noncompliance (teaching)

Implementation

Nasal route

- Have patient tilt head back, squeeze bulb to create a vacuum, and draw correct amount of sol into dropper, insert 2 gtt of sol into nostril; repeat in other nostril
- Store in light-resistant containers; do not expose to high temp or let sol come into contact with aluminum
- Give for <4 consecutive days
- Provide environmental humidification to decrease nasal congestion, dryness

Patient/family education

- Advise patient that stinging may occur for several applications; drying of mucosa may be decreased by environmental humidification
- Caution patient to notify prescriber if irregular pulse, insomnia, dizziness, or tremors occur
- Teach patient proper administration to avoid syst absorption
- Advise patient to rinse dropper with very hot water to prevent contamination

Evaluation

Positive therapeutic outcome

- Decreased nasal congestion

naproxen

(na-prox'en)

Apo-Naproxen ✤, Naxen, Novonaprox ✤, Naprosyn, naproxen sodium, Anaprox, Anaprox DS, Apo-Napro-Na ✤, Novonaprox Sodium ✤, Synflex ✤

Func. class.: Nonsteroidal antiinflammatory, nonopioid analgesic

Chem. class.: Propionic acid derivative

Pregnancy category **B**

Action: Inhibits prostaglandin synthesis by decreasing enzyme needed for biosynthesis; analgesic, antiinflammatory

Therapeutic Outcome: Decreased pain, inflammation

Uses: Mild to moderate pain, osteoarthritis, rheumatoid arthritis, gouty arthritis, juvenile arthritis, primary dysmenorrhea

Dosage and routes

Adult: PO 250-500 mg bid, not to exceed 1 g/day (base); 525 mg, then 275 mg q6-8h prn, not to exceed 1475 mg (sodium)

P *Child:* PO 10 mg/kg in 2 divided doses

Available forms: Naproxen, tab 250, 375, 500 mg; oral susp 125 mg/5 ml; naproxen sodium, tab 275, 550 mg

Side effects/adverse reactions

CNS: Dizziness, drowsiness, fatigue, tremors, confusion, insomnia, anxiety, depression
CV: Tachycardia, peripheral edema, palpitations, dysrhythmias
EENT: Tinnitus, hearing loss, blurred vision
GI: Nausea, anorexia, vomiting, diarrhea, jaundice, ***cholestatic hepatitis,*** constipation, flatulence, cramps, dry mouth, peptic ulcer, ***GI ulceration, bleeding, perforation***
GU: Nephrotoxicity: dysuria, hematuria, oliguria, azotemia
HEMA: Blood dyscrasias
INTEG: Purpura, rash, pruritus, sweating

Contraindications: Hypersensitivity, asthma, severe renal disease, severe hepatic disease, ulcer disease

Precautions: Pregnancy **B**, P lactation, children <2 yr, bleeding disorders, GI disorders, cardiac disorders, hypersensitivity to other antiinflammatory agents, G elderly

Pharmacokinetics

Absorption	Completely absorbed
Distribution	Crosses placenta, 99% protein binding
Metabolism	Liver, extensively
Excretion	Breast milk
Half-life	10-20 hr

Pharmacodynamics

	PO
Onset	1 hr
Peak	2-4 hr
Duration	<7 hr

N

Interactions

Drug/drug:

Individual drugs

Acetaminophen (long-term use): ↑ renal reactions
Alcohol: ↑ adverse reactions
Aspirin: ↓ effectiveness, ↑ adverse reactions
Cefamandole: ↑ bleeding
Cefoperazone: ↑ bleeding
Cefotetan: ↑ bleeding
Coumarin: ↑ anticoagulant effects
Digoxin: ↑ toxicity, levels
Insulin: ↓ insulin effect
Lithium: ↑ toxicity
Methotrexate: ↑ toxicity
Phenytoin: ↑ toxicity
Probenecid: ↑ toxicity
Sulfonylurea: ↑ toxicity
Valproic acid: ↑ bleeding

Drug classifications
Anticoagulants: ↑ risk of bleeding
Antihypertensives: ↓ effect of antihypertensives
Antineoplastics: ↑ risk of hematologic toxicity
β-Blockers: ↑ antihypertension
Cephalosporins: ↑ risk of bleeding
Diuretics: ↓ effectiveness of diuretics
Glucocorticoids: ↑ adverse reactions
Hypoglycemics, oral: ↓ hypoglycemic effect
NSAIDs: ↑ adverse reactions
Potassium supplements: ↑ adverse reactions
Radiation: ↑ risk of hematologic toxicity
Sulfonamides: ↑ toxicity

Lab test interferences

Increase: BUN, alkaline phosphatase
False increase: 5-HIAA, 17KGS

NURSING CONSIDERATIONS

Assessment

- Monitor liver function, renal function, other blood studies: AST (SGOT), ALT (SGPT), bilirubin, creatinine BUN, CBC, Hct, Hgb, pro-time if patient is on long term therapy
- Check I&O ratio; decreasing output may indicate renal failure (long-term therapy)
- Assess hepatotoxicity: dark urine, clay-colored stools, yellowing of the skin and sclera, itching, abdominal pain, fever, diarrhea if patient is on long-term therapy
- Assess for allergic reactions: rash, urticaria; if these occur, drug may have to be discontinued
- Assess for ototoxicity: tinnitus, ringing, roaring in ears; audiometric testing needed before, after long-term therapy
- Assess for visual changes: blurring, halos; may indicate corneal, retinal damage
- Check for edema in feet, ankles, legs
- Identify prior drug history; there are many drug interactions
- Monitor pain: location, duration, type, intensity before dose and 1 hour after; assess ROM before dose and after

Associated nursing diagnoses

- ✓ Pain (uses)
- ✓ Mobility, impaired (uses)
- ✓ Injury, risk for (adverse reactions)
- ✓ Knowledge deficit (teaching)

Implementation

PO route

- Administer to patient crushed or whole
- Give with food or milk to decrease gastric symptoms; give ½ hr ac or 2 hr pc for better absorption

Patient/family education

- Teach patient to report any symptoms of hepatotoxicity, renal toxicity, visual changes, ototoxicity, allergic reactions, bleeding (long-term therapy)
- Advise patient to take with 8 oz of water and sit upright for 30 min after dose to prevent ulceration
- Caution patient not to exceed recommended dosage; acute poisoning may result;

to take as prescribed, do not double dose
- Teach patient to read label on other OTC drugs; many contain other antiinflammatories; caution patient to avoid alcohol ingestion; GI bleeding may occur
- Inform patient that the therapeutic response takes 2 wk (arthritis)
- Teach patient to report tinnitus, confusion, diarrhea, sweating, hyperventilation, blurred vision, fever, joint aches

Evaluation

Positive therapeutic outcome
- Decreased pain
- Decreased inflammation
- Increased mobility

natamycin
(na-ta-mye'sin)
Natacyn
Func. class.: Antiinfective/ antifungal
Chem. class.: Tetraene polyene compound
Pregnancy category **B**

Action: Inhibits transport functions and cell permeability in susceptible organisms

Therapeutic Outcome: Absence of ocular infection

Uses: Fungal blepharitis, conjunctivitis, keratitis

Dosage and routes

Adult and child: Instill 1 gtt q1-2h × 3-4 days, then decrease to 1 gtt 8 times a day; duration of therapy 14-21 days

Available forms: Ophth susp 5%

Side effects/adverse reactions

EENT: Temporary visual haze, overgrowth of nonsusceptible organisms

Contraindication: Hypersensitivity

Precautions: Antibiotic hypersensitivity, pregnancy **B**; failure of keratitis to improve after 7-10 days suggests infection not caused by susceptible organism

Pharmacokinetics

Absorption	Minimal; not usually systemically absorbed
Distribution	Not distributed
Metabolism	Not metabolized unless systemically absorbed
Excretion	Not excreted
Half-life	Unknown

Pharmacodynamics

Onset	Unknown
Peak	Unknown
Duration	Unknown

Interactions

Drug/drug:

Drug classifications
Glucocorticoids: ↑ spreading infection

NURSING CONSIDERATIONS

Assessment

- Assess for eye infection: pain, drainage, redness, tearing, inflammation before, during, and after treatment

Associated nursing diagnoses

- ✓ Infection, risk for (uses)
- ✓ Knowledge deficit (teaching)

Implementation

Ophth route

• After washing hands, clean crusts or discharge from eye before application; pull down on lower lid; put i gtt in lower lid; patient should close eye and roll eye to spread medication, press on lacrimal sac to prevent absorption
• Store at room temp or refrigerate

Patient/family education

• Teach patient to use drug exactly as prescribed; to shake well before using; to use for prescribed time even if symptoms abate
• Advise patient not to use eye makeup, towels, washcloths, eye medication of others; reinfection may occur; that drug container tip should not be touched to eye
• Instruct patient to report itching, increased redness, burning, stinging, swelling or no improvements occur after 1 wk; drug should be discontinued and prescriber notified

Evaluation

Positive therapeutic outcome

• Absence of redness, inflammation, tearing

nedocromil

(ned-o-kroe'mil)
Func. class.: Antiasthmatic
Chem. class.: Mast cell stabilizer
Pregnancy category B

Action: Stabilizes the membrane of the sensitized mast cell, preventing release of chemical mediators after an antigen-IgE interaction

➔ **Therapeutic Outcome:** Reduced symptoms of asthma

Uses: Allergic rhinitis, severe perennial bronchial asthma, exercise-induced bronchospasm (prevention), prevention of acute bronchospasm induced by environmental pollutants, mastocytosis

Dosage and routes

Bronchospasm

P ***Adult and child >12 yr:*** 2 inh 2-4 times a day at regular intervals to provide 14 g/day

Bronchial asthma

P ***Adult and child >12 yr:*** same as above

Available forms: 1.75 mg nedocromil per activation in 16.2-g canisters providing at least 112 metered inh

Side effects/adverse reactions

CNS: Headache, dizziness, neuritis, dysphonia
EENT: Throat irritation, cough, nasal congestion, burning eyes, rhinitis

GI: Nausea, vomiting, anorexia, dry mouth, bitter taste

Contraindications: Hypersensitivity to this drug or lactose, status asthmaticus

Precautions: Pregnancy **B**, P lactation, children

Pharmacokinetics

Absorption	Poorly, 3% (inh)
Distribution	Unknown
Metabolism	Not usually metabolized
Excretion	Small amounts in bile, urine unchanged
Half-life	80 min

Pharmacodynamics

Onset	Unknown
Peak	15 min
Duration	4-6 hr

Interactions: None

NURSING CONSIDERATIONS

Assessment

- Monitor eosinophil count during treatment
- Assess respiratory status: respiratory rate, rhythm, characteristics, cough, wheezing, dyspnea

Associated nursing diagnoses

✓ Airway clearance, ineffective (uses)
✓ Knowledge deficit (teaching)

Implementation

Inh route

- Give by inh only
- Encourage patient to gargle, sip water to decrease irritation in throat

Patient/family education

- Instruct patient to clear mucus before using
- Teach patient proper inh technique: exhale; using inhaler, inhale deeply with head tipped back to open airway; remove, hold breath, exhale; repeat until all of drug is inhaled
- Inform patient that therapeutic effect may take up to 4 wk
- Teach patient that drug is preventive only, not restorative

Evaluation

Positive therapeutic outcome

- Decrease in asthmatic symptoms

N

nefazodone

(nef-az'oe-done)

Serzone

Func. class.: Second-generation antidepressant

Chem. class.: Phenylpiperazine

Pregnancy category **C**

Action: Selectively inhibits serotinin uptake by brain, potentiates behavioral changes, occupies central HT_2 receptors

Therapeutic Outcome: Decreased symptoms of depression after 2-3 wk

Uses: Major depression

Dosage and routes

Adult: PO 200 mg/day (100 mg bid); dosage may be increased to 300 mg/day (150 bid); max 600 mg/day

G *Elderly:* 100 mg/day (50 mg bid)

Available forms: Tab 100, 150, 200, 250 mg

Side effects/adverse reactions

CNS: Dizziness, headache, insomnia
CV: **Postenral hypotension**
GI: **Nausea, constipation, dry mouth**
EENT: **Blurred vision**
GU: **Urinary frequency,** retention, UTI
RESP: Pharyngitis, cough

Contraindications: Hypersensitivity to this drug or phenylpiperazines

Precautions: Pregnancy **C**, P lactation, children, elderly, G cardiovascular disease, seizure disorder

Pharmacokinetics

Absorption	Well absorbed
Distribution	Widely distributed; crosses placenta
Metabolism	Liver, extensively, to metabolites
Excretion	Kidneys, breast milk
Half-life	2-4 hr

Pharmacodynamics

Onset	Unknown
Peak	1-3 hr
Duration	Unknown

Interactions

Drug/drug:

Individual drugs
Alcohol: ↑ CNS depression
Drug classifications
Antihistamines, nonsedating: Fatal reaction
Benzodiazepines: ↑ plasma concentrations
Barbiturates: ↑ effects
CNS depressants: ↑ effects

Drug/smoking:

↑ metabolism, ↓ effects

NURSING CONSIDERATIONS

Assessment

- Monitor B/P (with patient lying, standing), pulse q4h; if systolic B/P drops 20 mm Hg hold drug, notify prescriber; take vital signs q4h in patients with cardiovascular disease
- Monitor blood studies: CBC, leukocytes, differential, cardiac enzymes if patient is receiving long-term therapy
- Monitor hepatic studies: AST (SGOT), ALT (SGPT), bilirubin
- Assess mental status: mood, sensorium, affect, suicidal tendencies; increase in psychiatric symptoms: depression, panic
- Monitor urinary retention, constipation; constipation is more likely to occur in the G elderly
- Assess for withdrawal symptoms: headache, nausea, vomiting, muscle pain, weakness; do not usually occur unless drug was discontinued abruptly
- Identify alcohol consumption; if alcohol is consumed, hold dose until AM

Associated nursing diagnoses

- ✓ Coping, ineffective individual (uses)
- ✓ Knowledge deficit (teaching)
- ✓ Noncompliance (teaching)

Implementation

PO route

- Give with food or milk for GI symptoms
- Give crushed if patient is unable to swallow medication whole
- Store at room temp; do not freeze

Patient/family education

- Teach patient that therapeutic effects may take 3-4 wk
- Teach patient to use caution in driving and other activities requiring alertness because of drowsiness, dizziness; to avoid rising quickly from sitting to standing, especially elderly G
- Teach patient to avoid alcohol ingestion, other CNS depressants
- Teach patient not to discontinue medication quickly after long-term use; may cause nausea, headache, malaise
- Teach patient to increase bulk in diet if constipation occurs, especially elderly G
- Teach patient to take gum, hard sugarless candy, or frequent sips of water for dry mouth

Evaluation

Positive therapeutic outcome

- Decrease in depression
- Absence of suicidal thoughts

Treatment of overdose:

ECG monitoring, induce emesis, lavage, activated charcoal, administer anticonvulsant

neomycin

(nee-oh-mye'sin)

Mycifradin Sulfate, Myciguent

Func. class.: Antiinfective

Chem. class.: Aminoglycoside

Pregnancy category **C**

Action: Interferes with protein synthesis in bacterial cell by binding to 30S ribosomal subunit causing inaccurate peptide sequence to form in protein chain, resulting in bacterial death

➔ Therapeutic Outcome: Bactericidal effects for *Pseudomonas aeruginosa, Escherichia coli, Enterobacter, enteropathogenic E. coli, Klebsiella pneumoniae, Proteus vulgaris*

Uses: Severe systemic infections of CNS, respiratory tract, GI tract, urinary tract, eye, bone, skin, soft tissues, also used for hepatic coma, preoperatively to sterilize bowel, infectious diarrhea; minor skin infections (top)

Dosage and routes

Severe systemic infections

Adult: IM 15 mg/kg/day in 4 divided doses; not to exceed 1 g/day

Hepatic coma

Adult: PO 4-12 g/day in divided doses times 5-6 days

P *Child:* 50-100 mg/kg/day in divided doses

Preoperative bowel sterilization

Adult: PO on 3rd day of a 3-day regimen; give 1 g early PM; repeat in 1 hr; repeat at hs (given with erythromycin); give saline cathartic before giving this drug

Skin infection

P *Adult and child:* Top 0.5% cream or ointment qd-tid

Available forms: Tab 500 mg; top 500 mg; oral sol 125 ml/5 ml; inj 500 mg

Side effects/adverse reactions

CNS: Confusion, depression, numbness, tremors, ***convulsions,*** muscle twitching, ***neurotoxicity,*** dizziness, vertigo

CV: Hypotension, hypertension, palpitations

EENT: ***Ototoxicity,*** deafness, visual disturbances, tinnitus

GI: Nausea, vomiting, anorexia, increased ALT (SGPT), AST (SGOT), bilirubin, hepatomegaly, ***hepatic necrosis,*** splenomegaly

GU: ***Oliguria, hematuria, renal damage, azotemia, renal failure, nephrotoxicity***

HEMA: ***Agranulocytosis, thrombocytopenia,*** leukopenia, eosinophilia, anemia

INTEG: Rash, burning, urticaria, photosensitivity, dermatitis, alopecia

Contraindications: Bowel obstruction (oral use), severe renal disease, hypersensitivity, P infants, children

Precautions: Mild renal disease, pregnancy **C**, hearing deficits, lactation, myasthenia gravis, Parkinson's disease

Pharmacokinetics

Absorption	Well absorbed (IM); minimally absorbed (top)
Distribution	Unknown
Metabolism	Liver, minimal
Excretion	Feces, unchanged
Half-life	2-3 hr

Pharmacodynamics

	IM
Onset	Rapid
Peak	1-2 hr
Duration	6-8 hr

Interactions

Drug/drug:

Individual drugs

Amphotericin B: ↑ Ototoxicity, neurotoxicity, nephrotoxicity

Cisplatin: ↑ Ototoxicity, neurotoxicity, nephrotoxicity

Ethacrynic acid: ↑ Ototoxicity, neurotoxicity, nephrotoxicity

Furosemide: ↑ Ototoxicity, neurotoxicity, nephrotoxicity

Mannitol: ↑ Ototoxicity, neurotoxicity, nephrotoxicity

Methoxyflurane: ↑ Ototoxicity, neurotoxicity, nephrotoxicity

Polymyxin: ↑ Ototoxicity, neurotoxicity, nephrotoxicity

Succinylcholine: ↑ Neuromuscular blockade, respiratory depression

Vancomycin: ↑ Ototoxicity, neurotoxicity, nephrotoxicity

Drug classifications

Aminoglycosides: ↑ Otoxicity, neurotoxicity, neurotoxicity
Anesthetics, inhalation: ↑ Neuromuscular blockade, respiratory depression
Nondepolarizing neuromuscular blockers: ↑ Neuromuscular blockade, respiratory depression

NURSING CONSIDERATIONS

Assessment

- Assess patient for previous sensitivity reaction
- Assess patient for signs and symptoms of infection: characteristics skin; obtain baseline information and during treatment
- Obtain C&S before beginning drug therapy to identify if correct treatment has been initiated
- Assess for allergic reactions: rash, urticaria, pruritus, chills, fever, joint pain

Associated nursing diagnoses

✓ Infection, risk for (uses)
✓ Knowledge deficit (teaching)
✓ Noncompliance (teaching)

Implementation

PO route

- Give as a preoperative medication before bowel surgery

Patient/family education

- Instruct patient to take all medication prescribed for the length of time ordered
- Advise patient to report headache, dizziness, symptoms of overgrowth of infection and loss of hearing, ringing or roaring in ears

Evaluation

Positive therapeutic outcome

- Reported improvement in symptoms of infection (top)

Treatment of overdose: Withdraw drug; hemodialysis; monitor serum levels of drug

neostigmine

(nee-oh-stig'meen)
neostigmine bromide, neostigmine methylsulfate, Prostigmin
Func. class.: Cholinergic stimulant; anticholinesterase
Chem. class.: Quaternary compound
Pregnancy category C

Action: Inhibits destruction of acetylcholine, which increases concentration at sites where acetylcholine is released; this facilitates transmission of impulses across the myoneural junction

➔ **Therapeutic Outcome:** Increased strength in myasthenia gravis, reversal of nondepolarizing muscular blockers

Uses: Myasthenia gravis, nondepolarizing neuromuscular blocker, antagonist, bladder distention, postoperative ileus

N

Dosage and routes

Myasthenia gravis

Adult: PO 15-375 mg/day; IM/**IV** 0.5-2 mg q1-3h

P *Child:* PO 2 mg/kg/day q3-4h

Nondepolarizing neuromuscular blocker antagonist

Adult: **IV** 0.5-2 mg slowly; may repeat if needed (give 0.6-1.2 mg atropine before this drug)

Abdominal distention/ postoperative ileus

Adult: IM/SC 0.25-1 mg q4-6h depending on condition

Available forms: Tab 15 mg; inj 1:1000, 1:2000, 1:4000

Side effects/adverse reactions

CNS: Dizziness, headache, sweating, weakness, ***convulsions,*** incoordination, ***paralysis,*** drowsiness, LOC
CV: Tachycardia, dysrhythmias, bradycardia, hypotension, AV block, ECG changes, ***cardiac arrest,*** syncope
EENT: Miosis, blurred vision, lacrimation, visual changes
GI: Nausea, diarrhea, vomiting, cramps, increased peristalsis, salivary and gastric secretions
GU: Frequency, incontinence, urgency
INTEG: Rash, urticaria, flushing
RESP: ***Respiratory depression, bronchospasm, constriction, laryngospasm, respiratory arrest,*** dyspnea

Contraindications: Obstruction of intestine, renal system, pregnancy **C**, bromide sensitivity, peritonitis

Precautions: Bradycardia, hypotension, seizure disorders, bronchial asthma, coronary occlusion, hyperthyroidism, dysrhythmias, peptic ulcer, megacolon, poor GI motility,
P lactation, children

Pharmacokinetics

Absorption	Poorly absorbed (PO), completely absorbed (IV)
Distribution	Unknown
Metabolism	Liver
Excretion	Kidneys
Half-life	40-90 min

Pharmacodynamics

	PO	IM	IV
Onset	45-75 min	10-30 min	4-8 min
Peak	Unknown	30 min	30 min
Duration	2½-4 hr	2½-4 hr	2-4 hr

Interactions

Drug/drug:

Individual drugs

Atropine: ↓ action of atropine
Mecamylamine: ↓ action of neostigmine
Polymyxin: ↓ action of neostigmine
Procainamide: ↓ action of neostigmine
Quinidine: ↓ action of neostigmine

Drug classifications
Antidepressants: ↑ antagonism
Antihistamines: ↑ antagonism
Cholinesterase inhibitors: ↑ toxicity
Phenothiazines: ↑ antagonism
Muscle relaxants, depolarizing: ↑ action of muscle relaxants

NURSING CONSIDERATIONS

Assessment

- Monitor VS, respiration during test
- Monitor for bradycardia, hypotension, bronchospasm, headache, dizziness, convulsions, respiratory depression; drug should be discontinued if toxicity occurs

Associated nursing diagnoses

✓ Breathing pattern, ineffective (uses)
✓ Knowledge deficit (teaching)

Implementation

PO route

- Give only after all other cholinergics have been discontinued
- Increased dosage may be needed if tolerance develops
- Give larger doses after exercise or fatigue
- Administer on empty stomach for better absorption
- Store at room temp

IV **IV route**

- Give direct **IV** undiluted, through Y-tube or 3-way stopcock; give 0.5 mg or less over 1 min
- Give only with atropine sulfate available for cholinergic crisis

Syringe compatibilities:
Glycopyrrolate, heparin, pentobarbital, or thiopental

Y-site compatibilities:
Heparin, hydrocortisone sodium succinate, potassium chloride

Additive compatibility:
Netilmicin

Patient/family education

- Teach patient to wear Medic Alert ID specifying myasthenia gravis, drugs taken, prescriber's phone number

Evaluation

Positive therapeutic outcome

- Increased muscle strength, hand grasp
- Improved gait
- Absence of labored breathing (if severe)

Treatment of overdose: Respiratory support, **IV** atropine 1-4 mg

N

netilmicin

(ne-til-mye'sin)
Netromycin
Func. class.: Antibiotic
Chem. class.: Aminoglycoside
Pregnancy category **D**

Action: Interferes with protein synthesis in bacterial cell by binding to 30S ribosomal subunit, causing inaccurate peptide sequence to form in protein chain, resulting in bacterial death

Therapeutic Outcome: Bactericidal effects for the organisms *Pseudomonas aeruginosa, Escherichia coli, Enterobacter, Citrobacter, Staphylococcus, Klebsiella pneumoniae, Proteus mirabilis, Serratia, Shigella, Salmonella, Acinetobacter, Neisseria*

Uses: Severe systemic infections of CNS, respiratory tract, GI tract, urinary tract, bone, skin, soft tissues

Dosage and routes

Normal renal function

P ***Adult and child >12 yr:*** IM/**IV** 3-6.5 mg/kg/day; may give q8-12h for severe infections

P ***Child and infant 6 wk-12 yr:*** IM/**IV** 5.5-8 mg/kg/day in divided doses q8-12h

P ***Neonate <6 wk:*** IM/**IV** 4-6.5 mg/kg/day in divided doses q12h

Available forms: Inj 100 mg/ml

Side effects/adverse reactions

CNS: Confusion, depression, numbness, tremors, ***convulsions,*** muscle twitching, ***neurotoxicity,*** dizziness, vertigo

CV: Hypotension, hypertension, palpitations

EENT: ***Ototoxicity,*** deafness, visual disturbances, tinnitus

GI: Nausea, vomiting, anorexia, increased ALT (SGPT), AST (SGOT), bilirubin, hepatomegaly, ***hepatic necrosis,*** splenomegaly

GU: ***Oliguria, hematuria, renal damage, azotemia, renal failure, nephrotoxicity***

HEMA: ***Agranulocytosis, thrombocytopenia, leukopenia, eosinophilia, anemia***

INTEG: Rash, burning, urticaria, dermatitis

Contraindications: Severe renal disease, hypersensitivity, pregnancy **D**

Precautions: Neonates, mild P renal disease, children <12 yr, lactation, myasthenia gravis, hearing deficit, Parkinson's disease, severe burns, cystic fibrosis

Pharmacokinetics

Absorption	Well absorbed (IM)
Distribution	Widely distributed in extracellular fluids, poor in CSF; crosses placenta
Metabolism	Liver, minimal
Excretion	Kidneys, unchanged (90%); breast milk
Half-life	2-3 hr; increased in renal disease

Pharmacodynamics

	IM	IV
Onset	Rapid	Immediate
Peak	1-2 hr	1-2 hr

Interactions

Drug/drug:

Individual drugs

Amphotericin B: ↑ Ototoxicity, neurotoxicity, nephrotoxicity

Cisplatin: ↑ Ototoxicity, neurotoxicity, nephrotoxicity

Ethacrynic acid: ↑ Ototoxicity, neurotoxicity, nephrotoxicity

Furosemide: ↑ Ototoxicity, neurotoxicity, nephrotoxicity

Mannitol: ↑ Ototoxicity, neurotoxicity, nephrotoxicity
Methoxyflurane: ↑ Ototoxicity, neurotoxicity, nephrotoxicity
Polymyxin: ↑ Ototoxicity, neurotoxicity, nephrotoxicity
Succinylcholine: ↑ Neuromuscular blockade, respiratory depression
Vancomycin: ↑ Ototoxicity, neurotoxicity, nephrotoxicity

Drug classifications
Anesthetics: ↑ Neuromuscular blockade, respiratory depression
Aminoglycosides: ↑ Otoxicity, neurotoxicity, nephrotoxicity
Nondepolarizing neuromuscular blockers: ↑ Neuromuscular blockade, respiratory depression

NURSING CONSIDERATIONS

Assessment

- Assess patient for previous sensitivity reaction
- Assess patient for signs and symptoms of infection including characteristics of wounds, sputum, urine, stool, WBC >10,000, fever; obtain baseline information and during treatment
- Obtain C & S before beginning drug therapy to identify if correct treatment has been initiated
- Assess for allergic reactions: rash, urticaria, pruritus, chills, fever, joint pain
- Identify urine output; if decreasing, notify prescriber (may indicate nephrotoxicity); also check for increased BUN, creatinine, urine CrCl <80 ml/min
- Monitor blood studies: AST (SGOT), ALT (SGPT), CBC, Hct, bilirubin, LDH, alkaline phosphatase, Coombs' test monthly if patient is on long-term therapy
- Monitor electrolytes: potassium, sodium, chloride monthly if patient is on long-term therapy
- Assess for overgrowth of infection: perineal itching, fever, malaise, redness, pain, swelling, drainage, rash, diarrhea, change in cough, sputum
- Obtain weight before treatment; calculation of dosage is usually based on ideal body weight, but may be calculated on actual body weight
- Monitor I&O ratio; perform urinalysis daily for proteinuria, cells, casts; report sudden change in urine output
- Monitor VS during inf; watch for hypotension, change in pulse
- Assess **IV** site for thrombophlebitis including pain, redness, swelling q30 min; change site if needed; apply warm compresses to discontinued site
- Obtain serum peak, drawn at 30-60 min after **IV** inf or 60 min after IM inj; trough level drawn just before next dose; blood level should be 2-4 times bacteriostatic level
- Monitor urine pH if drug is used for UTI; urine should be kept alkaline
- Monitor for dehydration: high sp gr, decrease in skin turgor, dry mucous membranes, dark urine
- Assess for vestibular dysfunction: nausea, vomiting, dizziness, headache; drug should be discontinued if severe; monitor deafness by audiometric testing, ringing,

N

roaring in ears, vertigo; assess hearing before, during, after treatment

Associated nursing diagnoses

- ✓ Infection, risk for (uses)
- ✓ Knowledge deficit (teaching)
- ✓ Noncompliance (teaching)
- ✓ Sensory-perceptual alteration: auditory (uses)

Implementation

IM route

• Give deeply in large muscle mass

IV **IV route**

• Dilute intermittent inf dose in 50-200 ml D_5W, $D_{10}W$, D_5/LR, D_5/0.9% NaCl, LR, 0.9% NaCl, 3% NaCl, 5% NaCl, or Ringer's; give over ½-2 hr

• Diluted sol is stable for 72 hr at room temp

Y-site incompatibilities: Furosemide, heparin

Y-site compatibilities: Aminophylline, calcium gluconate, melphalan, vinorelbine

Patient/family education

• Teach patient to report sore throat, bruising, bleeding, joint pain; may indicate blood dyscrasias (rare); ringing, roaring in the ears or a feeling of dullness in the head

• Advise patient to contact prescriber if vaginal itching, loose, foul-smelling stools, furry tongue occur; may indicate superinfection

Evaluation

Positive therapeutic outcome

• Absence of signs/symptoms of infection (WBC <10,000, temp WNL, absence of red, draining wounds)

• Reported improvement in symptoms of infection

Treatment of overdose: Withdraw drug; hemodialysis; exchange transfusion in the P newborn; monitor serum levels of drug; may give ticarcillin or carbenicillin

niacin (vitamin B_3/ nicotinic acid)/ niacinamide

(nye'a-sin) (nye-a-sin'a-mide)

Nia-Bid, Niac, Niacels, Niacin TD, SpaN Niacin, Niacin TR, Niacor, Nico-400, Nicobid, Nicolar, Nicotinex, nicotinic acid, Novaniacin ✣, Slo-Niacin, Tri-B_3 ✣, Vitamin B_3, Nicothamide

Func. class.: Vitamin B_3

Chem. class.: Water-soluble vitamin, lipid-lowering drug

Pregnancy category C

Action: Needed for conversion of fats, protein, carbohydrates by oxidation-reduction; acts directly on vascular smooth muscle, causing vasodilatation; high dosages decrease serum lipids

➔ Therapeutic Outcome: Decreasing cholesterol and

low-density lipoprotein levels, vitamin B_3 supplementation

Uses: Pellagra, hyperlipidemias, peripheral vascular disease

Dosage and routes

Niacin deficiency

Adult: PO up to 500 mg/day in divided doses; IM/SC 5-100 mg 5 or more times a day; **IV** 25-100 mg bid or tid

P *Child:* PO up to 300 mg/day in divided doses

Adjunct in hyperlipidemia

Adult: PO 500 mg qd in 3 divided doses pc; may be increased to 2 g/day

Pellagra

Adult: PO 300-500 mg, qd in divided doses

P *Child:* PO 100-300 mg qd in divided doses

Peripheral vascular disease

Adult: PO 250-800 mg qd in divided doses

Available forms: Nicotinic acid, tab 20, 25, 50, 100, 500 mg; time rel cap 125, 250, 300, 400, 500 mg; time rel tab 150 mg; elix 50 mg/5 ml; inj 100 mg/ml; nicotinamide, tab 50, 100, 500 mg; time rel tab 1000 mg

Side effects/adverse reactions

CNS: Paresthesias, headache, dizziness, anxiety
CV: Postural hypotension, vasovagal attacks, dysrhythmias, vasodilatation
EENT: Blurred vision, ptosis
GI: Nausea, vomiting, anorexia, flatulence, xerostomia, ***jaundice,*** diarrhea, peptic ulcer
GU: Hyperuricemia, ***glycosuria, hypoalbuminemia***
INTEG: Flushing, dry skin, rash, pruritus
RESP: Wheezing

Contraindications: Hypersensitivity, peptic ulcer, hepatic disease, lactation, hemorrhage, severe hypotension

Precautions: Glaucoma, cardiovascular disease, CAD, diabetes mellitus, gout, schizophrenia, pregnancy **C**

Pharmacokinetics

Absorption	Well absorbed (PO)
Distribution	Widely distributed
Metabolism	Converted to niacinamide
Excretion	Urine, unchanged (30%); breast milk
Half-life	45 min

Pharmacodynamics

	PO	IV
Onset	Unknown	Unknown
Peak	30-70 min	Unknown
Duration	Unknown	Unknown

Interactions

Drug/drug:

Individual drugs

Guanedrel: ↑ hypotension
Guanethidine: ↑ hypotension
Lovastatin: ↑ myopathy
Probenecid: ↑ uricosuric effects
Sulfinpyrazone: ↑ uricosuric effects

N

Lab test interferences

Increase: Bilirubin, alkaline phosphatase, liver enzymes, LDH, uric acid
Decrease: Cholesterol
False increase: Urinary catecholamines
False positive: Urine glucose

NURSING CONSIDERATIONS

Assessment

- Assess for niacin deficiency (pellagra): nausea, vomiting, stomatitis, confusion, hallucinations before and throughout treatment
- Assess nutrition: fat, protein, carbohydrates, nutritional analysis should be completed by dietician
- Monitor liver function studies: AST (SGOT), ALT (SGPT), bilirubin, alkaline phosphatase; blood glucose before and during treatment; liver dysfunction: clay-colored stools, itching, dark urine, jaundice
- Monitor niacin levels during administration of this drug
- Monitor cardiac status: rate, rhythm, quality; postural hypotension, dysrhythmias
- Monitor nutritional status: liver, yeast, legumes, organ meat, lean poultry; high-level niacin products should be included in the diet
- Assess for CNS symptoms: headache, paresthesias, blurred vision

Associated nursing diagnoses

✓ Nutrition, less than body requirements (uses)
✓ Knowledge deficit (teaching)
✓ Noncompliance (teaching)

Implementation

PO route

- Give with meals or milk for GI symptoms; do not crush, break, or chew time rel products

IV **IV route**

- Give by direct **IV** after diluting to 2 mg/ml at a rate of ≤2 mg/min
- Give by inf by adding 500 ml of 0.9% NaCl at a rate of ≤2 mg/min

Additive incompatibilities:

Acids (strong), alkalis, erythromycin, kanamycin, streptomycin

Additive compatibility:

TPN sol

Patient/family education

- Advise patient that flushing and increase in feelings of warmth will occur several hr after taking drug (PO); time rel product minimizes flushing
- Instruct patient to remain recumbent if postural hypotension occurs; to rise slowly from sitting or recumbent
- Caution patient to abstain from alcohol if drug is prescribed for hyperlipidemia
- Caution patient to avoid sunlight if skin lesions are present

Evaluation

Positive therapeutic outcome

- Decreased lipid levels
- Warm extremities
- Absence of numbness in extremities

nicardipine
(nye-card'i-peen)
Cardene, Cardene SR
Func. class.: Calcium channel blocker
Chem. class.: Dihydropyridine
Pregnancy category **C**

Action: Inhibits calcium ion influx across cell membrane during cardiac depolarization, produces relaxation of coronary vascular smooth muscle and peripheral vascular smooth muscle, dilates coronary arteries, increases myocardial oxygen delivery in patients with vasospastic angina

➔ Therapeutic Outcome: Decreased angina pectoris, decreased B/P in hypertension

Uses: Chronic stable angina pectoris, hypertension

Dosage and routes
Adult: PO 20 mg tid initially; may increase after 3 days (range 20-40 mg tid) or 30 mg bid sus rel, may increase to 60 mg bid

Available forms: Cap 20, 30 mg; sus rel cap 30, 45, 60 mg

Side effects/adverse reactions
CNS: Headache, fatigue, drowsiness, dizziness, anxiety, depression, weakness, insomnia, confusion, paresthesia, somnolence
CV: Dysrhythmia, edema, CHF, bradycardia, hypotension, palpitations, ***MI, pulmonary edema***
GI: Nausea, vomiting, diarrhea, gastric upset, constipation, ***hepatitis,*** abdominal cramps
GU: Nocturia, polyuria, ***acute renal failure***
INTEG: Rash, pruritus, urticaria, photosensitivity, hair loss
MISC: Blurred vision, flushing, nasal congestion, sweating, shortness of breath, gynecomastia, hyperglycemia, sexual difficulties

Contraindications: Sick sinus syndrome, 2nd- or 3rd-degree heart block, hypotension less than 90 mm Hg systolic, hypersensitivity

Precautions: CHF, hypotension, hepatic injury, pregnancy P C, lactation, children, renal G disease, elderly

N

Pharmacokinetics

Absorption	Well absorbed (PO); bioavailability poor
Distribution	Unknown
Metabolism	Liver, extensively
Excretion	Kidneys, minimal
Half-life	2-5 hr

Pharmacodynamics

	PO	PO–SUS REL
Onset	½ hr	Unknown
Peak	1-2 hr	2-6 hr
Duration	8 hr	10-12 hr

Interactions
Drug/drug:
Individual drugs
Alcohol: ↑ hypotension
Digoxin: ↑ digoxin levels, bradycardia, CHF

Phenobarbital: ↓ effectiveness
Phenytoin: ↓ effectiveness
Propranolol: ↑ toxicity

Drug classifications

Antihypertensives: ↑ hypotension
β-Adrenergic blockers: ↑ bradycardia, CHF
Nitrates: ↑ nitrates

NURSING CONSIDERATIONS

Assessment

- Assess fluid volume status (I & O ratio) and record weight, color, quality and sp gr of urine, skin turgor, adequacy of pulses, moist mucous membranes, bilateral lung sounds, peripheral pitting edema; dehydration symptoms of decreasing output, thirst, hypotension, dry mouth, and mucous membranes should be reported
- Monitor B/P and pulse

Associated nursing diagnoses

✓ Cardiac output, decreased (uses)
✓ Knowledge deficit (teaching)

Implementation

PO route

- Give ac, hs on an empty stomach 1 hr ac or 2 or more hr pc
- Store in tight container at room temp

Patient/family education

- Advise patient to avoid hazardous activities until stabilized on drug and dizziness is no longer a problem
- Instruct patient to limit caffeine consumption; to avoid alcohol and OTC drugs unless directed by a prescriber
- Instruct patient to comply in all areas of medical regimen: diet, exercise, stress reduction, drug therapy; to notify prescriber of irregular heart beat, shortness of breath, swelling of feet and hands, pronounced dizziness, constipation, nausea, hypotension
- Teach patient to use medication as directed even if feeling better; may be taken with other cardiovascular drugs (nitrates, β-blockers)
- Teach patient to take medication exactly as prescribed
- Advise patient to contact prescriber if anginal attacks continue or become worse

Evaluation

Positive therapeutic outcome

- Decreased angina attacks
- Decreased B/P

Treatment of overdose: Defibrillation, atropine for AV block, vasopressor for hypotension

nicotine polacrilex gum

(nik'o-teen)
Nicorette, Nicorette DS
Func. class.: Smoking deterrent
Chem. class.: Ganglionic cholinergic agonist
Pregnancy category **X**

Action: Agonist at nicotinic receptors in the peripheral and central nervous systems; acts at sympathetic ganglia, on chemoreceptors of the aorta and carotid bodies; also affects adrenalin-releasing catecholamines

Therapeutic Outcome: Decreased withdrawl efforts when smoking cessation is attempted

Uses: Deter cigarette smoking

Dosage and routes

Adult: Gum 1 piece chewed × 30 min as needed to abstain from smoking; not to exceed 30/day

Available forms: Gum 2 mg/piece of gum

Side effects/adverse reactions

CNS: Dizziness, vertigo, insomnia, headache, confusion, convulsions, depression, euphoria, numbness, tinnitus
CV: Dysrhythmias, tachycardia, palpitations, edema, flushing, hypertension
EENT: Jaw ache, irritation in buccal cavity
GI: Nausea, vomiting, anorexia, indigestion, diarrhea, abdominal pain, constipation, eructation
RESP: Breathing difficulty, cough, hoarseness, sneezing, wheezing

Contraindications: Hypersensitivity, immediate post-MI recovery period, severe angina pectoris, pregnancy **X**

Precautions: Vasospastic disease, dysrhythmias, diabetes mellitus, children, hyperthyroidism, pheochromocytoma, coronary disease, esophagitis, peptic ulcer, lactation, hepatic/renal disease

Pharmacokinetics

Absorption	Slowly absorbed, buccal cavity
Distribution	Unknown
Metabolism	Liver; some by lungs, kidneys
Excretion	Kidneys, unchanged (20%); breast milk
Half-life	1-2 hr

Pharmacodynamics

Onset	Rapid
Peak	½ hr
Duration	Unknown

Interactions

Drug/drug:

Individual drugs

Acetaminophen: ↑ effects of acetaminophen
Caffeine: ↑ effects of caffeine
Furosemide: ↑ effects of furosemide
Imipramine: ↑ effects of imipramine
Oxazepam: ↑ effects of oxazepam
Pentazocine: ↑ effects of pentazocine
Propranolol: ↑ effects of propranolol

NURSING CONSIDERATIONS

Assessment

- Assess for adverse reaction to gum: irritation of buccal cavity, dislike of taste, jaw ache
- Assess for withdrawal symptoms: headache, fatigue, drowsiness, restlessness, irritability, severe cravings for nicotine products before, during, and after treatment

• Obtain a nicotine assessment: brand of cigarettes, chewing tobacco, cigars, number of each used per day; what increases need or activities performed when each is used
• Gum should not be used if temporomandibular condition exists
• Assess for nicotine toxicity: GI symptoms (nausea, vomiting, diarrhea), cardiopulmonary symptoms (decreased B/P, dyspnea, change in pulse), weakness, abdominal cramping, headache, blurred vision, tinnitus; drug should be discontinued

Associated nursing diagnoses

✓ Coping, ineffective individual (uses)
✓ Knowledge deficit (teaching)
✓ Noncompliance (teaching)

Implementation

• Give only prescribed amount, or toxicity may occur
• Protect gum from light and heat

Patient/family education

• Instruct patient to chew gum slowly for 30 min to promote buccal absorption of the drug; do not chew over 45 min
• Advise patient to begin drug withdrawal after 3 mo use; do not exceed 6 mo
• Teach patient all aspects of drug; give package insert to patient and explain; caution patient not to exceed prescribed dose
• Inform patient that gum will not stick to dentures, dental appliances
• Caution patient that gum is as toxic as cigarettes; it is to be used only to deter smoking
• Caution patient not to use during pregnancy; birth defects may occur

Evaluation

Positive therapeutic outcome
• Decrease in urge to smoke
• Decreased need for gum after 3-6 mo

nicotine transdermal system

Habitrol, Nicoderm, Nicotrol, Prostep

Func. class.: Smoking deterrent

Chem. class.: Ganglionic cholinergic agonist

Pregnancy category **D**

Action: Binds to acetylcholine receptors at autonomic ganglia in the adrenal medulla, at neuromuscular junctions, and in the brain

⇒ Therapeutic Outcome: Decreased withdrawal efforts when smoking cessation is attempted

Uses: Deter cigarette smoking

Dosage and routes

Nicotrol

Adult: Transdermal 15 mg/day × 12 wk; 10 mg/day × 2 wk; 5 mg/day × 2 wk

Prostep

Adult: Transdermal 22 mg/day × 4-8 wk; 11 mg/day × 2-4 wk

Nicoderm/Habitrol

Adult: Transdermal 21 mg/day × 6 wk; 14 mg/day × 14 days; 7 mg/day × 14 days

Available forms: Transdermal patch delivering 7, 14, 21 mg; 15 mg, 10 mg, 5 mg, 22 mg, 11 mg/day patches depending on product

Side effects/adverse reactions

CNS: Abnormal dreams, *insomnia,* nervousness, *headache,* dizziness, paresthesia, poor concentration, weakness
EENT: Dry mouth, abnormal taste
GI: Diarrhea, dyspepsia, constipation, nausea, abdominal pain, vomiting, dry mouth, abnormal taste
INTEG: *Erythema, pruritus, burning at application site,* hypersensitivity, sweating, rash
MISC: Chest pain, dysmenorrhea
MS: Arthralgia, myalgia, back pain
RESP: Cough, sinusitis

Contraindications: Hypersensitivity, children, pregnancy **D**, nonsmokers, during immediate post-MI period, life-threatening dysrhythmias, severe or worsening angina pectoris

Precautions: Skin disease, angina pectoris, MI, renal or hepatic insufficiency, peptic ulcer, accelerated hypertension, serious cardiac dysrhythmias, hyperthyroidism, pheochromocytoma, insulin-dependent diabetes, elderly

Pharmacokinetics

Absorption	Slowly absorbed
Distribution	Unknown
Metabolism	Liver
Excretion	Kidneys, unchanged (20%)
Half-life	1-2 hr

Pharmacodynamics

Onset	Rapid
Peak	½ hr
Duration	Unknown

Interactions

Drug/drug:

Individual drugs

Acetaminophen: ↑ effects of acetaminophen
Caffeine: ↑ effects of caffeine
Furosemide: ↑ effects of furosemide
Imipramine: ↑ effects of imipramine
Oxazepam: ↑ effects of oxazepam
Pentazocine: ↑ effects of pentazocine
Propranolol: ↑ effects of propranolol

NURSING CONSIDERATIONS

Assessment

- Monitor for adverse reaction: irritation of buccal cavity, dislike of taste, jaw ache
- Assess for withdrawal symptoms: headache, fatigue, drowsiness, restlessness, irritability, severe cravings for nicotine products before, during, and after treatment
- Obtain a nicotine assessment: brand of cigarettes, chewing tobacco, cigars, number of each used per day; what

increases need or activities performed when each is used
- Assess for nicotine toxicity: GI symptoms (nausea, vomiting, diarrhea), cardiopulmonary symptoms (decreased B/P, dyspnea, change in pulse), weakness, abdominal cramping, headache, blurred vision, tinnitus; drug should be discontinued

Associated nursing diagnoses

✓ Coping, ineffective individual (uses)
✓ Knowledge deficit (teaching)
✓ Noncompliance (teaching)

Implementation

- Protect from heat
- Some patches are worn during the waking hr only (Nicotrol); other patches are worn 24 hr

Patient/family education

- Teach patient all aspects of drug; give package insert to patient and explain
- Caution patient that patch is as toxic as cigarettes; it is to be used only to deter smoking
- Caution patient not to use during pregnancy; birth defects may occur
- Caution patient to keep used and unused system out of reach of children and pets
- Instruct patient to apply once a day to a nonhairy, clean, dry area of skin on upper body or upper outer arm; some products are used during waking hr, some 24 hr/day
- Instruct patient to stop smoking immediately when beginning treatment with patch
- Teach patient to apply promptly after removing from protective patch; system may lose strength

Evaluation

Positive therapeutic outcome
- Decrease in urge to smoke
- Decreased need for gum after 3-6 mo

nifedipine

(nye-fed'i-peen)

Adalat, Adalat CC, Adalat P.A. ✤, Apo-Nifed ✤, Novo-Nifedin ✤, NuNifed ✤, nifedipine, Procardia, Procardia XL

Func. class.: Calcium channel blocker, antihypertensive

Chem. class.: Dihydropyridine

Pregnancy category C

Action: Inhibits calcium ion influx across cell membrane during cardiac depolarization, produces relaxation of coronary vascular smooth muscle and peripheral vascular smooth muscle, dilates coronary vascular arteries, increases myocardial oxygen delivery in patients with vasospastic angina

➔ **Therapeutic Outcome:** Decreased angina pectoris, decreased B/P in hypertension

Uses: Chronic stable angina pectoris, vasospastic angina, hypertension (sus rel only)

Investigational uses: Hypertension (acute), migraines, CHF, Raynaud's disease

Dosage and routes

Adult: PO immediate release, 10 mg tid; increase in 10-mg increments q4-6h, not to exceed 180 mg/24 hr or single dose of 30 mg

Adult: PO sus rel, 30-60 mg/day; may increase q7-14 days; doses >120 mg not recommended

Available forms: Cap 5 🍁, 10, 20 mg, sus rel tab 30, 60, 90 mg

Side effects/adverse reactions

CNS: *Headache,* fatigue, drowsiness, *dizziness,* anxiety, depression, weakness, insomnia, *lightheadedness,* paresthesia, tinnitus, blurred vision, nervousness
CV: Dysrhythmias, edema, ***CHF,*** hypotension, palpitations, ***MI, pulmonary edema,*** tachycardia
GI: *Nausea,* vomiting, diarrhea, gastric upset, constipation, increased liver function studies, dry mouth
GU: Nocturia, polyuria
INTEG: Rash, pruritus, *flushing,* photosensitivity, hair loss
MISC: Sexual difficulties, cough, fever, chills

Contraindication: Hypersensitivity

Precautions: CHF, hypotension, sick sinus syndrome, 2nd- or 3rd-degree heart block, hypotension less than 90 mm Hg systolic, hepatic injury, pregnancy **C**, lactation, P children, renal disease

Pharmacokinetics

Absorption	Well absorbed (PO)
Distribution	Unknown
Metabolism	Liver, extensively
Excretion	Unknown
Half-life	2-5 hr

Pharmacodynamics

	PO	PO–SUS REL
Onset	½ hr	Unknown
Peak	Unknown	Unknown
Duration	6-8 hr	24 hr

Interactions

Drug/drug:

Individual drugs
Alcohol: ↑ hypotension
Digoxin: ↑ digoxin levels, bradycardia, CHF
Propranolol: ↑ toxicity

Drug classifications
Antihypertensives: ↑ hypotension
β-Adrenergic blockers: ↑ bradycardia, CHF
Nitrates: ↑ nitrates

NURSING CONSIDERATIONS

Assessment

• Assess fluid volume status (I&O ratio) and record weight, distended red veins, crackles in lung, color, quality and sp gr of urine, skin turgor, adequacy of pulses, moist mucous membranes, bilateral lung sounds, peripheral pitting edema; dehydration symptoms of decreasing output, thirst, hypotension, dry mouth, and mucous membranes should be reported

N

• Monitor ALT (SGPT), AST (SGOT), bilirubin daily; if these are elevated, hepatotoxicity is suspected
• Monitor cardiac status: B/P, pulse, respirations, ECG

Associated nursing diagnoses

✓ Cardiac output, decreased (uses)
✓ Pain (uses)
✓ Knowledge deficit (teaching)

Implementation

PO route
• Give ac, at hs, or with meals for GI symptoms
• Store in tight container at room temp

Sublingual route
• Using a sterile needle puncture the cap and squeeze medication in buccal area (not an FDA-approved use)

Patient/family education

• Advise patient to avoid hazardous activities until stabilized on drug and dizziness is no longer a problem
• Instruct patient to limit caffeine consumption; to avoid alcohol and OTC drugs unless directed by prescriber
• Instruct patient to comply in all areas of medical regimen: diet, exercise, stress reduction, drug therapy; to notify prescriber of irregular heart beat, shortness of breath, swelling of feet and hands, pronounced dizziness, constipation, nausea, hypotension
• Teach patient to use as directed even if feeling better; may be taken with other cardiovascular drugs (nitrates, β-blockers)

Evaluation

Positive therapeutic outcome
• Decreased angina attacks
• Decreased B/P

Treatment of overdose: Defibrillation, atropine for AV block, vasopressor for hypotension

nimodipine

(ni-moe′dip-een)

Nimotop

Func. class.: Calcium channel blocker

Chem. class.: Dihydropyridine

Pregnancy category C

Action: Inhibits calcium ion influx across cell membrane during cardiac depolarization, produces relaxation of coronary vascular smooth muscle and peripheral vascular smooth muscle, dilates coronary vascular arteries, increases myocardial oxygen delivery in patients with vasospastic angina

➡ **Therapeutic Outcome:** Prevention of vascular spasm (subarachnoid hemorrhage)

Uses: Prevention of cerebral vascular spasm in subarachnoid hemorrhage

Dosage and routes

Adult: PO 20 mg tid initially; may increase after 3 days (range 20-40 mg tid)

Available forms: Cap 20, 30 mg; sus rel cap 30, 45, 60 mg

Side effects/adverse reactions

CNS: Headache, fatigue, drowsiness, dizziness, anxiety, depression, weakness, insomnia, confusion, paresthesia, somnolence
CV: Dysrhythmia, edema, CHF, bradycardia, hypotension, palpitations, ***MI, pulmonary edema***
GI: Nausea, vomiting, diarrhea, gastric upset, constipation, ***hepatitis,*** abdominal cramps
GU: Nocturia, polyuria, ***acute renal failure***
INTEG: Rash, pruritus, urticaria, photosensitivity, hair loss
MISC: Blurred vision, flushing, nasal congestion, sweating, shortness of breath, gynecomastia, hyperglycemia, sexual difficulties

Contraindications: Sick sinus syndrome, 2nd- or 3rd-degree heart block, hypotension less than 90 mm Hg systolic, hypersensitivity

Precautions: CHF, hypotension, hepatic injury, pregnancy P C, lactation, children, renal G disease, elderly

Pharmacokinetics

Absorption	Well absorbed (PO), bioavailability poor
Distribution	Crosses blood-brain barrier
Metabolism	Liver, extensively
Excretion	Kidneys
Half-life	1-2 hr

Pharmacodynamics

	PO
Onset	Unknown
Peak	1 hr
Duration	Unknown

Interactions

Drug/drug:

Individual drugs

Alcohol: ↑ hypotension
Digoxin: ↑ digoxin levels, bradycardia
Phenobarbital: ↓ effectiveness
Phenytoin: ↓ effectiveness
Propranolol: ↑ toxicity

Drug classifications

Antihypertensives: ↑ hypotension
β-Adrenergic blockers: ↑ bradycardia
Nitrates: ↑ nitrates

N

NURSING CONSIDERATIONS

Assessment

- Assess fluid volume status (I&O ratio) and record weight, distended red veins, crackles in lung, color, quality and sp gr of urine, skin turgor, adequacy of pulses, moist mucous membranes, bilateral lung sounds, peripheral pitting edema; dehydration symptoms of decreasing output, thirst, hypotension, dry mouth and mucous membranes should be reported
- Monitor B/P and pulse; if B/P drops 30 mm Hg, call prescriber
- Monitor ALT (SGPT), AST (SGOT), bilirubin daily; if these are elevated, hepatotoxicity is suspected

Associated nursing diagnoses

✓ Injury, risk for (uses)
✓ Knowledge deficit (teaching)

Implementation

PO route

- May puncture cap and dilute in water and give through gasogastric tube; flush tube with 0.90% NaCl
- Store in airtight container at room temp

Patient/family education

- Teach patient to comply in all areas of medical regimen: diet, exercise, stress reduction, drug therapy; to notify prescriber of irregular heart beat, shortness of breath, swelling of feet and hands, pronounced dizziness, constipation, nausea, hypotension

Evaluation

Positive therapeutic outcome

- Decreased angina
- Decreased B/P

Treatment of overdose:

Defibrillation, atropine for AV block, vasopressor for hypotension

nitroglycerin

(nye-troe-gli'ser-in)

Nitro-Bid IV, nitroglycerin, Tridil, Nitrostat, Nitro-Bid Plateau Caps, Nitrocine Timecaps, Nitroglyn, Nitrong, Nitro-Bid, Nitrol, Deponit, Minitran, Nitrodisc, Nitro-Dur, nitroglycerin transdermal, Nitrocine, Transderm-Nitro, Nitrolingual, Nitrogard

Func. class.: Coronary vasodilator, antianginal

Chem. class.: Nitrate

Pregnancy category **C**

Action: Decreases preload and afterload, which thus decreases left ventricular end-diastolic pressure and systemic vascular resistance; dilates coronary arteries and improves blood flow

➡ **Therapeutic Outcome:** Prevention of anginal attack

Uses: Chronic stable angina pectoris, prophylaxis of angina pain, CHF associated with acute MI, controlled hypotension in surgical procedures

Dosage and routes

Adult: SL dissolve tab under tongue when pain begins; may repeat q5 min until relief occurs; take no more than 3 tab/15 min; use 1 tab prophylactically 5-10 min before activities; sus rel cap q6-12h on empty stomach; top 1-2 in q8h; increase to 4 in q4h as

Pharmacodynamics

	SUS REL	SL	TRANS	IV	TRANSMUCOSAL	AEROSOL	TOP OINT
Onset	20-45 min	1-3 min	½-1 hr	Immediate	3 min	2 min	½-1 hr
Peak	Unknown	Unknown	Unknown	Unknown	Unknown	Unknown	Unknown
Duration	3-8 hr	½ hr	12-24 hr	Variable	10-30 min	½-1 hr	2-12 hr

needed; **IV** 5 μg/min, then increase by 5 μg/min q3-5 min; if no response after 20 μg/min, increase by 10-20 μg/min until desired response; trans apply a pad qd to a site free from hair

Available forms: Buccal tab 1, 2, 3 mg; aero 0.4 mg/meter spray; sus rel cap 2.5, 6.5, 9, 13 mg; sus rel tabs 2.6, 6.5, 9 mg; inj 0.5, 5 mg/ml; SL tab 0.15, 0.3, 0.4, 0.6 mg; trans oint 2%; trans syst 0.1, 0.2, 0.3, 0.4, 0.6 mg/24 hr; inj 25 mg/250 ml, 50 mg/250 ml, 50 mg/500 ml, 100 mg/250 ml, 200 mg/500 ml

Side effects/adverse reactions

CNS: Headache, flushing, dizziness
CV: Postural hypotension, tachycardia, ***collapse,*** syncope
GI: Nausea, vomiting
INTEG: Pallor, sweating, rash

Contraindications: Hypersensitivity to this drug or nitrites, severe anemia, increased intracranial pressure, cerebral hemorrhage

Precautions: Postural hypotension, pregnancy **C**, lactation

Pharmacokinetics

Absorption	Well absorbed (PO, buccal, SL)
Distribution	Unknown
Metabolism	Liver, extensively
Excretion	Kidney
Half-life	1-4 min

Interactions

Drug/drug:

Individual drugs
Alcohol: ↑ hypotension
Haloperidol: ↑ hypotension
Drug classifications
Antidepressants, tricyclic: ↓ absorption of SL, transmucosal
Antihistamines: ↓ absorption of SL, transmucosal
Antihypertensives: ↑ hypotension
β-Blockers: ↑ hypotension
Calcium channel blockers: ↑ hypotension
Phenothiazines: ↓ absorption of SL, transmucosal

NURSING CONSIDERATIONS

Assessment

- Monitor orthostatic B/P, pulse
- Assess pain: duration, time started, activity being performed, character; check for tolerance if taken over long period

N

- Monitor for headache, lightheadedness, decreased B/P; may indicate a need for decreased dosage

Associated nursing diagnoses

- ✓ Cardiac output, decreased (uses)
- ✓ Poisoning (uses)
- ✓ Tissue perfusion, decreased (uses)
- ✓ Knowledge deficit (teaching)
- ✓ Noncompliance (teaching)

Implementation

IV **IV route**

- Give **IV** diluted in amount specified D_5 or NS for inf; use glass inf bottles, non–polyvinyl chloride inf tubing; titrate to patient response; do not use filters

Syringe compatibility:
Heparin

Y-site compatibilities:
Amiodarone, amrinone, atracurium, diltiazem, dobutamine, dopamine, famotidine, haloperidol, lidocaine, nitroprusside, pancuronium, ranitidine, streptokinase, vecuronium

Y-site incompatibility:
Alteplase

Additive incompatibilities:
Manufacturer recommends that nitroglycerin not be admixed with other medications

SL route

- Keep tab in original container
- If 3 SL tab in 15 min do not relieve pain, consider diagnosis of MI
- SL tab should be held under tongue until dissolved (a few min); do not take anything by mouth when SL tab is in place

PO route

- Give 1 hr ac or 2 hr pc with 8 oz of water
- Sus rel tab should not be chewed or crushed

Transmucosal route

- Tab should be placed between cheek and gum line
- Do not take anything by PO when tab is in place

Top route

- Apply ointment using dose-measuring papers supplied; apply to an area without hair; ointment should cover 2-3 in area; may apply an occlusive dressing as directed
- Apply trans patches to area without hair; press hard to adhere; if patch becomes dislodged, apply a new one

Patient/family education

- Teach patient to place buccal tab between lip and gum above incisors or between cheek and gum; sus rel tab must be swallowed whole, do not chew; SL should be dissolved under tongue, do not swallow; aerosol should be sprayed under tongue, do not inhale; use inhaler only when lying down; do not inhale spray
- Instruct patient to avoid alcohol
- Advise patient that drug may cause headache; tolerance usually develops; use nonnarcotic analgesic
- Teach patient that drug may

be taken before stressful activity, exercise, sexual activity
- Inform patient that SL may sting when drug comes in contact with mucous membranes
- Caution patient to avoid hazardous activities if dizziness occurs
- Instruct patient to comply with complete medical regimen
- Advise patient to make position changes slowly to prevent fainting

Evaluation

Positive therapeutic outcome
- Decreased, prevention of anginal pain

nitroprusside

(nye-troe-pruss'ide)

Nitropress, Sodium nitroprusside

Func. class.: Antihypertensive

Chem. class.: Peripheral vasodilator

Pregnancy category **C**

Action: Directly relaxes arteriolar, venous smooth muscle, resulting in reduction in cardiac preload, afterload

Therapeutic Outcome: Decreased B/P in hypertensive crisis, decreased preload, afterload

Uses: Hypertensive crisis, to decrease bleeding by creating hypotension during surgery, acute CHF

Dosage and routes

Adult: **IV** inf dissolve 50 mg in 2-3 ml of D_5W, then dilute in 250-1000 ml of D5W; run at 0.5-8 μg/kg/min

Available forms: Inj 50 mg

Side effects/adverse reactions

CNS: Dizziness, headache, agitation, twitching, decreased reflexes, ***LOC,*** restlessness

CV: Palpitations, severe hypotension, dyspnea

EENT: Tinnitus, blurred vision

GI: Nausea, vomiting, abdominal pain

GU: Impotence

INTEG: Pain, irritation at inj site, sweating

MISC: Cyanide, thiocyanate toxicity

Contraindications: Hypersensitivity, hypertension (compensatory)

Precautions: Pregnancy **C**, P lactation, children, fluid, electrolyte imbalances, hepatic disease, renal disease, hypothyroidism, G elderly

Pharmacokinetics

Absorption	Complete bioavailability
Distribution	Not known
Metabolism	RBCs, tissues
Excretion	Kidneys
Half-life	Unknown

Pharmacodynamics

Onset	1-2 min
Peak	Rapid
Duration	1-10 min

Interactions

Drug/drug:

Drug classifications

Antihypertensives: ↑ hypotension

Ganglionic blockers: ↑ hypotension

NURSING CONSIDERATIONS

Assessment

- Monitor B/P q5 min × 2 hr, then q1h × 2 hr; monitor pulse q4h; monitor jugular venous distention q4h; ECG should be monitored continuously; monitor PCWP
- Monitor electrolytes, blood studies: potassium, sodium, chloride, CO_2, CBC, serum glucose, serum methemoglobin if pulmonary oxygen levels are decreased
- Check weight, I&O, edema in feet and legs daily; assess skin turgor, dryness of mucous membranes for hydration status
- Assess for signs of CHF: dyspnea, edema, wet rales
- Monitor for increased lactate, cyanide, thiocyanate levels
- Monitor for decrease in bicarbonate, Pco_2 and blood pH; acidosis may occur with this drug

Associated nursing diagnoses

✓ Tissue perfusion, altered (uses)
✓ Injury, risk for (adverse reactions)
✓ Knowledge deficit (teaching)

Implementation

IV **IV route**

- Give by cont inf after diluting 50 mg/2-3 ml of D_5W; further dilute in 250 ml of D_5W; use an inf pump only; wrap bottle with aluminum foil to protect from light; observe for color change in the inf; discard if highly discolored (blue, green, red); titrate to patient response; avoid extravasation

Additive incompatibilities:
Do not give with any other drugs

Syringe compatibility:
Heparin

Y-site compatibilities:
Amrinone, atracurium, dobutamine, dopamine, enalaprilat, famotidine, lidocaine, nitroglycerin, pancuronium, vecuronium

Patient/family education

- Patient should be taught to report headache, dizziness, loss of hearing, blurred vision, dyspnea, faintness; may indicate adverse reactions

Evaluation

Positive therapeutic outcome

- Decreased B/P in hypertension
- Absence of bleeding in surgery

Treatment of overdose:

Administer amyl nitrite inh until 3% sodium nitrate sol can be prepared for **IV** administration, then inject sodium thiosulfate **IV**; correct drop in BP with vasopressor

norfloxacin
(nor-flox'a-sin)
Chibroxin, Noroxin
Func. class.: Urinary anti-infective
Chem. class.: Fluoroquinolone antibacterial
Pregnancy category **C**

Action: Interferes with conversion of intermediate DNA fragments into high-molecular-weight DNA in bacteria

Therapeutic Outcome: Bactericidal action against the gram-positive *Staphylococcus epidermidis,* methicillin-resistant strains of *Staphylococcus aureus,* group D streptococci; gram-negative *Escherichia coli, Klebsiella pneumoniae, Enterobacter cloacae, Proteus mirabilis, P. vulgaris, Providencia rettgeri, Morganella morganii, Pseudomonas aeruginosa, Citrobacter freundii*

Uses: Adult UTIs (including complicated), uncomplicated gonorrhea, ocular infections

Dosage and routes

Uncomplicated infections

Adult: PO 400 mg bid × 7-10 days 1 hr ac or 2 hr pc

Complicated infections

Adult: PO 400 mg bid × 10-21 days; 400 mg qd × 7-10 days in impaired renal function

Uncomplicated gonorrhea

Adult: PO 800 mg as a single dose

Occular infection

P ***Adult and child:*** Ophth i gtt qid; may increase to i gtt q2h for severe infections

Available forms: Tabs 400 mg; ophth sol 3 mg/ml

Side effects/adverse reactions

CNS: Headache, dizziness, fatigue, somnolence, depression, insomnia
EENT: Visual disturbances
GI: Nausea, constipation, increased ALT (SGPT), AST (SGOT), flatulence, heartburn, vomiting, diarrhea, dry mouth
INTEG: Rash

Contraindications: Hypersensitivity to quinolones

Precautions: Pregnancy **C**, P lactation, children, renal disease, seizure disorders

Pharmacokinetics

Absorption	30% (PO)
Distribution	Concentration in urinary system
Metabolism	Liver (minimal)
Excretion	Kidneys, unchanged (30%)
Half-life	3-4 hr; increased in renal disease

Pharmacodynamics

	PO
Onset	Unknown
Peak	1 hr

Interactions

Drug/drug:

Individual drugs

Nitrofurantoin: ↓ effectiveness
Probenecid: ↑ blood levels

Sucralfate: ↓ absorption of norfloxacin
Theophylline: ↑ toxicity
Zinc sulfate: ↓ absorption of norfloxacin

Drug classifications
Antacids: ↓ absorption of norfloxacin
Anticoagulants, oral: ↑ effect of anticoagulants
Antineoplastics: ↓ norfloxacin levels
Iron salts: ↓ absorption of norfloxacin

Lab test interferences

Increase: AST (SGOT), ALT (SGPT), BUN, creatinine, alkaline phosphatase

NURSING CONSIDERATIONS

Assessment

- Assess patient for previous sensitivity reaction
- Assess patient for signs and symptoms of infection including characteristics of urine, WBC >10,000, temp; obtain baseline information before and during treatment
- Obtain C & S before beginning drug therapy to identify if correct treatment has been initiated
- Assess for allergic reactions: rash, urticaria, pruritus
- Monitor blood studies: AST (SGOT), ALT (SGPT), BUN, creatinine, alkaline phosphatase monthly if patient is on long-term therapy
- Assess bowel pattern qd; if severe diarrhea occurs, drug should be discontinued
- Assess for overgrowth of infection: perineal itching, fever, malaise, redness, pain, swelling, drainage, rash, diarrhea, change in cough, sputum

Associated nursing diagnoses

✓ Infection, risk for (uses)
✓ Diarrhea (adverse reactions)
✓ Injury, risk for (adverse reactions)
✓ Knowledge deficit (teaching)
✓ Noncompliance (teaching)

Implementation

PO route

- Give in equal intervals q12h around the clock to maintain proper blood levels; give with food to increase absorption of drug; do not give within 3 hr of other agents; drug interactions may occur; give with 8 oz of water
- Do not give with iron, zinc products, or antacids, which decrease absorption

Patient/family education

- Instruct patient to take all medication prescribed for the length of time ordered; drug must be taken around the clock to maintain blood levels; do not give medication to others; do not double doses; take any missed dose when remembered
- Advise patient to increase fluids to 2 L/day to prevent crystalluria
- Caution patient to avoid driving and other hazardous activities until response is known; dizziness, may occur
- Instruct patient to use sunglasses to prevent photophobia
- Have patient use hard candy, frequent sips of water for dry mouth
- Teach patient correct instillation procedure (ophth)

Evaluation

Positive therapeutic outcome
- Reported improvement in symptoms of infection
- Absence of red or itching eyes (ophth)

nortriptyline

(nor-trip'ti-leen)

Aventyl, Pamelor

Func. class.: Antidepressant, tricyclic

Chem. class.: Dibenzocycloheptene, secondary amine

Pregnancy category **C**

Action: Blocks reuptake of norepinephrine, serotonin into nerve endings, increasing action of norepinephrine, serotonin in nerve cells; has anticholinergic effects

➔ **Therapeutic Outcome:** Decreased symptoms of depression after 2-3 wk

Uses: Major depression

Investigational uses: Chronic pain management

Dosage and routes

Adult: PO 25 mg tid or qid; may increase to 150 mg/day; may give daily dose hs

Available forms: Cap 10, 25, 50, 75 mg; sol 10 mg/5 ml

Side effects/adverse reactions

CNS: Dizziness, drowsiness, confusion, headache, anxiety, tremors, stimulation, weakness, insomnia, nightmares, G EPS (elderly), increased psychiatric symptoms

CV: Orthostatic hypotension, ECG changes, tachycardia, ***hypertension,*** palpitations

EENT: Blurred vision, tinnitus, mydriasis

GI: Constipation, dry mouth, nausea, vomiting, ***paralytic ileus,*** increased appetite, cramps, epigastric distress, jaundice, ***hepatitis,*** stomatitis

GU: Retention, ***acute renal failure***

HEMA: ***Agranulocytosis, thrombocytopenia, eosinophilia, leukopenia***

INTEG: Rash, urticaria, sweating, pruritus, photosensitivity

Contraindications: Hypersensitivity to tricyclic antidepressants, recovery phase of MI, convulsive disorders, prostatic hypertrophy

Precautions: Suicidal patients, severe depression, increased intraocular pressure, narrow angle glaucoma, urinary retention, cardiac disease, hepatic disease, hyperthyroidism, electroshock therapy, elective surgery, pregnancy **C**

Pharmacokinetics

Absorption	Well absorbed
Distribution	Widely distributed; crosses placenta
Metabolism	Liver, extensively
Excretion	Kidneys, breast milk
Half-life	18-28 hr; steady state 4-19 days

N

Pharmacodynamics

	PO
Onset	Unknown
Peak	Unknown
Duration	Unknown

Interactions

Drug/drug:

Individual drugs

Alcohol: ↑ CNS depression
Cimetidine: ↑ levels, toxicity
Clonidine: Severe hypotension; avoid use
Disulfiram: Organic brain syndrome
Fluoxetine: ↑ levels, toxicity
Guanethidine: ↓ effects

Drug classifications

Analgesics: ↑ CNS depression
Anticholinergics: ↑ side effects
Antihistamines: ↑ CNS depression
Antihypertensives: May block antihypertensive effect
Barbiturates: ↑ effects
Benzodiazepines: ↑ effects
CNS depressants: ↑ effects
MAOI: Hypertensive crisis, convulsions
Oral contraceptives: ↑ effects, toxicity
Phenothiazines: ↑ toxicity
Sedative/hypnotics: ↑ CNS depression
Sympathomimetics, indirect-acting: ↓ effects

Drug/smoking:

↑ metabolism, ↓ effects

Lab test interferences

Increase: Serum bilirubin, blood glucose, alkaline phosphatase
Decrease: VMA, 5-HIAA, blood glucose
False increase: Urinary catecholamines

NURSING CONSIDERATIONS

Assessment

- Monitor B/P (with patient lying, standing), pulse q4h; if systolic B/P drops 20 mm Hg, hold drug, notify prescriber; take VS q4h of patients with cardiovascular disease
- Monitor blood studies: CBC, leukocytes, differential, cardiac enzymes if patient is receiving long-term therapy
- Monitor hepatic studies: AST (SGOT), ALT (SGPT), bilirubin
- Check weight weekly; appetite may increase with drug
- Assess ECG for flattening of T wave, bundle branch block, AV block, dysrhythmias in cardiac patients
- Assess for EPS primarily in G elderly: rigidity, dystonia, akathisia
- Assess mental status: mood, sensorium, affect, suicidal tendencies; increase in psychiatric symptoms: depression, panic
- Monitor urinary retention, constipation; constipation is P more likely to occur in children G or elderly
- Assess for withdrawal symptoms: headache, nausea, vomiting, muscle pain, weakness; do not usually occur unless drug was discontinued abruptly
- Identify alcohol consumption; if alcohol is consumed, hold dose until AM

Associated nursing diagnoses

✓ Coping, ineffective individual (uses)

- Injury, risk for (adverse reactions)
- Knowledge deficit (teaching)
- Noncompliance (teaching)

Implementation

PO route

- Give with food or milk for GI symptoms; mix conc with water, milk, fruit juice to disguise taste
- Give dose hs if oversedation occurs during day; may take entire dose hs; elderly may not tolerate once/day dosing
- Store at room temp; do not freeze

Patient/family education

- Teach patient that therapeutic effects may take 2-3 wk
- Teach patient to use caution in driving and other activities requiring alertness because of drowsiness, dizziness, blurred vision; to avoid rising quickly from sitting to standing, especially elderly
- Teach patient to avoid alcohol ingestion, other CNS depressants; teach patient not to discontinue medication quickly after long-term use; may cause nausea, headache, malaise
- Teach patient to wear sunscreen or large hat, since photosensitivity occurs
- Teach patient to increase fluids, bulk in diet if constipation, urinary retention occur, especially elderly
- Teach patient to take gum, hard sugarless candy, or frequent sips of water for dry mouth

Evaluation

Positive therapeutic outcome

- Decrease in depression
- Absence of suicidal thoughts

Treatment of overdose: ECG monitoring, induce emesis, lavage, activated charcoal, administer anticonvulsant

nystatin

(nis′ta-tin)

Mycostatin, Mycostatin Pastilles, Nadostine ♣, Nyaderm ♣, nystatin, Nystex; topical: Mycostatin, Nilstat, Nodostine ♣, Nyoderm ♣, Nystatin, Nystex; vaginal: Mycostatin, Nilstat, Nadostine ♣, Nyoderm ♣, O-V Statin

Func. class.: Antiinfective

Chem. class.: Antifungal

Pregnancy category **B; A** vaginal

Action: Interferes with fungal DNA replication; binds sterols in fungal cell membrane, which increases permeability, resulting in leaking of cell nutrients

Therapeutic Outcome: Fungistatic/fungicidal against *Candida* organisms

Uses: *Candida* species causing oral, vaginal, intestinal infections; vag: cutaneous vulvovaginal candidiasis, top: mucocutaneous fungal infections, infant eczema, pruritus ani and vulvae

N

Dosage and routes

Oral infection

Adult: Susp 400,000-600,000 U qid

P ***Child and infants >3 mo:*** Susp 250,000-500,000 U qid

P ***Newborn and premature infants:*** Susp 100,000 U qid

GI infection

Adult: PO 500,000-1,000,000 U tid

Top

P ***Adult and child:*** Top apply to affected area bid-tid × 14 days

Vag: 1-2 tabs (100,000 U each) inserted into vagina

Available forms: Tab 500,000 U; powder 50 mill, 150 mill, 500 mill, 1 bill, 2 bill, 5 bill U; susp 100,000 U; cream, oint, powder, spray, vag tab 100,000 U; vag cream, lotion 2%

Side effects/adverse reactions

GI: Nausea, vomiting, anorexia, diarrhea, cramps
INTEG: Rash, urticaria, stinging, burning

Contraindication: Hypersensitivity

Precautions: Pregnancy **B**, lactation

Pharmacokinetics	
Absorption	Poorly absorbed
Distribution	Unknown
Metabolism	Not metabolized
Excretion	Feces, unchanged
Half-life	Unknown

Pharmacodynamics	
Onset	Rapid
Peak	Unknown
Duration	6-12 hr

Interactions: None

NURSING CONSIDERATIONS

Assessment

- Assess for allergic reaction: rash, urticaria; drug may have to be discontinued
- Assess for predisposing factors for Candidal infection: antibiotic therapy, pregnancy, diabetes mellitus, sexual partner infection (vag infections), AIDS

Associated nursing diagnoses

✓ Skin integrity, impaired (uses)
✓ Infection, risk for (uses)
✓ Knowledge deficit (teaching)

Implementation

PO route
- Give oral susp dose by placing ½ in each cheek, swish for several min, then swallow; shake susp before use
- Store oral susp, in refrigerator, tab in tight, light-resistant containers at room temp

Top route
- Administer by moistening lesions with a swab coated with cream or ointment; use enough medication to cover lesions completely; give after cleansing with soap, water before each application; dry well

Vag route
- Insert vag tab high into vagina with applicator provided; administer in gravid client 3-6 wk before term to

decrease candidiasis in the newborn
• Store at room temp in dry place; protect from light, air, heat

Patient/family education

• Instruct patient that long-term therapy may be needed to clear infection; to complete entire course of medication
• Teach patient proper hygiene: use no commercial mouthwashes for mouth infection
• Advise patient to avoid getting preparation on hands
• Instruct patient to wear light-day pad for vag preparations to avoid soiling clothing; to avoid sexual contact during treatment to minimize reinfection
• Instruct patient to notify prescriber if irritation occurs; drug may have to be discontinued
• Inform patient that relief from itching may occur after 24-72 hr

Top

• Advise patient to discontinue use and notify prescriber if irritation occurs
• Teach patient to apply with glove to prevent further infection; drug may stain
• Caution patient not to use occlusive dressings; to avoid use of OTC creams, ointments, lotions unless directed by prescriber

Evaluation

Positive therapeutic outcome

• Culture negative for *Candida*
• Decrease in size, number of lesions
• Decreased itching, white patches on vulva (vag)

ofloxacin

(o-flox'a-sin)

Floxin, Floxin IV, Ocuflox

Func. class.: Antiinfective
Chem. class.: Fluoroquinolone

Pregnancy category C

Action: Interferes with conversion of intermediate DNA fragments into high-molecular-weight DNA in bacteria

Therapeutic Outcome: Bactericidal action against the following gram-positive pathogens: *Staphylococcus epidermidis,* methicillin-resistant strains of *S. aureus, Streptococcus pyogenes, S. pneumoniae;* gram-negative pathogens *Escherichia coli, Klebsiella* species, *Enterobacter, Salmonella, Shigella, Proteus vulgaris, Providencia stuartii, P. rettgeri, Morganella morganii, Pseudomonas aeruginosa, Serratia, Haemophilus* species, *Acinetobacter, Neisseria gonorrhoeae, N. meningitidis, Yersinia, Vibrio, Brucella, Campylobacter,* and *Aeromonas* species; anaerobic pathogens: *Bacteroides fragilis intermedius, Clostridium perfrigens, Gardnerella vaginalis, Peptococcus niger, Peptostreptococcus* species; *Chlamydia pneumoniae, C. trachomatis, Legionella pneumoniae, Mycobacterium tuberculosis, Mycoplasma pneumoniae*

Uses: Treatment of lower respiratory tract infections

O

(pneumonia, bronchitis), genitourinary infections (prostatitis, UTIs), skin and skin structure infections, conjunctivitis (ophth)

Dosage and routes

Lower respiratory tract infection/skin and skin structure infections

Adult: PO/**IV** 200-400 mg q12h × 10 days

Cervicitis, urethritis

Adult: PO/**IV** 300 mg q12h × 7 days

Prostatitis

Adult: PO 300 mg q12h × 6 wk

Acute, uncomplicated gonorrhea

Adult: PO/**IV** 400 mg as a single dose

Conjunctivitis

P *Adult and child:* Ophth 1-2 gtt q2-4h × 2 days, then qid × 5 days

Available forms: Tab 200, 300, 400 mg; inj 200, 400 mg; ophth sol 0.3%

Side effects/adverse reactions

CNS: Dizziness, headache, fatigue, somnolence, depression, insomnia, lethargy, malaise

EENT: Visual disturbances

GI: Diarrhea, nausea, vomiting, anorexia, flatulence, heartburn, dry mouth, increased AST (SGOT), ALT (SGPT), abdominal pain, constipation

INTEG: Rash, pruritus

Contraindication: Hypersensitivity to quinolones

Precautions: Pregnancy **C**, P lactation, children, elderly, G renal disease, seizure disorders, excessive sunlight

Pharmacokinetics

Absorption	Well absorbed (PO)
Distribution	Widely distributed
Excretion	Kidneys, unchanged; breast milk
Half-life	5-9 hr; increased in renal disease

Pharmacodynamics

	PO	IV	OPHTH
Onset	Rapid	Rapid	Unknown
Peak	1-2 hr	Inf end	Unknown

Interactions

Drug/drug:

Individual drugs

Nitrofurantoin: ↓ effectiveness

Probenecid: ↑ blood levels

Sucralfate: ↓ absorption of ofloxacin

Theophylline: ↑ toxicity

Zinc sulfate: ↓ absorption of ofloxacin

Drug classifications

Antacids: ↓ absorption of ofloxacin

Anticoagulants, oral: ↑ effect of anticoagulants

Antineoplastics: ↓ ofloxacin levels

Iron salts: ↓ absorption of ofloxacin

Lab test interferences

Increase: AST (SGOT), ALT (SGPT), BUN, creatinine, alkaline phosphatase

NURSING CONSIDERATIONS

Assessment

- Assess patient for previous sensitivity reaction
- Assess patient for signs and symptoms of infection including characteristics of wounds, sputum, urine, stool, WBC >10,000, fever; obtain baseline information before and during treatment
- Obtain C&S before beginning drug therapy to identify if correct treatment has been initiated
- Assess for allergic reactions: rash, urticaria, pruritus
- Monitor blood studies: AST (SGOT), ALT (SGPT), CBC, serum glucose monthly if patient is on long-term therapy
- Assess bowel pattern qd; if severe diarrhea occurs, drug should be discontinued
- Assess for overgrowth of infection: perineal itching, fever, malaise, redness, pain, swelling, drainage, rash, diarrhea, change in cough, sputum
- Assess for CNS symptoms: seizures, vertigo, drowsiness, agitation, confusion, tremors

Associated nursing diagnoses

- ✓ Infection, risk for (uses)
- ✓ Diarrhea (adverse reactions)
- ✓ Injury, risk for (adverse reactions)
- ✓ Knowledge deficit (teaching)
- ✓ Noncompliance (teaching)

Implementation

PO route

- Give in equal intervals q12h around the clock to maintain proper blood levels; do not give within 3 hr of other agents, since drug interactions are possible: give with 8 oz of water
- Do not give with iron, aluminum, zinc products or antacids, which decrease absorption and form insoluble chelate

IV **IV route**

- For intermittent inf, dilute to 4 mg/ml with D_5W, D_5/0.9% NaCl, 0.9% NaCl, D_5/LR, sodium bicarbonate, sodium lactate, D_5/Plasmalyte 56; give over 1 hr or more

Patient/family education

- Instruct patient to take all medication prescribed for the length of time ordered; drug must be taken around the clock to maintain blood levels; do not give medication to others
- Teach patient to use sunscreen when outdoors to decrease phototoxicity
- Advise patient to increase fluids to 2 L/day to prevent crystalluria
- Caution patient to avoid driving and other hazardous activities until response is known; dizziness, confusion, drowsiness may occur

O

Evaluation

Positive therapeutic outcome

- Absence of signs/symptoms of infection (WBC <10,000, temp WNL)
- Reported improvement in symptoms of infection

- Absence of red or itching eyes (ophth)

omeprazole

(oh-mep'ra-zole)

Losec ♣, Prilosec

Func. class.: Antisecretory compound

Chem. class.: Benzimidazole

Pregnancy category C

Action: Suppresses gastric secretion by inhibiting hydrogen/potassium ATPase enzyme system in the gastric parietal cell; characterized as a gastric acid pump inhibitor, since it blocks the final step of acid production

Therapeutic Outcome: Absence of duodenal ulcers; decreased gastroesophageal reflux

Uses: Gastroesophageal reflux disease (GERD), severe erosive esophagitis, poorly responsive systemic GERD, pathologic hypersecretory conditions (Zollinger-Ellison syndrome, systemic mastocytosis, multiple endocrine adenomas); possibly effective for treatment of duodenal ulcers

Dosage and routes

Severe erosine esophagitis/poorly responsive gastroesophageal reflux disease

Adult: PO 20 mg qd × 4-8 wk

Pathologic hypersecretory conditions

Adult: PO 60 mg/day; may increase to 120 mg tid; daily doses >80 mg should be divided

Available forms: Sus rel cap 20 mg

Side effects/adverse reactions

CNS: ***Headache, dizziness, asthenia***

CV: Chest pain, angina, tachycardia, bradycardia, palpitations, peripheral edema

EENT: Tinnitus, taste perversion

GI: *Diarrhea, abdominal pain, vomiting, nausea, constipation, flatulence, acid regurgitation,* abdominal swelling, anorexia, irritable colon, esophageal candidiasis, dry mouth

GU: UTI, frequency, increased creatinine, ***proteinuria, hematuria,*** testicular pain, glycosuria

HEMA: ***Pancytopenia, thrombocytopenia, neutropenia, leukocytosis,*** anemia

INTEG: Rash, dry skin, urticaria, pruritus, alopecia

META: Hypoglycemia, increased hepatic enzymes, weight gain

MISC: *Back pain,* fever, fatigue, malaise

RESP: *Upper respiratory tract infections, cough,* epistaxis

Contraindications: Hypersensitivity

Precautions: Pregnancy **C**, P lactation, children

Pharmacokinetics

Absorption	Rapidly absorbed (PO)
Distribution	Protein binding (95%); gastric parietal cells
Metabolism	Liver, extensively
Excretion	Kidneys, feces
Half-life	½-1 hr; increased in the elderly, hepatic disease

G

Pharmacodynamics

Onset	1 hr
Peak	½-3½ hr
Duration	3-4 days

Interactions

Drug/drug:

Individual drugs

Ampicillin: ↓ absorption of omeprazole

Diazepam: ↑ serum levels of diazepam

Ketoconazole: ↓ absorption of ketoconazole

Phenytoin: ↑ serum levels of phenytoin

Warfarin: ↑ bleeding tendencies

Drug classification

Iron products: ↓ absorption of iron

NURSING CONSIDERATIONS

Assessment

- Assess GI system: bowel sounds q8h, abdomen for pain and swelling, anorexia
- Monitor hepatic enzymes: AST (SGOT), ALT (SGPT), increased alkaline phosphatase during treatment

Associated nursing diagnoses

✓ Pain (uses)

✓ Knowledge deficit (teaching)

Implementation

PO route

- Give before patient eats; patient should swallow cap whole; do not open, chew, or crush; may give with antacids

Patient/family education

- Advise patient to report severe diarrhea; drug may have to be discontinued
- Caution patient to avoid driving and other hazardous activities until response to drug is known
- Caution patient to avoid alcohol, salicylates, ibuprofen; may cause GI irritation

Evaluation

Positive therapeutic outcome

- Absence of epigastric pain, swelling, fullness

O

ondansetron

(on-dan'sa-tron)

Zofran

Func. class.: Antiemetic

Chem. class.: 5-HT receptor antagonist

Pregnancy category **B**

Action: Prevents nausea, vomiting by blocking serotonin peripherally, centrally, and in the small intestine

➔ **Therapeutic Outcome:** Control of nausea, vomiting

Uses: Prevention of nausea, vomiting associated with cancer chemotherapy and prevention of postopertive nausea, vomiting

Dosage and routes

Adult: **IV** 0.15 mg/kg infused over 15 min, 30 min before start of cancer chemotherapy; 0.15 mg/kg is given 4 hr and 8 hr after first dose; dilute in 50 ml of D_5W or 0.9% NaCl before giving

Prevention of nausea/ vomiting associated with cancer chemotherapy

Adult: PO 8 mg tid; give first dose 30 min before chemotherapy, subsequent doses 4, 8 hr after first dose; give 8 mg tid × 1-2 days after chemotherapy completion

Prevention of postoperative nausea/vomiting

Adult: **IV** 4 mg undiluted over >30 sec

Available forms: Inj 2 mg/ ml; tab 4, 8 mg

Side effects/adverse reactions

CNS: Headache
GI: Diarrhea, constipation, increased AST (SGOT), ALT (SGPT)
MISC: Rash, ***bronchospasm***

Contraindication: Hypersensitivity

P G **Precautions:** Pregnancy **B**, lactation, children, elderly

Pharmacokinetics

Absorption	Completely absorbed (IV)
Distribution	Unknown
Metabolism	Liver, extensively
Excretion	Kidneys
Half-life	3.5-4.7 hr

Pharmacodynamics

	IV/PO
Onset	Unknown
Peak	Unknown
Duration	Unknown

Interactions: Unknown

NURSING CONSIDERATIONS

Assessment

- Assess for absence of nausea, vomiting during chemotherapy
- Assess for hypersensitivity reaction: rash, bronchospasm

Associated nursing diagnoses

✓ Knowledge deficit (teaching)
✓ Noncompliance (teaching)

Implementation

IV **IV route**

- Give **IV** after diluting a single dose in 50 ml 0.9% NaCl or D_5W, 0.45%; give over 15 min
- Store at room temp for 48-hr dilution

Y-site compatibilities:

Amikacin, aztreonam, bleomycin, carboplatin, carmustine, cefazolin, ceforanide, cefotazime, cefoxitin, ceftazidime, ceftizoxime, cefuroxime, chlorpromazine, cimetidine, cisplatin, clindamycin, cyclophosphamide, cytarabine, dacarbazine, dactinomycin, daunorubicin, dexamethasone sodium phosphate, diphenhydramine, doxorubicin, doxycycline, droperidol, etoposide, famotidine, floxuridine, fluconazole, fludarabine, gentamicin, haloperidol, heparin, hydrocortisone sodium succinate, hydromorphone, hydroxyzine, ifosfamide, imipenem/cilastatin, magnesium sulfate, mannitol, mechlorethamine, melphalan, meperidine, mesna, methotrexate, metoclopramide, miconazole, mitomycin, mitoxantrone, morphine, paclitaxel, pentostatin, potassium chloride, prochlorperazine edisylate, ranitidine, streptozocin, teniposide, ticarcillin, ticar cillin/clavulanate, vancomycin, vinblastine, vincristine, vinorelbine, zidovudine

Y-site incompatibilities:

Acyclovir, aminophylline, amphotericin B, ampicillin, ampicillin/sulbactam, cefoperazone, furosemide, ganciclovir, lorazepam, methylprednisolone sodium succinate, mezlocillin, piperacillin, sargramostim, sodium bicarbonate

Solution compatibilities:

May also be diluted with D_5W, Lactated Ringers, D_5/0.9% NaCl, D_5/0.45% NaCl,

Patient/family education

- Instruct patient to report diarrhea, constipation, rash, or changes in respirations
- Teach patient reason for medication and expected results

Evaluation

Positive therapeutic outcome
- Absence of nausea, vomiting during cancer chemotherapy

oral contraceptives

Func. class.: Hormone
Chem. class.: Estrogen/progestin combinations
Pregnancy category **X**

Action: Prevents ovulation by suppressing FSH, LH; **monophasic:** estrogen/progestin (fixed dose) used during a 21-day cycle; ovulation is inhibited by suppression of FSH and LH; thickness of cervical mucus and endometrial lining prevents pregnancy; **biphasic:** ovulation is inhibited by suppression of FSH and LH; alteration of cervical mucus, endometrial lining prevents pregnancy; **triphasic:** ovulation is inhibited by suppression of FSH and LH; change of cervical mucus, endometrial lining prevents pregnancy; variable doses of estrogen/progestin combinations may be similar to natural hormonal fluctuations; **progestin-only pill and implant:** change of cervical mucus and endometrial lining prevents pregnancy; ovulation may be suppressed

Therapeutic Outcome: Prevention of pregnancy, decreased severity of endometriosis, hypermenorrhea

Uses: To prevent pregnancy, endometriosis, hypermenorrhea

Dosage and routes

Adult: PO 1 qd starting on day 5 of menstrual cycle; day 1 is 1st day of period

20/21-tab packs

Adult: PO 1 qd starting on day 7 of menstrual cycle; day 1 is 1st day of period; then on 20 or 21 days, off 7 days

28-tab packs

Adult: PO 1 qd continuously

Biphasic

Adult: 1 qd × 10 days, then next color 1 qd × 11 days

Triphasic

Adult: 1 qd; check package insert for each brand

Implant

Adult: Subdermal 6 cap implanted during the first wk of menses

Endometriosis

Adult: PO 1 qd × 20 days from day 5 to day 24 of cycle

Adult: PO 1 qd; check package insert for specific instructions

Available forms: Check specific brand

Side effects/adverse reactions

CNS: Depression, fatigue, dizziness, nervousness, anxiety, headache
CV: Increased B/P, thromboembolic conditions, fluid retention, edema
EENT: Optic neuritis, retinal thrombosis, cataracts
ENDO: Decreased glucose tolerance, increased TBG, PBI, T_4, T_3
GI: Nausea, vomiting, cramps, diarrhea, bloating, constipation, change in appetite, ***cholestatic jaundice***
GU: Breakthrough bleeding, amenorrhea, spotting, dysmenorrhea, galactorrhea, endocervical hyperplasia, vaginitis, cystitis-like syndrome, breast change
HEMA: Increased fibrinogen, clotting factor
INTEG: Chloasma, melasma, acne, rash, urticaria, erythema, pruritus, hirsutism, alopecia, photosensitivity

Contraindications: Pregnancy **X**, lactation, reproductive cancer, thrombophlebitis, MI, hepatic tumors, hepatic disease, CAD, women 40 yr and over, CVA

Precautions: Depression, hypertension, renal disease, seizure disorders, lupus erythematosus, rheumatic disease, migraine headache, amenorrhea, irregular menses, breast cancer (fibrocystic), gallbladder disease, diabetes mellitus, heavy smoking, acute mononucleosis, sickle cell disease

Pharmacokinetics

Absorption	Well absorbed
Distribution	Unknown
Metabolism	Liver, extensively
Excretion	Kidneys
Half-life	Unknown

Pharmacodynamics

	PO	IM	IMPLANT
Onset	1 mo	1 mo	1 mo
Peak	1 mo	1 mo	1 mo
Duration	1 mo	3 mo	5 yr

Interactions

Drug/drug:

Individual drugs

Aminocaproic acid: ↑ clotting
Bromocriptine: ↓ effectiveness of bromocriptine
Carbamazepine: ↓ effectiveness of oral contraceptive
Chenodiol: ↓ effectiveness of oral contraceptive
Chloramphenicol: ↓ effectiveness of oral contraceptive
Dantrolene: ↑ hepatic toxicity (estrogen only)
Dihydroergotamine: ↓ effectiveness of oral contraceptive
Griseofulvin: ↓ effectiveness of oral contraceptive
Mineral oil: ↓ effectiveness of oral contraceptive
Phenylbutazone: ↓ effectiveness of oral contraceptive
Phenytoin: ↓ effectiveness of oral contraceptive
Primidone: ↓ effectiveness of oral contraceptive
Rifampin: ↓ effectiveness of oral contraceptive
Warfarin: ↑ or ↓ effect of warfarin

Drug classifications

Analgesics: ↓ action of oral contraceptives
Antibiotics: ↓ action of oral contraceptives
Anticonvulsants: ↓ action of oral contraceptives
Antihistamines: ↓ action of oral contraceptives
Glucocorticoids: ↓ action of oral contraceptives
Oral anticoagulants: ↓ action of oral anticoagulants
Tricyclic antidepressants: ↑ toxicity

Lab test interferences

Increase: Pro-time; clotting factors VII, VIII, IX, X; TBG, PBI, T_4, platelet aggregation, BSP, triglycerides, bilirubin, AST (SGOT), ALT (SGPT)
Decrease: T_3, antithrombin III, folate, metyrapone test, GTT, 17-OHCS

NURSING CONSIDERATIONS

Assessment

- Assess for reproductive changes: change in breasts, tumors, positive Pap smear; drug should be discontinued if changes occur
- Monitor glucose, thyroid function, liver function tests, B/P

Associated nursing diagnoses

- ✓ Injury, risk for (adverse reactions)
- ✓ Body image disturbance (adverse reactions)
- ✓ Knowledge deficit (teaching)
- ✓ Noncompliance (teaching)

Implementation

PO route

- If GI symptoms occur, medication may be taken with food; take at same time each day

Implant route

- Inject 6 cap subdermally
- Implant is effective for 5 yr, should be removed after that

IM route

- Administer deep in large muscle mass after shaking susp well; ensure pregnancy has not occurred if inj are 2 wk or more apart

Patient/family education

- Teach patient about detection of clots using Homans' sign; teach monitoring technique for heat, redness, pain, swelling
- Teach patient to use sunscreen or to avoid sunlight; photosensitivity can occur
- Teach patient to take at same time each day to ensure equal drug level; to take another tab as soon as possible if one is missed; teach patient that after drug is discontinued, pregnancy may not occur for several mo
- Instruct patient to report GI symptoms that occur after 4 mo
- Advise patient to use another birth control method during first 3 wk of oral contraceptive use
- Teach patient to report abdominal pain, change in vision, shortness of breath, change in menstrual flow, spotting, breakthrough bleeding, breast lumps, swelling, headache, severe leg pain, mental changes; that continuing medical care is needed: PAP smear and gynecologic examinations q6 mo
- Teach patient to notify physicians and dentist of oral contraceptive use

Evaluation

Positive therapeutic outcome

- Absence of pregnancy
- Decreased severity of endometriosis
- Decreased severity of hypermenorrhea

oxacillin

(ox-a-sill'in)

Bactocill, oxacillin sodium, Prostaphilin

Func. class.: Broad-spectrum antiinfective

Chem. class.: Penicillinase-resistant penicillin

Pregnancy category **B**

Action: Interferes with cell wall replication of susceptible organisms; osmotically unstable cell wall swells, bursts from osmotic pressure

Uses: Infections caused by penicillinase-producing staphylococci, streptococci; respiratory tract, skin, skin structure urinary tract, bone, joint infections, sinusitis, endocarditis, septicemia, meningitis

➔ Therapeutic Outcome: Bactericidal effects for gram-positive cocci *Staphylococcus aureus, Streptococcus pneumoniae,* infections caused by penicillinase-producing *staphylococci*

Dosage and routes

Adult: PO 2-6 g/day in divided doses q4-6h; IM/**IV** 2-12 g/day in divided doses q4-6h

P *Child:* PO 50-100 mg/kg/day in divided doses q6h; IM/**IV** 50-100 mg/kg/day in divided doses q4-6h

Available forms: Cap 250, 500 mg; powder for oral susp 250 mg/5 ml; powder for inj

250, 500 mg, 1, 2, 4, 10 g; inf 1, 2 g

Side effects/adverse reactions

CNS: Lethargy, hallucinations, anxiety, depression, twitching, ***coma, convulsions***
GI: Nausea, vomiting, diarrhea, increased AST (SGOT), ALT (SGPT), abdominal pain, glossitis, colitis
GU: Oliguria, proteinuria, hematuria, vaginitis, moniliasis, glomerulonephritis
HEMA: Anemia, increased bleeding time, ***bone marrow depression, granulocytopenia***

Contraindications: Hypersensitivity to penicillins

Precautions: Pregnancy **B**, hypersensitivity to cephalosporins, neonates

P

Pharmacokinetics

Absorption	Rapid, incomplete (PO); well absorbed (IM); completely (IV)
Distribution	Widely distributed; crosses placenta
Metabolism	Liver
Excretion	Kidneys, unchanged (51%); breast milk
Half-life	20-50 min; increased in severe hepatic disease

Pharmacodynamics

	PO	IM	IV
Onset	Rapid	Rapid	Rapid
Peak	½-1 hr	½ hr	Inf end

Interactions

Drug/drug:

Individual drugs

Aspirin: ↑ oxacillin levels, ↓ renal excretion
Chloramphenicol: ↑ half-life of chloramphenicol, ↓ effectiveness of oxacillin
Cholestyramine: ↓ effectiveness of oxacillin
Colestipol: ↓ effectiveness of oxacillin
Probenecid: ↑ oxacillin levels, ↓ renal excretion

Drug classifications

Erythromycins: ↓ antimicrobial effectiveness
Oral anticoagulants: ↑ anticoagulant effects
Oral contraceptives: ↓ contraceptive effectiveness
Tetracyclines: ↓ antimicrobial effectiveness

Drug/food:

Food, carbonated drinks, citrus fruit juices: ↓ absorption

Lab test interferences

False positive: Urine glucose, urine protein

O

NURSING CONSIDERATIONS

Assessment

- Assess patient for previous sensitivity reaction to penicillins or other cephalosporins; cross-sensitivity between penicillins and cephalosporins is common
- Assess patient for signs and symptoms of infection including characteristics of wounds, sputum, urine, stool, WBC >10,000, fever; obtain baseline information and during treatment
- Obtain C&S before beginning drug therapy to identify if correct treatment has been initiated
- Assess for allergic reactions:

rash, urticaria, pruritus, chills, fever, joint pain; angioedema may occur a few days after therapy begins; epinephrine, resuscitation equipment should be available for anaphylactic reaction

- Assess urine output; if decreasing, notify prescriber (may indicate nephrotoxicity); also check for increased BUN, creatinine
- Monitor blood studies: AST (SGOT), ALT (SGPT), CBC, Hct, bilirubin, LDH, alkaline phosphatase, Coombs' test monthly if patient is on long-term therapy
- Monitor electrolytes: potassium, sodium, chloride monthly if patient is on long-term therapy
- Assess bowel pattern qd; if severe diarrhea occurs, drug should be discontinued; may indicate pseudomembranous colitis
- Monitor for bleeding: ecchymosis, bleeding gums, hematuria, stool guaiac daily if on long-term therapy
- Assess for overgrowth of infection: perineal itching, fever, malaise, redness, pain, swelling, drainage, rash, diarrhea, change in cough, sputum

Associated nursing diagnoses

- ✓ Infection, risk for (uses)
- ✓ Diarrhea (adverse reactions)
- ✓ Injury, risk for (adverse reactions)
- ✓ Knowledge deficit (teaching)
- ✓ Noncompliance (teaching)

Implementation

PO route

- Give in even doses around the clock; if GI upset occurs, give with food; drug must be given for 10-14 days to ensure organism death and prevent superinfection; store in tight container
- Shake susp; store in refrigerator for 2 wk, 1 wk at room temp

IM route

- Reconstitute 250 mg/1.4 ml, 500 mg/2.7-2.8 ml, 1 g/5.7 ml, 2 g/11.4-11.5 ml, 4 g/21.8-23 ml of sterile water for a conc of 250 mg/1.5 ml; store unused portion in refrigerator for 1 wk or 3 days at room temp
- Inject deeply in large muscle mass

IV **IV route**

- Reconstitute 250 mg/1.4 ml, 500 mg/2.7-2.8 ml, 1 g/5.7 ml, 2 g/11.4-11.5 ml, 4 g/21.8-23 ml of sterile water for a conc of 250 mg/1.5 ml; store unused portion in refrigerator for 1 week or 3 days at room temp
- Give direct **IV** by diluting reconstituted sol with 250-500 mg/5 ml, 1 g/10 ml, 2 g/20 ml, 4 g/40 ml of sterile water or 0.9% NaCl, give over 10 min
- Give by intermittent inf by diluting to a conc of 0.5-40 mg/ml with D_5W, 0.9% NaCl, D_5/0.9% NaCl, LR; give over 6 hr or less

Y-site incompatibility:

Verapamil

Y-site compatibilities:

Acyclovir, cyclophosphamide, famotidine, fluconazole, foscarnet, heparin, hydrocortisone sodium succinate, hydromorphone, labetalol, magnesium sulfate, meperidine, morphine, perphenazine, potassium chloride, vitamin B with C, zidovudine

Additive incompatibilities: Cytarabine, tetracycline

Additive compatibilities: Cephapirin, chloramphenicol, dopamine, potassium chloride, sodium bicarbonate

Patient/family education

- Teach patient to report sore throat, bruising, bleeding, joint pain; may indicate blood dyscrasias (rare)
- Advise patient to contact prescriber if vaginal itching, loose, foul-smelling stools, furry tongue occur; may indicate superinfection
- Instruct patient to take all medication prescribed for the length of time ordered
- Advise patient to notify prescriber of diarrhea with blood or pus, which may indicate pseudomembranous colitis

Evaluation

Positive therapeutic outcome

- Absence of signs/symptoms of infection (WBC <10,000, temp WNL, absence of red, draining wounds)
- Reported improvement in symptoms of infection

Treatment of anaphylaxis: Withdraw drug, maintain airway, administer epinephrine, aminophylline, O_2, **IV** corticosteroids

oxaprozin

(ox-a-proe′zin)

Daypro

Func. class.: Nonsteroidal antiinflammatory

Chem. class.: Propionic acid derivative

Pregnancy category **C**

Action: Inhibits prostaglandin synthesis by decreasing an enzyme needed for biosynthesis; analgesic, antiinflammatory

➔ **Therapeutic Outcome:** Decreased pain, inflammation

Uses: Acute and long-term management of osteoarthritis, rheumatoid arthritis

Dosage and routes

Adult: PO 600-1200 mg qd; maximum dose 1800 mg/day or 26 mg/kg, whichever is lower in divided doses

Available forms: Tab 600 mg

Side effects/adverse reactions

CNS: Dizziness, headache, drowsiness, fatigue, tremors, confusion, insomnia, anxiety, malaise, depression

CV: Tachycardia, peripheral edema, palpitations, dysrhythmias

EENT: Tinnitus, hearing loss, blurred vision

GI: Nausea, *anorexia,* vomiting, *diarrhea,* jaundice, ***cholestatic hepatitis,*** constipation, flatulence, *cramps,* dry mouth, peptic ulcer, ***bleeding,*** melena, gastroenteritis

O

GU:* *Nephrotoxicity: dysuria, hematuria, oliguria, azotemia
HEMA: Increased bleeding time
INTEG: Purpura, rash, pruritus, sweating, photosensitivity
SYST:* *Anaphylaxis, angioneurotic edema

Contraindications: Hypersensitivity, asthma, patients in whom aspirin and iodides have induced symptoms of allergic reactions or asthma

Precautions: Pregnancy **C** 1st and 2nd trimester, lactation, P children, bleeding disorders, GI disorders, cardiac disorders, hypersensitivity to other antiinflammatory agents, severe renal G and hepatic disease, elderly

Pharmacokinetics	
Absorption	Well absorbed (PO)
Distribution	Unknown
Metabolism	Liver, extensively
Excretion	Breast milk
Half-life	40-50 hr

Pharmacodynamics	
Onset	Unknown
Peak	2 hr
Duration	Unknown

Interactions
Drug/drug:
Individual drugs
Acetaminophen (long-term use): ↑ renal reactions
Alcohol: ↑ adverse reactions
Aspirin: ↓ effectiveness, ↑ adverse reactions
Coumarin: ↑ anticoagulant effects
Digoxin: ↑ toxicity, levels
Insulin: ↑ insulin effect
Lithium: ↑ toxicity
Methotrexate: ↑ toxicity
Sulfonylurea: ↑ toxicity
Drug classifications
Anticoagulants: ↑ risk of bleeding
Antihypertensives: ↓ effect of antihypertensives
Antineoplastics: ↑ risk of hematologic toxicity
β-Blockers: ↑ antihypertension
Cephalosporins: ↑ risk of bleeding
Glucocorticoids: ↑ adverse reactions
Hypoglycemics: ↓ hypoglycemic effect
Diuretics: ↓ effectiveness of diuretics
NSAIDs: ↑ adverse reactions
Potassium supplements: ↑ adverse reactions
Radiation: ↑ risk of hematologic toxicity
Sulfonamides: ↑ toxicity

Lab test interferences
Increase: BUN, alkaline phosphatase
False increase: 5-HIAA, 17KGS

NURSING CONSIDERATIONS
Assessment
- Assess for pain and ROM: intensity, location, duration
- Monitor blood studies: alkaline phosphatase, LDH, AST (SGOT), ALT (SGPT), and bleeding time (may be increased)

Associated nursing diagnoses
✓ Pain (uses)
✓ Mobility, impaired (uses)

✓ Injury, risk for (adverse reactions)
✓ Knowledge deficit (teaching)

Implementation

PO route

- Give with food or milk to decrease gastric symptoms

Patient/family education

- Teach patient that drug must be continued for prescribed time to be effective; to avoid aspirin, alcoholic beverages
- Instruct patient to use caution when driving; drowsiness, dizziness may occur
- Teach patient to take with a full glass of water to enhance absorption; do not crush, break, or chew; patient should sit upright for 30 min to prevent stomach irritation and ulceration
- Instruct patient to use sunscreen and protective clothing to prevent burns
- Advise patient to report to prescriber severe abdominal pain, rash, itching, yellowing of skin or eyes, depression

Evaluation

Positive therapeutic outcome

- Decreased pain
- Decreased inflammation
- Increased mobility

oxazepam

(ox-az'e-pam)
Apo-Oxazepam ♣, Novoxapam ♣, oxazepam, Ox-Pam ♣, Serax, Zapex ♣
Func. class.: Sedative/hypnotic; antianxiety
Chem. class.: Benzodiazepine
Pregnancy category **D**
Controlled substance schedule **IV**

Action: Depresses subcortical levels of CNS, including limbic system, reticular formation; potentiates GABA

➔ **Therapeutic Outcome:** Decreased anxiety, successful alcohol withdrawal, relaxation

Uses: Anxiety, alcohol withdrawal

Dosage and routes

Anxiety

Adult: PO 10-30 mg tid-qid

Alcohol withdrawal

Adult: PO 15-30 mg tid-qid

Available forms: Cap 10, 15, 30 mg; tab 15 mg

Side effects/adverse reactions

CNS: Dizziness, drowsiness, confusion, headache, anxiety, tremors, fatigue, depression, insomnia, hallucinations, paradoxic excitement, transient amnesia
CV: Orthostatic hypotension,

O

ECG changes, tachycardia, hypotension
EENT: ***Blurred vision,*** tinnitus, mydriasis
GI: Nausea, vomiting, anorexia
INTEG: Rash, dermatitis, itching

Contraindications: Hypersensitivity to benzodiazepines, narrow angle glaucoma, psychosis, pregnancy **D**, child <12 yr

Precautions: Elderly, debilitated, hepatic disease, renal disease

Pharmacokinetics

Absorption	Well absorbed (PO)
Distribution	Widely distributed; crosses placenta, blood-brain barrier
Metabolism	Liver
Excretion	Kidneys, breast milk
Half-life	5-15 hr

Pharmacodynamics

Onset	½-1½ hr
Peak	Unknown
Duration	6-12 hr

Interactions

Drug/drug:

Individual drugs

Alcohol: ↑ CNS depression
Cimetidine: ↑ action
Fluoxetine: ↑ action
Levodopa: ↓ action of levodopa
Metoprolol: ↑ action
Phenytoin: ↓ effect
Propoxyphene: ↑ action
Theophylline: ↓ sedative effects

Drug classifications

Analgesics, opioid: ↑ CNS depression
Antidepressants: ↑ CNS depression
Antihistamines: ↑ CNS depression
Oral contraceptives: ↑ effect

Lab test interferences

Increase: AST (SGOT), ALT (SGPT), serum bilirubin
False increase: 17-OHCS
Decrease: RAIU

NURSING CONSIDERATIONS

Assessment

- Assess mental status: mood, sensorium, anxiety, affect, sleeping pattern, drowsiness, dizziness, especially elderly; physical dependency, withdrawal symptoms: anxiety, panic attacks, agitation, convulsions, headache, nausea, vomiting, muscle pain, weakness; suicidal tendencies; indications of increasing tolerance and abuse
- Monitor B/P with patient lying, standing, pulse; if systolic B/P drops 20 mm Hg, hold drug, notify prescriber
- Monitor blood studies: CBC during long-term therapy; blood dyscrasias have occurred rarely; decreased hematocrit, neutropenia may occur
- Monitor hepatic studies: AST (SGOT), ALT (SGPT), bilirubin, creatinine LDH, alkaline phosphatase
- Monitor I&O; indicate renal dysfunction

Associated nursing diagnoses

✓ Anxiety (uses)
✓ Depression (uses)
✓ Injury, risk for (adverse reactions)

✓ Knowledge deficit (teaching)

Implementation

PO route

- Give with food or milk for GI symptoms; tab may be crushed if patient is unable to swallow medication whole; give sugarless gum, hard candy, frequent sips of water for dry mouth

Patient/family education

- Teach patient that drug may be taken with food or fluids; tab may be crushed or swallowed whole
- Caution patient not to use for everyday stress or longer than 3 mo unless directed by prescriber; not to take more than prescribed amount; may be habit forming; not to double doses or skip doses
- Advise patient to avoid OTC preparations unless approved by prescriber; alcohol and CNS depressants will increase CNS depression
- Caution patient to avoid driving and activities that require alertness, since drowsiness may occur; to avoid alcohol and other psychotropic medications; to rise slowly or fainting may occur, especially G elderly; that drowsiness may worsen at beginning of treatment
- Caution patient not to discontinue medication abruptly after long-term use; withdrawal symptoms include vomiting, cramping, tremors, seizures

Evaluation

Positive therapeutic outcome

- Decreased anxiety, restlessness, sleeplessness (short-term treatment only)

Treatment of overdose: Lavage, VS, supportive care

oxtriphylline

(ox-trye'fi-lin)

Apo-Oxtriphylline ✦, Choledyl, Choledyl SA, Novotriphyl ✦, oxtriphylline

Func. class.: Bronchodilator, spasmolytic

Chem. class.: Choline salt of theophylline

Pregnancy category **C**

Action: Relaxes smooth muscle of respiratory system by blocking phosphodiesterase, which increases cAMP; 64% theophylline

➔ **Therapeutic Outcome:** Bronchodilatation with ease of breathing

Uses: Acute bronchial asthma, reversible bronchospasm in chronic bronchitis and COPD

Dosage and routes

P *Adult and child >12 yr:* PO 200 mg qid or sus action q12h

P *Child 2-12 yr:* PO 4 mg/kg q6h; may be increased to desired response, therapeutic level

Available forms: Elix 100 mg/5 ml; syr 50 mg/5 ml; tab 100, 200, 400, 600 mg; sus action tab 400, 600 mg

O

Side effects/adverse reactions

CNS: Anxiety, restlessness, insomnia, dizziness, ***convulsions****,* headache, lightheadedness
CV: Palpitations, sinus tachycardia, hypotension
GI: Nausea, vomiting, anorexia, diarrhea, bitter taste, dyspepsia
INTEG: Flushing, urticaria, alopecia
RESP: Increased rate

Contraindications: Hypersensitivity to xanthines, tachydysrhythmias

G **Precautions:** Elderly, CHF, cor pulmonale, hepatic disease, active peptic ulcer disease, diabetes mellitus, hyperthy-
P roidism, hypertension, children, pregnancy **C**, glaucoma, prostatic hypertrophy

Pharmacokinetics

Absorption	Well absorbed (PO); slow (PO-SA)
Distribution	Widely distributed; crosses placenta
Metabolism	Liver to caffeine
Excretion	Kidneys, breast milk
Half-life	3-13 hr; increased in renal disease, CHF

Pharmacodynamics

	PO	PO-SA
Onset	15-60 min	Unknown
Peak	1-5 hr	4-8 hr
Duration	6-8 hr	8-12 hr

Interactions

Drug/drug:

Individual drugs
Allopurinol: ↓ metabolism, ↑ toxicity
Carbamazepine: ↑ or ↓ oxtriphylline levels
Cimetidine: ↓ metabolism, ↑ toxicity
Disulfiram: ↓ metabolism, ↑ toxicity
Erythromycin: ↓ metabolism, ↑ toxicity
Halothane: ↑ risk of dysrhythmias
Interferon: ↓ metabolism, ↑ toxicity
Isoniazid: ↑ or ↓ oxtriphylline level
Ketoconazole: ↑ metabolism, ↓ effect
Lithium: ↓ effect of lithium
Mexiletine: ↓ metabolism, ↑ toxicity
Phenytoin: ↑ metabolism, ↓ effect
Rifampin: ↑ metabolism, ↓ effect
Thiabendazole: ↓ metabolism, ↑ toxicity

Drug classifications
Barbiturates: ↓ effect of oxtriphylline
β-Adrenergic blockers: ↓ metabolism, ↑ toxicity
Diuretics, loop: ↑ or ↓ oxtriphylline levels
Fluoroquinolones: ↓ metabolism, ↑ toxicity
Glucocorticoids: ↓ metabolism, ↑ toxicity
Sympathomimetics: ↑ CNS, CV adverse reactions

Drug/smoking:

↑ metabolism, ↓ effect

Drug/food:

Caffeinated foods (cola, coffee, tea, chocolate): ↑ CNS, CV adverse reactions

Lab test interferences

Increase: Plasma free fatty acids

NURSING CONSIDERATIONS

Assessment

• Monitor blood levels (therapeutic level is 10-20 μg/ml); toxicity may occur with small increase above 20 μg/ml, G especially elderly; check whether theophylline was given recently (24 hr)

• Monitor I&O; diuresis can occur; dehydration may result G in elderly or children

P • Monitor respiratory rate, rhythm, depth; auscultate lung fields bilaterally; notify prescriber of abnormalities

• Monitor allergic reactions: rash, urticaria; if these occur, drug should be discontinued

Associated nursing diagnoses

✓ Airway clearance, ineffective (uses)
✓ Activity intolerance (uses)
✓ Injury, risk for (uses, adverse reactions)
✓ Knowledge deficit (teaching)

Implementation

PO route

• Give PO pc to decrease GI symptoms; absorption may be affected with a full glass of water; do not crush or chew enteric coated or SA tab

Patient/family education

• Teach patient to take doses as prescribed, not to skip dose; to check OTC medications, current prescription medications for ephedrine, which will increase CNS stimulation; not to drink alcohol or caffeine products (tea, coffee, chocolate, colas)

• Caution patient to avoid hazardous activities; dizziness may occur

• Instruct patient if GI upset occurs, to take drug with 8 oz water or food

• Advise patient to remain in bed 15-20 min after rec supp is inserted to prevent loss

• Teach patient to notify prescriber of change in smoking habit; a change in dosage may be required

• Teach patient to increase fluids to 2L/day to decrease viscosity of secretions

Evaluation

Positive therapeutic outcome

• Decreased dyspnea
• Clear lung fields bilaterally

oxybutynin

(ox-i-byoo'ti-nin)

Ditropan, oxybutynin chloride

Func. class.: Spasmolytic, urinary

Chem. class.: Synthetic tertiary amine

Pregnancy category **C**

Action: Relaxes smooth muscles in urinary tract by inhibiting acetylcholine at postganglionic sites

➡ **Therapeutic Outcome:** Decreased symptoms of urgency, nocturia, incontinence

Uses: Antispasmodic for neurogenic bladder

O

Dosage and routes

Adult: PO 5 mg bid-tid, not to exceed 5 mg qid

P *Child >5 yr:* PO 5 mg bid, not to exceed 5 mg tid

Available forms: Syrup 5 mg/5 ml; tab 5 mg

Side effects/adverse reactions

CNS: Anxiety, restlessness, dizziness, ***convulsions,*** headache, drowsiness, confusion
CV: Palpitations, sinus tachycardia, hypotension
EENT: Blurred vision, increased intraocular tension, dry mouth, throat
GI: Nausea, vomiting, anorexia, abdominal pain, constipation
GU: Dysuria, retention, hesitancy
HEMA: ***Leukopenia, eosinophilia***
INTEG: Urticaria, dermatitis

Contraindications: Hypersensitivity, GI obstruction, GI hemorrhage, GU obstruction, glaucoma, severe colitis, myasthenia gravis, unstable CV status in acute hemorrhage

Precautions: Pregnancy **C**, lactation, suspected glaucoma, P children <12 yr

Pharmacokinetics

Absorption	Rapidly absorbed (PO)
Distribution	Unknown
Metabolism	Liver
Excretion	Unknown
Half-life	Unknown

Pharmacodynamics

Onset	½-1 hr
Peak	3-4 hr
Duration	6-10 hr

Interactions

Drug/drug:

Individual drugs

Alcohol: ↑ CNS depression
Disopyramide: ↑ anticholinergic effects
Haloperidol: ↑ anticholinergic effects

Drug classifications

Analgesics, narcotic: ↑ CNS depressants
Antidepressants: ↑ anticholinergic effects
Antihistamines: ↑ CNS depression
Phenothiazines: ↑ anticholinergic effects
Sedative/hypnotics: ↑ CNS depressants

NURSING CONSIDERATIONS

Assessment

- Assess for allergic reactions: rash, urticaria; if these occur, drug should be discontinued
- Assess urinary patterns: distention, nocturia, frequency, urgency, incontinence; catheterization may be required to remove residual urine

Associated nursing diagnoses

✓ Urinary elimination, altered patterns (uses)
✓ Pain (uses)
✓ Knowledge deficit (teaching)

Implementation

PO route

- May be given with meals or

fluids or given on an empty stomach

Patient/family education

- Advise patient to avoid hazardous activities until response to drug is known; dizziness may occur
- Caution patient to avoid OTC medication with alcohol or other CNS depressants
- Advise patient to prevent photophobia by wearing sunglasses
- Caution patient to stay cool, since overheating may occur
- Teach patient to use frequent rinsing of mouth, sips of water

Evaluation

Positive therapeutic outcome

- Absence of dysuria, frequency, nocturia, incontinence

oxycodone

(ox-i-koe'done)

Roxicodone Supeudol ✤; oxycodone/aspirin: Endodan ✤, Oxycodan ✤, Percodan, Percodan-Demi, Roxiprin; oxycodone/acetaminophen: Endocet ✤, Oxycocet ✤, Percocet, Roxicet, Roxilox, Tylox

Func. class.: Narcotic analgesic

Chem. class.: Opiate, semisynthetic derivative

Pregnancy category B

Controlled substance schedule II

Action: Inhibits ascending pain pathways in CNS, increases pain threshold, alters pain perception

➔ Therapeutic Outcome: Decreased pain

Uses: Moderate to severe pain

Dosage and routes

Adult: PO 5 mg q4-6h or 10 mg tid or qid prn

Available forms: Oxycodone: supp 10, 20 mg; tabs 5 mg; oral sol conc 20 mg/ml; oxycodone with acetaminophen: tab 5 mg/325 mg; cap 5 mg/500 mg; oral sol 5 mg/325 mg/5 ml; oxycodone with aspirin: 2.44 mg/325 mg, 4.88/325 mg

Side effects/adverse reactions

CNS: Drowsiness, dizziness, confusion, headache, sedation, euphoria

CV: Palpitations, bradycardia, change in B/P

EENT: Tinnitus, blurred vision, miosis, diplopia

GI: Nausea, vomiting, anorexia, constipation, cramps

GU: Increased urinary output, dysuria, urinary retention

INTEG: Rash, urticaria, bruising, flushing, diaphoresis, pruritus

RESP: Respiratory depression

Contraindications: Hypersensitivity, addiction (narcotic)

Precautions: Addictive personality, pregnancy **B**, lactation, increased intracranial pressure, MI (acute), severe heart disease, respiratory depression, hepatic disease, renal disease, child <18 yr

Pharmacokinetics

Absorption	Well absorbed
Distribution	Widely distributed; crosses placenta
Metabolism	Liver, extensively
Excretion	Kidneys, breast milk
Half-life	2-3 hr

Pharmacodynamics

	PO	REC
Onset	10-15 min	Unknown
Peak	½-1 hr	Unknown
Duration	4-6 hr	4-6 hr

Interactions

Drug/drug:

Individual drugs

Alcohol: ↑ respiratory depression, hypotension, sedation
Nalbuphine: ↓ analgesia
Pentazocine: ↓ analgesia

Drug classifications

Antihistamines: ↑ respiratory depression, hypotension
CNS depressants: ↑ respiratory depression, hypotension
MAOI: Do not use 2 wk before oxycodone
Phenothiazines: ↑ respiratory depression, hypotension
Sedative/hypnotics: ↑ respiratory depression, hypotension

Lab test interferences

Increase: Amylase

NURSING CONSIDERATIONS

Assessment

- Monitor VS after parenteral route; note muscle rigidity, drug history, liver, kidney function tests, respiratory dysfunction: respiratory depression, character, rate, rhythm; notify prescriber if respirations are <10/min
- Monitor CNS changes: dizziness, drowsiness, hallucinations, euphoria, LOC, pupil reaction
- Monitor allergic reactions: rash, urticaria

Associated nursing diagnoses

- ✓ Pain (uses)
- ✓ Sensory-perceptual alteration: visual, auditory (adverse reactions)
- ✓ Breathing pattern, ineffective (adverse reactions)
- ✓ Injury, risk for (adverse reactions)
- ✓ Knowledge deficit (teaching)

Implementation

- Give with antiemetic if nausea, vomiting occur
- Give when pain is beginning to return; determine dosage interval by patient response; continuous dosing of medication is more effective than when given prn
- Medication should be slowly withdrawn after long-term use to prevent withdrawal symptoms
- Store in light-resistant container at room temp

PO route

- May be given with food or milk to lessen GI upset

Rec route

- Store supp in the refrigerator; run under warm water before insertion

Patient/family education

- Advise patients to avoid CNS depressants: alcohol, sedative/hypnotics
- Discuss with patient that dizziness, drowsiness, and confusion are common; to avoid getting up without assistance
- Discuss in detail all aspects of the drug, including purpose and what to expect
- Advise patient to make position changes slowly to lessen orthostatic hypotension

Evaluation

Positive therapeutic outcome
- Decreased pain

Treatment of overdose:
Narcan 0.2-0.8 **IV**, O_2, **IV** fluids, vasopressors

oxymetazoline

(ox-i-met-az'oh-leen)

Afrin, Afrin Children's Nose Drops, Allerest 12-Hour Nasal, Chlorphed-LA, Coricidin Nasal Mist, Dristan Long Lasting, Duramist Plus, Duration, Genasal, NTZ Long-Acting Nasal, Nafrine ✱, Neo-Synephrine 12 Hour, Nostrilla, oxymetazoline HCl, Sinarest 12-Hour, Sinex Long-Acting, Twice-A-Day Nasal, 4-Way Long Acting Nasal

Func. class.: Nasal decongestant

Chem. class.: Sympathomimetic amine

Pregnancy category C

Action: Produces vasoconstriction (rapid, long-acting) of arterioles, thereby decreasing fluid exudation, mucosal engorgement by stimulation of α-adrenergic receptors in vascular smooth muscle

➡ **Therapeutic Outcome:** Absence of nasal congestion

Uses: Nasal congestion

Dosage and routes

P ***Adult and child >6 yr:*** Instill 2-3 gtt or sprays to each nostril bid

P ***Child 2-6 yr:*** Instill 2-3 gtt or sprays 0.025% sol bid, not to exceed 3 days

Available forms: Nasol sol 0.025%, 0.05%

Side effects/adverse reactions

CNS: Anxiety, restlessness, tremors, weakness, insomnia, dizziness, fever, headache
EENT: Irritation, burning, sneezing, stinging, dryness, rebound congestion
GI: Nausea, vomiting, anorexia
INTEG: Contact dermatitis

Contraindications: Hypersensitivity to sympathomimetic amines

P G **Precautions:** Child <6 yr, elderly, diabetes, cardiovascular disease, hypertension, hyperthyroidism, increased intracranial pressure, prostatic hypertrophy, pregnancy **C**, glaucoma

Interactions

Drug/drug:

Individual drugs

Mecamylamine: ↑ hypotension
Methyldopa: ↑ hypotension
Reserpine: ↑ hypotension

Drug classifications

β-Adrenergic blockers: ↑ hypertension
MAOI: ↑ hypertension

NURSING CONSIDERATIONS

Assessment

- Assess for redness, swelling, pain in nasal passages before and during treatment
- Assess for syst absorption: hypertension, tachycardia; notify prescriber; syst absorption occurs at high doses or after prolonged use

Associated nursing diagnoses

- ✓ Airway clearance, ineffective (uses)
- ✓ Knowledge deficit (teaching)
- ✓ Noncompliance (teaching)

Implementation

Nasal route

- Have patient tilt head back, squeeze bulb to create a vacuum, and draw correct amount of sol into dropper; insert 2 gtt of sol into nostril; repeat in other nostril
- Store in light-resistant container; do not expose to high temp or let sol come into contact with aluminum
- Give for <4 consecutive days
- Provide environmental humidification to decrease nasal congestion, dryness

Patient/family education

- Advise patient that stinging may occur for several applications; drying of mucosa may be decreased by environmental humidification
- Caution patient to notify prescriber if irregular pulse, insomnia, dizziness, or tremors occur
- Teach patient proper administration to avoid syst absorption
- Advise patient to rinse dropper with very hot water to prevent contamination

Evaluation

Positive therapeutic outcome

- Decreased nasal congestion

oxymorphone

(ox-i-mor'fone)

Numorphan

Func. class.: Narcotic analgesic

Chem. class.: Opiate, semisynthetic phenanthrene derivative

Pregnancy category **B**

Controlled substance schedule **II**

Action: Depresses pain impulse transmission at the spinal cord level by interacting with opioid receptors

➔ Therapeutic Outcome: Decreased pain

Uses: Moderate to severe pain

Dosage and routes

Adult: IM/SC 1-1.5 mg q4-6h prn; **IV** 0.5 mg q4-6h prn; rec 2.5-5 mg q4-6h prn

Labor analgesia

Adult: IM 0.5-1 mg

Available forms: Inj 1, 1.5 mg/ml; supp 5 mg

Side effects/adverse reactions

CNS: *Drowsiness, dizziness, confusion, headache, sedation, euphoria*

CV: Palpitations, bradycardia, change in B/P

EENT: Tinnitus, blurred vision, miosis, diplopia

GI: *Nausea, vomiting, anorexia, constipation, cramps*

GU: Increased urinary output, dysuria, urinary retention

INTEG: *Rash,* urticaria, bruising, flushing, diaphoresis, pruritus

RESP: Respiratory depression

Contraindications: Hypersensitivity, addiction (narcotic)

Precautions: Addictive personality, pregnancy **B**, lactation, increased intracranial pressure, MI (acute), severe heart disease, respiratory depression, hepatic disease, renal disease, P child <18 yr

Pharmacokinetics

Absorption	Well absorbed (rec, IM, SC); completely absorbed (IV)
Distribution	Widely distributed; crosses placenta
Metabolism	Liver, extensively
Excretion	Kidneys
Half-life	2½-4 hr

Pharmacodynamics

	IM/SC	IV	REC
Onset	15 min	10 min	30 min
Peak	1-1½ hr	15-30 min	Unknown
Duration	2-6 hr	3-4 hr	3-6 hr

Interactions

Drug/drug:

Individual drugs

Alcohol: ↑ respiratory depression, hypotension, sedation

Nalbuphine: ↓ analgesia

Pentazocine: ↓ analgesia

O

Drug classifications
Antihistamines: ↑ respiratory depression, hypotension
CNS depressants: ↑ respiratory depression, hypotension
MAOI: Do not use 2 wk before oxymorphone
Sedative/hypnotics: ↑ respiratory depression, hypotension

Lab test interferences

Increase: Amylase, lipase

NURSING CONSIDERATIONS

Assessment

- Monitor VS after parenteral route; note muscle rigidity, drug history, liver, kidney function tests, respiratory dysfunction: respiratory depression, character, rate, rhythm; notify prescriber if respirations are <10/min
- Monitor CNS changes: dizziness, drowsiness, hallucinations, euphoria, LOC, pupil reaction
- Monitor allergic reactions: rash, urticaria

Associated nursing diagnoses

✓ Pain (uses)
✓ Sensory-perceptual alteration: visual, auditory (adverse reactions)
✓ Breathing pattern, ineffective (adverse reactions)
✓ Injury, risk for (adverse reactions)
✓ Knowledge deficit (teaching)

Implementation

- Give with antiemetic if nausea, vomiting occur
- Give when pain is beginning to return; determine dosage interval by patient response; continuous dosing of medication is more effective than when given prn
- Medication should be slowly withdrawn after long-term use to prevent withdrawal symptoms
- Store in light-resistant container at room temp

Rec route
- Store in refrigerator

IV **IV route**
- Give by direct **IV** undiluted over 2-3 min

Y-site compatibilities:

Glycopyrrolate, hydroxyzine, ranitidine

Patient/family education

- Advise patients to avoid CNS depressants: alcohol, sedative/hypnotics
- Discuss with patient that dizziness, drowsiness, and confusion are common; to avoid getting up without assistance
- Discuss in detail all aspects of the drug, including purpose and what to expect
- Advise patient to make position changes slowly to lessen orthostatic hypotension

Evaluation

Positive therapeutic outcome
- Decreased pain

Treatment of overdose:

Naloxone (Narcan) 0.2-0.8 **IV**, O_2, **IV** fluids, vasopressors

oxytocin

(ox-i-toe'sin)

Pitocin, Syntocinon

Func. class.: Oxytocic hormone

Chem. class.:

Pregnancy category **N/A**

Action: Acts directly on myofibrils, producing uterine contraction; stimulates breast milk letdown

Therapeutic Outcome: Stimulation of labor, control of bleeding; stimulation of milk letdown

Uses: Stimulation, induction of labor; missed or incomplete abortion, postpartum bleeding, postpartum breast engorgement, initial milk letdown

Dosage and routes

Labor induction

Adult: **IV** 0.5-2 μU/min, increase by 1-2 μU q15-60 min until regular contractions occur, then decrease dosage

Postpartum hemorrhage

Adult: **IV** 10 U infused at 20-40 μU/min

Adult: IM 10 U after placenta delivery

Incomplete abortion

Adult: **IV** 10 U at a rate of 20-40 μU/min

Fetal stress test

Adult: **IV** 0.5 μU/min; increase q20 min until 3 contractions occur at 10 min; not to exceed 20 μU only with fetal monitoring

Milk letdown

Adult: Instill 1 spray into one or both nostrils q2-3 min before breastfeeding; instill 3 gtt into one or both nostrils q2-3 min before breastfeeding

Available forms: Nasal spray 40 U/ml; inj 10 U/ml

Side effects/adverse reactions

CNS: Hypertension, ***convulsions, tetanic contractions***

CV: Hypotension, dysrhythmias, increased pulse, bradycardia, tachycardia, PVC

FETUS: Dysrhythmias, jaundice, hypoxia, ***intracranial hemorrhage***

GI: Anorexia, nausea, vomiting, constipation

GU: ***Abruptio placentae, decreased uterine blood flow***

HEMA: Increased hyperbilirubinemia

INTEG: Rash

RESP: Asphyxia

Contraindications: Hypersensitivity, PIH, cephalopelvic disproportion, fetal distress, hypertonic uterus

Precautions: Cervical/uterine surgery, uterine sepsis, primipara >35 yr, 1st, 2nd stage of labor

Pharmacokinetics

Absorption	Well absorbed (nasal); completely absorbed (IV)
Distribution	Widely distributed (extracellular fluid)
Metabolism	Liver, rapidly
Excretion	Kidneys
Half-life	3-12 min

O

Pharmacodynamics

	NASAL	IV	IM
Onset	5 min	Rapid	3-7 min
Peak	Unknown	Unknown	Unknown
Duration	20 min	1 hr	1 hr

Interactions

Drug/drug:

Individual drugs

Cyclopropane anesthesia: ↑ hypotension

Drug classifications

Vasopressors: ↑ hypertension

NURSING CONSIDERATIONS

Assessment

- Assess labor contractions: fetal heart tones, frequency, duration, intensity of contractions; if fetal heart tones increase or decrease significantly or if contractions are longer than 1 min, notify prescriber; turn patient on left side to increase oxygen to fetus
- Assess for water intoxication: confusion, anuria, drowsiness, headache; notify prescriber
- Watch for fetal distress, acceleration, deceleration, fetal presentation, pelvic dimensions
- Monitor B/P, pulse, respiratory rate, rhythm, depth
- Monitor I&O ratio
- Provide an environment conducive to letdown reflex

Associated nursing diagnoses

✓ Breastfeeding (uses)
✓ Injury, risk for (uses)
✓ Knowledge deficit (teaching)

Implementation

IV **IV route**

- Use an inf pump; rotate sol for mixing; have magnesium sulfate available
- For labor induction administer after diluting 10 U/1 L of D_5W, 0.9% NaCl, 0.45% NaCl, LR, Ringer's for a conc of 10 μU/ml; start at 1-2 μU/min (0.1-0.2 ml); may increase by 1-2 μU/min q15-30 min until labor begins
- For threatened abortion administer after diluting 10 U/500 ml of D_5W, $D_{10}W$, 0.9% NaCl, 0.45% NaCl, LR, Ringer's for a conc of 20 μU/ml; give at 10-40 μU/m
- For postpartum bleeding administer after diluting 10-40 U/L of D_5W, $D_{10}W$, 0.9% NaCl, 0.45% NaCl, LR, Ringer's for a conc of 10-40 μU/ml; may titrate to response

Additive incompatibilities:

Fibrinolysin, warfarin

Additive compatibilities:

Chloramphenicol, metaraminol, netilmicin, sodium bicarbonate, tetracycline, thiopental, verapamil

Y-site compatibilities:

Heparin, insulin hydrocortisone, meperidine, morphine, potassium chloride, vitamin B with C

Nasal route

- Have patient clear nasal passages before use; use product while holding upright

Patient/family education

Nasal route

- Advise patient to blow nose

before administering; not to overuse
• Teach patient to report increased blood loss, abdominal cramps, increased temp or foul-smelling lochia
• Advise patient that contractions will be similar to menstrual cramps, gradually increasing in intensity

Evaluation

Positive therapeutic outcome
• Stimulation of milk letdown (nasal)
• Induction of labor
• Decreased postpartum bleeding

paclitaxel
(pa-kli-tax'el)
Taxol
Func. class.: Miscellaneous antineoplastic
Chem. class.: Natural diterpene, antimicrotubule
Pregnancy category **D**

Action: Inhibits the reorganization of the microtubule network needed for interphase and mitotic cellular functions; also causes abnormal bundles of microtubules during cell cycle and multiple esters of microtubules during mitosis

Therapeutic Outcome: Prevention of rapidly growing malignant cells

Uses: Metastatic carcinoma of the ovary unresponsive to other treatment

Dosage and routes

Adults: **IV** inf 135 mg/m^2 given over 24 hr q 3 wk

Available forms: Inj 30 mg/5 ml vial

Side effects/adverse reactions

CV: Bradycardia, hypotension, abnormal ECG
GI: Nausea, vomiting, diarrhea, mucositis; increased bilirubin, alkaline phosphatase, AST (SGOT)
HEMA: Neutropenia, leukopenia, thrombocytopenia, anemia, bleeding, infections
INTEG: Alopecia
MS: Arthralgia, myalgia
NEURO: Peripheral neuropathy
*SYST: Hypersensitivity reactions, **anaphylaxis***

Contraindications: Hypersensitivity to paclitaxel or other drugs with polyoxyethylated castor oil, neutropenia of <1500/mm^3, pregnancy **D**

P Precautions: Children, lactation, hepatic disease, cardiovascular disease, CNS disorder

Pharmacokinetics	
Absorption	Completely absorbed (IV)
Distribution	89%-98% protein binding
Metabolism	Liver, extensively
Excretion	Unknown
Half-life	5-17 hr

Pharmacodynamics	
Onset	Unknown
Peak	1-2 wk
Duration	3 wk

P

Interactions

Drug/drug:

Individual drugs

Cisplatin: ↑ myleosuppression
Ketoconazole: ↑ toxicity

NURSING CONSIDERATIONS

Assessment

- Assess CNS changes: confusion, paresthesias, psychosis, tremors, seizures, neuropathies; drug should be discontinued
- Check buccal cavity q8h for dryness, sores or ulceration, white patches, oral pain, bleeding, dysphagia; obtain prescription for viscous lidocaine (Xylocaine) to use in mouth
- Assess symptoms indicating severe allergic reaction: rash, pruritus, urticaria, purpuric skin lesions, itching, flushing
- Monitor CBC, differential, platelet count weekly; withhold drug if WBC count is <4000/mm^3 or platelet count is <100,000/mm^3, notify prescriber of results
- Monitor renal function studies: BUN, creatinine, serum uric acid, urine CrCl before and during therapy; check I&O ratio; report fall in urine output to <30 ml/hr
- Monitor temp q4h (may indicate beginning of infection)
- Monitor liver function tests before and during therapy (bilirubin, AST [SGOT], ALT [SGPT], LDH) as needed or monthly; check for yellowing of skin and sclera, dark urine, clay-colored stools, itchy skin, abdominal pain, fever, diarrhea
- Assess for bleeding: hematuria, stool guaiac, bruising or petechiae, mucosa or orifices q8h; check for inflammation of mucosa, breaks in skin
- Assess effects of alopecia on body image; discuss feelings about body changes

Associated nursing diagnoses

- ☑ Injury, risk for (adverse reactions)
- ☑ Body image disturbance (adverse reactions)
- ☑ Infection, risk for (adverse reactions)
- ☑ Knowledge deficit (teaching)

Implementation

- Give fluids **IV** or PO before chemotherapy to hydrate patient
- Give antacid before oral agent; give drug after evening meal, before hs; provide antiemetic 30-60 min before giving drug and prn to prevent vomiting; administer antibiotics for prophylaxis of infection
- Give top or syst analgesics for pain to lessen effects of stomatitis
- Give liq diet: carbonated beverages; gelatin may be added if patient is not nauseated or vomiting
- Encourage patient to rinse mouth tid-qid with water, club soda; brush teeth bid-qid with soft brush or cotton-tipped applicators for stomatitis; use unwaxed dental floss

Patient/family education

- Inform patient that contraceptive measures are recommended during therapy and >4 mo after; teratogenic effects are possible

• Teach patient to avoid use of products containing aspirin or ibuprofen, razors, commercial mouthwash, since bleeding may occur; to report symptoms of bleeding (hematuria, tarry stools)
• Instruct patient to report signs of anemia (fatigue, headache, irritability, faintness, shortness of breath) and CNS reactions (confusion, psychosis, nightmares, seizures, severe headaches)
• Inform patient that hair may be lost during treatment; a wig or hair piece may make patient feel better; new hair may be different in color, texture
• Inform patient that receiving vaccinations during therapy may cause serious reactions

Evaluation

Positive therapeutic outcome
• Prevention of rapid division of malignant cells

pamidronate
(pam-i-drone′ate)
Aredia
Func. class.: Bone resorption inhibitor
Chem. class.: Bisphosphonate
Pregnancy category **C**

Action: Absorbs calcium phosphate crystals in bone and may directly block dissolution of hydroxyapatite crystals of bone; inhibits bone resorption, apparently without inhibiting bone formation and mineralization

➡ **Therapeutic Outcome:** Serum calcium at normal level

Uses: Moderate to severe hypercalcemia associated with malignancy with or without bone metastases

Dosage and routes

Adult: **IV** inf 60-90 mg in moderate hypercalcemia, 90 mg in severe hypercalcemia given over 24 hr

Available forms: Inj 30 mg pamidronate disodium and 470 mg of mannitol

Side effects/adverse reactions

CNS: Fatigue
CV: Hypertension, fluid overload, dysrhythmias, tachycardia
GI: Abdominal pain, anorexia, constipation, nausea, vomiting
GU: UTI, fluid overload
INTEG: Redness, swelling, induration, pain on palpation at site of catheter insertion
META: Anemia, hypokalemia, hypomagnesemia, hypophosphatemia
MS: Bone pain

Contraindications: Hypersensitivity to bisphosphonates

P **Precautions:** Children, nursing mothers, pregnancy **C**, renal dysfunction

P

Pharmacokinetics

Absorption	Rapidly cleared from circulation
Distribution	Mainly to bones
Metabolism	Unknown
Excretion	Kidneys, unchanged (50%)
Half-life	Biphasic 1½ hr; 27 hr; from bone to 300 days

Pharmacodynamics

Onset	1 day
Peak	1 wk
Duration	Unknown

Interactions: None

NURSING CONSIDERATIONS

Assessment

• Assess for hypocalcemia: Chuostek's, Trousseau's sign, paresthesia, twitching, laryngospasm
• Monitor manifestations of hypocalcemia: personality changes, anxiety, disturbances, depression, psychosis; nausea, vomiting, constipation, abdominal pain from muscle spasm; decreased contractility, decreased cardiac output, hypotension, lengthened ST segment, prolonged QT interval; scaling eczema, alopecia, hyperpigmentation; tetany, muscle twitching, cramping, grimacing, seizure, altered deep tendon reflexes, spasm
• Monitor for manifestations of hypomagnesemia: agitation; muscle twitching, paresthesia, hyperactive reflexes, positive Babinski reflex, dysphagia, nystagmus, seizures, tetany; nausea, vomiting, diarrhea, anorexia, abdominal distention; ectopy, tachycardia, broad, flat or inverted T waves, depressed ST segment, prolonged QT, decreased cardiac output, hypotension
• Monitor manifestations of hypokalemia: acidic urine, reduced urine osmolality, nocturia, polyuria, polydipsia; hypotension, broad T wave, U wave, ectopy, tachycardia, weak pulse; muscle weakness, altered LOC, drowsiness, apathy, lethargy, confusion, depression; anorexia, nausea, cramps, constipation, distention, paralytic ileus; hypoventilation, respiratory muscle weakness
• Assess fluid volume status: check I&O ratio and record, assess for distended red veins, crackles in lung, color, quality and sp gr of urine, skin turgor, adequacy of pulses, moist mucous membranes, bilateral lung sounds, peripheral pitting edema
• Monitor electrolytes: phosphorus, potassium, sodium, calcium, magnesium; also include BUN, creatinine, CBC, platelets, hemoglobin
• Assess B/P before and during therapy
• Assess for pain: in joints or on exertion, duration and characteristics; analgesics may be ordered
• Assess for phlebitis at **IV** site: swelling, redness, pain, warmth

Associated nursing diagnoses

✓ Injury, risk for (uses, adverse reactions)
✓ Fluid excess (side effects)
✓ Knowledge deficit (teaching)

Implementation

IV **IV route**

• Give by **IV** inf after recon-

stituting by adding 10 ml of sterile water for inj to each vial, then adding to 1000 ml of sterile 0.45%, 0.9% NaCl, D_5W, run over 24 hr
• Store inf sol for up to 24 hr at room temp
• Reconstituted sol with sterile water may be stored under refrigeration for up to 24 hr

Additive incompatibilities:

Calcium products, sol

Evaluation

Positive therapeutic outcome
• Decreased calcium levels to normal

pancrelipase

(pan-kre-li'pase)
Catozym, Cotazym Capsules, Cotazym-S Capsules, Creon Capsules, Ilozyme, Ku-Zyme HP Capsules, Pancrease Capsules, Pancrease MT 4, Pancrease MT 10, Pancrease MT 16, Ultrase MT 12, Ultrase MT 20, Ultrase MT 24, Viokase Powder, Viokase Tablets, Zymase
Func. class.: Digestant
Chem. class.: Pancreatic enzyme (bovine/porcine)
Pregnancy category **C**

Action: Pancreatic enzyme needed for proper pancreatic functioning

Therapeutic Outcome: Increases protein, fat, carbohydrate digestion

Uses: Exocrine pancreatic secretion insufficiency, cystic fibrosis (digestive aid), steatorrhea, pancreatic enzyme deficiency

Dosage and routes

P *Adult and child:* PO 1-3 cap/tab ac or with meals, or 1 cap/tab with snack or 1-2 powder packets ac

Available forms: Tab 8000, 11,000, 30,000 U; cap 8000, 30,000 U; enteric coated cap 4000, 5000, 20,000, 25,000 U; powder 16,800 U

Side effects/adverse reactions

GI: Anorexia, nausea, vomiting, diarrhea
GU: Hyperuricuria, hyperuricemia

Contraindications: Allergy to pork, chronic pancreatic disease

Precautions: Pregnancy **C**

Pharmacokinetics	
Absorption	Unknown
Distribution	Unknown
Metabolism	Unknown
Excretion	Unknown
Half-life	Unknown

Pharmacodynamics	
Onset	Unknown
Peak	Unknown
Duration	Unknown

P

Interactions

Drug/drug:

Individual drugs

Cimetidine: ↓ absorption of pancrelipase

Oral iron: ↓ absorption of pancrelipase

Drug classifications

Antacids: ↓ absorption of pancrelipase

Drug/food:

Alkaline foods: ↓ enteric coating

Lab test interferences

Increase: Uric acid (serum, urine)

NURSING CONSIDERATIONS

Assessment

- Monitor I&O ratio; watch for increasing urinary output
- Monitor fecal fat, nitrogen, pro-time, during treatment
- Monitor for polyuria, polydipsia, polyphagia (may indicate diabetes mellitus)
- Assess for allergy to pork; patient may also be sensitive to this drug
- Assess for appropriate weight, height, development; there may be a developmental lag
- Check stools for steatorrhea, which signifies undigested fat content

Associated nursing diagnoses

✓ Nutrition, altered: less than body requirements (uses)
✓ Knowledge deficit (teaching)

Implementation

PO route

- Give after antacid or cimetidine; decreased pH inactivates drug
- P Give powder mixed in prepared fruit for infants, children
- Give whole, not crushed or chewed (enteric coated)
- Administer low-fat diet to decrease GI symptoms
- Store in tight container at room temp

Patient/family education

- Teach patient to take tab with 8 oz or more water, not to let tab sit in mouth; have patient take tab sitting up only
- Advise patient to notify prescriber of allergic reactions, abdominal pain, cramping, or hematuria

Evaluation

Positive therapeutic outcome

- Absence of steatorrhea
- Improved digestion of carbohydrates, proteins, fat

pancuronium

(pan-cure-oh'nee-yum)

pancuronium bromide, Pavulon

Func. class.: Neuromuscular blocker (nondepolarizing)

Chem. class.: Synthetic curariform

Pregnancy category C

Action: Inhibits transmission of nerve impulses by binding with cholinergic receptor sites, antagonizing action of acetylcholine; no analgesic response

→ Therapeutic Outcome:
Paralysis of all skeletal muscles

Uses: Facilitation of endotracheal intubation, skeletal muscle relaxation during mechanical ventilation, surgery, or general anesthesia

Dosage and routes
Adult: **IV** 0.04-0.1 mg/kg, then 0.01 mg/kg q30-60 min

P *Child >10 yr:* **IV** 0.04-0.1 mg/kg, then 1/5 initial dose q30-60 min

Available forms: Inj 1, 2 mg/ml

Side effects/adverse reactions
CV: Bradycardia, tachycardia, increased, decreased B/P, ventricular extrasystoles
EENT: Increased secretions
INTEG: Rash, flushing, pruritus, urticaria, sweating, salivation
MS: Weakness to prolonged skeletal muscle relaxation
RESP: Prolonged apnea, bronchospasm, cyanosis, respiratory depression

Contraindications: Hypersensitivity to bromide ion

Precautions: Pregnancy **C**, renal disease, cardiac disease,
P lactation, children <2 yr, electrolyte imbalances, dehydration, neuromuscular disease, respiratory disease

Pharmacokinetics

Absorption	Complete bioavailability (IV)
Distribution	Extracellular space; crosses placenta
Metabolism	Plasma
Excretion	Kidneys, unchanged
Half-life	2 hr

Pharmacodynamics

Onset	30-45 sec
Peak	3-5 min
Duration	35-40 min

Interactions
Drug/drug:
Individual drugs
Clindamycin: ↑ paralysis length and intensity
Colistin: ↑ paralysis length and intensity
Lidocaine: ↑ paralysis length and intensity
Lithium: ↑ paralysis length and intensity
Magnesium: ↑ paralysis length and intensity
Polymyxin B: ↑ paralysis length and intensity
Procainamide: ↑ paralysis length and intensity
Quinidine: ↑ paralysis length and intensity
Succinylcholine: ↑ paralysis length and intensity

Drug classifications
Aminoglycosides: ↑ paralysis length and intensity
β-Blockers: ↑ paralysis length and intensity
Diuretics, potassium-losing: ↑ paralysis length and intensity
General anesthesia: ↑ paralysis length and intensity

P

NURSING CONSIDERATIONS

Assessment

- Monitor vital signs (B/P, pulse, respirations, airway) until fully recovered; note rate, depth, pattern of respirations, strength of hand grip; patient should be intubated before use
- Monitor for electrolyte imbalances (potassium, magnesium) before drug is used; electrolyte imbalances may lead to increased action of this drug
- Monitor for recovery: decreased paralysis of face, diaphragm, leg, arm, rest of body; residual weakness and respiratory problems may occur during recovery period
- Assess for hypersensitive reactions: rash, fever, respiratory distress, pruritus; drug should be discontinued

Associated nursing diagnoses

✓ Breathing pattern, ineffective (uses)
✓ Communication, impaired verbal (adverse reactions)
✓ Fear (adverse reactions)
✓ Knowledge deficit (teaching)

Implementation

IV **IV route**

- Use peripheral nerve stimulator (anesthesiologist) to determine neuromuscular blockade; deep tendon reflexes should be monitored during extended periods
- Give direct **IV** undiluted over 1-2 min, or diluted in D_5W or 0.9% NaCl and give as an inf at prescribed rate; titrate to patient response; should be administered only by qualified person, usually an anesthesiologist; do not administer IM
- Store in light-resistant area
- Give anticholinesterase to reverse neuromuscular blockade

Syringe compatibility:
Heparin

Y-site compatibilities:
Aminophylline, cefazolin, cefuroxime, cimetidine, cotrimoxazole, dobutamine, dopamine, epinephrine, esmolol, fentanyl, gentamicin, heparin, hydrocortisone sodium succinate, isoproterenol, lorazepam, midazolam, morphine, nitroglycerin, ranitidine, sodium nitroprusside, sulfamethoxazole/trimethoprim, vancomycin

Y-site incompatibility:
Diazepam

Additive compatibility:
Verapamil

Additive incompatibility:
Barbiturates

Patient/family education

- Provide reassurance if communication is difficult during recovery from neuromuscular blockade
- Provide explanation to patients regarding all procedures or treatments; patient will remain conscious if anesthesia is not given also

Evaluation

Positive therapeutic outcome

- Paralysis of jaw, eyelid, head, neck, rest of body as evaluated by peripheral nerve stimulator

Treatment of overdose: Edrophonium or neostigmine, atropine; monitor VS; may require mechanical ventilation

papaverine

(pa-pav'er-een)

Cerespan, Genabid, Papaverine HCl, Pavabid HP Capsulets, Pavabid Plateau Caps, Pavarine Spancaps, Pavased, Pavatine, Pavatym, Paverolan Lanacaps

Func. class.: Peripheral vasodilator

Chem. class.: Opium alkaloid (no narcotic activity)

Pregnancy category C

Action: Relaxes all smooth muscle; inhibits cyclic nucleotide phosphodiesterase, which increases intracellular cAMP, causing vasodilatation

Uses: Arterial spasm resulting in cerebral and peripheral ischemia, myocardial ischemia associated with vascular spasm or dysrhythmias, angina pectoris, peripheral pulmonary embolism, visceral spasm as in ureteral, biliary, GI colic PVD

Investigational uses: Male impotence caused by organic condition

Dosage and routes

Adult: PO 100-300 mg 3-5 times day; sus rel cap 150-300 mg q8-12h; IM/**IV** 30-120 mg q3h prn; Intracavernosal (IC) 30 mg/0.5-1 mg phentolamine or 60 mg alone

Available forms: Sus rel cap 150, 200, 300 mg; tab 30, 60, 100, 150, 200, 300 mg; inj 30 mg/ml

Side effects/adverse reactions

CNS: Headache, dizziness, drowsiness, sedation, vertigo, malaise

CV: ***Tachycardia,*** increased B/P

GI: Nausea, anorexia, abdominal pain, constipation, diarrhea, jaundice, altered liver enzymes, ***hepatotoxicity***

INTEG: *Flushing, sweating,* rash

RESP: Increased depth of respirations

Contraindications: Hypersensitivity, complete AV heart block

Precautions: Cardiac dysrhythmias, glaucoma, pregnancy **C**, lactation, drug dependency, children

P

Pharmacokinetics

Absorption	Variable
Distribution	90% bound to plasma protein
Metabolism	Liver
Excretion	Kidneys to inactive metabolite
Half-life	½-2 hr

Pharmacodynamics

	PO	PO–SUS REL	IV	IM	IC
Onset	30 min	Erratic	Unkn	Unkn	10 min
Peak	1-2 hr	Unkn	Unkn	Unkn	Unkn
Duration	3-4 hr	3 hr	4 hr	3 hr	4 hr

Interactions

Drug/drug:

Individual drugs

Levodopa: ↓ effect of levodopa

Drug classifications

α-Adrenergic agonists: ↓ vasodilatation

Vasodilators: ↑ hypotension

NURSING CONSIDERATIONS

Assessment

- Monitor B/P, pulse, respiratory rate, rhythm, character during treatment until stable; take B/P with patient lying, standing; orthostatic hypotension is common
- Monitor hepatic tests, AST (SGOT), ALT (SGPT), bilirubin; liver enzymes may increase
- Monitor hepatic hypersensitivity reaction: nausea, vomiting, jaundice; drug should be discontinued if this occurs

Associated nursing diagnoses

✓ Tissue perfusion, altered (uses)
✓ Knowledge deficit (teaching)

Implementation

PO route

- Give with meals to reduce GI upset
- Do not crush, chew, or break sus rel form

IV **IV route**

- Administer analgesic if headache develops
- Give **IV** undiluted or diluted in equal amount of sterile water; give 30 mg or less/2 min through Y-tube or 3-way stopcock
- Store at room temp

Syringe compatibility:

Phentolamine

Solution/additive compatibilities:

0.9% NaCl, 0.45% NaCl, D_5W, $D_{10}W$, D_5/0.9% NaCl, D_5/0.45% NaCl, D_5/0.25% NaCl, Ringer's inj, phentolamine

Solution/additive incompatibilities:

LR inj, aminophylline, alkaline sol, bromides, iodides

Patient/family education

- Advise patient that medication is not cure, may have to be taken continuously depending on condition; therapeutic response may not be evident for 2-3 mo
- Instruct patient that it is necessary to quit smoking to prevent excessive vasoconstriction
- Caution patient to avoid hazardous activities until stabilized on medication; dizziness may occur
- Advise patient to notify prescriber if nausea, flushing, sweating, headache, or jaundice occurs

Evaluation

Positive therapeutic outcome

- Ability to walk without pain

- Increased pulse volume
- Increased temp in extremities
- Oriented, long- and short-term memory improved
- Erection in men with impotence

Treatment of overdose: Discontinue medication

paroxetine
(par-ox'e-teen)
Paxil
Func. class.: Antidepressant, serotonin reuptake inhibitor
Chem. class.: Phenylpiperidine derivative
Pregnancy category B

Action: Inhibits CNS neuron reuptake of serotonin but not of norepinephrine or dopamine

Therapeutic Outcome: Relief of depression

Uses: Major depressive disorder

Dosage and routes

Adult: PO 20 mg qd in AM; after 4 wk if no clinical improvement is noted, dosage may be increased by 10 mg/day weekly to desired response; not to exceed 50 mg/day; G decrease dosage for elderly, max 40 mg/day

Available forms: Tab 20, 30 mg

Side effects/adverse reactions

CNS: Headache, nervousness, insomnia, drowsiness, anxiety, tremor, dizziness, fatigue, sedation, abnormal dreams, agitation, apathy, euphoria, hallucinations, delusions, psychosis
CV: Vasodilatation, postural hypotension, palpitations
EENT: Visual changes, rhinitis, oropharyngeal disorder
GI: Nausea, diarrhea, constipation, dry mouth, anorexia, dyspepsia, vomiting, taste changes, flatulence, decreased appetite
GU: Dysmenorrhea, decreased libido, urinary frequency, UTI, amenorrhea, cystitis, impotence, *abnormal ejaculation, male genital disorders*
INTEG: Sweating, rash
MS: Pain, arthritis, myalgia, myopathy, myasthenia
RESP: Infection, pharyngitis, nasal congestion, sinus headache, sinusitis, cough, dyspnea
SYST: Asthenia, fever, chills

Contraindications: Hypersensitivity, patients taking MAOIs

Precautions: Pregnancy **B**, P lactation, children, elderly, G seizure history, patients with history of mania, renal and hepatic disease

P

Pharmacokinetics

Absorption	Well absorbed (PO)
Distribution	Widely distributed; crosses blood-brain barrier
Metabolism	Liver, mostly
Excretion	Kidneys, unchanged (2%); breast milk
Half-life	2 days

Pharmacodynamics

Onset	Unknown
Peak	6-8 hr
Duration	Unknown

Interactions

Drug/drug:

Individual drugs

Alcohol: ↑ CNS depression
Digoxin: ↓ effect of digoxin
Phenytoin: ↓ effect of paroxetine
Procycline: ↓ metabolism
Quinidine: ↓ metabolism

Drug classifications

Antidepressants: ↓ metabolism
Antidysrhythmics, IC: ↓ metabolism
Barbiturates: ↑ effects
Benzodiazepines: ↑ effects
CNS depressants: ↑ effects
MAOI: Hypertensive crisis, convulsions; do not use together
Phenothiazines: ↓ metabolism

Lab test interferences

Increase: Serum bilirubin, blood glucose, alkaline phosphatase
Decrease: VMA, 5-HIAA, blood glucose
False increase: Urinary catecholamines

NURSING CONSIDERATIONS

Assessment

- Assess mental status: mood, sensorium, affect, suicidal tendencies; increase in psychiatric symptoms: depression, panic
- Assess for withdrawal symptoms: headache, nausea, vomiting, muscle pain, weakness; do not usually occur unless drug was discontinued abruptly
- Monitor B/P (with patient lying, standing), pulse q4h; if systolic B/P drops 20 mm Hg, hold drug, notify prescriber; take VS q4h in patients with cardiovascular disease
- Monitor blood studies: CBC, leukocytes, differential, cardiac enzymes if patient is receiving long-term therapy
- Monitor hepatic studies: AST (SGOT), ALT (SGPT), bilirubin
- Check weight weekly; appetite may increase with drug
- Assess ECG for flattening of T wave, bundle branch block, AV block, dysrhythmias in cardiac patients
- Assess for EPS primarily in G elderly: rigidity, dystonia, akathisia
- Monitor urinary retention, constipation; constipation is P more likely to occur in children G or elderly
- Identify alcohol consumption; if alcohol is consumed, hold dose until AM

Associated nursing diagnoses

✓ Coping, ineffective individual (uses)
✓ Injury, risk for (adverse reactions)

☑ Knowledge deficit (teaching)
☑ Noncompliance (teaching)

Implementation

PO route

- Give with food or milk for GI symptoms; store at room temp; do not freeze

Patient/family education

- Advise patient that therapeutic effects may take 1-4 wk
- Teach patient to use caution in driving and other activities requiring alertness because of drowsiness, dizziness, blurred vision; to avoid rising quickly from sitting to standing, especially elderly
- Caution patient to avoid alcohol ingestion, other CNS depressants, and OTC medication unless prescribed
- Caution patient not to discontinue medication quickly after long-term use; may cause nausea, anxiety, headache, malaise; do not double doses if one is missed
- Advise patient to use gum, hard sugarless candy, or frequent sips of water for dry mouth; if dry mouth continues an artificial saliva may be used

Evaluation

Positive therapeutic outcome

- Decrease in depression
- Absence of suicidal thoughts

pegaspargase

(peg-as′per-gase)

Colaspase, Elspar, Kidrolase ✱

Func. class.: Antineoplastic

Chem. class.: Escherichia coli enzyme

Pregnancy category **D**

Action: Indirectly inhibits protein synthesis in tumor cells; without amino acid, DNA, RNA synthesis is halted; asparagine, protein synthesis is halted; G_1 phase of cell cycle specific; a nonvesicant

Therapeutic Outcome: Prevention of rapidly growing malignant cells

Uses: Acute lymphocytic leukemia in combination with other antineoplastics unresponsive to other agents

Dosage and routes

In combination

Adult: **IV** 1000 IU/kg/day × 10 days given over 30 min; IM 6000 IU/m²/day

Sole induction

Adult: **IV** 200 IU/kg/day × 28 days

Available forms: Inj 10,000 IU

Side effects/adverse reactions

CNS: Neuritis, dizziness, headache, ***coma,*** depression, fatigue, confusion, hallucinations

CV: Chest pain

P

ENDO: Hyperglycemia
GI: *Nausea, vomiting, anorexia, cramps, stomatitis,* ***hepatotoxicity, pancreatitis***
GU: Urinary retention, ***renal failure,*** glycosuria, polyuria, azotemia, uric acid neuropathy
HEMA: Thrombocytopenia, leukopenia, myelosuppression, anemia, decreased clotting factors
INTEG: *Rash,* urticaria, chills, fever
RESP: Fibrosis, pulmonary infiltrate
SYST: Anaphylaxis, hypersensitivity

Contraindications: Hypersensitivity, infants, pregnancy **D**, lactation, pancreatitis

Precautions: Renal disease, hepatic disease

Pharmacokinetics

Absorption	Complete bioavailability (IV)
Distribution	Intravascular spaces
Metabolism	Unknown
Excretion	Reticuloendothelial system
Half-life	Unknown

Pharmacodynamics

Onset	Unknown
Peak	Unknown
Duration	Unknown

Interactions
Drug/drug:
Individual drugs
Methotrexate: Blocking action of methotrexate
Vincristine: ↑ neurotoxicity

Drug classifications
Hepatotoxic agents: ↑ hepatotoxic agents
Glucocorticosteroids: ↑ hyperglycemia

Lab test interferences
Decrease: Thyroid function tests
Increase: BUN

NURSING CONSIDERATIONS
Assessment

- Assess for signs and symptoms of pancreatitis (nausea, vomiting, severe abdominal pain), anaphylaxis (bronchospasm, dyspnea), cyanosis; monitor amylase, glucose
- Assess symptoms indicating severe allergic reaction: rash, pruritus, urticaria, purpuric skin lesions, itching, flushing; monitor for joint pain, bronchospasm, hypotension; epinephrine and crash carts should be nearby
- Monitor for frequency of stools, characteristics: cramping, acidosis; signs of dehydration: rapid respirations, poor skin turgor, decreased urine output, dry skin, restlessness, weakness
- Monitor CBC, differential, platelet count weekly; withhold drug if WBC count is <4000/mm^3 or platelet count is <100,000/mm^3; notify physician of results; also assess PT, PTT and thrombin time, which may be increased
- Monitor renal function studies: BUN, creatinine, serum uric acid, urine CrCl before and during therapy; check I&O ratio; report fall in urine output to <30 ml/hr; patient should be well hydrated

with 2-3 L/day to prevent urate deposits
- Monitor temp q4h (may indicate beginning of infection)
- Monitor liver function tests before and during therapy (bilirubin, AST [SGOT], ALT [SGPT], LDH) as needed or monthly; check for yellowing of skin and sclera, dark urine, clay-colored stools, itchy skin, abdominal pain, fever, diarrhea; also monitor cholesterol, alkaline phosphatase
- Assess for bleeding: hematuria, stool guaiac, bruising or petechiae, mucosa or orifices q8h; check for inflammation of mucosa, breaks in skin
- Identify edema in feet, joint pain, stomach pain, shaking

Associated nursing diagnoses

- ✓ Injury, risk for (adverse reactions)
- ✓ Infection, risk for (adverse reactions)
- ✓ Knowledge deficit (teaching)

Implementation

- Preparation by trained personnel is required in controlled environment
- Give fluids **IV** or PO before chemotherapy to hydrate patient
- Provide antiemetic 30-60 min before giving drug and PRN to prevent vomiting; administer antibiotics for prophylaxis of infection
- Provide a liq diet: carbonated beverages; gelatin may be added if patient is not nauseated or vomiting

Intradermal route

- After intradermal skin testing and desensitization, give 0.1 ml (2 IU) intradermally after reconstituting with 5 ml sterile water or 0.9% NaCl for inj; then add 0.1 ml of reconstituted drug to 9.9 ml diluent (20 IU/ml); observe for 1 hr, check for wheal; desensitization may be required

IV **IV route**

- For direct **IV** dilute 10,000 IU/5 ml sterile water for inj or 0.9% NaCl without preservatives; give through 5-μm filter if fibers are present; do not use if cloudy or discolored, give over 30 min through Y-site of full-flowing **IV** of 0.9% NaCl or D_5W; run **IV** sol for at least 2 hr after direct administration
- Give **IV** inf using 21G, 23G, 25G needle; administer by slow **IV** inf via Y-tube or 3-way stop cock of flowing D_5W or NS inf over 30 min after diluting 10,000 IU/5 ml of sterile water or 0.9% NaCl (no preservatives) to 2000 IU/ml; filter may be necessary if fibers are present
- Provide allopurinol or sodium bicarbonate to reduce uric acid levels, alkalinization of urine

IM route

- Dilute 10,000 IU/2 ml 0.9% NaCl with preservatives; give 2 ml or less per site

Patient/family education

- Advise patient that contraceptive measures are recommended during therapy; drug is teratogenic
- Teach patient to avoid use of products containing aspirin or ibuprofen, razors, commercial mouthwash, since bleeding may occur; to report symptoms

P

of bleeding (hematuria, tarry stools)
- Teach patient to report signs of anemia (fatigue, headache, irritability, faintness, shortness of breath)
- Tell patient to avoid crowds and persons with respiratory tract infections to prevent patient infection
- Advise patient to avoid vaccinations, since serious reactions can occur

Evaluation

Positive therapeutic outcome
- Prevention of rapid division of malignant cells

pemoline
(pem'oh-leen)
Cylert, Cylert Chewable
Func. class.: Cerebral stimulant
Chem. class.: Oxazolidinone derivative
Pregnancy category **B**
Controlled substance schedule **IV**

Action: Exact mechanism unknown; may act through dopaminergic mechanisms; produces CNS stimulation and a paradoxic effect in ADHD

Therapeutic Outcome: Increased alertness, increased attention span, decreased hyperactivity (ADHD)

Uses: Attention deficit hyperactivity disorder for children >6 yr

Investigational uses: Schizophrenia, fatigue, depression

Dosage and routes

P *Child >6 yr:* 37.5 mg in AM, increasing by 18.75 mg/wk, not to exceed 112.5 mg/day

Available forms: Tab 18.75, 37.5, 75 mg; chewable tab 37.5 mg

Side effects/adverse reactions

CNS: ***Hyperactivity, insomnia, restlessness,*** dizziness, depression, headache, stimulation, irritability, aggressiveness, hallucinations, ***seizures, Gilles de la Tourette's disorder,*** drowsiness, dyskinetic movements
CV: Tachycardia
GI: Nausea, ***anorexia,*** diarrhea, abdominal pain, increased liver enzymes, hepatitis, jaundice, weight loss
MISC: Rashes, growth suppression in children

Contraindications: Hypersensitivity, hepatic insufficiency

Precautions: Renal disease, pregnancy **B**, lactation, drug abuse, P child <6 yr, psychosis, tics, seizure disorders

Pharmacokinetics

Absorption	Well absorbed (PO)
Distribution	Widely distributed; crosses placenta
Metabolism	Liver
Excretion	Kidneys, pH dependent; increased pH, increased reabsorption
Half-life	12 hr; increased when urine is alkaline

Pharmacodynamics

Onset	Unknown
Peak	2-4 hr
Duration	8 hr

Interactions

Drug/drug:

Drug classifications

Adrenergics: ↑ stimulation
Decongestants: ↑ stimulation
Stimulants, CNS: ↑ stimulation

Drug/food:

Caffeine (coffee, teas, chocolate): ↑ stimulation

NURSING CONSIDERATIONS

Assessment

- Monitor VS, B/P, since this drug may reverse antihypertensives; check patients with cardiac disease more often for increased B/P
- Monitor height and weight q3 mo, since growth rate in children may be decreased; appetite is suppressed; weight loss is common during the first few mo of treatment
- Monitor mental status: mood, sensorium, affect, stimulation, insomnia; aggressiveness may occur; depression with crying spells may occur after drug has worn off
- Assess for tolerance; should not be used for extended time except in ADHD; dosage should be diminished gradually to prevent withdrawal symptoms
- In children or adults with ADHD, monitor for improved organizational skills, attention span, attending to tasks, impulse control, socialization, and ability to get along better with others
- Assess for withdrawal symptoms: headache, nausea, vomiting, muscle pain, weakness; drug tolerance will develop after long-term use; dosage should not be increased if tolerance develops.

Associated nursing diagnoses

- ✓ Thought processes, altered (uses, adverse reactions)
- ✓ Coping, impaired individual (uses)
- ✓ Knowledge deficit (teaching)
- ✓ Family coping, impaired individual (uses)

Implementation

PO route

- Give at least 6 hr before hs to avoid sleeplessness; titrate to patient's response; lowest dosage should be used to control symptoms
- Provide gum, hard candy, frequent sips of water for dry mouth at beginning of treatment; these symptoms tend to lessen with time

Patient/family education

- Teach patient to decrease caffeine consumption (coffee, tea, cola, chocolate), which may increase irritability and stimulation; to avoid OTC preparations unless approved by prescriber; to avoid alcohol ingestion; these may cause serious drug interactions
- Instruct patient to taper off drug over several wk, or de-

pression, increased sleeping, lethargy may occur

- Caution patient to avoid hazardous activities until stabilized on medication
- Instruct patient not to double doses if medication is missed; prescriber may suggest drug holidays (ADHD) during the school year to assess progress and determine continued drug necessity
- Teach patient/family to notify prescriber if significant side effects occur: tremors, insomnia, palpitations, restlessness; drug changes may be needed
- Inform patient that if dry mouth occurs to use frequent sips of water, sugarless gum, hard candy during beginning therapy; dry mouth lessens with continued treatment
- Advise patient to get needed rest; patients will feel more tired at end of day; to take last dose at least 6 hr before hs to avoid insomnia

Evaluation

Positive therapeutic outcome

- Decreased activity in ADHD

Treatment of overdose: Administer fluids, hemodialysis, peritoneal dialysis, antihypertensives for increased B/P; ammonium chloride for increased excretion

penicillin G benzathine

(pen-i-sill'in)

Bicillin L-A, Megacillin ✤, Permapen, Bicillin C-R, Bicillin C-R 900/300

Func. class.: Broad-spectrum antiinfective

Chem. class.: Natural penicillin

Pregnancy category B

Action: Interferes with cell wall replication of susceptible organisms; osmotically unstable cell wall swells and bursts from osmotic pressure

Uses: Respiratory tract infections, scarlet fever, erysipelas, otitis media, pneumonia, skin and soft tissue infections, gonorrhea; prevention of rheumatic fever, glomerulonephritis

➔ Therapeutic Outcome: Bactericidal effects on the gram-positive cocci *Staphylococcus, Streptococcus pyogenes, S. viridans, S. faecalis, S. bovis, S. pneumoniae;* gram-negative cocci *Neisseria gonorrhoeae;* gram-positive bacilli *Bacillus anthracis, Clostridium perfringens, C. tetani, Corynebacterium diphtheriae, Listeria monocytogenes;* gram-negative bacilli *Escherichia coli, Proteus mirabilis, Salmonella, Shigella, Enterobacter, Streptobacillus moniliformis,* spirochete *Treponema pallidum; Actinomyces*

Dosage and routes

Early syphilis

Adult: IM 2.4 million U in single dose

Congenital syphilis

P *Child <2 yr:* IM 50,000 U/kg in single dose

Prophylaxis of rheumatic fever, glomerulonephritis

P *Adult and child >60 lb:* IM 1.2 million U in single dose q mo or 600,000 U q2 wk

P *Child <60 lb:* IM 600,000 U in single dose

Upper respiratory tract infections (group A streptococcal)

Adult: IM 1.2 million U in single dose; PO 400,000-600,000 U q4-6h

P *Child >27 kg:* IM 900,000 U in single dose

P *Child <27 kg:* IM 300,000-600,000 U in single dose

Available forms: Inj 300,000, 600,000 U/ml; tabs 200,000 U

Side effects/adverse reactions

CNS: Lethargy, hallucinations, anxiety, depression, twitching, ***coma, convulsions***

GI: Nausea, vomiting, diarrhea, increased AST (SGOT), ALT (SGPT), abdominal pain, glossitis, colitis

GU: Oliguria, proteinuria, hematuria, vaginitis, moniliasis, glomerulonephritis

HEMA: Anemia, increased bleeding time, ***bone marrow depression, granulocytopenia***

META: Hyperkalemia, hypokalemia, alkalosis, hypernatremia

MISC: Local pain, tenderness and fever with IM inj

Contraindications: Hypersensitivity to penicillins; neonates P

Precautions: Hypersensitivity to cephalosporins, pregnancy **B**

Pharmacokinetics

Absorption	Delayed; prolonged drug levels
Distribution	Widely distributed; crosses placenta
Metabolism	Liver, minimally
Excretion	Kidneys, unchanged; breast milk
Half-life	½-1 hr

Pharmacodynamics

Onset	Slow
Peak	12-24 hr
Duration	1-4 wk

Interactions

Drug/drug:

Individual drugs

Aspirin: ↑ penicillin levels, ↓ renal excretion

Chloramphenicol: ↑ half-life of chloramphenicol, ↓ effectiveness of penicillin

Probenecid: ↑ penicillin levels, ↓ renal excretion

Drug classifications

Erythromycins: ↓ antimicrobial effectiveness

Oral anticoagulants: ↑ anticoagulant effects

Oral contraceptives: ↓ contraceptive effectiveness

Tetracyclines: ↓ antimicrobial effectiveness

Lab test interferences

False positive: Urine glucose, urine protein

NURSING CONSIDERATIONS

Assessment

- Assess patient for previous sensitivity reaction to penicillins or other cephalosporins; cross-sensitivity between penicillins and cephalosporins is common
- Assess patient for signs and symptoms of infection including characteristics of wounds, sputum, urine, stool, WBC >10,000, earache, fever; obtain baseline information and during treatment
- Obtain C & S before beginning drug therapy to identify if correct treatment has been initiated
- Assess for allergic reactions: rash, urticaria, pruritus, chills, fever, joint pain; angioedema may occur a few days after therapy begins; epinephrine, resuscitation equipment should be available for anaphylactic reaction
- Identify urine output; if decreasing, notify prescriber (may indicate nephrotoxicity); also check for increased BUN, creatinine
- Monitor blood studies: AST (SGOT), ALT (SGPT), CBC, Hct, bilirubin, LDH, alkaline phosphatase, Coombs' test monthly if patient is on long-term therapy
- Monitor electrolytes: potassium, sodium, chloride monthly if patient is on long-term therapy
- Assess bowel pattern daily; if severe diarrhea occurs, drug should be discontinued; may indicate pseudomembranous colitis
- Monitor for bleeding: ecchymosis, bleeding gums, hematuria, stool guaiac daily if on long-term therapy
- Assess for overgrowth of infection: perineal itching, fever, malaise, redness, pain, swelling, drainage, rash, diarrhea, change in cough, sputum

Associated nursing diagnoses

- ✓ Infection, risk for (uses)
- ✓ Diarrhea (adverse reactions)
- ✓ Injury, risk for (adverse reactions)
- ✓ Knowledge deficit (teaching)
- ✓ Noncompliance (teaching)

Implementation

PO route

- Give in even doses around the clock; if GI upset occurs, give with food; drug must be given for 10-14 days to ensure organism death and prevent superinfection
- Shake susp

IM route

- Do not give **IV**
- Give deep in large muscle mass
- Reconstitute with 0.9% NaCl, sterile water for inj, D_5W; refrigerate unused portion

Patient/family education

- Teach patient to report sore throat, bruising, bleeding, joint pain; may indicate blood dyscrasias (rare)
- Advise patient to contact prescriber if vaginal itching, loose, foul-smelling stools, furry tongue occur; may indicate superinfection
- Instruct patient to take all medication prescribed for the length of time ordered

• Advise patient to notify prescriber of diarrhea with blood or pus, which may indicate pseudomembranous colitis

Evaluation

Positive therapeutic outcome
• Absence of signs/symptoms of infection (WBC <10,000, temp WNL, absence of red, draining wounds, earache)
• Reported improvement in symptoms of infection

Treatment of anaphylaxis: Withdraw drug, maintain airway, administer epinephrine, aminophylline, O_2, **IV** corticosteroids

penicillin G potassium

Acrocillin, Burcillin-G, Deltapen, Megacillin ✦, Novopen G ✦, Pentids, Pfizerpen

Func. class.: Broad-spectrum antiinfective

Chem. class.: Natural penicillin

Pregnancy category **B**

Action: Interferes with cell wall replication of susceptible organisms; osmotically unstable cell wall swells and bursts from osmotic pressure

Uses: Emphysema, gangrene, anthrax, gonorrhea, mastoiditis, meningitis, osteomyelitis, pneumonia, tetanus, UTIs, prophylactically in rheumatic fever

Therapeutic Outcome: Bactericidal effects for the non–penicillinase-producing gram-positive cocci *Staphylococcus aureus, Streptococcus pyogenes, S. viridans, S. faecalis, S. bovis, S. pneumoniae;* gram-negative cocci *Neisseria gonorrhoeae, N. meningitidis;* gram-positive bacilli *Bacillus anthracis, Clostridium perfringens, C. tetani, Corynebacterium diphtheriae, Listeria monocytogenes;* gram-negative bacilli *Bacteroides, Fusobacterium nucleatum, Pasteurella multocida, Streptobacillus moniliformis;* spirochetes *Treponema pallidum, T. pertenue, Borrelia recurrentis, Leptospira icterohaemorrhagiae; Actinomyces*

Dosage and routes

Pneumococcal/streptococcal infections (mild to moderate)

Adult: PO 400,000-500,000 U q6-8h × 10 days (streptococcal infections) or afebrile × 2 days (pneumococcal infections); IM/**IV** 1.2-24 million U in divided doses q4h

P *Child <12 yr:* PO 25,000-90,000 U/kg/day in 3-6 divided doses; IM/**IV** 25,000-300,000 μ/kg/day in individual doses q4h

Prevention of recurrence of rheumatic fever

Adult: PO 200,000-250,000 U bid continuously

P *Child <12 yr:* PO 25,000-90,000 U/kg/day in 3-6 divided doses

P

Vincent's gingivitis/ pharyngitis

Adult: PO 400,000-500,000 U q6-8h

Available forms: Tab 200,000, 250,000, 400,000, 500,000, 800,000 U; powder for oral sol 200,000, 400,000 U/5 ml; inj

Side effects/adverse reactions

CNS: Lethargy, hallucinations, anxiety, depression, twitching, ***coma, convulsions***
GI: Nausea, vomiting, diarrhea, increased AST (SGOT) and ALT (SGPT), abdominal pain, glossitis, colitis
HEMA: Anemia, ***increased bleeding time, bone marrow depression, granulocytopenia***
META: ***Hyperkalemia, hypokalemia, alkalosis, hypernatremia***

Contraindications: Hypersensitivity to penicillins; neonates P

Precautions: Hypersensitivity to cephalosporins, pregnancy **B**

Pharmacokinetics

Absorption	Variably absorbed (PO); well absorbed (IM)
Distribution	Widely distributed; crosses placenta
Metabolism	Liver, minimally
Excretion	Kidneys unchanged; breast milk
Half-life	½-1 hr

Pharmacodynamics

	PO	IM	IV
Onset	Rapid	Rapid	Rapid
Peak	1 hr	¼-½ hr	Immediate

Interactions

Drug/drug:

Individual drugs

Aspirin: ↑ penicillin levels, ↓ renal excretion
Cholestyramine: ↓ effectiveness of penicillin
Chloramphenicol: ↑ half-life of chloramphenicol, ↓ effectiveness of penicillin
Colestipol: ↓ effectiveness of penicillin
Probenecid: ↑ penicillin levels, ↓ renal excretion

Drug classifications

Erythromycins: ↓ antimicrobial effectiveness
Oral anticoagulants: ↑ anticoagulant effects
Oral contraceptives: ↓ contraceptive effectiveness
Tetracyclines: ↓ antimicrobial effectiveness

Drug/food:

Food, carbonated drinks, citrus fruit juices: ↓ absorption

Lab test interferences

False positive: Urine glucose, urine protein

NURSING CONSIDERATIONS

Assessment

- Assess patient for previous sensitivity reaction to penicillins or other cephalosporins; cross-sensitivity between penicillins and cephalosporins is common
- Assess patient for signs and symptoms of infection including characteristics of wounds, sputum, urine, stool, WBC >10,000, earache, fever; obtain baseline information and during treatment

• Obtain C&S before beginning drug therapy to identify if correct treatment has been initiated
• Assess for allergic reactions: rash, urticaria, pruritus, chills, fever, joint pain; angioedema may occur a few days after therapy begins; epinephrine, resuscitation equipment should be available for anaphylactic reaction
• Identify urine output; if decreasing, notify prescriber (may indicate nephrotoxicity); also check for increased BUN, creatinine
• Monitor blood studies: AST (SGOT), ALT (SGPT), CBC, Hct, bilirubin, LDH, alkaline phosphatase, Coombs' test monthly if patient is on long-term therapy
• Monitor electrolytes: potassium, sodium, chloride monthly if patient is on long-term therapy
• Assess bowel pattern daily; if severe diarrhea occurs, drug should be discontinued; may indicate pseudomembranous colitis
• Monitor for bleeding: ecchymosis, bleeding gums, hematuria, stool guaiac daily if on long-term therapy
• Assess for overgrowth of infection: perineal itching, fever, malaise, redness, pain, swelling, drainage, rash, diarrhea, change in cough, sputum

Associated nursing diagnoses

✓ Infection, risk for (uses)
✓ Diarrhea (adverse reactions)
✓ Injury, risk for (adverse reactions)
✓ Knowledge deficit (teaching)
✓ Noncompliance (teaching)

Implementation

PO route
• Give in even doses around the clock; if GI upset occurs, give with food; drug must be given for 10-14 days to ensure organism death and prevent superinfection
• Shake susp

IM route
• Reconstitute with D_5W, 0.9% NaCl, sterile water for inj; shake well
• Give deep in large muscle mass; massage
• Do not give SC; may cause severe pain
• If injected near a nerve, loss of function and severe pain may occur

IV **IV route**
• Change **IV** sites q48h to prevent pain and phlebitis
• Give by intermittent inf by diluting 3 million U or less/50 ml or more; dilute 3 million U or more/100 ml D_5W, $D_{10}W$, 0.45% NaCl, 0.9% NaCl, LR, Ringer's or any combination run over 1-2 hr (adult), 15-30 P min (child)
• Give by cont inf by diluting and infusing over 24 hr

Syringe incompatibility:

Metoclopramide

Syringe compatibility:

Heparin

Additive incompatibilities:

Aminoglycosides, aminophylline, amphotericin B, chlorpromazine, dopamine, floxacillin, hydroxyzine, metaraminol, oxytetracycline, pentobarbital,

P

prochlorperazine mesylate, promazine, tetracycline, thiopental

Additive compatibilities:

Asorbic acid, calcium chloride, calcium gluconate, cephapirin, chloramphenicol, cimetidine, clindamycin, colistimethate, corticotropin, dimenhydrinate, diphenhydramine, ephedrine, erythromycin, furosemide, hydrocortisone sodium succinate, kanamycin, lidocaine, magnesium sulfate, methicillin, methylprednisolone sodium succinate, metronidazole, polymyxin B, prednisolone sodium phosphate, potassium chloride, procaine, prochlorperazine edisylate, verapamil

Y-site compatibilities:

Acyclovir, amiodarone, cyclophosphamide, enalaprilat, esmolol, fluconazole, foscarnet, heparin, hydromorphone, labetalol, magnesium sulfate, meperidine, morphine, perphenazine, potassium chloride, verapamil, vitamin B with C

Patient/family education

- Teach patient to report sore throat, bruising, bleeding, joint pain; may indicate blood dyscrasias (rare)
- Advise patient to contact prescriber if vaginal itching, loose, foul-smelling stools, furry tongue occur; may indicate superinfection
- Instruct patient to take all medication prescribed for the length of time ordered
- Advise patient to notify prescriber of diarrhea with blood or pus, which may indicate pseudomembranous colitis

Evaluation

Positive therapeutic outcome

- Absence of signs/symptoms of infection (WBC <10,000, temp WNL, absence of red, draining wounds, earache)
- Reported improvement in symptoms of infection

Treatment of anaphylaxis: Withdraw drug, maintain airway, administer epinephrine, aminophylline, O_2, **IV** corticosteroids

penicillin G procaine

Ayercillin ✦, Crysticillin A.S., Duracillin A.S., Wycillin, Pfizerpen-AS

Func. class.: Broad-spectrum long-acting antiinfective

Chem. class.: Natural penicillin

Pregnancy category **B**

Action: Interferes with cell wall replication of susceptible organisms; osmotically unstable cell wall swells and bursts from osmotic pressure

Uses: Empyema, gangrene, anthrax, gonorrhea, mastoiditis, meningitis, osteomyelitis, pneumonia, tetanus, UTIs, prophylactically in rheumatic fever

➡ Therapeutic Outcome: Bactericidal effects for the gram-positive cocci *Staphylococcus aureus, Streptococcus pyogenes, S. viridans, S. faecalis, S. bovis, S. pneumoniae;* gram-negative cocci *Neisseria gonorrhoeae, N. meningitidis;* gram-positive bacilli *Bacillus anthracis, Clostridium perfringens, C. tetani, Corynebacterium diphtheriae, Listeria monocytogenes;* gram-negative bacilli *Bacteroides, Fusobacterium nucleatum, Pasteurella multocida, Streptobacillus moniliformis;* spirochetes *Treponema pallidum, T. pertenue, Borrelia recurrentis, Leptospira icterohaemorrhagiae; Actinomyces*

Dosage and routes

Moderate to severe infections

P *Adult and child:* IM 600,000-1.2 million U in one or two doses/day × 10 days to 2 wk

P *Newborn:* IM 50,000 U/kg single dose

Gonorrhea

P *Adult and child >12 yr:* IM 4.8 million units in two inj given 30 min after probenecid 1 g

Pneumonia (pneumococcal)

P *Adult and child >12 yr:* IM 300,000-600,000 U q6-12h

Available forms: Inj 300,000, 500,000, 600,000 U/ml, 600,000 U/1.2 ml, 1.2 million U/dose, 2.4 million U/dose

Side effects/adverse reactions

CNS: Lethargy, hallucinations, anxiety, depression, twitching, ***coma, convulsions***
GI: Nausea, vomiting, diarrhea, increased AST (SGOT), ALT (SGPT), abdominal pain, glossitis, colitis
GU: ***Oliguria, proteinuria, hematuria, vaginitis, moniliasis, glomerulonephritis***
HEMA: Anemia, increased bleeding time, ***bone marrow depression, granulocytopenia***
META: Hyperkalemia, hypokalemia, alkalosis, hypernatremia

Contraindications: Hypersensitivity to penicillins, procaine, P neonates

Precautions: Hypersensitivity to cephalosporins, pregnancy **B**

Pharmacokinetics

Absorption	Delayed; prolonged drug levels
Distribution	Widely distributed; crosses placenta
Metabolism	Liver, minimally
Excretion	Kidneys, unchanged; breast milk
Half-life	½-1 hr

Pharmacodynamics

Onset	Slow
Peak	1-4 hr
Duration	15 hr

Interactions

Drug/drug:

Individual drugs
Aspirin: ↑ penicillin levels, ↓ renal excretion
Chloramphenicol: ↑ half-life of chloramphenicol, ↓ effectiveness of penicillin
Probenecid: ↑ penicillin levels, ↓ renal excretion
Drug classifications
Erythromycins: ↓ antimicrobial effectiveness

P

Oral anticoagulants: ↑ anticoagulant effects
Oral contraceptives: ↓ contraceptive effectiveness
Tetracyclines: ↓ antimicrobial effectiveness

Lab test interferences

False positive: Urine glucose, urine protein

NURSING CONSIDERATIONS

Assessment

- Assess patient for previous sensitivity reaction to penicillins or other cephalosporins; cross-sensitivity between penicillins and cephalosporins is common
- Assess patient for signs and symptoms of infection including characteristics of wounds, sputum, urine, stool, WBC >10,000, earache, fever; obtain baseline information and during treatment
- Obtain C & S before beginning drug therapy to identify if correct treatment has been initiated
- Assess for allergic reactions: rash, urticaria, pruritus, chills, fever, joint pain; angioedema may occur a few days after therapy begins; epinephrine, resuscitation equipment should be available for anaphylactic reaction
- Identify urine output; if decreasing, notify prescriber (may indicate nephrotoxicity); also check for increased BUN, creatinine
- Monitor blood studies: AST (SGOT), ALT (SGPT), CBC, Hct, bilirubin, LDH, alkaline phosphatase, Coombs' test monthly if patient is on long-term therapy
- Monitor electrolytes: potassium, sodium, chloride monthly if patient is on long-term therapy
- Assess bowel pattern daily; if severe diarrhea occurs, drug should be discontinued; may indicate pseudomembranous colitis
- Monitor for bleeding: ecchymosis, bleeding gums, hematuria, stool guaiac daily if on long-term therapy
- Assess for overgrowth of infection: perineal itching, fever, malaise, redness, pain, swelling, drainage, rash, diarrhea, change in cough, sputum

Associated nursing diagnoses

- ✓ Infection, risk for (uses)
- ✓ Diarrhea (adverse reactions)
- ✓ Injury, risk for (adverse reactions)
- ✓ Knowledge deficit (teaching)
- ✓ Noncompliance (teaching)

Implementation

IM route

- Do not give **IV**
- Give deeply in large muscle mass
- Reconstitute with 0.9% NaCl, sterile water for inj, D_5W; refrigerate unused portion
- Shake medication before administering
- IM route may include procaine reactions: fear of death, depression, convulsions, anxiety, confusion, hallucinations

Patient/family education

- Teach patient to report sore throat, bruising, bleeding,

joint pain; may indicate blood dyscrasias (rare)
- Advise patient to contact prescriber if vaginal itching, loose, foul-smelling stools, furry tongue occur; may indicate superinfection
- Advise patient to notify prescriber of diarrhea with blood or pus, which may indicate pseudomembranous colitis

Evaluation

Positive therapeutic outcome
- Absence of signs/symptoms of infection (WBC <10,000, temp WNL, absence of red, draining wounds, earache)
- Reported improvement in symptoms of infection

Treatment of anaphylaxis: Withdraw drug, maintain airway, administer epinephrine, aminophylline, O_2, **IV** corticosteroids

penicillin G sodium

Crystapen ✦, Pfizerpen
Func. class.: Broad-spectrum antiinfective
Chem. class.: Natural penicillin
Pregnancy category **B**

Action: Interferes with cell wall replication of susceptible organisms; osmotically unstable cell wall swells and bursts from osmotic pressure

Uses: Empyema, gangrene, anthrax, gonorrhea, mastoiditis, meningitis, osteomyelitis, pneumonia, tetanus, UTIs, prophylactically in rheumatic fever

Therapeutic Outcome: Bactericidal effects for the non–penicillinase-producing gram-positive cocci *Staphylococcus aureus, Streptococcus pyogenes, S. viridans, S. faecalis, S. bovis, S. pneumoniae;* gram-negative cocci *Neisseria gonorrhoeae, N. meningitidis;* gram-positive bacilli *Bacillus anthracis, Clostridium perfringens, C. tetani, Corynebacterium diphtheriae, Listeria monocytogenes;* gram-negative bacilli *Bacteroides, Fusobacterium nucleatum, Pasteurella multocida, Streptobacillus moniliformis;* spirochetes *Treponema pallidum, T. pertenue, Borrelia recurrentis, Leptospira icterohaemorrhagiae; Actinomyces*

Dosage and routes

Moderate to severe infections

Adult: IM/**IV** 12 million-30 million U/day in divided doses q4h

P *Child:* IM/**IV** 25,000-300,000 U/day in divided doses q4-12h

Dental surgery prophylaxis for endocarditis

Adult: IM/**IV** 2 million U 30-60 min before procedure, then 1 million U 6 hr after procedure

Available forms: Inj 1 million, 5 million, 20 million U

P

Side effects/adverse reactions

CNS: Lethargy, hallucinations, anxiety, depression, twitching, ***convulsions***
GI: Nausea, vomiting, diarrhea, increased AST (SGOT), ALT (SGPT), abdominal pain, glossitis, colitis
GU: ***Oliguria, proteinuria, hematuria,*** vaginitis, moniliasis, ***glomerulonephritis***
HEMA: Anemia, increased bleeding time, ***bone marrow depression, granulocytopenia***
META: Hyperkalemia, hypokalemia, alkalosis, hypernatremia

Contraindications: Hypersensitivity to penicillins, neonates P

Precautions: CHF caused by sodium retention, pregnancy **B**

Pharmacokinetics

Absorption	Well absorbed
Distribution	Widely distributed; crosses placenta
Metabolism	Liver, minimally
Excretion	Kidneys, unchanged; breast milk
Half-life	½-1 hr

Pharmacodynamics

	IM	IV
Onset	Rapid	Rapid
Peak	1-3 hr	Rapid

Interactions
Drug/drug:
Individual drugs
Aspirin: ↑ penicillin levels, ↓ renal excretion
Cholestyramine: ↓ effectiveness of penicillin
Chloramphenicol: ↑ half-life of chloramphenicol, ↓ effectiveness of penicillin
Colestipol: ↓ effectiveness of penicillin
Probenecid: ↑ penicillin levels, ↓ renal excretion

Drug classifications
Erythromycins: ↓ antimicrobial effectiveness
Oral anticoagulants: ↑ anticoagulant effects
Oral contraceptives: ↓ contraceptive effectiveness
Tetracyclines: ↓ antimicrobial effectiveness

Drug/food:

Food, carbonated drinks, citrus fruit juices: ↓ absorption

Lab test interferences

False positive: Urine glucose, urine protein

NURSING CONSIDERATIONS
Assessment

- Assess patient for previous sensitivity reaction to penicillins or other cephalosporins; cross-sensitivity between penicillins and cephalosporins is common
- Assess patient for signs and symptoms of infection including characteristics of wounds, sputum, urine, stool, WBC >10,000, earache, fever; obtain baseline information and during treatment
- Obtain C & S before beginning drug therapy to identify if correct treatment has been initiated
- Assess for allergic reactions: rash, urticaria, pruritus, chills, fever, joint pain; angioedema

may occur a few days after therapy begins; epinephrine, resuscitation equipment should be available for anaphylactic reaction
- Identify urine output; if decreasing, notify prescriber (may indicate nephrotoxicity); also check for increased BUN, creatinine
- Monitor blood studies: AST (SGOT), ALT (SGPT), CBC, Hct, bilirubin, LDH, alkaline phosphatase, Coombs' test monthly if patient is on long-term therapy
- Monitor electrolytes: potassium, sodium, chloride monthly if patient is on long-term therapy
- Assess bowel pattern daily; if severe diarrhea occurs, drug should be discontinued; may indicate pseudomembranous colitis
- Monitor for bleeding: ecchymosis, bleeding gums, hematuria, stool guaiac daily if on long-term therapy
- Assess for overgrowth of infection: perineal itching, fever, malaise, redness, pain, swelling, drainage, rash, diarrhea, change in cough, sputum

Associated nursing diagnoses

- ✓ Infection, risk for (uses)
- ✓ Diarrhea (adverse reactions)
- ✓ Injury, risk for (adverse reactions)
- ✓ Knowledge deficit (teaching)
- ✓ Noncompliance (teaching)

Implementation

IM route

- Reconstitute with 0.9% NaCl, D_5W, sterile water
- May be diluted with lidocaine (1%, 2%) to prevent pain from inj (IM only); use lidocaine without epinephrine only
- Shake after reconstitution; give deep in large muscle mass; massage
- Do not give SC; severe pain may occur
- Inj near nerves can result in severe pain and loss of function of nerve that was injected

IV **IV route**

- Change **IV** sites q48h to prevent phlebitis and pain at site
- Give by intermittent inf by diluting 3 million U or less/50 ml or more; or doses of 73 million U/100 ml D_5W, 0.9% NaCl; give over 1-2 hr (adult) P or 30 min (child)
- Give by cont inf by diluting in compatible sol and run over 24 hr

Syringe incompatibilities:

Oxytetracycline, tetracycline

Syringe compatibilities:

Aminoglycosides, chloramphenicol, cimetidine, colistimethate, gentamicin, heparin, kanamycin, lincomycin, polymyxin B, streptomycin

Additive incompatibilities:

Amphotericin B, bleomycin, cephalothin, chlorpromazine, cytarabine, floxacillin, hydroxyzine, methylprednisolone sodium succinate, oxytetracycline, prochlorperazine, promethazine

Additive compatibilities:

Calcium chloride, calcium gluconate, chloramphenicol,

P

clindamycin, colistimethate, diphenhydramine, erythromycin, furosemide, gentamicin, hydrocortisone sodium succinate, kanamycin, methicillin, polymyxin B, prednisolone, procaine, ranitidine, verapamil, vitamin B with C

Patient/family education

• Teach patient to report sore throat, bruising, bleeding, joint pain; may indicate blood dyscrasias (rare)
• Advise patient to contact prescriber if vaginal itching, loose, foul-smelling stools, furry tongue occur; may indicate superinfection
• Advise patient to notify prescriber of diarrhea with blood or pus, which may indicate pseudomembranous colitis

Evaluation

Positive therapeutic outcome
• Absence of signs/symptoms of infection (WBC <10,000, temp WNL, absence of red, draining wounds, earache)
• Reported improvement in symptoms of infection

Treatment of anaphylaxis: Withdraw drug, maintain airway, administer epinephrine, aminophylline, O_2, **IV** corticosteroids

penicillin V potassium

Pen-Vee K ✱, Deltapen-VK, V-Cillin K, Veetids, PVFK ✱, Apo-Pen-VK ✱, Novopen-VK ✱, Ledercillin-VK, Uticillin-VK, Betapen-VK, Penapar-VK, Robicillin-VK

Func. class.: Broad-spectrum antiinfective
Chem. class.: Natural penicillin

Pregnancy category **B**

Action: Interferes with cell wall replication of susceptible organisms; osmotically unstable cell wall swells and bursts from osmotic pressure

Uses: Emphysema, gangrene, anthrax, gonorrhea, mastoiditis, meningitis, osteomyelitis, pneumonia, tetanus, UTIs, prophylactically in rheumatic fever

Therapeutic Outcome: Bactericidal effects for gram-positive cocci *Staphylococcus aureus, Streptococcus pyogenes, S. viridans, S. faecalis, S. bovis, S. pneumoniae;* gram-negative cocci *Neisseria gonorrhoeae, N. meningitidis;* gram-positive bacilli *Bacillus anthracis, Clostridium perfringens, C. tetani, Corynebacterium diphtheriae, Listeria monocytogenes;* gram-negative bacillus *Streptobacillus moniliformis;* spirochete *Treponema pallidum; Actinomyces*

Dosage and routes

Pneumococcal/staphylococcal infections

Adult: PO 250-500 mg q6h

P *Child <12 yr:* PO 15-50 mg/kg/day in divided doses q6-8h

Streptococcal infections

Adult: PO 125-250 mg q6-8h × 10 days

Prevention of recurrence of rheumatic fever/chorea

Adult: PO 125-250 mg bid continuously

Vincent's infection of oropharynx

Adult: PO 500 mg q6h

Available forms: Tab 125, 250, 500 mg; film-coated tab 250, 500 mg; powder for oral susp 125, 250 mg/5 ml

Side effects/adverse reactions

CNS: Lethargy, hallucinations, anxiety, ***depression,*** twitching, ***coma, convulsions***
GI: Nausea, vomiting, diarrhea, increased AST (SGOT), ALT (SGPT), abdominal pain, glossitis, colitis
GU: Oliguria, proteinuria, hematuria, vaginitis, moniliasis, glomerulonephritis
HEMA: Anemia, increased bleeding time, ***bone marrow depression, granulocytopenia***
META: Hyperkalemia, hypokalemia, alkalosis

Contraindications: Hypersensitivity to penicillins, P neonates

Precautions: Hypersensitivity to cephalosporins, pregnancy **B**

Pharmacokinetics

Absorption	Widely absorbed
Distribution	Widely distributed; crosses placenta
Metabolism	Liver, minimally
Excretion	Kidneys, unchanged; breast milk
Half-life	½-1 hr

Pharmacodynamics

Onset	Rapid
Peak	½-1 hr

Interactions

Drug/drug:

Individual drugs

Aspirin: ↑ penicillin levels, ↓ renal excretion
Cholestyramine: ↓ effectiveness of penicillin
Chloramphenicol: ↑ half-life of chloramphenicol, ↓ effectiveness of penicillin
Colestipol: ↓ effectiveness of penicillin
Probenecid: ↑ penicillin levels, ↓ renal excretion

Drug classifications

Erythromycins: ↓ antimicrobial effectiveness
Oral anticoagulants: ↑ anticoagulant effects
Oral contraceptives: ↓ contraceptive effectiveness
Tetracyclines: ↓ antimicrobial effectiveness

Drug/food:

Food, carbonated drinks, citrus fruit juices: ↓ absorption

Lab test interferences

False positive: Urine glucose, urine protein

P

NURSING CONSIDERATIONS

Assessment

- Assess patient for previous sensitivity reaction to penicillins or other cephalosporins; cross-sensitivity between penicillins and cephalosporins is common
- Assess patient for signs and symptoms of infection including characteristics of wounds, sputum, urine, stool, WBC >10,000, earache, fever; obtain baseline information and during treatment
- Obtain C & S before beginning drug therapy to identify if correct treatment has been initiated
- Assess for allergic reactions: rash, urticaria, pruritus, chills, fever, joint pain; angioedema may occur a few days after therapy begins; epinephrine, resuscitation equipment should be available for anaphylactic reaction
- Identify urine output; if decreasing, notify prescriber (may indicate nephrotoxicity); also check for increased BUN, creatinine
- Monitor blood studies: AST (SGOT), ALT (SGPT), CBC, Hct, bilirubin, LDH, alkaline phosphatase, Coombs' test monthly if patient is on long-term therapy
- Monitor electrolytes: potassium, sodium, chloride monthly if patient is on long-term therapy
- Assess bowel pattern daily; if severe diarrhea occurs, drug should be discontinued; may indicate pseudomembranous colitis
- Monitor for bleeding: ecchymosis, bleeding gums, hematuria, stool guaiac daily if on long-term therapy
- Assess for overgrowth of infection: perineal itching, fever, malaise, redness, pain, swelling, drainage, rash, diarrhea, change in cough, sputum

Associated nursing diagnoses

✓ Infection, risk for (uses)
✓ Diarrhea (adverse reactions)
✓ Injury, risk for (adverse reactions)
✓ Knowledge deficit (teaching)
✓ Noncompliance (teaching)

Implementation

PO route

- Give in even doses around the clock; if GI upset occurs, give with food; drug must be given for 10-14 days to ensure organism death and prevent superinfection; store in tight container
- Shake susp; store in refrigerator for 2 wk or for 1 wk at room temp

Patient/family education

- Teach patient to report sore throat, bruising, bleeding, joint pain; may indicate blood dyscrasias (rare)
- Advise patient to contact prescriber if vaginal itching, loose, foul-smelling stools, furry tongue occur; may indicate superinfection
- Instruct patient to take all medication prescribed for the length of time ordered
- Advise patient to notify prescriber of diarrhea with blood or pus, which may indicate pseudomembranous colitis

Evaluation

Positive therapeutic outcome
- Absence of signs/symptoms of infection (WBC <10,000, temp WNL, absence of red, draining wounds, earache)
- Reported improvement in symptoms of infection

Treatment of anaphylaxis:
Withdraw drug, maintain airway, administer epinephrine, aminophylline, O_2, **IV** corticosteroids

pentamidine
(pen-tam'i-deen)
Nebupent, Pentam 300, Pentacarinat ✱, Pneumopent ✱
Func. class.: Antiprotozoal
Chem. class.: Aromatic diamide derivative
Pregnancy category **C**

Action: Interferes with DNA/RNA synthesis in protozoa; has direct effect on islet cells in the pancreas

Therapeutic Outcome: Protozoa death

Uses: *Pneumocystis carinii* infections

Investigational uses: Babesiosis, leishmaniasis, African trypanosomiasis

Dosage and routes
P *Adult and child:* **IV**/IM 4 mg/kg/day × 2 wk; neb 600 mg/6 ml NS via specific nebulizer given q4 wk for prevention

Available forms: Inj; aerosol 300 mg/vial

Side effects/adverse reactions
CNS: Disorientation, hallucinations, dizziness, confusion
CV: Hypotension, ventricular tachycardia, ECG abnormalities
GI: Nausea, vomiting, anorexia, increased AST (SGOT), ALT (SGPT), ***acute pancreatitis,*** metallic taste
GU: Acute renal failure, increased serum creatinine, renal toxicity
HEMA: Anemia, ***leukopenia, thrombocytopenia***
INTEG: Sterile abscess, pain at inj site, pruritus, urticaria, rash
META: Hyperkalemia, hypocalcemia, *hypoglycemia, hyperglycemia*
MISC: Fatigue, chills, night sweats
RESP: Cough, shortness of breath, ***bronchospasm*** (with aerosol)

Precautions: Blood dyscrasias, hepatic disease, renal disease, diabetes mellitus, cardiac disease, hypocalcemia, pregnancy **C**, hypertension, hypotension, P lactation, children

Pharmacokinetics

Absorption	Well absorbed (IM); minimally absorbed (inh); completely absorbed (IV)
Distribution	Widely distributed; does not appear in CSF
Metabolism	Not known
Excretion	Kidneys, unchanged (up to 30%)
Half-life	6½-9½ hr; increased in renal disease

Pharmacodynamics

	IM	IV	INH
Onset	Unknown	Unknown	Unknown
Peak	½-1 hr	Inf end	Unknown

Interactions
Drug/drug:
Individual drugs
Amphotericin B: ↑ nephrotoxicity
Cisplatin: ↑ bone marrow depression
Colistin: ↑ nephrotoxicity
Methoxyflurane: ↑ bone marrow depression
Polymyxin B: ↑ bone marrow depression
Vancomycin: ↑ bone marrow depression
Drug classifications
Aminoglycosides: ↑ nephrotoxicity
Antineoplastics: ↑ nephrotoxicity, bone marrow depression
Radiation: ↑ nephrotoxicity, bone marrow depression

NURSING CONSIDERATIONS
Assessment
- Assess any patient with compromised renal system: drug is excreted slowly in poor renal system function; toxicity may occur rapidly
- Assess patient for infection including increased temp, thick sputum, WBC >10,000; monitor these signs of infection throughout treatment; obtain C&S before beginning therapy; treatment may begin after culture is obtained
- Assess respiratory system including rate, rhythm, bilateral lung sounds, shortness of breath, wheezing, dyspnea
- Monitor ECG for cardiac dysrhythmias; ECG and pulse should be checked frequently during treatment, since cardiotoxicity can occur
- Assess for hypoglycemia including nausea, tremors, anxiety, chills, diaphoresis, headache, hunger, cold, pale skin; this side effect can last for several mo after treatment is completed
- Monitor for hyperglycemia including flushed, dry skin, acetone breath, thirst, anorexia, drowsiness, polyuria; this side effect can last for several mo after treatment is completed
- Monitor renal studies including BUN, urinalysis, creatinine; obtain at baseline and frequently during treatment; nephrotoxicity may occur; check I&O, report hematuria, oliguria
- Monitor blood studies including blood glucose, CBC, platelets; blood glucose fluctuations are common; anemia, leukopenia, thrombocytopenia can occur
- Monitor liver studies including AST (SGOT), ALT (SGPT), alkaline phosphatase, bilirubin before beginning treatment and every 3 days during therapy
- Monitor calcium before beginning treatment and every 3 days during therapy; hypocalcemia may occur

Associated nursing diagnoses
✓ Infection, risk for (uses)
✓ Knowledge deficit (teaching)

Implementation

IM route

- Reconstitute 300 mg/3 ml sterile water for inj; give deep in large muscle mass; IM is a painful route

IV **IV route**

- For intermittent inf reconstitute 300 mg/3-5 ml sterile water for inj, D_5W; withdraw dose and further dilute in 50-250 ml D_5W; diluted sol is stable for 48 hr; discard unused sol; give over 1 hr or more

Y-site incompatibilities:
Foscarnet, fluconazole

Y-site compatibility:
Zidovudine

Inh route

- Dilute 300 mg/600 ml sterile water for inj; put reconstituted sol into nebulizer; do not use with other drugs or sol precipitate may occur; stable for 48 hr at room temp; protect from light; administer over 30-45 min

Patient family education

- Teach patient to report sore throat, fever, fatigue; could indicate superinfection
- Advise patient not to drink alcohol or take aspirin, since gastric bleeding may occur
- Teach patient to make position changes slowly to prevent orthostatic hypotension

Evaluation

Positive therapeutic outcome

- Decreased signs and symptoms of protozoan infections
- Decreased signs and symptoms of *Pneumocystis carinii* pneumonia in HIV infections

pentazocine

(pen-taz'oh-seen)
Talwin, Talwin NX
Func. class.: Narcotic analgesic
Chem. class.: Synthetic benzomorphan (agonist/ antagonist)
Pregnancy category **C**
Controlled substance schedule **IV**

Action: Inhibits ascending pain pathways in limbic system, thalamus, midbrain, hypothalamus by binding to opiate receptor sites, altering pain perception and response

➔ **Therapeutic Outcome:** Relief of pain

Uses: Moderate to severe pain

Dosage and routes

Adult: PO 50-100 mg q3-4h prn, not to exceed 600 mg/day; **IV**/IM/SC 30 mg q3-4h prn, not to exceed 360 mg/day

Available forms: SC, IM, IV 30 mg/ml; tab 50 mg

Side effects/adverse reactions

CNS: Drowsiness, dizziness, confusion, headache, sedation, euphoria, hallucinations, dreaming
CV: Palpitations, bradycardia, change in B/P, tachycardia, increased B/P (high doses)
EENT: Tinnitus, blurred vision, miosis (high doses), diplopia

P

GI: Nausea, vomiting, anorexia, constipation, cramps
GU: Urinary retention
INTEG: Rash, urticaria, bruising, flushing, diaphoresis, pruritus, severe irritation at inj sites
RESP: Respiratory depression

Contraindications: Hypersensitivity, addiction (narcotic)

Precautions: Addictive personality, pregnancy **C**, lactation, increased intracranial pressure, MI (acute), severe heart disease, respiratory depression, hepatic disease, renal disease, seizure disorder, P child <18 yr

Pharmacokinetics

Absorption	Well absorbed (PO, SC, IM); completely absorbed (IV)
Distribution	Widely distributed; crosses placenta
Metabolism	Liver, extensively
Excretion	Kidneys, small amounts (unchanged)
Half-life	2-3 hr

Pharmacodynamics

	PO	SC/IM	IV
Onset	15-30 min	15-30 min	Rapid
Peak	1-3 hr	1-2 hr	15 min
Duration	3 hr	2-4 hr	1 hr

Interactions
Drug/drug:

Individual drugs
Alcohol: ↑ respiratory depression, hypotension, sedation

Drug classifications
Antihistamines: ↑ respiratory depression, hypotension
CNS depressants: ↑ respiratory depression, hypotension
MAOI: Use cautiously; results are unpredictable
Phenothiazines: ↑ respiratory depression, hypotension
Opioid agonists: ↑ opioid withdrawals (dependency)
Sedative/hypnotics: ↑ respiratory depression, hypotension

Lab test interferences
Increase: Amylase, lipase

NURSING CONSIDERATIONS
Assessment
- Assess pain characteristics: location, intensity, type of pain before medication administration and following treatment
- Monitor VS after parenteral route; note muscle rigidity, drug history, liver, kidney function tests, respiratory dysfunction: respiratory depression, character, rate, rhythm; notify prescriber if respirations are <10/min
- Monitor CNS changes: dizziness, drowsiness, hallucinations, euphoria, LOC, pupil reaction
- Monitor allergic reactions: rash, urticaria

Associated nursing diagnoses
- ✓ Pain (uses)
- ✓ Sensory-perceptual alteration: visual, auditory (adverse reactions)
- ✓ Breathing pattern, ineffective (adverse reactions)
- ✓ Knowledge deficit (teaching)

Implementation
- Give by inj (IM, **IV**), only when resuscitative equipment

available; give slowly to prevent rigidity
• Store in light-resistant area at room temp

PO route
• Tab made in the United States contain naloxone 0.5 mg to prevent abuse if the PO preparation is used **IV**

IM route
• Give deeply in large muscle mass; rotate inj sites

IV **IV route**
• Give by direct **IV** after diluting 5 mg/ml of sterile water for inj; give 5 mg or less over 1 min

Syringe incompatibilities:
Glycopyrrolate, heparin, pentobarbital, other barbiturates

Syringe compatibilities:
Atropine, benzquinamide, butorphanol, chlorpromazine, cimetidine, dimenhydrinate, diphenhydramine, droperidol, fentanyl, hydromorphone, hydroxyzine, meperidine, metoclopramide, morphine, perphenazine, prochlorperazine edisylate, promazine, promethazine, propiomazine, ranitidine, scopolamine

Y-*site incompatibility:*
Nafcillin

Y-*site compatibilities:*
Heparin, hydrocortisone sodium succinate, potassium chloride, vitamin B with C

Additive incompatibilities:
Aminophylline, amobarbital, pentobarbital, phenobarbital, secobarbital, sodium bicarbonate

Patient/family education
• Teach patient to report any symptoms of CNS changes, allergic reactions
• Advise patients to avoid CNS depressants: alcohol, sedative/hypnotics for at least 24 hr after taking this drug
• Discuss with patient that dizziness, drowsiness, and confusion are common; to avoid getting up without assistance
• Discuss in detail all aspects of the drug
• Instruct patient to change position slowly to prevent orthostatic hypotension
• Teach patient to turn, cough, deep breathe after surgery to prevent atelectasis

Evaluation
Positive therapeutic outcome
• Relief of pain

Treatment of overdose:
Naloxone (Narcan) 0.2-0.8 **IV**, O_2, **IV** fluids, vasopressors

P

pentobarbital
(pen-toe-bar′bi-tal)
Nembutal, Nembutal Sodium, Nembutal Sodium Solution, Nova-Rectal ✤, pentobarbital sodium, Pentogen ✤
Func. class.: Sedative/hypnotic barbiturate
Chem. class.: Barbitone, short acting
Pregnancy category **D**
Controlled substance schedule **II** (USA), schedule **G** (Canada)

Action: Depresses activity in brain cells, primarily in reticular activating system in brainstem; also selectively depresses neurons in posterior hypothalamus, limbic structures; may decrease cerebral blood flow, intracranial pressure (**IV**) and cerebral edema; may potentiate GABA, an inhibitory neurotransmitter

Therapeutic Outcome: Sedation, sleep

Uses: Insomnia, sedation, preoperative medication, increased intracranial pressure, dental anesthetic

Dosage and routes

Adult: PO 100-200 mg hs; IM 150-200 mg hs; **IV** 100 mg initially, then up to 500 mg; rec 120-200 mg hs

P *Child:* IM 3-5 mg, not to exceed 100 mg

P *Child 2 mo-1 yr:* rec 30 mg

P *Child 1-4 yr:* rec 30-60 mg

P *Child 5-12 yr:* rec 60 mg

P *Child 12-14 yr:* rec 60-120 mg

Available forms: Cap 50, 100 mg; elix 18.2 mg/5 ml; powder, rec supp 30, 60, 120, 200 mg; inj 50 mg/ml

Side effects/adverse reactions

CNS: Lethargy, drowsiness, hangover, dizziness, paradoxic G stimulation in elderly and P children, lightheadedness, dependence, ***CNS depression,*** mental depression, slurred speech

CV: Hypotension, bradycardia

GI: Nausea, vomiting, diarrhea, constipation

HEMA: ***Agranulocytosis, thrombocytopenia, megaloblastic anemia*** (long-term treatment)

INTEG: ***Rash,*** urticaria, pain, abscesses at inj site, angioedema, thrombophlebitis, ***Stevens-Johnson syndrome***

RESP: Depression, apnea, laryngospasm, bronchospasm

Contraindications: Hypersensitivity to barbiturates, respiratory depression, addiction to barbiturates, severe liver, renal impairment, porphyria, uncontrolled pain

Precautions: Anemia, pregnancy **D**, lactation, hepatic disease, renal disease, hyper- G tension, elderly, acute/chronic pain

Pharmacokinetics

Absorption	Well absorbed
Distribution	Widely distributed; crosses placenta, enters breast milk
Metabolism	Liver
Excretion	Kidneys, unchanged (minimally)
Half-life	15-48 hr

Pharmacodynamics

	PO	IM	IV	REC
Onset	15-30 min	10-25 min	Immediate	Slow
Peak	3-4 hr	Unknown	1 min	Unknown
Duration	4-6 hr	1-4 hr	15 min	4-6 hr

Interactions:

Drug/drug:

Individual drugs

Alcohol: ↑ CNS depression
Chloramphenicol: ↓ effectiveness
Cyclosporine: ↓ effectiveness
Dacarbazine: ↓ effectiveness
Cyclophosphamide: ↑ hematologic toxicity
Quinidine: ↓ effectiveness
Valproic acid: ↑ sedation

Drug classifications

Anticoagulants: ↓ effectiveness
Antidepressants: ↑ CNS depression
Antihistamines: ↑ CNS depression
Glucocorticoids: ↓ effectiveness
MAOI: ↑ CNS depression
Narcotics: ↑ CNS depression
Oral contraceptives: ↓ effectiveness
Sedative/hypnotics: ↑ CNS depression
Tricyclics antidepressants: ↓ effectiveness

NURSING CONSIDERATIONS

Assessment

- Assess mental status: mood, sensorium, affect, memory G (long, short), especially elderly; if using as a hypnotic, assess sleep patterns during therapy; drug suppresses REM sleep with dreaming; withdrawal insomnia may occur after short-term use; do not start using drug again; insomnia will improve in 1-3 nights; may experience increased dreaming
- Monitor for respiratory dysfunction: respiratory depression, character, rate, rhythm (when using **IV**); hold drug if respirations are <10/min or if pupils are dilated; also check VS q30 min after parenteral route for 2 hr
- Assess for blood dyscrasias: fever, sore throat, bruising, rash, jaundice, epistaxis (long-term treatment only)
- Assess seizure activity including type, location, duration, and character; provide seizure precaution
- Assess for pain in postoperative patients; pain threshold is lowered when patients are taking this medication

Associated nursing diagnoses

✓ Injury, risk for (side effects)
✓ Knowledge deficit (teaching)

Implementation

- Administer only after removal of cigarettes, to prevent fires
- Reserve use until after trying conservative measures for insomnia

PO route

- Give 30 min before hs for expected sleeplessness
- May dilute elixir in juice, milk, or water if needed
- Give on empty stomach for best absorption

IM route

- Give deeply in muscle mass (gluteal) to minimize irritation to tissues; split inj of >5 ml into two since irritation to tissues may occur; do not administer SC

IV **IV route**

- Use large vein to prevent extravasation; if extravasation occurs, use moist heat to the area and 5% procaine sol injected into area; give at 50 mg/1 min or more

P

• Give **IV** only with resuscitative equipment available (and only by qualified personnel)

Syringe compatibilities:
Aminophylline, ephedrine, hydromorphone, neostigmine, scopolamine, sodium bicarbonate, thiopental

Syringe incompatibilities:
Benzquinamide, butorphanol, chlorpromazine, cimetidine, dimenhydrinate, diphenhydramine, droperidol, fentanyl, glycopyrrolate, hydroxyzine, meperidine, midazolam, nalbuphine, pentazocine, perphenazine, prochlorperazine, promazine, promethazine, ranitidine

Y-site compatibilities:
Acyclovir, regular insulin

Additive compatibilities:
Amikacin, aminophylline, calcium chloride, cephapirin, chloramphenicol, dimenhydrinate, erythromycin lactobionate, lidocaine, thiopental, verapamil

Additive incompatibilities:
Chlorpheniramine, codeine, ephedrine, erythromycin gluceptate, regular insulin, levorphanol, hydrocortisone, sodium succinate, hydroxyzine, methadone, norepinephrine, pentazocine, penicillin G potassium, phenytoin, promazine, promethazine, streptomycin, triflupromazine, vancomycin

Patient/family education

• Teach patient to carry ID card or Medic Alert bracelet stating name, drugs taken, condition, prescriber's name, phone number
• Caution patient to avoid driving and other activities that require alertness
• Caution patient to avoid alcohol ingestion and CNS depressants; increased sedation may occur
• Teach patient not to discontinue medication quickly after long-term use; taper off over several wk

Evaluation

Positive therapeutic outcome
• Improved sleeping patterns
• Decreased seizure activity
• Improved energy

Treatment of overdose:
Lavage, activated charcoal, warming blanket, vital signs, hemodialysis

pentostatin
(pen′toe-sta-tin)
Nipent
Func. class.: Antineoplastic, enzyme inhibitor
Chem. class.: Streptomyces antibioticus derivative
Pregnancy category **C**

Action: Inhibits the enzyme adenosine deaminase (ADA), which is able to block DNA synthesis and some RNA synthesis

➡ Therapeutic Outcome:
Prevention of rapidly growing malignant cells

Uses: α-Interferon–refractory hairy cell leukemia

Dosage and routes

Adult: **IV** 4 mg/m^2 every other wk; may be given **IV** bol or diluted in a larger volume and given over 20-30 min

Available forms: Inj 10 mg/vial

Side effects/adverse reactions

CNS: Headache, anxiety, confusion, depression, dizziness, insomnia, nervousness, paresthesia
GI: Nausea, vomiting, anorexia, diarrhea, constipation, flatulence, stomatitis, elevated liver function tests
GU: ***Hematuria,*** dysuria, increased BUN/creatinine
HEMA: ***Leukopenia, anemia, thrombocytopenia, ecchymosis, lymphadenopathy,*** petechiae
INTEG: Rash, eczema, dry skin, pruritus, sweating, herpes simplex/zoster
RESP: Cough, upper respiratory tract infection, bronchitis, dyspnea, epistaxis, pneuomonia, pharyngitis, rhinitis, sinusitis
SYST: Fever, infection, fatigue, pain, allergic reaction, chills, ***death, sepsis,*** chest pain, flu syndrome

Contraindications: Hypersensitivity to this drug or mannitol

Precautions: Renal disease, pregnancy **C**, lactation, children, bone marrow depression

Pharmacokinetics

Absorption	Completely absorbed (IV)
Distribution	Unknown; low protein binding
Metabolism	Unknown
Excretion	Kidneys
Half-life	5-7 hr; increased in renal disease

Pharmacodynamics

Onset	4-5 mo
Peak	Unknown
Duration	1½-34 mo

Interactions

Drug/drug:

Individual drugs
Fludarabine: Fatal pulmonary reaction
Vidarabine: ↑ adverse reactions

NURSING CONSIDERATIONS

Assessment

- Assess CNS changes: confusion, paresthesias, psychosis, tremors, seizures, neuropathies; drug should be discontinued
- Assess for toxicity: facial flushing, epistaxis, increased pro-time, thrombocytopenia; drug should be discontinued
- Assess acidosis, signs of dehydration: rapid respirations, poor skin turgor, decreased urine output, dry skin, restlessness, weakness
- Check buccal cavity q8h for dryness, sores or ulceration, white patches, oral pain, bleeding, dysphagia; obtain prescription for viscous lidocaine (Xylocaine) to use in mouth
- Assess symptoms indicating

severe allergic reaction: rash, pruritus, urticaria, purpuric skin lesions, itching, flushing

- Assess tachypnea, ECG changes, dyspnea, edema, fatigue; respiratory and cardiovascular reaction can be severe
- Monitor CBC, differential, platelet count weekly; withhold drug if WBC count is <4000/mm^3 or platelet count is <100,000/mm^3, notify prescriber of results
- Monitor renal function studies: BUN, creatinine, serum uric acid, urine CrCl before and during therapy; I&O ratio; report fall in urine output to <30 ml/hr
- Monitor temp q4h (may indicate beginning of infection)
- Monitor liver function tests before and during therapy (bilirubin, AST [SGOT], ALT [SGPT], LDH) as needed or monthly; check for yellowing of skin and sclera, dark urine, clay-colored stools, itchy skin, abdominal pain, fever, diarrhea
- Assess for bleeding: hematuria, stool guaiac, bruising or petechiae, mucosa or orifices q8h; check for inflammation of mucosa, breaks in skin
- Assess effects of alopecia on body image; discuss feelings about body changes

Associated nursing diagnoses

- ✓ Injury, risk for (adverse reactions)
- ✓ Body image disturbance (adverse reactions)
- ✓ Infection, risk for (adverse reactions)
- ✓ Knowledge deficit (teaching)

Implementation

- Give fluids **IV** or PO before chemotherapy to hydrate patient
- Give antacid before oral agent, antiemetic 30-60 min before giving drug and prn to prevent vomiting; administer antibiotics for prophylaxis of infection
- Give top or syst analgesics for pain to lessen effects from stomatitis
- Give liq diet: carbonated beverages; gelatin may be added if patient is not nauseated or vomiting
- Encourage patient to rinse mouth tid-qid with water, club soda; brush teeth bid-qid with soft brush or cotton-tipped applicators for stomatitis; use unwaxed dental floss

IV IV route

- Preparation should be done by personnel knowledgeable in preparing antineoplastics wearing gloves, gown, mask in biologic cabinet
- Give by direct **IV** by reconstituting 10 mg/5 ml of sterile water for inj (2 mg/ml); shake well
- Give over 5 min
- Give by intermittent inf after diluting 10 mg/25-50 ml of 0.9% NaCl, D_5W; give over 30 min
- Diluted sol should be used within 8 hr at room temp

Y-site compatibilities:

Fludarabine, melphalan, ondansetron, paclitaxel, sargramostin

Solution compatibilities:

D_5W, 0.9% NaCl, Ringer's inj

Patient/family education

- Teach patient to avoid use of products containing aspirin or ibuprofen, razors, commercial mouthwash, since bleeding may occur; to report symptoms of bleeding (hematuria, tarry stools)
- Advise patient to report signs of anemia (fatigue, headache, irritability, faintness, shortness of breath); CNS reactions including confusion, psychosis, nightmares, seizures, severe headaches
- Inform patient that hair may be lost during treatment; a wig or hair piece may make patient feel better; new hair may be different in color, texture
- Advise patient to use sunscreen and protective clothing to prevent photosensitive reactions

Evaluation

Positive therapeutic outcome

- Prevention of rapid division of malignant cells
- Decreased bone marrow hairy cells

pentoxifylline

(pen-tox-if′i-lin)

Trental

Func. class.: Hemorheologic agent

Chem. class.: Dimethylxanthine derivative

Pregnancy category **C**

Action: Decreases blood viscosity, stimulates prostacyclin formation, increases blood flow by increasing flexibility of RBCs; decreases RBC hyperaggregation; reduces platelet aggregation, decreases fibrinogen concentration

Therapeutic Outcome: Decreased claudication and improved blood flow

Uses: Intermittent claudication related to chronic occlusive vascular disease

Dosage and routes

Adult: PO 400 mg tid with meals

Available forms: Cont rel tab 400 mg

Side effects/adverse reactions

CNS: Headache, anxiety, *tremors,* confusion, *dizziness*
CV: Angina, dysrhythmias, palpitations, hypotension, chest pain, dyspnea, edema
EENT: Blurred vision, earache, increased salivation, sore throat, conjunctivitis
GI: Dyspepsia, nausea, vomiting, anorexia, bloating, belching, constipation, cholecystitis, dry mouth, thirst, bad taste
INTEG: Rash, pruritus, urticaria, brittle fingernails
MISC: Epistaxis, flulike symptoms, laryngitis, nasal congestion, ***leukopenia,*** malaise, weight changes

Contraindications: Hypersensitivity to this drug or xanthines

Precautions: Pregnancy **C**, angina pectoris, cardiac disease,

P

P lactation, children, impaired renal function

Pharmacokinetics

Absorption	Well absorbed (PO)
Distribution	Unknown
Metabolism	Liver, degradation
Excretion	Kidneys
Half-life	½-1 hr

Pharmacodynamics

Onset	Unknown
Peak	1 hr
Duration	Unknown

Interactions

Drug/drug:

Individual drugs

Aspirin: ↑ bleeding
Cefamandole: ↑ bleeding
Cefoperazone: ↑ bleeding
Cefotetan: ↑ bleeding
Heparin: ↑ bleeding
Plicamycin: ↑ bleeding
Valproic acid: ↑ bleeding
Warfarin: ↑ bleeding

Drug classifications

Antihypertensives: ↑ hypotension
Nitrates: ↑ hypotension
NSAIDs: ↑ bleeding

NURSING CONSIDERATIONS

Assessment

- Monitor B/P, respirations in patient taking antihypertensives
- Assess for intermittent claudication during treatment

Associated nursing diagnoses

- ✓ Pain (uses)
- ✓ Activity intolerance (uses)
- ✓ Knowledge deficit (teaching)
- ✓ Noncompliance (teaching)

Implementation

PO route

- Give with meals to prevent GI upset; tab should not be crushed or chewed

Patient/family education

- Teach patient that therapeutic response may take 2-4 wk
- Advise patient that decreased fats, cholesterol, increased exercise, decreased smoking are necessary to correct condition
- Instruct patient to observe feet for arterial insufficiency
- Instruct patient to use cotton socks, well-fitted shoes; not to go barefoot
- Advise patient to watch for bleeding, bruises, petechiae, epistaxis

Evaluation

Positive therapeutic outcome

- Decreased pain, cramping
- Increased ambulation

permethrin

(per-meth'ren)

Elimite, Nix, Nix Dermal Cream

Func. class.: Pediculicide
Chem. class.: Synthetic pyrethroid

Pregnancy category **B**

Action: Disrupts sodium channel current in parasite's nerve cell resulting in delayed repolarization and paralysis

Uses: Lice, nits, ticks, flea nits, scabies

Dosage and routes

Lice (head)

P ***Adult and child:*** Wash hair, towel dry; apply liberally to hair; leave on 10 min; rinse with water

Scabies

P ***Adult and child:*** Top 5% cream should be applied and massaged to all skin surfaces; cream should be left on for 8-14 hr then washed off

Available forms: Liq 1%; cream 5%

Side effects/adverse reactions

INTEG: Pruritus, burning, stinging, rash, tingling, numbness, edema

Contraindication: Hypersensitivity

Precautions: Head rash, P children, lactation, pregnancy **B**

Pharmacokinetics

Absorption	Small amounts
Distribution	Unknown
Metabolism	Inactivated by enzymes
Excretion	Unknown
Half-life	Unknown

Pharmacodynamics

	TOP
Onset	10 min
Peak	Unknown
Duration	Unknown

Interactions: None

NURSING CONSIDERATIONS

Assessment

- Assess head, hair for lice and nits before and after treatment; if scabies are present, check all skin surfaces
- Identify source of infection: school, family members, sexual contacts

Associated nursing diagnoses

- ✓ Self-care deficit (uses)
- ✓ Skin integrity, impaired (uses)
- ✓ Knowledge deficit (teaching)

Implementation

Top route

- Apply to body areas, scalp only; do not apply to face, lips, mouth, eyes, any mucous membrane, anus, or meatus
- Give top corticosteroids as ordered to decrease contact dermatitis; provide antihistamines
- Give lotions of menthol or phenol to control itching
- Give top antibiotics for infection
- Provide isolation until areas on skin, scalp have cleared and treatment is completed
- Remove nits by using a fine-toothed comb rinsed in vinegar after treatment; use gloves

Patient/family education

- Advise patient to wash all inhabitants' clothing, using insecticide; preventive treatment may be required of all persons living in same house, using lotion or shampoo to decrease spread of infection; use rubber gloves when applying drug

P

• Instruct patient that itching may continue for 4-6 wk; that drug must be reapplied if accidently washed off, or treatment will be ineffective
• Advise patient not to apply to face; if accidental contact with eyes occurs, flush with water
• Advise patient that sexual contacts should be treated simultaneously

Evaluation

Positive therapeutic outcome
• Decreased crusts, nits, brownish trails on skin
• Decreased itching papules in skinfolds
• Decreased itching after several wk

Treatment of ingestion: Gastric lavage, saline laxatives, **IV** diazepam for convulsions

perphenazine

(per-fen'a-zeen)

Apo-Perphenazine ♣, Trilafon, perphenazine, Phenazine ♣, PMS Perphenazine ♣

Func. class.: Antipsychotic/neuroleptic

Chem. class.: Phenothiazine piperidine

Pregnancy category **C**

Action: Depresses cerebral cortex, hypothalamus, limbic system, which control activity, aggression; blocks neurotransmission produced by dopamine at synapse; exhibits strong α-adrenergic, anticholinergic blocking action; as antiemetic inhibits medullary chemoreceptor trigger zone; mechanism for antipsychotic effects is unclear

Therapeutic Outcome: Decreased signs and symptoms of psychosis; decreased nausea and vomiting

Uses: Psychotic disorders, schizophrenia, nausea, vomiting

Dosage and routes

Nausea/vomiting/alcoholism

P ***Adult and child >12 yr:*** IM 5-10 mg prn, max 15 mg in ambulatory patients, 30 mg in hospitalized patients; PO 8-16 mg/day in divided doses, up to 24 mg; **IV** not to exceed 5 mg; give diluted or slow **IV** drip

Psychiatric use in hospitalized patients

Adults: PO 8-16 mg bid-qid, gradually increased to desired dose, not to exceed 64 mg/day; IM 5 mg q6h, not to exceed 30 mg/day

P ***Child >12 yr:*** PO 6-12 mg in divided doses

Nonhospitalized patients

Adult: PO 4-8 mg tid; IM 5 mg q6h

Available forms: Tab 2, 4, 8, 16 mg; oral sol 16 mg/5ml; inj 5 mg/ml

Side effects/adverse reactions

CNS: EPS: pseudoparkinsonism, akathisia, dystonia,

*tardive dyskinesia, **seizures, headache***
CV: Orthostatic hypotension, ***cardiac arrest,*** ECG changes, ***tachycardia***
EENT: Blurred vision, glaucoma
GI: Dry mouth, nausea, vomiting, anorexia, constipation, diarrhea, jaundice, weight gain
GU: Urinary retention, urinary frequency, enuresis, impotence, amenorrhea, gynecomastia
HEMA: Anemia, ***leukopenia, leukocytosis, agranulocytosis***
INTEG: Rash, photosensitivity, dermatitis
RESP: ***Laryngospasm,*** dyspnea, ***respiratory depression***

Contraindications: Hypersensitivity, blood dyscrasias, coma, P child <12 yr, brain damage, bone marrow depression

Precautions: Pregnancy **C**, lactation, seizure disorders, hypertension, hepatic disease, cardiac disease

Pharmacokinetics

Absorption	Variably absorbed (PO); well absorbed (IM)
Distribution	Widely distributed; high concentrations in CNS; crosses placenta
Metabolism	Liver, extensively; GI mucosa
Excretion	Kidneys

Pharmacodynamics

	PO	IM	IV
Onset	Erratic	10 min	Rapid
Peak	2-4 hr	1-2 hr	Unknown
Duration	6-12 hr	6-12 hr	Unknown

Interactions

Drug/drug:

Individual drugs

Alcohol: ↑ effects of both drugs, oversedation
Aluminum hydroxide: ↓ absorption
Bromocriptine: ↓ antiparkinson activity
Disopyramide: ↑ anticholinergic effects
Epinephrine: ↑ toxicity
Guanethidine: ↓ antihypertensive response
Levodopa: ↓ antiparkinson activity
Lithium: ↓ perphenazine levels, ↑ EPS, masking of lithium toxicity
Magnesium hydroxide: ↓ absorption
Norepinephrine: ↓ vasoresponse, ↑ toxicity
Phenobarbital: ↓ effectiveness, ↑ metabolism

Drug classifications

Antacids: ↓ absorption
Anticholinergics: ↑ anticholinergic effects
Antidepressants: ↑ CNS depression
Antidiarrheals, adsorbent: ↓ absorption
Antihistamines: ↑ CNS depression
Antihypertensives: ↑ hypotension
Antithyroid agents: ↑ agranulocytosis
Barbiturate anesthetics: ↑ CNS depression
β-Adrenergics: ↑ effects of both drugs
General anesthetics: ↑ CNS depression
MAOI: ↑ CNS depression
Narcotics: ↑ CNS depression
Sedative/hypnotics: ↑ CNS depression

P

Lab test interferences

Increase: Liver function tests, cardiac enzymes, cholesterol, blood glucose, prolactin, bilirubin, PBI, cholinesterase, iodine, alkaline phosphatase, leukocytes, granulocytes, platelets
Decrease: Hormones (blood and urine)
False positive: Pregnancy tests, PKU
False negative: Urinary steroids, 17-OHCS

NURSING CONSIDERATIONS

Assessment

- Assess mental status: orientation, mood, behavior, presence and type of hallucinations before initial administration and monthly; this drug should significantly reduce psychotic behavior
- Check for swallowing of PO medication; check for hoarding or giving medication to other patients
- Monitor I&O ratio; palpate bladder if low urinary output occurs, especially in elderly; urinalysis recommended before, during prolonged therapy
- Monitor bilirubin, CBC, liver function studies monthly
- Assess affect, orientation, LOC, reflexes, gait, coordination, sleep pattern disturbances
- Monitor B/P with patient sitting, standing, and lying; take pulse and respirations q4h during initial treatment; establish baseline before starting treatment; report drops of 30 mm Hg; obtain baseline ECG, Q wave and T wave changes
- Check for dizziness, faintness, palpitations, tachycardia on rising; severe orthostatic hypotension is common
- Identify for neuroleptic malignant syndrome: hyperpyrexia, muscle rigidity, increased CPK, altered mental status; drug should be discontinued
- Assess for EPS including akathisia (inability to sit still, no pattern to movements), tardive dyskinesia (bizarre movements of the jaw, mouth, tongue, extremities), pseudoparkinsonism (ragged tremors, pill rolling, shuffling gate); an antiparkinsonian drug should be prescribed
- Assess for constipation, urinary retention daily; if these occur, increase bulk, water in diet

Associated nursing diagnoses

✓ Thought processes, altered (uses)
✓ Coping, ineffective individual (uses)
✓ Knowledge deficit (teaching)
✓ Noncompliance (teaching)

Implementation

PO route

- Administer drug in liq form mixed in glass of juice or cola if hoarding is suspected; do not mix in caffeine drinks, tannics, pectins
- Administer decreased dose in elderly, in whom metabolism is slowed
- Administer PO with full glass of water, milk; or give with food to decrease GI upset
- Store in airtight, light-resistant container; oral sol in amber bottle

IM route

- Inject in deep muscle mass;

do not give SC; do not administer sol with a precipitate

IV route

• Give by direct **IV** after diluting with 0.9% NaCl to a conc of 0.5 mg/1 ml; administer at 1 mg/min; may be further diluted and given as an inf

Syringe incompatibilities:

Midazolam, opium alkaloids, pentobarbital, thiethylperazine

Syringe compatibilities:

Atropine, butorphanol, chlorpromazine, cimetidine, dimenhydrinate, diphenhydramine, droperidol, fentanyl, meperidine, metoclopramide, morphine, pentazocine, prochlorperazine, promethazine, scopolamine

Y-site compatibilities:

Acyclovir, amikacin, ampicillin, azlocillin, cefamandole, cefazolin, ceforanide, cefotaxime, cefoxitin, cefuroxime, cephalothin, cephapirin, chloramphenicol, clindamycin, co-trimoxazole, doxycycline, erythromycin lactobionate, famotidine, gentamicin, kanamycin, metronidazole, mezlocillin, minocycline, moxalactam, nafcillin, oxacillin, penicillin G potassium, piperacillin, tetracycline, ticarcillin, tacarcillin/clavulanate, tobramycin, vancomycin

Additive incompatibility:

Cefoperazone

Additive compatibilities:

Ascorbic acid, ethacrynate, netilmicin

Patient/family education

• Teach patient to use good oral hygiene; frequent rinsing of mouth, sugarless gum for dry mouth

• Advise patient to avoid hazardous activities until drug response is determined, dizziness, blurred vision may occur

• Inform patient that orthostatic hypotension occurs often and to rise from sitting or lying position gradually; to remain lying down after IM inj for at least 30 min; tell patient to avoid hot tubs, hot showers, tub baths, since hypotension may occur; teach patient that in hot weather heat stroke may occur; take extra precautions to stay cool

• Teach patient to avoid abrupt withdrawal of this drug, or EPS may result; drug should be withdrawn slowly

• Teach patient to avoid OTC preparations (cough, hay fever, cold) unless approved by prescriber, since serious drug interactions may occur; avoid use with alcohol, CNS depressants; increased drowsiness may result

• Caution patient to use a sunscreen and sunglasses to prevent burns

• Teach patient about EPS and necessity of meticulous oral hygiene, since oral candidiasis may occur

• Instruct patient to take antacids 2 hr before or after taking this drug

• Teach patient to report sore throat, malaise, fever, bleeding, mouth sores; if these occur, CBC should be drawn and drug discontinued

• Teach that urine may turn pink or red

P

Evaluation

Positive therapeutic outcome

- Decrease in emotional excitement, hallucinations, delusions, paranoia
- Reorganization of patterns of thought, speech

Treatment of overdose: Lavage if orally ingested; provide airway; *do not induce vomiting or use epinephrine*

phenazopyridine

(fen-az-eh-peer'i-deen)

Azo-Standard, Baridium, Eridium, Geridium, Phenazo ✤, Phenazodine, phenazopyridine HCl, Pyridiate, Pyridium, Urodine, Urogesic, Viridium

Func. class.: Nonnarcotic analgesic

Chem. class.: Azodye

Pregnancy category B

Action: Exerts analgesic, anesthetic action on the urinary tract mucosa

Uses: Urinary tract irritation, infection (for symptoms only of pain, burning, itching) used with urinary antiinfectives

Dosage and routes

Adult: PO 100-200 mg tid

P *Child 6-12 yr:* PO 12 mg/kg/24 hr in divided doses × 2 days

Available forms: Tab 95, 100, 200 mg

Side effects/adverse reactions

CNS: Headache, vertigo

GI: Nausea, vomiting, GI bleeding, diarrhea, heartburn, anorexia, ***hepatic toxicity***

GU: Renal toxicity, orange-red urine

HEMA: Thrombocytopenia, agranulocytosis, leukopenia, neutropenia, hemolytic anemia, methemoglobinemia

INTEG: Rash, urticaria, skin pigmentation

Contraindications: Hypersensitivity, hepatic disease

Precautions: Pregnancy **B**, renal disease

Pharmacokinetics	
Absorption	Well absorbed (PO)
Distribution	Unknown; crosses placenta
Metabolism	Unknown
Excretion	Kidneys, unchanged
Half-life	Unknown

Pharmacodynamics	
Onset	Unknown
Peak	5-6 hr
Duration	8 hr

Interactions: None

Lab test interferences

Interfere: Bilirubin, urinary glucose tests, urinalysis, PSP excretion, urinary ketones, steroids, proteins

False positive: Clinitest

NURSING CONSIDERATIONS

Assessment

- Assess urinary status: burning, pain, itching, urgency,

frequency, hematuria before, during and after completion of drug therapy
- Monitor liver function studies: AST (SGOT), ALT (SGPT), bilirubin if patient is on long-term therapy
- Assess for hepatotoxicity: dark urine, clay-colored stools, yellowing of skin and sclera, itching, abdominal pain, fever, diarrhea if patient is on long-term therapy
- Assess for allergic reactions: rash, urticaria; if these occur, drug may have to be discontinued

Associated nursing diagnoses

✓ Pain (uses)
✓ Urinary elimination, altered patterns (uses)
✓ Knowledge deficit (teaching)

Implementation

PO route
- Give to patient crushed or whole; chew tab may be chewed
- Give with food or milk to decrease gastric symptoms

Patient/family education

- Advise patient to report any symptoms of hepatotoxicity
- Caution patient not to exceed recommended dosage and to take with meals; to read label on other OTC drugs; may contain aspirin
- Teach patient not to discontinue after pain is relieved but continue to take concurrent prescribed antibiotic until finished
- Inform patient urine may turn red-orange, may stain clothing

Evaluation

Positive therapeutic outcome
- Decrease in pain, burning, itching when urinating

Treatment of overdose:
Methylene blue 1-2 mg/kg **IV** or 100-200 mg vitamins C PO

phenelzine
(fen′el-zeen)
Nardil
Func. class.: Antidepressant, MAOI
Chem. class.: Hydrazine
Pregnancy category **C**

Action: Increases concentrations of endogenous epinephrine, norepinephrine, serotonin, dopamine in storage sites in CNS by inhibition of MAO; increased concentration reduces depression

➔ **Therapeutic Outcome:** Decreased symptoms of depression after 2-3 wk

Uses: Depression, when uncontrolled by other means

Dosage and routes
Adult: PO 45 mg/day in divided doses; may increase to 60 mg/day; dosage should be reduced to 15 mg/day, not to exceed 90 mg/day

Available forms: Tab 15 mg

P

Side effects/adverse reactions

CNS: Dizziness, drowsiness, confusion, headache, anxiety, tremors, stimulation, weakness, hyperreflexia, mania, insomnia, fatigue, weight gain
CV: Orthostatic hypotension, hypertension, dysrhythmias, hypertensive crisis
EENT: Blurred vision
ENDO: SIADH-like syndrome
GI: Constipation, dry mouth, nausea, vomiting, *anorexia,* diarrhea, weight gain
GU: Change in libido, frequency
HEMA: Anemia
INTEG: Rash, flushing, increased perspiration

Contraindications: Hypersensitivity to MAOIs, elderly, hypertension, CHF, severe hepatic disease, pheochromocytoma, severe renal disease, severe cardiac disease

Precautions: Suicidal patients, convulsive disorders, severe depression, schizophrenia, hyperactivity, diabetes mellitus, pregnancy **C**

Pharmacokinetics	
Absorption	Well absorbed
Distribution	Crosses placenta
Metabolism	Liver, extensively
Excretion	Kidneys, breast milk
Half-life	Unknown

Pharmacodynamics	
Onset	Unknown
Peak	Unknown
Duration	Unknown

Interactions

Drug/drug:

Individual drugs
Alcohol: ↑ CNS depression
Clonidine: Severe hypotension; avoid use
Guanethidine: ↓ effects

Drug classifications
Analgesics: ↑ CNS depression
Anticholinergics: ↑ side effects
Antihistamines: ↑ CNS depression
Antihypertensives: May block antihypertensive effect
Barbiturates: ↑ effects
Benzodiazepines: ↑ effects
CNS depressants: ↑ effects
Oral contraceptives: ↑ effects, toxicity
Phenothiazines: ↑ toxicity
Sedative/hypnotics: ↑ CNS depression
Sympathomimetics, indirect-acting: ↑ pressor effect

Drug/food:

Tyramine-containing foods: Hypertensive crisis

NURSING CONSIDERATIONS

Assessment

- Monitor B/P (with patient lying, standing), pulse q4h; if systolic B/P drops 20 mm Hg, hold drug, notify prescriber; take VS q4h in patients with cardiovascular disease
- Monitor hepatic studies: AST (SGOT), ALT (SGPT), bilirubin if patient is on long-term therapy
- Check weight weekly; appetite may increase with drug
- Assess ECG for flattening of T wave, bundle branch block, AV block, dysrhythmias in cardiac patients

• Assess mental status: mood, sensorium, affect, suicidal tendencies; increase in psychiatric symptoms: depression, panic
• Monitor urinary retention, constipation; constipation is G more likely to occur in elderly
• Assess for withdrawal symptoms: headache, nausea, vomiting, muscle pain, weakness; do not usually occur unless drug was discontinued abruptly
• Identify alcohol consumption; if alcohol is consumed, hold dose until AM

Associated nursing diagnoses

✓ Coping, ineffective individual (uses)
✓ Injury, risk for (adverse reactions)
✓ Knowledge deficit (teaching)
✓ Noncompliance (teaching)

Implementation

PO route
• Give with food or milk for GI symptoms; crush if patient is unable to swallow medication whole and mix with food or fluids
• Store at room temp; do not freeze

Patient/family education

• Teach patient that therapeutic effects may take 2-3 wk
• Advise patient to use caution in driving and other activities requiring alertness because of drowsiness, dizziness, blurred vision; to avoid rising quickly from sitting to standing, espe- G cially elderly
• Caution patient to avoid alcohol ingestion, other CNS depressants; serious reaction can occur
• Advise patient not to discontinue medication quickly after long-term use: may cause nausea, headache, malaise, sweating, hallucinations
• Instruct patient to increase fluids, bulk in diet if constipation, urinary retention occur, G especially elderly; a stool softener may be ordered
• Teach patient to take gum, hard sugarless candy, or frequent sips of water for dry mouth
• Teach patient that therapeutic effects may take 1-4 wk
• Teach patient to avoid alcohol ingestion, CNS depressants, OTC medications: cold, weight loss, hay fever, cough syrup
• Teach patient not to discontinue medication quickly after long-term use
• Teach patient to avoid high-tyramine foods: cheese (aged), sour cream, beer, wine, pickled products, liver, raisins, bananas, figs, avocados, meat tenderizers, chocolate, yogurt; increased caffeine
• Teach patient to report headache, palpitations, neck stiffness

Evaluation

Positive therapeutic outcome
• Decrease in depression
• Absence of suicidal thoughts

Treatment of overdose:

Lavage, activated charcoal, monitor electrolytes, VS, diazepam **IV**, sodium bicarbonate

P

phenobarbital

(fee-noe-bar'bit-tal)
Barbita, Luminal, Phenobarbital, phenobarbital sodium, Solfoton
Func. class.: Anticonvulsant, sedative/hypnotic
Chem. class.: Barbiturate
Pregnancy category **D**
Controlled substance schedule **IV**

Action: Depresses activity in brain cells primarily in reticular activating system in brainstem; also selectively depresses neurons in posterior hypothalamus, limbic structures; able to decrease seizure activity by inhibition of impulses in CNS; decreases motor activity

Therapeutic Outcome: Sedation, anticonvulsant, improved energy

Uses: All forms of epilepsy, status epilepticus, febrile P seizures in children, sedation, insomnia

Investigational uses: Hyperbilirubinemia, chronic cholestasis

Dosage and routes

Seizures

Adult: PO 100-200 mg/day in divided doses tid or total dose hs

P *Child:* PO 4-6 mg/kg/day in divided doses q12h; may be given as single dose

Status epilepticus

Adult: **IV** inf 10 mg/kg; run no faster than 50/mg/min; may give up to 20 mg/kg

P *Child:* **IV** inf 5-10 mg/kg; may repeat q10-15 min up to 20 mg/kg; run no faster than 50 mg/min

Insomnia

Adult: PO/IM 100-320 mg

P *Child:* PO/IM 3-6 mg/kg

Sedation:

Adult: PO 30-120 mg/day in 2-3 divided doses

P *Child:* PO 6 mg/kg/day in 3 divided doses

Preoperative sedation

Adult: IM 100-200 mg 1-1½ hr before surgery

P *Child:* PO 6 mg/kg/day in 3 divided doses

Hyperbilirubinemia

P *Neonate:* PO 7 mg/kg/day on days 1-5 after birth; IM 5 mg/kg/day on day 1, then PO on days 2-7 after birth

Chronic cholestasis

Adult: PO 90-180 mg/day in 2-3 divided doses

P *Child <12 yr:* PO 3-12 mg/kg/day in 2-3 divided doses

Available forms: Cap 16 mg; elix 15, 20 mg/5 ml; tab 8, 15, 16, 30, 32, 60, 65, 100 mg; inj 30, 60, 130 mg/ml

Side effects/adverse reactions

CNS: Paradoxic excitement G (elderly), drowsiness, leth-

argy, *hangover headache*, flushing, hallucinations, coma
GI: Nausea, vomiting, diarrhea, constipation
INTEG: Rash, urticaria, Stevens-Johnson syndrome, angioedema, local pain, swelling, necrosis, thrombophlebitis

Contraindications: Hypersensitivity to barbiturates, porphyria, hepatic disease, respiratory disease, nephritis, hyperthyroidism, diabetes mellitus, G elderly, lactation, pregnancy **D**

Precaution: Anemia

Pharmacokinetics

Absorption	Slow (70%-90%) (PO/IM/IV)
Distribution	Not known; crosses placenta
Metabolism	Liver (75%)
Excretion	Kidneys (25% unchanged)
Half-life	2-6 days

Pharmacodynamics

	PO	IM	IV
Onset	30-60 min	10-30 min	5 min
Peak	Unknown	Unknown	30 min
Duration	6-8 hr	4-6 hr	4-6 hr

Interactions

Drug/drug:

Individual drugs

Alcohol: ↑ CNS depression
Chloramphenicol: ↓ effectiveness
Cyclosporine: ↓ effectiveness
Cytophosphamide: ↑ hematologic toxicity
Dacarbazine: ↓ effectiveness
Quinidine: ↓ effectiveness
Valproic acid: ↑ sedation

Drug classifications

Anticoagulants: ↓ effectiveness
Antidepressants: ↑ CNS depression
Antihistamines: ↑ CNS depression
Glucocorticoids: ↓ effectiveness
MAOI: ↑ CNS depression
Narcotics ↑ CNS depression
Oral contraceptives: ↓ effectiveness
Sedative/hypnotics: ↑ CNS depression
Tricyclic antidepressants: ↓ effectiveness

NURSING CONSIDERATIONS

Assessment

- Assess mental status: mood, sensorium, affect, memory G (long, short), especially elderly; if using as a hypnotic, assess sleep patterns during therapy; drug suppresses REM sleep with dreaming
- Withdrawal insomnia may occur after short-term use; do not start using drug again; insomnia improves in 1-3 nights; may experience increased dreaming
- Assess respiratory dysfunction: respiratory depression, character, rate, rhythm when using **IV**; hold drug if respirations are <10/min or if pupils are dilated; also check VS q30 min after parenteral route for 2 hr
- Assess for barbiturate toxicity: hypotension, pulmonary constriction, cold, clammy skin, cyanosis of lips, CNS depression, nausea, vomiting,

P

hallucinations, delirium, weakness, coma, pupillary constriction; mild symptoms occur in 8-12 hr without drug
• Assess for pain in postoperative patients; pain threshold is lowered when patients are taking this medication
• Assess for blood dyscrasias: fever, sore throat, bruising, rash, jaundice, epistaxis (long-term treatment only)
• Assess seizure activity including type, location, duration, and character; provide seizure precaution

Associated nursing diagnoses

✓ Sleep pattern disturbance (uses)
✓ Injury, risk for (adverse reactions)
✓ Knowledge deficit (teaching)

Implementation

• Give medication after removal of cigarettes to prevent fires
• Give medication after trying conservative measures for insomnia

PO route
• Tab may be crushed and mixed with food if swallowing is difficult; also may be mixed with other fluids 30-60 min before hs for expected sleeplessness; on empty stomach for best absorption

IM route
• Give in deep muscle mass (gluteal) to minimize irritation to tissues
• Split inj of >5 ml into two, since irritation to tissues may occur

IV **Direct IV route**
• Use large vein to prevent extravasation; if extravasation occurs, use moist heat to the area and 5% procaine sol injected into area; give at 65 mg or less/min; titrate to patient response

Syringe compatibility:

Heparin

Syringe incompatibilities:

Benzquinamide, ranitidine

Y-site incompatibility:

Hydromorphone

Solution compatibilities:

D_5W, $D_{10}W$, 0.45% NaCl, 0.9% NaCl, Ringer's, dextrose/saline combinations, dextrose/Ringer's, dextrose/LR combinations, sodium lactate

Additive compatibilities:

Amikacin, aminophylline, calcium chloride, calcium gluceptate, cephapirin, colistimethate, dimenhydrinate, polymyxin B, sodium bicarbonate, thiopental, verapamil

Additive incompatibilities:

Cephalothin, chlorpromazine, codeine, ephedrine, hydralazine, hydrocortisone sodium succinate, hydroxyzine, insulin, levorphanol, meperidine, methadone, morphine, norepinephrine, pentazocine, procaine, prochlorazine mesylate, promazine, promethazine, streptomycin, vancomycin

Patient/family education

- Teach patient that hangover is common
- Instruct patient that drug is indicated only for short-term treatment of insomnia and is probably ineffective after 2 wk
- Inform patient that physical dependency may result when used for extended time (45-90 days depending on dosage)
- Teach patient to avoid driving and other activities requiring alertness
- Caution patient to avoid alcohol ingestion and CNS depressants; serious CNS depression may result
- Instruct patient not to discontinue medication quickly after long-term use; may cause seizures; drug should be tapered over 1 wk; take exactly as prescribed
- Emphasize the need to tell all prescribers that a barbiturate is being taken
- Teach the patient to make position changes slowly; orthostatic hypotension may occur
- Teach patient that response may take from 4 days to 2 wk of therapy
- Instruct patient to notify prescriber immediately if bruising, bleeding occur, which may indicate blood dyscrasias

Evaluation

Positive therapeutic outcome

- Improved sleeping patterns
- Decreased seizure activity
- Sedative preoperatively

Treatment of overdose:

Lavage, activated charcoal, warming blanket, VS, hemodialysis, alkalinize urine, give **IV** volume expanders, **IV** fluids

phenolphthalein

(fee-nol-thay'leen)

Alophen, Correctol, Espotabs, Evac-U-Gen, Evac-U-Lax, Ex-Lax, Feen-A-Mint, Lax-Pills, Modane, Medilax, Phenolax, Prulet

Func. class.: Laxative, stimulant/irritant

Chem. class.: Diphenylmethane

Pregnancy category C

Action: Directly acts on intestinal smooth muscle by increasing motor activity; thought to irritate colonic intramural plexus; increases fluid in small intestine; alters fluid and electrolytes; action requires presence of bile

Therapeutic Outcome: Decreased constipation

Uses: Constipation, preparation for bowel surgery or examination

Dosage and routes

Adult: PO 30-270 mg hs

P *Child >6 yr:* 30-60 mg/day

P *Child 2-5 yr:* 15-20 mg/day

Available forms: Tab 60, 90, 97.2, 130 mg; chew tab 65, 90, 97.2 mg; chew gum 97.2 mg; wafers 64.8 mg; chew wafers 80 mg

Side effects/adverse reactions

GI: Nausea, vomiting, an-

orexia, diarrhea, abdominal cramps, rectal burning
INTEG: Rash, urticaria, ***Stevens-Johnson syndrome***
META: Hypokalemia, electrolyte and fluid imbalances

Contraindications: Hypersensitivity, GI obstructions, abdominal pain, nausea/vomiting, fecal impaction, rectal fissures, hemorrhoids (ulcerated)

Precautions: Pregnancy **C**, lactation

Pharmacokinetics

Absorption	Minimally absorbed (15%)
Distribution	Unknown
Metabolism	Not metabolized
Excretion	Kidneys, feces
Half-life	Unknown

Pharmacodynamics

Onset	6-8 hr
Peak	Unknown
Duration	3-4 days

Interactions

Drug/drug:

Drug classifications

Oral drugs (any): ↓ absorption

Lab test interferences

Interfere: BSP test

NURSING CONSIDERATIONS

Assessment

- Monitor blood, urine electrolytes if used often by patient; check I&O ratio to identify fluid loss
- Assess for cramping, rec bleeding, nausea, vomiting; if these symptoms occur, drug should be discontinued; identify cause of constipation; identify whether fluids, bulk, or exercise is missing from lifestyle
- Assess stool for color, consistency, amount, presence of flatulence

Associated nursing diagnoses

- ✓ Constipation (uses)
- ✓ Diarrhea (adverse reaction)
- ✓ Knowledge deficit (teaching)
- ✓ Noncompliance (teaching)

Implementation

PO route

- Chew well before swallowing; follow with 4 oz of water to prevent undissolved tab entering small intestine
- Give with 8 oz water (tab); administer on empty stomach for more rapid results; do not give at hs

Patient/family education

- Discuss with the patient that adequate fluid consumption is necessary
- Teach patient that normal bowel movements do not always occur daily
- Caution patient not to use in presence of abdominal pain, nausea, vomiting; tell patient to notify prescriber if constipation is unrelieved or if symptoms of electrolyte imbalance occur (muscle cramps, pain, weakness, dizziness, excessive thirst)
- Teach patient not to use laxatives for long-term therapy; bowel tone will be lost and will decrease

• Shake susp well as needed
• Teach patient not to take at hs as a laxative; may interfere with sleep; also can cause problems with lipid pneumonia
• Teach patient not to use with food or vitamin preparations; delays digestion and absorption of fat-soluble vitamins

Evaluation

Positive therapeutic outcome
• Decreased constipation in 8-10 hr

phenoxybenzamine
(fen-ox-ee-ben'za-meen)
Dibenzyline
Func. class.: Antihypertensive
Chem. class.: α-Adrenergic blocker
Pregnancy category **C**

Action: α-Adrenergic blocker that binds to α-adrenergic receptors, dilating peripheral blood vessels; lowers peripheral resistance, lowers blood pressure

Therapeutic Outcome: Decreased symptoms of pheochromocytoma or peripheral vascular disease

Uses: Pheochromocytoma

Investigational uses: Peripheral vascular disease

Dosage and routes

Adult: PO 10 mg qd; increase by 10 mg qod; usual range 20-40 mg bid-tid

P ***Child:*** PO 0.2 mg/kg or 6 mg/m^2/day; max 10 mg; may increase at 4-day intervals; maintenance dosage 0.4-1.2 mg/kg/day or 12-36 mg/m^2/day given in divided doses tid or qid

Available forms: Cap 10 mg

Side effects/adverse reactions

CNS: Dizziness, flushing, drowsiness, sedation, weakness, confusion, headache, malaise
CV: Postural hypotension, tachycardia, palpitations
EENT: Nasal congestion, dry mouth, miosis
GI: Dry mouth, nausea, vomiting, diarrhea
GU: Inhibition of ejaculation
INTEG: Allergic contact dermatitis

Contraindications: Hypersensitivity, CHF, angina, cerebral vascular insufficiency, coronary arteriosclerosis

Precautions: Severe renal disease, severe pulmonary disease, pregnancy **C**

Pharmacokinetics	
Absorption	Variable
Distribution	Unknown
Metabolism	Liver
Excretion	Unknown
Half-life	24 hr

Pharmacodynamics	
Onset	2 hr
Peak	4-6 hr
Duration	3-4 days

P

Interactions

Drug/drug:

Individual drugs
Alcohol: ↑ hypotension
Ephedrine: Blocks antihypertensive effect
Levodopa: ↑ hypotension
Norepinephrine: ↓ pressor effect
Phenylephrine: ↑ pressor effects

Drug classifications
Antidepressants, tricyclic: ↑ hypotension
Antihypertensives: ↑ hypotension
Amphetamines: ↑ pressor effect
Nitrates: ↑ hypotension
MAOI: Block antihypertensive effect

Lab test interferences

Increase: Urinary norepinephrine, VMA

NURSING CONSIDERATIONS

Assessment

- Monitor B/P, orthostatic hypotension, syncope; monitor urinary catecholamines

Associated nursing diagnoses

✓Cardiac output, decreased (uses)
✓Injury, potential for (side effects)
✓Knowledge deficit (teaching)
✓Noncompliance (teaching)

Implementation

PO route
- Store in tight container at 86° F (30° C) or less
- Severe hypotension may occur after 1st dose of this medication; decreased hypotension may be prevented by reducing or discontinuing diuretic therapy 3 days before beginning benzapril therapy

Patient/family education

- Teach patient not to discontinue drug abruptly
- Teach patient not to use OTC products (cough, cold, allergy) unless directed by prescriber
- Teach patient the importance of complying with dosage schedule, even if feeling better
- Emphasize the need to rise slowly to sitting or standing position to minimize orthostatic hypotension
- Teach patient to notify prescriber of mouth sores, sore throat, fever, swelling of hands or feet, irregular heartbeat, chest pain
- Caution patient to report excessive perspiration, dehydration, vomiting, diarrhea; may lead to fall in B/P
- Caution patient that drug may cause dizziness, fainting, lightheadedness; may occur during 1st few days of therapy
- Teach patient how to take B/P and normal readings for age group

Evaluation

Positive therapeutic outcome
- Decreased B/P in hypertension
- Increased peripheral pulses

Treatment of overdose:

Administer **IV** saline, norepinephrine, elevate legs, discontinue drug

phentolamine
(fen-tole'a-meen)
Regitine, Rogitine ♣
Func. class.: Antihypertensive
Chem. class.: α-Adrenergic blocker
Pregnancy category **C**

Action: α-Adrenergic blocker, binds to α-adrenergic receptors, dilating peripheral blood vessels, lowering peripheral resistances, lowering blood pressure

➔ **Therapeutic Outcome:** Decreased B/P, reversal of vasoconstriction (dermal necrosis)

Uses: Hypertension, pheochromocytoma, prevention, treatment of dermal necrosis following extravasation of norepinephrine or dopamine

Dosage and routes

Treatment of hypertensive episodes in pheochromocytoma

Adult: **IV**/IM 5 mg; repeat if necessary

P *Child:* **IV**/IM 1 mg; repeat if necessary

Diagnosis of pheochromocytoma

Adult: **IV** 2.5 mg;, if negative, repeat with 5 mg **IV**

P *Child:* **IV** 0.5 mg; if negative, repeat with 1 mg **IV**

Prevention of dermal necrosis

Adult: **IV** 10 mg/100 ml of **IV** fluids with norepinephrine

Impotence (adjunct)

Adult: Intracavernosal 0.5-1 mg with 30 mg papaverine given 1, 2, or 3 treatments/wk

Available forms: Inj 5 mg/ml; tab 25, 50 mg (only injectable form available in US)

Side effects/adverse reactions

CNS: *Dizziness,* flushing, weakness
CV: *Hypotension, tachycardia, angina, dysrhythmias,* ***MI***
EENT: Nasal congestion
GI: ***Dry mouth, nausea, vomiting, diarrhea, abdominal pain***

Contraindications: Hypersensitivity, MI, coronary insufficiency, angina

Precautions: Pregnancy **C**, lactation

Pharmacokinetics

Absorption	Well absorbed (IM); completely absorbed (**IV**)
Distribution	Unknown
Metabolism	Unknown
Excretion	Kidneys, unchanged (10%)
Half-life	Unknown

Pharmacodynamics

	IM	IV	INTRA-CAVERN-OSAL
Onset	Unknown	Rapid	Unknown
Peak	20 min	2 min	5-10 min
Duration	½-1 hr	½ hr	4 hr

P

Interactions

Drug/drug:

Individual drugs

Epinephrine: ↑ effects of epinephrine, hypotension
Guanethidine: ↑ hypotension, bradycardia
Guanadrel: ↑ hypotension, bradycardia
Dopamine: ↓ peripheral vasoconstriction
Ephedrine: ↓ pressor effect
Phenylephrine: ↓ pressor effect
Metaraminol: ↓ pressor effect
Methoxamine: ↑ effects of methoxamine, hypotension

Drug classifications

α-Adrenergics: Antagonistic effect
Antihypertensives: ↑ effects of antihypertensives

NURSING CONSIDERATIONS

Assessment

- Monitor B/P, orthostatic hypotension, syncope, pulse and ECG until stable

Associated nursing diagnoses

✓ Cardiac output, decreased (uses)
✓ Injury, potential for (adverse reactions)
✓ Knowledge deficit (teaching)
✓ Noncompliance (teaching)

Implementation

- Give with vasopressor nearby

IV route

- Give by direct **IV** after diluting 5 mg/1 ml sterile water for inj or 0.9% NaCl; give 5 mg or less/min
- Give by cont inf by further diluting 5-10 mg/500 ml D_5W

Y-site compatibility:

Amiodarone

Syringe compatibility:

Papaverine

Additive compatibilities:

Dobutamine, verapamil

Prevention of dermal necrosis

- Add 10 mg/L to norepinephrine in **IV** sol

Patient/family education

- Caution patient not to discontinue drug abruptly
- Teach patient not to use OTC products (cough, cold, allergy) unless directed by prescriber
- Teach patient the importance of complying with dosage schedule, even if feeling better
- Emphasize the need to rise slowly to sitting or standing position to minimize orthostatic hypotension
- Teach patient to notify prescriber of mouth sores, sore throat, fever, swelling of hands or feet, irregular heartbeat, chest pain
- Caution patient to report excessive perspiration, dehydration, vomiting, diarrhea; may lead to fall in B/P
- Caution patient that drug may cause dizziness, fainting, lightheadedness; may occur during 1st few days of therapy
- Teach patient how to take B/P, and normal readings for age group

Evaluation

Positive therapeutic outcome

- Decreased B/P in hypertension

- Resolution of impotence
- Prevention of dermal necrosis

Treatment of overdose: Administer norepinephrine; discontinue drug

phenylephrine

(fen-ill-ef'rin)

AK-Dilate Ophthalmic, AK-Nefrin Ophthalmic, Alconefrin, Alconefrin-25, Alconefrin-50, Duration, Isopto Frin, Neo-Synephrine, Neo-Synephrine 2.5%, Neo-Synephrine 10% Plain, Neo-Synephrine Viscous, Nostril, Phenylephrine HCl, 2.5% Mydfrin Ophthalmic, Phenoptic, Relief, Rhinall-10 Prefrin, Sinex, St Joseph Measured Dose

Func. class.: Adrenergic, direct acting; ophthalmic vasoconstrictor

Chem. class.: Direct sympathomimetic amine (α-agonist)

Pregnancy category C

Action: Powerful and selective receptor agonist causing contraction of blood vessels, vasoconstriction of eye arterioles; decreases eye engorgement by stimulation of α-adrenergic receptors

Therapeutic Outcome: Increased B/P, decreased nasal congestion, decreased eye irritation

Uses: Hypotension, paroxysmal, supraventricular tachycardia, shock, B/P maintenance during spinal anesthesia, top ocular vasoconstrictor in uveitis, open angle glaucoma, preoperatively, diagnostic procedures, refraction without cycloplegia, nasal congestion

Dosage and routes

Eye irritation

Adult: Instill 2 gtt of a 0.12% sol; may repeat q3-4h

Refraction/ophthalmoscopic exam

Adult: Sol 1 gtt of 2.5%

Uveitis/glaucoma/surgery

P ***Adult and child:*** Instill 1 gtt of a 2.5% or 10% sol in upper surface of cornea

Nasal congestion

Adult: Instill 2-3 gtt or sprays to nasal mucosa bid (0.25%-1%); top apply to nasal mucosa q3-4h prn

P ***Child 6-12 yrs:*** Instill 1-2 gtt or sprays (0.25%) q3-4h prn

P ***Child <6 yrs:*** Instill 2-3 gtt or sprays (0.125%) q3-4h prn

Hypotension

Adult: SC/IM 2-5 mg; may repeat q10-15 min if needed **IV** 0.1-0.5 mg; may repeat q10-15 min if needed

PVCs

Adult: **IV** bol 0.5 mg given rapidly, not to exceed prior

P

dose by >0.1 mg; total dose > 1 mg

Shock

Adult: **IV** inf 10 mg/500 ml D_5W given 100-180 gtt/min, then 40-60 gtt/min titrated to B/P

Available forms: Sol 10%, 2.5%, 1%, 0.12%, 0.125%, 0.16%, 0.2%, 0.25%, 0.5%; jelly 0.5%; inj **IV**, SC, IM, 1% (10 mg/ml)

Side effects/adverse reactions

CNS: ***Headache, dizziness, weakness, anxiety, tremor, insomnia***
CV: Reflex bradycardia, *hypertension, dysrhythmias,* ***tachycardia, CV collapse,*** palpitations, ectopic beats, angina
EENT: Stinging, lacrimation, blurred vision, conjunctival allergy
GI: Nausea, vomiting
INTEG: Necrosis, tissue sloughing with extravasation, ***gangrene***

Contraindications: Hypersensitivity, narrow angle glaucoma, ventricular fibrillation, tachydysrhythmias, pheochromocytoma

Precautions: Severe hypertension, diabetes, hyperthyroidism, G elderly, severe arteriosclerosis, cardiac disease, P infants, pregnancy **C**, lactation, arterial embolism, peripheral vascular disease, bradycardia, myocardial disease

Pharmacokinetics

Absorption	Well absorbed (IM); completely absorbed (IV); minimally absorbed (nasal, ophth)
Distribution	Unknown
Metabolism	Liver
Excretion	Unknown
Half-life	Unknown

Pharmacodynamics

	IV	SC/IM	NASAL	OPTIC
Onset	Rapid	15 min	Unknown	Min
Peak	Unknown	Unknown	Unknown	1 hr
Duration	20-30 min	45-60 min	½-4 hr	½-7 hr

Interactions

Drug/drug:

Individual drugs
Bretylium: ↑ dysrhythmias
Guanethidine: ↑ pressor effect
Mecamylamine: ↑ hypotension
Methyldopa: ↑ hypotension
Reserpine: ↑ hypotension

Drug classifications
Antidepressants, tricyclic: ↑ pressor effect
β-Blockers: ↑ pressor effect
General anesthetics: ↑ dysrhythmias
H_1 antihistamines: ↑ pressor effect
MAOI: ↑ pressor effect
Oxytocics: ↑ B/P

NURSING CONSIDERATIONS

Assessment

Syst route
- Monitor I&O ratio, notify prescriber if output <30 ml/hr
- Monitor ECG during administration continuously; if B/P increases, drug is decreased

• Monitor B/P and pulse q5 min after parenteral route; CVP or PWP during inf if possible
• Assess for paresthesias and coldness of extremities; peripheral blood flow may decrease

Nasal route
• Assess for redness, swelling, pain in nasal passages

Associated nursing diagnoses

✓ Tissue perfusion, altered (uses)
✓ Cardiac output, decreased (uses)
✓ Knowledge deficit (teaching)

Implementation

IV **IV route**
• Give plasma expanders for hypovolemia
• Give **IV** after diluting 1 mg/9 ml sterile water for inj; give dose over 30-60 sec; may be diluted 10 mg/500 ml of D_5W or NS; titrate to patient response; low normal B/P; check for extravasation; check site for infiltration; use inf pump
• Store reconstituted sol in refrigerator for no longer than 24 hr
• Do not use discolored sol

Y-site compatibilities:

Amrinone, famotidine, zidovudine

Additive compatibilities:

Chloramphenicol, dobutamine, lidocaine, potassium chloride, sodium bicarbonate

Nasal route
• Use no more than q4h for <4 consecutive days
• Use environmental humidification to decrease nasal congestion, dryness
• Store in light-resistant container; do not expose to high temp

Ophth route
• Store in tight, light-resistant container; do not use discolored sol

Patient/family education

• Inform patient of reason for drug administration and expected result
• Advise patient to report pain at inf site immediately
• Instruct patient to report change in vision, blurring, loss of sight; breathing trouble, sweating, flushing

Ophth route
• Teach patient method of instill: tilt head backward, hold dropper over eye, drop medication inside lower lid; using pressure on inside corner of eye hold 1 min; do not touch dropper to eye
• Teach patient that blurred vision will decrease with repeated use of drug
• Advise patient to notify prescriber of headache, spots, redness, pain; discontinue use
• Advise patient to use sunglasses if photophobia occurs
• Instruct patient to use exactly as prescribed

Nasal route
• Inform patient that stinging may occur for a few applications; drying of mucosa may be decreased by environmental humidification
• Teach patient to notify prescriber if irregular pulse, insomnia, dizziness, or tremors occur
• Teach patient proper admin-

P

istration to avoid syst absorption

Evaluation

Positive therapeutic outcome
- Increased B/P with stabilization
- Decreased nasal congestion
- Decreased eye irritation

phenytoin ⊶
(fen'i-toyn)
Diphenylhydantoin, Dilantin, Dilantin Capsules, Diphenylan, Phenytoin Oral Suspension
Func. class.: Anticonvulsant/antidysrhythmic (IB)
Chem. class.: Hydantoin
Pregnancy category **D**

Action: Inhibits spread of seizure activity in motor cortex by altering ion transport; increases AV conduction to decrease dysrhythmias

➡ **Therapeutic Outcome:** Decreased seizures, absence of dysrhythmias

Uses: Generalized tonic-clonic seizures, status epilepticus, nonepileptic seizures associated with Reye's syndrome or after head trauma, migraines, trigeminal neuralgia, Bell's palsy, ventricular dysrhythmias uncontrolled by antidysrhythmics

Dosage and routes

Seizures

Adult: **IV** loading dose 900 mg-1.5 g run at 50 mg/min; if patient has received phenytoin, 100-300 mg run at 50 mg/min; PO loading dose 900 mg-1.5 g divided tid, then 300 mg/day (extended) or divided tid (extended/prompt)

P *Child:* **IV** loading dose 15 mg/kg run at 50 mg/min; if patient has received phenytoin, 5-7 mg/kg run at 50 mg/min; may repeat in 30 min; PO loading dose of 15 mg/kg divided q8-12h, then 5-7 mg/kg in divided doses q12h

Status epilepticus

Adult: **IV** 15-20 mg/kg, max 25-50 mg/min; may give 100 mg q6-8h thereafter

P *Child:* **IV** 15-20 mg/kg given 1-3 mg/kg/min

Neuritic pain

Adult: PO 200-400 mg/day in divided doses

Ventricular dysrhythmias

Adult: PO loading dose 1 g divided over 24 hr, then 500 mg/day × 2 days; **IV** 250 mg given over 5 min until dysrhythmias subside or 1 g is given, or 100 mg q15 min until dysrhythmias subside or 1 g is given

P *Child:* PO 3-8 mg/kg or 250 mg/m^2/day as single dose or divided in 2 doses; **IV** 3-8 mg/kg given over several min, or 250 mg/m^2/day as single dose or divided in 2 doses

Available forms: Susp 30, 125 mg/5 ml; chew tab 50 mg; inj 50 mg/ml; ext rel cap 100 mg; prompt cap 30, 100 mg

Side effects/adverse reactions

CNS: Drowsiness, dizziness, insomnia, paresthesias, depression, suicidal tendencies, aggression, headache, confusion, slurred speech
CV: Hypotension, ***ventricular fibrillation***
EENT: Nystagmus, diplopia, blurred vision
GI: Nausea, vomiting, constipation, anorexia, weight loss, ***hepatitis,*** jaundice, gingival hyperplasia
GU: ***Nephritis,*** urine discoloration
HEMA: ***Agranulocytosis, leukopenia, aplastic anemia, thrombocytopenia, megaloblastic anemia***
INTEG: Rash, ***lupus erythematosus, Stevens-Johnson syndrome,*** hirsutism
SYST: Hypocalcemia

Contraindications: Hypersensitivity, psychiatric condition, pregnancy **D**, bradycardia, SA and AV block, Stokes-Adams syndrome

Precautions: Allergies, hepatic disease, renal disease

Pharmacokinetics

Absorption	Slowly absorbed from GI tract; erratic (IM)
Distribution	Crosses placenta
Metabolism	Liver, extensively
Excretion	Kidneys, minimally; enters breast milk
Half-life	22 hr

Pharmacodynamics

	PO	PO–EXT REL	IM	IV
Onset	2-24 hr	2-24 hr	Erratic	1-2 hr
Peak	1.5-3 hr	4-12 hr	Erratic	Unknown
Duration	6-12 hr	12-36 hr	12-24 hr	12-24 hr

Interactions

Drug/drug:

Individual drugs

Alcohol: ↑ CNS depression
Carbamazepine: ↓ effectiveness
Chloramphenicol: ↑ blood level
Cimetidine: ↓ metabolism, ↑ action, blood level
Disulfiram: ↓ metabolism, ↑ action
Felbamate: ↑ blood level
Fluconazole: ↑ blood level
Isoniazid: ↓ metabolism, ↑ action
Ketoconazole: ↓ metabolism, ↑ action
Metronidazole: ↑ blood level
Miconazole: ↑ blood level
Omeprazole: ↑ blood level
Phenylbutazone: ↑ blood level
Valproic acid: ↑ seizures
Warfarin: ↓ blood level of phenytoin

Drug classifications

Anticonvulsants: ↑ CNS depression
Antidepressants: ↑ CNS depression
Antihistamines: ↑ CNS depression
Barbiturates: ↑ CNS depression, ↓ effect of phenytoin
Benzodiazepines: ↑ blood levels
General anesthetics: ↑ CNS depression

P

Hypnotics: ↑ CNS depression
Narcotics: ↑ CNS depression
Oral contraceptives: ↓ metabolism, ↑ action
Sedatives: ↑ CNS depression
Sulfonamides: ↑ blood levels

Lab test interferences

Decrease: Dexamethasone, metyrapone test serum, PBI, urinary steroids
Increase: Glucose, alkaline phosphatase, BSP

NURSING CONSIDERATIONS

Assessment

- Assess drug level: toxic level 30-50 μg/ml
- Assess mental status: mood, sensorium, affect, memory **G** (long, short), especially elderly
- Assess for blood dyscrasias: fever, sore throat, bruising, rash, jaundice, epistaxis (long-term treatment only)
- Assess seizure activity including type, location, duration, and character; provide seizure precaution
- Assess renal studies: urinalysis, BUN, urine creatinine
- Monitor blood studies: RBC, Hct, Hgb, reticulocyte counts weekly for 4 wk then monthly; also check thyroid function tests, serum calcium
- Monitor hepatic studies: ALT (SGPT), AST (SGOT), bilirubin, creatinine
- Assess for signs of physical withdrawal if medication suddenly discontinued
- Assess eye problems: need for ophth examinations before, during, after treatment (slit lamp, fundoscopy, tonometry)
- Assess allergic reaction: red raised rash; if this occurs, drug should be discontinued
- Monitor for toxicity: bone marrow depression, nausea, vomiting, ataxia, diplopia, cardiovascular collapse, slurred speech, confusion

Associated nursing diagnoses

- ✓ Injury, risk for (uses, adverse reactions)
- ✓ Knowledge deficit (teaching)
- ✓ Noncompliance (teaching)

Implementation

PO route

- Give with meals to decrease GI upset
- Chew tab can be crushed or chewed; cap can be opened and mixed with foods or fluids; cap and tab are not interchangeable
- Shake oral susp well; use measuring devise for correct dose

IV **IV route**

- Administer by direct **IV** after diluting with special diluent provided (1 ml/50 mg, 2.2 ml/100 mg, 5.2 ml/250 mg); shake; place vial in warm water to dissolve powder; give through Y-tube or 3-way stopcock; inject slowly <50 mg/min
- Give intermittent **IV** after diluting to a conc of 1-10 mg/ml
- Clear **IV** tubing first with 0.9% NaCl sol; use in-line filter; discard 4 hr after preparation; inject into large veins to prevent purple glove syndrome

Y-site incompatibilities:

Enalaprilat, potassium chloride, vitamin B with C

Y-site compatibilities:

Esmolol, famotodine, foscarnet

Patient/family education

- Teach patient to carry ID card or Medic Alert bracelet stating name, drugs taken, condition, prescriber's name and phone number
- Advise patient to avoid driving and other activities that require alertness until drug response is known; dizziness, drowsiness can occur
- Advise patient to avoid alcohol ingestion and CNS depressants unless approved by prescriber; increased sedation may occur
- Teach patient not to discontinue medication quickly after long-term use; taper off over several wk
- Advise patient that urine may turn pink, red, or brown, which is normal
- Caution patient to avoid antacids within 2-3 hr of taking phenytoin
- To prevent gingival hyperplasia, instruct patient in proper oral hygiene; a dentist should be seen routinely

Evaluation

Positive therapeutic outcome

- Decreased seizure activity
- Decreased dysrhythmias
- Relief of pain

physostigmine

(fi-zoe-stig'meen)

Antilerium, Isopto Eserine Solution, Eserine Sulfate Ointment, Fisostin

Func. class.: Antidote, reversible anticholinesterine, miotic

Chem. class.: Tertiary amine; cholinesterase inhibitor

Pregnancy category **C**

Action: Increases concentration of acetylcholine at cholinergic transmission sites, causing prolonged, exaggerated action; produces constriction of ciliary muscles, iris sphincter, causing iris to be pulled away from anterior chamber angle, aiding in aqueous humor drainage

Therapeutic Outcome: Treatment of anticholinergic overdose, alzheimer disease, glaucoma

Uses: To reverse CNS effects of diazepam; anticholinergic, tricyclic antidepressant; Alzheimer's disease, hereditary ataxia, wide angle glaucoma

Dosage and routes

Overdose of anticholinergics

Adult: IM/**IV** 2 mg; give no more than 1 mg/min; may repeat

P *Child:* IM/**IV** inj 0.02 mg/kg, not more than 0.5 mg/min; may repeat at 5-10 min

P

intervals until max dose of 2 mg

Postanesthesia

Adult: IM/**IV** 0.5-1 mg; give no more than 1 mg/min (**IV**); can repeat at 10-30 min intervals

P *Adult and child:* Instill ¼-inch strip of 0.25% oint in conjunctival sac; instill 1-2 gtt of a 0.25%-0.5% sol in conjunctival sac qd-qid

Available forms: Inj IM, **IV** 1 mg/ml; oint 0.25% (sulfate); sol 0.25% (salicylate)

Side effects/adverse reactions

CNS: ***Convulsions,*** headache, dizziness, sweating, weakness, incoordination, ***paralysis,*** hallucinations, delirium, drowsiness
CV: Hypertension, hypotension, bradycardia, irregular pulse, syncope
EENT: Blurred vision, conjunctivitis, allergic reactions, rhinorrhea, salivation, eye and brow pain, lacrimation, twitching of eyelids
GI: Nausea, vomiting, abdominal cramps, diarrhea, increased salivary and gastric secretions
GU: Frequency, incontinence, urgency
INTEG: Rash, urticaria
RESP: Bronchospasm, dyspnea, ***pulmonary edema, respiratory depression, constriction***

Contraindications: Hypotension, obstruction of intestine or renal system, asthma, gangrene, CV disease, choline esters, depolarizing neuromuscular blocking agents, diabetes, hypersensitivity, inflammatory disease of iris or ciliary body

Precautions: Epilepsy, parkinsonism, bradycardia, pregnancy **C**, asthma, bronchitis, diabetes mellitus, CV disease, seizure disorders, bronchial asthma, coronary occlusion, hyperthyroidism, dysrhythmias, peptic ulcer, megacolon, poor GI motility, Parkinson's disease, bradycardia, lactation

Pharmacokinetics

Absorption	Well absorbed
Distribution	Widely distributed; crosses blood-brain barrier
Metabolism	By cholinesterase
Excretion	Kidneys, unknown
Half-life	Unknown

Pharmacodynamics

	MIOSIS	INTRAOCULAR PRES	IV/IM
Onset	20-30 min	Unknown	Unknown
Peak	Unknown	2-6 hr	5 min
Duration	12-36 hr	12-36 hr	45-60 min

Interactions

Drug/drug:

Individual drugs

Decamethonium: ↑ action
Succinylcholine: ↑ action
Procainamide: ↓ action
Quinidine: ↓ action

Drug classifications

Aminoglycosides: ↓ action
Anesthetics: ↓ action
Neuromuscular blockers: ↓ action

NURSING CONSIDERATIONS

Assessment

- Monitor VS, respiration q8h
- Monitor I&O ratio; check for urinary retention or incontinence
- Drug should be discontinued if toxicity occurs

Associated nursing diagnoses

✓ Mobility, impaired physical (uses)
✓ Breathing pattern, ineffective (uses)
✓ Knowledge deficit (teaching)

Implementation

IV **IV route**

- Give **IV** undiluted through Y-tube or 3-way stopcock; give 1 mg or less/1-3 min or 0.5 mg or less over 1 min or more P (child)
- Give only with atropine sulfate available for cholinergic crisis
- Give only after all other cholinergics have been discontinued
- Give increased doses if tolerance occurs
- Store at room temp

Ophth route

- Give topically to conjunctival sac
- Give immediately after reconstituting; discard unused portion
- Give only clear sol, never pink or brown

Patient/family education

Ophth route

- Advise patient to report change in vision, blurring, or loss of sight, trouble breathing, sweating, flushing
- Teach patient method of instillation, including pressure on lacrimal sac for 1 min, not to touch dropper to eye
- Advise patient that long-term therapy may be required
- Advise patient that blurred vision will decrease with repeated use of drug
- Advise patient that drug is often irritating to eye, rarely tolerated for prolonged periods
- Advise patient that drug may be prescribed for bedtime use to prevent nocturnal rise in ocular tension
- Inform patient that maximal effect of top application is reached in 30 min, may last 12-36 hr
- Inform patient to observe eyes for irritation, development of cataracts

Evaluation

Positive therapeutic outcome

- Decreased intraocular pressure
- Alert

Treatment of overdose: Can cause cholinergic crisis; atropine is an antagonist

P

phytonadione

(fye-toe-na-dye'one)
AquaMEPHYTON, Konakion, Mephyton, vitamin K_1

Func. class.: Vitamin K_1, fat-soluble vitamin

Pregnancy category **C**

Action: Needed for adequate blood clotting (factors II, VII, IX, X)

➡ Therapeutic Outcome: Prevention of bleeding

Uses: Vitamin K malabsorption, hypoprothrombinemia, prevention of hypoprothrombinemia caused by oral anticoagulants, prevention of hemorrhagic disease of the newborn

Dosage and routes

Hypoprothrombinemia caused by vitamin K malabsorption

Adult: PO/IM 2-25 mg; may repeat or increase to 50 mg

Child: PO/IM 5-10 mg

Infants: PO/IM 2 mg

Prevention of hemorrhagic disease of the newborn

Neonate: SC/IM 0.5-1 mg after birth; repeat in 6-8 hr if required

Hypoprothrombinemia caused by oral anticoagulants

Adult: PO/SC/IM 2.5-10 mg, may repeat 12-48 hr after PO dose or 6-8 hr after SC/IM dose, based on PT

Available forms: Tab 5 mg; inj 2 mg, 10 mg/ml; aqueous colloidal (IM, **IV**); inj aqueous dispersion 2, 10 mg/ml (IM)

Side effects/adverse reactions

CNS: Headache, ***brain damage*** (large doses)
GI: Nausea, decrease liver function tests
HEMA: Hemolytic anemia, hemoglobinuria, hyperbilirubinemia
INTEG: Rash, urticaria

Contraindications: Hypersensitivity, severe hepatic disease, last few wk of pregnancy

Precautions: Pregnancy **C**, neonates

Pharmacokinetics

Absorption	Well absorbed (PO, IM, SC)
Distribution	Crosses placenta
Metabolism	Liver, rapidly
Excretion	Breast milk
Half-life	Unknown

Pharmacodynamics

	PO	SC/IM
Onset	6-12 hr	1-2 hr
Peak	Unknown	6 hr
Duration	Unknown	14 hr

Interactions

Drug/drug:

Individual drugs

Cholestyramine: ↓ action of phytonadione
Mineral oil: ↓ action of phytonadione
Sucralfate: ↓ phytonadione absorption

Drug classifications

Antiinfectives: ↑ phytonadione need
Oral anticoagulants: ↓ action of phytonadine
Salicylates: ↑ phytonadione need

NURSING CONSIDERATIONS

Assessment

• Monitor pro-time during treatment (2-sec deviation from control time, bleeding time, and clotting time); monitor for bleeding, pulse, and BP
• Assess nutritional status: liver (beef), spinach, tomatoes,

coffee, asparagus, broccoli, cabbage, lettuce, greens
- Assess for bleeding or bruising: hematuria, black tarry stools, hematemesis

Associated nursing diagnoses

✓ Nutrition, altered: less than body requirements (uses)
✓ Tissue perfusion, altered (uses)
✓ Knowledge deficit (teaching)

Implementation

IV **IV route**
- Give **IV** after diluting with D_5 NS 10 ml or more; give 1 mg/min or more
- Give **IV** only when other routes not possible (deaths have occurred)
- Store in tight, light-resistant container

Patient/family education

- Teach patient not to take other supplements, unless directed by prescriber; to take this medication as directed
- Teach patient necessary foods to be included in diet high in vitamin K
- Advise patient to avoid IM inj, hard toothbrush, flossing; use electric razor until treatment is terminated
- Instruct patient to report symptoms of bleeding, bruising, nosebleeds, blood in urine, heavy menstruation, black tarry stools
- Caution patient not to use OTC medications unless approved by prescriber
- Stress the need for periodic lab tests to monitor coagulation levels
- Stress the need for patient to wear identification with condition, treatment, and medication taken

Evaluation

Positive therapeutic outcome
- Decreased bleeding tendencies
- Decreased pro-time
- Decreased clotting time

pilocarpine

(pye-loe-kar′peen)

Adsorbocarpine, Akarpine, Isopto Carpine, Ocu-Carpine Ocusert-Pilo, Pilagan, Pilocar, pilocarpine HCl, Pilopine HS, Piloptic-1, Piloptic-2, Pilostat, Pilopto-Carpine

Func. class.: Direct-acting miotic

Chem. class.: Cholinergic agonist

Pregnancy category **C**

P

Action: Acts directly on cholinergic receptor sites; induces miosis, spasm of accommodation, fall in intraocular pressure, caused by stimulation of ciliary, pupillary sphincter muscles, which leads to pulling away of iris from filtration angle, resulting in increased outflow of aqueous humor

➔ **Therapeutic Outcome:** Reduction of intraocular pressure

Uses: Primary glaucoma, early stages of wide angle glaucoma (less useful in advanced stages), chronic open angle glaucoma, acute narrow angle glaucoma before emergency surgery; also neutralizes mydriatics used during eye exam; may be used alternately with mydriatics to break adhesions between iris and lens

Dosage and routes

P ***Adult and child:*** Instill 1-2 gtt of 1% or 2% sol in eye q6-8h; instill 20-40 µg/hr (Ocusert) in cul-de-sac of eye

Available forms: Ophth sol 0.25, 0.5, 1, 2, 3, 4, 6, 8, 10%; Ocusert Pilo 20, 40 µg/hr system; 4% gel

Side effects/adverse reactions

CV: Hypotension, tachycardia
EENT: Blurred vision, browache, twitching of eyelids, eye pain with change in focus
GI: Nausea, vomiting, abdominal cramps, diarrhea
GU: Bladder tightness
RESP: Bronchospasm

Contraindication: Hypersensitivity

Precautions: Bronchial asthma, hypertension, pregnancy **C**, bradycardia, hyperthyroidism, coronary artery disease, obstruction of GI/urinary tracts (or if strength of walls of these structures in question, peptic ulcers), epilepsy, parkinsonism, asthma

Pharmacokinetics

Absorption	Minimally absorbed
Distribution	Minimally distributed
Metabolism	None
Excretion	Lacrimation
Half-life	Short

Pharmacodynamics

Onset	45 min-1 hr
Peak	1-12 hr
Duration	4-24 hr

NURSING CONSIDERATIONS

Assessment

- Assess heart, respiratory rate, B/P, lung sounds, changes in respiratory rate; if these occur, notify prescriber

Associated nursing diagnoses

✓ Sensory-perceptual alteration: visual (uses)
✓ Knowledge deficit (teaching)

Implementation

Ophth route

- Use reconstituted sol immediately; discard unused portion

Patient/family education

- Instruct patient to report change in vision, blurring or loss of sight, trouble breathing, sweating, flushing
- Teach patient method of instillation, including pressure on lacrimal sac for 1 min, and not to touch dropper to eye; use demonstration, return demonstration
- Advise patient that blurred vision will decrease with repeated use of drug
- Caution patient not to drive

during first few days of treatment; visual changes may occur including impaired night vision, eye and brow ache

Evaluation

Positive therapeutic outcome

- Decreasing intraocular pressure
- Miosis during ocular surgery

pindolol

(pin'doe-lole)

Visken

Func. class.: Antihypertensive

Chem. class.: Nonselective β-blocker

Pregnancy category **B**

Action: Competitively blocks stimulation of β-adrenergic receptor within vascular smooth muscle; produces chronotropic, inotropic activity (decreases rate of SA node discharge, increases recovery time), slows conduction of AV node, decreases heart rate, which decreases O_2 consumption in myocardium; also decreases renin-aldosterone-angiotensin system and at high doses inhibits β_2 receptors in bronchial system

Therapeutic Outcome: Increased B/P in hypertension, heart rate

Uses: Mild to moderate hypertension

Investigational uses: Mitral valve prolapse, hypertrophic cardiomyopathy, angina pectoris

Dosage and routes

Adult: PO 5 mg bid; usual dose 15 mg/day (5 mg tid); may increase by 10 mg/day q3-4 wk to a max of 60 mg/day

Available forms: Tab 5, 10 mg

Side effects/adverse reactions

CNS: Insomnia, dizziness, hallucinations, anxiety, fatigue

CV: Hypotension, bradycardia, ***CHF,*** edema, chest pain, palpitations, claudication, tachycardia, ***AV block***

EENT: Visual changes, sore throat, *double vision,* dry burning eyes

GI: Nausea, vomiting, ***ischemic colitis,*** diarrhea, *abdominal pain,* ***mesenteric arterial thrombosis***

GU: Impotence, frequency

HEMA: Agranulocytosis, thrombocytopenia, purpura

INTEG: Rash, alopecia, pruritus, fever

MISC: Joint pain, muscle pain

RESP: ***Bronchospasm,*** *dyspnea,* cough, rales

Contraindications: Hypersensitivity to β-blockers, cardiogenic shock, 2nd-, 3rd-degree heart block, sinus bradycardia, CHF, cardiac failure, bronchial asthma

Precautions: Major surgery, pregnancy **B**, lactation, diabetes mellitus, renal disease,

P

thyroid disease, COPD, well-compensated heart failure, CAD, nonallergic bronchospasm

Pharmacokinetics

Absorption	Well absorbed
Distribution	Crosses placenta; some penetration in CNS
Metabolism	Liver, moderately (60%-65%)
Excretion	Kidneys, unchanged (30%-45%)
Half-life	3-4 hr

Pharmacodynamics

	PO
Onset	Unknown
Peak	2-4 hr
Duration	8-24 hr

Interactions

Drug/drug:

Individual drugs

Alcohol: ↑ hypotension (large amounts)
Epinephrine: α-Adrenergic stimulation
Hydralazine: ↑ hypotension, bradycardia
Indomethacin: ↓ antihypertensive effect
Insulin: ↑ hypoglycemia
Methyldopa: ↑ hypotension, bradycardia
Phenytoin (IV): ↑ cardiac depression
Prazosin: ↑ hypotension, bradycardia
Reserpine: ↑ hypotension, bradycardia
Thyroid: ↓ effectiveness
Verapamil: ↑ cardiac depression

Drug classifications

Antihypertensives: ↑ hypertension
β_2-Agonist: ↓ bronchodilatation
Cardiac glycosides: ↑ bradycardia
Nitrates: ↑ hypotension
Theophyllines: ↓ bronchodilatation

Lab test interferences

False increase: Urinary catecholamines

NURSING CONSIDERATIONS

Assessment

- Monitor B/P during beginning treatment, periodically thereafter; pulse q4h; note rate, rhythm, quality: apical/radial pulse before administration; notify prescriber of any significant changes (pulse <50 bpm)
- Check for baselines in renal, liver function tests before therapy begins
- Assess for edema in feet, legs daily; monitor I&O, daily weight; check for jugular vein distention, rales bilaterally, dyspnea (CHF)
- Monitor skin turgor, dryness of mucous membranes for hydration status, especially G elderly

Associated nursing diagnoses

- ✓ Cardiac output, decreased (uses)
- ✓ Injury, potential for (adverse reactions)
- ✓ Knowledge deficit (teaching)
- ✓ Noncompliance (teaching)

Implementation

PO route

- Given ac, hs, tab may be crushed or swallowed whole;

give with food to prevent GI upset reduced dosage in renal

- Store protected from light, moisture; place in cool environment

Patient/family education

- Teach patient not to discontinue drug abruptly; taper over 2 wk; may cause precipitate angina if stopped abruptly
- Teach patient not to use OTC products containing α-adrenergic stimulants (such as nasal decongestants, cold preparations); to avoid alcohol, smoking, and to limit sodium intake as prescribed
- Teach patient how to take pulse and B/P at home; advise when to notify prescriber
- Instruct patient to comply with weight control, dietary adjustments, modified exercise program
- Tell patient to carry/wear Medic Alert ID to identify drug being taken, allergies; tell patient drug controls symptoms but does not cure
- Caution patient to avoid hazardous activities if dizziness, drowsiness present
- Teach patient to report symptoms of CHF: difficult breathing, especially on exertion or when lying down, night cough, swelling of extremities or bradycardia, dizziness, confusion, depression, fever
- Teach patient to take drug as prescribed, not to double doses, skip doses; take any missed doses as soon as remembered if at least 4 hr until next dose

Evaluation

Positive therapeutic outcome

- Decreased B/P in hypertension (after 1-2 wk)

Treatment of overdose:

Lavage, **IV** atropine for bradycardia, **IV** theophylline for bronchospasm, digitalis, O_2, diuretic for cardiac failure, hemodialysis, **IV** glucose for hyperglycemia, **IV** diazepam (or phenytoin) for seizures

pipecuronium

(pip-e-kyoor'oh'nee-um)

Arduran

Func. class.: Neuromuscular blocker (nondepolarizing)

Chem. class.: Synthetic curariform

Pregnancy category **C**

Action: Inhibits transmission of nerve impulses by binding with cholinergic receptor sites, antagonizing action of acetylcholine; no analgesic response

Therapeutic Outcome: Paralysis of all skeletal muscles

Uses: Facilitation of endotracheal intubation, skeletal muscle relaxation during mechanical ventilation, surgery, or general anesthesia

Dosage and routes

Adult: **IV** dosage is individualized; in patients with normal renal function who are not obese, initial dose is 70-85

P

μg/kg; maintenance dose ranges from 10-15 μg/kg

P *Child 1-14 yr:* **IV** 57 μg/kg

P *Child 3 mo-1 yr:* **IV** 40 μg/kg

Available forms: Inj 10-mg vials

Side effects/adverse reactions

CNS: Hypesthesia, CNS depression
CV: Bradycardia, tachycardia, increased or decreased B/P, ventricular extrasystole, ***myocardial ischemia, cardiovascular accident, thrombosis, atrial fibrillation***
EENT: Increased secretions
GU: ***Anuria***
INTEG: Rash, urticaria
META: Hypoglycemia, hyperkalemia, increased creatinine
MS: Weakness to prolonged skeletal muscle relaxation
RESP: ***Prolonged apnea, bronchospasm, cyanosis, respiratory depression***

Contraindications: Hypersensitivity to bromide ion

Precautions: Pregnancy **C**, renal disease, cardiac disease, P lactation, children <3 mo, fluid and electrolyte imbalances, neuromuscular diseases, respiratory disease, obesity

Pharmacokinetics

Absorption	Complete bioavailability (IV)
Distribution	Unknown
Metabolism	Unknown
Excretion	Kidneys, unchanged (>75%)
Half-life	1½ hr; increased in renal disease

Pharmacodynamics

Onset	30-45 sec
Peak	3-5 min
Duration	1-2 hr

Interactions

Drug/drug:

Individual drugs

Clindamycin: ↑ paralysis length and intensity
Colistin: ↑ paralysis length and intensity
Lidocaine: ↑ paralysis length and intensity
Lithium: ↑ paralysis length and intensity
Magnesium: ↑ paralysis length and intensity
Polymyxin B: ↑ paralysis length and intensity
Procainamide: ↑ paralysis length and intensity
Quinidine: ↑ paralysis length and intensity
Succinylcholine: ↑ paralysis length and intensity

Drug classifications

Aminoglycosides: ↑ paralysis length and intensity
β-Blockers: ↑ paralysis length and intensity
Diuretics, potassium-losing: ↑ paralysis length and intensity
General anesthesia: ↑ paralysis length and intensity

NURSING CONSIDERATIONS

Assessment

- Monitor vital signs (B/P, pulse, respirations, airway) until fully recovered; rate, depth, pattern of respirations, strength of hand grip; patient should be intubated before use
- Monitor for electrolyte imbalances (potassium, magnesium) before drug is used;

electrolyte imbalances may lead to increased action of this drug
- Monitor for recovery: decreased paralysis of face, diaphragm, leg, arm, rest of body; residual weakness and respiratory problems may occur during recovery period
- Assess for hypersensitive reactions: rash, fever, respiratory distress, pruritus; drug should be discontinued

Associated nursing diagnoses

- ✓ Breathing pattern, ineffective (uses)
- ✓ Communication, impaired verbal (adverse reactions)
- ✓ Fear (adverse reactions)
- ✓ Knowledge deficit (teaching)

Implementation

IV route

- Use peripheral nerve stimulator (anesthesiologist) to determine neuromuscular blockade; deep tendon reflexes should be monitored during extended periods
- Give **IV** after reconstituting with 0.9% NaCl, D_5W, D_5/0.9% NaCl, LR, sterile water for inj; sol with benzyl alcohol should not be used for newborns; should be administered only by qualified person, usually an anesthesiologist; do not administer IM
- Store in light-resistant area (powder); refrigerate unused portions (sterile water); use within 24 hr

Patient/family education

- Provide reassurance if communication is difficult during recovery from neuromuscular blockade
- Provide explanation to patients regarding all procedures or treatments; patient will remain conscious if anesthesia is not given also

Evaluation

Positive therapeutic outcome

- Paralysis of jaw, eyelid, head, neck, rest of body as evaluated by peripheral nerve stimulator

Treatment of overdose: Edrophonium or neostigmine, atropine, monitor VS; may require mechanical ventilation

piperacillin

(pi-per′a-sill-in)

Pipracil

Func. class.: Broad-spectrum antiinfective

Chem. class.: Extended-spectrum penicillin

Pregnancy category **B**

Action: Interferes with cell wall replication of susceptible organisms; osmotically unstable cell wall swells and bursts from osmotic pressure

Uses: Respiratory tract, skin, skin structure, urinary tract, bone, and joint infections; gonorrhea, pneumonia, endocarditis, septicemia, meningitis, sinusitis; infections caused by penicillinase-producing staphylococci, streptococci; may be combined with an aminoglycoside for *Pseudomonas* infection

Therapeutic Outcome: Bactericidal effects for gram-

P

positive cocci *Staphylococcus aureus, Streptococcus pyogenes, S. viridans, S. faecalis, S. bovis, S. pneumoniae;* gram-negative cocci *Neisseria gonorrhoeae, N. meningitidis;* gram-positive bacilli *Clostridium perfringens, C. tetani;* gram-negative bacilli *Bacteroides, Fusobacterium nucleatum, Escherichia coli, Klebsiella, Proteus mirabilis, Morganella morganii, P. vulgaris, P. rettgeri, Enterobacter, Citrobacter, Pseudomonas aeruginosa, Serratia, Acinetobacter, Peptococcus, Peptostreptococcus, Eubacterium*

Dosage and routes

Systemic infections

P *Adult and child >12 yr:* IM/**IV** 100-300 mg/kg/day in divided doses q4-6h

Prophylaxis of surgical infections

Adult: **IV** 2 g 30-60 min before procedure; may be repeated during or after surgery

Available forms: Inj 2, 3, 4, 40 g; inf 2, 3, 4 g

Side effects/adverse reactions

CNS: Lethargy, hallucinations, anxiety, depression, twitching, ***coma, convulsions***
GI: Nausea, vomiting, diarrhea, increased AST (SGOT), ALT (SGPT), abdominal pain, glossitis, colitis
GU: ***Oliguria, proteinuria, hematuria, vaginitis, moniliasis, glomerulonephritis***
HEMA: Anemia, increased bleeding time, ***bone marrow depression***
META: Hypokalemia, hypernatremia

Contraindications: Hypersensitivity to penicillins; P neonates

Precautions: Pregnancy **B**; hypersensitivity to cephalosporins, CHF

Pharmacokinetics

Absorption	Well absorbed (80%)
Distribution	Widely distributed; crosses placenta
Metabolism	Not metabolized
Excretion	Kidneys, unchanged (90%); bile (10%); breast milk
Half-life	0.7-1.3 hr

Pharmacodynamics

	IM	IV
Onset	Rapid	Rapid
Peak	30-50 min	Inf end

Interactions

Drug/drug:

Individual drugs

Aminoglycosides: ↓ half-life in renal disease
Amphotericin B: ↑ hypokalemia
Aspirin: ↑ piperacillin levels, ↓ renal excretion
Cholestyramine: ↓ effectiveness of piperacillin
Chloramphenicol: ↑ half-life of chloramphenicol, ↓ effectiveness of piperacillin
Colestipol: ↓ effectiveness of piperacillin
Diuretics: ↑ hypokalemia
Glucocorticoids: ↑ hypokalemia
Hepatotoxic agents: ↑ hepatotoxicity
Probenecid: ↑ piperacillin levels, ↓ renal excretion

Drug classifications
Erythromycins: ↓ antimicrobial effectiveness
Lithium: ↓ excretion, ↑ toxicity
Oral anticoagulants: ↑ anticoagulant effects
Oral contraceptives: ↓ contraceptive effectiveness
Tetracyclines: ↓ antimicrobial effectiveness

Drug/food:

Food, carbonated drinks, citrus fruit juices: ↓ absorption

Lab test interferences

False positive: Urine glucose, urine protein

NURSING CONSIDERATIONS

Assessment

- Assess patient for previous sensitivity reaction to penicillins or other cephalosporins; cross-sensitivity between penicillins and cephalosporins is common
- Assess patient for signs and symptoms of infection including characteristics of wounds, sputum, urine, stool, WBC >10,000, fever; obtain baseline information and during treatment
- Obtain C&S before beginning drug therapy to identify if correct treatment has been initiated
- Assess for allergic reactions: rash, urticaria, pruritus, chills, fever, joint pain; angioedema may occur a few days after therapy begins; epinephrine, resuscitation equipment should be available for anaphylactic reaction
- Identify urine output; if decreasing, notify prescriber (may indicate nephrotoxicity); also check for increased BUN, creatinine
- Monitor blood studies: AST (SGOT), ALT (SGPT), CBC, Hct, bilirubin, LDH, alkaline phosphatase, Coombs' test monthly if patient is on long-term therapy
- Monitor electrolytes: potassium, sodium, chloride monthly if patient is on long-term therapy
- Assess bowel pattern daily; if severe diarrhea occurs, drug should be discontinued; may indicate pseudomembranous colitis
- Monitor for bleeding: ecchymosis, bleeding gums, hematuria, stool guaiac daily if on long-term therapy
- Assess for overgrowth of infection: perineal itching, fever, malaise, redness, pain, swelling, drainage, rash, diarrhea, change in cough, sputum

Associated nursing diagnoses

- ✓ Infection, risk for (uses)
- ✓ Diarrhea (adverse reactions)
- ✓ Injury, risk for (adverse reactions)
- ✓ Knowledge deficit (teaching)
- ✓ Noncompliance (teaching)

Implementation

IM route
- Reconstitute 2 g/4 ml, 3 g/6 ml, 4 g/7.8 gm with sterile water, 0.9% NaCl, bacteriostatic water, 0.5% or 1% lidocaine without epinephrine
- Inject deep in large muscle mass, massage; split inj over 2 g into 2 inj

P

IV **IV route**

- Reconstitute with 5 ml or more 0.9% NaCl, bacteroistatic water; shake sol to dissolve
- Change **IV** sites q48h to prevent phlebitis and pain
- Give direct **IV** over 3-5 min
- Give by intermittent inf by diluting in 50 ml or more D_5W, 0.9% NaCl, D_5/0.9% NaCl, LR give over 20-30 min by Y-site; discontinue primary inf during intermittent inf

Syringe compatibility:
Heparin

Y-site incompatibilities:
Ondansetron, fluconazole, sargramostim, vinorelbine

Y-site compatibilities:
Acyclovir, aldesleukin, ciprofloxacin, cyclophosphamide, enalaprilat, esmolol, famotidine, fludarabine, foscarnet, hydromorphone, labetalol, magnesium sulfate, melphalan, merperidine, morphine, perphenazine, verapamil, zidovudine

Additive incompatibility:
Aminoglycosides

Additive compatibilities:
Ciprofloxacin, clindamycin, hydrocortisone sodium succinate, potassium chloride, verapamil

Patient/family education

- Teach patient to report sore throat, bruising, bleeding, joint pain; may indicate blood dyscrasias (rare)
- Advise patient to contact prescriber if vaginal itching, loose, foul-smelling stools, furry tongue occur; may indicate superinfection
- Advise patient to notify prescriber of diarrhea with blood or pus, which may indicate pseudomembranous colitis

Evaluation

Positive therapeutic outcome

- Absence of signs/symptoms of infection (WBC <10,000, temp WNL, absence of red, draining wounds)
- Reported improvement in symptoms of infection

Treatment of anaphylaxis: Withdraw drug, maintain airway, administer epinephrine, aminophylline, O_2, **IV** corticosteroids

piperacillin/tazobactam

Pipracil

Func. class.: Broad-spectrum antiinfective

Chem. class.: Extended-spectrum penicillin

Pregnancy category **B**

Action: Interferes with cell wall replication of susceptible organisms; osmotically unstable cell wall swells and bursts from osmotic pressure

➔ **Therapeutic Outcome:** Bactericidal effects for piperacillin-resistant β-lactamase, *Escherichia coli, Staphylococcus aureus, Bacteroides fragilis, Haemophilus influenzae*

Uses: Respiratory tract, skin, skin structure, urinary tract, bone, and joint infections; gonorrhea, pneumonia, infections from penicillinase-producing staphylococci, streptococci

Dosage and routes

Adult: **IV** 3 g piperacillin with 0.375 g tazaobactam q6h before procedure; may be repeated during or after surgery

Available forms: 2 g/0.25 g; 3 g/0.375 g; 4 g/0.5 g

Side effects/adverse reactions

CNS: Headache, insomnia, agitation, dizziness
CV: Chest pain, edema, hypertension
EENT: Rhinitis
INTEG: Rash
MISC: Fever, superinfection
RESP: Dyspnea

Contraindications: Hypersensitivity to penicillins, cephalosporins, tazobactam; neonates

Precautions: Pregnancy **B,** CHF, renal disease, lactation, sodium restriction

Pharmacodynamics	
Absorption	Well absorbed (80%)
Distribution	Widely distributed; crosses placenta
Metabolism	Not metabolized
Excretion	Kidneys, unchanged (90%); bile (10%); breast milk
Half-life	0.7-1.3 hr

Pharmacodynamics	
Onset	Rapid
Peak	Inf end

Interactions

Drug/drug:

Individual drugs

Aminoglycosides: ↓ half-life in renal disease
Amphotericin B: ↑ hypokalemia
Aspirin: ↑ piperacillin levels, ↑ renal excretion
Cholestyramine: ↓ effectiveness of piperacillin
Chloramphenicol: ↑ half-life of chloramphenicol, ↓ effectiveness of piperacillin
Colestipol: ↓ effectiveness of piperacillin
Diuretics: ↑ hypokalemia
Glucocorticoids: ↑ hypokalemia
Hepatotoxic agents: ↑ hepatotoxicity
Probenecid: ↑ piperacillin levels, ↓ renal excretion

Drug classifications

Erythromycins: ↓ antimicrobial effectiveness
Lithium: ↓ excretion, ↑ toxicity
Oral anticoagulants: ↑ anticoagulant effects
Oral contraceptives: ↓ contraceptive effectiveness
Tetracyclines: ↓ antimicrobial effectiveness

Drug/food:

Food, carbonated drinks, citrus fruit juices: ↓ absorption

Lab test interferences

False positive: Urine glucose, urine protein

NURSING CONSIDERATIONS

Assessment

- Assess patient for previous sensitivity reaction to penicillins or other cephalosporins, cross-sensitivity between penicillins and cephalosporins is common

- Assess patient for signs and symptoms of infection including characteristics of wounds, sptum, urine, stool, WBC >10,000, fever; obtain baseline information and during treatment
- Obtain C&S before beginning drug therapy to identify if correct treatment has been initiated
- Assess for allergic reactions: rash, urticaria, pruritus, chills, fever, joint pain; angioedema may occur a few days after therapy begins; epinephrine, resuscitation equipment should be available for anaphylactic reaction
- Identify urine output; if decreasing, notify prescriber (may indicate nephrotoxicity); also check for increase BUN, creatinine
- Monitor blood studies: AST (SGOT), ALT (SGPT), CBC, Hct, bilirubin, LDH, alkaline phosphatase, Coombs' test monthly if patient is on long-term therapy
- Monitor electrolytes: potassium, sodium, chloride monthly if patient is on long-term therapy
- Assess bowel pattern daily; if severe diarrhea occurs, drug should be discontinued; may indicate pseudomembranous colitis
- Monitor for bleeding: ecchymosis, bleeding gums, hematuria, stool guaiac daily if on long-term therapy
- Assess for overgrowth of infection: perineal itching, fever, malaise, redness, pain, swelling, drainage, rash, diarrhea, change in cough, sputum

Associated nursing diagnoses

- ✓ Infection, risk for (uses)
- ✓ Diarrhea (adverse reactions)
- ✓ Injury, risk for (adverse reactions)
- ✓ Knowledge deficit (teaching)
- ✓ Noncompliance (teaching)

Implementation

IV route

- Reconstitute with 5 ml or more 0.9% NaCl, bacteroistatic water; shake sol to dissolve
- Give by intermittent inf by diluting in 50 ml or more D_5W, 0.9% NaCl, $D_5/0.9\%$ NaCl, LR; give over 20-30 min by Y-site; discontinue primary inf during intermittent inf
- Change **IV** sites q48h to prevent phlebitis and pain
- Give direct **IV** over 3-5 min

Syringe compatibility:
Heparin

Y-site incompatibilities:
Ondansetron, fluconazole, sargramostim, vinorelbine

Y-site compatibilities:
Acyclovir, aldesleukin, ciprofloxacin, cyclophosphamide, enalaprilat, esmolol, famotidine, fludarabine, foscarnet, hydromorphone, labetalol, magnesium sulfate, melphalan, merperidine, morphine, perphenazine, verapamil, zidovudine

Additive incompatibility:
Aminoglycosides

Additive compatibilities:
Ciprofloxaxin, clindamycin, hydrocortisone sodium succinate, potassium chloride, verapamil

Patient/family education
- Teach patient to report sore throat, bruising, bleeding, joint pain; may indicate blood dyscrasias (rare)
- Advise patient to contact prescriber if vaginal itching, loose, foul-smelling stools, furry tongue occur; may indicate superinfection
- Advise patient to notify prescriber of diarrhea with blood or pus, which may indicate pseudomembranous colitis

Evaluation
Positive therapeutic outcome
- Absence of signs/symptoms of infection (WBC <10,000, temp WNL, absence of red, draining wounds)
- Reported improvement in symptoms of infection

Treatment of anaphylaxis: Withdraw drug, maintain airway, administer epinephrine, aminophylline, O_2, **IV** corticosteroids

pirbuterol
(peer-byoo'ter-ole)
Maxair
Func. class.: Bronchodilator
Chem. class.: β-Adrenergic agonist
Pregnancy category **C**

Action: Relaxes bronchial smooth muscle by direct action on β_2-adrenergic receptors, with increased levels of cAMP and increased bronchodilatation, diuresis, and cardiac and CNS stimulation

Therapeutic Outcome: Bronchodilatation with ease of breathing

Uses: Reversible bronchospasm (prevention, treatment), including asthma, may be given with theophylline or steroids

Dosage and routes
P *Adult and child >12 yr:* Aerosol 1-2 inh (0.4 mg) q4-6h; do not exceed 12 inh/day

Available forms: Aerosol delivers 0.2 mg pirbuterol/actuation

Side effects/adverse reactions
CNS: Tremors, anxiety, insomnia, headache, dizziness, stimulation, restlessness, hallucinations, drowsiness, irritability
CV: Palpitations, tachycardia, hypertension, angina, hypotension, dysrhythmias
EENT: Dry nose and mouth, irritation of nose, throat
GI: Gastritis, nausea, vomiting, anorexia
MS: Muscle cramps
RESP: ***Bronchospasm,*** dyspnea, coughing

Contraindications: Hypersensitivity to sympathomimetics, tachycardia

P

Precautions: Lactation, pregnancy **C**, cardiac disorders, hyperthyroidism, diabetes mellitus, prostatic hypertrophy

Pharmacokinetics

Absorption	Minimally absorbed (inh)
Distribution	Unknown
Metabolism	Liver
Excretion	Unknown
Half-life	2 hr

Pharmacodynamics

Onset	5-15 min
Peak	1-1½ hr
Duration	5 hr

Interactions

Drug/drug:

Drug classifications

β-Adrenergic blockers: Block therapeutic effect
Bronchodilators, aerosol: ↑ action of bronchodilator
MAOI: ↑ chance of hypertensive crisis
Sympathomimetics: ↑ adrenergic side effects

NURSING CONSIDERATIONS

Assessment

- Monitor respiratory function: vital capacity, FEV, ABGs, lung sounds, heart rate, rhythm (baseline)
- Monitor for evidence of allergic reactions; paradoxic bronchospasm; withhold dose; notify prescriber

Associated nursing diagnoses

✓ Airway clearance, ineffective (uses)
✓ Gas exchange, impaired (uses)
✓ Knowledge deficit (teaching)

Implementation

Aerosol route

- Give after shaking; have patient exhale, place mouthpiece in mouth, inhale slowly, hold breath, remove, exhale slowly; allow at least 1 min between inh
- Store in light-resistant container; do not expose to temp over 86° F (30° C)

Patient/family education

- Advise patient not to use OTC medications; extra stimulation may occur; to use this medication before other medications and allow at least 1 min between each to prevent overstimulation
- Teach patient use of inhaler; review package insert with patient; to avoid getting aerosol in eyes; blurring may result; to wash inhaler in warm water and dry daily; to avoid smoking, smoke-filled rooms, persons with respiratory tract infections
- Teach patient that paradoxic bronchospasm may occur and to stop drug immediately and notify prescriber; to limit caffeine products such as chocolate, coffee, tea, and colas
- Instruct patient on administration of dose; not to use more than prescribed; serious side effects may occur

Evaluation

Positive therapeutic outcome

- Absence of dyspnea, wheezing after 1 hr
- Improved airway exchange
- Improved ABGs

Treatment of overdose: Administer a β_2-adrenergic blocker

piroxicam
(peer-ox'i-kam)
Apo-Piroxicam ♣, Feldene, Novopirocam ♣
Func. class.: Nonsteroidal antiinflammatory
Chem. class.: Oxicam derivative
Pregnancy category **C**

Action: Inhibits prostaglandin synthesis by decreasing an enzyme needed for biosynthesis; analgesic, antiinflammatory

➔ **Therapeutic Outcome:** Decreased pain, inflammation

Uses: Mild to moderate pain, osteoarthritis, rheumatoid arthritis

Dosage and routes
Adult: PO 20 qd or 10 mg bid

Available forms: Cap 10, 20 mg

Side effects/adverse reactions
GI: Nausea, anorexia, vomiting, diarrhea, jaundice, ***cholestatic hepatitis,*** constipation, flatulence, cramps, dry mouth, peptic ulcer, ***bleeding, ulceration, perforation***
CNS: Dizziness, *drowsiness,* fatigue, tremors, confusion, insomnia, anxiety, depression, *headache*
CV: Tachycardia, peripheral edema, palpitations, dysrhythmias
EENT: Tinnitus, hearing loss, blurred vision
GU: ***Nephrotoxicity: dysuria, hematuria, oliguria, azotemia***
HEMA: ***Blood dyscrasias***
INTEG: Purpura, rash, pruritus, sweating, photosensitivity

Contraindications: Hypersensitivity, asthma, severe renal disease, severe hepatic disease, ulcer disease, cardiac disease

Precautions: Pregnancy **C**, P lactation, children, bleeding disorders, GI disorders, cardiac disorders, hypersensitivity to other antiinflammatory agents

Pharmacokinetics

Absorption	Well absorbed
Distribution	Unknown
Metabolism	Liver, extensively
Excretion	Kidneys, minimal; breast milk
Half-life	50 hr

Pharmacodynamics

	PO
Onset	1 hr
Peak	Unknown
Duration	Unknown

Interactions
Drug/drug:
Individual drugs
Acetaminophen (long-term use): ↑ renal reactions

P

Alcohol: ↑ adverse reactions
Aspirin: ↓ effectiveness, ↑ adverse reactions
Coumarin: ↑ anticoagulant effects
Digoxin: ↑ toxicity, levels
Insulin: ↓ insulin effect
Lithium: ↑ toxicity
Methotrexate: ↑ toxicity
Phenytoin: ↑ toxicity
Probenecid: ↑ toxicity
Sulfonylurea: ↑ toxicity

Drug classifications

Anticoagulants: ↑ risk of bleeding
Antihypertensives: ↓ effect of antihypertensives
Antineoplastics: ↑ risk of hematologic toxicity
β-Blockers: ↑ antihypertension
Cephalosporins: ↑ risk of bleeding
Glucocorticoids: ↑ adverse reactions
Hypoglycemics: ↓ hypoglycemic effect
Diuretics: ↓ effectiveness of diuretics
NSAIDs: ↑ adverse reactions
Potassium supplements: ↑ adverse reactions
Radiation: ↑ risk of hematologic toxicity
Sulfonamides: ↑ toxicity

Lab test interferences

Increase: Serum potassium, liver function studies
Decrease: Hct, Hgb, blood glucose

NURSING CONSIDERATIONS

Assessment

- Monitor blood counts during therapy; watch for decreasing platelets; if low, therapy may need to be discontinued, restarted after hematologic recovery; check for blood dyscrasia (thrombocytopenia): bruising, fatigue, bleeding, poor healing

Associated nursing diagnoses

- ✓ Pain (uses)
- ✓ Mobility, impaired (uses)
- ✓ Knowledge deficit (teaching)
- ✓ Injury, risk for (adverse reactions)

Implementation

PO route

- Administer to patient whole; give with food or milk to decrease gastric symptoms

Patient/family education

- Teach patient that drug must be continued for prescribed time to be effective; to avoid aspirin, alcoholic beverages and other OTC medications unless approved by prescriber
- Caution patient to report bleeding, bruising, fatigue, malaise, since blood dyscrasias do occur
- Instruct patient to use caution when driving; drowsiness, dizziness may occur
- Teach patient to take with a full glass of water to enhance absorption; do not crush, break, or chew

Evaluation

Positive therapeutic outcome

- Decreased pain
- Decreased inflammation
- Increased mobility

plasma protein fraction

Plasmanate, Plasma Plex, Plasmatein, PPF Protenate

Func. class.: Blood derivative

Chem. class.: Human plasma in sodium chloride

Pregnancy category **C**

Action: Exerts similar oncotic pressure as human plasma, expands blood volume, shifts water from extravascular space to intravascular space

Therapeutic Outcome: Shift of fluid from extravascular into intravascular space

Uses: Hypovolemic shock, hypoproteinemia, ARDS, preoperative cardiopulmonary bypass, acute liver failure, nephrotic syndrome

Dosage and routes

Hypovolemia

Adult: **IV** inf 250-500 ml (12.5-25 g protein), not to exceed 10 ml/min

P *Child:* **IV** inf 22-33 ml/kg at 5-10 ml/min

Hypoproteinemia

Adult: **IV** inf 1000-1500 ml qd, not to exceed 8 ml/min

Available forms: Inj 50 mg/ml

Side effects/adverse reactions

CNS: Fever, chills, headache, paresthesias, flushing

CV: Fluid overload, hypotension, erratic pulse

GI: Nausea, vomiting, increased salivation

INTEG: Rash, urticaria, cyanosis

RESP: Altered respirations, dyspnea, pulmonary edema

Contraindications: Hypersensitivity, CHF, severe anemia, renal insufficiency

Precautions: Decreased salt intake, decreased cardiac reserve, lack of albumin deficiency, hepatic disease, renal disease, pregnancy **C**

Pharmacokinetics

Absorption	Completely absorbed (IV)
Distribution	Intravascular space
Metabolism	Unknown
Excretion	Unknown
Half-life	Unknown

Pharmacodynamics

Onset	15-30 min
Peak	Unknown
Duration	Unknown

Interactions: None

Lab test interferences

False increase: Alkaline phosphatase

NURSING CONSIDERATIONS

Assessment

- Monitor blood studies: Hct, Hgb; electrolytes, serum protein, if serum protein declines, dyspnea, hypoxemia can result
- Monitor B/P (decreased), pulse (erratic), respiration during inf; CVP, pulmonary

P

wedge pressure (increases if overload occurs)
- Monitor I&O ratio; urinary output may decrease
- Assess for allergy: fever, rash, itching, chills, flushing, urticaria, nausea, vomiting, or hypotension requires discontinuation of inf; use new lot if therapy reinstituted
- Monitor for increased CVP reading: distended neck veins indicate circulatory overload; SOB, anxiety, insomnia, expiratory rales, frothy blood-tinged cough, cyanosis indicate pulmonary overload

Associated nursing diagnoses

✓ Fluid volume deficit (uses)
✓ Cardiac output, decreased (uses)
✓ Fluid volume excess (adverse reactions)

Implementation

IV **IV route**
- Give by **IV**; no dilution required; use inf pump, large-gauge needle (≥20 G); discard unused portion; infuse slowly within 4 hr of opening
- Provide adequate hydration before administration
- When storing, check type of albumin, date; may have to refrigerate

Additive compatibilities: Carbohydrate and electrolyte sol, whole blood, packed red blood cells, chloramphenicol, tetracycline

Additive incompatibilities: Protein hydrolysate sol, amino acids solution, alcohol, norepinephrine

Patient/family education

- Explain reason for and expected result of medication

Evaluation

Positive therapeutic outcome
- Increased B/P
- Decreased edema
- Increased serum albumin

plicamycin

(plik-a-mi′cin)

Mithramycin, Mithracin

Func. class.: Antineoplastic, antibiotic; hypocalcemic

Chem. class.: Crystalline aglycone

Pregnancy category X

Action: Inhibits DNA, RNA, protein synthesis; derived from *Streptomyces plicatus;* replication is decreased by binding to DNA; demonstrates calcium-lowering effect not related to its tumoricidal activity; also acts on osteoclasts and blocks action of parathyroid hormone; a vesicant

⇒ **Therapeutic Outcome:** Prevention of rapidly growing malignant cells, decreased calcium levels

Uses: Testicular cancer, hypercalcemia, hypercalciuria, symptomatic treatment of advanced neoplasms

Dosage and routes

Testicular tumors

Adult: **IV** 25-30 μg/kg/day × 8-10 days, not to exceed 30 μg/kg/day

Hypercalcemia/ hypercalciuria

Adult: **IV** 25 μg/kg/day × 3-4 days; repeat at intervals of 1 wk

Available forms: Inj 2.5 mg/vial powder

Side effects/adverse reactions

CNS: Drowsiness, weakness, lethargy, headache, flushing, fever, depression
GI: Nausea, vomiting, anorexia, diarrhea, stomatitis, increased liver enzymes
GU: Increased BUN, creatinine, ***proteinuria***
HEMA: Hemorrhage, thrombocytopenia, decreased pro-time, WBC count
INTEG: Rash, cellulitis, ***extravasation,*** facial flushing
META: Decreased serum calcium, potassium, phosphorus

Contraindications: Hypersensitivity, thrombocytopenia, bone marrow depression, bleeding disorders, pregnancy **X**

Precautions: Renal disease, hepatic disease, electrolyte imbalances

Pharmacokinetics

Absorption	Completely absorbed (IV)
Distribution	Crosses blood-brain barrier; concentration in bone, liver, renal system
Metabolism	Unknown
Excretion	Kidneys
Half-life	Unknown

Pharmacodynamics

	IV
Onset	Unknown
Peak	Unknown
Duration	Unknown

Interactions

Drug/drug:

Individual drugs

Aspirin: ↑ risk of bleeding
Dextran: ↑ risk of bleeding
Heparin: ↑ risk of bleeding
Radiation: ↑ toxicity, bone marrow suppression
Sulfinpyrazone: ↑ risk of bleeding
Valproic acid: ↑ risk of bleeding

Drug classifications

Anticoagulants, oral: ↑ risk of bleeding
Antineoplastics: ↑ toxicity, bone marrow suppression
Cephalosporins: ↑ risk of bleeding
Hepatotoxic agents: ↑ hepatotoxicity
Neurotoxic agents: ↑ neurotoxicity
NSAIDs: ↑ risk of bleeding
Thrombolytics: ↑ risk of bleeding

NURSING CONSIDERATIONS

Assessment

- Assess buccal cavity q8h for dryness, sores or ulceration, white patches, oral pain, bleeding, dysphagia; obtain prescription for viscous lidocaine (Xylocaine)
- Assess symptoms indicating severe allergic reaction: rash, pruritus, urticaria, purpuric skin lesions, itching, flushing
- Monitor CBC, differential, platelet count weekly; withhold

P

drug if WBC count is <4000/mm^3 or platelet count is <100,000/mm^3; notify prescriber of results if WBC <20,000/mm^3, platelets <150,000/mm^3

- Monitor renal function studies: BUN, creatinine, serum uric acid, urine CrCl before and during therapy; I&O ratio; report fall in urine output to <30 ml/hr
- Monitor temp q4h (may indicate beginning of infection)
- Monitor liver function tests before and during therapy (bilirubin, AST [SGOT], ALT [SGPT], LDH) as needed or monthly; check for yellowing of skin and sclera, dark urine, clay-colored stools, itchy skin, abdominal pain, fever, diarrhea
- Assess for bleeding: hematuria, stool guaiac, bruising or petechiae, mucosa or orifices q8h; check for inflammation of mucosa, breaks in skin

Associated nursing diagnoses

- ✓ Injury, risk for (adverse reactions)
- ✓ Body image disturbance (adverse reactions)
- ✓ Infection, risk for (adverse reactions)
- ✓ Knowledge deficit (teaching)

Implementation

- Avoid contact with skin; very irritating; wash completely to remove
- Give fluids **IV** or PO before chemotherapy to hydrate patient
- Give antacid before oral agent; give drug after evening meal, before hs; provide antiemetic 30-60 min before giving drug and prn to prevent vomiting; administer antibiotics for prophylaxis of infection
- Give top or syst analgesics for pain
- Give in AM so drug can be eliminated before hs
- Provide liq diet: carbonated beverages; gelatin may be added if patient is not nauseated or vomiting
- Encourage patient to rinse mouth tid-qid with water, club soda; brush teeth bid-qid with soft brush or cotton-tipped applicators for stomatitis; use unwaxed dental floss

IV **IV route**

- Drug should be prepared by experienced personnel using proper precautions
- Give **IV** direct by **IV** push over 20-30 min
- Give **IV** intermittent inf by diluting 2.5 mg/4.9 ml of sterile water; (1 ml = 500 μg); dilute single dose in 1000 ml of D_5W run over 4-6 hr; give slow **IV** inf using 20 G, 21 G needle
- Administer EDTA for extravasation; apply ice compress

Patient/family education

- Teach patient to avoid use of products containing aspirin or ibuprofen, razors, commercial mouthwash, since bleeding may occur; to report symptoms of bleeding (hematuria, tarry stools)
- Caution patient to report signs of anemia (fatigue, headache, irritability, faintness, shortness of breath)
- Advise patient to report any changes in breathing or cough-

ing even several mo after treatment; to avoid crowds or persons with respiratory tract and other infections
• Advise patient that hair may be lost during treatment; a wig or hair piece may make patient feel better; new hair may be different in color, texture
• Caution patient not to have any vaccinations without the advice of the prescriber; serious reactions can occur
• Advise patient contraception is needed during treatment and for several mo after completion of therapy

Evaluation

Positive therapeutic outcome
• Prevention of rapid division of malignant cells

polymyxin B

(pol-ee-mix'in)
Aerosporin, polymyxin B Sulfate
Func. class.: Antiinfective
Chem. class: Polymyxin
Pregnancy category **B**

Action: Interferes with phospholipids, penetrates cell wall; immediately changes bacterial membrane, causing leakage of essential metabolites

➡ **Therapeutic Outcome:** Bactericidal against *Pseudomonas aeruginosa, Enterobacter aerogenes, Klebsiella pneumoniae, Escherichia coli, Haemophilus influenzae*

Uses: Serious infections or when other antibiotics cannot be used; septicemia, meningitis, UTI, ophth infections (ophth route)

Dosage and routes

P *Adult and child:* **IV** inf 15,000-25000 U/kg/day in divided doses q12h, or 25,000 U/kg/day in divided doses q4-8h

P. aeruginosa/H. influenzae

P *Adult and child >2 yr:* INTRATHECAL 50,000 U/day × 3-4 days, then 50,000 U/qod × 2 wks after CSF negative, glucose normal

P *Child < 2 yr:* IT 20,000 U/day × 3-4 days, then 25,000 U/qod × 2 wk after CSF negative

Ocular infections

Adult: Ophth 1-3 gtt qh; may be increased if needed

Available forms: Inj 500,000 U; powder for ophth sol 500,000 U/20-50 ml

P

Side effects/adverse reactions

CNS: Dizziness, confusion, weakness, drowsiness, paresthesia, slurred speech, ***coma, seizures,*** headache, stiff neck, fever
EENT (OPHTH): itching, burning, stinging, vision changes
GU: ***Proteinuria, hematuria, azotemia, leukocyturia***
INTEG: Urticaria, pain at inj site, phlebitis, flushing
RESP: ***Paralysis***
SYST: ***Anaphylaxis, superinfection***

Contraindications: Hypersensitivity, severe renal disease

Precaution: Pregnancy **B**

Pharmacokinetics

Absorption	Well absorbed (IM); completely absorbed (IV)
Distribution	Widely distributed
Metabolism	Unknown
Excretion	Kidneys, unchanged (50%-60%)
Half-life	4½-6 hr; increased in renal disease

Pharmacodynamics

	IM	IV	OPHTH
Onset	Rapid	Rapid	Unknown
Peak	1-2 hr	Inf end	Unknown

Interactions

Drug/drug:

Individual drugs

Tubocurarine: ↑ skeletal muscle relaxation

Succinylcholine: ↑ skeletal muscle relaxation

Gallamine: ↑ skeletal muscle relaxation

Drug classifications

Aminoglycosides: ↑ nephrotoxicity

Anesthetics: ↑ skeletal muscle relaxation

Neuromuscular blockers: ↑ skeletal muscle relaxation

NURSING CONSIDERATIONS

Assessment

- Assess patient for previous sensitivity reaction
- Assess patient for signs and symptoms of infection including characteristics of wounds, sputum, urine, stool, WBC >10,000, fever; obtain baseline information before and during treatment
- Obtain C&S before beginning drug therapy to identify if correct treatment has been initiated
- Assess for allergic reactions: rash, urticaria, pruritus
- Identify urine output; if decreasing, notify prescriber (may indicate nephrotoxicity); also check for increased BUN, creatinine
- Monitor blood studies: AST (SGOT), ALT (SGPT), CBC, Hct, bilirubin, LDH, alkaline, phosphatase, Coombs' test monthly if patient is on long-term therapy
- Assess bowel pattern daily; if severe diarrhea occurs, drug should be discontinued
- Assess for overgrowth of infection: perineal itching, fever, malaise, redness, pain, swelling, drainage, rash, diarrhea, change in cough, sputum
- Assess for CNS symptoms: insomnia, vertigo, headaches, agitation, confusion

Associated nursing diagnoses

- ✓ Infection, risk for (uses)
- ✓ Diarrhea (adverse reactions)
- ✓ Injury, risk for (adverse reactions)
- ✓ Knowledge deficit (teaching)
- ✓ Noncompliance (teaching)

Implementation

IV **IV route**

- For intermittent inf dilute to 4 mg/ml of D_5W, D_5/0.9% NaCl, 0.9% NaCl, D_5/LR, sodium bicarbonate, sodium lactate, D_5/Plasma-Lyte 56; give over 1 hr or more

Y-site compatibility:
Esmolol

Additive compatibilities:
Amikacin, colistimethate, diphenhydramine, erythromycin lactobionate, hydrocortisone sodium succinate, kanamycin, methicillin, penicillin G potassium, sodium

Additive incompatibilities:
Amphotericin B, cefazolin, cephalothin, chloramphenicol, heparin, magnesium sulfate, prednisolone sodium phosphate

• For direct **IV** dissolve 500,000 U of polymyxin B in 10 ml of 0.9% NaCl for a conc of 50,000 U/ml

Patient/family education

• Teach patient reason for medication and expected results

Evaluation

Positive therapeutic outcome
• Absence of signs/symptoms of infection (WBC <10,000, temp WNL)
• Reported improvement in symptoms of infection
• Absence of red or itching eyes (ophth)

potassium bicarbonate/potassium acetate/ potassium chloride/ potassium gluconate/ potassium phosphate

Effer-K, K-Lyte, K-Lyte DS, Klorvess, Tri-K, Twin-K, Cena-K, Gen-K, K^+10, K-Tab, K-Norm, K-Dur 10, K-Dur 20, K-Lyte/Cl, K-Lease, K^+ Care, Kaon-Cl, Kaon-Cl-10, Kaochlor, Kaochlor S-F, Kato, Kay Ciel, Klor, Klor-Con, Klor-Con 8, Klor-Con 10, Klor-Con/25, Klortrix, Klorvess, Micro-K, Micro KLS, Potachlor, Potage, Potasalan, Potassium Chloride, Rum-K, Slow-K, Ten-K, Urocit-K, Kao-Nor, Kaylixir, K-G Elixir, My-K Elixir, Potassium Gluconate

Func. class.: Electrolyte
Chem. class.: Potassium

Pregnancy category **C**

P

Action: Needed for adequate transmission of nerve impulses and cardiac contraction, renal function, intracellular ion maintenance

Uses: Prevention and treatment of hypokalemia

Therapeutic Outcome: Potassium level 3.0-5.0

Dosage and routes

Potassium bicarbonate

Adult: PO dissolve 25-50 mEq in water qd-qid

Potassium acetate—hypokalemia

P ***Adult and child:*** PO 40-100 mEq/day in divided doses × 2-4 days

Hypokalemia (prevention)

P ***Adult and child:*** PO 20 mEq/day in 2-4 divided doses

Potassium chloride

Adult: PO 40-100 mEq in divided doses tid-qid; **IV** 20 mEq/hr when diluted as 40 mEq/1000 ml, not to exceed 150 mEq/day

Potassium gluconate

Adult: PO 40-100 mEq in divided doses tid-qid

Potassium phosphate

Adult: **IV** 1 mEq/hr in sol of 60 mEq/L, not to exceed 150 mEq/day; PO 40-100 mEq/day in divided doses

Available forms: Tab for sol 6.5, 25 mEq; inj for prep of **IV** 2, 4 mEq; ext rel cap 8, 10 mEq; powder for sol 3.3, 5, 6.7, 10, 13.3 mEq/5 ml; tab 4, 13.4 mEq; ext rel tab 6.7, 8, 10 mEq; inj for prep of **IV** 1.5, 2, 2.4, 3, 3.2 mEq/ml; elix 6.7 mEq/5 ml; tab 2, 5 mEq; oral sol 2.375 mEq/5 ml; inj for prep of **IV** 4.4, 4.7 mEq/ml

Side effects/adverse reactions

CNS: Confusion
CV: Bradycardia, ***cardiac depression, dysrhythmias, arrest, peaking T waves, lowered R and depressed RST, prolonged PR interval, widened QRS complex***
GI: Nausea, vomiting, cramps, pain, *diarrhea,* ulceration of small bowel
GU: Oliguria
INTEG: Cold extremities, rash

Contraindications: Renal disease (severe), severe hemolytic disease, Addison's disease, hyperkalemia, acute dehydration, extensive tissue breakdown

Precautions: Cardiac disease, potassium-sparing diuretic therapy, systemic acidosis, pregnancy **C**

Pharmacokinetics	
Absorption	Well absorbed (PO)
Distribution	To cells
Metabolism	Unknown
Excretion	Kidneys
Half-life	Unknown

Pharmacodynamics	
Onset	Unknown
Peak	Unknown
Duration	Unknown

Interactions

Drug/drug:

Drug classification

Angiotensin converting enzyme inhibitors: ↑ hyperkalemia
Potassium-sparing diuretics: ↑ hyperkalemia

NURSING CONSIDERATIONS

Assessment

• Assess ECG for peaking T waves, lowered R, depressed RST, prolonged PR interval, widening QRS complex,

hyperkalemia; drug should be reduced or discontinued
- Monitor potassium level during treatment (3.5-5.0 mg/dl is normal level)
- Monitor I&O ratio; watch for decreased urinary output; notify prescriber immediately; check urinary pH in patients receiving the drug as a urinary acidifier
- Assess cardiac status: rate, rhythm, CVP, PWP, PAWP if being monitored directly

Associated nursing diagnoses

✓ Nutrition, altered: less than body requirements (uses)
✓ Knowledge deficit (teaching)

Implementation

IV **IV route**
- Give through large-bore needle to decrease vein inflammation; check for extravasation; administer in large vein, avoiding scalp vein

P in child
- After diluting in large volume of **IV** sol give as an **IV** inf slowly to prevent toxicity; never give **IV** bolus or IM

PO route
- Give with or pc; dissolve effervescent tab, powder in 8 oz cold water or juice; do not give IM, SC
- Store at room temp

Patient/family education

- Teach patient to add potassium-rich foods to diet; bananas, orange juice, avocados, whole grains, broccoli, carrots, prunes, cocoa after this medication is discontinued
- Advise patient to avoid OTC products: antacids, salt substitutes, analgesics, vitamin preparations, unless specifically directed by prescriber
- Advise patient to report hyperkalemia symptoms (lethargy, confusion, diarrhea, nausea, vomiting, fainting, decreased output) or continued hypokalemia symptoms (fatigue, weakness, polyuria, polydipsia, cardiac changes)
- Tell patient to take cap with full glass of liq; to dissolve powder or tab completely in at least 120 ml water or juice; not to chew time rel or ext rel preparations
- Emphasize importance of regular follow-up

Evaluation

Positive therapeutic outcome
- Absence of fatigue, muscle weakness, and decreased thirst and urinary output, cardiac changes
- Potassium level normal

potassium iodide

Pima, Iosat, Thyro-Block, SSKI

Func. class.: Expectorant

Pregnancy category **D**

P

Action: Increases respiratory tract fluid by decreasing surface tension, adhesiveness, which increases removal of mucus

Uses: Bronchial asthma, emphysema, bronchitis, nuclear radiation protection

Therapeutic Outcome: Radiation protection, resolution of asthma symptoms, emphysema

Dosage and routes

Adult: PO 0.3-0.6 ml q4-6h

P *Child:* PO 0.25-1 ml saturated sol bid-qid

Radiation protection

Adult: PO 0.13 ml SSKI before or after initial exposure

P *Infant <1 yr:* Half adult dose

Available forms: Sol 1 g/ml; oral syr 325 mg/5 ml; tab 130 mg ✦

Side effects/adverse reactions

CNS: Frontal headache, ***CNS depression,*** fever, parkinsonism

EENT: Burning mouth, throat, eye irritation, swelling of eyelids

ENDO: Iodism, goiter, myxedema

GI: Gastric irritation

INTEG: Angioedema, rash

RESP: Pulmonary edema

Contraindications: Hypersensitivity to iodides, pulmonary TB, pregnancy **D**, hyperthyroidism, hyperkalemia, acute bronchitis

Precautions: Hypothyroidism, cystic fibrosis, lactation

Pharmacokinetics	
Absorption	To GI tract
Distribution	Thyroid gland; crosses placenta
Metabolism	Thyroid gland
Excretion	Thyroid gland
Half-life	Unknown

Pharmacodynamics	
Onset	24-48 hr
Peak	10-15 days
Duration	Variable

Interactions

Drug/drug:

Individual drugs

Lithium: ↑ hypothyroid symptoms

Drug classifications

Antithyroid agents: ↑ hypothyroidism

Lab test interferences

Interfere: Urinary 17-OHCS

NURSING CONSIDERATIONS

Assessment

- Monitor pulse, B/P, temp
- Monitor I&O ratio; check for edema that indicates hypothyroidism: puffy hands, feet, periorbit
- Monitor weight daily with same clothing, scale, time of day
- Monitor T_3, T_4, which is increased; serum TSH, which is decreased; free thyroxine index, which is increased if dosage is too low; discontinue drug 3-4 days before RAIU
- Assess for overdose: peripheral edema, heat intolerance, diaphoresis, palpitations, dysrhythmias, severe tachycardia, increased temp, delirium, CNS irritability
- Assess for hypersensitivity: rash; enlarged cervical lymph nodes indicate drug may have to be discontinued
- Assess for hypoprothrombinemia: bleeding, petechiae, ecchymosis

• Assess for clinical response: after 3 wk should include increased weight, pulse; decreased T_4

Associated nursing diagnoses

✓ Knowledge deficit (teaching)

Implementation

PO route

• Give strong iodine sol after diluting with water or juice to improve taste; give through straw to prevent tooth discoloration; with meals to decrease GI upset
• Encourage fluids to 3-4 L/day unless contraindicated
• Give at same time each day to maintain drug level; give lowest dosage that relieves symptoms; discontinue before RAIU

Patient/family education

• Advise patient to abstain from breastfeeding after delivery
• Instruct patient to keep graph of weight, pulse, mood
• Caution patient to avoid OTC products that contain iodine; seafood, other iodine products may be restricted
• Advise patient not to discontinue this medication abruptly; thyroid crisis may occur; stress patient response
• Teach patient that response may take several mo if thyroid is large
• Caution patient not to discontinue drug; notify prescriber if fever, rash, metallic taste, swelling of throat, burning of mouth, throat, sore gums, teeth, severe GI distress, enlargement of thyroid, cold symptoms occur

Evaluation

Positive therapeutic outcome

• Weight gain
• Decreased pulse, T_4
• Decreased size of thyroid gland

pralidoxime

(pra-li-dox'eem)

Protopam Chloride

Func. class.: Cholinesterase reactivator

Chem. class.: Quaternary ammonium oxide

Pregnancy category **C**

Action: Reactivated enzyme metabolizes and inactivates acetylcholine at both muscarinic and nicotinic sites in the periphery

➔ **Therapeutic Outcome:** Prevention of death from organophosphate poisoning

Uses: Cholinergic crisis in myasthenia gravis, organophosphate poisoning antidote early, relief of paralysis of respiratory muscles; used as an adjunct to systemic atropine administration

Dosage and routes

Anticholinesterase overdose

Adult: **IV** 1-2 g, then 250 mg q5 min until desired response

Organophosphate poisoning

Adult: **IV** inf 1-2 g/100 ml

P

0.9% NaCl over 15-30 min; may repeat in 1 hr; PO 1-3 g q5h

P *Child:* **IV** inf 20-40 mg/kg/dose diluted in 100 ml 0.9% NaCl over 15-30 min

Available forms: Inj 600 mg/2 ml; tab 500 mg; emergency kit 1 g/20-ml vial

Side effects/adverse reactions

CNS: Dizziness, headache, drowsiness, blurred vision, diplopia, impaired accommodation
CV: Tachycardia
GI: Nausea
MS: Weakness, muscle rigidity
RESP: Hyperventilation, ***laryngospasm***

Contraindications: Hypersensitivity, carbamate insecticide poisoning

Precautions: Myasthenia gravis, pregnancy **C**, renal P insufficiency, children, lactation

Pharmacokinetics

Absorption	Variably absorbed (PO), well absorbed (IM), completely absorbed (IV)
Distribution	Widely distributed (extracellular water)
Metabolism	Liver
Excretion	Kidneys, unchanged (90%)
Half-life	1½ hr

Pharmacodynamics

	PO	IV	IM
Onset	Unknown	Unknown	Unknown
Peak	2-3 hr	5-15 min	10-20 min
Duration	Unknown	Unknown	Unknown

Interactions

Drug/drug:

Individual drugs

Aminophylline: Do not use together
Morphine: Do not use together
Reserpine: Do not use together
Succinylcholine: Do not use together
Theophylline: Do not use together

Drug classifications

Analgesics, narcotic: Do not use together
Barbiturates: Do not use together
Sedative/hypnotics: Do not use together

NURSING CONSIDERATIONS

Assessment

- Monitor liver function studies: AST (SGOT), ALT (SGPT), CPK; liver function enzymes and CPK return to normal levels in 10-14 days
- Assess insecticide that was ingested including amount ingested, time, and if patient used any products to counteract effect; treatment should begin within 24 hr to be completely effective
- Assess for neurologic and muscular effects: weakness, pale skin, hypertension, tachycardia, muscle cramping, twitching; these reactions are the effect of anticholinesterase
- Monitor B/P, VS, I&O ratio; observe for decreased urinary output for 48-72 hr after poisoning to determine atropine toxicity from poisoning effects
- Monitor respiratory status:

rate, rhythm, characteristics, tidal volume, vital capacity

Associated nursing diagnoses

✓ Injury, risk for (uses)
✓ Airway clearance, ineffective (uses)

Implementation

IV route

- Give **IV** after diluting 1 g/20 ml sterile water for inj; give directly over 5 min
- Further dilute/100 ml 0.9% NaCl; may be given as an inf over 15-30 min
- Give **IV** slowly after dilution with sterile water; rapid administration may lead to tachycardia, hypertension, rigidity, laryngospasm
- Give concurrent atropine 2-4 mg **IV** or IM if cyanosis is present to block accumulated acetylcholine in respiratory center; repeat q5-10 min until toxicity occurs: dry mouth, flushing, tachycardia, delirium, hallucinations
- Give only with edrophonium (Tensilon) available for myasthenia gravis patient
- Give only with emergency equipment available

Patient/family education

- Explain purpose of drug and expected results

Evaluation

Positive therapeutic outcome

- Decreased effects of organophosphate poisoning
- Decreased effects of anticholesterase overdose

pramoxine

(pra-mox'een)

Fleet Relief, Prax, ProctoFoam, Tronolane, Tronothane

Func. class.: Topical anesthetic

Pregnancy category C

Action: Inhibits conduction of nerve impulses from sensory nerves

Therapeutic Outcome: Resolution of pain, itching

Uses: Pruritus, sunburn, toothache, sore throat, cold sores, oral pain, rectal pain and irritation

Dosage and routes

Adult and child: Top apply q3-4h; rec apply 1 full applicator bid-tid and after each BM

Available forms: Cream 1%; rec oint 1%; rec aero foam; cream supp 1%

Side effects/adverse reactions

INTEG: Rash, irritation, sensitization

Contraindications: Hypersensitivity, infants <1 yr, application to large areas

Precautions: Child <6 yr, sepsis, pregnancy **C**, denuded skin

P

Pharmacokinetics

Absorption	Poorly absorbed
Distribution	Unknown
Metabolism	Unknown
Excretion	Unknown
Half-life	Unknown

Pharmacodynamics

Onset	1 min
Peak	Unknown
Duration	½-1 hr

Interactions: None

NURSING CONSIDERATIONS

Assessment

- Assess pain: location, duration, characteristics before and after administration
- Assess for infection: redness, drainage, inflammation; this drug should not be used until infection is treated

Associated nursing diagnoses

✓ Pain (uses)
✓ Knowledge deficit (teaching)

Implementation

- Store in tight, light-resistant container; do not freeze, puncture, or incinerate aerosol container

Patient/family education

- Teach patient to avoid contact with eyes
- Instruct patient not to use for prolonged periods: use for <1 wk; if condition remains, prescriber should be contacted

Evaluation

Positive therapeutic outcome
- Decreased redness, swelling, pain

pravastatin
(pra'va-sta-tin)
Pravachol
Func. class.: Antilipidemic
Pregnancy category **X**

Action: Inhibits biosynthesis of VLDL, LDL, which are responsible for cholesterol development, by the enzyme HMG-CoA reductase

Therapeutic Outcome: Decreasing cholesterol levels and LDL, increased HDLD

Uses: As an adjunct in primary hypercholesterolemia types IIa, IIb

Dosage and routes

Adult: PO 10-20 mg qd at hs (range 10-40 mg qd); G elderly may require the lowest dosage

Available forms: Tab 10, 20 mg

Side effects/adverse reactions

CNS: Headache, dizziness, psychic disturbances
EENT: Lens opacities, common cold, rhinitis, cough
GI: Nausea, constipation, diarrhea, dyspepsia, flatus, abdominal pain, heartburn, ***liver dysfunction,*** pancreatitis, ***hepatitis***
INTEG: Rash, pruritus
MS: Muscle cramps, myalgia, ***myositis, rhabdomyolysis***

Contraindications: Hypersensitivity, pregnancy **X**, lactation, active liver disease

Precautions: Past liver disease, alcoholism, severe acute infections, trauma, hypotension, uncontrolled seizure disorders, severe metabolic disorders, electrolyte imbalances

Pharmacokinetics

Absorption	Poorly absorbed, erratic (PO)
Distribution	Unknown
Metabolism	Liver, extensively
Excretion	Feces (70%-75%); kidneys, unchanged (10%), breast milk (minimal)
Half-life	2 hr

Pharmacodynamics

Onset	Unknown
Peak	1-1½ hr
Duration	Unknown

Interactions

Drug/drug:

Individual drugs

Cholestyramine: ↑ action
Colestipol: ↑ action
Cyclosporine: ↑ risk of myopathy, rhabdomyolysis
Erythromycin: ↑ risk of myopathy, rhabdomyolysis
Gemfibrozil: ↑ risk of myopathy, rhabdomyolysis
Niacin: ↑ risk of myopathy, rhabdomyolysis

Drug/food:

↑ levels of lovastatin

Lab test interferences

Increase: CPK, liver function tests

NURSING CONSIDERATIONS

Assessment

- Assess nutrition: fat, protein, carbohydrates; nutritional analysis should be completed by dietician before treatment
- Monitor triglycerides, cholesterol at baseline and throughout treatment; LDL and VLDL should be watched closely; if increased, drug should be discontinued

Associated nursing diagnoses

- ✓ Knowledge deficit (teaching)
- ✓ Noncompliance (teaching)

Implementation

PO route

- Give at hs only; give 1 hr before or 4 hr after bile acid sequestrants
- Store in cool environment in tight, light-resistant container

Patient/family education

- Inform patient that compliance is needed for positive results to occur; not to double doses or skip doses
- Teach patient that risk factors should be decreased: high-fat diet, smoking, alcohol consumption, absence of exercise
- Advise patient to notify prescriber of weakness, tenderness, or limited mobility
- Explain to patient that contraception is necessary, since drug produces teratogenic effects

Evaluation

Positive therapeutic outcome

- Decreased cholesterol serum triglyceride levels and improved ratio with HDL

P

prazepam

(praz'e-pam)

Centrax

Func. class.: Sedative/hypnotic; antianxiety agent

Chem. class.: Benzodiazepine

Pregnancy category **D**

Controlled substance schedule **IV**

Action: Depresses subcortical levels of CNS, including limbic system, reticular formation; potentiates GABA

Therapeutic Outcome: Decreased anxiety, relaxation, sedation

Uses: Anxiety

Dosage and routes

Adult: PO 10 mg tid; 20-60 mg in divided doses or 20 mg at hs

G *Elderly:* PO 10-15 mg/day in divided doses

Available forms: Cap 5, 10, 20 mg; tab 10 mg

Side effects/adverse reactions

CNS: Dizziness, drowsiness, confusion, headache, anxiety, tremors, stimulation, fatigue, insomnia, weakness

CV: Orthostatic hypotension, ***ECG changes, tachycardia,*** hypotension, palpitations, syncope

EENT: Blurred vision, tinnitus, mydriasis

GI: Constipation, dry mouth, nausea, vomiting, anorexia, diarrhea

INTEG: Rash, dermatitis, itching

Contraindications: Hypersensitivity to benzodiazepines, narrow angle glaucoma, psychosis, pregnancy **D**, P child <18 yr

G **Precautions:** Elderly, debilitated, hepatic disease, renal disease

Pharmacokinetics

Absorption	Slowly absorbed (PO)
Distribution	Widely distributed; crosses placenta, blood-brain barrier
Metabolism	Liver, extensively to active metabolites
Excretion	Kidneys, breast milk
Half-life	5-15 hr; active metabolite 30-100 hr

Pharmacodynamics

Onset	Unknown
Peak	6 hr
Duration	Up to 48 hr

Interactions

Drug/drug:

Individual drugs

Alcohol: ↑ CNS depression
Cimetidine: ↑ action
Disulfiram: ↑ action
Fluoxetine: ↑ action
Isoniazid: ↑ action
Ketoconazole: ↑ action
Levodopa: ↓ action of levodopa
Metoprolol: ↑ action
Propoxyphene: ↑ action
Propranolol: ↑ action
Rifampin: ↓ action of prazepam

Theophylline: ↓ sedative effects
Valproic acid: ↑ action

Drug classifications

Analgesics, opioid: ↑ CNS depression
Antidepressants: ↑ CNS depression
Antihistamines: ↑ CNS depression
Barbiturates: ↓ effect of prazepam
Oral contraceptives: ↑ effect

Lab test interferences

Increase: AST (SGOT), ALT (SGPT), serum bilirubin
False increase: 17-OHCS
Decrease: RAIU

NURSING CONSIDERATIONS

Assessment

- Assess mental status: mood, sensorium, anxiety, affect, sleeping pattern, drowsiness, G dizziness, especially elderly; physical dependency, withdrawal symptoms: anxiety, panic attacks, agitation, convulsions, headache, nausea, vomiting, muscle pain, weakness; suicidal tendencies; for indications of increasing tolerance and abuse
- Monitor B/P (with patient lying, standing), pulse; if systolic B/P drops 20 mm Hg, hold drug, notify prescriber
- Monitor hepatic studies: AST (SGOT), ALT (SGPT), bilirubin, creatinine LDH, alkaline phosphatase
- Monitor I&O; indicate renal dysfunction

Associated nursing diagnoses

✓ Anxiety (uses)
✓ Depression (uses)
✓ Injury, risk for (adverse reactions)
✓ Knowledge deficit (teaching)

Implementation

PO route

- Give with food or milk for GI symptoms; tab may be crushed if patient is unable to swallow medication whole; provide sugarless gum, hard candy, frequent sips of water for dry mouth

Patient/family education

- Teach patient that drug may be taken with food or fluids, and tab may be crushed or swallowed whole
- Advise patient not to use for everyday stress or longer than 3 mo unless directed by prescriber; not to take more than prescribed amount; may be habit forming; not to double doses or skip doses
- Caution patient to avoid OTC preparations unless approved by prescriber; alcohol and CNS depressants will increase CNS depression
- Advise patient to avoid driving, activities that require alertness, since drowsiness may occur; to avoid alcohol and other psychotropic medications; to rise slowly or fainting may occur, especially G elderly; that drowsiness may worsen at beginning of treatment
- Instruct patient not to discontinue medication abruptly after long-term use; withdrawal symptoms include vomiting, cramping, tremors, seizures

P

Evaluation

Positive therapeutic outcome

- Decreased anxiety, restlessness, sleeplessness (short-term treatment only)

Treatment of overdose: Lavage, VS, supportive care

prazosin ⚷

(pra'zoe-sin)

Minipress, prazosin

Func. class.: Antihypertensive

Chem. class.: α_1-Adrenergic blocker

Pregnancy category C

Action: Peripheral blood vessels dilate, peripheral resistance drops; reduction in blood pressure results from α-adrenergic receptors being blocked

Therapeutic Outcome: Decreased B/P in hypertension; decreased cardiac preload, afterload

Uses: Hypertension

Investigational uses: Benign prostatic hypertrophy to decreased urine outflow obstruction

Dosage and routes

Hypertension

Adult: PO 1 mg bid or tid, increasing to 20 mg qd in divided doses if required, usual range 6-15 mg/day, not to exceed 1 mg initially; max 20-40 mg/day

Benign prostatic hypertrophy

Adult: PO 1-5 mg bid

Available forms: Cap 1, 2, 5 mg

Side effects/adverse reactions

CNS: *Dizziness, headache, drowsiness,* anxiety, depression, vertigo, weakness, fatigue

CV: *Palpitations, orthostatic hypotension,* tachycardia, edema, rebound hypertension

EENT: Blurred vision, epistaxis, tinnitus, dry mouth, red sclera

GI: *Nausea,* vomiting, diarrhea, constipation, abdominal pain

GU: Urinary frequency, incontinence, impotence, priapism, water and sodium retention

Contraindications: Hypersensitivity

Precautions: Pregnancy **C**, P children

Pharmacokinetics

Absorption	60% (PO)
Distribution	Widely distributed
Metabolism	Liver, extensively
Excretion	Kidneys, unchanged (10%), bile (90%)
Half-life	2-3 hr

Pharmacodynamics

Onset	2 hr
Peak	1-3 hr
Duration	6-12 hr

Interactions

Drug/drug:

Individual drugs

Alcohol: ↑ hypotension
Indomethacin: ↓ effect
Nitroglycerin: ↑ hypotension

Drug classifications

Antihypertensives: ↑ hypotension
β-Blockers: ↑ hypotension
Nitrates: ↑ hypotension

Lab test interferences

Increase: Urinary norepinephrine, VMA

NURSING CONSIDERATIONS

Assessment

- Monitor B/P, orthostatic hypotension, syncope; check for edema in feet, legs daily; monitor I&O, weight daily; notify prescriber of changes
- Assess for allergic reactions: rash, fever, pruritus, urticaria; drug should be discontinued if antihistamines fail to help
- Assess for orthostatic hypotension; tell patient to rise slowly from sitting or lying position

Associated nursing diagnoses

- ✓ Cardiac output, decreased (uses)
- ✓ Injury, risk for (adverse reactions)
- ✓ Knowledge deficit (teaching)
- ✓ Noncompliance (teaching)

Implementation

PO route

- Severe hypotension may occur after 1st dose of this medication; decreased hypotension may be prevented by reducing or discontinuing diuretic therapy 3 days before beginning prazosin therapy
- Store in airtight container at 86° F (30° C) or less

Patient/family education

- Instruct patient not to discontinue drug abruptly; stress the importance of complying with dosage schedule, even if feeling better; if dose is missed, take as soon as remembered; take at same time each day
- Advise patient not to use OTC products (cough, cold, allergy) unless directed by prescriber; also to avoid large amounts of caffeine
- Emphasize the need to rise slowly to sitting or standing position to minimize orthostatic hypotension
- Teach patient to notify prescriber of mouth sores, sore throat, fever, swelling of hands or feet, irregular heartbeat, chest pain
- Caution patient to report excessive perspiration, dehydration, vomiting, diarrhea; may lead to fall in B/P
- Caution patient that drug may cause dizziness, fainting, light headedness; may occur during 1st few days of therapy; to avoid hazardous activities
- Teach patient how to take B/P and normal readings for age group; instruct to take B/P q7 days

Evaluation

Positive therapeutic outcome

- Decreased B/P in hypertension

Treatment of overdose:

Administer volume expanders or vasopressors, discontinue drug, place in supine position

P

prednisolone

(pred-niss'oh-lone)

Articulose-50, Delta-Cortef, Prednisolone, Prelone, Key-Pred 25, Key-Pred 50, Predaject-50, Predalone 50, Predcor-25, Predcor-50, Prednisolone Acetate, Hydeltrasol, Key-Pred-SP, Pediapred, Hydeltra-T.B.A., Predalone-T.B.A., Prednisol TBA

Func. class.: Corticosteroid

Chem. class.: Intermediate-acting glucocorticoid

Pregnancy category **C**

Action: Decreases inflammation by suppressing migration of polymorphonuclear leukocytes, fibroblasts; reversal to increase capillary permeability and lysosomal stabilization, minimal mineralocorticoid

➔ **Therapeutic Outcome:** Decreased inflammation, decreased adrenal insufficiency

Uses: Severe inflammation, immunosuppression, neoplasms

Dosage and routes

Adult: PO 2.5-15 mg bid-qid; IM 2-30 mg (acetate, phosphate) q12h; **IV** 2-30 mg (phosphate) q12h, 2-30 mg in joint or soft tissue (phosphate), 4-40 mg in joint of lesion (tebutate), 0.25-1 ml/wk in joints (acetate-phosphate)

Available forms: Tab 5 mg; inj 25, 50, 100 mg/ml acetate; inj 20 mg/ml tebutate; inj 20 mg/ml phosphate; inj 80 mg/ml acetate/phosphate

Side effects/adverse reactions

CNS: ***Depression,*** flushing, sweating, headache, mood changes

CV: Hypertension, ***circulatory collapse, thrombophlebitis, embolism,*** tachycardia

EENT: Fungal infections, increased intraocular pressure, blurred vision

GI: Diarrhea, nausea, abdominal distention, ***GI hemorrhage,*** increased appetite, ***pancreatitis***

HEMA: ***Thrombocytopenia***

INTEG: Acne, poor wound healing, ecchymosis, petechiae

MS: Fractures, osteoporosis, weakness

Contraindications: Psychosis, hypersensitivity, idiopathic thrombocytopenia, acute glomerulonephritis, amebiasis, fungal infections, nonasthmatic bronchial disease, **P** child <2 yr

Precautions: Pregnancy **C**, diabetes mellitus, glaucoma, osteoporosis, seizure disorders, ulcerative colitis, CHF, myasthenia gravis

Pharmacokinetics

Absorption	Well absorbed (PO, IM), completely absorbed (IV)
Distribution	Widely distributed; crosses placenta
Metabolism	Liver, extensively
Excretion	Kidney, breast milk
Half-life	2-4 hr

Pharmacodynamics

	PO	IM (phosphate)	IV	IA/IL
Onset	1 hr	Rapid	Rapid	Slow
Peak	2 hr	1 hr	Unknown	Unknown
Duration	1½ days	Unknown	Unknown	Up to 1 mo

Interactions

Drug/drug:

Individual drugs
Alcohol: ↑ GI effects
Amphotericin B: ↑ hypokalemia
Aspirin: ↑ GI effects
Insulin: ↑ need for insulin
Mezlocillin: ↑ hypokalemia
Phenytoin: ↓ action, ↑ metabolism
Piperacillin: ↑ hypokalemia
Rifampin: ↓ action, ↑ metabolism
Ticarcillin: ↑ hypokalemia
Drug classifications
Barbiturates: ↓ action, ↑ metabolism
Diuretics: ↑ hypokalemia
Hypoglycemia agents: ↑ need for hypoglycemic agents

Lab test interferences

Increase: Cholesterol, sodium, blood glucose, uric acid, calcium, urine glucose
Decrease: Calcium, potassium, T_4, T_3, thyroid ^{131}I uptake test, urine 17-OHCS, 17-KS, PBI
False negative: Skin allergy tests

NURSING CONSIDERATIONS

Assessment

- Monitor potassium, blood sugar, urine glucose while patient is on long-term therapy; hypokalemia and hyperglycemia may occur
- Monitor weight daily; notify prescriber of weekly gain >5 lb; monitor I&O ratio; be alert for decreasing urinary output and increasing edema
- Monitor B/P q4h, pulse; notify prescriber if chest pain occurs
- Monitor plasma cortisol levels during long-term therapy (normal level; 138-635 nmol/L SI units when drawn at 8 AM)
- Assess adrenal function periodically for HPA axis suppression
- Assess infection: increased temp, WBC even after withdrawal of medication; drug masks infection symptoms
- Assess for potassium depletion: paresthesias, fatigue, nausea, vomiting, depression, polyuria, dysrhythmias, weakness, edema, hypertension, cardiac symptoms
- Assess mental status: affect, mood, behavioral changes, aggression
- Monitor temp; if fever develops, drug should be discontinued
- Assess for systemic absorption: increased temp, inflammation, irritation (top)

Associated nursing diagnoses

✓ Infection, risk for (adverse reactions)
✓ Knowledge deficit (teaching)
✓ Noncompliance (teaching)

Implementation

IV IV route

- Give by direct **IV** only so-

P

dium phosphate product; give over >1 min; may be given by IV inf in D_5W, 0.9% NaCl
- Give after shaking susp (parenteral)
- Give titrated dose; use lowest effective dosage

Y-site compatibilities:
Potassium chloride, vitamin B with C

Additive compatibilities:
Ascorbic acid, cephalothin, cytarabine, erythromycin lactobionate, fluorouracil, heparin, methicillin, penicillin G potassium, penicillin G sodium, vitamin B with C

Additive incompatibilities:
Calcium, gluceptate, methotrexate, polymyxin B sulfate

IM route
- Give IM inj deep in large mass; rotate sites; avoid deltoid; use 21 G needle
- Give in one dose in AM to prevent adrenal suppression; avoid SC administration; may damage tissue

PO route
- Give with food or milk to decrease GI symptoms

Patient/family education
- Advise patient that ID as steroid user should be carried
- Advise patient to notify prescriber if therapeutic response decreases; dosage adjustment may be needed
- Caution patient not to discontinue abruptly; adrenal crisis can result
- Caution patient to avoid OTC products: salicylates, alcohol in cough products, cold preparations unless directed by prescriber
- Teach patient all aspects of drug usage including cushingoid symptoms
- Teach patient symptoms of adrenal insufficiency: nausea, anorexia, fatigue, dizziness, dyspnea, weakness, joint pain
- Advise patient that long-term therapy may be needed to clear infection (1-2 mo depending on type of infection)

Evaluation
Positive therapeutic outcome
- Decreased inflammation

prednisone 🔑
(pred′ni-sone)
Apo-Prednisone ✤, Deltasone, Liquid Pred, Meticorten, Orasone, Panasol-S, Prednicen-M, Prednisone, Sterapred, Winpred

Func. class.: Corticosteroid

Chem. class.: Intermediate-acting glucocorticoid

Pregnancy category C

Action: Decreases inflammation by suppressing migration of polymorphonuclear leukocytes, fibroblasts; reversal to increase capillary permeability and lysosomal stabilization

➡ **Therapeutic Outcome:** Decreased inflammation, decreased adrenal insufficiency

Uses: Severe inflammation, immunosuppression, neoplasms, multiple sclerosis, collagen disorders, dermatologic disorders

Dosage and routes

Adult: PO 1.5-2.5 mg bid-qid, then qd or qod; maintenance up to 250 mg/day

Nephrosis

P *Child 18 mo-4 yr:* 7.5-10 mg qid initially

P *Child 4-10 yr:* 15 mg qid initially

P *Child >10 yr:* 20 mg qid initially

Multiple sclerosis

Adult: PO 200 mg/day × 1 wk, then 80 mg qod × 1 mo

Available forms: Tab 1, 2.5, 5, 10, 20, 25, 50 mg; oral sol 5 mg/5 ml; syr 5 mg/5 ml

Side effects/adverse reactions

CNS: Depression, flushing, sweating, headache, mood changes

CV: Hypertension, ***circulatory collapse, thrombophlebitis, embolism,*** tachycardia

EENT: Fungal infections, increased intraocular pressure, blurred vision

GI: Diarrhea, nausea, abdominal distention, ***GI hemorrhage,*** increased appetite, ***pancreatitis***

HEMA: ***Thrombocytopenia***

INTEG: Acne, poor wound healing, ecchymosis, petechiae

MS: Fractures, osteoporosis, weakness

Contraindications: Psychosis, hypersensitivity, idiopathic thrombocytopenia, acute glomerulonephritis, amebiasis, fungal infections, nonasthmatic bronchial disease, P child <2 yr, AIDS, TB

Precautions: Pregnancy **C**, diabetes mellitus, glaucoma, osteoporosis, seizure disorders, ulcerative colitis, CHF, myasthenia gravis, renal disease, esophagitis, peptic ulcer

Pharmacokinetics

Absorption	Well absorbed (PO)
Distribution	Widely distributed; crosses placenta
Metabolism	Liver, extensively
Excretion	Kidney, breast milk
Half-life	3-4 hr

Pharmacodynamics

Onset	Unknown
Peak	1-2 hr
Duration	1½ days

P

Interactions

Drug/drug:

Individual drugs

Alcohol: ↑ GI effects

Amphoterican B: ↑ hypokalemia

Aspirin: ↑ GI effects

Insulin: ↑ need for insulin

Mezlocillin: ↑ hypokalemia

Ticarcillin: ↑ hypokalemia

Drug classifications

Diuretics: ↑ hypokalemia

Hypoglycemic agents: ↑ need for hypoglycemic agents

Lab test interferences

Increase: Cholesterol, sodium, blood glucose, uric acid, calcium, urine glucose
Decrease: Calcium, potassium, T_4, T_3, thyroid ^{131}I uptake test, urine 17-OHCS, 17-KS, PBI
False negative: Skin allergy tests

NURSING CONSIDERATIONS

Assessment

- Monitor potassium, blood sugar, urine glucose while on long-term therapy; hypokalemia and hyperglycemia may occur
- Monitor weight daily; notify prescriber of weekly gain >5 lb; monitor I&O ratio; be alert for decreasing urinary output and increasing edema
- Monitor B/P q4h, pulse; notify prescriber if chest pain occurs
- Monitor plasma cortisol levels during long-term therapy (normal level 138-635 nmol/L when drawn at 8 AM)
- Assess adrenal function periodically for HPA axis suppression
- Assess infection: increased temp, WBC even after withdrawal of medication; drug masks infection symptoms
- Assess for potassium depletion: paresthesias, fatigue, nausea, vomiting, depression, polyuria, dysrhythmias, weakness, edema, hypertension, cardiac symptoms
- Assess mental status: affect, mood, behavioral changes, aggression
- Monitor temp; if fever develops, drug should be discontinued
- Assess for systemic absorption: increased temp, inflammation, irritation (top)

Associated nursing diagnoses

✓ Infection, risk for (adverse reactions)
✓ Knowledge deficit (teaching)
✓ Noncompliance (teaching)

Implementation

PO route

- Give with food or milk to decrease GI symptoms; use measuring device for liq route

Patient/family education

- Advise patient that ID as steroid user should be carried
- Advise patient to notify prescriber if therapeutic response decreases; dosage adjustment may be needed
- Caution patient not to discontinue abruptly; adrenal crisis can result
- Caution patient to avoid OTC products: salicylates, alcohol in cough products, cold preparations unless directed by prescriber
- Teach patient all aspects of drug usage including cushingoid symptoms
- Teach patient symptoms of adrenal insufficiency: nausea, anorexia, fatigue, dizziness, dyspnea, weakness, joint pain
- Advise patient that long-term therapy may be needed to clear infection (1-2 mo depending on type of infection)

Evaluation

Positive therapeutic outcome

- Decreased inflammation

primidone

(pri′mi-done)

Apo-Primidone ✦, Myidone, Mysoline, primidone, Sertan ✦

Func. class.: Anticonvulsant

Chem. class.: Barbiturate derivative

Pregnancy category D

Action: Raises seizure threshold by conversion of drug to phenobarbital; decreases neuron firing

➔ **Therapeutic Outcome:** Reduction in seizure activity

Uses: Generalized tonic-clonic (grand mal), complex-partial, psychomotor seizures

Dosage and routes

P *Adult and child >8 yr:* PO 250 mg/day; may increase by 250 mg/wk, not to exceed 2 g/day in divided doses qid

P *Child <8 yr:* PO 125 mg/day; may increase by 125 mg/wk, not to exceed 1 g/day in divided doses qid

Available forms: Tab 50, 250 mg; susp 250 mg/5 ml; chew tab 125 mg*

Side effects/adverse reactions

CNS: Stimulation, drowsiness, dizziness, confusion, sedation, headache, flushing, hallucinations, coma, psychosis, ataxia, *vertigo*

EENT: Diplopia, nystagmus, edema of eyelids

GI: Nausea, vomiting, anorexia, hepatitis

GU: Impotence, polyuria

HEMA: Thrombocytopenia, leukopenia, neutropenia, eosinophilia, megaloblastic anemia, decreased serum folate level, lymphadenopathy

INTEG: Rash, edema, alopecia, lupuslike syndrome

Contraindications: Hypersensitivity, porphyria, pregnancy **D**

Precautions: COPD, hepatic disease, renal disease, hyperactive children P

Pharmacokinetics	
Absorption	60%-80%
Distribution	Widely distributed; crosses placenta
Metabolism	Liver, converted to phenobarbital + PEMA
Excretion	Kidneys, breast milk
Half-life	3-24 hr

Pharmacodynamics	
Onset	Unknown
Peak	4 hr
Duration	Unknown

Interactions

Drug/drug:

Individual drugs

Acebutolol: ↓ effectiveness
Alcohol: ↑ CNS depression
Chloramphenicol: ↓ effectiveness
Doxycycline: ↑ half-life
Griseofulvin: ↓ effectiveness
Metoprolol: ↓ effectiveness
Phenobarbital: ↑ toxicity

Propranolol: ↓ effectiveness
Quinidine: ↓ effectiveness
Timolol: ↓ effectiveness

Drug classifications

Antidepressants, tricyclic: ↑ CNS depression
Antihistamines: ↑ CNS depression
Glucocorticoids: ↓ effectiveness
Narcotics: ↑ CNS depression
Oral contraceptives: ↓ effectiveness
Phenothiazines: ↓ CNS depression
Sedative/hypnotics: ↑ CNS depression

Lab test interferences

False increase: Sulfobromophthalein

NURSING CONSIDERATIONS

Assessment

- Assess mental status: mood, sensorium, affect, memory G (long, short), especially elderly
- Assess for blood dyscrasias: fever, sore throat, bruising, rash, jaundice, epistaxis (long-term treatment only)
- Assess seizure activity including type, location, duration, and character; provide seizure precaution
- Assess renal studies: urinalysis, BUN, urine creatinine
- Monitor blood studies: RBC, Hct, Hgb, reticulocyte counts weekly for 4 wk then monthly
- Monitor hepatic studies: ALT (SGPT), AST (SGOT), bilirubin, creatinine
- Monitor drug levels during initial treatment
- Assess for signs of physical withdrawal if medication suddenly discontinued
- Assess eye problems: need for ophthalmic examinations before, during, after treatment (slit lamp, fundoscopy, tonometry)
- Assess allergic reaction: red raised rash; if this occurs, drug should be discontinued
- Monitor for toxicity: bone marrow depression, nausea, vomiting, ataxia, diplopia, cardiovascular collapse

Associated nursing diagnoses

✓ Injury, risk for (side effects)
✓ Knowledge deficit (teaching)

Implementation

PO route

- May give with food to decrease gastric irritation
- May crush tab and mix with food or fluid

Patient/family education

- Teach patient to carry ID card or Medic Alert bracelet stating name, drugs taken, condition, prescriber's name, phone number
- Advise patient to avoid driving and other activities that require alertness
- Caution patient to avoid alcohol and CNS depressants; increased sedation may occur
- Teach patient not to discontinue medication quickly after long-term use; taper off over several wk

Evaluation

Positive therapeutic outcome

- Decreased seizure activity

probenecid

(proe-ben'e-sid)

Benemid, Benuryl ✦, Probalan, probenecid

Func. class.: Uricosuric; antigout

Chem. class.: Sulfonamide derivative

Pregnancy category **B**

Action: Inhibits tubular reabsorption of urates, with increased excretion of uric acids

➔ **Therapeutic Outcome:** Decreased uric acid levels

Uses: Hyperuricemia in gout, gouty arthritis; adjunct to cephalosporin or penicillin treatment (gonorrhea)

Dosage and routes

Gonorrhea

Adult: PO 1 g with 3.5 g ampicillin or 1 g 30 min before 4.8 million U of aqueous penicillin G procaine injected into 2 sites IM

Gout/gouty arthritis

Adult: PO 250 mg bid for 1 wk, then 500 mg bid, not to exceed 2 g/day; maintenance 500 mg/day × 6 mo

Adjunct in penicillin/cephalosporin treatment

P ***Adult and child >50 kg:*** PO 500 mg qid

P ***Child <50 kg:*** PO 25 mg/kg, then 40 mg/kg in divided doses qid

Available forms: Tab 0.5 g

Side effects/adverse reactions

CNS: Drowsiness, headache

CV: Bradycardia

GU: Glycosuria, thirst, frequency, ***nephrotic syndrome***

GI: Gastric irritation, nausea, vomiting, anorexia, ***hepatic necrosis***

INTEG: Rash, dermatitis, pruritus, fever

META: Acidosis, hypokalemia, hyperchloremia, hyperglycemia

RESP: ***Apnea,*** irregular respirations

Contraindications: Hypersensitivity, severe hepatic disease, blood dyscrasias, severe renal disease, CrCl <50 mg/min, history of uric acid calculus

Precautions: Pregnancy **B**, severe respiratory disease, P lactation, cardiac edema, child <2 yr

Pharmacokinetics

Absorption	Well absorbed (PO)
Distribution	Crosses placenta
Metabolism	Liver
Excretion	Kidneys
Half-life	8-17 hr

Pharmacodynamics

Onset	½ hr
Peak	2-4 hr
Duration	8 hr

Interactions

Drug/drug:

Individual drugs

Aspirin: ↑ uricosuric effect
Acyclovir: ↑ toxicity
Methotrexate: ↑ toxicity
Nitrofurantoin: ↑ toxicity

Clofibrate: ↑ effect
Dapsone: ↑ effect
Heparin: ↑ effect
Penicillamine: ↑ effect
Zidovudine: ↑ effect

Drug classifications
Barbiturates: ↑ effect
Benzodiazepher: ↑ effect
Cephalosporins: ↑ levels
Fluoroquinolones: ↑ levels
NSAIDs: ↑ toxicity
Penicillins: ↑ levels

Lab test interferences

Increase: Alkaline phosphatase, AST (SGOT), ALT (SGPT)
False positive: RBC, Hgb

NURSING CONSIDERATIONS

Assessment

- Monitor I&O ratio; observe for decrease in urinary output; increase fluids to 2-3 L/day; urine may be alkalized with sodium bicarbonate acetazolamide
- Assess mobility, joint pain, and swelling in the joints
- Monitor CBC, urine pH, uric acid and BUN, creatinine before and periodically during treatment

Associated nursing diagnoses

✓ Pain, chronic (uses)
✓ Mobility, impaired (uses)
✓ Knowledge deficit (teaching)

Implementation

PO route
- Give with food or antacid to decrease GI upset
- Reduce dosage gradually if uric acid levels are normal after 6 mo

Patient/family education

- Advise patient to increase fluids to 2-3 L/day
- Caution patient to avoid salicylates; probenecid levels will be decreased
- Advise patient to report any pain, redness, or hard area, usually in legs
- Instruct patient in importance of complying with medical regimen including weight loss program, diet restrictions, and alcohol intake

Evaluation

Positive therapeutic outcome
- Decreased pain in joints
- Normal serum uric acid levels
- Increased duration of antiinfectives

probucol

(proe′byoo-kole)
Lorelco
Func. class.: Antilipemic
Chem. class.:
Pregnancy category **B**

Action: Inhibits biosynthesis of VLDL, LDL, which are responsible for cholesterol development

➔ **Therapeutic Outcome:** Decreasing cholesterol and LDL levels, decreased pruritus

Uses: Severe hypercholesterolemia when other treatment is unsuccessful

Dosage and routes

Adult: PO 500 mg bid with breakfast, supper

Available forms: Tab 250, 500 mg

Side effects/adverse reactions

CNS: *Insomnia,* dizziness, palpitations, paresthesias, syncope
CV: Palpitations, dysrhythmias, ***MI,*** prolonged QT interval
EENT: Visual disturbances, ptosis, tinnitus
GI: *Nausea, vomiting, diarrhea,* flatulence, anorexia

Contraindication: Hypersensitivity

Precautions: Dysrhythmias, pregnancy **B,** lactation, P children

Pharmacokinetics

Absorption	Limited
Distribution	Fatty tissue
Metabolism	Unknown
Excretion	Feces
Half-life	3 wk

Pharmacodynamics

Onset	Unknown
Peak	Unknown
Duration	Unknown

Interactions

Drug/drug:

Individual drugs
Clofibrate: ↑ HDLs
Drug classification
Anticoagulants, oral: ↓ absorption
Anticholinergics: ↑ cardiovascular effects
Antidepressants, tricyclic: ↑ cardiovascular effects
β-**Blockers:** ↑ cardiovascular effects
Cardiac glycosides: ↓ absorption
Diuretics, thiazide: ↓ absorption
Phenothiazines: ↑ cardiovascular effects

Drug/food:

↑ absorption

Lab test interferences

Increase: Liver function studies, cloride, phosphate

NURSING CONSIDERATIONS

Assessment

- Assess nutrition: fat, protein, carbohydrates; nutritional analysis should be completed by dietician before treatment
- Monitor bowel pattern daily; diarrhea may be a problem
- Monitor triglycerides, cholesterol at baseline and throughout treatment; LDL and VLDL should be watched closely; if increased, drug should be discontinued

Associated nursing diagnoses

- ✓ Diarrhea (adverse reactions)
- ✓ Knowledge deficit (teaching)
- ✓ Noncompliance (teaching)

Implementation

PO route

- Give drug with meals; increased absorption will result

Patient/family education

- Inform patient that compli-

P

ance is needed for positive results to occur; not to double doses

- Tell patient that risk factors should be decreased: high-fat diet, smoking, alcohol consumption, absence of exercise
- Advise patient to notify prescriber if the GI symptoms of diarrhea, abdominal or epigastric pain, nausea, vomiting occur; or if chills, fever, sore throat occur

Evaluation

Positive therapeutic outcome

- Decreased cholesterol and serum triglyceride levels and improved ratio with HDL

procainamide

(proe'kane-ah-mide)

Procan SR, Promine, procainamide, Pronestyl, Pronestyl-SR

Func. class.: Antidysrhythmic (Class IA)

Chem. class.: Procaine HCl amide analog

Pregnancy category **C**

Action: Prolongs action potential duration and effective refractory period; reduces disparity in refractory between normal and infarcted myocardium; prevents increased myocardial excitability and conduction contractility

Therapeutic Outcome: Prevention of dysrhythmias

Uses: PVCs, atrial fibrillation, PAT, ventricular tachycardia, atrial dysrhythmias, ventricular tachycardia

Dosage and routes

Atrial fibrillation/PAT

Adult: PO 1-1.25 g; may give another 750 mg if needed; if no response, 500 mg-1g q2h until desired response; maintenance 50 mg/kg in divided doses q6h

Ventricular tachycardia

Adult: PO 1 g; maintenance 50 mg/kg/day given in 3-hr intervals; sus rel tab 500 mg-1.25 g q6h

Other dysrhythmias

Adult: **IV** bol 100 mg q5 min, given 25-50 mg/min, not to exceed 500 mg; or 17 mg/kg total, then **IV** inf 2-6 mg/min

Available forms: Cap 250, 375, 500 mg; tab 250, 375, 500 mg; sus rel tab 250, 500, 750, 1000 mg; inj IV 100, 500 mg/ml

Side effects/adverse reactions

CNS: Headache, dizziness, confusion, psychosis, restlessness, irritability, weakness
*CV: Hypotension, **heart block, cardiovascular collapse, arrest***
GI: Nausea, vomiting, anorexia, diarrhea, hepatomegaly
HEMA: SLE syndrome, ***agranulocytosis, thrombocytopenia, neutropenia, hemolytic anemia***
INTEG: Rash, urticaria, edema, swelling (rare), pruritus

Contraindications: Hypersensitivity, myasthenia gravis, severe heart block

Precautions: Pregnancy **C**, lactation, children, renal disease, liver disease, CHF, respiratory depression

Pharmacokinetics

Absorption	Well absorbed (PO, IM)
Distribution	Rapidly distributed
Metabolism	Liver
Excretion	Kidneys, unchanged (50%-70%)
Half-life	2½-4½ hr; increased in renal disease

Pharmacodynamics

	PO	PO–ext rel	IV	IM
Onset	½ hr	Unknown	Rapid	½-1 hr
Peak	1-1½ hr	Unknown	½-1 hr	½-1 hr
Duration	3 hr	Up to 8 hr	3-4 hr	3 hr

Interactions

Drug/drug:

Individual drugs

Atropine: ↑ anticholinergic effect
Digoxin: ↑ blood levels, toxicity
Disopyramide: ↑ levels, toxicity
Flecainide: ↑ levels, toxicity
Lidocaine: Bradycardia, arrest
Haloperidol: ↑ anticholinergic effect
Mexiletine: ↑ levels, toxicity
Phenytoin: ↑ blood levels
Quinidine: ↑ levels, toxicity
Warfarin: ↑ level, bleeding

Drug classifications

β-Blockers: ↑ dysrhythmias, arrest
Calcium channel blockers: ↑ dysrhythmias, arrest
Phenothiazines: ↑ anticholinergic effect

Lab test interferences

Increase: CPK

NURSING CONSIDERATIONS

Assessment

- Assess for oxygenation or perfusion deficit: decreased B/P, chest pain, dizziness, loss of consciousness
- Assess respiratory status: auscultate lung fields for bibasilar crackles in patients with advanced CHF
- Monitor I&O ratio; electrolytes: potassium, sodium, chloride; watch for decreasing urinary output, possible retention
- Monitor liver function studies: AST (SGOT), ALT (SGPT), bilirubin, alkaline phosphatase
- Monitor ECG continuously to determine drug effectiveness; measure PR, QRS, QT intervals; check for PVCs, other dysrhythmias; check B/P continuously for hypotension, hypertension; for rebound hypertension after 1-2 hr; prolonged PR/QT intervals, QRS complex; if QT or QRS increases by 50% or more, withhold next dose, notify prescriber
- Monitor for dehydration or hypovolemia
- Monitor for CNS symptoms: confusion, psychosis, numbness, depression, involuntary movements; if these occur, drug should be discontinued
- Monitor blood levels (therapeutic level 3-10 μg/ml), ANA

titer; notify prescriber of abnormal results
• Assess cardiac rate, respiration: rate, rhythm, character, chest pain, ventricular tachycardia, supraventricular tachycardia or fibrillation

Associated nursing diagnoses

- ✓ Cardiac output, decreased (uses)
- ✓ Impaired gas exchange (adverse reactions)
- ✓ Knowledge deficit (teaching)

Implementation

PO route
• Give on an empty stomach with a full glass of water
• May be given with meals if GI irritation occurs; absorption will be decreased
• Tab may be crushed and mixed with fluid or foods for patients with swallowing difficulties; do not break, chew, or crush sus-rel tab

IM route
• Give deep in large muscle mass

IV **IV route**
• Give by direct **IV** after diluting 100 mg/10 ml of D_5W or sterile water for inj; give 50 mg/min or less
• Give by intermittent inf after diluting to a conc of 2-4 mg/ml 200 mg up to 1 g/50-500 ml D_5W; give over 30 min (2-6 mg/min maintenance); use inf pump for correct dosage
• Do not use dark sol or if precipitate is present

Solution compatibilities:
D_5W, D_5/0.9% NaCl, 0.45% NaCl, 0.9% NaCl, water for inj

Y-site compatibilities:
Amiodarone, famotidine, heparin, hydrocortisone sodium succinate, potassium chloride, ranitidine, vitamin B with C

Y-site incompatibility:
Milrinone

Additive compatibilities:
Amiodarone, dobutamine, lidocaine, netilmicin, verapamil

Additive incompatibilities:
Esmolol, ethacrynate, milrinone

Patient/family education

• Advise patient to report side effects immediately to prescriber; to take exactly as prescribed; if dose is missed take when remembered if within 3-4 hr of next dose, do not double doses
• Caution patient that dark glasses may be needed for photophobia; to use sunscreen or stay out of sun to prevent burns; avoid temp extremes; impairment of heat-regulating mechanism can occur
• Advise patient to complete follow-up appointment with prescriber including pulmonary function studies, chest-x-ray
• Instruct patient that dry mouth may be relieved by frequent sips of water, hard candy, sugarless gum
• Caution patient to make position changes from lying to standing slowly to prevent orthostatic hypotension

Evaluation

Positive therapeutic outcome
• Decreased PVCs, ventricular tachycardia

Treatment of overdose:
O_2, artificial ventilation, ECG, administer dopamine for circulatory depression, administer diazepam or thiopental for convulsions, isoproterenol

procarbazine
(proe-kar'ba-zeen)
Matulane, Natulan ✦
Func. class.: Antineoplastic, alkylating agent
Chem. class.: Hydrazine derivative
Pregnancy category **D**

Action: Inhibits DNA, RNA, protein synthesis, cell cycle S phase specific; has multiple sites of action; a nonvesicant

➔ **Therapeutic Outcome:** Prevention of rapidly growing malignant cells

Uses: Lymphoma, Hodgkin's disease, cancers resistant to other therapy

Investigational uses: Brain, lung malignancies, other lymphomas, multiple myeloma, malignant melanoma, polycythemia vera

Dosage and routes
Adult: PO 2-4 mg/kg/day for first wk; maintain dosage of 4-6 mg/kg/day until platelets and WBC fall; after recovery, 1-2 mg/kg/day

P *Child:* PO 50 mg/day for 7 days, then 100 mg/m^2 until desired response, leukopenia, or thrombocytopenia occurs; 50 mg/day is maintenance after bone marrow recovery

Available forms: Cap 50 mg

Side effects/adverse reactions
CNS: Headache, dizziness, insomnia, hallucinations, confusion, coma, pain, chills, fever, sweating, paresthesias
EENT: Retinal hemorrhage, nystagmus, photophobia, diplopia
GI: *Nausea, vomiting,* anorexia, diarrhea, constipation, dry mouth, stomatitis
GU: Azoospermia, cessation of menses
HEMA: ***Thrombocytopenia, anemia, leukopenia, myelosuppression, bleeding tendencies,*** purpura, petechiae, epistaxis
INTEG: *Rash,* pruritus, dermatitis, alopecia, herpes, hyperpigmentation
MS: Arthralgias, myalgias
RESP: Cough, pneumonitis

Contraindications: Hypersensitivity, thrombocytopenia, bone marrow depression, pregnancy **D**

Precautions: Renal disease, hepatic disease, radiation therapy

P

Pharmacokinetics

Absorption	Well absorbed (PO)
Distribution	Widely distributed; crosses blood-brain barrier
Metabolism	Liver
Excretion	Kidneys
Half-life	1 hr

Pharmacodynamics

Onset	Unknown
Peak	Unknown
Duration	Unknown

Interactions

Drug/drug:

Individual drugs

Alcohol: ↑ CNS depressant, disulfiram reaction
Guanedrel: ↑ hypertensive crisis
Guanethidine: ↑ hypertensive crisis
Levodopa: ↑ hypertensive crisis
Meperidine: Avoid use; paradoxic reactions
Radiation: ↑ toxicity, bone marrow suppression
Reserpine: ↑ hypertensive crisis

Drug classifications

Antidepressants: ↑ hypertensive crisis
Antihistamines: ↑ CNS depression
Antineoplastics: ↑ toxicity bone marrow suppression
CNS depressants: ↑ CNS depression
Local anesthetics: ↑ hypertensive crisis
MAOI: ↑ seizures, temperature
Narcotic analgesics: ↑ CNS depression
Sedative/hypnotics: ↑ CNS depression
Sympathomimetic amines: ↑ hypertensive crisis
Vasoconstrictors: ↑ hypertensive crisis

NURSING CONSIDERATIONS

Assessment

- Monitor CBC, differential, platelet count weekly; withhold drug if WBC is <4000 or platelet count is <75,000; notify prescriber of results if WBC <20,000/mm^3, platelets <150,000/mm^3
- Monitor pulmonary function tests, chest x-ray films before, during therapy; chest film should be obtained q2 wk during treatment; check for dyspnea, rales, unproductive cough, chest pain, tachypnea
- Monitor renal function studies: BUN, serum uric acid, urine CrCl before, during therapy; I&O ratio; report fall in urine output of 30 ml/hr; for decreased hyperuricemia
- Monitor for cold, fever, sore throat (may indicate beginning infection); identify edema in feet, joint and stomach pain, shaking; prescriber should be notified
- Assess for bleeding: hematuria, guaiac, bruising or petechiae, mucosa or orifices q8h, no rectal temp

Associated nursing diagnoses

✓ Injury, risk for (adverse reactions)
✓ Body image disturbance (adverse reactions)

☑ Infection, risk for (adverse reactions)
☑ Knowledge deficit (teaching)

Implementation

PO route

• Give with foods, fluids for GI upset; open cap and give with food/fluids for swallowing difficulty; administer as directed

Patient/family education

• Teach patient to avoid use of products containing aspirin or ibuprofen, razors, commercial mouthwash, since bleeding may occur; to report symptoms of bleeding (hematuria, tarry stools)
• Caution patient to report signs of anemia (fatigue, headache, irritability, faintness, shortness of breath)
• Advise patient to report any changes in breathing or coughing even several mo after treatment; to avoid crowds and persons with respiratory tract or other infections
• Inform patient hair loss is common; discuss the use of wigs or hair pieces
• Caution patient not to have any vaccinations without the advice of the prescriber; serious reactions can occur
• Advise patient contraception is needed during treatment and for several mo after the completion of therapy

Evaluation

Positive therapeutic outcome

• Absence of swelling at night
• Increased appetite, increased weight

prochlorperazine

(proe-klor-pair'a-zeen)

Chlorpazine, Compa-Z, Compazine, Contranzine, Provazin ✱, Stemetil ✱, Ultrazine

Func. class.: Antiemetic/antipsychotic

Chem. class.: Phenothiazine, piperazine derivative

Pregnancy category **C**

Action: Depresses cerebral cortex, hypothalamus, limbic system, which control activity aggression; blocks neurotransmission produced by dopamine at synapse; exhibits a strong α-adrenergic, anticholinergic blocking action; mechanism for antipsychotic effects is unclear; acts centrally by blocking chemoreceptor trigger zone, which in turn acts on vomiting center

➔ **Therapeutic Outcome:** Decreased nausea, vomiting, decreased signs and symptoms of psychosis

Uses: Nausea, vomiting, psychosis

Dosage and routes

Postoperative nausea/vomiting

Adult: IM 5-10 mg 1-2 hr before anesthesia; may repeat in 30 min; **IV** 5-10 mg 15-30 min before anesthesia; **IV** inf 20 mg/L D_5W or NS 15-30 min before anesthesia, not to exceed 40 mg/day

P

Severe nausea/vomiting

Adult: PO 5-10 mg tid-qid; sus rel 15 mg qd in AM or 10 mg q12h; rec 25 mg/bid; IM 5-10 mg; may repeat q4h, not to exceed 40 mg/day

P ***Child 18-39 kg:*** PO 2.5 mg tid or 5 mg bid; do not exceed 15 mg/day; IM 0.132 mg/kg

P ***Child 14-17 kg:*** PO/rec 2.5 mg bid-tid, not to exceed 10 mg/day; IM 0.132 mg/kg

P ***Child 9-13 kg:*** PO/rec 2.5 mg qd-bid, not to exceed 7.5 mg/day; IM 0.132 mg/kg

Available forms: Syr 5 mg/ml; inj 5 mg/ml; tab 5, 10, 25 mg; sus rel cap 10, 15, 30 mg; supp 2.5, 5, 25 mg

Side effects/adverse reactions

CNS: Euphoria, depression, EPS, restlessness, tremor, dizziness, ***neuroleptic malignant syndrome***

CV: Circulatory failure, tachycardia

GI: Nausea, vomiting, anorexia, dry mouth, diarrhea, constipation, weight loss, metallic taste, cramps, hepatitis

RESP: Respiratory depression

Contraindications: Hypersensitivity to phenothiazines, coma, seizure, encephalopathy, bone marrow depression

P G **Precautions:** Children <2 yr, pregnancy **C**, elderly

Pharmacokinetics

Absorption	Variably absorbed (PO); well absorbed (IM)
Distribution	Widely distributed; high concentration in CNS; crosses placenta
Metabolism	Liver, extensively; GI mucosa
Excretion	Kidneys, breast milk
Half-life	Unknown

Pharmacodynamics

	PO	PO–EXT REL	REC	IM	IV
Onset	½ hr	½ hr	1 hr	10-20 min	4-5 min
Peak	Unkn	Unkn	Unkn	Unkn	Unkn
Duration	3-4 hr	10-12 hr	3-4 hr	3-4 hr	3-4 hr

Interactions

Drug/drug:

Individual drugs

Alcohol: ↑ effects of both drugs, oversedation
Aluminum hydroxide: ↓ absorption
Bromocriptine: ↓ antiparkinsonian activity
Disopyramide: ↑ anticholinergic effects
Epinephrine: ↑ toxicity
Guanethidine: ↓ antihypertensive response
Levodopa: ↓ antiparkinsonian activity
Lithium: ↓ prochlorperizine levels, ↑ extrapyramidal symptoms, masking of lithium toxicity
Magnesium hydroxide: ↓ absorption
Norepinephrine: ↓ vasoresponse, ↑ toxicity
Phenobarbital: ↓ effectiveness, ↑ metabolism

Drug classifications

Antacids: ↓ absorption
Anticholinergics: ↑ anticholinergic effects
Antidepressants: ↑ CNS depression
Antidiarrheals, adsorbent: ↓ absorption
Antihistamines: ↑ CNS depression
Antihypertensives: ↑ hypotension
Antithyroid agents: ↑ agranulocytosis
Barbiturate anesthetics: ↑ CNS depression
β-Adrenergics: ↑ effects of both drugs
General anesthetics: ↑ CNS depression
MAOI: ↑ CNS depression
Narcotics: ↑ CNS depression
Sedative/hypnotics: ↑ CNS depression

Lab test interferences

Increase: Liver function tests, cardiac enzymes, cholesterol, blood glucose, prolactin, bilirubin, PBI, cholinesterase, ^{131}I, alkaline phosphatase, leukocytes, granulocytes, platelets
Decrease: Hormones (blood and urine)
False positive: Pregnancy tests, PKU, urine bilirubin
False negative: Urinary steroids, 17-OHCS, pregnancy tests

NURSING CONSIDERATIONS

Assessment

- Assess mental status: orientation, mood, behavior, presence and type of hallucinations before initial administration and monthly; this drug should significantly reduce psychotic behavior
- Check for swallowing of PO medication; check for hoarding or giving of medication to other patients
- Monitor I&O ratio; palpate bladder if low urinary output G occurs, especially in elderly; urinalysis recommended before, during prolonged therapy
- Monitor bilirubin, CBC, liver function studies monthly
- Assess affect, orientation, LOC, reflexes, gait, coordination, sleep pattern disturbances
- Monitor B/P with patient sitting, standing, and lying; take pulse and respirations q4h during initial treatment; establish baseline before starting treatment; report drops of 30 mm Hg; obtain baseline ECG, Q wave and T wave changes
- Check for dizziness, faintness, palpitations, tachycardia on rising; severe orthostatic hypotension is common
- Identify neuroleptic malignant syndrome: hyperpyrexia, muscle rigidity, increased CPK, altered mental status; drug should be discontinued
- Assess for EPS including akathisia (inability to sit still, no pattern to movements), tardive dyskinesia (bizarre movements of the jaw, mouth, tongue, extremities), pseudoparkinsonism (ragged tremors, pill rolling, shuffling gate); an antiparkinsonism drug should be prescribed
- Assess for constipation, urinary retention daily; if these occur, increase bulk, water in diet

P

Associated nursing diagnoses

- ✓ Thought processes, altered (uses)
- ✓ Coping, ineffective individual (uses)
- ✓ Knowledge deficit (teaching)
- ✓ Noncompliance (teaching)

Implementation

PO route

- Give drug in liq form mixed in glass of juice or cola if hoarding is suspected; do not mix in caffeine drinks, tannics, pectins
- Give decreased dosage in G elderly since metabolism is slowed
- Give PO with full glass of water, milk; or give with food to decrease GI upset
- Store in airtight, light-resistant container; oral sol in amber bottle
- Do not crush or chew sus rel cap

IM route

- Inject slowly in deep muscle mass; do not give SC; aspirate to avoid **IV** administration; do not administer sol with a precipitate; have patient lie down afterward for at least 30 min

IV **IV route**

- Give by direct **IV** after diluting **IV** using 0.9% NaCl to 1 mg/1 ml; administer at 1 mg/min or less
- Administer by intermittent inf after diluting 20 mg/L or less LR, Ringer's, dextrose, saline, or any combination

Syringe incompatibilities:

Dimenhydrinate, midazolam, pentobarbital, thiopental

Syringe compatibilities:

Atropine, butorphanol, chlorpromazine, cimetidine, diamorphine, diphenhydramine, droperidol, fentanyl, glycopyrrolate, hydroxyzine, meperidine, metoclopramide, nalbuphine, pentazocine, perphenazine, prochlorperazine, promazine, promethazine, ranitidine, scopolamine

Y-site incompatibility:

Foscarnet

Y-site compatibilities:

Amsacrine, fluconazole, fludarabine, gentamicin, heparin, hydrocortisone, kanamycin, melphalan, metronidazole, mezlocillin, minocycline, moxalactam, nafcillin, ondansetron, oxacillin, paclitaxel, penicillin G potassium, piperacillin, potassium chloride, sargramostim, tetracycline, ticarcillin, ticarcilin/clavulanate, tobramycin, vancomycin, vinorelbine, vitamin B with C

Additive incompatibilities:

Aminophylline, amphotericin B, ampicillin, calcium gluceptate, cefoperazone, cephalothin, chloramphenicol, chlorothiazide, floxacillin, furosemide, hydrocortisone sodium succinate, methohexital sodium, penicillin G sodium, phenobarbital, thiopental

Additive compatibilities:

Amikacin, ascorbic acid, dexamthasone, dimenhydrinate, erthromycin, ethacrynate, lidocaine, nafcillin, netilmicin, sodium bicarbonate, vitamin B with C

Patient/family education

• Teach patient to use good oral hygiene; frequent rinsing of mouth, sugarless gum for dry mouth
• Caution patient to avoid hazardous activities until drug response is determined; dizziness, blurred vision may occur
• Inform patient that orthostatic hypotension occurs often and to rise from sitting or lying position gradually; to remain lying down after IM inj for at least 30 min; tell patient to avoid hot tubs, hot showers, tub baths, since hypotension may occur; tell patient that in hot weather heat stroke may occur; take extra precautions to stay cool
• Advise patient to avoid abrupt withdrawal of this drug, or EPS may result; drug should be withdrawn slowly
• Teach patient to avoid OTC preparations (cough, hay fever, cold) unless approved by prescriber, since serious drug interactions may occur; avoid use with alcohol, CNS depressants; increased drowsiness may occur; avoid activities requiring mental alertness
• Instruct patient to use a sunscreen and sunglasses to prevent burns
• Teach patient about EPS and necessity of meticulous oral hygiene, since oral candidiasis may occur
• Advise patient to take antacids 2 hr before or after taking this drug
• Advise patient to report sore throat, malaise, fever, bleeding, mouth sores; if these occur, CBC should be drawn and drug discontinued
• Teach patient not to double or skip doses
• Teach patient urine may turn pink to reddish brown
• Instruct patient to report dark urine, clay-colored stools, bleeding, bruising, rash, blurred vision

Evaluation

Positive therapeutic outcome
• Relief of nausea and vomiting
• Decrease in emotional excitement, hallucinations, delusions, paranoia
• Reorganization of patterns of thought, speech

Treatment of overdose:
Lavage if orally ingested; provide airway; *do not induce vomiting or use epinephrine*

progesterone
(proe-jess'ter-one)
Femotrone, Progestasert, progesterone, Progestilin ♣, Gesterol 50, Progesterone in Oil
Func. class.: Progestogen
Chem. class.: Progesterone derivative
Pregnancy category **X**

Action: Inhibits secretion of pituitary gonadotropins, which prevents follicular maturation, ovulation; stimulates growth of mammary tissue; antineoplastic action against endometrial cancer

Therapeutic Outcome: Decreased abnormal uterine

bleeding, absence of amenorrhea

Uses: Contraception, amenorrhea, premenstrual syndrome, abnormal uterine bleeding

Dosage and routes

Amenorrhea/uterine bleeding

Adult: IM 5-10 mg qd × 6-8 doses

Contraception

Adult: Insert 1 in uterine cavity; active for 1 yr

PMS

Adult: Rec supp/vag supp 200-400 mg

Available forms: Inj 25, 50, 100 mg/ml; IU system 38 mg; rec supp, vag supp

Side effects/adverse reactions

CNS: Dizziness, headache, migraines, depression, fatigue
CV: Hypotension, thrombophlebitis, edema, ***thromboembolism, stroke, pulmonary embolism, MI***
EENT: Diplopia
GI: *Nausea,* vomiting, anorexia, cramps, increased weight, ***cholestatic jaundice***
GU: Amenorrhea, cervical erosion, breakthrough bleeding, dysmenorrhea, vaginal candidiasis, breast changes, *gynecomastia, testicular atrophy, impotence,* endometriosis, ***spontaneous abortion***
INTEG: Rash, urticaria, acne, hirsutism, alopecia, oily skin, seborrhea, purpura, melasma
META: Hyperglycemia

Contraindications: Breast cancer, hypersensitivity, thromboembolic disorders, reproductive cancer, genital bleeding (abnormal, undiagnosed), cerebral hemorrhage, pregnancy **X**

Precautions: Lactation, hypertension, asthma, blood dyscrasias, gallbladder disease, CHF, diabetes mellitus, bone disease, depression, migraine headache, convulsive disorders, hepatic disease, renal disease, family history of breast or reproductive tract cancer

Pharmacokinetics

Absorption	Unknown
Distribution	Unknown
Metabolism	Unknown
Excretion	Breast milk
Half-life	Unknown

Pharmacodynamics

	IM	REC	VAG
Onset	Unknown	Unknown	Unknown
Peak	Unknown	Unknown	Unknown
Duration	24 hr	24 hr	24 hr

Interactions

Drug/drug:

Individual drugs

Bromocriptine: ↓ effectiveness of bromocriptine

Lab test interferences

Increase: Alkaline phosphatase, nitrogen (urine), pregnanediol, amino acids, factors VII, VIII, IX, X
Decrease: GTT, HDL

NURSING CONSIDERATIONS

Assessment

- Monitor B/P at beginning of treatment and periodically; check weight daily; notify prescriber of weekly weight gain >5 lb
- Monitor I&O ratio: be alert for decreasing urinary output, increasing edema, hypertension
- Assess liver function studies: ALT (SGPT), AST (SGOT), bilirubin periodically during long-term therapy
- Assess edema, hypertension, cardiac symptoms, jaundice
- Assess mental status: affect, mood, behavioral changes, depression
- Assess hypercalcemia

Associated nursing diagnoses

- ✓ Sexual dysfunction (uses)
- ✓ Tissue perfusion, altered (adverse reactions)
- ✓ Injury, risk for (adverse reactions)
- ✓ Knowledge deficit (teaching)

Implementation

IM route

- Store in dark area
- Give titrated dose; use lowest effective dosage; give oil sol deep in large muscle mass; rotate sites; use after warming to dissolve crystals

Patient/family education

- Teach patient to report breast lumps, vaginal bleeding, edema, jaundice, dark urine, clay-colored stools, dyspnea, headache, blurred vision, abdominal pain, numbness or stiffness in legs, chest pain
- Teach patient to report suspected pregnancy

Evaluation

Positive therapeutic outcome

- Decreased abnormal uterine bleeding
- Absence of amenorrhea
- Prevented pregnancy

promazine

(proe′ma-zeen)

Promanyl ✦, promazine, Prozine, Sparine

Func. class.: Antipsychotic/neuroleptic

Chem. class.: Phenothiazine, aliphatic

Pregnancy category C

Action: Depresses cerebral cortex, hypothalamus, limbic system, which control activity, aggression; blocks neurotransmission produced by dopamine at synapse; exhibits a strong α-adrenergic, anticholinergic blocking action; as antiemetic, inhibits medullary chemoreceptor trigger zone; mechanism for antipsychotic effects is unclear

➔ **Therapeutic Outcome:** Decreased signs and symptoms of psychosis, absence of nausea, vomiting

Uses: Psychotic disorders, schizophrenia, nausea, vomiting, alcohol withdrawal

Dosage and routes

Psychosis

Adult: PO 10-200 mg q4-6h;

max dose 1000 mg/day; IM 50-150 mg, followed in 30 min with additional dose up to a total dose of 300 mg

P *Child >12 yr:* PO 10-25 mg q4-6h

Nausea/vomiting

Adult: PO 25-50 mg q4-6h; IM 50 mg; **IV** not recommended, but may use in conc of <25 mg/ml

Available forms: Tab 25, 50, 100 mg; inj 25, 50 mg/ml

Side effects/adverse reactions

CNS: Extrapyramidal symptoms: pseudoparkinsonism, akathisia, dystonia, tardive dyskinesia, drowsiness, headache, ***seizures, neuroleptic malignant syndrome***

CV: Orthostatic hypotension, ***cardiac arrest,*** ECG changes, ***tachycardia***

EENT: Blurred vision, glaucoma, dry eyes

GI: Dry mouth, nausea, vomiting, anorexia, constipation, diarrhea, jaundice, weight gain

GU: Urinary retention, urinary frequency, enuresis, impotence, amenorrhea, gynecomastia

HEMA: Anemia, ***leukopenia, leukocytosis, agranulocytosis***

INTEG: Rash, photosensitivity, dermatitis

RESP: ***Laryngospasm,*** dyspnea, ***respiratory depression***

Contraindications: Hypersensitivity, blood dyscrasias, coma, P child <12 yr, brain damage, bone marrow depression, glaucoma

Precautions: Pregnancy **C**, lactation, seizure disorders, hypertension, hepatic disease, cardiac disease

Pharmacokinetics

Absorption	Variably absorbed (PO); well absorbed (IM); completely absorbed (IV)
Distribution	Widely distributed; high concentrations in CNS; crosses placenta
Metabolism	Liver, extensively
Excretion	Kidneys, breast milk
Half-life	Unknown

Pharmacodynamics

	PO	IM
Onset	½ hr	Up to ½ hr
Peak	2-4 hr	Unknown
Duration	4-6 hr	4-6 hr

Interactions

Drug/drug:

Individual drugs

Alcohol: ↑ effects of both drugs, oversedation

Aluminum hydroxide: ↓ absorption

Bromocriptine: ↓ antiparkinsonian activity

Disopyramide: ↑ anticholinergic effects

Epinephrine: ↑ toxicity

Guanethidine: ↓ antihypertensive response

Levodopa: ↓ antiparkinsonian activity

Lithium: ↓ promazine levels, ↑ EPS, masking of lithium toxicity

Magnesium hydroxide: ↓ absorption

Norepinephrine: ↓ vasoresponse, ↑ toxicity
Phenobarbital: ↓ effectiveness, ↑ metabolism

Drug classifications
Antacids: ↓ absorption
Anticholinergics: ↑ anticholinergic effects
Antidepressants: ↑ CNS depression
Antidiarrheals, adsorbent: ↓ absorption
Antihistamines: ↑ CNS depression
Antihypertensives: ↑ hypotension
Antithyroid agents: ↑ agranulocytosis
Barbiturate anesthetics: ↑ CNS depression
β-Adrenergics: ↑ effects of both drugs
General anesthetics: ↑ CNS depression
MAOI: ↑ CNS depression
Narcotics: ↑ CNS depression
Sedative/hypnotics: ↑ CNS depression

Lab test interferences

Increase: Liver function tests, cardiac enzymes, cholesterol, blood glucose, prolactin, bilirubin, PBI, cholinesterase, iodine, alkaline phosphatase, leukocytes, granulocytes, platelets
Decrease: Hormones (blood and urine)
False positive: Pregnancy tests, PKU, urine bilirubin
False negative: Urinary steroids, 17-OHCS

NURSING CONSIDERATIONS

Assessment

- Assess mental status: orientation, mood, behavior, presence and type of hallucinations before initial administration and monthly; this drug should significantly reduce psychotic behavior
- Check for swallowing of PO medication; check for hoarding or giving of medication to other patients
- Monitor I&O ratio; palpate bladder if low urinary output G occurs, especially in elderly; urinalysis recommended before, during prolonged therapy
- Monitor bilirubin, CBC, liver function studies monthly
- Assess affect, orientation, LOC, reflexes, gait, coordination, sleep pattern disturbances
- Monitor B/P with patient sitting, standing and lying, take pulse and respirations q4h during initial treatment; establish baseline before starting treatment; report drops of 30 mm Hg; obtain baseline ECG, Q wave and T wave changes
- Check for dizziness, faintness, palpitations, tachycardia on rising; severe orthostatic hypotension is common
- Identify for neuroleptic malignant syndrome: hyperpyrexia, muscle rigidity, increased CPK, altered mental status; drug should be discontinued
- Assess for EPS including akathisia (inability to sit still, no pattern to movements), tardive dyskinesia (bizarre movements of the jaw, mouth, tongue, extremities), pseudoparkinsonism (ragged tremors, pill rolling, shuffling gate); an antiparkinsonian drug should be prescribed
- Assess for constipation, urinary retention daily; if these occur, increase bulk, water in diet

P

Associated nursing diagnoses

✓Thought processes, altered (uses)
✓Coping, ineffective individual (uses)
✓Knowledge deficit (teaching)
✓Noncompliance (teaching)

Implementation

PO route

- Give decreased dosage in G elderly since metabolism is slowed
- Give PO with full glass of water, milk; or give with food to decrease GI upset
- Store in airtight, light-resistant container

IM route

- Inject in deep muscle mass; do not give SC; do not administer sol with a precipitate; patient should remain recumbent for at least 30 min to prevent severe hypotension

Patient/family education

- Teach patient to use good oral hygiene; frequent rinsing of mouth, sugarless gum for dry mouth
- Advise patient to avoid hazardous activities until drug response is determined; dizziness, blurred vision may occur
- Inform patient that orthostatic hypotension occurs often and to rise from sitting or lying position gradually; to remain lying down after IM injection for at least 30 min; tell patient to avoid hot tubs, hot showers, tub baths, since hypotension may occur; tell patient that in hot weather heat stroke may occur; take extra precautions to stay cool
- Caution patient to avoid abrupt withdrawal of this drug, or EPS may result; drug should be withdrawn slowly
- Teach patient to avoid OTC preparations (cough, hay fever, cold) unless approved by prescriber, since serous drug interactions may occur; avoid use with alcohol, CNS depressants; increased drowsiness may occur
- Caution patient to use a sunscreen and sunglasses to prevent burns
- Teach patient about EPS and necessity of meticulous oral hygiene, since oral candidiasis may occur
- Instruct patient to take antacids 2 hr before or after taking this drug
- Teach patient to report sore throat, malaise, fever, bleeding, mouth sores; if these occur, CBC should be drawn and drug discontinued
- Teach that urine may turn pink or red

Evaluation

Positive therapeutic outcome

- Decrease in emotional excitement, hallucinations, delusions, paranoia
- Reorganization of patterns of thought, speech

Treatment of overdose:

Lavage if orally ingested; provide airway; *do not induce vomiting or use epinephrine*

promethazine

(proe-meth'a-zeen)

Anergan 25, Anergan 50, Histanil ✱, Mallergan, Pentazine, Phenameth, Phenazine 25, Phenazine 50, Phenergan, Phenergan Fortis, Phenergan Plain, Phenoject-50, PMS promethazine ✱, Pro 50, Prometh-50, Promethazine HCl, Prorex 25, Prorex 50, Prothazine Plain, Remsed, V-Gan 25, V-Gan 50

Func. class.: Antihistamine, H_1-receptor antagonist; antiemetic; sedative/hypnotic

Chem. class.: Phenothiazine derivative

Pregnancy category C

Action: Acts on blood vessels, GI, respiratory system by competing with histamine for H_1-receptor site; decreases allergic response by blocking histamine; also acts on chemoreceptor trigger zone to decrease vomiting; increases CNS stimulation, has anticholinergic response

➡ Therapeutic Outcome: Absence of allergy symptoms and rhinitis, absence of nausea/vomiting, sedation

Uses: Motion sickness, rhinitis, allergy symptoms, sedation, nausea, preoperative and postoperative sedation

Dosage and routes

Nausea

Adult: PO/IM/**IV**/rec 10-25 mg; may repeat 12.5-25 mg q4-6h

P *Child >2 yr:* PO/IM/**IV**/rec 0.25-0.5 mg/kg q4-6h

Motion sickness

Adult: PO 25 mg bid; give 30-60 min before departure

P *Child >2 yr:* PO/IM/rec 12.5-25 mg bid; give 30-60 min before departure

Allergy/rhinitis

Adult: PO 12.5 mg qid, or 25 mg hs

P *Child >2 yr:* PO 6.25-12.5 mg tid or 25 mg hs

Sedation

Adult: PO/IM/**IV**/rec 25-50 mg hs

P *Child >2 yr:* PO/IM/rec/**IV** 12.5-25 mg hs

Sedation (preoperative/postoperative)

Adult: PO/IM/**IV** 25-50 mg

P *Child >2 yr:* PO/IM/**IV** 12.5-25 mg

Available forms: Tab 12.5, 25, 50 mg; supp 12.5, 25, 50 mg; inj 25, 50 mg/ml

Side effects/adverse reactions

CNS: Dizziness, drowsiness, poor coordination, fatigue, anxiety, euphoria, confusion, paresthesia, neuritis

CV: Hypotension, palpitations, tachycardia

EENT: Blurred vision, dilated pupils, tinnitus, nasal

P

stuffiness, dry nose, throat, mouth, photosensitivity
GI: Constipation, dry mouth, nausea, vomiting, anorexia, diarrhea
GU: Retention, dysuria, frequency
HEMA: Thrombocytopenia, agranulocytosis, hemolytic anemia
INTEG: Rash, urticaria, photosensitivity
RESP: Increased thick secretions, wheezing, chest tightness

Contraindications: Hypersensitivity to H_1-receptor antagonist, acute asthma attack, lower respiratory tract disease

Precautions: Increased intraocular pressure, renal disease, cardiac disease, hypertension, bronchial asthma, seizure disorder, stenosed peptic ulcers, hyperthyroidism, prostatic hypertrophy, bladder neck obstruction, pregnancy **C**

Pharmacokinetics

Absorption	Well absorbed (PO, IM); erratically absorbed (rec)
Distribution	Widely distributed; crosses the blood-brain barrier, placenta
Excretion	Kidneys, breast milk
Half-life	Unknown

Pharmacodynamics

	PO	IM	IV	REC
Onset	20 min	20 min	3-5 min	20 min
Peak	Unkn	Unkn	Unkn	Unkn
Duration	4-6 hr	4-6 hr	4-6 hr	4-6 hr

Interactions

Drug/drug:

Individual drugs
Alcohol: ↑ CNS depression
Atropine: ↑ anticholinergic reactions
Disopyramide: ↑ anticholinergic reactions
Haloperidol: ↑ anticholinergic reactions
Quinidine: ↑ anticholinergic reactions
Drug classifications
Antidepressants: ↑ anticholinergic reactions
Antihistamines: ↑ anticholinergic reactions
CNS depressants: ↑ CNS depression
MAOI: ↑ anticholinergic effect
Narcotics: ↑ CNS depression
Phenothiazines: ↑ anticholinergic reactions
Sedative/hypnotics: ↑ CNS depression

Lab test interferences

False negative: Skin allergy tests (discontinue antihistamines 3 days before testing)
Increase: Serum glucose

NURSING CONSIDERATIONS

Assessment

- Assess respiratory status: rate, rhythm, increase in bronchial secretions, wheezing, chest tightness; provide fluids to 2 L/day to decrease secretion thickness
- Monitor I&O ratio: be alert for urinary retention, frequency, dysuria, especially G elderly; drug should be discontinued if these occur
- Monitor CBC during long-term therapy; blood dyscrasias may occur but are rare

Associated nursing diagnoses

- ✓ Airway clearance, ineffective (uses)
- ✓ Injury, risk for (adverse reactions)
- ✓ Knowledge deficit (teaching)
- ✓ Noncompliance (teaching, overuse)

Implementation

PO route

• Give with meals to decrease GI upset

• Store in tight, light-resistant container

IM route

• Give IM inj in large muscle mass; aspirate to avoid **IV** administration; do not give SC; necrosis may occur

IV **IV route**

• Give IV directly; give 25 mg or less over 1 min; rapid drop in B/P may occur with rapid administration

Syringe incompatibilities:

Dimenhydrinate, heparin, pentobarbital, thiopental

Syringe compatibilities:

Atropine, butorphanol, chlorpromazine, cimetidine, diphenhydramine, droperidol, fentanyl, glycopyrrolate, hydromorphone, hydroxyzine, meperidine, metoclopromide, midazolam, morphine, pentazocine, perphenazine, prochlorperazine, promazine, ranitidine, scopolamine

Y-site incompatibilities:

Cefoperazone, foscarnet, heparin

Y-site compatibilities:

Amsacrine, fluconazole, fludarabine, melphalan, ondansetron, sargramostim, vinorelbine

Additive compatibilities:

Amikacin, ascorbic acid, netilmicin, vitamin B with C

Additive incompatibilities:

Aminophylline, carbenicillin, chloramphenicol, chlorothiazide, floxacillin, furosemide, heparin, hydrocortisone sodium succinate, methicillin, methohexital, penicillin G, pentobarbital, phenobarbital, thiopental

Patient/family education

• Inform patient that a false negative result may occur with skin testing; these procedures should not be scheduled until 3 days after discontinuing use

• Advise patient to take 30 min before departure to prevent motion sickness

• Caution patient to avoid hazardous activities, activities requiring alertness, since dizziness may occur; instruct patient to request assistance with ambulation

• Advise patient to avoid alcohol, other depressants; serious CNS depression may occur

• Teach all aspects of drug use; to notify prescriber if confusion, sedation, hypotension occur; to avoid driving and other hazardous activity if drowsiness occurs; to avoid alcohol and other CNS depressants that may potentiate effect

• Advise patient to take 1 hr ac or 2 hr pc to facilitate absorption

- Caution patient not to exceed recommended dosage; dysrhythmias may occur
- Inform patient hard candy, gum, frequent rinsing of mouth may be used for dryness

Evaluation

Positive therapeutic outcome
- Absence of motion sickness
- Absence of nausea, vomiting

Treatment of overdose: Administer ipecac syrup or lavage, diazepam, vasopressors, barbiturates (short-acting)

propantheline
(proe-pan'the-leen)
Norpanth, Pro-Banthine, Propanthel ✦, propantheline bromide
Func. class.: GI anticholinergic; antimuscarinic
Chem. class.: Synthetic quaternary ammonium compound
Pregnancy category C

Action: Inhibits muscarinic actions of acetylcholine at postganglionic parasympathetic neuroeffector sites

Therapeutic Outcome: Absence of peptic ulcer disease symptoms

Uses: Treatment of peptic ulcer disease, irritable bowel syndrome, duodenography, urinary incontinence

Investigational uses: Antispasmodic uses

Dosage and routes

Adult: PO 15 mg tid ac, 30 mg hs
G *Elderly:* PO 7.5 mg tid ac

Antispasmodic
P *Child:* PO 2-3 mg/kg/day

Antisecretory
P *Child:* PO 1.5 mg/kg/day in 3-4 divided doses

Available forms: Tab 7.5, 15 mg

Side effects/adverse reactions

CNS: *Confusion, stimulation* G *in elderly,* headache, insomnia, dizziness, drowsiness, anxiety, weakness, hallucinations
CV: Palpitations, tachycardia
EENT: *Blurred vision,* photophobia, mydriasis, cycloplegia, increased ocular tension
GI: *Dry mouth, constipation,* ***paralytic ileus,*** heartburn, nausea, vomiting, dysphagia, absence of taste
GU: Hesitancy, retention, impotence
INTEG: Urticaria, rash, pruritus, anhidrosis, fever, allergic reactions

Contraindications: Hypersensitivity to anticholinergics, narrow angle glaucoma, GI obstruction, myasthenia gravis, paralytic ileus, GI atony, toxic megacolon

Precautions: Hyperthyroidism, CAD, dysrhythmias, CHF, ulcerative colitis, hypertension, hiatal hernia, hepatic disease, renal disease, pregnancy **C**, urinary retention, prostatic hypertrophy

Pharmacokinetics

Absorption	Moderately absorbed (PO)
Distribution	Unknown
Metabolism	Unknown
Excretion	Unknown
Half-life	Unknown

Pharmacodynamics

Onset	½ hr
Peak	2-6 hr
Duration	4-6 hr

Interactions

Drug/drug:

Individual drugs

Amantadine: ↑ anticholinergic effect
Atropine: ↑ anticholinergic effect
Disopyramide: ↑ anticholinergic effect
Haloperidol: ↑ anticholinergic effect
Potassium chloride, oral: ↑ GI lesions
Quinidine: ↑ anticholinergic effect

Drug classifications

Antacids: ↓ absorption of propantheline
Anticholinergics: ↑ anticholinergic effect
Antidepressants, tricyclic: ↑ anticholinergic effect
Antihistamines: ↑ anticholinergic effect
Phenothiazines: ↑ anticholinergic effect

NURSING CONSIDERATIONS

Assessment

- Assess for the pain of peptic ulcer disease before, during, and after treatment

Associated nursing diagnoses

- ✓ Pain (uses)
- ✓ Constipation (adverse reactions)
- ✓ Thought processes, impaired (adverse reactions)
- ✓ Knowledge deficit (teaching)

Implementation

PO route

- Give 30 min ac and at hs; do not give with antacids; separate by at least 1 hr

Patient/family education

- Teach patient to report blurred vision, chest pain, allergic reactions
- Advise patient not to perform strenuous activity in high temp; heat stroke may result due to decreased perspiration
- Instruct patient to take as prescribed; not to skip doses
- Instruct patient to report change in vision; blurring or loss of sight; drug should be discontinued
- Advise patient not to operate machinery or drive if dizziness occurs
- Caution patient not to take OTC products without approval of prescriber

Evaluation

Positive therapeutic outcome

- Decreased pain in peptic ulcer disease

P

propofol

(proe-po'foel)

Disoprofol, Diprivan

Func. class.: General anesthetic

Pregnancy category **B**

Action: Produces dose-dependent CNS depression and amnesia; action is unknown

Therapeutic Outcome: Anesthesia, induction, maintenance

Uses: Induction or maintenance of anesthesia as part of balanced anesthetic technique; monitored anesthesia care (MAC) for intubated, ventilated patients

Dosage and routes

Induction

P *Adult:* **IV** 2-2.5 mg/kg; approximately 40 mg q10 sec until induction onset, then 100-200 µg/kg/min maintenance

G *Elderly:* 1-1.5 mg/kg, approximately 20 mg q10 sec until induction onset, then 500-1000 µg/kg/min maintenance

Maintenance

Adult: 0.1-0.2 mg/kg/min (6-12 mg/kg/hr)

G *Elderly:* 0.05-0.1 mg/kg/min (3-6 mg/kg/hr)

Intermittent bolus

Adult: Increments of 25-50 mg as needed

Critical care sedation

Adult: **IV** 5 mg/kg over 5 min; may give 5-10 µg/kg/min over 5-10 min until desired response

Available forms: Inj 10 mg/ml in 20 ml amp

Side effects/adverse reactions

CNS: Movement, headache, jerking, fever, dizziness, shivering, tremor, confusion, somnolence, paresthesia, agitation, abnormal dreams, euphoria, fatigue

CV: Bradycardia, hypotension, hypertension, PVC, PAC, tachycardia, abnormal ECG, ST segment depression, ***asystole***

EENT: Blurred vision, tinnitus, eye pain, strange taste

GI: Nausea, vomiting, abdominal cramping, dry mouth, swallowing, hypersalivation

GU: Urine retention, green urine

INTEG: Flushing, phlebitis, hives, burning/stinging at inj site

MS: Myalgia

RESP: ***Apnea,*** *cough, hiccups,* dyspnea, hypoventilation, sneezing, wheezing, tachypnea, hypoxia

Contraindications: Hypersensitivity, hyperlipidemia

G **Precautions:** Elderly, respiratory, depression, severe respiratory disorders, cardiac dysrhythmias, pregnancy **B**, labor
P and delivery, lactation, children

Pharmacokinetics

Absorption	Completely absorbed (IV)
Distribution	Rapidly, widely distributed; crosses placenta
Metabolism	Liver by conjugation (inactive metabolites)
Excretion	Kidneys (70%)
Half-life	Biphasic: 1-8 min, 5-10 hr

Pharmacodynamics

Onset	40 sec
Peak	Unknown
Duration	3-5 min

Interactions

Drug/drug:

Individual drugs

Alcohol: ↑ CNS depression

Drug classifications

Antipsychotics: ↑ CNS depression
Inhalation anesthetics: ↑ CNS depression
Narcotics: ↑ CNS depression
Sedative/hypnotics: ↑ CNS depression
Skeletal muscle relaxants: ↑ CNS depression

NURSING CONSIDERATIONS

Assessment

- Monitor inj site for redness, pain, swelling
- Assess degree of amnesia in elderly; may be increased
- Assess anterograde amnesia and sedation throughout and after using
- Assess VS for recovery period in patient: respirations, pulse, B/P

Associated nursing diagnoses

- ✓ Breathing pattern, ineffective (adverse reactions)
- ✓ Injury, risk for (adverse reactions)
- ✓ Knowledge deficit (teaching)

Implementation

IV IV route

- Give after diluting with D_5W mixed in lipid base; use only glass containers when mixing; not stable in plastic
- Give alone; do not mix with other agents before using; use only when resuscitative equipment available; should be administered only by qualified persons trained in anesthesia
- Store in light-resistant area at room temp

Y-*site incompatibilities:*

Blood, blood products

Additive incompatibilities:

Do not admix with other medications

Patient/family education

- Caution patient to avoid hazardous activities until drowsiness, weakness subside
- Teach patient that amnesia occurs; events may not be remembered

Evaluation

Positive therapeutic outcome

- Induction of sedation, general anesthesia

Treatment of overdose:

Discontinue drug; administer vasopressor agents or anticholinergics, artificial ventilation

P

propoxyphene

(proe-pox'i-feen)

Darvin, Darvon-N, Dolene, Doraphen, Doxaphene, Novapropoxyn ✤, Profene, Pro-Pox, Propoxycon, propoxyphene HCl; **propoxyphene/ acetaminophen:** Darvocet-N, Dolene AP, Doxapap-N, D-Pox, E-Lor, Genagesia, Pancet Propacet, Pro-Pox with APAP; **propoxyphene with APAP,** Wygesic; **propoxyphene/aspirin/ caffeine:** Benophene, Cotanal, Darvon Compound-65, Darvon-N Compound ✤, Doraphen Compound, Doxaphene Compound, Margesic A-C, Novopropoxy Compound ✤, Pro-Pox Plus

Func. class.: Nonnarcotic analgesics

Chem. class.: Synthetic opiate

Pregnancy category C

Controlled substance schedule IV

Action: Depresses pain impulse transmission at the spinal cord level by interacting with opioid receptors

➔ **Therapeutic Outcome:** Decreased pain

Uses: Mild to moderate pain

Dosage and routes

Adult: PO 65 mg q4h prn (HCl)

Adult: PO 100 mg q4h prn (napsylate)

Available forms: Propoxyphene HCl: cap 65 mg, tab 65 mg ✤; Propoxyphene napsylate: tab 50, 100 mg; cap 100 mg ✤, oral susp 50 mg/ 5 ml; propoxyphene HCl/ acetaminophen: tab 65 mg/ 650 mg; propoxyphene napsylate/acetaminophen: tab 50 mg/325 mg, 100 mg/650 mg; propoxyphene/aspirin/ caffeine: cap 65 mg/389 mg/ 32.4 mg

Side effects/adverse reactions

CNS: Drowsiness, dizziness, confusion, headache, sedation, euphoria, ***convulsions, hyperthermia***

CV: Palpitations, bradycardia, change in B/P, ***dysrhythmias***

EENT: Tinnitus, blurred vision, miosis, diplopia

GI: Nausea, vomiting, anorexia, constipation, cramps

GU: Urinary retention, dysuria

INTEG: Rash, urticaria, bruising, flushing, diaphoresis, pruritus

RESP: Respiratory depression

Contraindications: Hypersensitivity to ASA products (some preparations), addiction (narcotic)

Precautions: Addictive personality, pregnancy **C**, lactation, increased intracranial pressure, MI (acute), severe heart disease, respiratory depression, hepatic disease, renal disease, child <18 yr

Pharmacokinetics

Absorption	Well absorbed
Distribution	Widely distributed; crosses placenta
Metabolism	Liver, extensively
Excretion	Kidneys, breast milk
Half-life	6-12 hr

Pharmacodynamics

Onset	15-30 min
Peak	2-3 hr
Duration	4-6 hr

Interactions

Drug/drug:

Individual drugs

Alcohol: ↑ respiratory depression, hypotension, sedation
Nalbuphine: ↓ analgesia
Pentazocine: ↓ analgesia

Drug classifications

Antihistamines: ↑ respiratory depression, hypotension
CNS depressants: ↑ respiratory depression, hypotension
MAOI: Use ↓ dosage; reaction is unpredictable
Sedative/hypnotics: ↑ respiratory depression, hypotension

Drug/smoking:

↓ analgesic effect

Lab test interferences

Increase: Amylase

NURSING CONSIDERATIONS

Assessment

• Assess pain: location, duration, intensity before and 1 hr after administration
• Monitor CNS changes: dizziness, drowsiness, euphoria, LOC, pupil reaction
• Monitor allergic reactions: rash, urticaria

Associated nursing diagnoses

✓ Pain (uses)
✓ Sensory-perceptual alteration: visual, auditory (adverse reactions)
✓ Breathing pattern, ineffective (adverse reactions)
✓ Injury, risk for (adverse reactions)
✓ Knowledge deficit (teaching)

Implementation

• Give with antiemetic if nausea, vomiting occur
• Give when pain is beginning to return; determine dosage interval by patient response; continuous dosing of medication is more effective than when given prn
• Medication should be slowly withdrawn after long-term use to prevent withdrawal symptoms
• Store in light-resistant container at room temp

PO route

• May be given with food or milk to lessen GI upset

Patient/family education

• Teach patient to avoid CNS depressants: alcohol, sedative/hypnotics for at least 24 hr after taking this drug
• Discuss with patient that dizziness, drowsiness, and confusion are common; to avoid getting up without assistance
• Discuss in detail all aspects of the drug, including purpose

P

and what to expect after anesthesia
- Advise patient to make position changes slowly to lessen orthostatic hypotension

Evaluation

Positive therapeutic outcome
- Decreased pain

Treatment of overdose: Narcan 0.2-0.8 **IV**, O_2, **IV** fluids, vasopressors

propranolol

(proe-pran'oh-lole)

Apo-Propranolol ♣, Detensol ♣, Inderal, Inderal LA, Inderal 10, Inderal 20, Inderal 40, Inderal 60, Inderal 80, propranolol HCl, Propranolol Intensol, Novo-pranol ♣

Func. class.: Antihypertensive, antianginal

Chem. class.: β-Adrenergic blocker

Pregnancy category **C**

Action: Competitively blocks stimulation of β-adrenergic receptor within vascular smooth muscle; produces chronotropic, inotropic activity (decreases rate of SA node discharge, increases recovery time), slows conduction of AV node, decreased heart rate, which decreases O_2 consumption in myocardium; also decreases renin-aldosterone-angiotensin system at high doses, inhibits β_2-receptors in bronchial system (high doses)

Therapeutic Outcome: Decreased B/P, heart rate

Uses: Chronic stable angina pectoris, hypertension, supraventricular dysrhythmias, migraine, prophylaxis, MI, pheochromocytoma, essential tremor, tetralogy of Fallot, cyanotic spells

Investigational uses: Mitral valve prolapse, anxiety, dysrhythmias associated with thyrotoxicosis

Dosage and routes

Dysrhythmias

Adult: PO 10-30 mg tid-qid; **IV** bol 0.5-3 mg over 1 mg/min; may repeat in 2 min; may repeat q4h thereafter

Hypertension

Adult: PO 40 mg bid or 80 mg qd (ext rel) initially; usual dosage 120-240 mg/day bid-tid or 120-160 mg qd (ext rel)

Angina

Adult: PO 80-320 mg in divided doses bid-qid or 80 mg qd (ext rel); usual dosage 160 mg qd (ext rel)

MI prophylaxis

Adult: PO 180-240 mg/day tid-qid starting 5 days to 3 wk after MI

Pheochromocytoma

Adult: PO 60 mg/day × 3 days preoperatively in divided doses or 30 mg/day in divided doses (inoperable tumor)

Migraine

Adult: PO 80 mg/day (ext

rel) or in divided doses; may increase to 160-240 mg/day in divided doses

Essential tremor

Adult: PO 40 mg bid; usual dosage 120 mg/day

Available forms: Ext rel cap 60, 80, 120, 160 mg; tab 10, 20, 40, 60, 90 mg; inj 1 mg/ml; oral sol 4 mg, 8 mg/ml; conc oral sol 80 mg/ml

Side effects/adverse reactions

CNS: Depression, hallucinations, dizziness, fatigue, lethargy, paresthesia, bizarre dreams, disorientation
CV: Bradycardia, hypotension, ***CHF,*** palpitations, AV block, peripheral vascular insufficiency, vasodilatation
EENT: Sore throat, ***laryngospasm,*** blurred vision, dry eyes
GI: Nausea, vomiting, diarrhea, colitis, constipation, cramps, dry mouth, hepatomegaly, gastric pain, acute pancreatitis
GU: Impotence, decreased libido, UTIs
HEMA: ***Agranulocytosis, thrombocytopenia***
INTEG: Rash, pruritus, fever
META: Hyperglycemia, hypoglycemia
MISC: Facial swelling, weight change, Raynaud's phenomenon
MS: Joint pain, arthralgia, muscle cramps, pain
RESP: Dyspnea, respiratory dysfunction, *bronchospasm*

Contraindications: Hypersensitivity to this drug, cardiac failure, cardiogenic shock, 2nd- or 3rd-degree heart block, bronchospastic disease, sinus bradycardia, CHF

Precautions: Diabetes mellitus, pregnancy **C**, renal disease, lactation, hyperthyroidism, COPD, hepatic disease, P children, myasthenia gravis, peripheral vascular disease, hypotension, CHF

Pharmacokinetics

Absorption	Well absorbed (PO); slowly absorbed (ext rel); completely absorbed (IV)
Distribution	Widely distributed; crosses blood-brain barrier
Metabolism	Liver, extensively
Excretion	Kidneys
Half-life	3-5 hr; ext rel 8-11 hr

Pharmacodynamics

	PO	PO–ext rel	IV
Onset	½ hr	Unknown	Rapid
Peak	1-1½ hr	6 hr	1 min
Duration	6-12 hr	24 hr	4-6 hr

P

Interactions

Drug/drug:

Individual drugs
Alcohol: ↑ hypotension (large amounts)
Epinephrine: α-Adrenergic stimulation
Hydralazine: ↑ hypotension, bradycardia
Indomethacin: ↓ antihypertensive effect
Insulin: ↑ hypoglycemia
Methyldopa: ↑ hypotension, bradycardia
Phenytoin (IV): ↑ myocardial depression

Prazosin: ↑ hypotension, bradycardia
Reserpine: ↑ hypotension, bradycardia
Thyroid: ↓ effectiveness
Verapamil: ↑ myocardial depression

Drug classifications

Antihypertensive: ↑ hypertension
Cardiac glycosides: ↑ bradycardia
Nitrates: ↑ hypotension
Theophyllines: ↓ bronchodilatation

Lab test interferences

False increase: Urinary catecholamines

NURSING CONSIDERATIONS

Assessment

- Monitor B/P during beginning treatment, periodically thereafter; pulse q4h; note rate, rhythm, quality; check apical/radial pulse before administration; notify prescriber of any significant changes (pulse <50 bpm)
- Check for baselines in renal, liver function tests before therapy begins and periodically thereafter
- Assess for edema in feet, legs daily; monitor I&O, weight daily; check for jugular vein distention, rales bilaterally; dyspnea (CHF)
- Monitor skin turgor, dryness of mucous membranes for hydration status, especially G elderly

Associated nursing diagnoses

✓ Cardiac output, decreased (uses)
✓ Injury, potential for (adverse reactions)
✓ Knowledge deficit (teaching)
✓ Noncompliance (teaching)

Implementation

PO route

- Given ac, hs, tab may be crushed or swallowed whole; do not crush or chew ext rel cap; give with food to prevent GI upset; reduce dosage in renal dysfunction
- Store protected from light, moisture; placed in cool environment

IV **IV route**

- Give by direct **IV** undiluted or diluted 1 mg/10 ml D_5W for inj; administer over 1 min or more
- Give by intermittent inf after diluting in 50 ml D_5W, 0.9% NaCl, D_5/0.45% NaCl, D_5/0.9% NaCl, LR; administer over 15 min

Syringe compatibilities:
Amrione, benzquinamide, milrinone

Y-site incompatibility:
Diazoxide

Y-site compatibilities:
Amrione, heparin, hydrocortisone sodium succinate, meperidine, milrinone, morphine, potassium chloride, vitamin B with C

Additive compatibilities:
Dobutamine, verapamil

Solution compatibilities:
0.9% NaCl, 0.45 NaCl, Ringer's, D_5W, D_5/0.9% NaCl, D_5/0.45% NaCl

Patient/family education

- Teach patient not to discontinue drug abruptly, taper over 2 wk; may cause precipitate angina if stopped abruptly
- Teach patient not to use OTC products containing α-adrenergic stimulants (such as nasal decongestants, cold preparations); to avoid alcohol, smoking and to limit sodium intake as prescribed
- Teach patient how to take pulse and B/P at home; advise when to notify prescriber
- Instruct patient to comply with weight control, dietary adjustments, modified exercise program
- Instruct patient to carry/wear Medic Alert ID to identify drug being taken, allergies; tell patient drug controls symptoms but does not cure
- Caution patient to avoid hazardous activities if dizziness, drowsiness is present
- Teach patient to report symptoms of CHF: difficult breathing, especially on exertion or when lying down, night cough, swelling of extremities or bradycardia, dizziness, confusion, depression, fever
- Teach patient to take drug as prescribed, not to double doses, skip doses; take any missed doses as soon as remembered if at least 8 hr until next dose

Evaluation

Positive therapeutic outcome

- Decreased B/P in hypertension (after 1-2 wk)
- Decreased tremors
- Absence of dysrhythmias
- Decreased migraine headaches

Treatment of overdose:

Lavage, **IV** atropine for bradycardia, **IV** theophylline for bronchospasm, digitalis, O_2, diuretic for cardiac failure, hemodialysis, **IV** glucose for hyperglycemia, **IV** diazepam (or phenytoin) for seizures

propylthiouracil

(proe-pill-thye-oh-yoor'a-sill)

propylthiouracil, Propyl-Thyracil ✤, PTU

Func. class.: Thyroid hormone antagonist (antithyroid)

Chem. class.: Thioamide

Pregnancy category **D**

Action: Blocks synthesis peripherally of T_3, T_4, inhibits organification of iodine

Therapeutic Outcome: Decreased T_3, T_4 levels, hyperthyroid symptoms

Uses: Preparation for thyroidectomy, thyrotoxic crisis, hyperthyroidism, thyroid storm

Dosage and routes

Thyrotoxic crisis

P *Adult and child:* PO same as hyperthyroidism with iodine and propranolol

Preparation for thyroidectomy

Adult: 600-1200 mg/day

P *Child:* 10 mg/kg/day in divided doses

P

Hyperthyroidism

Adult: PO 100 mg tid increasing to 300 mg q8h if condition is severe; continue to euthyroid state, then 100 mg qd-tid

P ***Child >10 yr:*** PO 100 mg tid; continue to euthyroid state, then 25 mg tid to 100 mg bid

P ***Child 6-10 yr:*** PO 50-150 mg in divided doses q8h

P ***Neonates:*** PO 10 mg/kg/day in divided doses

Available forms: Tab 50 mg

Side effects/adverse reactions

CNS: Drowsiness, headache, vertigo, fever, paresthesias, neuritis

GI: Nausea, diarrhea, vomiting, ***jaundice, hepatitis,*** loss of taste

GU: Nephritis

HEMA: Agranulocytosis, leukopenia, thrombocytopenia, hypothrombinemia, lymphadenopathy, bleeding, vasculitis, periarteritis

INTEG: Rash, urticaria, pruritus, alopecia, hyperpigmentation, lupuslike syndrome

MS: Myalgia, arthralgia, nocturnal muscle cramps

Contraindications: Hypersensitivity, pregnancy **D**, lactation

Precautions: Infection, bone marrow depression, hepatic disease

Pharmacokinetics

Absorption	Rapidly absorbed (PO)
Distribution	Crosses placenta; concentration in thyroid gland
Metabolism	Liver
Excretion	Urine, bile, breast milk
Half-life	1-2 hr

Pharmacodynamics

Onset	30-40 min
Peak	Unknown
Duration	2-4 hr

Interactions

Drug/drug:

Individual drugs

Heparin: ↑ anticoagulant effect

Lithium: ↑ antithyroid effect

Radiation: ↑ bone marrow depression

Drug classifications

Antineoplastics: ↑ bone marrow depression

Oral anticoagulants: ↑ anticoagulant effect

Phenothiazines: ↑ agranulocytosis

Lab test interferences

Increases: Pro-time, AST (SGOT), ALT (SGPT), alkaline phosphatase

NURSING CONSIDERATIONS

Assessment

- Monitor pulse, B/P, temp; I&O ratio; check for edema (puffy hands, feet, periorbits); indicates hypothyroidism
- Check weight daily with same clothing, scale, time of day

• Monitor T_3, T_4, which are increased; check serum TSH, which is decreased; assess free thyroxine index, which is increased if dosage is too low; discontinue drug 3-4 wk before RAIU
• Monitor blood work: CBC for blood dyscrasias (leukopenia, thrombocytopenia, agranulocytosis); liver function tests
• Assess overdose (peripheral edema, heat intolerance, diaphoresis, palpitations, dysrhythmias, severe tachycardia, increased temp, delirium, CNS irritability); drug should be discontinued
• Assess for hypersensitivity (rash, enlarged cervical lymph nodes); drug may have to be discontinued
• Assess for hypoprothrombinemia (bleeding, petechiae, ecchymosis)
• Monitor clinical response: after 3 wk should include increased weight, decreased pulse, decreased T_4
• Assess for bone marrow depression: sore throat, fever, fatigue

Associated nursing diagnoses

✓ Knowledge deficit (teaching)
✓ Noncompliance (teaching)

Implementation

PO route
• Give with meals to decrease GI upset
• Give at same time each day to maintain drug level
• Give lowest dosage that relieves symptoms
• Store in light-resistant container
• Increase fluids to 3-4 L/day, unless contraindicated

Patient/family education

• Advise patient to abstain from breastfeeding after delivery; drug appears in breast milk
• Teach patient to take pulse daily and to keep graph of weight, pulse, mood
• Advise patient to report redness, swelling, sore throat, mouth lesions, which indicate blood dyscrasias
• Caution patient to avoid OTC products that contain iodine; that seafood, other iodine-containing foods may be restricted by prescriber
• Caution patient not to discontinue this medication abruptly; thyroid crisis may occur; stress patient response
• Teach patient that response may take several mo if thyroid is large
• Teach patient symptoms/signs of overdose: periorbital edema, cold intolerance, mental depression; notify prescriber at once
• Teach patient symptoms of inadequate dose: tachycardia, diarrhea, fever, irritability; prescriber should be notified to adjust dosage
• Teach patient to take medication exactly as prescribed, not to skip or double doses; missed doses should be taken when remembered up to 1 hr before next dose
• Instruct patient to carry identification (Medic Alert) indicating medication taken and condition being treated

P

Evaluation

Positive therapeutic outcome
- Weight gain
- Decreased pulse
- Decreased T_4
- Decreased B/P

protamine

(proe'ta-meen)
Func. class.: Heparin antagonist
Chem. class.: Low-molecular-weight protein
Pregnancy category **C**

Action: Binds heparin, making it ineffective

Therapeutic Outcome: Prevention of heparin overdose

Uses: Heparin overdose; neutralizes heparin in procedures

Dosage and routes

P *Adult and child:* **IV** 1 mg of protamine/90-115 U heparin given; administer slowly over 1-3 min; give undiluted to 1%, not to exceed 50 mg/10 min

Available forms: Inj 10 mg/ml

Side effects/adverse reactions

CNS: Lassitude
CV: Hypotension, bradycardia, ***circulatory collapse***
GI: Nausea, vomiting, anorexia
INTEG: *Rash*, dermatitis, urticaria
HEMA: Bleeding, ***anaphylaxis***
RESP: Dyspnea, ***pulmonary edema, severe respiratory distress***

Contraindication: Hypersensitivity

Precautions: Pregnancy **C**, P lactation, children, allergy to fish

Pharmacokinetics	
Absorption	Completely absorbed (IV)
Distribution	Unknown
Metabolism	Unknown
Excretion	Unknown
Half-life	Unknown

Pharmacodynamics	
Onset	5 min
Peak	Unknown
Duration	2 hr

Interactions: None

NURSING CONSIDERATIONS

Assessment

- Monitor blood studies (Hct, platelets, occult blood stools) q3 mo
- Monitor coagulation tests (APTT, ACT) 15 min after dose, then in several hr
- Monitor VS, B/P, pulse q 30 min, plus 3 hr after dose
- Assess for skin rash, urticaria, dermatitis
- Assess for allergy to fish; use with caution in these patients

Associated nursing diagnoses

- ✓ Injury, risk for (uses)
- ✓ Tissue perfusion, altered (uses)
- ✓ Knowledge deficit (teaching)

Implementation

IV route

- Give by direct **IV** after diluting 50 mg/5 ml sterile bacteriostatic water for inj; shake; give 20 mg or less over 1-3 min
- Give by intermittent inf after further diluting with equal volume of NaCl or D_5W and run over 2-3 hr; titrate to APTT, ACT; use inf pump
- Store at 36° to 46° F (2°-8° C)

Additive incompatibilities:

Penicillins, cephalosporins

Additive compatibilities:

Cimetidine, verapamil

Patient/family education

- Explain reason for medication and expected results
- Caution patient to avoid contact activities that may result in bleeding

Evaluation

Positive therapeutic outcome

- Reversal of heparin overdose

pseudoephedrine

(soo-doe-e-fed'rin)

Allerid, Children's Sudafed, Decofed Syrup, DeFed-60, Dorcol Children's Decongestant, Drixoral Non-Drowsy Formula, Eltor ✤, Efidac/24, Genaphed, Halofed, Myfedrine, Novafed, Pedia Care Infant's Decongestant, Pseudoephedrine HCl, Pseudogest Decongestant, Pseudo Syrup, Sinustat, Sudafed, Sudafed 12 hour, Sudrin

Func. class.: Adrenergic

Chem. class.: Substituted phenylethylamine

Pregnancy category **B**

Action: Primary activity through α-adrenergic effects on respiratory mucosal membranes reducing congestion hyperemia, edema; minimal bronchodilatation secondary to β-adrenergic effects

Therapeutic Outcome: Decreased nasal congestion, swelling

Uses: Nasal decongestant, otitis media adjustment, adjunct with antihistamines

Dosage and routes

Adult and child >12 yr: PO 60 mg q6h; ext rel 60-120 mg q12h or q24h

Child 6-12 yr: PO 30 mg q6h, not to exceed 120 mg/day

P

P *Child 2-6 yr:* PO 15 mg q6h, not to exceed 60 mg/day

Available forms: Ext rel cap 120, 240 mg; oral sol 15 mg, 30 mg/5 ml; drops 7.5 mg/ 0.8 ml; tab 30, 60 mg; cap 60 mg; ext rel tabs 120 mg

Side effects/adverse reactions

CNS: Tremors, anxiety, insomnia, headache, dizziness, anxiety, hallucinations, ***seizures***
CV: Palpitations, tachycardia, hypertension, chest pain, ***dysrhythmias***
EENT: Dry nose, irritation of nose and throat
GI: Anorexia, nausea, vomiting, dry mouth
GU: Dysuria

Contraindications: Hypersensitivity to sympathomimetics, narrow angle glaucoma

Precautions: Pregnancy **B**, cardiac disorders, hyperthyroidism, diabetes mellitus, prostatic hypertrophy

Pharmacokinetics

Absorption	Well absorbed (PO)
Distribution	Enters CSF, crosses placenta
Metabolism	Liver, partially
Excretion	Kidneys, unchanged (75%); breast milk
Half-life	7 hr

Pharmacodynamics

	PO	PO–EXT REL
Onset	15-30 min	1 hr
Peak	Unknown	Unknown
Duration	4-6 hr	12 hr

Interactions

Drug/drug:

Individual drugs
Methyldopa: ↓ effect of pseudoephedrine
Rauwolfia: ↓ effect of pseudoephedrine
Drug classifications
β-Blockers: Hypertensive crisis
MAOI: Hypertensive crisis
Urinary acidifiers: ↓ effect of pseudoephedrine
Urinary alkalizers: ↑ effect of pseudoephedrine

NURSING CONSIDERATIONS

Assessment

- Monitor for nasal congestion; auscultate lung sounds; check for tenacious bronchial secretions; children with otitis media should be assessed for eustachian tube congestion
- Monitor B/P and pulse throughout treatment

Associated nursing diagnoses

✓ Airway clearance, ineffective (uses)
✓ Knowledge deficit (teaching)

Implementation

PO route
- Give ext rel cap and tab whole; do not crush, break or chew
- Give several hr before hs if insomnia occurs
- Store at room temp

Patient/family education

- Teach patient reason for drug administration and expected results
- Instruct patient not to use continuously, or more than

recommended dose; rebound congestion may occur
- Advise patient to check with prescriber before using other drugs, as drug interactions may occur
- Advise patient to avoid taking near bedtime; stimulation can occur
- Caution patient not to use if stimulation, restlessness, tremors occur

Evaluation

Positive therapeutic outcome
- Decreased nasal congestion

psyllium

(sill'i-um)

Cillium, Effer-Syllium, Fiberall, Fiberall Natural Flavor and Orange Flavor, Hydrocil Instant Powder, Karacil ✤, Konsyl-D, Metamucil, Metamucil Instant Mix Lemon Lime, Metamucil Instant Mix Orange, Metamucil Orange Flavor, Metamucil Sugar Free, Metamucil Sugar Free Orange Flavor, Modane Bulk, Natural Vegetable Reguloid, Perdiem, Pro-Lax, Prodiem Plain ✤, Reguloid Natural, Reguloid Orange, Reguloid Sugar Free Orange, Reguloid Sugar Free Regular, Serutan, Siblin, Syllact, V-Lax

Func. class.: Laxative, bulk-forming

Chem. class.: Psyllium colloid

Pregnancy category **C**

Action: Promotes peristalsis by combining with water in the intestine to form a gel-like substance that is easily evacuated

➔ **Therapeutic Outcome:** Decreased constipation, decreased diarrhea in colitis

Uses: Chronic constipation, ulcerative colitis, irritable bowel syndrome

Dosage and routes

Adult: PO 1-2 tsp in 8 oz water bid or tid, then 8 oz water or 1 premeasured packet in 8 oz water bid or tid, then 8 oz water

P *Child >6 yr:* 1 tsp in 4 oz water hs

Available forms: Chew pieces 1.7 g/piece; powder 309, 390, 430, 450, 486, 500, 600, 630, 654, 672, 791, 919, 950 mg/g, 1 g/g; granules 2.5 g/dose

Side effects/adverse reactions

GI: Nausea, vomiting, anorexia, diarrhea, cramps, intestinal/esophageal blockage

Contraindications: Hypersensitivity, intestinal obstruction, abdominal pain, nausea/vomiting, fecal impaction

Precautions: Pregnancy **C**

Pharmacokinetics

Absorption	None
Distribution	None
Excretion	Feces
Half-life	Unknown

Pharmacodynamics

Onset	12-24 hr
Peak	2-4 days
Duration	Unknown

Interactions

Drug/drug:

Drug classifications

Cardiac glycosides: ↓ absorption of cardiac glycosides
Oral anticoagulants: ↓ absorption of oral anticoagulants
Salicylates: ↓ absorption of salicylates

Lab test interferences

Increase: Blood glucose

NURSING CONSIDERATIONS

Assessment

- Monitor blood, urine electrolytes if used often by patient; check I&O ratio to identify fluid loss
- Assess for cramping, rec bleeding, nausea, vomiting; if these symptoms occur, drug should be discontinued; identify cause of constipation; identify whether fluids, bulk, or exercise is missing from lifestyle
- Assess stool for color, consistency, amount, presence of flatulence

Associated nursing diagnoses

✓ Constipation (uses)
✓ Knowledge deficit (teaching)
✓ Noncompliance (teaching)

Implementation

PO route

- Give alone for better absorption; give after mixing with water immediately before use; administer with 8 oz water or juice followed by another 8 oz of fluid
- Administer in AM or PM (oral dose)

Patient/family education

- Discuss with patient that adequate fluid consumption is necessary
- Teach patient that normal bowel movements do not always occur daily
- Caution patient not to use in presence of abdominal pain, nausea, vomiting; tell patient to notify prescriber if constipation is unrelieved or if symptoms of electrolyte imbalance occur (muscle cramps, pain, weakness, dizziness, excessive thirst)
- Teach patient not to use laxatives for long-term therapy; bowel tone will be lost and will decrease
- Shake susp well as needed
- Teach patient not to take at hs as a laxative; may interfere with sleep; also problems with lipid pneumonia
- Teach patient not to use with food or vitamin preparations; delays digestion and absorption of fat-soluble vitamins

Evaluation

Positive therapeutic outcome

- Decreased constipation in 12-24 hr

pyrazinamide

(peer-a-zin'a-mide)
PMS Pyrazinamide ✤,
pyrazinamide,
Tebrazid ✤
Func. class.: Antitubercular agent
Chem. class.: Pyrazinoic acid amine/nicoturimide analog
Pregnancy category C

Action: Bactericidal interference with lipid; nucleic acid biosynthesis is possible

Therapeutic Outcome: Bactericidal for *Mycobacterium* species

Uses: Tuberculosis, as an adjunct when other drugs are not feasible

Dosage and routes

Adult: PO 20-35 mg/kg/day qd or individed doses, not to exceed 3 g/day

P *Child:* PO 15-30 mg/kg/day qd or divided bid; max 1.5 g/day

Available forms: Tab 500 mg

Side effects/adverse reactions

CNS: Headache
GI: ***Hepatotoxicity,*** abnormal liver function tests, peptic ulcer
GU: Urinary difficulty, increased uric acid
HEMA: Hemolytic anemia
INTEG: Photosensitivity, urticaria

Contraindications: Hypersensitivity

Precautions: Pregnancy **C**,
P child <13 yr

Pharmacokinetics

Absorption	Well absorbed (PO)
Distribution	Widely distributed
Metabolism	Liver, extensively
Excretion	Kidneys, breast milk
Half-life	9-10 hr

Pharmacodynamics

Onset	Unknown
Peak	2 hr
Duration	9½ hr; metabolites 12 hr

Interactions: None

NURSING CONSIDERATIONS

Assessment

- C & S studies should be taken before treatment begins, and periodically during treatment
- Monitor serum uric acid, which may be elevated and cause gout symptoms
- Monitor liver studies weekly: ALT (SGPT), AST (SGOT), bilirubin; hepatic status: decreased appetite, jaundice, dark urine, fatigue
- Monitor renal status: before treatment and monthly thereafter: BUN, creatinine, output, sp gr, urinalysis
- Monitor mental status often: affect, mood, behavioral changes; psychosis may occur

Associated nursing diagnoses

✓ Infection, risk for (uses)
✓ Diarrhea (adverse reactions)

- ☑ Injury, risk for (adverse reactions)
- ☑ Knowledge deficit (teaching)
- ☑ Noncompliance (teaching)

Implementation

PO route
- Give with meals to decrease GI symptoms
- Give antiemetic if vomiting occurs
- May be given with other antituberculars

Patient/family education

- Instruct patient that compliance with dosage schedule, duration is necessary; that scheduled appointments must be kept or relapse may occur
- Advise diabetic patient to use blood glucose monitor to obtain correct result
- Advise patient to report weakness, fatigue, loss of appetite, nausea, vomiting, yellowing of skin or eyes, tingling/numbness of hands/feet

Evaluation

Positive therapeutic outcome
- Decreased symptoms of TB
- Sputum culture negative × 3

pyridostigmine

(peer-id-oh-stig′meen)
Mestinon, Mestinon SR ✥, Mestinon Timespan, Regonol
Func. class.: Cholinergic, anticholinesterase
Chem. class.: Tertiary amine carbamate
Pregnancy category **C**

Action: Inhibits destruction of acetylcholine, which increases concentration at sites where acetylcholine is released; this facilitates transmission of impulses across myoneural junction

➔ Therapeutic Outcome: Decreased action of nondepolarizing muscle relaxant; increased muscle strength in myasthenia gravis

Uses: Nondepolarizing muscle relaxant antagonist, myasthenia gravis

Dosage and routes

Myasthenia gravis
Adult: PO 60-180 mg bid-qid, not to exceed 1.5 g/day; IM/**IV** 1/30 of PO dose; sus rel 180-540 mg qd or bid at intervals of at least 6 hr

Nondepolarizing neuromuscular blocker antagonist
Adult: 0.6-1.2 mg **IV** atropine, then 10-30 mg

Available forms: Tab 60 mg; sus rel tab 180 mg; syr 60 mg/5 ml; inj 5 mg/ml

Side effects/adverse reactions

CNS: Dizziness, headache, sweating, weakness, ***convulsions,*** uncoordination, paralysis, drowsiness, LOC
EENT: Miosis, blurred vision, lacrimation, visual changes
CV: Tachycardia, dysrhythmias, bradycardia, AV block, hypotension, ECG changes, ***cardiac arrest,*** syncope

GI: Nausea, diarrhea, vomiting, cramps, increased salivary and gastric secretions, peristalsis
GU: Frequency, incontinence, urgency
INTEG: Rash, urticaria, flushing
RESP: Respiratory depression, bronchospasm, constriction, laryngospasm, respiratory arrest

Contraindications: Bradycardia, hypotension, obstruction of intestine, or renal system, bromide sensitivity

Precautions: Seizure disorders, bronchial asthma, coronary occlusion, hyperthyroidism, dysrhythmias, peptic ulcer, megacolon, poor GI motility, pregnancy **C**

Pharmacokinetics

Absorption	Poorly absorbed (PO)
Distribution	Widely distributed; crosses placenta
Metabolism	Liver, plasma cholinesterase
Excretion	Kidneys
Half-life	2 hr (IV); 4 hr (PO)

Pharmacodynamics

	PO	IM/IV	PO–SUS REL
Onset	20-30 min	2-15 min	½-1 hr
Peak	Unknown	Unknown	Unknown
Duration	3-6 hr	2-4 hr	3-6 hr

Interactions

Drug/drug:

Individual drugs

Digitalis: Bradycardia
Magnesium: ↓ action of pyridostigmine
Mecamylamine: ↓ action of pyridostigmine
Polymyxin: ↓ action of pyridostigmine
Procainamide: ↓ action of pyridostigmine
Quinidine: ↓ action of pyridostigmine

Drug classifications

Antihistamines: ↑ antagonism
Antidepressants: ↑ antagonism
Phenothiazines: ↑ antagonism
Muscle relaxants, depolarizing: ↑ action of muscle relaxants
Cholinesterase inhibitors: ↑ toxicity

NURSING CONSIDERATIONS

Assessment

- Monitor VS, respiration ↑ B/P during test and at baseline
- Monitor diabetic patient carefully, since this drug lowers blood glucose

Associated nursing diagnoses

✓ Breathing pattern, ineffective (uses)
✓ Knowledge deficit (teaching)

Implementation

IV **IV route**

- Give **IV** undiluted, give through Y-tube or 3-way stopcock; give 0.5 mg or less /min
- Give only when atropine sulfate available for cholinergic crisis

Syringe compatibility:
Glycopyrrolate

P

Y-site compatibilities:
Heparin, hydrocortisone sodium succinate, potassium chloride, vitamin B with C

PO route
- Give only after all other cholinergics have been discontinued
- Give increased doses if tolerance occurs
- Give larger doses after exercise or fatigue
- Give on empty stomach for better absorption
- Store at room temp

Patient/family education
- Advise patient to wear Medic Alert ID specifying myasthenia gravis, drugs taken

Evaluation
Positive therapeutic outcome
- Increased muscle strength, hand grasp
- Improved gait
- Absence of labored breathing (if severe)

Treatment of overdose: Discontinue drug, atropine 1-4 mg **IV**

pyridoxine (vitamin B_6)
(peer-i-dox'een)
Beesix, Nestrex, pyridoxine HCl, Vitamin B_6, Rodex TD, Hexa-Betalin ♣
Func. class.: Vitamin B_6, water soluble
Pregnancy category A

Action: Needed for fat, protein, carbohydrate metabolism; enhances glycogen release from liver and muscle tissue; needed as coenzyme for metabolic transformations of a variety of amino acids

Uses: Vitamin B_6 deficiency associated with the following: inborn errors of metabolism, seizures, cycloserine, hydralazine penicillamine, isoniazid therapy, oral contraceptives, alcoholism, polyneuritis

Dosage and routes
Vitamin B_6 deficiency
Adult: PO/IM/**IV** 2.5-10 mg until corrected, then 2-5 mg qd
P *Child:* PO/IM/**IV** 100 mg until desired response, or 2.5-10 mg/day × 3 wk, then 2-5 mg qd

Inborn errors of metabolism
Adult: IM/**IV**/PO 600 mg or less qd, then 50 mg qd for life
P *Child:* IM/PO/**IV** 100 mg, then 2-10 mg IM or 10-100 mg PO qd

Deficiency caused by isoniazid, cycloserine, hydralazine, penicillamine
Adult: PO 100 mg qd × 3 wk, then 50 mg qd
P *Child:* PO dose titrated to patient response

Prevention of deficiency caused by isoniazid, cycloserine, hydralazine, penicillamine
Adult: PO 10-50 mg qd
P *Child:* PO 0.5-1.5 mg qd
P *Infant:* PO 0.1-0.5 mg qd

Available forms: Tab 10, 25, 50, 100, 200, 250, 500 mg; time rel tab 100, 150, 500 mg; inj 100 mg/ml; time rel cap 100, 150 mg

Side effects/adverse reactions

CNS: Paresthesia
INTEG: Pain at inj site

Contraindication: Hypersensitivity

Precautions: Pregnancy **A**, P lactation, children, Parkinson's disease

Pharmacokinetics

Absorption	Well absorbed (PO)
Distribution	Stored in liver, muscle, brain; crosses placenta
Metabolism	Unknown
Excretion	Kidneys, unchanged (not used)
Half-life	Unknown

Pharmacodynamics

	PO/IM/IV
Onset	Unknown
Peak	Unknown
Duration	Unknown

Interactions
Drug/drug:
Individual drugs
Chloramphenicol: ↓ effects of pyridoxine
Cycloserine: ↓ effects of pyridoxine
Hydralazine: ↓ effects of pyridoxine
Isoniazid: ↓ effects of pyridoxine
Levodopa: ↓ effects of levodopa
Penicillamine: ↓ effects of pyridoxine
Drug classifications
Immunosuppressants: ↓ effects of pyridoxine
Oral contraceptives: ↓ effects of pyridoxine

Lab Test Interferences

False increase: Urobilinogen

NURSING CONSIDERATIONS

Assessment

- Monitor pyridoxine levels throughout treatment
- Assess nutritional status: yeast, liver, legumes, bananas, green vegetables, whole grains
- Assess for pyridoxine (B_6) deficiency: nausea, vomiting, dermatitis, cheilosis, seizures, irritability, dermatitis before and during treatment

Associated nursing diagnoses

☑ Nutrition: less then body requirements (uses)
☑ Knowledge deficit (teaching)
☑ Noncompliance (teaching, overuse)

Implementation

IV **IV route**
- Give **IV** undiluted or added to most **IV** sol; give 50 mg or less/1 min if undiluted

IM route
- Rotate sites; burning or stinging at site may occur; give by Z-track to minimize pain
- Store in tight, light-resistant container

Additive incompatibilities:

Erythromycin, iron salts, kanamycin, riboflavin, streptomycin

P

PO route
- Ext rel cap and tab should be swallowed whole; do not break, crush, or chew

IM/SC route
- Administer in different site each time to avoid pain

Patient/family education
- Teach patient to avoid other vitamin supplements unless directed by prescriber
- Advise patient to increase meat, bananas, potatoes, lima beans, whole grain cereals in diet which are high in vitamin B_6
- Caution patient not to increase dosage, since serious reactions may occur

Evaluation
Positive therapeutic outcome
- Absence of nausea, vomiting, anorexia, skin lesions, glossitis, stomatitis, edema, convulsions, restlessness, paresthesia

pyrimethamine
(peer-i-meth'a-meen)
Daraprim, Fansidar (with sulfadoxine)
Func. class.: Antimalarial, antiprotozol
Chem. class.: Folic acid antagonist
Pregnancy category **C**

Action: Inhibits folic acid metabolism in parasite; prevents transmission by stopping growth of fertilized gametes

➔ **Therapeutic Outcome:** Prevention of malaria

Uses: Malaria prophylaxis, antiprotozoal action against *Plasmodium vivax*

Investigational uses: *Pneumocystis carinii* pneumonia as an adjunct

Dosage and routes
Prophylaxis of malaria

Adult: PO 1 tab qwk or 2 tab q2 wk (Fansidar)

P *Child 9-14 yr:* PO ¾ tab qwk or 1½ tab q2 wk (Fansidar)

P *Child >10 yr:* PO 25 mg qwk

P *Child 4-10 yr:* PO 12.5 mg qwk

P *Child 4-8 yr:* PO ½ tab qwk or 1 tab q2 wk (Fansidar)

P *Child <4 yr:* PO ¼ tab qwk or ½ tab q2 wk (Fansidar)

P *Child <4 yr:* PO 6.25 mg qwk

Acute attacks of malaria

Adult: PO 2-3 tab as a single dose (Fansidar) alone or with quinine or primaquine

P *Child 9-14 yr:* 2 tab

P *Child 4-8 yr:* 1 tab

P *Child <4 yr:* ½ tab

Toxoplasmosis

Adult: PO 100 mg, then 25 mg qd × 4-5 wk, with 1 g sulfadiazine q6h

P *Child:* PO 1 mg/kg, then 0.25 mg/kg qd × 4-5 wk, with sulfadiazine 100 mg/kg/day in divided doses q6h

Available forms: Tab 25 mg; combo tab 500 mg sulfadoxine/25 mg pyrimethamine

Side effects/adverse reactions

CNS: Stimulation, irritability, ***convulsions,*** tremors, ataxia, fatigue
GI: Nausea, vomiting, cramps, anorexia, diarrhea, atrophic glossitis, gastritis
HEMA: Thrombocytopenia, leukopenia, pancytopenia, megaloblastic anemia, decreased folic acid, ***agranulocytosis***
INTEG: Skin eruptions, photosensitivity
RESP: Respiratory failure

Contraindications: Hypersensitivity, chloroquine-resistant malaria, megaloblastic anemia caused by folate deficiency

Precautions: Blood dyscrasias, seizure disorder, pregnancy **C**, lactation, G6PD disease, renal/hepatic disease

Pharmacokinetics

Absorption	Well absorbed (PO)
Distribution	Widely; crosses placenta
Metabolism	Liver, extensively
Excretion	Kidnes, unchanged (30%); breast milk
Half-life	4 days

Pharmacodynamics

Onset	Unknown
Peak	2 hr
Duration	Unknown

Interactions

Drug/drug:

Individual drugs
Folic acid: ↑ synergistic action
Drug classifications
Antiinfectives: ↑ bone marrow suppression

NURSING CONSIDERATIONS

Assessment

- C & S studies should be taken before treatment begins and periodically during treatment
- Monitor serum uric acid, which may be elevated and cause gout symptoms
- Monitor liver studies weekly: ALT (SGPT), AST (SGOT), bilirubin; hepatic status: decreased appetite, jaundice, dark urine, fatigue
- Monitor renal status: before therapy and monthly thereafter: BUN, creatinine, output, sp gr, urinalysis
- Monitor mental status often: affect, mood, behavioral changes; psychosis may occur

Associated nursing diagnoses

- ✓ Infection, risk for (uses)
- ✓ Diarrhea (adverse reactions)
- ✓ Injury, risk for (adverse reactions)
- ✓ Knowledge deficit (teaching)
- ✓ Noncompliance (teaching)

P

Implementation

PO route

- Give with meals to decrease GI symptoms
- Give antiemetic if vomiting occurs

Patient/family education

- Instruct patient that compliance with dosage schedule, duration is necessary; that scheduled appointments must be kept or relapse may occur
- Advise diabetic patient to use blood glucose monitor to obtain correct result
- Advise patient to report

weakness, fatigue, loss of appetite, nausea, vomiting, yellowing of skin or eyes, sore throat, glossitis

Evaluation

Positive therapeutic outcome
- Decreased symptoms of toxolasmosis
- Decreased symptoms of *Pneumocystis carinii* pneumonia

quazepam

(kway'ze-pam)

Doral

Func. class.: Sedative-hypnotic

Chem. class.: Benzodiazepine derivative

Pregnancy category **X**

Controlled substance schedule **IV (USA)**

Action: Depresses subcortical levels of CNS, including limbic system, reticular formation; potentiates GABA (gamma aminobutryic acid)

➔ **Therapeutic Outcome:** Decreased insomnia

Uses: Insomnia (short-term)

Dosage and routes

Adult: PO 15 mg hs; then 7.5-15 mg hs

G ***Elderly:*** PO 15 mg hs × 2 days, then 7.5 mg hs

Available forms: Tab 7.5, 15 mg

Side effects/adverse reactions

CNS: Lethargy, drowsiness, daytime sedation, dizziness, confusion, lightheadedness, headache, anxiety, irritability, weakness, tremor, depression
CV: Chest pain, pulse changes, palpitations, tachycardia
GI: Nausea, vomiting, diarrhea, heartburn, abdominal pain, constipation, anorexia, taste alteration
HEMA: Leukopenia, granulocytopenia (rare)
MISC: Joint pain, congestion, dermatitis, sweating

Contraindications: Hypersensitivity to benzodiazepines, pregnancy **X**, lactation

Precautions: Hepatic disease, renal disease, suicidal individuals, drug abuse, G elderly, psychosis, P child <18 yr, lactation, depression, pulmonary insufficiency

Pharmacokinetics

Absorption	Well absorbed (PO)
Distribution	Crosses placenta, >95% bound to plasma proteins
Metabolism	Liver—extensively, to active metabolite
Excretion	Kidneys
Half-life	39 hr, active metabolite 70-75 hr

Pharmacodynamics

	PO
Onset	15-45 min
Peak	2 hr
Duration	8 hr

Interactions

Drug/drug:

Individual drugs

Alcohol: ↑ CNS depression
Cimetidine: ↑ action
Fluoxetine: ↑ action
Levodopa: ↓ action of levodopa
Propoxyphene: ↑ action
Rifampin: ↓ action of quazepam
Valproic acid: ↑ action

Drug classifications

Analgesics, opioid: ↑ CNS depression
Antidepressants: ↑ CNS depression
Antihistamines: ↑ CNS depression
Barbiturates: ↓ effect of quazepam
Oral contraceptives: ↑ effect of quazepam

Lab test interferences

Increase: AST (SGOT)/ALT (SGPT), serum bilirubin
False increase: 17-OHCS
Decrease: RAIU

NURSING CONSIDERATIONS

Assessment

- Assess patient's mental status: mood, sensorium, anxiety, affect, sleeping pattern, drowsiness, dizziness, especially G elderly; physical dependency, withdrawal symptoms: anxiety, panic attacks, agitation, convulsions, headache, nausea, vomiting, muscle pain, weakness; suicidal tendencies; for indications of increasing tolerance and abuse
- Monitor B/P (lying, standing), pulse; if systolic B/P drops 20 mm Hg, hold drug, notify prescriber
- Monitor blood studies: CBC during long-term therapy; blood dycrasias have occurred rarely; decreased hematocrit, neutropenia may occur
- Monitor hepatic studies: AST (SGOT), ALT (SGPT), bilirubin, creatinine LDH, alk phosphatase
- Monitor I&O; indicate renal dysfunction

Associated nursing diagnoses

✓ Anxiety (uses)
✓ Depression (uses)
✓ Injury, risk for (adverse reactions)
✓ Knowledge deficit (teaching)

Implementation

PO route

- Give with food or milk for GI symptoms; tab may be crushed and mixed with foods or fluids if patient is unable to swallow medication whole
- Give sugarless gum, hard candy, frequent sips of water for dry mouth

Patient/family education

- Inform patient that drug may be taken with food or fluids and that tab may be crushed or swallowed whole
- Caution patient not to use for everyday stress or longer than 3 mo unless directed by prescriber; not to take more than prescribed amount; may be habit-forming; not to double doses or skip doses
- Advise patient to avoid OTC preparations unless approved by health care prescriber; alcohol and CNS depressants will increase CNS depression

Q

• Caution patient to avoid driving, activities that require alertness because drowsiness may occur; to avoid alcohol ingestion or other psychotropic medications; to rise slowly or fainting may occur, especially G elderly; that drowsiness may worsen at beginning of treatment

• Advise patient not to discontinue medication abruptly after long-term use; withdrawal symptoms include vomiting, cramping, tremors, seizures

Evaluation

Positive therapeutic outcome

• Decreased anxiety, restlessness, sleeplessness (short-term treatment only)

Treatment of overdose: Lavage, VS, supportive care

quinapril

(kwin'a-pril)

Accupril

Func. class.: Antihypertensive

Chem. class.: Angiotensin-converting enzyme (ACE) inhibitor

Pregnancy category D

Action: Selectively suppresses renin-angiotensin-aldosterone system; inhibits ACE, prevents conversion of angiotensin I to angiotensin II; results in dilation of arterial, venous vessels

➡ **Therapeutic Outcome:** Decreased B/P in hypertension

Uses: Hypertension, alone or in combination with thiazide diuretics

Dosage and routes

Hypertension

Adult: PO 10 mg qd initially, then 20-80 mg/day divided bid or qd

Congestive heart failure

Adult: PO 2.5 mg initially, then 5-40 mg/day maintenance dose given qd or in 2 divided doses

Available forms: Tab 5, 10, 20, 40 mg

Side effects/adverse reactions

CNS: Headache, dizziness, fatigue, somnolence, depression, malaise, nervousness, vertigo

CV: Hypotension, postural hypotension, syncope, palpitations, angina pectoris, MI, tachycardia, vasodilation

GI: Nausea, constipation, vomiting, gastritis, GI hemorrhage, dry mouth

GU: Increased BUN, creatinine, decreased libido, impotence, urinary tract infection

HEMA: Thrombocytopenia, agranulocytosis

INTEG: ***Angioedema,*** rash, sweating, photosensitivity, pruritus

META: Hyperkalemia

MISC: Back pain, amblyopia, pharyngitis

MS: Arthralgia, arthritis, myalgia

RESP: Cough, bronchitis

Contraindications: Hypersensitivity to ACE inhibitors, P pregnancy **D**, children

Precautions: Impaired renal and liver function, dialysis patients, hypovolemia, blood dyscrasias, COPD, asthma, G elderly, lactation

Pharmacokinetics

Absorption	Well absorbed (PO)
Distribution	Unknown, crosses placenta
Metabolism	Unknown
Execution	Unknown
Half-life	2 hr

Pharmacodynamics

	PO
Onset	½-1 hr
Peak	2-6 hr
Duration	12-24 hr

Interactions

Drug/drug:

Individual drugs

Alcohol: ↑ hypotension (large amounts)
Allopurinol: ↑ hypersensitivity
Hydralazine: ↑ toxicity
Indomethacin: ↓ antihypertensive effect
Lithium: ↑ serum levels
Prazosin: ↑ toxicity

Drug classifications

Adrenergic blockers: ↑ hypotension
Antacids: ↓ absorption
Antihypertensives: ↑ hypotension
Diuretics: ↑ hypotension
Diuretics, potassium-sparing: ↑ toxicity
Ganglionic blockers: ↑ hypotension
Potassium supplements: ↑ toxicity
Sympathomimetics: ↑ toxicity

Lab test interferences

False positive: Urine acetone

NURSING CONSIDERATIONS

Assessment

- Monitor blood studies: neutrophils, decreased platelets
- Monitor B/P, check for orthostatic hypotension, syncope; if changes occur dosage change may be required
- Monitor renal studies: protein, BUN, creatinine; watch for increased levels that may indicate nephrotic syndrome and renal failure; monitor renal symptoms: polyuria, oliguria, frequency, dysuria
- Establish baselines in renal, liver function tests before therapy begins
- Check potassium levels throughout treatment, although hyperkalemia rarely occurs
- Check for edema in feet, legs daily
- Assess for allergic reactions: rash, fever, pruritus, urticaria; drug should be discontinued if antihistamines fail to help

Associated nursing diagnoses

- ✓ Cardiac output, decreased (uses)
- ✓ Injury, risk for physical (adverse reactions)
- ✓ Knowledge deficit (teaching)
- ✓ Noncompliance (teaching)

Q

Implementation

PO route

- Store in airtight container at 86° F (30° C) or less
- Severe hypotension may occur after 1st dose of this medication; may be prevented by reducing or discontinuing diuretic therapy 3 days before beginning quinapril therapy

Patient/family education

- Advise patient not to discontinue drug abruptly; advise patient to tell all persons associated with his care
- Teach patient not to use OTC products (cough, cold, allergy) unless directed by physician; serious side effects can occur
- Inform patient that xanthines such as coffee, tea, chocolate, cola can prevent action of drug
- Caution patient on the importance of complying with dosage schedule, even if feeling better; to continue with medical regimen to decrease B/P: exercise, cessation of smoking, decreasing stress, diet modifications
- Emphasize the need to rise slowly to sitting or standing position to minimize orthostatic hypotension; not to exercise in hot weather or increased hypotension can occur
- Teach patient to notify prescriber of mouth sores, sore throat, fever, swelling of hands or feet, irregular heartbeat, chest pain, coughing, shortness of breath
- Caution patient to report excessive perspiration, dehydration, vomiting, diarrhea; may lead to fall in B/P
- Caution patient that drug may cause dizziness, fainting, light headedness; may occur during 1st few days of therapy; to avoid activities that may be hazardous
- Teach patient how to take B/P, and normal readings for age group

Evaluation

Positive therapeutic outcome

- Decreased B/P in hypertension

Treatment of overdose: 0.9% NaCl **IV** INF, hemodialysis

quinidine gluconate/ quinidine polygalacturonase/ quinidine sulfate 🔑

(kwin'i-deen)

Apo-Quinidine ♣, Cin-Quin, Duraquin, Novoquinidin ♣, Quinaglute, Quinalan, quinidine gluconate; Cardioquin; Quinidex Extentabs, quinidine sulfate, Quinora

Func. class.: Antidysrhythmic (Class IA)

Chem. class.: Quinine dextro isomer

Action: Prolongs action, potential duration, and effective refractory period, thus decreasing myocardial excitability; anticholinergic properties

Therapeutic Outcome: Treatment of dysrhythmias

Uses: PVCs, atrial fibrillation, PAT, ventricular tachycardia, atrial dysrhythmias

Investigational uses: Malaria/**IV** quinidine gluconate

Dosage and routes

Quinidine sulfate

Atrial fibrillation/flutter

Adult: PO 200 mg q2-3h × 5-8 doses; may increase qd until sinus rhythm is restored; max 4 g/day given only after digitalization

Paroxysmal supraventricular tachycardia

Adult: PO 400-600 mg q2-3h, then 200-300 mg q6-8h or 300-600 mg q8-12h (sus rel)

Premature atrial/ventricular contraction

Adult: PO 200-300 mg q6-8h or 300-600 mg (sus rel) q8-12h, not to exceed 4 g/day

P *Child:* PO 6mg/kg or 180 mg/m^2 5/day

Quinidine gluconate

Adult: PO 324-660 mg q6-12h (sus rel); IM 600 mg, then 400 mg q2h; **IV** give 16 mg/min

Quinidine polygalacteronate

Adult: PO 275-825 mg q3-4h × 4 doses, then increase by 137.5-275 mg; repeat up to 4 × until dysrhythmia decreases

P *Child:* PO 8.25 mg/kg (247.5 mg/m^2) 5/day

Available forms: (Gluconate) tab sus rel 324, 330 mg; inj gluconate 80 mg/ml; (Sulfate) tab 200, 300 mg; tab sus rel 300 mg; (polygalacturonase) tab 275 mg

Side effects/adverse reactions

CNS: Headache, dizziness, involuntary movement, confusion, psychosis, restlessness, irritability, syncope, excitement

CV: Hypotension, bradycardia, PVCs, ***heart block, cardiovascular collapse, arrest***

EENT: Cinchonism: tinnitus, blurred vision, hearing loss, mydriasis, disturbed color vision

GI: Nausea, vomiting, anorexia, *diarrhea,* ***hepatotoxicity***

HEMA: ***Thrombocytopenia,*** hemolytic anemia, agranulocytosis, hypoprothrombinemia

INTEG: Rash, urticaria, angioedema, swelling, photosensitivity

RESP: Dyspnea, ***respiratory depression***

Contraindications: Hypersensitivity, blood dyscrasias, severe heart block, myasthenia gravis

Precautions: Pregnancy **C**, P lactation, children, renal disease, K imbalance, liver disease, CHF, respiratory depression

Q

Pharmacodynamics

	PO (SULFATE)	PO-SR	PO (GLUCONATE)	PO (POLYGALACTERONASE)	IM	IV
Onset	½ hr	Unknown	Unknown	Unknown	½ hr	5 min
Peak	1-1½ hr	4 hr	4 hr	6 hr	½-1½ hr	Unknown
Duration	6-8 hr	8-12 hr	6-8 hr	8-12 hr	6-8 hr	6-8 hr

Pharmacokinetics

Absorption	Well absorbed (PO, IM), slowly absorbed (sus-rel)
Distribution	Widely distributed, crosses placenta
Metabolism	Liver
Excretion	Kidney unchanged, breast milk
Half-life	6-8 hr

Interactions

Drug/drug:

Individual drugs

Amiodarone: ↑ toxicity
Cimetidine: ↑ effects of quinidine
Coumadin: ↑ levels of coumadin
Digoxin: ↑ blood levels, ↑ toxicity
Nifedipine: ↓ effects of quinidine
Phenytoin: ↓ effects of quinidine
Propranolol: ↑ effects of quinidine
Rifampin: ↓ effects of quinidine
Verapamil: ↑ effects of quinidine

Drug classifications

Anticoagulants (oral): ↑ levels of anticoagulant
Anticholinergics: ↑ vagolytic effects
Antacids: ↑ effects of quinidine
Barbiturates: ↓ effects of quinidine
Thiazide diuretics: ↑ effects of quinidine
Antidysrhythmics: ↑ cardiac depression
Phenothiazines: ↑ cardiac depression

Lab test interferences

Increase: CPK

NURSING CONSIDERATIONS

Assessment

- Monitor ECG continuously to determine drug effectiveness, measure PR, QRS, QT intervals, check for PVCs, other dysrhythmias; monitor B/P continuously for hypotension, hypertension; for rebound hypertension after 1-2 hr; check for dehydration or hypovolemia
- Monitor I&O ratio; electrolytes: [K (potassium), Na (sodium), Cl (Chloride)]; check weight daily; check for signs of CHG or pulmonary toxicity: dyspnea, fatigue, cough, fever, chest pain; if these occur, drug should be discontinued
- Monitor liver function studies: AST (SGOT), ALT (SGPT), bilirubin, alk phosphatase
- Assess for CNS symptoms:

confusion, psychosis, numbness, depression, involuntary movements; if these occur, drug should be discontinued
• Monitor cardiac rate, respiration: rate, rhythm, character, chest pain; watch for ventricular tachycardia, supraventricular tachycardia, or fibrillation that indicates toxicity

Associated nursing diagnoses

✓ Cardiac output, decreased (uses)
✓ Impaired gas exchange (adverse reactions)
✓ Knowledge deficit (teaching)

Implementation

PO route
• Give on an empty stomach with a full glass of water
• May be given with meals if GI irritation occurs, absorption will be decreased
• Tab may be crushed and mixed with fluid or foods for patients with swallowing difficulties; do not break, chew or crush sus rel tab

IV **IV route**
• Give by intermittent inf after diluting 800 mg/50 ml D_5W (Gluconate) (16 mg/ml) give at 1 ml/min or less using an inf pump for correct dose
• Do not use colored sol or sol with precipitate
• Diluted quinidine is stable for 24 hr at room temp

Y-site compatibilities:

Diazepam, milrinone

Y-site incompatibility:

Furosemide

Additive compatibilities:

Bretylium, cimetidine, milrinone, verapamil

Additive incompatibilities:

Amiodarone

Patient/family education

• Instruct patient to report adverse effects immediately to prescriber
• Caution patient that dark glasses may be needed for photophobia; to use sunscreen, protective clothing, or stay out of sun to prevent burns
• Instruct patient to complete follow-up appointment with health care provider including pulmonary function studies, chest x-ray, ophth and otoscopic examinations

Treatment of overdose:

O_2, artificial ventilation, ECG, administer dopamine for circulatory depression, administer diazepam or thiopental for convulsions, isoproterenol

ramipril

(ra-mi′pril)
Altace
Func. class.: Antihypertensive
Chem. class.: Angiotensin-converting enzyme (ACE) inhibitor
Pregnancy category **D**

Action: Selectively suppresses renin-angiotensin-aldosterone system; inhibits ACE; prevents conversion of angiotensin I to angiotensin II; results in dila-

R

tion of arterial, venous vessels

➔ **Therapeutic Outcome:** Decreased B/P in hypertension

Uses: Hypertension, alone or in combination with thiazide diuretics

Dosage and routes

Adult: PO 2.5 mg qd initially, then 2.5-20 mg/day divided bid or qd; renal impairment: 1.25 mg qd with CrCl <40 ml/min/1.73 m^2, increase as needed to max or 5 mg/day

Available forms: Cap 1.25, 2.5, 5, 10 mg

Side effects/adverse reactions

CNS: *Headache, dizziness,* anxiety, insomnia, paresthesia, fatigue, depression, malaise, vertigo, ***convulsions,*** hearing loss

CV: *Hypotension,* chest pain, palpitations, angina, syncope, dysrhythmia

GI: Nausea, constipation, vomiting, dyspepsia, dysphagia, anorexia, diarrhea, abdominal pain

GU: ***Proteinuria,*** increased BUN, creatinine, impotence

HEMA: Decreased Hct, Hgb, ***eosinophilia, leukopenia***

INTEG: ***Angioedema,*** rash, sweating, photosensitivity, pruritus

META: Hyperkalemia

MS: Arthralgia, arthritis, myalgia

RESP: Cough, dyspnea

Contraindications: Hypersensitivity to ACE inhibitors, pregnancy **D**, lactation, P children

Precautions: Impaired renal and liver function, dialysis patients, hypovolemia, blood dyscrasias, COPD, asthma, G elderly

Pharmacokinetics

Absorption	Well absorbed
Distribution	Not known, crosses placenta
Metabolism	Liver, extensively
Half-life	Ramipril (5 hr), ramiprilat (24 hr)

Pharmacodynamics

	PO
Onset	½-1 hr
Peak	6-8 hr
Duration	24-72 hr

Interactions

Drug/drug:

Individual drugs

Alcohol: ↑ hypotension (large amounts)
Allopurinol: ↑ hypersensitivity
Digoxin: ↑ serum levels
Hydralazine: ↑ toxicity
Indomethacin: ↓ antihypertensive effect
Lithium: ↑ serum levels
Prazosin: ↑ toxicity

Drug classifications

Adrenergic blockers: ↑ hypotension
Antacids: ↓ absorption
Antihypertensives: ↑ hypotension
Diuretics: ↑ hypotension
Diuretics, potassium sparing: ↑ toxicity

Ganglionic blockers: ↑ hypotension
Potassium supplements: ↑ toxicity
Sympathomimetics: ↑ toxicity

Lab test interferences
False positive: Urine acetone

NURSING CONSIDERATIONS
Assessment
- Monitor blood studies: neutrophils, decreased platelets
- Monitor B/P, check for orthostatic hypotension, syncope; if changes occur, dosage may need to be changed
- Monitor renal studies: protein, BUN, creatinine; watch for increased levels that may indicate nephrotic syndrome and renal failure; monitor renal symptoms: polyuria, oliguria, frequency, dysuria
- Establish baselines in renal, liver function tests before therapy begins
- Check potassium levels throughout treatment, although hyperkalemia rarely occurs
- Check for edema in feet, legs daily
- Assess for allergic reactions: rash, fever, pruritus, urticaria; drug should be discontinued if antihistamines fail to help

Associated nursing diagnoses
✓ Cardiac output, decreased (uses)
✓ Injury, risk for (side effects)
✓ Knowledge deficit (teaching)
✓ Noncompliance (teaching)

Implementation
PO route
- Store in air-tight container at 86° F (30° C) or less
- Severe hypotension may occur after 1st dose of this medication; decreased hypotension may be prevented by reducing or discontinuing diuretic therapy 3 days before beginning benazepril therapy
- Give **IV** inf of 0.9% NaCl (as ordered) to expand fluid volume if severe hypotension occurs

Patient/family education
- Caution patient not to discontinue drug abruptly; advise patient to tell all persons associated with his care
- Teach patient not to use OTC products (cough, cold, allergy) unless directed by physician; serious side effects can occur—xanthines such as coffee, tea, chocolate, cola can prevent action of drug.
- Instruct patient on the importance of complying with dosage schedule, even if feeling better; to continue with medical regimen to decrease B/P: exercise, cessation of smoking, decreasing stress, diet modifications
- Emphasize the need to rise slowly to sitting or standing position to minimize orthostatic hypotension; not to exercise in hot weather because increased hypotension can occur
- Teach patient to notify prescriber of mouth sores, sore throat, fever, swelling of hands or feet, irregular heartbeat, chest pain, coughing, shortness of breath

• Caution patient to report excessive perspiration, dehydration, vomiting, diarrhea; may lead to fall in B/P
• Caution patient that drug may cause dizziness, fainting, light headedness; may occur during 1st few days of therapy; to avoid activities that may be hazardous
• Teach patient how to take B/P, and normal readings for age group

Evaluation

Positive therapeutic outcome
• Decreased B/P in hypertension

Treatment of overdose: 0.9% NaCl **IV** inf, hemodialysis

ranitidine

(ra-nit-ti-deen)
Apo-Ranitidine ✦, Zantac, Zantac-C ✦
Func. class.: H_2 histamine receptor antagonist
Pregnancy category **B**

Action: Inhibits histamine at H_2 receptor site in the gastric parietal cells, which inhibits gastric acid secretion

Therapeutic Outcome: Healing of duodenal ulcers or gastric ulcers; prevention of duodenal ulcers; decreases symptoms of GERD or Zollinger-Ellison syndrome

Uses: Short-term treatment of duodenal and gastric ulcers and maintenance; management of gastroesophageal reflux disease (GERD) Zollinger-Ellison syndrome

Investigational uses: Prevention of aspiration pneumonitis, stress ulcers, upper GI bleeding

Dosage and routes

Adult: PO 150 mg bid, 300 mg hs; IM 50 mg q6-8h; **IV** bol 50 mg diluted to 20 ml over 5 min q6-8h; **IV** int inf 50 mg/100 ml D_5 over 15-20 min, q6-8h

Available forms: Tab 150, 300 mg; inj 0.5, 25 mg/ml; cap ✦ 150, 300 mg; syr 15 mg/ml

Side effects/adverse reactions

CNS: Headache, sleeplessness, dizziness, confusion, agitation, depression, hallucination
CV: Tachycardia, bradycardia, PVCs
EENT: Blurred vision, increased ocular pressure
GI: Constipation, abdominal pain, diarrhea, nausea, vomiting, ***hepatotoxicity***
GU: Impotence, gynecomastia
INTEG: Urticaria, rash, fever

Contraindications: Hypersensitivity

Precautions: Pregnancy **B**, P lactation, child <12 yr, hepatic disease, renal disease

Pharmacokinetics

Absorption	Well absorbed (PO, IM), completely absorbed (IV)
Distribution	Widely distributed, crosses placenta
Metabolism	Liver (30%)
Excretion	Kidneys unchanged (70%)
Half-life	2-3 hr, ↑ renal disease

Pharmacodynamics

	PO	IV/IM
Onset	Unknown	Unknown
Peak	2-3 hr	15 min
Duration	8-12 hr	8-12 hr

Interactions

Drug/drug:

Individual drugs

Ketoconazole: ↓ absorption of ranitidine

Drug classifications

Antacids: ↓ absorption of ranitidine

Drug/smoking:

↓ effectiveness

Lab test interferences

Increase: Alk phosphatase, AST (SGOT), creatinine
False positive: Gastric bleeding test

NURSING CONSIDERATIONS

Assessment

- Assess patient with ulcers or suspected ulcers: epigastric or abdominal pain, hematemesis, occult blood in stools, blood in gastric aspirate prior to and throughout treatment, monitor gastric pH (5 should be maintained)
- Monitor I&O ratio, BUN, creatinine, CBC with differential monthly

Associated nursing diagnoses

✓ Pain (uses)
✓ Knowledge deficit (teaching)

Implementation

PO route

- May be given with or without meals
- Give antacids 1 hr before or 1 hr after this drug

IV **IV route**

Direct **IV**

- Give by direct **IV** after diluting 50 mg/20 ml of 0.9% D_5W, NaCl given over 5 min or more

Intermittent inf

- Give by intermittent inf over 15 min after diluting 50 mg/100 ml D_5W, 0.9% NaCl

Continuous inf

- Give by continuous inf for a concentration 150 mg/250 ml, give 6.25 mg/hr
- Give Zollinger-Ellison patients up to a conc of 2.5 mg/ml at 1 mg/kg/hr initially

Syringe compatibilities:

Atropine, cyclizine, dexameth asone, dimenhydrinate, diphenhydramine, fentanyl, glycopyrrolate, hydromorphone, meperidine, metoclopramide, morphine, nalbuphine, oxmorphone, pentazocine, perphenizine, prochloperizine, promethazine, scopolamine, thiethyl perazine

Syringe incompatibilities:

Hydroxyzine, methotrimeprazine, midazolam, pentobarbital, phenobarbital

R

Y-site compatibilities:
Acyclovir, aminophylline, atracurium, bretylium, dobutamine, dopamine, enalaprilat, esmolol, fludarabine, foscarnet, heparin, labetalol, meperidine, morphine, nitroglycerin, ondansetron, pancuronium, procainamide, sargramostim, vecuronium, zidovudine

Additive compatibilities:
Amikacin, chloramphenicol, doxycycline, furosemide, gentamicin, heparin, lidocaine, penicillin G sodium, potassium chloride, ticarcillin, tobramycin, vancomycin

Additive incompatibilities:
Amphotericin B, clindamycin

Patient/family education
- Caution patient that gynecomastia, impotence may occur and are reversible after treatment is discontinued
- Advise patient to avoid driving, other hazardous activities until stabilized on this medication; drowsiness or dizziness may occur
- Caution patient to avoid black pepper, caffeine, alcohol, harsh spices, extremes in temp of food; tell patient to avoid OTC preparations: aspirin, cough, cold preparations because condition may worsen
- Inform patient that smoking decreases the effectiveness of the drug; that smoking cessation should be considered
- Instruct patient that drug must be continued for prescribed time to be effective and taken exactly as prescribed; doses should not be doubled; a missed dose should be taken when remembered up to 1 hr before next dose
- Advise patient to report bruising, fatigue, malaise; blood dyscrasias may occur
- Inform patient to report diarrhea, black tarry stools, sore throat, rash, dizziness, confusion, rash or delirium to prescriber immediately

Evaluation

Positive therapeutic outcome
- Decreased pain in abdomen
- Healing of ulcers
- Absence of gastroesophageal reflex

reserpine
(re-ser′peen)

Novoreserpine ✤, Reserfia ✤, Serpalan, Serpasil

Func. class.: Antihypertensive

Chem. class.: Antiadrenergic agent (peripherally acting)

Pregnancy category D

Action: Inhibits norepinephrine release, depleting norepinephrine stores in adrenergic nerve endings

➔ Therapeutic Outcome: Decreased B/P

Uses: Hypertension

Dosage and routes

Hypertension

Adult: PO 0.25-0.5 mg qd × 1-2 wk, then 0.1-0.25 mg qd for maintenance

P *Child:* PO 0.07 mg/kg or 2 mg/m^2 given with hydralazine IM q12-24h

Available forms: Tab 0.1, 0.2, 0.25, 1 mg

Side effects/adverse reactions

CNS: *Drowsiness, fatigue, lethargy, dizziness,* depression, anxiety, headache, increased dreaming, nightmares, convulsions, parkinsonism, EPS (high doses)
CV: *Bradycardia,* chest pain, dysrhythmias, prolonged bleeding time, ***thrombocytopenia,*** purpura
EENT: Lacrimation, miosis, blurred vision, ptosis, dry mouth, epistaxis
GI: Nausea, vomiting, cramps, peptic ulcer, dry mouth, increased appetite, anorexia
GU: Impotence, dysuria, nocturia, Na and H_2O retention, edema, breast engorgement, galactorrhea, gynecomastia
INTEG: Rash, purpura, alopecia, flushing, warm feeling, pruritus, ecchymosis
RESP: ***Bronchospasm,*** dyspnea, cough, rales

Contraindications: Hypersensitivity, depression, suicidal patients, active peptic ulcer disease, ulcerative colitis, pregnancy **D**, Parkinson's disease

Precautions: Lactation, seizure disorders, renal disease

Pharmacokinetics

Absorption	40%-50%
Distribution	Widely distributed, crosses placenta
Metabolism	Liver
Excretion	Feces 50% unabsorbed drug, kidneys small amounts
Half-life	11 days

Pharmacodynamics

	PO
Onset	Unknown
Peak	4 hr
Duration	1-6 wk

Interactions

Drug/drug:

Individual drugs
Alcohol: ↑ CNS depression

Drug classifications
Amphetamines: ↓ hypotensive effects
Anesthetics: ↑ CNS depression
Antidepressants, tricyclic: ↓ hypotensive effects
β-blockers: ↑ bradycardia
Cardiac glycosides: ↑ bradycardia
Diuretics: ↑ hypotensive effects
Hypnotics: ↑ CNS depression
Narcotics: ↑ CNS depression
Nitrates: ↑ hypotensive effects
Sedatives: ↑ CNS depression

R

Lab test interferences

Increase: VMA excretion, 5-HIAA excretion, prolactin
Interferences: 17-OHCS, 17-KS

NURSING CONSIDERATIONS

Assessment

• Monitor B/P, orthostatic hypotension, syncope; check

for edema in feet, legs daily; check I&O; monitor for weight daily; notify prescriber of changes
- Assess for allergic reactions: rash, fever, pruritus, urticaria; drug should be discontinued if antihistamines fail to help
- Assess for orthostatic hypotension, tell patient to rise slowly from sitting or lying position

Associated nursing diagnoses

✓ Cardiac output, decreased (uses)
✓ Injury, risk for (adverse reactions)
✓ Knowledge deficit (teaching)
✓ Noncompliance (teaching)

Implementation

PO route
- Store in tight container at 86° F (30° C) or less
- May be used in combination with other antihypertensives
- May be given with food to prevent GI symptoms

Patient/family education

- Caution patient not to discontinue drug abruptly and about the importance of complying with dosage schedule, even if feeling better; if dose is missed take as soon as remembered; take dose at same time each day
- Teach patient not to use OTC products (cough, cold, allergy) unless directed by prescriber and to avoid large amounts of caffeine
- Emphasize the need to rise slowly to sitting or standing position to minimize orthostatic hypotension
- Teach patient to notify prescriber of swelling of hands or feet, irregular heartbeat, chest pain
- Caution patient to report excessive perspiration, dehydration, vomiting, diarrhea; may lead to fall in B/P
- Caution patient that drug may cause dizziness, fainting, light headedness; may occur during 1st few days of therapy; to avoid hazardous activities
- Teach patient how to take B/P, and normal readings for age group; to take B/P q7 days

Evaluation

Positive therapeutic outcome
- Decreased B/P in hypertension

Treatment of overdose:

Administer volume expanders or vasopressors; discontinue drug; place patient in supine position

Rh_o (d) immune globulin, human

HypoRho-D, MICRhoGAM, Mini-Gamulin RH, Hypo Rho-D Mini-Dose, Gamulin Rh, Rhesonatin, RhoGAM

Func. class.: IgG, Immunizing agent

Pregnancy category **C**

Action: Suppresses immune response of nonsensitized Rh_o (D or D^u)-negative patients who are exposed to Rh_o (D or D^u)-positive blood

Therapeutic Outcome: Absence of Rh factor and transfusion error

Uses: Prevention of isoimmunization in Rh-negative women exposed to Rh-positive blood given after abortions, miscarriages, amniocentesis

Dosage and routes

After delivery

Adult: IM 1 vial of fetal packed RBCs <15 ml, or 2 vials of fetal packed RBCs >15 ml; given within 72 hr of delivery or miscarriage

Before delivery

Adult: IM 1 vial (standard dose) at 26-28 wk, 1 vial (standard dose) 72 hr after delivery

Pregnancy termination <13 wk

Adult: IM 1 vial (micro dose) within 72 hr

Pregnancy termination >13 wk

Adult: IM 1 vial (standard dose) within 72 hr

Fetal-maternal hemorrhage

Adult: IM packed RBCs volume of hemorrhage/15 = needed vials (standard dose)

Transfusion error

Adult: IM—Give within 72 hr

Available forms: Inj single-dose vial (50 μg/vial-microdose, 300 μg/vial-standard)

Side effects/adverse reactions

CNS: Lethargy
INTEG: Irritation at inj site, fever
MS: Myalgia

Contraindications: Previous immunization with this drug, Rh_o (O)-positive/D^u-positive patient

Precautions: Pregnancy **C**

Pharmacokinetics	
Absorption	Well absorbed (IM)
Distribution	Unknown
Metabolism	Unknown
Excretion	Unknown
Half-life	Unknown

Pharmacodynamics	IM
Onset	Rapid
Peak	Unknown
Duration	Unknown

Interactions

Drug/drug:

Live virus vaccines: ↓ antibody response to vaccine

NURSING CONSIDERATIONS

Assessment

- Assess for allergies, reactions to immunizations; previous immunization with this drug
- Obtain type and cross-match of mother's blood and of neonate's cord blood. Neonate must be Rh_o(D)-positive, mother must be Rh_o(D)-negative and (D^u)-negative, medication should be given if there is a doubt

Associated nursing diagnoses

✓ Knowledge deficit (teaching)

R

Implementation

IM route

- Give after sending newborn's cord blood to lab after delivery for cross, match, type
- Give IM in deltoid; aspirate to prevent **IV** administration
- Give only equal lot numbers of drug, cross match
- Give only MICrhoGAM for abortions or miscarriages <13 wk unless fetus or father is Rh-negative
- Store in refrigerator

Patient/family education

- Teach patient how drug works; that drug must be given after subsequent deliveries if subsequent babies are Rh-positive

Evaluation

Positive therapeutic outcome

- Prevention of Rh_o(D) sensitization in transfusion error
- Prevention of erythroblastosis fetalis in subsequent Rh_o(D)-positive neonates

ribavarin

(rye-ba-vye'rin)

Virazole

Func. class.: Synthetic antiviral

Chem. class.: Tricyclic amine

Pregnancy category **X**

Action: Prevents replication of DNA and RNA synthesis

Therapeutic Outcome: Resolution of severe lower respiratory tract infections

Uses: Severe lower respiratory **P** tract infections in infants and children

Investigational uses: Influenza A or B (early)

Dosage and routes

P ***Infant/young children:*** Inh 300 ml of 200 mg/ml sol by mist × 12-18 h/day

Available forms: Powder for reconstitution for aerosol: 6 g/vial

Side effects/adverse reactions

CNS: Dizziness, faintness
CV: Hypotension, cardiac arrest
EENT: Eye irritation, conjunctivitis, blurred vision, photosensitivity
INTEG: Rash

Contraindications: Hypersen- **P** sitivity, lactation, child <1 yr, pregnancy **X**

Precautions: Epilepsy, hepatic disease, renal disease

Pharmacokinetics

Absorption	Inh (syst)
Distribution	To respiratory tract
Metabolism	Liver
Excretion	Respiratory tract
Half-life:	9½ hr

Pharmacodynamics

	INH
Onset	Unknown
Peak	Inh end
Duration	Unknown

Interactions

Drug/drug:

Individual drugs

Zidovudine: ↓ antiviral action, ↑ toxicity

Drug classification

Cardiac glycosides: ↑ toxicity

NURSING CONSIDERATIONS

Assessment

- Assess allergies before initiation of treatment, reaction of each medication; list allergies on chart in bright red letters
- Monitor respiratory status: rate, character, wheezing, tightness in chest
- Obtain C&S test results before starting treatment

Associated nursing diagnoses

✓ Infection, risk for (uses)
✓ Gas exchange, impaired (uses)
✓ Knowledge deficit (teaching)

Implementation

Inh route

- Give by the viratek SPAG (SPAG-2), do not use other inh equipment
- May be given by an oxygen hood for infants or a face mask may be attached to the SPAG-2
- Reconstitute 6 g sterile water for inj or inh, place sol in the Erlenmeyer flask and dilute further to 20 mg/ml

Patient/family education

- Teach patient and parents aspects of drug therapy

Evaluation

Positive therapeutic outcome
- Absence of RSV (respiratory syncytical virus)

riboflavin (vitamin B_2)

(rye'boo-flay-vin)

Func. class.: Vitamin B_2, water soluble

Pregnancy category A

Action: Needed for respiratory reactions (catalyzes proteins) and for normal vision

Therapeutic Outcome: Prevention or treatment of riboflavin deficiency

Uses: Vit B_2 deficiency or polyneuritis; cheilosis adjunct with thiamine

Dosage and routes

P ***Adult and child >12 yr:*** PO 5-50 mg qd in divided doses

P ***Child <12 yr:*** PO 2-10 mg qd, then 0.6 mg/1000 calories ingested

Available forms: Tab 10, 25, 50, 100 mg

Side effects/adverse reactions

GU: Yellow discoloration of urine (large doses)

P **Contraindications:** Child <12 yr

Precautions: Pregnancy **A**

R

Pharmacokinetics

Absorption	Well absorbed (by active transport)
Distribution	60% protein bound, widely distributed, crosses placenta
Metabolism	Unknown
Excretion	Kidneys (unchanged), excess amounts
Half-life	1-1½ hr

Pharmacodynamics

	PO
Onset	Unknown
Peak	Unknown
Duration	Unknown

Interactions

Drug/drug:

Individual drugs

Alcohol: ↑ riboflavin need
Probenicid: ↑ riboflavin need
Tetracycline: ↓ action of tetracycline

Drug classifications

Antidepressants, tricyclic: ↑ riboflavin need
Phenothiazines: ↑ riboflavin need

Lab test interferences

May cause false elevations of urinary catecholamines, urobilinogen

NURSING CONSIDERATIONS

Assessment

- Assess patient's nutritional status: liver, eggs, dairy products, yeast, whole grain, green vegetables
- Assess for vitamin B_2 deficiency: photophobia, cheilosis, stomatitis, ocular swelling

Associated nursing diagnoses

✓ Nutrition: less than body requirements (uses)
✓ Knowledge deficit (teaching)

Implementation

PO route

- Give with food for better absorption
- Store in tight, light-resistant container

Patient/family education

- Inform patient that urine may turn bright yellow
- Instruct patient about addition of needed foods that are rich in riboflavin

Evaluation

Positive therapeutic outcome

- Absence of headache, GI problems, cheilosis, skin lesions, depression, burning, itchy eyes, anemia

rifabutin

(riff'a-byoo-tin)
Mycobutin
Func. class.: Antimycobacterial
Chem. class.: Rifamycin S derivative
Pregnancy category **B**

Action: Inhibits DNA-dependent RNA polymerase in susceptible strains

➔ **Therapeutic Outcome:** Antimycobacterial death of *E. coli, B. subtilis,* and *M. avium*

Uses: Prevention of *M. avium* complex in patients with advanced HIV infection

Dosage and routes

Adult: 300 mg qd (may take as 150 mg bid)

Available forms: Cap 150 mg

Side effects/adverse reactions

CNS: Headache, fatigue, anxiety, confusion, insomnia
GI: Nausea, vomiting, anorexia, diarrhea, heartburn, hepatitis
GU: Hematuria
HEMA: Hemolytic anemia, eosinophilia, thrombocytopenia, leukopenia
INTEG: Rash
MISC: Flulike syndrome, shortness of breath, chest pressure
MS: Asthenia, arthralgia, myalgia

Contraindications: Hypersensitivity, active TB

Precautions: Pregnancy **B**, lactation, hepatic disease, P blood dyscrasias, children

Pharmacokinetics

Absorption	Well absorbed (PO)
Distribution	Widely distributed
Metabolism	Liver
Excretion	Kidney
Half-life	45 hr

Pharmacodynamics

	PO
Onset	Unknown
Peak	2-3 hr

Interactions

Drug/drug:

Individual drugs
Alcohol: ↑ toxicity
Carbamazepine: ↑ toxicity
Cycloserine: ↑ toxicity
Ethionamide: ↑ toxicity
Rifampin: ↑ toxicity

Drug classifications
Antacids, aluminum: ↓ absorption

NURSING CONSIDERATIONS

Assessment

- Assess for active tuberculosis: chest x-ray, sputum culture, blood culture, biopsy of lymph nodes, obtain PPD test. Drug should be given only for Mycobacterium avium complex (MAC) and never for TB
- Monitor CBC for neutropenia, thrombocytopenia, eosinophilia

Associated nursing diagnoses

✓ Infection, risk for (uses)
✓ Diarrhea (adverse reaction)
✓ Injury, risk for (adverse reaction)
✓ Knowledge deficit (teaching)
✓ Noncompliance (teaching)

Implementation

PO route

- Give with meals to decrease GI symptoms; better to take on empty stomach 1 hr ac or 2 hr pc; high fat food slows absorption
- Give antiemetic if vomiting occurs

Patient/family education

- Caution patient that compliance with dosage schedule and duration is necessary

R

- Instruct patient that scheduled appointments must be kept or relapse may occur
- Instruct patient to notify prescriber if hepatitis, neutropenia, or thrombocytopenia occurs: sore throat, fever, bleeding, bruising, yellow sclera, anorexia, nausea, vomiting, fatigue, weakness
- Advise patient that urine, feces, saliva, sputum, sweat, tears, may be colored red-orange; soft contact lens may become permanently stained
- Caution patients using oral contraceptives to use a nonhormonal method of birth control because rifabutin may decrease efficiency of oral contraceptives

Evaluation

Positive therapeutic outcome

- Decreased symptoms of *M. avium* in patients with HIV

rifampin

(rif'am-pin)

Rifadin, Rifampicin, Rimactane, Rofact ♣

Func. class.: Antitubercular

Chem. class.: Rifamycin B derivative

Pregnancy category **C**

Action: Inhibits DNA-dependent polymerase, decreases replication

➡ **Therapeutic Outcome:** Bactericidal against the following organisms: mycobacteria, *Staphylococcus aureus, Hemophilus influenzae, Neisseria meningitides, Legionella pneumophilia*

Uses: Pulmonary tuberculosis, meningococcal carriers (prevention)

Dosage and routes

Tuberculosis

Adult: PO/**IV** 600 mg/day as single dose 1 hr ac or 2 hr pc or 10 mg/kg/day

P *Child >5 yr:* PO/**IV** 10-20 mg/kg/day as single dose 1 hr ac or 2 hr pc, not to exceed 600 mg/day, with other antituberculars

Meningococcal carriers

Adult: PO/**IV** 600 mg bid × 2 days

P *Child >5 yr:* PO/**IV** 10 mg/kg bid × 2 days, not to exceed 600 mg/dose

P *Infant 3 mo-1 yr:* 5 mg/kg PO bid for 2 days

Available forms: Caps 150, 300 mg; inj 600 mg/vial

Side effects/adverse reactions

CNS: Headache, fatigue, anxiety, drowsiness, confusion

EENT: Visual disturbances

GI: Nausea, vomiting, anorexia, diarrhea, ***pseudomembranous colitis,*** *heartburn,* sore mouth and tongue, pancreatitis

GU: ***Hematuria, acute renal failure, hemoglobinuria***

HEMA: ***Hemolytic anemia, eosinophilia, thrombocytopenia, leukopenia***

INTEG: Rash, pruritus, urticaria
MISC: Flulike syndrome, menstrual disturbances, edema, shortness of breath
MS: Ataxia, weakness

Contraindications: Hypersensitivity

Precautions: Pregnancy **C**, lactation, hepatic disease, blood dyscrasias

Pharmacokinetics

Absorption	Well absorbed (PO), completely absorbed (IV)
Distribution	Widely distributed, crosses placenta
Metabolism	Liver—extensively
Excretion	Feces
Half-life	3 hr

Pharmacodynamics

	PO	IV
Onset	Rapid	Rapid
Peak	2-3 hr	Inf end

Interactions
Drug/drug:
Individual drugs
Alcohol: ↑ toxicity
Chloramphenicol: ↓ effect of chloramphenicol
Disopyramide: ↓ effect of disopyramide
Fluconazole: ↓ effect of fluconazole
Isoniazid: ↑ toxicity
Ketoconazole: ↑ toxicity
Miconazole: ↑ toxicity
Phenytoin: ↓ effect of phenytoin
Quinidine: ↓ effect of quinidine
Theophylline: ↓ effect of theophylline
Tocainide: ↓ effect of tocainide
Verapamil: ↓ effect of verapamil
Drug classifications
Analgesics, narcotic: ↓ effect
Glucocorticoids: ↓ effect
Oral contraceptives: ↓ effect

NURSING CONSIDERATIONS
Assessment
- Monitor liver studies qwk: ALT (SGPT), AST (SGOT), bilirubin
- Renal status: before, qmo: BUN, creatinine, output, specific gravity, urinalysis
- Mental status often: affect, mood, behavioral changes; psychosis may occur
- Hepatic status: decreased appetite, jaundice, dark urine, fatigue
- Assess for infection: sputum culture, lung sounds
- C&S tests should be performed prior to beginning treatment, during, and after therapy is completed

Associated nursing diagnoses
✓ Infection, risk for (uses)
✓ Diarrhea (adverse reactions)
✓ Injury, risk for (adverse reactions)
✓ Knowledge deficit (teaching)
✓ Noncompliance (teaching)

Implementation
PO route
- Administer with meals to decrease GI symptoms; better to take on empty stomach 1 hr ac or 2 hr pc

R

IV **IV route**

Intermittent **IV**

- Give by intermittent inf after reconstituting 600 mg/10 ml of sterile water for inj, agitate gently. Dilute further in 100 or 500 ml 0.9% NaCl or D_5W; give 100 ml/30 min or 500 ml/3 hr
- Do not mix with other drugs or sols

Patient/family education

- Instruct patient that compliance with dosage schedule, duration is necessary
- Instruct patient that scheduled appointments must be kept or relapse may occur
- Instruct patient to notify prescriber if hepatitis, neutropenia, or thrombocytopenia occurs: sore throat, fever, bleeding, bruising, yellow sclera, anorexia, nausea, vomiting, fatigue, weakness
- Advise patient that urine, feces, saliva, sputum, sweat, tears, may be colored red-orange; soft contact lens may be permanently stained
- Caution patient that patients using oral contraceptives should use a nonhormonal method of birth control because rifabutin may decrease the efficiency of oral contraceptives

Evaluation

Positive therapeutic outcome

- Decreased symptoms of TB

rimantadine

(ri-man'ti-deen)

Flumadine

Func. class.: Synthetic antiviral

Chem. class.: Tricyclic amine

Pregnancy category C

Action: Prevents uncoating of nucleic acid in viral cell, preventing penetration of virus to host; causes release of dopamine from neurons

➔ **Therapeutic Outcome:** Prevention of influenza type A

Uses: Prophylaxis or treatment of influenza type A

Dosage and routes

Influenza type A prophylaxis

Adult: PO 100 mg bid; in renal hepatic disease, lower dose to 100 mg/day

P *Child: <10 yr:* PO 5 mg/kg/day, not to exceed 150 mg

Treatment

Adult: PO 100 mg bid; in renal or hepatic disease, lower dose to 100 mg/day; start treatment at onset of symptoms, continue for at least 1 wk

Available forms: Tab 100 mg; syr 50 mg/5 ml

Side effects/adverse reactions

CNS: Headache, dizziness, fatigue, depression, hallucinations, tremors, ***convulsions,***

insomnia, poor concentration, asthenia, gait abnormalities
CV: Pallor, palpitations, hypertension
EENT: Tinnitus, taste abnormality, eye pain
GI: Nausea, vomiting, constipation, dry mouth, anorexia, abdominal pain, diarrhea, dyspepsia
INTEG: Rash

Contraindications: Hypersensitivity, lactation, child <1 yr, pregnancy **C**

P

Precautions: Epilepsy, hepatic disease, renal disease

Pharmacokinetics

Absorption	Minimally absorbed (PO)
Distribution	Widely distributed, crosses placenta, CSF concentration 50% plasma
Metabolism	Liver
Excretion	95% unchanged—kidneys
Half-life	2-3.5 hr, increased in renal disease

Pharmacodynamics

	PO	IV
Onset	Unknown	Rapid
Peak	1½-2½	Inf end

Interactions
Drug/drug:
Individual drugs
Amphotericin B: ↑ neurotoxicity, nephrotoxicity
Interferon: ↑ neurotoxicity, nephrotoxicity
Methotrexate: ↑ neurotoxicity, nephrotoxicity
Probenecid: ↑ neurotoxicity, nephrotoxicity

Drug classification
Aminoglycosides: ↑ neurotoxicity, nephrotoxicity

NURSING CONSIDERATIONS
Assessment
- Assess allergies before initiation of treatment, patient's reaction to each medication; list allergies on chart in bright red letters
- Monitor respiratory status: rate, character, wheezing, tightness in chest

Associated nursing diagnoses
✓ Infection, risk for (uses)
✓ Knowledge deficit (teaching)

Implementation
- Give before exposure to influenza; continue for 10 days after contact
- Give at least 4 hr before hs to prevent insomnia
- Administer pc for better absorption, to decrease GI symptoms; cap may be opened and mixed with food for easy swallowing
- Give in divided doses to prevent CNS disturbances: headache, dizziness, fatigue, drowsiness
- Store in tight, dry container

R

Patient/family education
- Instruct patient about aspects of drug therapy: need to report dyspnea, dizziness, poor concentration, behavioral changes
- Advise patient to avoid hazardous activities if dizziness occurs
- Caution patient to discuss with prescriber before taking

OTC medications, or alcohol —serious drug interactions may result

Evaluation

Positive therapeutic outcome
• Absence of fever, malaise, cough, dyspnea

Treatment of overdose: Withdraw drug, maintain airway, administer epinephrine, aminophylline, O_2, **IV** corticosteroids, physostigmine

risperidone
(res-pare'a-done)
Risperdal
Func. class: Antipsychotic/neuroleptic
Chem. class.: Benzisoxazole derivative
Pregnancy category **C**

Action: Unknown; may be mediated through both dopamine type 2 (D_2) and serotinin type 2 (5-HT_2) antagonism

Therapeutic Outcome: Decreased hallucination and disorganized thought

Uses: Psychotic disorders

Dosage and routes

Adult: PO 1 mg bid, with incremental increases of 1 mg bid on days 2 and 3 to a dose of 3 mg bid by day 3; then do not increase dose for at least 1 wk

Available forms: Tab 1, 2, 3, 4 mg

Side effects/adverse reactions

CNS: *Extrapyrimidal symptoms, pseudoparkinsonism, akathisia, dystonia, tardive dyskinesia, drowsiness, insomnia, agitation, anxiety, headache,* ***neuroleptic malignant syndrome***
CV: Orthostatic hypotension, ***tachycardia***
EENT: Blurred vision
GI: *Nausea,* vomiting, *anorexia, constipation,* jaundice, weight gain
RESP: Rhinitis

Contraindications: Hypersensitivity, lactation, seizure disorders

P **Precautions:** Children, renal disease, pregnancy **C,** hepatic G disease, elderly, breast cancer

Pharmacokinetics

Absorption	Unknown
Distribution	Unknown
Metabolism	Liver, extensively
Excretion	Unknown
Half-life	Unknown

Pharmacodynamics

	PO
Onset	Unknown
Peak	Unknown
Duration	Up to 12 hr

Interactions

Drug/drug:

Individual drugs
Alcohol: ↑ effects of both drugs, oversedation
Lithium: ↑ extrapyramidel symptoms, masking of lithium toxicity

Drug classifications

Antidepressants: ↑ CNS depression
Antihistamines: ↑ CNS depression
Barbiturate anesthetics: ↑ CNS depression
General anesthetics: ↑ CNS depression
MAO inhibitors: ↑ CNS depression
Narcotics: ↑ CNS depression
Sedative/hypnotics: ↑ CNS depression

Lab test interferences

Increase: Liver function tests, cardiac enzymes, cholesterol, blood glucose, prolactin, bilirubin, PBI, cholinesterase. I, alk phosphatase, leukocytes, granulocytes, platelets
Decrease: Hormones (blood and urine)
False positive: Pregnancy tests, PKU, urine bilirubin
False negative: Urinary steroids, 17-OCHS

NURSING CONSIDERATIONS

Assessment

- Assess mental status: orientation, mood, behavior, presence and type of hallucinations before initial administration and monthly; this drug should significantly reduce psychotic behavior
- Check that patient swallows all PO medication; check for hoarding or giving of medication to other patients
- Monitor I&O ratio, palpate bladder if low urinary output occurs, especially in elderly; urinalysis recommended before, during prolonged therapy
- Monitor bilirubin, CBC, liver function studies monthly
- Assess affect, orientation, LOC, reflexes, gait, coordination, sleep pattern disturbances
- Monitor B/P with patient in sitting, standing, and lying positions; take pulse and respirations q4h during initial treatment; establish baseline before starting treatment; report drops of 30 mm Hg; obtain baseline ECG; and Q-wave and T-wave changes
- Check for dizziness, faintness, palpitations, tachycardia on rising; severe orthostatic hypotension is common
- Identify for neuroleptic malignant syndrome: hyperpyrexia, muscle rigidity, increased CPK, altered mental status; drug should be discontinued
- Assess for extrapyramidal symptoms including akathisia (inability to sit still, no pattern to movements), tardive dyskinesia (bizarre movements of the jaw, mouth, tongue, extremities) pseudoparkinsonism (rigidity, tremors, pill rolling, shufling gait); an antiparkinson drug should be prescribed
- Assess for constipation, urinary retention daily; if these occur, increase bulk, water in diet

Associated nursing diagnoses

- ✓ Thought processes, altered (uses)
- ✓ Coping, ineffective individual (uses)
- ✓ Knowledge deficit (teaching)
- ✓ Noncompliance (teaching)

Implementation

PO route
- PO with full glass of water, milk; or give with food to decrease GI upset
- Store in airtight, light-resistant container

Patient/family education
- Teach patient to use good oral hygiene; frequent rinsing of mouth, sugarless gum for dry mouth
- Caution patient to avoid hazardous activities until drug response is determined—dizziness, blurred vision may occur
- Inform patient that orthostatic hypotension occurs often—patient should rise from sitting or lying position gradually and remain lying down for at least 30 min after IM inj
- Instruct patient to avoid hot tubs, hot showers, tub baths—hypotension may occur
- Inform patient that heat stroke may occur in hot weather, and to take extra precautions to stay cool
- Advise patient to avoid abrupt withdrawal of this drug, or extrapyramidal symptoms may result; drug should be withdrawn slowly
- Teach patient to avoid OTC preparations (cough, hayfever, cold) unless approved by prescriber—serious drug interactions may occur; avoid use with alcohol, CNS depressants because increased drowsiness may occur

Evaluation

Positive therapeutic outcome
- Decrease in emotional excitement, hallucinations, delusions, paranoia
- Reorganization of patterns of thought, speech

Treatment of overdose: Lavage, provide airway

roeuronium
(roe-ure-own-i-um)

Zemuron

Func. class.: Neuromuscular blocker (nondepolarizing)

Chem. class.: Biquaternary ammonium ester

Pregnancy category B

Action: Inhibits transmission of nerve impulses by binding with cholinergic receptor sites, antagonizing action of acetylcholine

➡ **Therapeutic Outcome:** Skeletal muscle paralysis after anesthesia

Uses: Facilitation of endotracheal intubation, skeletal muscle relaxation during mechanical ventilation, surgery, or general anesthesia

Dosage and routes
Adult: **IV** bol 600 μg/kg, may repeat with 75-225 μg/kg

Available forms: Inj **IV**

Side effects/adverse reactions
CV: Bradycardia, tachycardia, increase, decrease B/P
EENT: Increased secretions
INTEG: Rash, flushing, pruritus, urticaria

RESP: Prolonged apnea, bronchospasm, cyanosis, respiratory depression

Contraindications: Hypersensitivity

Precautions: Pregnancy **B,** cardiac disease, lactation, P children >2 yr, electrolyte imbalances, dehydration, neuromuscular disease, respiratory disease

Pharmacokinetics

Absorption	Complete bioavailability (IV)
Distribution	Unknown
Metabolism	Plasma
Excretion	Unknown
Half-life	71-203 min

Pharmacodynamics

	IV
Onset	Unknown
Peak	Unknown
Duration	30 min

Interactions

Drug/drug

Individual drugs

Phenylephrine: Blocking of roeuronium

Drug classifications

Anesthetics: ↑ effect of roeuronium

NURSING CONSIDERATIONS

Assessment

• Monitor for electrolyte imbalances (potassium, magnesium), before drug is used; electrolyte imbalances may lead to increased action of this drug

• Monitor vital signs (B/P, pulse, respirations, airway) until patient recovers fully; rate, depth, pattern of respirations, strength of hand grip; patient should be intubated before use

• Monitor recovery: decreased paralysis of face, diaphragm, leg, arm, rest of body; residual weakness and respiratory problems may occur during recovery period

• Monitor allergic reactions: rash, fever, respiratory distress, pruritus; drug should be discontinued

Associated nursing diagnoses

✓ Breathing pattern, ineffective (uses)

✓ Communication, impaired verbal (adverse reactions)

✓ Fear (adverse reactions)

✓ Knowledge deficit (teaching)

Implementation

IV **IV route**

• Using peripheral nerve stimulator by anesthesiologist to determine neuromuscular blockade; deep tendon reflexes should be monitored during extended periods

• Give **IV** undiluted by direct **IV** over 1 min (only by qualified person, usually an anesthesiologist); do not administer IM

• Maintenance is given q20-45 min after 1st dose; titrate to patient response

• Store in light-resistant area

Patient/family education

• Reassure patient if communication is difficult during recovery from neuromuscular blockade

R

- Explain all procedures or treatments to patient; patient will remain conscious if anesthetic is not given at the same time

Evaluation

Positive therapeutic outcome

- Paralysis of jaw, eyelid, head, neck, rest of body as evaluated by peripheral nerve stimulator

Treatment of overdose: Edrophonium or neostigmine, atropine, monitor VS; may require mechanical ventilation

salmeterol

(sal-met'er-ole)

Serevent

Func. class.: Adrenergic β_2 agonist

Pregnancy category **C**

Action: Causes bronchodilation by action on β_2 (pulmonary) receptors by increasing levels of cAMP, which relaxes smooth muscle; with very little effect on heart rate, maintains improvement in FEV from 3 to 12 hr; prevents nocturnal asthma symptoms

➔ **Therapeutic Outcome:** Ease of breathing

Uses: Prevention of exercise-induced asthma, bronchospasm

Dosage and routes

Adult: Inh 2 puffs bid (AM and PM)

Available forms: Aerosol

Side effects/adverse reactions

CNS: *Tremors, anxiety,* insomnia, headache, dizziness, stimulation, restlessness, hallucinations, flushing, irritability

CV: Palpitations, tachycardia, hypertension, angina, hypotension, dysrhythmias

EENT: Dry nose, irritation of nose and throat

GI: Heartburn, nausea, vomiting

MS: Muscle cramps

RESP: Bronchospasm

Contraindications: Hypersensitivity to sympathomimetics, tachydysrhythmias, severe cardiac disease

Precautions: Lactation, pregnancy **C**, cardiac disorders, hyperthyroidism, diabetes mellitus, hypertension, prostatic hypertrophy, narrow-angle glaucoma, seizures

Pharmacokinetics

Absorption	Unknown
Distribution	Unknown
Metabolism	Unknown
Excretion	Unknown
Half-life	Unknown

Pharmacodynamics

	AEROSOL
Onset	5-15 min
Peak	4 hr
Duration	12 hr

Interactions

Drug/drug:

Drug classifications

Beta-adrenergic blockers: Block therapeutic effect

Bronchodilators, aerosol: ↑ action of bronchodilator
MAOI: ↑ chance of hypertensive crisis
Sympathomimetics: ↑ adrenergic side effects

NURSING CONSIDERATIONS

Assessment

• Monitor respiratory function: vital capacity, forced expiratory volume, ABGs, lung sounds, heart rate, rhythm (baseline)

Associated nursing diagnoses

✓ Airway clearance, ineffective (uses)
✓ Impaired gas exchange (uses)
✓ Knowledge deficit (teaching)

Implementation

Aerosol route

• Shake aerosol container, ask patient to exhale, then place mouthpiece in mouth, inhale slowly, hold breath, remove, exhale slowly; allow at least 1 min between inh
• Store in light-resistant container, do not expose to temp over 86° F (30° C)

Patient/family education

• Caution patient not to use OTC medications because extra stimulation may occur
• Instruct patient to use this medication before other medications and to allow at least 1 min between each, to prevent overstimulation
• Teach patient how to use inhaler; review package insert with patient; to avoid getting aerosol in eyes; blurring may result; to wash inhaler in warm water qd and dry; to avoid smoking, smoke-filled rooms, and persons with respiratory infections
• Instruct patient on administration of dose, not to use more than prescribed; serious side effects may occur

Evaluation

Positive therapeutic outcome

• Absence of dyspnea, wheezing
• Improved airway exchange
• Improved ABGs

Treatment of overdose: Administer a β_2-adrenergic blocker

salsalate

(sal-sa'late)

Amigesic, Argesic-SA, Arthra-G, Disalcid, Mono-Gesic, Salflex, Salsalate, Salsitab

Func. class.: Nonnarcotic analgesic; nonsteroidal antiinflammatory agent
Chem. class.: Salicylate

Pregnancy category **C**

S

Action: Blocks formation of peripheral prostaglandins, which cause pain and inflammation; antipyretic action results from inhibition of hypothalamic heat-regulating center; does not inhibit platelet aggregation

➔ **Therapeutic Outcome:** Decreased pain, inflammation

Uses: Mild to moderate pain or fever, including arthritis, juvenile rheumatoid arthritis

Dosage and routes

Adult: PO 3 g/day in divided doses

Available forms: Cap 500 mg; tab 500, 750 mg

Side effects/adverse reactions

CNS: Stimulation, drowsiness, dizziness, confusion, ***convulsions,*** headache, flushing, hallucinations, coma
CV: Rapid pulse, ***pulmonary edema***
EENT: Tinnitus, hearing loss
ENDO: Hypoglycemia, hyponatremia, hypokalemia, alteration in acid-base balance
GI: Nausea, vomiting, GI bleeding, diarrhea, heartburn, anorexia, ***hepatotoxicity***
HEMA: Thrombocytopenia, agranulocytosis, leukopenia, neutropenia, hemolytic anemia, increased pro-time
INTEG: Rash, urticaria, bruising
RESP: Wheezing, hyperpnea

Contraindications: Hypersensitivity to salicylates, NSAIDs, GI bleeding, bleeding disorders, P children <3 yr, Vitamin K deficiency

Precautions: Anemia, hepatic disease, renal disease, Hodgkin's disease, pregnancy **C**, lactation

Pharmacokinetics

Absorption	Absorbed in small intestine
Distribution	Rapidly and widely distributed, crosses placenta
Metabolism	Not metabolized
Excretion	Unchanged—kidneys
Half-life	2-3 hr (low doses), 15-30 hr (high doses)

Pharmacodynamics

	PO
Onset	30 min
Peak	1-3 hr
Duration	3-6 hr

Interactions

Drug/drug:

Individual drugs

Alcohol: ↑ bleeding
Cefamandole: ↑ bleeding
Furosemide: ↑ toxic effects
Heparin: ↑ bleeding
Insulin: ↑ effects
Methotrexate: ↑ effects
PABA: ↑ toxic effects
Phenytoin: ↑ effects
Plicamycin: ↑ bleeding
Probenecid: ↓ effects
Spironolactone: ↓ effects
Sulfinpyrazone: ↓ effects
Valproic acid: ↑ effects, ↑ bleeding
Vancomycin: ↑ ototoxicity

Drug classifications

Antacids: ↓ effects of aspirin
Anticoagulants: ↑ effects
Carbonic anhydrase inhibitors: ↑ toxic effects
Nonsteroidal antiinflammatories: ↑ gastric ulcers
Penicillins: ↑ effects
Salicylates: ↓ blood sugar levels
Steroids: ↓ effects of aspirin, ↑ gastric ulcers

Sulfonylamides: ↓ effects
Urinary acidifiers: ↑ salicylate levels
Urinary alkalizers: ↓ effects of aspirin

Lab test interferences

Increase: Coagulation studies, liver function studies, serum uric acid, amylase, CO_2, urinary protein
Decrease: Serum potassium, PBI, cholesterol, blood glucose
Interfere: Urine catecholamines, pregnancy test

NURSING CONSIDERATIONS

Assessment

- Monitor liver function studies: AST (SGOT), ALT (SGPT), bilirubin, creatinine if patient is on long-term therapy
- Monitor renal function studies: BUN, urine creatinine if patient is on long-term therapy
- Monitor blood studies: CBC, Hct, Hgb, pro-time if patient is on long-term therapy
- Check I&O ratio; decreasing output may indicate renal failure if patient is on long-term therapy
- Assess hepatotoxicity: dark urine, clay-colored stools, yellowing of the skin and sclera, itching, abdominal pain, fever, diarrhea if patient is on long-term therapy
- Assess for allergic reactions: rash, urticaria; if these occur, drug may have to be discontinued
- Assess for ototoxicity: tinnitus, ringing, roaring in ears; audiometric testing needed before, after long-term therapy
- Assess for visual changes: blurring, halos; corneal, retinal damage
- Check edema in feet, ankles, legs
- Identify prior drug history; many drug interactions are possible
- Monitor pain: location, duration, type, intensity, prior to dose and 1 hr after
- Monitor musculoskeletal status: ROM prior to dose
- Identify fever, length of time, and related symptoms

Associated nursing diagnoses

☑ Pain (uses)
☑ Mobility, impaired physical mobility (uses)
☑ Knowledge deficit (teaching)
☑ Injury, risk for (side effects)

Implementation

PO route

- Administer to patient crushed or whole; chewable tab may be chewed
- Give with food or milk to decrease gastric symptoms; give 30 min ac or 2 hr pc; absorption may be slowed
- Give antacids 1-2 hr after enteric products

Patient/family education

- Advise patient to report any symptoms of hepatotoxicity, renal toxicity, visual changes, ototoxicity, allergic reactions, bleeding (long-term therapy)
- Instruct patient to take with 8 oz of water and sit upright for ½ hr after dose
- Caution patient not to exceed recommended dosage; acute poisoning may result
- Advise patient to read label

S

on other OTC drugs; many contain aspirin
- Inform patient that the therapeutic response takes 2 wk (arthritis)
- Teach patient to report tinnitus, confusion, diarrhea, sweating, hyperventilation
- Caution patient to avoid alcohol ingestion; GI bleeding may occur
- Inform patient that patients who have allergies may develop allergic reactions

Evaluation

Positive therapeutic outcome
- Decreased pain
- Decreased inflammation

Treatment of overdose: Lavage, activated charcoal, monitor electrolytes, VS

sargramostim

(sar-gram'oh-stim)
Leukine, Prokine, rhu GM-CSF, recombinant human
Func. class.: Biologic modifier
Chem. class.: Granulocyte/macrophage colony stimulating factor
Pregnancy category **C**

Action: Stimulates proliferation and differentiation of hematopoietic progenitor cells (granulocyte, macrophage)

Uses: Acceleration of myeloid recovery in patients with non-Hodgkin's lymphoma, acute lymphoblastic leukemia, autologous bone marrow transplantation in Hodgkin's disease; bone marrow transplantation failure or engraftment delay

Dosage and routes

Myeloid reconstitution after autologous bone marrow transplantation
Adult: **IV** 250 μg/m²/day × 3 wk; give over 2 hr, 2-4 hr after autologous bone marrow inf, and not less than 24 hr after last dose of antineoplastics and 12 hr after last dose of radiotherapy, bone marrow transplantation failure, or engraftment delay

Acceleration of myeloid recovery
Adult: **IV** 250 μg/m²/day × 14 days; give over 2 hr; may repeat in 7 days, may repeat 500 μg/m²/day × 14 days after another 7 days if no improvement

Available forms: Powder for inj lyophilized 250, 500 μg

Side effects/adverse reactions

CNS: Fever, malaise, CNS disorder, weakness, chills
CV: Supraventricular tachycardia, peripheral edema, pericardial effusion
GI: Nausea, vomiting, diarrhea, anorexia, ***GI hemorrhage***, stomatitis, ***liver damage***
GU: Urinary tract disorder, abnormal kidney function
HEMA: ***Blood dyscrasias, hemorrhage***
INTEG: Alopecia, rash, peripheral edema

MS: Bone pain
RESP: Dyspnea

Contraindications: Hypersensitivity to GM-CSF, yeast products; excessive leukemic myeloid blast in the bone marrow or peripheral blood

Precautions: Pregnancy **C**, P lactation, children; renal, hepatic, lung disease; cardiac disease; pleural, pericardial effusions

Pharmacokinetics

Absorption	Completely absorbed (IV)
Distribution	Unknown
Metabolism	Unknown
Excretion	Unknown
Half-life	2 hr

Pharmacodynamics

	IV
Onset	Rapid
Peak	2 hr
Duration	Unknown

Interactions

Drug/drug:

Individual drugs

Lithium: ↑ myeloproliferation

Drug classifications

Antineoplastics: Do not use together

Corticosteroids: ↑ myeloproliferation

NURSING CONSIDERATIONS

Assessement

- Monitor blood studies: CBC, differential count before treatment and twice weekly; leukocytosis may occur (WBC >50,000 cells/mm^3, ANC >20,000 cells/mm^3)
- Monitor renal and hepatic studies before treatment: BUN, creatinine, urinalysis; AST (SGOT), ALT (SGPT), alk phosphatase; monitoring is needed twice a week in renal, hepatic disease
- Assess for hypersensitive reactions/rashes, and local inj site reactions; usually transient
- Assess for increased fluid retention in cardiac disease

Associated nursing diagnoses

✓ Infection, risk for (uses)
✓ Knowledge deficit (teaching)

Implementation

IV **IV route**

Intermittent IV

- Reconstitute with 1 ml sterile water for inj without preservative; do not reenter vial; discard unused portion; direct reconstitution sol at side of vial; rotate contents; do not shake
- Give by intermittent inf after diluting in 0.9% NaCl inj to prepare **IV** inf; if final conc is <10 μg/ml, add human albumin to make a final conc of 0.1% to the NaCl before adding sargramostim to prevent absorption; for a final conc of 0.1% albumin, add 1 mg human albumin/1 ml 0.9% NaCl inj; run over 2 hr; give within 6 hr after reconstitution
- Store in refrigerator; do not freeze

Y-site compatibilities:

Amikacin, aminophylline, aztreonam, bleomycin, butorphanol, calcium gluconate, carboplatin, carmustine, cefazolin, ceforanide, cefotaxime,

S

cefotetan, ceftizoxime, ceftriaxone, cefuroxime, cimetidine, cisplatin, clindamycin, cyclophosphamide, cytarabine, dacarbazine, dactinomycin, dexamethasone sodium phosphate, diphenhydramine, doxorubicin, doxycycline, droperidol, etoposide, famotidine, floxuridine, fluconazole, fluorouracil, furosemide, gentamicin, heparin, ifosfamide, magnesium sulfate, mannitol, mechlorethamine, meperidine, mesna, methotrexate, metoclopramide, metronidazole, mezlocillin, miconazole, minocycline, mitoxantrone, netilmicin, pentostatin, potassium chloride, prochlorperazine, promethazine, ranitidine, teniposide, ticarcillin, ticarcillin/clavulanate, trimethoprim/sulfamethoxazole, vancomycin, vinblastine, vincristine, zidovudine

Y-site incompatibilities:
Acyclovir, ampicillin, ampicillin/sulbactam, cefonicid, cefoperazine, ceftazidime, chlorpromazine, ganciclovir, haloperidol, hydrocortisone, hydromorphone, hydroxyzine, idarubicin, imipenem/cilastatin, lorazepam, methylprednisolone sodium succinate, mitomycin, morphine, nalbuphine, ondansetron, piperacillin, sodium bicarbonate, tobramycin

Patient/family education
- Teach patient reason for medication and expected results
- Advise patient to notify nurse or prescriber of side effects

Evaluation
Positive therapeutic outcome
- WBC and differential recovery
- Absence of infection

scopolamine
(skoe-pol'a-meen)
Transderm-Scop, Isopoto-Hyoscine, Transderm-V ✦, Triptol
Func. class.: Antiemetic, anticholinergic, mydriatic
Chem. class.: Belladonna alkaloid
Pregnancy category C

Action: Inhibits acetylcholine at receptor sites in autonomic nervous system, which controls secretions, free acids in stomach; blocks central muscarinic receptors, which decreases involuntary movements; blocks response of iris sphincter muscle, muscle of accommodation of ciliary body to cholinergic stimulation, resulting in dilation, paralysis of accommodation

➔ Therapeutic Outcome: Absence of vomiting, secretions (preop), involuntary movements

Uses: Reduction of secretions before surgery, calm delirium, motion sickness, uveitis, iritis, cycloplegia, mydriasis; prevention of motion sickness, parkinson symptoms

Dosage and routes

Ophth

Adult: Instill 1-2 gtt before refraction or 1-2 gtt qd-tid for iritis or uveitis

P ***Child:*** Instill 1 gtt bid × 2 days before refraction

Prevention of motion sickness

Adult: Patch 1 placed behind ear 4-5 hr before travel

P Not recommended for children

Parkinson symptoms

Adult: IM/SC/**IV** 0.3-0.6 mg tid-qid diluted using dilution provided

P ***Child:*** SC 0.006 mg/kg tid-qid or 0.2 mg/m^2

Preoperatively

Adult: SC 0.4-0.6 mg

Available forms: Sol 0.25%; patch 0.5 mg delivered in 72 hr; inj 0.3, 0.4, 0.86, 1 mg/ml

Side effects/adverse reactions

CNS: Confusion, anxiety, restlessness, irritability, delusions, hallucinations, headache, sedation, depression, incoherence, dizziness, excitement, delirium, flushing, weakness

CV: Palpitations, tachycardia, postural hypotension, paradoxical bradycardia

EENT: Blurred vision, photophobia, dilated pupils, difficulty swallowing, mydriasis, cycloplegia

GI: Dryness of mouth, constipation, nausea, vomiting, abdominal distress, ***paralytic ileus***

GU: Hesitancy, retention

INTEG: Urticaria

MISC: Suppression of lactation, nasal congestion, decreased sweating

Contraindications: Hypersensitivity, narrow-angle glaucoma, myasthenia gravis, GI/GU obstruction, hypersensitivity to belladonna, barbiturates

Precautions: Pregnancy **C**, G elderly, lactation, prostatic hypertrophy, CHF, hypertension, P dysrhythmia, children, gastric ulcer

Pharmacokinetics

Absorption	Well absorbed (IM, SC, Trans)
Distribution	Crosses placenta, blood-brain barrier
Metabolism	Liver
Excretion	Unknown
Half-life	8 hr

Pharmacodynamics

	SC/IM	IV	TRANS	INSTILL
Onset	30-45 min	10-15 min	4-5 hr	Unknown
Peak	1 hr	1 hr	Unknown	20-30 min
Duration	6 hr	4 hr	72 hr	3-7 days

Interactions

Drug/drug:

Individual drugs

Alcohol: ↑ CNS depression

Quinidine: ↑ anticholinergic effect

Drug classifications

Antidepressants: ↑ anticholinergic effect

Antihistamines: ↑ anticholinergic effect

S

Narcotics: ↑ anticholinergic effect
Phenothiazines: ↑ anticholinergic effect
Tricyclics: ↑ anticholinergic effect

NURSING CONSIDERATIONS

Assessment

- Assess for eye pain; discontinue use (opticue)
- Monitor I&O ratio; retention commonly causes decreased urinary output
- Assess for Parkinsonism, extrapyramidal symptoms: shuffling gait, muscle rigidity, involuntary movements
- Assess for urinary hesitancy, retention; palpate bladder if retention occurs
- Assess for constipation; increase fluids, bulk, exercise if this occurs
- Assess for tolerance over long-term therapy; dose may have to be increased or changed
- Assess mental status: affect, mood, CNS depression, worsening of mental symptoms during early therapy

Associated nursing diagnoses

✓ Fluid volume deficit (uses)
✓ Knowledge deficit (teaching)

Implementation

IV **SC/IM/IV** route
- Administer parenteral dose with patient recumbent to prevent postural hypotension

IV **IV route**
- Give by direct **IV** after diluting with sterile water; give slowly

Syringe compatibilities:

Benzquinamide, butorphanol, chlorpromazine, cimetidine, dimenhydrinate, diphenhydramine, droperidol, fentanyl, hydromorphone, hydroxyzine, meperidine, metoclopramide, midazolam, morphine, nalbuphine, pentazocine, pentobarbital, perphenazine, prochlorperazine, promazine, promethazine, ranitidine, thiopental

Y-*site compatibilities:*

Heparin, hydrocortisone sodium succinate, potassium chloride, vitamin B with C

Patient/family education

- Tell patient to avoid hazardous activities, activities requiring alertness; dizziness may occur

Trans route
- Instruct patient to wash, dry hands before and after applying to surface behind ear; to change patch q72h; to apply at least 4 hr before traveling
- Advise patient to discontinue use if blurred vision, severe dizziness, drowsiness occurs—another type of antiemetic may be used
- Instruct patient to read labels of all OTC medications; if any scopolamine is found in product, avoid use
- Advise patient to keep medication out of children's reach
- Caution patient to report change in vision; blurring or loss of sight; trouble breathing; inhibition of sweating; flushing

Ophth route
- Teach patient method of instill: pressure on lacrimal sac

for 1 min; do not touch dropper to eye
- Inform patient that blurred vision will decrease with repeated use of drug
- Advise patient to wait 5 min to use other drops; blink more than usual
- Caution patient not to discontinue this drug abruptly; to taper off over 1 wk

Evaluation

Positive therapeutic outcome
- Decrease in inflammation, cycloplegic refraction
- Decreased secretions
- Absence of motion sickness

secobarbital

(see-koe-bar'bi-tal)

secobarbital sodium, Secogen Sodium ♣, Seconal Sodium, Seconal Sodium Pulvules, Seral ♣, Secretin-Ferring

Func. class.: Sedative/hypnotic-barbiturate

Chem. class.: Barbitone (short-acting)

Pregnancy category D

Controlled substance schedule II (USA), schedule G (Canada)

Action: Depresses activity in brain cells primarily in reticular activating system in brainstem; selectively depresses neurons in posterior hypothalamus, limbic structures; decreases seizure activity by inhibition of epileptic activity in CNS

➔ **Therapeutic Outcome:** Sedation, anticonvulsant, improved energy

Uses: Insomnia, sedation, preoperative medication, status epilepticus, acute tetanus convulsions

Dosage and routes

Insomnia

Adult: PO/IM 100-200 mg hs

P *Child:* IM 3-5 mg/kg, not to exceed 100 mg, not to inject >5 ml in one site; rec 4-5 mg/kg

Sedation/preoperatively

Adult: PO 200-300 mg 1-2 hr preoperatively

P *Child:* PO 50-100 mg 1-2 hr preoperatively; rec 4-5 mg/kg 1-2 hr preoperatively

Status epilepticus

P *Adult and child:* IM/**IV** 250-350 mg

Acute psychotic agitation

P *Adult and child:* IM/**IV** 5.5 mg/kg q3-4h

Available forms: Cap 50, 100 mg; tab 100 mg, inj 50 mg/ml; powder, rec supp 200 mg

Side effects/adverse reactions

CNS: Lethargy, drowsiness, hangover, dizziness, paradoxical stimulation in the elderly (G) and children (P), light-headedness, dependency, CNS depression, mental depression, slurred speech

CV: Hypotension, bradycardia

S

GI: Nausea, vomiting, diarrhea, constipation
HEMA: Agranulocytosis, thrombocytopenia, megaloblastic anemia (long-term treatment)
INTEG: ***Rash,*** urticaria, pain, abscesses at inj site, angioedema, thrombophlebitis, ***Stevens-Johnson syndrome***
RESP: Depression, ***apnea, laryngospasm, bronchospasm***

Contraindications: Hypersensitivity to barbiturates, respiratory depression, addiction to barbiturates, severe liver impairment, porphyria, uncontrolled severe pain

Precautions: Anemia, pregnancy **D**, lactation, hepatic disease, renal disease, hypertension, G elderly, acute/chronic pain

Pharmacokinetics

Absorption	Slow (70%-90%) (PO), IV complete
Distribution	Not known, crosses placenta
Metabolism	Liver (75%)
Excretion	Kidneys (25% unchanged)
Half-life	2-6 days

Pharmacodynamics

	PO	IM	IV
Onset	30-60 min	10-30 min	5 min
Peak	Unknown	Unknown	30 min
Duration	6-8 hr	4-6 hr	4-6 hr

Interactions

Drug/drug:

Individual drugs

Alcohol: ↑ CNS depression
Chloramphenicol: ↓ effectiveness
Cyclosporine: ↓ effectiveness
Cytophosphamide: ↑ hematologic toxicity
Dacarbazine: ↓ effectiveness
Quinidine: ↓ effectiveness
Valproic acid: ↑ sedation

Drug classifications

Anticoagulants: ↓ effectiveness
Antidepressants: ↑ CNS depression
Antihistamines: ↑ CNS depression
Glucocorticoids: ↓ effectiveness
MAOI: ↑ CNS depression
Narcotics: ↑ CNS depression
Oral contraceptives: ↓ effectiveness
Sedatives/hypnotics: ↑ CNS depression
Tricyclics: ↓ effectiveness

NURSING CONSIDERATIONS

Assessment

- Assess patient's mental status: mood, sensorium, affect, memory (long, short), G especially in elderly patients. If using as a hypnotic, assess sleep patterns during therapy. Drug suppresses REM sleep with dreaming. Withdrawal insomnia may occur after short-term use; do not start using drug again—insomnia will improve in 1-3 nights; patient may experience increased dreaming.
- Monitor patient for respiratory dysfunction: respiratory depression, character, rate, rhythm (when using **IV**). Hold drug if resp are <10/min or if pupils are dilated. Also check VS q30 min after parenteral route for 2 hr
- Assess patient for barbiturate

toxicity: hypotension; pulmonary constriction; cold, clammy skin; cyanosis of lips; CNS depression; nausea; vomiting; hallucinations; delirium; weakness; coma; pupillary constriction, mild symptoms may occur in 8-12 hr without drug
• Assess patient for blood dyscrasias: fever, sore throat, bruising, rash, jaundice, epistaxis (long-term treatment only)
• Assess for pain in postoperative patients; pain threshold is lowered when patients are taking this medication

Associated nursing diagnoses

✓ Sleep pattern disturbance (uses)
✓ Injury, risk for (adverse reactions)
✓ Knowledge deficit (teaching)

Implementation

• Administer after removal of cigarettes, to prevent fires
• Administer after trying conservative measures for insomnia

PO route
• Tab may be crushed and mixed with food if swallowing is difficult. Also may be mixed with other fluids ½-1 hr before hs for expected sleeplessness; on empty stomach for best absorption

IM route
• Give in deep muscle mass (gluteal) to minimize irritation to tissues
• Split inj of >5 ml into two because irritation to tissues may occur

IV **Direct IV route**
• Use large vein to prevent extravasation; if extravasation occurs, use moist heat to the area and procaine sol 5% inj into area
• Give at rate of 65 mg or less/min; titrate to patient response

Syringe compatibilities:

Heparin

Syringe incompatibilities:

Benzquinamide, dimenhydrinate, diphenhydramine, erythromycin gluceptate, hydroxyzine, kanamycin, oxytetracycline, phenytoin, prochlorperazine, promazine, promethazine, ranitidine, tetracycline

Solution compatibilities:

D_5W, $D_{10}W$, 0.45% NaCl, 0.9% NaCl, Ringer's sol, dextrose/saline combinations, dextrose/Ringer's or dextrose/lactated Ringer's combinations

Additive compatibilities:

Amikacin, aminophylline, calcium chloride, calcium gluceptate, cephapirin, colistimethate, dimenhydrinate, polymyxin B, sodium bicarbonate, thiopental, or verapamil

S

Additive incompatibilities:

Cephalothin, chlorpromazine, codeine, ephedrine, hydralazine, hydrocortisone sodium succinate, hydroxyzine, insulin, levorphanol, meperidine, methadone, morphine, norepinephrine, pentazocine, procaine, prochlorazine mesylate, premazine, promethazine, streptomycin, or vancomycin

Patient/family education

- Teach patient that hangover is common
- Instruct patient that drug is indicated only for short-term treatment of insomnia and is probably ineffective after 2 wk
- Inform patient that physical dependency may result when used for extended time (45-90 days depending on dose)
- Caution patient to avoid driving or other activities requiring alertness
- Caution patient to avoid alcohol ingestion or CNS depressants; serious CNS depression may result
- Instruct patient not to discontinue medication quickly after long-term use; drug should be tapered over 1 wk
- Emphasize the need to tell all prescribers that a barbiturate is being taken
- Inform patient that withdrawal insomnia may occur after short-term use; patient should not start using drug again—insomnia will improve in 1-3 nights; patient may experience increased dreaming
- Inform patient that effects may take 2 nights for benefits to be noticed; teach patient alternate measures to improve sleep: reading, exercise several hours before hs, warm bath, warm milk, TV, self-hypnosis, deep breathing
- Teach patient to make position changes slowly; orthostatic hypotension may occur
- Instruct patient to notify prescriber immediately if bruising or bleeding occur, which may indicate blood dycrasias

Evaluation

Positive therapeutic outcome

- Improved sleeping patterns
- Decreased seizure activity
- Improved energy

Treatment of overdose: Lavage, activated charcoal, warming blanket, vital signs, hemodialysis, alkalinize urine; give **IV** volume expanders, **IV** fluids

selegiline

(se-le'ji-leen)

Eldepryl, SD-Deprenyl

Func. class.: Antiparkinson agent

Chem. class.: Levorotatory acetylenic derivative of phenethylamine

Pregnancy category C

Action: Increased dopaminergic activity by inhibition of MAO type B activity; not fully understood

➡ Therapeutic Outcome: Decreased symptoms of Parkinson's disease

Uses: Adjunct management of Parkinson's disease in patients being treated with levodopa/carbidopa who have responded poorly to therapy

Dosage and routes

Adult: PO 10 mg/day in divided doses 5 mg at breakfast and lunch; after 2-3 days begin to reduce the dose of levodopa/carbidopa 10%-30%

Available forms: Tab 5 mg

Side effects/adverse reactions

CNS: Increased tremors, chorea, restlessness, blepharospasm, increased bradykinesia, grimacing, tardive dyskinesia, dystonic symptoms, involuntary movements, increased apraxia, hallucinations, dizziness, mood changes, nightmares, delusions, lethargy, apathy, overstimulation, sleep disturbances, headache, migraine, numbness, muscle cramps, confusion, anxiety, tiredness, vertigo, personality change, back/leg pain
CV: Orthostatic hypotension, hypertension, dysrhythmia, palpitations; angina pectoris, hypotension, tachycardia, edema, sinus bradycardia, syncope
EVENT: Diploplia, dry mouth, blurred vision, tinnitus
GI: Nausea, vomiting, constipation, weight loss, anorexia, diarrhea, heartburn, rectal bleeding, poor appetite, dysphagia
GU: Slow urination, nocturia, prostatic hypertrophy, hesitation, retention, frequency, sexual dysfunction
INTER: Increased sweating, alopecia, hematoma, rash, photosensitivity, facial hair
RESP: Asthma, shortness of breath

Contraindications: Hypersensitivity

Precautions: Pregnancy **C**, P lactation, children

Pharmacokinetics

Absorption	Well absorbed (PO)
Distribution	Widely distributed
Metabolism	Rapidly, liver
Excretion	Metabolites-N-desmethyldeprenyl, amphetamine, methamphetamine
Half-life	Unknown

Pharmacodynamics

	PO
Onset	Unknown
Peak	½-2 hr
Duration	Unknown

Interactions

Drug/drug:

Individual drugs

Meperidine: Do not use—fatal reaction
Levodopa/carbidopa: ↑ side effects
Fluoxetine: ↑ adverse reactions

Drug classifications

Narcotics: Do not use—fatal reaction

Drug/food:

Tyramine foods: ↑ hypertension

Lab test interferences

False positive: Urine ketones, urine glucose
False negative: Urine glucose (glucose oxidase)
False increase: Uric acid, urine protein
Decrease: VMA

NURSING CONSIDERATIONS

Assessment

- Monitor B/P, respiration throughout treatment

S

• Assess mental status: affect, mood, behavioral changes, depression; perform suicide assessment
• Assess for decreased Parkinson's symptoms: rigidity, unsteady gait, weakness, tremors; these should decrease in severity

Associated nursing diagnoses

✓ Physical mobility, impaired (uses)
✓ Knowledge deficit (teaching)

Implementation

PO route
• Adjust dosage to patient response
• Give with meals; limit protein taken with drug
• Give at doses <10 mg/day because of risks associated with nonselective inhibition of MAO

Patient/family education

• Caution patient to change positions slowly to prevent orthostatic hypotension
• Advise patient to report side effects: twitching, eye spasms —may indicate overdose
• Caution patient to use drug exactly as prescribed; if drug is discontinued abruptly, parkinsonian crisis may occur
• Instruct patient to avoid foods high in tyramine: cheese, pickled products, wine, beer, large amounts of caffeine
• Instruct patient not to exceed recommended dose of 10 ml—might precipitate a hypertensive crisis; report severe headache or other unusual symptoms

Evaluation

Positive therapeutic outcome
• Decreased symptoms of Parkinson's disease

Treatment of overdose:

IV fluids for hypertension, **IV** dilute pressure agent for B/P titration

senna

(sin'na)

Black Draught, Dr. Caldwell Senna Laxative, Fletcher's Castoria, Gentlax, Senexon, Senna-Gen, Senokot, Senokotxtra, Senolax

Func. class.: Laxative-stimulant

Chem. class.: Anthraquinone

Pregnancy category C

Action: Stimulates peristalsis by action on Auerbach's plexus; softens feces by increasing water and electrolytes in large intestine

Therapeutic Outcome: Decreased constipation

Uses: Acute constipation; bowel preparation for surgery or examination

Dosage and routes

Adult: PO 1-8 tab (Senokot)/day or 1/2 to 4 tsp of granules added to water or juice; rec supp 1-2 hs; syr 1-4 tsp hs (1 tsp = 4 ml), 7.5-15 ml; (Black Draught) 3/4 oz dissolved in 2.5 oz liq given between 2-4

PM the day before procedure (X-Prep)

P *Child >27 kg:* ½ adult dose; do not use Black Draught for children

P *Child 1 mo-1 yr:* Syr 1.25-2.5 ml (Senokot) hs

Available forms: Supp 625 mg, 30 mg sennosides; powder 662 mg/g, 6, 15 mg sennosides/3 g; tab 8.6 sennosides, 180 mg

Side effects/adverse reactions

GI: *Nausea, vomiting, anorexia, abdominal cramps,* diarrhea, flatulence
GU: Pink-red or brown-black discoloration of urine
META: Hypocalcemia, enteropathy, alkalosis, hypokalemia, ***tetany***

Contraindications: Hypersensitivity, GI bleeding, intestinal obstruction, CHF, lactation, abdominal pain, nausea/vomiting, appendicitis, acute surgical abdomen

Precautions: Pregnancy **C**

Pharmacokinetics

Absorption	Minimally absorbed (PO)
Distribution	Unknown
Metabolism	Not metabolized
Excretion	Kidneys, feces
Half-life	Unknown

Pharmacodynamics

	PO	REC
Onset	6-24 hr	Unknown
Peak	Unknown	Unknown
Duration	3-4 days	Unknown

Interactions

Drug/drug:

Drug classifications

Oral drugs: ↓ absorption

Individual drugs

Disulfiram: Do not use together

NURSING CONSIDERATIONS

Assessment

- Monitor blood, urine electrolytes if used often by patient; check I&O ratio to identify fluid loss
- Assess cramping, rec bleeding, nausea, vomiting; if these symptoms occur, drug should be discontinued; identify cause of constipation; identify whether fluids, bulk, or exercise is missing from life-style
- Assess for Mg toxicity: thirst, confusion, decrease in reflexes
- Monitor blood ammonia level (30-70 mg/100 ml); monitor for clearing of confusion, lethargy, restlessness, irritability (hepatic encephalopathy)
- Monitor blood, urine electrolytes if drug is used often by patient

Associated nursing diagnoses

- ✓ Bowel elimination, altered: constipation (uses)
- ✓ Bowel elimination, altered; diarrhea (side effects)
- ✓ Knowledge deficit (teaching)
- ✓ Noncompliance (teaching)

Implementation

PO route

- Administration on empty stomach produces more rapid results

S

- Give with a full glass of water in AM or PM (oral dose); evacuation occurs 6-12 hr later
- Dissolve granules in water or juice before administration
- Shake oral sol before giving

Patient/family education

- Discuss with the patient that adequate fluid consumption is necessary
- Inform patient that normal bowel movements do not always occur daily
- Teach patient not to use in presence of abdominal pain, nausea, vomiting; tell patient to notify prescriber if constipation is unrelieved or if symptoms of electrolyte imbalance occur: muscle cramps, pain, weakness, dizziness, excessive thirst

Evaluation

Positive therapeutic outcome

- Decreased constipation in 8-10 hr

sertraline

(ser'tra-leen)

Zoloft

Func. class.: Antidepressant

Pregnancy category B

Action: Inhibits serotonin reuptake in the CNS, thus increasing action of serotonin; does not affect dopamine, norepinephrine

Therapeutic Outcome: Relief of depression

Uses: Major depression

Dosage and routes

Adult: PO 50 mg qd; may increase to a maximum of 200 mg/day, do not change dose at intervals of <1 wk; administer qd in AM or PM

Available forms: Tab 50, 100 mg

Side effects/adverse reactions

CNS: *Insomnia, agitation, somnolence, dizziness, headache, tremor, fatigue,* paresthesia, twitching, confusion, ataxia, fever
CV: Palpitations, chest pain, hypotension
EENT: Vision abnormalities
GI: *Diarrhea, nausea,* constipation, anorexia, *dry mouth,* dyspepsia, *vomiting,* flatulence
GU: *Male sexual dysfunction,* micturition disorder
INTEG: Increased sweating, rash, hot flashes

Contraindications: Hypersensitivity

Precautions: Pregnancy **B**, G lactation, elderly, hepatic, renal disease, epilepsy

Pharmacokinetics

Absorption	Well absorbed (PO)
Distribution	Unknown
Metabolism	Liver, extensively
Excretion	Feces (14%)
Half-life	25 hr

Pharmacodynamics

	PO
Onset	Unknown
Peak	6-10 hr
Duration	Unknown

Interactions

Drug/drug:

Individual drugs

Alcohol: ↑ CNS depression
Warfarin: ↑ effect of warfarin

Drug classifications

MAOI: Hypertensive crisis, convulsions, do not use together

Lab test interferences

Increase: Serum bilirubin, blood glucose, alk phosphatase
Decrease: VMA, 5-HIAA
False increase: Urinary catecholamines

NURSING CONSIDERATIONS

Assessment

- Assess mental status: mood, sensorium, affect, suicidal tendencies; increase in psychiatric symptoms: depression, panic
- Identify alcohol consumption; if alcohol is consumed, hold dose until AM

Associated nursing diagnoses

✓ Coping, ineffective individual (uses)
✓ Injury, risk for (adverse reactions)
✓ Knowledge deficit (teaching)
✓ Noncompliance (teaching)

Implementation

PO route

- Administer dosage hs if oversedation occurs during day; may take entire dose hs
- Store at room temp; do not freeze

Patient/family education

- Teach patient that therapeutic effects may take 2-3 wk
- Instruct patient to use caution in driving or other activities requiring alertness because of drowsiness, dizziness, blurred vision; to avoid rising quickly from sitting to standing, especially elderly [G]
- Advise patient to avoid alcohol ingestion, other CNS depressants
- Teach patient not to discontinue medication quickly after long-term use: may cause nausea, headache, malaise
- Caution patient to wear sunscreen or large hat because photosensitivity can occur
- Teach patient to increase fluids, bulk in diet if constipation, urinary retention occur, especially elderly [G]
- Instruct patient to take gum, hard sugarless candy, or frequent sips of water for dry mouth

Evaluation

Positive therapeutic outcome

- Decrease in depression
- Absence of suicidal thoughts

Treatment of overdose:

ECG monitoring, induce emesis, lavage, activated charcoal, administer anticonvulsant

silver sulfadiazine (topical)

(sul-fa-dye'a-zeen)
Flamazine ✤, Silvadene, SSD, Thermazene
Func. class.: Local anti-infective
Chem. class.: Sulfonamide
Pregnancy category **C**

Action: Interferes with bacterial cell wall synthesis, broad spectrum

➔ Therapeutic Outcome: Bacteriocidal for organisms (gram-positive/gram-negative pathogens)

Uses: Burns (2nd, 3rd degree); prevention of wound sepsis

Dosage and routes

P *Adult and child:* Top apply 1% cream qd-bid 1½ mm thick to all burned areas

Available forms: Cream 10 mg/g

Side effects/adverse reactions

HEMA: Reversible leukopenia
INTEG: Rash, urticaria, stinging, burning, itching, pain, skin necrosis, erythema

Contraindications: Hypersensitivity, P child <2 mo

Precautions: Impaired renal function, pregnancy **C**, impaired hepatic function, lactation

Pharmacokinetics

Absorption	Small amount systemically (top)
Distribution	Unknown
Metabolism	Unknown
Excretion	Kidneys—unchanged
Half-life	Unknown

Pharmacodynamics

	TOP
Onset	Rapid
Peak	Unknown
Duration	Unknown

Interactions

Drug/drug:

Individual drugs

Deoxyribonuclease: Inactivates deoxyribonuclease
Fibrinolysin: Inactivates fibrinolysin

NURSING CONSIDERATIONS

Assessment

- Assess for infection/sepsis in all burned areas: drainage, fever, >WBCs, odor; culture of burns should be performed
- Assess for allergic reaction: burning, stinging, swelling, redness, itching
- Monitor renal function studies; check for crystalluria; CBC tests should be performed to identify leukopenia

Associated nursing diagnoses

✓ Infection, risk for (uses)
✓ Skin integrity, impaired (uses)
✓ Knowledge deficit (teaching)

Implementation

Top route

- Apply using aseptic technique; use sterile gloves
- Apply enough medication to cover burns completely; keep burns covered with medication at all times
- Apply after cleansing debris before each application; bathe daily
- Give analgesic before application if needed, pain may be severe
- Store medication at room temp in dry place

Patient/family education

- Inform patient that drug may be continued until graft can be done

Evaluation

Positive therapeutic outcome

- Relief or prevention of infection

simethicone

(si-meth'i-kone)

Extra Strength Gas-X, Flatulex Gas Relief, Gas-X, Major Con, Mylanta Gas, Mylicon, Mylicon 80, Ovol ✦, Phazyme, Phazyme 95, Phazyme 125

Func. class.: Antiflatulent

Pregnancy category **C**

Action: Disperses, prevents gas pockets in GI system. Does not decrease gas production

➔ **Therapeutic Outcome:** Belching or flatus

Uses: Flatulence

Dosage and routes

P *Adult and child >12 yr:* PO 40-100 mg pc, hs

Available forms: Chew tab 40, 80 mg; tab 50, 60, 95, 125 mg; drops 40 mg/0.6 ml; cap 125 mg

Side effects/adverse reactions

GI: Belching, rectal flatus

Contraindications: Hypersensitivity

Precautions: Pregnancy **C**

Pharmacokinetics

Absorption	None
Distribution	None
Metabolism	None
Excretion	None
Half-life	Unknown

Pharmacodynamics

	PO
Onset	Rapid
Peak	Unknown
Duration	3 hr

Interactions: None

NURSING CONSIDERATIONS

Assessment

- Identify the reason for excess gas production; decreased bowel sounds, recent surgery, other GI conditions

Associated nursing diagnoses

✓ Pain (uses)
✓ Knowledge deficit (teaching)

Implementation

PO route

- Give pc and hs
- Shake suspension well before administration
- Chewable tab should be chewed and not swallowed whole

Patient/family education

- Caution patient that tab must be chewed; to shake suspension well before pouring

Evaluation

Positive therapeutic outcome

- Absence of flatulence

simvastatin

(sim-va-stat-in)

Zocor

Func. class.: Antihyperlipidemic

Chem. class.: Synthetically derived fermentation product

Pregnancy category **X**

Action: Inhibits HMG-COA reductase enzyme, which reduces cholesterol synthesis; this enzyme is needed for cholesterol production

➡ **Therapeutic Outcome:** Decreasing cholesterol levels and low-density lipoproteins, increased high-density lipoproteins

Uses: As an adjunct in primary hypercholesterolemia (types IIa, IIb), mixed hyperlipidemia

Dosage and routes

Adult: PO 5-10 mg qd in PM initially, usual range 5-40 mg/day qd in PM, not to exceed 40 mg/day; dosage adjustments may be made at 4-wk intervals or more

Available forms: Tab 5, 10, 20, 40 mg

Side effects/adverse reactions

CNS: Headache, tremor, vertigo, peripheral neuropathy
EENT: Lens opacities
GI: Nausea, constipation, diarrhea, dyspepsia, flatus, abdominal pain, heartburn, ***liver dysfunction***
INTEG: Rash, pruritus, alopecia
MS: Muscle cramps, myalgia, ***myositis, rhabdomyolysis***

Contraindications: Hypersensitivity, pregnancy **X**, lactation, active liver disease

Precautions: Past liver disease, alcoholism, severe acute infections, trauma, hypotension, uncontrolled seizure disorders, severe metabolic disorders, electrolyte imbalances

Pharmacokinetics	
Absorption	85% (PO)
Distribution	Unknown
Metabolism	Liver—extensively
Excretion	70% feces, 20% kidneys
Half-life	Unknown

Pharmacodynamics

	PO
Onset	Unknown
Peak	1-2½ hr
Duration	Unknown

Interactions

Drug/drug:

Individual drugs

Cholestyramine: ↑ action
Colestipol: ↑ action
Cyclosporine: ↑ risk of myopathy, rhabdomyolysis
Erythromycin: ↑ risk of myopathy
Gemfibrozil: ↑ risk of myopathy, rhabdomyolysis
Niacin: ↑ risk of myopathy
Warfarin: ↑ risk of bleeding

Drug/food:

↑ levels of lovastatin

Lab test interferences

Increased: CPK, liver function tests

NURSING CONSIDERATIONS

Assessment

- Assess nutrition: fat, protein, carbohydrates; nutritional analysis should be completed by dietitian before treatment is initiated
- Monitor bowel pattern daily; diarrhea may be a problem
- Monitor triglycerides, cholesterol baseline and throughout treatment. LDL and VLDL should be watched closely; if it increases, drug should be discontinued

Associated nursing diagnoses

✓ Diarrhea (adverse reactions)
✓ Knowledge deficit (teaching)
✓ Noncompliance (teaching)

Implementation

PO route

- Give 30 min before AM and PM meals

Patient/family education

- Inform patient that compliance is needed for positive results to occur; not to double doses
- Advise patient to lower risk factors: high-fat diet, smoking, alcohol consumption, absence of exercise
- Advise patient to notify health care prescriber if the GI symptoms of diarrhea, abdominal or epigastric pain, nausea, vomiting occur; or if chills, fever, sore throat occur

Evaluation

Positive therapeutic outcome

- Decreased cholesterol levels, serum triglycerides and improved ratio with high-density lipoproteins (HDLs)

sodium bicarbonate

Arm and Hammer Pure Baking Soda, Bell/ans, Citrocarbonate, soda mint

Func. class.: Alkalinizer; antacid

Pregnancy category **C**

Action: Orally neutralizes gastric acid, which forms water, NaCl, CO_2; increases plasma bicarbonate, which buffers H^+

S

ion concentration; reverses acidosis **IV**

Therapeutic Outcome: Correction of acidosis, gastric acid neutralization

Uses: Acidosis (metabolic), cardiac arrest, alkalinization (systemic/urinary); antacid (PO)

Dosage and routes

Acidosis, metabolic

P ***Adult and child:*** **IV** inf 2-5 mEq/kg over 4-8 hr depending on CO_2, pH

Cardiac arrest

P ***Adult and child:*** **IV** bol 1 mEq/kg, then 0.5 mEq/kg q10 min, then doses based on ABGs

P ***Infant:*** **IV** inf not to exceed 8 mEq/kg/day based on ABGs (4.2% sol)

Alkalinization of urine

Adult: PO 325 mg-2 g qid or 48 mEq/kg (4 g), then 12-24 mEq q4hr

P ***Child:*** PO 12-120 mg/kg/day (1-10 mEq/kg)

Antacid

Adult: PO 300 mg-2 g chewed, taken with water qd-qid

Available forms: Tab 300, 325, 600, 650 mg; inj 4%, 4.2%, 5%, 7.5%, 8.4%

Side effects/adverse reactions

CNS: Irritability, headache, confusion, stimulation, tremors, *twitching, hyperreflexia,* ***tetany,*** weakness, ***convulsions*** caused by alkalosis
CV: Irregular pulse, ***cardiac arrest,*** water retention, edema, weight gain
GI: Flatulence, *belching, distention,* ***paralytic ileus,*** acid rebound
GU: Calculi
META: Alkalosis
RESP: Shallow, slow respirations, cyanosis, ***apnea***

Contraindications: Hypertension, peptic ulcer, renal disease, hypocalcemia

Precautions: CHF, cirrhosis, toxemia, renal disease, pregnancy **C**

Pharmacokinetics

Absorption	Unknown
Distribution	Widely distributed—extracellular fluids
Metabolism	Unknown
Excretion	Kidneys
Half-life	Unknown

Pharmacodynamics

	PO	IV
Onset	2 min	Rapid
Peak	½ hr	Rapid
Duration	1-3 hr	Unknown

Interactions

Drug/drug:

Individual drugs

Flecainide: ↑ effects
Ketoconazole: ↓ absorption of ketocanazole
Methenamine: ↓ effect of methenamine
Mexiletine: ↑ blood level of mexiletine

Quinidine: ↑ effects

Drug classifications

Amphetamines: ↑ effects
Anorexants: ↑ effects
Barbiturates: ↓ effects of barbiturates
Corticosteroids: ↑ sodium, potassium
Fluoroquinolones: ↑ crystalluria
Salicylates: ↓ effect of salicylate

Lab test interferences

Increase: Urinary urobilinogen
False positive: Urinary protein, blood lactate

NURSING CONSIDERATIONS

Assessment

- Assess respiratory and pulse rate, rhythm, depth, lung sounds; notify prescriber of abnormalities
- Monitor fluid balance (I&O, weight qd, edema); notify prescriber of fluid overload
- Monitor electrolytes: blood pH, PO_2, HCO_3, during beginning treatment; ABGs frequently during emergencies
- Monitor urine pH, urinary output, during beginning treatment
- Monitor extravasation with **IV** administration (tissue sloughing, ulceration, and necrosis)
- Assess for alkalosis: irritability, confusion, twitching, hyperreflexia, stimulation, slow respirations, cyanosis, irregular pulse
- Monitor manifestations of hypokalemia: *Renal:* acidic urine, reduced urine osmolality, nocturia, polyuria, polydipsia; *Cardiac:* hypotension, broad T wave, U wave, ectopy, tachycardia, weak pulse; *Neurologic:* muscle weakness, altered LOC, drowsiness, apathy, lethargy, confusion, depression; *GI:* anorexia, nausea, cramps, constipation, distension, paralytic ileus; *Respiratory:* hypoventilation, respiratory muscle weakness
- Monitor for manifestations of hyponatremia: *CV:* ↑ B/P, cold, clammy skin, hypo or hypervolemia; *GI:* anorexia, nausea, vomiting, diarrhea, abdominal cramps; *Neuro:* lethargy, increased ICP, confusion, headache, seizures, coma, fatigue, tremors, hyperreflexia
- Assess for milk-alkali syndrome: confusion, headache, nausea, vomiting, anorexia, urinary stones, hypercalcemia

Associated nursing diagnoses

- ✓ Gas exchange, impaired (uses)
- ✓ Fluid volume excess (adverse reactions)
- ✓ Knowledge deficit (teaching)

Implementation

PO route

- Tab must be chewed and taken with 8 oz of water
- Dissolve effervescent tab in water
- May be used to neutralize gastric acid in peptic ulcer disease, given 1 and 3 hr pc and hs

IV **IV route**

- Give **IV** bol in cardiac arrest, may be repeated q10min

S

• Give by intermittent or continuous inf in prepared sol or diluted in an equal amount of any dextrose/saline combination; administer 2-5mEq/kg over 4-8 hr, not to exceed 50mEq/hr; slower rate in children

Syringe compatibilities:
Milrinone, pentobarbital

Syringe incompatibilities:
Glycopyrrolate, metoclopramide, thiopental

Y-*site compatibilities:*
Acyclovir, famotidine, fludarabine, indomethacin sodium trihydrate, insulin, melphan, morphine, paclitaxel, potassium chloride, tolazoline, vitamin B with C

Y-*site incompatibilities:*
Amrinone, calcium chloride, indarubicin, sargramostim, verapamil, vinorelbine

Additive compatibilities:
Amikacin, aminophylline, amobarbital, amphotericin B, atropine, bretylium, calcium chloride, calcium gluceptate, carbenicillin, cefoxitin, ceftazine, cephalothin, cephapirin, chloramphenicol, chlorothiazide, cimetidine, clindamycin, cytarabine, droperidol/fentanyl, ergonovine maleate, erythromycin, floxacillin, furosemide, heparin, hyaluronidase, hydrocortisone sodium succinate, kanamycin, lidocaine, metaraminol, methotrexate, methyldopate, multivitamins, nafcillin, netilmicin, nizatidine, oxacillin, oxytocin, phenobarbital, phenylephrine, phenytoin, phytonadione, potassium chloride, prochlorperazine, sodium iodide, thiopental, verapamil

Additive incompatibilities:
Amoxicillin, ascorbic acid, carboplatin, carmustine, cefotaxime, cisplatin, codeine, dobutamine, epinephrine, hydromorphone, impenem cilastatin, insulin, isoproterenol, labetalol, levorphanol, magnesium sulfate, methadone, morphine, norepinephrine, pentazocine, pentobarbital, procaine, secobarbital, streptomycin, succinylcholine, tetracycline, vitamin B with C

Patient/family education

• Instruct patient to chew antacid tab and drink 8 oz water; not to take antacid with milk because milk-alkali syndrome may result; not to use antacid for more than 2 wk
• Advise patient to notify prescriber if indigestion is accompanied by chest pain; dyspnea; diarrhea; dark, tarry stools
• Teach patient about sodium-restricted diet; to avoid use of baking soda for indigestion

Evaluation

Positive therapeutic outcome
• ABGs, electrolytes, blood pH, HCO_3 normal levels
• Decreased gastric pain

sodium biphosphate

Fleet Enema, Phospho-Soda

Func. class.: Laxative, saline

Pregnancy category **C**

Action: Increases water absorption in the small intestine by osmotic action; laxative effect occurs by increased peristalsis and water retention

Therapeutic Outcome: Absence of constipation

Uses: Constipation, bowel or rectal preparation for surgery, examination

Dosage and routes

Adult: PO 20-30 ml (phospho-soda)

P *Child:* PO 5-15 ml (phospho-soda)

P *Adult and child >12 yr:* Rec ÷ enema (118 ml)

P *Child 2-12 yr:* Rec ½ enema (59 ml)

Available forms: Enema 7 g/phosphate and 19 g/biphosphate/118 ml; oral sol 18 g phosphate/48 g biphosphate/100 ml

Side effects/adverse reactions

GI: Nausea, cramps, diarrhea

META: Electrolyte, fluid imbalances

Contraindications: Hypersensitivity, rectal fissures, abdominal pain, nausea/vomiting, appendicitis, acute surgical abdomen, ulcerated hemorrhoids, Na-restricted diets (Sal-Hepatica, PhosphoSoda)

Precautions: Pregnancy **C**

Pharmacokinetics

Absorption	Up to 20% (Rec)
Distribution	Unknown
Metabolism	Unknown
Excretion	Kidneys
Half-life	Unknown

Pharmacodynamics

	PO	REC
Onset	½-3 hr	5 min
Peak	Unknown	Unknown
Duration	Unknown	Unknown

Interactions: None

NURSING CONSIDERATIONS

Assessment

- Assess stools: color, amount, consistency
- Assess for bowel pattern, bowel sounds (frequency, intensity), flatulence, distention, increased temp, dietary patterns (fluid, bulk), exercise
- Assess for cramping, rec bleeding, nausea, vomiting; if these symptoms occur, drug should be discontinued

Associated nursing diagnoses

✓ Constipation (uses)

✓ Knowledge deficit (teaching)

Implementation

PO route

- Give on empty stomach
- Mix oral sol in cold water
- Alone for better absorption; do not take within 1 hr of other drugs

S

Patient/family education

- Advise patient not to use laxatives or enema for long-term therapy; bowel tone will be lost
- Teach patient that normal bowel movements do not always occur daily
- Caution patient not to use in presence of abdominal pain, nausea, vomiting
- Caution patient to notify prescriber if constipation is unrelieved or if symptoms of electrolyte imbalance occur: muscle cramps, pain, weakness, dizziness, excessive thirst
- Instruct patient to maintain adequate fluid consumption to help prevent constipation

Evaluation

Positive therapeutic outcome

- Decrease in constipation

sodium polystyrene sulfonate

(po-lee-stye'reen)

Kayexalate, SPS Suspension

Func. class.: Potassium-removing resin

Chem. class.: Cation exchange resin

Pregnancy category C

Action: Removes potassium by exchanging sodium for potassium in body; occurs primarily in large intestine

Therapeutic Outcome: Potassium levels within accepted range

Uses: Hyperkalemia in conjunction with other measures

Dosage and routes

Adult: PO 15 g qd-qid; rec enema 30-50 g/100 ml of sorbitol warmed to body temp q6h

P ***Child:*** PO/Rec 1 mEq of K exchanged/g of resin, approximate dose 1g/kg q6hr

Available forms: Susp, 15 g polystyrene sulfonate, 21.5 ml sorbitol, 15 g (65 mEq) sodium/60 ml; powder 15 g/4 level tsp

Side effects/adverse reactions

GI: *Constipation,* anorexia, nausea, vomiting, diarrhea (sorbitol), ***fecal impaction,*** gastric irritation

META: Hypocalcemia, hypokalemia, hypomagnesemia, sodium retention

Precautions: Pregnancy **C**, renal failure, CHF, severe edema, severe hypertension

Pharmacokinetics

Absorption	None
Distribution	None
Metabolism	None
Excretion	Feces
Half-life	Unknown

Pharmacodynamics

	PO	REC
Onset	2-12 hr	2-12 hr
Peak	Unknown	Unknown
Duration	6-24 hr	4-6 hr

Interactions

Drug classifications

Antacids, calcium or magnesium: ↓ effect of sodium polystyrene
Laxatives: ↓ effect of sodium polystyrene

NURSING CONSIDERATIONS

Assessment

- Assess bowel function daily: amount of stool, color, characteristics
- Assess hypotension: confusion, irritability, muscular pain, weakness
- Monitor manifestations of hypokalemia: *Renal:* acidic urine, reduced urine osmolality, nocturia, polyuria, polydipsia; *Cardiac:* hypotension, broad T wave, U wave, ectopy, tachycardia, weak pulse; *Neuro:* muscle weakness, altered LOC, drowsiness, apathy, lethargy, confusion, depression; *GI:* anorexia, nausea, cramps, constipation, distension, paralytic ileus; *Respiratory:* hypoventilation, respiratory muscle weakness
- Monitor for manifestations of hypocalcemia: *CNS:* personality changes, anxiety, disturbances, depression, psychosis, nausea, vomiting, *GI:* constipation, abdominal pain from muscle spasm; *CV:* decreased contractility, decreased cardiac output, hypotension, lengthened ST segment, prolonged QT interval; *INTEG:* scaling eczema, alopecia, hyperpigmentation; *NEURO:* tetany, muscle twitching, cramping grimacing, seizure, altered deep tendon reflexes, spasm
- Monitor for manifestations of hypomagnesemia; *CNS:* agitation; *NEURO:* muscle twitching, paresthesias, hyperactive reflexes, positive Babinski reflex, dysphagia, nystagmus, seizures, tetany; *GI:* nausea, vomiting, diarrhea, anorexia, abdominal distention; *Cardiac:* ectopy; tachycardia, broad, flat, or inverted T waves; depressed ST segment; prolonged QT; decreased cardiac output; hypotension
- Monitor electrolytes: potassium, sodium, calcium, magnesium

Associated nursing diagnoses

- ✓ Constipation (adverse reactions)
- ✓ Diarrhea (adverse reactions)
- ✓ Knowledge deficit (teaching)

Implementation

PO route

- Give oral dose as susp mixed with H_2O or syr (20-100 ml)
- Give mild laxative as ordered to prevent constipation and fecal impaction; sorbitol as ordered to prevent constipation

Rec route

- Give by retention enema after mixing with warm water; introduce by gravity, continue stirring, flush with 100 ml of fluid, clamp, and leave in place for at least ½-1 hr
- Complete irrigation of colon after enema with 1-2 qt of nonsodium sol, drain
- Store freshly prepared sol for 24 hr at room temp

S

Patient/family education

- Explain reason for medication and expected results

Evaluation

Positive therapeutic outcome
- Potassium level normal

somatropin (human growth hormone)/somatrem

(soe-ma-troe′pin)

Humatrope ✤/Protropin

Func. class.: Pituitary hormone

Chem. class.: Growth hormone

Pregnancy category **C**

Action: Stimulates growth; similar to natural growth hormone—both preparations are developed by recombinant DNA technique

Therapeutic Outcome: Increase in height as a result of skeletal growth in pituitary growth hormone deficiency

Uses: Pituitary growth hormone deficiency (hypopituitary dwarfism)

Dosage and routes

Somatropin

P *Child:* IM/SC 2 IU 3 ×/wk, less than 48 hr between doses, may give 4 IU if growth is <1 inch/6 mo

Somatrem

P *Child:* IM/SC up to 0.1 mg/kg 3 ×/wk

Available forms: Inj 5 mg (13 IU)/vial, 10 mg (26 IU)/vial (somatrem); inj 2 mg (5 IU)/vial ✤, 5 mg (13 IU)/vial (somatropin)

Side effects/adverse reactions

CNS: Headache, growth of intracranial tumor

ENDO: Hyperglycemia, ketosis, hypothyroidism

GU: Hypercalciuria

INTEG: Rash, urticaria, pain, inflammation at injection site

SYST: Antibodies to growth hormone

Contraindications: Hypersensitivity to benzyl alcohol, closed epiphyses, intracranial lesions

Precautions: Diabetes mellitus, hypothyroidism, pregnancy **C**

Pharmacokinetics

Absorption	Well absorbed (SC/IM)
Distribution	Unknown
Metabolism	Unknown
Half-life	15-60 min

Pharmacodynamics

	IM/SC (GROWTH)
Onset	Unknown
Peak	Unknown
Duration	7 days

Interactions

Drug/drug:

Drug classifications

Androgens: ↑ epiphyseal closure

Glucocorticosteroids: ↓ growth, ↓ somatropin response

Thyroid hormones: ↑ epiphyseal closure

NURSING CONSIDERATIONS

Assessment

- Identify growth hormone antibodies if patient fails to respond to therapy
- Monitor thyroid function tests: T_3, T_4, T_7, TSH to identify hypothyroidism
- Assess for allergic reaction: rash, itching, fever, nausea, wheezing
- Assess for hypercalciuria: urinary stones; groin, flank pain; nausea, vomiting, frequency, hematuria, chills
- P • Monitor growth rate of child at intervals during treatment

Associated nursing diagnoses

✓ Body image disturbance (uses)
✓ Knowledge deficit (teaching)

Implementation

- Store in refrigerator for <1 mo; if reconstituted, <1 wk; do not use discolored or cloudy sol

IM route

- Rotate inj site after reconstituting 10 IU/5 m; bacteriostatic H_2O for inj, do not shake (somatrem)

Patient/family education

- Explain reason for medication and expected results
- Advise patient that routine follow up is needed to monitor growth rate
- Instruct parents on procedure for medication preparation and inj use—request demonstration, return demonstration; provide written instructions

Evaluation

Positive therapeutic outcome

- Growth in children until epiphyseal plates close

sotalol

(soe-ta'lole)

Betapace, Sotacar ♣

Func. class.: Antidysrhythmic, group II, III

Chem. class.: Nonselective β-blocker

Pregnancy category **C**

Action: Competitively blocks stimulation of β-adrenergic receptor within vascular smooth muscle; produces chronotropic, inotropic activity (decreases rate of SA node discharge, increases recovery time), slows conduction of AV node, decreases heart rate, which decreases O_2 consumption in myocardium; also decreases renin-aldosterone-angiotensin system at high doses, inhibits β-2 receptors in bronchial system (high doses)

➔ **Therapeutic Outcome:** Decreased B/P, heart rate, AV conduction

Uses: Life-threatening ventricular dysrhythmias

Dosage and routes

Adult: PO initial 80 mg bid, may increase to total of 240-320 mg/day

S

Available forms: Tab 80, 160, 240 mg

Side effects/adverse reactions

CNS: Dizziness, mental changes, drowsiness, fatigue, headache, catatonia, depression, anxiety, nightmares, paresthesia, lethargy, insomnia, decreased concentration
CV: Orthostatic hypotension, bradycardia, CHF, chest pain, ventricular dysrhythmias, AV block, peripheral vascular insufficiency, palpitations
EENT: Tinnitus, visual changes, sore throat, double vision, dry, burning eyes
GI: Nausea, vomiting, diarrhea, dry mouth, flatulence, constipation, anorexia
HEMA: ***Agranulocytosis, thrombocytopenic purpura (rare), thrombocytopenia, leukopenia***
INTEG; Rash, alopecia, urticaria, pruritus, fever
MS: Joint pain, arthralgia, muscle cramps, pain
RESP: ***Bronchospasm,*** dyspnea, wheezing, nasal stuffiness, pharyngitis
OTHER: Facial swelling, decreased exercise tolerance, weight change, Raynaud's disease

Contraindications: Hypersensitivity to β-blockers, cardiogenic shock, heart block (2nd or 3rd degree) sinus bradycardia, CHF, bronchial asthma, congenital or acquired long QT syndrome

Precautions: Major surgery, pregnancy **C**, lactation, diabetes mellitus, renal disease, thyroid disease, COPD, well-compensated heart failure, CAD, nonallergic bronchospasm, electrolyte disturbances, bradycardia, cardiac dysrhythmias, peripheral vascular disease

Pharmacokinetics

Absorption	Variably (30%)
Distribution	Crosses placenta, minimal penetration in CNS
Excretion	70% unchanged—kidneys
Half-life	10-24 hr, ↑ in renal disease

Pharmacodynamics

	PO
Onset	Several hr
Peak	Unknown
Duration	Unknown

Interactions

Drug/drug:

Individual drugs

Digoxin: ↑ blood levels, ↑ toxicity
Disopyramide: ↑ levels, ↑ toxicity
Flecainide: ↑ levels, ↑ toxicity
Lidocaine: Bradycardia, arrest
Mexiletine: ↑ levels, ↑ toxicity
Phenytoin: ↑ blood levels
Procainamide: ↑ levels, ↑ toxicity
Quinidine: ↑ levels, ↑ toxicity
Warfarin: ↑ level, ↑ bleeding

Drug classifications

Beta blockers: ↑ dysrhythmias, arrest
Calcium channel blockers: ↑ dysrhythmias, arrest

Lab test interferences

False increase: Urinary catecholamines

NURSING CONSIDERATIONS

Assessment

- Monitor B/P during beginning treatment, periodically thereafter; pulse q4hr; note rate, rhythm, quality: apical/radial pulse before administration; notify prescriber of any significant changes (pulse <50 bpm)
- Check for baselines in renal, liver function tests before therapy begins
- Assess for edema in feet, legs daily, monitor I&O, daily weight; check for jugular vein distention, rales, bilaterally, dyspnea (CHF)
- Monitor skin turgor, dryness of mucous membranes for hydration status, especially in G elderly

Associated nursing diagnoses

✓ Cardiac output, decreased (uses)
✓ Injury, risk for (adverse reactions)
✓ Knowledge deficit (teaching)
✓ Noncompliance (teaching)

Implementation

PO route

- Given ac, hs, tab may be crushed or swallowed whole; give with food to prevent GI upset; reduce dosage in renal dysfunction
- Store protected from light, moisture; placed in cool environment

Patient/family education

- Teach patient not to discontinue drug abruptly, taper over 2 wk; may cause precipitate angina if stopped abruptly
- Teach patient not to use OTC products containing α-adrenergic stimulants (such as nasal decongestants, cold preparations); to avoid alcohol and smoking and to limit sodium intake as prescribed
- Teach patient how to take pulse and B/P at home, advise when to notify prescriber
- Instruct patient to comply with weight control, dietary adjustments, modified exercise program
- Caution patient to carry/wear Medic Alert ID to identify drug begin taken, allergies
- Inform patient that drug controls symptoms but does not cure
- Caution patient to avoid hazardous activities if dizziness, drowsiness is present
- Teach patient to report symptoms of CHF: difficulty breathing, especially on exertion or when lying down; night cough; swelling of extremities; bradycardia; dizziness; confusion; depression; fever
- Teach patient to take drug as prescribed, not to double or skip doses; take any missed doses as soon as remembered if at least 4 hr until next dose

Evaluation

Positive therapeutic outcome

- Absence of dysrhythmias

Treatment of overdose:

Lavage; **IV** atropine for bradycardia; **IV** theophylline for bronchospasm; digitalis, O_2, diuretic for cardiac failure; hemodialysis; **IV** glucose for hyperglycemia; **IV** diazepam (or phenytoin) for seizures

S

spectinomycin

(spek-ti-noe-mye'sin)

Trobicin

Func. class.: Antibiotic

Chem. class.: Aminocyclitol

Pregnancy category **B**

Action: Inhibits bacterial synthesis by binding to 30S subunit on ribosome

Therapeutic Outcome: Treatment and resolution of gonococcal infection

Uses: Gonorrhea, gonococcal urethritis, cervicitis, proctitis

Dosage and routes

P *Adult and child >45 kg:* IM 2-4 g as single dose

P *Child <45 kg:* 40 mg/kg single dose

Available forms: Powder for inj IM 2, 4 g

Side effects/adverse reactions

CNS: Dizziness, chills, fever, insomnia, headache, anxiety

GI: ***Nausea,*** vomiting, increased BUN

GU: Decreased urine output

HEMA: Anemia

INTEG: ***Pain at injection site,*** urticaria, rash, pruritus, fever

Contraindications: Hypersensitivity, syphilis

Precautions: Pregnancy **B,** P infants, children

Pharmacokinetics

Absorption	Well absorbed (IM)
Distribution	Unknown
Metabolism	Liver
Excretion	Kidneys
Half-life	1⅔-2½ hr

Pharmacodynamics

	IM
Onset	Rapid
Peak	1 hr

NURSING CONSIDERATIONS

Assessment

- Monitor gonorrhea culture after treatment
- Monitor I&O ratio; report decreased output
- Monitor liver studies: AST (SGOT), ALT (SGPT), serum alk phosphatase following multiple doses
- Monitor blood studies: Hct, Hgb, BUN if multiple diagnoses given
- Monitor serologic test for gonorrhea 3 mo after treatment
- Assess for allergies before treatment, reaction of each medication

Associated nursing diagnoses

✓ Infection, risk for (uses)

✓ Knowledge deficit (teaching)

Implementation

IM route

- Give after shaking vial; IM in deep muscle mass; with 20-gauge needle; no more than 5 ml per site
- Store at room temp; reconstituted sol should be discarded after 24 hr

Evaluation

Positive therapeutic outcome
• Negative gonorrhea culture after treatment

spironolactone

(speer'on-oh-lak'tone)
Aldactone, Novospiroton, Sincomen
Func. class: Potassium-sparing diuretic
Chem. class.: Aldosterone antagonist
Pregnancy category **D**

Action: Competes with aldosterone at receptor sites in the distal tubule in the renal system, resulting in excretion of sodium, chloride, water, bicarbonate, and calcium. Potassium, phosphate and hydrogen are retained.

➔ **Therapeutic Outcome:** Diuretic and antihypertensive effect while retaining potassium; lowered aldosterone levels

Uses: Edema, hypertension, diuretic induced hypokalemia, primary hyperaldosteronism (diagnosis, short-term treatment, long-term treatment), nephrotic syndrome, cirrhosis of the liver with ascites

Dosage and routes

Edema/Hypertension

Adult: PO 25-200 mg/qd in single or divided doses

P *Child:* PO 3.3 mg/kg/day in single or divided doses

Hypokalemia

Adult: PO 25-100 mg/day; if PO, K supplements are unable to be used

Primary hyperaldosteronism diagnosis

Adult: PO 400 mg/day × 4 days depending on the test, then 100-400 mg/day maintenance

Available forms: Tab 25, 50, 100 mg

Side effects/adverse reactions

CNS: Headache, confusion, drowsiness, lethargy, ataxia
CV: Dysrythmias
ELECT: Hyperchloremic metabolic acidosis, ***hyperkalemia,*** hyponatremia
ENDO: Impotence, gynecomastia, irregular menses, amenorrhea, postmenopausal bleeding, hirsutism, deepening voice
GI: Diarrhea, cramps, bleeding, gastritis, vomiting
HEMA: Decreased WBCs, platelets

Contraindications: Hypersensitivity, anuria, severe renal disease, hyperkalemia, pregnancy **D**

G **Precautions:** Dehydration, hepatic disease, lactation, elderly

Pharmacokinetics

PO

Absorption	GI tract; well absorbed
Distribution	Crosses placenta
Metabolism	Liver to canrenone (active metabolite)
Excretion	Renal; breast milk
Half-life	12-24 hr (canrenone)

S

Pharmacodynamics

	PO
Onset	24-48 hr
Peak	48-72 hr
Duration	Unknown

Interaction

Drug/drug:

Individual drugs

Aspirin: ↓ action of spironolactone

Digitalis: ↑ action

Lithium: ↑ action, toxicity

Drug classifications

ACE inhibitors: ↑ hyperkalemia

Antihypertensives: ↑ action

Diuretics, potassium-sparing: ↑ hyperkalemia

Nonsteroidal anti-inflammatories: ↓ antihypertensive reaction, adverse reactions

Potassium products: ↑ hyperkalemia

Salt substitutes: ↑ hyperkalemia

Drug/food:

Potassium foods: ↑ hyperkalemia

Lab test interferences

False increase: Urinary catecholamines

Inteference: Glucose, insulin tolerance tests

NURSING CONSIDERATIONS

Assessment

- Monitor manifestations of hyperkalemia: *MS:* fatigue, muscle weakness; *CARDIAC:* arrhythmias hypotension, *NEURO:* paresthesias, confusion, *RESP:* dyspnea
- Monitor for manifestations of hyponatremia: *CV:* ↑ B/P, cold, clammy skin, hypo or hypervolemia; *GI:* anorexia, nausea, vomiting, diarrhea, abdominal cramps; *NEURO:* lethargy, increased ICP, confusion headache, seizures, coma, fatigue, tremors, hyperreflexia
- Monitor for manifestations of hyperchloremia: *NEURO:* weakness, lethargy, coma; *RESP:* deep rapid breathing
- Assess fluid volume status: I&O ratios and record, count or weigh diapers as appropriate, weight, distended red veins, crackles in lung, color, quality and sp gr of urine, skin turgor, adequacy of pulses, moist mucous membranes, bilateral lung sounds, peripheral pitting edema. Dehydration symptoms of decreasing output, thirst, hypotension, dry mouth and mucous membranes should be reported.
- Monitor electrolytes: potassium, sodium, calcium, magnesium; also include BUN, ABGs, uric acid, CBC, blood sugar

Associated nursing diagnoses

- ☑ Urinary elmination, altered (adverse reactions)
- ☑ Fluid volume deficit (adverse reactions)
- ☑ Fluid volume excess (uses)
- ☑ Knowledge deficit (teaching)

Implementation

- Give in AM to avoid interference with sleep

PO route

- With food, if nausea occurs,

absorption may be increased; take at same time each day

Patient/family education

General

- Teach patient to take the medication early in the day to prevent nocturia
- Instruct the patient to take with food or milk if GI symptoms of nausea and anorexia occur
- Teach patient to maintain a record of weight on a weekly basis and notify prescriber of weight loss of >5 lbs
- Caution patient that this drug causes an increase in potassium levels, that foods high in potassium should be avoided. Refer to dietician for assistance planning
- Teach patient not to use alcohol, or any over-the-counter medications without prescriber's approval; serious drug reactions may occur
- Emphasize the need to contact prescriber immediately if muscle cramps, weakness, nausea, dizziness, or numbness ocurs
- Teach patient to take own B/P and pulse and record
- Advise patient that dizziness and confusion may occur; avoid driving or other hazardous activities if alertness is decreased
- Teach patient to continue taking medication even if feeling better; this drug controls symptoms but does not cure the condition
- Advise patient with hypertension to continue other treatment (exercise, weight loss, relaxation techniques, cessation of smoking)

Evaluation

Positive therapeutic outcome

- Prevention of hypokalemia (diuretic use)
- Decreased edema
- Decreased B/P
- Decreased aldosterone levels
- Increased diuresis

Treatment of overdose:

- Lavage if taken orally, monitor electrolytes
- Administer sodium bicarbonate for K^2 6.5 mEq/L
- Monitor hydration, CV, renal status

stavudine

(sta'vu-deen)

Zerit

Func. class.: Antiviral

Chem. class.: Primidone Nucleoside

Pregnancy category **C**

Action: Prevents replication of HIV by the inhibition of the enzyme reverse transcriptase

➔ **Therapeutic Outcome:** Decreasing diarrhea, fatigue, night sweats; increased body weight

Uses: Treatment of advanced HIV infection for patients who have not responded to other antivirals

Dosage and routes

Adult >60 kg: PO 40 mg q12h up to 2 mg/kg/day

Adult <60 kg: 30 mg q12h

S

Available forms: Cap 15, 20, 30, 40 mg

Side effects/adverse reactions

CNS: ***Peripheral neuropathy***
GI: ***Hepatotoxicity***
HEMA: ***Bone marrow suppression***, anemia
INTEG: Rash
MS: Myalgia

Contraindications: Hypersensitivity to this drug or zidovudine, didanosine, zalcitabine; severe peripheral neuropathy

Precautions: Advanced HIV infections, pregnancy, lactation, bone marrow suppression, renal disease, liver disease, folic acid or B_{12} deficiency

Pharmacokinetics

Absorption	Rapidly absorbed (PO) 82% bioavailability
Distribution	Cerebrospinal fluid
Metabolism	Unknown
Excretion	Kidneys, breast milk
Half-life	Elimination: 1-1.6 hr, intracellular: 3-3.5 hr

Pharmacodynamics

	PO
Onset	Unknown
Peak	1 hr
Duration	Unknown

Interactions

Drug/drug:

Drug classifications

Myelosuppressants: ↑ myelosuppressor

NURSING CONSIDERATIONS

Assessment

- Monitor liver studies: AST (SGOT), ALT (SGPT)
- Monitor blood studies: WBC, diff, RBC, Hct, Hgb, platelets
- Monitor renal studies: urinalysis, protein, blood
- Obtain C&S before drug therapy; drug may be taken as soon as culture is taken; C&S may be taken after therapy
- Monitor bowel pattern before, during treatment
- Monitor fluid overload; drug requires large volume to stay in sol
- Assess for weakness, tremors, confusion, dizziness, psychosis; if these occur, drug may have to be decreased or discontinued

Associated nursing diagnoses

- ✓ Infection, risk for (uses)
- ✓ Knowledge deficit (teaching)

Implementation

PO route

- Give with or without meals, absorption does not appear to be lowered when taken with food

Patient/family education

- Teach patient signs of peripheral neuropathy: burning, weakness, pain, pricking feeling in the extremities
- Caution patient that this drug should not be given with antineoplastics
- Inform patient that GI complaints and insomnia resolve after 3-4 wk of treatment

• Inform patient that drug is not cure for AIDS, but will control symptoms
• Advise patient to call prescriber if sore throat, swollen lymph nodes, malaise, fever occur—may indicate presence of other infections
• Caution patient that even with drug administration, patient is still infective and may pass AIDS virus on to others
• Caution patient that follow-up visits must be continued because serious toxicity may occur, blood counts must be done q2wk
• Teach patient that drug must be taken q4hr around clock even during night
• Caution patient that serious drug interactions may occur if OTC products are ingested; check with prescriber first if taking aspirin, acetaminophen, indomethacin
• Inform patient that other drugs may be necessary to prevent other infections
• Inform patient that drug may cause fainting or dizziness

Evaluation

Positive therapeutic outcome
• Decreased symptoms of HIV

streptokinase 🔑

(strep-toe-kye'nase)
Kabikinase, Streptase
Func. class.: Thrombolytic enzyme
Chem. class.: β-hemolytic streptococcus filtrate (purified)
Pregnancy category **C**

Action: Activates conversion of plasminogen to plasmin (fibrinolysin): plasmin breaks down clots (fibrin), fibrinogen, factors V, VII; occlusion of venous access lines

➔ **Therapeutic Outcome:** Lysis of emboli, or thrombosis in various parts of the body

Uses: Deep vein thrombosis, pulmonary embolism, arterial thrombosis, arterial embolism, arteriovenous cannula occlusion, lysis of coronary artery thrombi after MI, acute evolving transmural MI

Dosage and routes

Lysis of coronary artery thrombi
Adult: CC 20,000 IU, then 2000 IU/min over 1 hr as **IV** INF

Arteriovenous cannula occlusion
Adult: **IV** INF 250,000 IU/2 ml sol into occluded limb of cannula run over ½ hr; clamp for 2 hr; aspirate contents; flush with NaCl sol and reconnect

Thrombosis/embolism
Adult: **IV** INF 250,000 IU over ½ hr, then 100,000 IU/hr for 72 hr for deep thrombosis; 100,000 IU/hr over 24-72 hr for pulmonary embolism

Acute evolving transmural MI
Adult: **IV** INF 1,500,000 IU diluted to a volume of 45 ml; give within 1 hr

S

Available forms: Inj 250,000, 600,000, 750,000 IU

Side effects/adverse reactions

CNS: Headache, fever
EENT: Periorbital edema
GI: Nausea
HEMA: Decreased Hct, ***bleeding***
INTEG: Rash, urticaria, phlebitis at **IV** inf site, itching, flushing
MS: Low back pain
RESP: Altered respirations, SOB, ***bronchospasm***
SYST: ***GI, GU, intracranial retroperitoneal bleeding, surface bleeding, anaphylaxis***

Contraindications: Hypersensitivity, active bleeding, intraspinal surgery, neoplasms of the CNS, ulcerative colitis, enteritis, severe hypertension, severe renal disease, hepatic disease, hypocoagulation, COPD, subacute bacterial endocarditis, rheumatic valvular disease, cerebral embolism/thrombosis/hemorrhage, intraarterial diagnostic procedure or surgery (10 days), recent major surgery

Precautions: Arterial emboli from left side of heart, pregnancy **C**

Pharmacokinetics

Absorption	Completely absorbed (IV)
Distribution	Unknown
Metabolism	>80%—liver, rapidly cleared by reticuloendothelial system
Excretion	Kidneys
Half-life	35 min

Pharmacodynamics

	IV
Onset	Immediate
Peak	Rapid
Duration	<12 hr

Interaction

Drug/drug:

Individual drugs
Aspirin: ↑ bleeding
Dipyridamole: ↑ bleeding
Heparin: ↑ bleeding
Plicamycin: ↑ bleeding
Valproic acid: ↑ bleeding

Drug classifications
Cephalosporins: ↑ bleeding
Anticoagulants, oral: ↑ bleeding
Nonsteroidal antiinflammatories: ↑ bleeding

Lab test interferences

Increase: PT, APTT, TT

NURSING CONSIDERATIONS

Assessment

- Monitor VS, B/P, pulse, respirations (including peripheral), neurologic signs, temp at least q4h; temp >104° F (40° C) indicates internal bleeding; monitor rhythm closely; ventricular dysrhythmias may occur with hyperfusion; monitor heart, breath sounds, neuro status, peripheral pulses
- Assess for bleeding during first hr of treatment: hematuria, hematemesis, bleeding from mucous membranes, epistaxis, ecchymosis; guaiac, all body fluids, stools; blood studies (Hct, platelets, PTT, PT, TT, APTT) before starting therapy; PT or APTT must be less than 2 × control before

starting therapy TT or PT q3-4h during treatment

- Assess allergy: fever, rash, itching, chills; mild reaction may be treated with antihistamines; report to prescriber
- Monitor ECG on monitor, watch for segment changes, changes in rhythm; sinus bradycardia, ventricular tachycardia, accelerated idioventricular rhythm may occur as a result of reperfusion (coronary thrombosis)
- Monitor ABGs, respiratory rate, (depth, characteristics), pulse, B/P, hemodynamics (pulmonary embolism)
- Monitor peripheral pulses, assess Homan's sign, check for redness, swelling q hr; notify health care prescriber of changes; B/P should not be taken in extremities (deep vein thrombosis)
- Check catheter for ability to aspirate blood from port; patient must exhale and hold breath when inserting and removing syringe to prevent air embolism (catheter/cannula occlusion)

Associated nursing diagnoses

- ✓ Tissue perfusion, altered (uses)
- ✓ Injury, risk for (adverse reactions)
- ✓ Impaired gas exchange (uses)
- ✓ Knowledge deficit (teaching)

Implementation

IV **IV route**

- Give after reconstituting with provided diluent; add appropriate amount of sterile water for inj (no preservatives) 20 mg vial/20 ml or 50 mg vial/50 ml to make 1 mg/ml, mix by slow inversion or dilute with NaCl, D_5W to a concentration of 0.5 mg/ml; further dilution, 1.5 to <0.5 mg/ml may result in precipitation of drug; use 18-gauge needle; flush line with NaCl after administration; reconstituted **IV** solution within 8 hr; within 6 hr of coronary occlusion for best results
- Give **IV** loading dose over 30 min to avoid hypotension
- **IV** after dilution with 4-5 g/250 ml NS, D_5W, LR, give over 1 hr; may give by continuous inf after loading dose(s) of 1 g/hr diluted in 50-100 ml of compatible sol; use inf pump; do not give by direct **IV**
- Give heparin therapy after thrombolytic therapy is discontinued, TT, ACT, or APTT less than 2 × control (about 3-4 hr)
- Avoid invasive procedures, injection, taking temp via rec route
- Apply pressure for 30 sec to minor bleeding sites; 30 min to sites of atrial puncture, followed by pressure dressing; inform prescriber if this does not attain hemostasis; apply pressure dressing
- Store powder at room temp or refrigerate; protect from excessive light

Y-site incompatibilities:

Dobutamine, dopamine, heparin, nitroglycerine

Y-site compatibility:

Lidocaine

Additive incompatibilities:

Do not mix with other medications

S

Patient/family education

- Teach patient reason for medication, signs and symptoms of bleeding, allergic reactions, when to notify prescriber
- Explain that patient is to remain on bed rest to avoid injury

Evaluation

Positive therapeutic outcome

- Lysis of thrombi or emboli

streptomycin

(strep-toe-mye'sin)

Func. class.: Antiinfective, antitubercular

Chem. class.: Aminoglycoside

Pregnancy category B

Action: Interferes with protein synthesis in bacterial cell by binding to ribosomal subunit, causing inaccurate peptide sequence to form in protein chain, resulting in bacterial death

Therapeutic Outcome: Bactericidal effects for the following organisms: sensitive strains of *M. tuberculosis,* nontuberculous infections caused by sensitive strains of *Y. pestus, Brucella, H. influenzae, K. pneumoniae, E. coli, E. aerogenes, S. viridans, F. tularensis, Proteus*

Uses: Active TB; used in combination for streptococcal and enterococcal infections; endocarditis, tularemia, plague

Dosage and routes

Tuberculosis

Adult: IM 1 g qd × 2-3 mo, then 1 g 2-3 ×/week given with other antitubercular drugs

P ***Child:*** IM 20-40 mg/kg/day in divided doses given with other antitubercular drugs; max 15 mg/kg/day

Streptococcal endocarditis

Adult: IM 1 g q12h × 1 wk with penicillin, then 500 mg bid × 1 wk

Enterococcal endocarditis

Adult: IM 1 g q12h × 2 wk, then 500 mg q12h × 4 wk with penicillin max 15 mg/kg/day

Available forms: Inj 1, 5 g: 400 mg/ml

Side effects/adverse reactions

CNS: Confusion, depression, numbness, tremors, ***convulsions,*** muscle twitching, ***neurotoxicity***
CV: Hypotension, myocarditis, palpitations
EENT: ***Ototoxicity,*** deafness, visual disturbances
GI: *Nausea, vomiting, anorexia,* increased ALT (SGPT), AST (SGOT), bilirubin, hepatomegaly, ***hepatic necrosis,*** splenomegaly
GU: ***Oliguria, hematuria, renal damage, azotemia, renal failure, nephrotoxicity***
HEMA: ***Agranulocytosis, thrombocytopenia, leukopenia, eosinophilia, anemia***
INTEG: *Rash,* burning urticaria, dermatitis, alopecia

Contraindications: Severe renal disease, hypersensitivity

Precautions: Neonates, mild renal disease, pregnancy **B**, myasthenia gravis, lactation, G hearing deficits, elderly, Parkinson's disease

Pharmacokinetics

Absorption:	Well absorbed (IM)
Distribution	Widely distributed in extracellular fluids, poorly distributed in CSF; crosses placenta
Metabolism	Minimal—liver
Excretion	Mostly unchanged (>90%) kidneys
Half-life	2-2½ hr, increase in renal disease

Pharmacodynamics

	IM
Onset	Rapid
Peak	1-2 hr

Interactions

Drug/drug:

Individual drugs

Amphotericin B: ↑ Ototoxicity, neurotoxicity, nephrotoxicity
Cisplatin: ↑ Ototoxicity, neurotoxicity, nephrotoxicity
Ethacrynic acid: ↑ Ototoxicity, neurotoxicity, nephrotoxicity
Furosemide: ↑ Ototoxicity, neurotoxicity, nephrotoxicity
Mannitol: ↑ Ototoxicity, neurotoxicity, nephrotoxicity
Methoxyflurane: ↑ Ototoxicity, neurotoxicity, nephrotoxicity
Polymyxin: ↑ Ototoxicity, neurotoxicity, nephrotoxicity
Succinylcholine: ↑ Neuromuscular blockade, respiratory depression
Vancomycin: ↑ Ototoxicity, neurotoxicity, nephrotoxicity

Drug classifications

Anesthetics: ↑ Neuromuscular blockade, respiratory depression
Aminoglycosides: ↑ Ototoxicity, neurotoxicity, nephrotoxicity
Nondepolarizing neuromuscular blockers: ↑ Neuromuscular blockade, respiratory depression
Penicillins: Inactivated in renal disease

NURSING CONSIDERATIONS

Assessment

- Assess patient for previous sensitivity reaction
- Assess patient for signs and symptoms of infection including characteristics of sputum, urine, stool WBC >10,000, temp
- Obtain baseline information before and during treatment
- Complete C&S testing before and beginning drug therapy—this will identify if correct treatment has been initiated
- Assess for allergic reactions: rash, urticaria, pruritus, chills, fever, joint pain; angioedema may occur a few days after therapy begins—epinephrine, resuscitation equipment should be on unit for anaphylactic reaction
- Identify urine output; if decreasing, notify prescriber (may indicate nephrotoxicity); also, increased BUN, creatinine, urine CrCl <80 ml/min
- Monitor blood studies: AST (SGOT), ALT (SGPT), CBC, Hct, bilirubin, LDH, alk phosphatase, Coombs' test monthly

S

if patient is on long-term therapy
• Monitor electrolytes: potassium, sodium, chloride monthly if patient is on long-term therapy
• Monitor for bleeding: ecchymosis, bleeding gums, hematuria, stool guaiac daily if on long-term therapy
• Assess for overgrowth of infection: perineal itching, fever, malaise, redness, pain, swelling, drainage, rash, diarrhea, change in cough, sputum
• Obtain weight before treatment; calculation of dosage is usually based on ideal body weight, but may be calculated on actual body weight
• Monitor I&O ratio; urinalysis daily for proteinuria, cells, casts; report sudden change in urine output
• Obtain serum peak 60 min after IM inj, trough level drawn just before next dose; blood level should be 2-4 times bacteriostatic level
• Monitor for deafness by audiometric testing, ringing, roaring in ears, vertigo; assess hearing before, during, after treatment
• Monitor for dehydration: high sp gr, decrease in skin turgor, dry mucous membranes, dark urine
• Monitor for overgrowth of infection including increased temp, malaise, redness, pain, swelling, perineal itching, diarrhea, stomatitis, change in cough, sputum

Associated nursing diagnoses

✓ Infection, risk for (uses)
✓ Diarrhea (adverse reactions)
✓ Injury, risk for (adverse reactions)
✓ Knowledge deficit (teaching)
✓ Noncompliance (teaching

Implementation

IM route
• Give deeply in large muscle mass
• Reconstitute with 4.2-4.5 ml sterile water for inj or 0.9% NaCl/1 g (200 mg/ml); 3.2-3.5 ml/1 g (250 mg/ml); 17 ml/5 g (250 mg/ml) (500 mg/ml); give at 500 mg/ml or less

Syringe incompatibility:
Heparin

Patient/family education

• Teach patient to report sore throat, bruising, bleeding, joint pain, (may indicate blood dyscrasias—rare), ringing, roaring in the ears
• Advise patient to contact prescriber if vaginal itching, loose, foul-smelling stools, furry tongue occur—may indicate superimposed infection

Evaluation

Positive therapeutic outcome
• Absence of signs/symptoms of infection
• Reported improvement in symptoms of infection

Treatment of overdose:
Withdraw drug, hemodialysis, monitor serum levels of drug, may give ticarcillin or carbenicillin

streptozocin
(strep-toe-zoe'sin)
Zanosar
Func. class.: Antineoplastic alkylating agent
Chem. class.: Nitrosourea
Pregnancy category C

Action: Alkylates DNA, RNA; inhibits enzymes that allow synthesis of amino acids in proteins; is also responsible for cross-linking DNA strands; activity is not specific to phase of cell cycle

Therapeutic Outcome: Prevention of rapidly growing malignant cells, decreased calcium levels

Uses: Metastatic islet cell carcinoma of pancreas

Investigational uses: Prevention of spread of Hodgkins' disease, metastatic carcinoid tumor, pancreatic adenocarcinoma colon malignancies

Dosage and routes
Adult: **IV** 500 mg/m^2 × 5 days q6 wk until desired response; alternate with 1 g/m^2 qwk × 2 wk, not to exceed 1.5 g/m^2 in 1 dose

Available forms: Inj 1 g

Side effects/adverse reactions
CNS: Confusion, depression, lethargy
GI: Nausea, vomiting, diarrhea, weight loss, ***hepatotoxicity***
GU: ***Azotemia, anuria,*** hypophosphatemia, glycosuria, renal tubular acidosis, ***renal toxicity***
HEMA: ***Thrombocytopenia, leukopenia, pancytopenia***

Contraindications: Hypersensitivity

Precautions: Radiation therapy, children, lactation, pregnancy **C**, hepatic disease, renal disease

Pharmacokinetics

Absorption	Complete bioavailability
Distribution	Rapid, crosses placenta
Metabolism	Liver, kidneys—extensively
Excretion	<20% kidneys unchanged
Half-life	35-40 min

Pharmacodynamics

	IV
Onset	Unknown
Peak	Unknown
Duration	Unknown

Interactions
Drug/drug:
Individual drugs
Doxorubicin: ↑ toxicity
Phenytoin: ↑ toxicity
Radiation: ↑ toxicity, bone marrow suppression
Drug classifications
Aminoglycosides: ↑ risk of nephrotoxicity
Antineoplastics: ↑ toxicity, bone marrow suppression
Live virus vaccines: ↓ antibody response

NURSING CONSIDERATIONS
Assessment
- Assess symptoms indicating

severe allergic reaction: rash, pruritus, urticaria, purpuric skin lesions, itching, flushing
- Monitor CBC, differential, platelet count weekly; withhold drug if WBC count is <4000/mm^3 or platelet count is <100,000/mm^3, notify prescriber of results if WBC <20,000/mm^3, platelets </50,800/mm^3
- Monitor renal function studies: BUN, creatinine, serum uric acid, urine CrCl before and during therapy; I&O ratio; report fall in urine output to <30 ml/hr
- Monitor temp q4hr (may indicate beginning of infection)
- Monitor liver function tests before and during therapy [bilirubin, AST (SGOT), ALT (SGPT), LDH] as needed or monthly; yellowing of skin, sclera, dark urine, clay-colored stools, itchy skin, abdominal pain, fever, diarrhea
- Assess for bleeding: hematuria, stool guaiac, bruising or petechiae, mucosa or orifices q8hr; inflammation of mucosa, breaks in skin
- Identify edema in feet, joint pain, stomach pain, shaking; health care prescriber should be notified
- Identify inflammation of mucosa, breaks in skin

Associated nursing diagnoses

- ✓ Injury, risk for (adverse reactions)
- ✓ Body image disturbance (adverse reactions)
- ✓ Infection, risk for (adverse reactions)
- ✓ Knowledge deficit (teaching)

Implementation

- Hypoglycemia may occur, have **IV** dextrose available
- Give fluids **IV** or PO before chemotherapy to hydrate patient
- Give antiemetic 30-60 min before giving drug to prevent vomiting, and prn
- Give antibiotics for prophylaxis of infection
- Give topical or systemic analgesics for pain
- Provide liq diet: carbonated beverages; gelatin may be added if patient is not nauseated or vomiting
- Provide rinsing of mouth tid-qid with water, club soda; brushing of teeth bid-qid with soft brush or cotton-tipped applicators for stomatitis; use unwaxed dental floss

IV **IV route**
- Give **IV** after diluting 1 g/9.5 ml 0.9% NaCl or D_5 (100 mg/ml)
- May be further diluted with 10-200 ml 0.9% NaCl, D_5W give over prescribed rate, usually 15 min

Patient/family education

- Inform patient that contraceptive measures are recommended during therapy
- Caution patient to avoid use of products containing aspirin or ibuprofen, razors, commercial mouthwash—bleeding may occur; to report symptoms of bleeding (hematuria, tarry stools)
- Instruct patient to report signs of anemia, (fatigue, headache, irritability, faintness, shortness of breath)
- Caution patient not to have any vaccinations without the

advice of the prescriber, serious reactions can occur

Evaluation

Positive therapeutic outcome
- Prevention of rapid division of malignant cells

succimer
(sux'i-mer)
Chemet
Func. class: Heavy metal antagonist
Chem. class.: Chelating agent
Pregnancy category **C**

Action: Binds with ions of lead to form a water-soluble complex that is excreted by kidneys

➔ **Therapeutic Outcome:** Removal of lead from the body

Uses: Lead poisoning in children with lead levels above 45 µg/dl; may be beneficial in mercury, arsenic poisoning

Dosage and routes

Child: PO 10 mg/kg or 350 mg/m^2 q8h × 5 days, then 10 mg/kg or 350 mg/m^2 q12h × 2 wk; another course may be required depending on lead levels; allow 2 wk between courses

Available forms: Cap 100 mg

Side effects/adverse reactions

CNS: Drowsiness, dizziness, paresthesia, sensorimotor neuropathy
EENT: Otitis media, watery eyes, film in eyes, plugged ears
GI: Nausea, vomiting, diarrhea, metallic taste, anorexia
GU: ***Proteinuria,*** decreased urination, voiding difficulties
HEMA: ***Increased platelets, intermittent eosinophilia***
INTEG: Rash, urticaria, pruritus
META: Increased AST (SGOT), ALT (SGPT), alk phosphatase, cholesterol
RESP: Sore throat, rhinorrhea, nasal congestion, cough
SYST: Back, stomach, head, rib flank pain; abdominal cramps; chills; fever; flulike symptoms, head cold; headache

Contraindications: Hypersensitivity

Precautions: Pregnancy **C,** P lactation, children <1 yr

Pharmacokinetics	
Absorption	Rapidly absorbed (PO)
Distribution	Unknown
Metabolism	Liver—extensively
Excretion	Kidneys—unchanged
Half-life	2 days

Pharmacodynamics	
Onset	Up to 2 hr
Peak	2-4 hr
Duration	8-12 hr

Interactions

Drug/drug:

Drug classifications
Heavy metal antagonist, others: Do not use together

S

NURSING CONSIDERATIONS

Assessment

- Assess VS, B/P, pulse, respirations, weigh daily
- Monitor I&O, kidney function studies, BUN, creatinine, CrCl; watch for decreasing urine output
- Assess neuro status: watch for paresthesias, beginning convulsions
- Monitor urine: pH, albumin, casts, blood, coproporphyrins, calcium
- Assess for febrile reactions that may occur 4-8 hr following drug therapy
- Monitor for cardiac abnormalities: dysrhythmias, hypotension, tachycardia
- Assess for allergic reactions (rash, urticaria); if these occur, drug should be discontinued

Associated nursing diagnoses

✓ Poisoning, risk for (uses)
✓ Injury, risk for (uses, adverse reactions)
✓ Knowledge deficit (teaching)

Implementation

PO route

- Give PO whole or cap contents mixed with food or fluid

Patient/family education

- Explain reason for medication and expected results
- Provide a referral to health department to assess lead levels in home or workplace

Evaluation

Positive therapeutic outcome

- Decreased symptoms of lead intoxication
- Decreased lead level <50 μg/dl

succinylcholine

(suk-sin-ill-koe'leen)

Anectine, Anectine Flo-Pack, Quelicin, succinylcholine chloride, Sucostrin, Suxamethonium

Func. class.: Neuromuscular blocker (depolarizing—ultra short)
Chem. class.:

Pregnancy category **C**

Action: Inhibits transmission of nerve impulses by binding with cholinergic receptor sites, antagonizing action of acetylcholine; causes release of histamine

➡ **Therapeutic Outcome:** Paralysis of skeletal muscles

Uses: Facilitation of endotracheal intubation, skeletal muscle relaxation during orthopedic manipulations

Dosage and routes

Adult: **IV** 25-75 mg, then 2.5 mg/min as needed; IM 2.5 mg/kg, not to exceed 150 mg

P *Child:* **IV**/IM 1-2 mg/kg, not to exceed 150 mg IM

Available forms: Inj 20, 50, 100 mg/ml; powder for inj 100/vial; powder for inf 500 mg/vial, 1 g/vial

Side effects/adverse reactions

CV: Bradycardia, tachycardia; increased, decreased B/P, ***sinus arrest, dysrhythmias***
EENT: Increased secretions, increased IOP
HEMA: Myoglobulinemia
INTEG: Rash, flushing, pruritus, urticaria
MS: Weakness, muscle pain, fasciculation, prolonged relaxation
RESP: Prolonged apnea, bronchospasm, cyanosis, respiratory depression

Contraindications: Hypersensitivity, malignant hyperthermia, decreased plasma pseudocholinesterase, penetrating eye injuries, acute narrow-angle glaucoma

Precautions: Pregnancy **C**, cardiac disease, severe burns, fractures—fasciculation may increase damage—lactation, P children <2 yr, electrolyte imbalances, dehydration, neuromuscular disease, respiratory disease, collagen diseases, glaucoma, eye surgery, penetrating eye wounds, G elderly or debilitated patients

Pharmacokinetics

Absorption	Well absorbed (IM)
Distribution	Widely distributed, crosses placenta
Metabolism	Plasma (90%)
Excretion	Hydrolyzed in urine (active/inactive metabolites)
Half-life	Unknown

Pharmacodynamics

	IV	IM
Onset	1 min	2-3 min
Peak	2-3 min	Unknown
Duration	6-10 min	10-30 min

Interactions

Drug/drug:

Individual drugs

Clindamycin: ↑ neuromuscular blockage
Ecothiphate: ↑ paralysis
Enflurane: ↑ neuromuscular blockage
Isofluorophate: ↑ paralysis
Isoflurane: ↑ neuromuscular blockage
Lincomycin: ↑ neuromuscular blockage
Quinidine: ↑ neuromuscular blockage

Drug classifications

Aminoglycosides: ↑ neuromuscular blockage
Beta blockers: ↑ neuromuscular blockage
Local anesthetics: ↑ neuromuscular blockage
Magnesium salts: ↑ neuromuscular blockage
Polymyxin antibiotics: ↑ neuromuscular blockage
Diuretics, potassium-losing: ↑ neuromuscular blockage

S

NURSING CONSIDERATIONS

Assessment

- Assess for electrolyte imbalances (potassium, magnesium); may lead to increased action of this drug
- Monitor vital signs (B/P, pulse, respirations, airway) until fully recovered; rate, depth, pattern of respirations, strength of hand grip

• Monitor I&O ratio; check for urinary retention, frequency, hesitancy
• Assess for recovery: decreased paralysis of face, diaphragm, leg, arm, rest of body
• Assess for allergic reactions: rash, fever, respiratory distress, pruritus; drug should be discontinued if these occur

Associated nursing diagnoses

✓ Communication, impaired verbal (adverse reactions)
✓ Breathing pattern, ineffective (uses)

Implementation

IV **IV route**
• Use nerve stimulator by anesthesiologist to determine neuromuscular blockade
• Give anticholinesterase to reverse neuromuscular blockade
• Give by **IV** inf; dilute 1-2 mg/ml in D_5, isotonic saline sol, give 0.5-10 mg/min, titrate to patient response; may be given directly over 1 min

Syringe compatibility:

Heparin

Y-site compatibilities:

Potassium chloride, vitamin B with C

Additive compatibilities:

Amikacin, cephapirin, isoproterenol, meperidine, methyldopate, morphine, norepinephrine, scopolamine

Additive incompatibilities:

Barbiturates, nafcillin, sodium bicarbonate

IM route
• Give deep IM, preferably high in deltoid muscle
• Store in refrigerator; store powder at room temp; close container tightly

Patient/family education

• Explain reason for medication and expected results
• Provide reassurance if communication is difficult during recovery from neuromuscular blockade; postoperative stiffness is normal, soon subsides

Evaluation

Positive therapeutic outcome
• Paralysis of jaw, eyelid, head, neck, rest of body

Treatment of overdose:

Edrophonium or neostigmine, atropine, monitor VS; may require mechanical ventilation

sucralfate

(soo-kral'fate)
Carafate, Sulcrate ♣
Func. class.: Protectant; antiulcer
Chem. class.: Aluminum hydroxide/sulfated sucrose
Pregnancy category **B**

Action: Forms a complex that adheres to ulcer site, adsorbs pepsin

Therapeutic Outcome: Healing of ulcers

Uses: Duodenal ulcer

Investigational uses: Gastric ulcers, gastroesophageal reflux

Dosage and routes

Adult: PO 1 g qid 1 hr ac, hs

Available forms: Tab 1 g; oral susp 500 mg/5 ml ✤

Side effects/adverse reactions

CNS: Drowsiness, dizziness
GI: ***Dry mouth, constipation,*** nausea, gastric pain, vomiting
INTEG: Urticaria, rash, pruritus

Contraindications: Hypersensitivity

Precautions: Pregnancy **B**, lactation, children

Pharmacokinetics

Absorption	Minimally absorbed
Distribution	Unknown
Metabolism	Not metabolized
Excretion	Feces (90%)
Half-life	6-20 hr

Pharmacodynamics

	PO
Onset	½ hr
Peak	Unknown
Duration	5 hr

Interactions

Drug/drug:

Individual drugs

Phenytoin: ↓ absorption
Tetracycline: ↓ absorption

Drug classifications

Fluoroquinolones: ↓ absorption
Fat-soluble vitamins: ↓ absorption

NURSING CONSIDERATIONS

Assessment

- Monitor gastric pH (>5 should be maintained)

Associated nursing diagnoses

- ✓ Pain, chronic (uses)
- ✓ Pain (uses)
- ✓ Constipation (adverse reactions)
- ✓ Knowledge deficit (teaching)

Implementation

PO route

- Give on empty stomach 1 hr ac and hs
- Storage at room temp

Patient/family education

- Advise patient to avoid black pepper, caffeine, alcohol, harsh spices, extremes in temp of food—may aggravate condition
- Instruct patient to take medication on empty stomach
- Caution patient to take full course of therapy
- Caution patient to avoid antacids within ½ hr of drug or 1 hr after this drug

Evaluation

Positive therapeutic outcome

- Absence of pain or GI complaints

sufentanil
(soo-fen'ta-nil)
Sufenta
Func. class.: Narcotic analgesic
Chem. class.: Opiate, synthetic
Pregnancy category **C**
Controlled substance schedule **II**

Action: Inhibits ascending pain pathways in CNS, increases pain threshold, alters pain perception

➔ **Therapeutic Outcome:** Anesthesia, decreased pain

Uses: Primary anesthetic, adjunct to general anesthetic

Dosage and routes
Primary anesthetic
Adult: **IV** 8-30 μg/kg given with 100% O_2, a muscle relaxant

Adjunct
Adult: **IV** 1-8 μg/kg given with nitrous oxide/O_2

Available forms: Inj 50 μg/ml

Side effects/adverse reactions
CNS: Drowsiness, dizziness, confusion, headache, sedation, euphoria
CV: Palpitations, bradycardia, change in B/P
EENT: Tinnitus, blurred vision, miosis, diplopia
GI: Nausea, vomiting, anorexia, constipation, abdominal cramps
GU: Increased urinary output, dysuria, urinary retention
INTEG: Rash, urticaria, bruising, flushing, diaphoresis, pruritus
RESP: Respiratory depression

Contraindications: Hypersensitivity, addiction (narcotic)

Precautions: Addictive personality, pregnancy **C,** lactation, increased intracranial pressure, MI (acute), severe heart disease, respiratory depression, hepatic disease, renal disease, P child <18 yr

Pharmacokinetics

Absorption	Completely absorbed (IV)
Distribution	Crosses placenta
Metabolism	Liver—extensively, small intestines—small amount
Excretion	Kidneys, breast milk
Half-life	1-2 hr

Pharmacodynamics

	IV
Onset	Immediate
Peak	Unknown
Duration	5 min

Interactions
Drug/drug:
Individual drugs
Alcohol: ↑ respiratory depression, hypotension, ↑ sedation
Cimetidine: ↑ recovery
Erythromycin: ↑ recovery
Nalbuphine: ↓ analgesia
Pentazocine: ↓ analgesia

Drug classifications
Antihistamines: ↑ respiratory depression, hypotension
CNS depressants: ↑ respiratory depression, hypotension
MAOI: Do not use 2 wk before alfentanil
Phenothiazines: ↑ respiratory depression, hypotension
Sedative/hypnotics: ↑ respiratory depression, hypotension

Lab test interferences

Increase: Amylase

NURSING CONSIDERATIONS

Assessment

- Monitor VS after parenteral route; note muscle rigidity, drug history, liver, kidney function tests
- Monitor respiratory dysfunction: respiratory depression, character, rate, rhythm; notify prescriber if respirations are <10/min
- Monitor for CNS changes: dizziness, drowsiness, hallucinations, euphoria, LOC, pupil reaction
- Monitor allergic reactions: rash, urticaria

Associated nursing diagnoses

✓ Pain (uses)
✓ Sensory perceptual alteration: visual, auditory (adverse reactions)
✓ Breathing pattern, ineffective (adverse reactions)
✓ Knowledge deficit (teaching)

Implementation

- Give by inj (IM, **IV**), only with resuscitative equipment available; give slowly to prevent rigidity
- Give **IV** undiluted by anesthesiologist or diluted as an inf in 0.9% NaCl
- Store in light-resistant area at room temp

Patient/family education

- Advise patient to report any symptoms of CNS changes, allergic reactions
- Caution patient to avoid CNS depressants: alcohol, sedative/hypnotics for at least 24 hr after this drug
- Discuss with patient that dizziness, drowsiness, and confusion are common, to avoid getting up without assistance
- Discuss in detail all aspects of the drug

Evaluation

Positive therapeutic outcome
- Maintenance of anesthesia

Treatment of overdose:

Narcan 0.2-0.8 **IV**, O_2, **IV** fluids, vasopressors

sulfacetamide sodium (ophthalmic)

(sul-fa-seet'a-mide)

AK-Sulf, Bleph-10 Liquifilm, Bleph-10 S.O.P., Isopto Cetamide, Ophthacet, Sodium Sulamyd, sodium sulfacetamide 10%, sodium sulfacetamide 15%, sodium sulfacetamide 30%, SOSS-10, Sulfair 15

Func. class.: Antiinfective, ophthalmic

Chem. class.: Sulfonamide

Pregnancy category **C**

Action: Inhibits folic acid synthesis by preventing PABA use, which is necessary for bacterial growth

➔ **Therapeutic Outcome:** Bactericidal action against susceptible organisms

Uses: Conjunctivitis, superficial eye infections, corneal ulcers, prophylaxis against infection after removal of foreign matter from the eye

Dosage and routes

Adult and child: Instill 1-2 gtt q2-3h; Top apply ½-1 inch oint into conjunctival sac qid-tid and hs

Available forms: Ophth sol 10%, 15%, 30%; ophth oint 10%

Side effects/adverse reactions

EENT: Burning, stinging, swelling

Contraindications: Hypersensitivity

Precautions: Antibiotic hypersensitivity, pregnancy **C**

Pharmacokinetics

Absorption	Minimally absorbed
Distribution	None
Metabolism	None
Excretion	None
Half-life	Not known

Pharmacodynamics

	OPHTH
Onset	Rapid
Peak	Unknown
Duration	1-4 hr

Interactions

Drug/drug:

Individual drugs

Gentamicin, ophth: ↑ Antagonism

Mild silver nitrate: Incompatible with this drug

Silver nitrate: Incompatible with this drug

NURSING CONSIDERATIONS

Assessment

- Assess for allergy: itching, lacrimation, redness, swelling
- Asses for eye infection: discharge, pain, redness, baseline and during treatment

Associated nursing diagnoses

☑ Knowledge deficit (teaching)
☑ Infection, risk for (uses)

Implementation

Ophth route
• Administer after washing hands, cleanse crusts or discharge from eye before application; have patient tilt head back or lie down; instill after pulling lower lid down and place in conjunctival sac; wait at least 5 min before instilling other eye drops
• Store at room temp

Patient/family education

• Advise patient to use drug exactly as prescribed; not to use eye makeup, towels, washcloths, eye medication of others; reinfection may occur
• Teach patient that drug container tip should not be touched to eye; reinfection of the eye may occur
• Advise patient to report itching,
increased redness, burning, stinging; drug should be discontinued
• Caution patient that drug may cause blurred vision when ointment is applied

Evaluation

Positive therapeutic outcome
• Absence of redness, inflammation, tearing

sulfamethoxazole
(sul-fa-meth-ox'a-zole)
Apo-Sulfamethoxazole ♣, Gantanol, Gantanol DS
Func. class.: Antiinfective
Chem. class.: Sulfonamide, intermediate-acting
Pregnancy category **C**

Action: Interferes with bacterial biosynthesis of proteins by competitive antagonism of PABA

➔ **Therapeutic Outcome:** Bactericidal action against susceptible organisms: Streptococci and staphylococci, *Clostridium perfringens, Clostridium tetani, Nocardia asteroides;* active against gram-negative pathogens, including *Enterobacter, Escherichia coli, Klebsiella, Proteus mirabilis, Proteus vulgaris, Salmonella, Shigella*

Uses: UTIs, lymphogranuloma venereum, systemic infections

Dosage and routes

Adult: PO 2 g, then 1 g bid or tid for 7-10 days
P *Child >2 mo:* PO 50-60 mg/kg then 25-30 mg/kg bid, not to exceed 75 mg/kg/day

Lymphogranuloma venereum
Adult: PO 1 g bid × 14 days

Available forms: Tab 500 mg; oral susp 500 mg/5 ml

Side effects/adverse reactions

CNS: Headache, insomnia, hallucinations, depression, vertigo, fatigue, anxiety, convulsions, drug fever, chills, drowsiness
CV: Allergic myocarditis
GI: Nausea, vomiting, abdominal pain, stomatitis, ***hepatitis,*** glossitis, pancreatitis, diarrhea, ***enterocolitis,*** anorexia

S

GU: Renal failure, toxic nephrosis, increased BUN, creatinine, crystalluria, hematuria, proteinuria
HEMA: Leukopenia, thrombocytopenia, agranulocytosis, hemolytic anemia, aplastic anemia
INTEG: Rash, dermatitis, urticaria, ***Stevens-Johnson syndrome,*** erythema, photosensitivity, alopecia
SYST: Anaphylaxis

Contraindications: Hypersensitivity to sulfonamides, sulfonylureas, thiazide and loop diuretics, salicylates, pregnancy at term

Precautions: Pregnancy **C**, lactation, impaired hepatic function, severe allergy, bronchial asthma

Pharmacokinetics

Absorption	Well absorbed
Distribution	Widely distributed, crosses placenta
Metabolism	Liver, large amounts
Excretion	Unchanged kidneys (20%), enters breast
Half-life	7-12 hr

Pharmacodynamics

	PO
Onset	1 hr
Peak	3-4 hr

Interactions
Drug/drug:
Individual drugs
Cyclosporine: ↑ nephrotoxicity
Methotrexate: ↑ toxicity
Phenytoin: ↑ folic acid deficiency

Drug classifications
Anticoagulants, oral: ↑ effects of anticoagulant
Hypoglycemics, oral: ↑ effects of hypoglycemics
Thiazide diuretics: ↑ thrombocytopenia

Lab test interferences
False positive: Urinary glucose test

NURSING CONSIDERATIONS
Assessment
- Assess patient for previous sensitivity reaction
- Assess patient for signs and symptoms of infection including characteristics of wounds, sputum, urine, stool, WBC >10,000, elevated temp; obtain baseline information before and during treatment
- Complete C & S studies before beginning drug therapy to identify if correct treatment has been initiated
- Assess for allergic reactions: rash, urticaria, pruritus, chills, fever, joint pain; angioedema may occur a few days after therapy begins. Epinephrine, resuscitation equipment should be on unit for anaphylactic reaction—AIDS patients are more susceptible
- Monitor blood studies: CBC, Hct, bilirubin, alk phosphatase, monthly if patient is on long-term therapy
- Monitor for bleeding: ecchymosis, bleeding gums, hematuria, stool guaiac daily if patient is on long-term therapy
- Assess for overgrowth of infection: perineal itching, fever, malaise, redness, pain, swelling, drainage, rash, diarrhea, change in cough, sputum

Associated nursing diagnoses

- ✓ Infection, risk for (uses)
- ✓ Diarrhea (adverse reactions)
- ✓ Injury, risk for (adverse reactions)
- ✓ Knowledge deficit (teaching)
- ✓ Noncompliance (teaching)

Implementation

PO route

- Give around the clock to maintain proper blood levels; give with food to increase absorption of drug; do not give within 3 hr of other agents, drug actions may occur
- Give with 8 oz of water to prevent crystalluria
- Shake liq preparation well before giving; use calibrated device for proper dosing

Patient/family education

- Teach patient to report sore throat, bruising, bleeding, joint pain—may indicate blood dyscrasias (rare)
- Advise patient to contact prescriber if vaginal itching, loose, foul-smelling stools, furry tongue occur—may indicate superinfection; report itching, rash, pruritus, urticaria
- Instruct patient to take all medication prescribed for the length of time ordered; drug must be taken around the clock to maintain blood levels; do not give medication to others

Evaluation

Positive therapeutic outcome

- Absence of signs/symptoms of infection (WBC <10,000, temp WNL, absence of urinary pain, hematuria)
- Reported improvement in symptoms of infection

sulfasalazine

(sul-fa-sal'a-zeen)

Azulfidine, Azulfidine EN-Tabs, Salazopyrin ✤, sulfasalazine

Func. class.: Antiinflammatory

Chem. class.: Sulfonamide

Pregnancy category **C**

Action: Prodrug to deliver sulfapyridine and 5-aminosalicylic acid to colon

➔ **Therapeutic Outcome:** Treatment of ulcerative colitis

Uses: Ulcerative colitis

Dosage and routes

Adult: PO 3-4 g/day in divided doses; maintenance 1.5-2 g/day in divided doses q6h

Child >2 yr: PO 40-60 mg/kg/day in 4-6 divided doses, then 20-30 mg/kg/day in 4 doses, max 2 g/day

Available forms: Tab 500 mg; oral susp 250 mg/5 ml; enteric-coated tab 500 mg

Side effects/adverse reactions

CNS: Headache, confusion, insomnia, hallucinations, depression, vertigo, fatigue, anxiety, ***convulsions,*** drug fever, chills

CV: ***Allergic myocarditis***

GI: Nausea, vomiting, abdominal pain, stomatitis, ***hepatitis,*** glossitis, pancreatitis, diarrhea
GU: Renal failure, toxic nephrosis, increased BUN, creatinine, crystalluria

Contraindications: Hypersensitivity to sulfonamides or salicylates, pregnancy at term, P child <2 yr intestinal, urinary obstruction

Precautions: Pregnancy **C,** lactation, impaired hepatic function, severe allergy, bronchial asthma, impaired renal function

Pharmacokinetics

Absorption	Partially absorbed (PO)
Distribution	Crosses placenta
Metabolism	Liver
Excretion	Kidneys, breast milk
Half-life	5-10 hr

Pharmacodynamics

	PO
Onset	1 hr
Peak	1½-6 hr
Duration	Unknown

Interactions

Drug/drug:

Individual drugs
Digoxin: ↓ effectiveness
Folic acid: ↓ effectiveness
Methotrexate: ↓ renal excretion
Phenytoin: ↓ hepatic clearance
Drug classifications
Hypoglycemics, oral: ↑ toxicity
Anticoagulants, oral: ↑ toxicity

Drug/food:

Iron, folic acid will be poorly absorbed

Lab test interferences

False positive: Urinary glucose test

NURSING CONSIDERATIONS

Assessment

- Monitor I&O ratio; note color, amount, character, pH of urine if drug administered for urinary tract infections; output should be 800 ml less than intake; if urine is highly acidic, alkalization may be needed
- Monitor kidney function studies: BUN, creatinine, urinalysis if on long-term therapy
- Monitor blood dyscrasias: skin rash, fever, sore throat, bruising, bleeding, fatigue, joint pain
- Assess for allergic reaction: rash, dermatitis, urticaria, pruritus, dyspnea, bronchospasm

Associated nursing diagnoses

✓ Injury, risk for (uses)
✓ Knowledge deficit (teaching)

Implementation

PO route

- Give with full glass of water to maintain adequate hydration; increase fluids to 2 L/day to decrease crystallization in kidneys
- Give medication after C&S; repeat C&S after full course of medication completed
- Give with resuscitative equipment available; severe allergic reaction may occur

• Give total daily dose in evenly spaced doses and after meals to help minimize GI intolerance
• Store in tight, light-resistant container at room temp

Patient/family education

• Advise patient to take each oral dose with full glass of H_2O to prevent crystalluria
• Teach patient to complete full course of treatment to prevent superimposed infection
• Teach patient to avoid sunlight or to use sunscreen to prevent burns
• Teach patient to avoid OTC medication (aspirin, Vit C) unless directed by prescriber
• Caution patient to use alternative contraceptive measures; decreased effectiveness of oral contraceptives may result
• Advise patient to notify prescriber if skin rash, sore throat, fever, mouth sores, unusual bruising, bleeding occur

Evaluation

Positive therapeutic outcome
• Absence of fever, mucus in stools

sulfinpyrazone

(sul-fin-peer'a-zone)
Antazone ♣, Antiple, Anturan ♣, Anturane, Apo-Sulfinpyrazone ♣, Novopyrazone ♣
Func. class.: Uricosuric
Chem. class.: Pyrazolone
Pregnancy category **C**

Action: Inhibits tubular reabsorption of urates, with increased excretion of uric acid; inhibits prostaglandin synthesis, which decreases platelet aggregation

Therapeutic Outcome: Decreased uric acid levels, absence of platelet aggregation

Uses: Inhibition of platelet aggregation, gout

Dosage and routes

Inhibition of platelet aggregation
Adult: PO 200 mg qid

Gout/gouty arthritis
Adult: PO 100-200 mg bid × 1 wk, then 200-400 mg bid, not to exceed 800 mg/day

Available forms: Tab 100 mg; cap 200 mg

Side effects/adverse reactions

CNS: Dizziness, ***convulsions, coma***
EENT: Tinnitus
GI: *Gastric irritation, nausea, vomiting, anorexia,* ***hepatic necrosis,*** GI bleeding
GU: Renal calculi, hypoglycemia
HEMA: ***Agranulocytosis*** (rare)
INTEG: Rash, dermatitis, pruritus, fever, photosensitivity
RESP: ***Apnea,*** irregular respirations

Contraindications: Hypersensitivity to pyrazolone derivatives, severe hepatic disease, blood dyscrasias, severe renal disease, CrCl <50 mg/min, active peptic ulcer, GI inflammation, renal calculi

Precautions: Pregnancy **C**, lactation

Pharmacokinetics

Absorption	Well absorbed (PO)
Distribution	Unknown
Metabolism	Liver
Excretion	Feces (metabolites/ active drug)
Half-life	3 hr

Pharmacodynamics

	PO
Onset	Unknown
Peak	1-2 hr
Duration	4-6 hr

Interactions

Drug/drug:

Individual drugs:

Aspirin: ↑ risk of bleeding
Cefamandole: ↑ risk of bleeding
Cefoperazone: ↑ risk of bleeding
Cefotetan: ↑ risk of bleeding
Nitrofurantoin: ↑ of sulfinpyrazone
Plicamycin: ↑ risk of bleeding
Theophylline: ↓ of sulfinpyrazone
Valproic acid: ↑ risk of bleeding
Verapamil: ↓ effect of sulfinpyrazone

Drug classifications

Antiinflammatories: ↑ risk of bleeding
Anticoagulants: ↑ risk of bleeding
Salicylates: ↓ effect of sulfinpyrazone
Thrombolytics: ↑ risk of bleeding

Lab test interferences

Increase: Alk phosphatase, AST (SGPT) /ALT (SGOT)
False positive: RBC, Hgb

NURSING CONSIDERATIONS

Assessment

- Monitor I&O ratio; observe for decrease in urinary output; increase fluids to 2-3 L/day
- Monitor CBC, platelets, reticulocytes before, during therapy (q3mo)
- Assess mobility, joint pain, and swelling in the joints

Associated nursing diagnoses

✓ Pain, chronic (uses)
✓ Immobility, impaired physical (uses)
✓ Knowledge deficit (teaching)

Implementation

PO route

- Give with food or antacid to decrease GI upset
- Reduce dose gradually if uric acid levels are normal after 6 mo

Patient/family education

- Advise patient to increase fluids to 3-4 L/day
- Caution patient to avoid alcohol, OTC preparations that contain alcohol—skin rashes may occur
- Advise patient to report any pain, redness, or hard area, usually in legs
- Instruct patient on importance of complying with medical regimen; bone marrow depression may occur

Evaluation

Positive therapeutic outcome
- Decreased pain in joints
- Normal serum uric acid levels
- Increased duration of anti-infectives

sulfisoxazole
(sul-fi-sox'a-zole)
Gantrisin, Novosoxazole ♣, sulfisoxazole
Func. class.: Antiinfective
Chem. class.: Sulfonamide, short-acting
Pregnancy category **C**

Action: Interferes with bacterial biosynthesis of proteins by competitive antagonism of PABA

Therapeutic Outcome: Bactericidal action against susceptible organisms; gram-positive pathogens, including *Streptococci* and *Staphylococci, Clostridium perfringens, Clostridium tetani, Nocardia asteroides;* active against gram-negative pathogens, including *Enterobacter, Escherichia coli, Klebsiella, Proteus mirabilis, Proteus vulgaris, Salmonella, Shigella*

Uses: Urinary tract, systemic infections; chancroid; trachoma; toxoplasmosis; acute otitis media; lymphogranuloma venereum, eye infections

Dosage and routes

Adult: PO 2-4 g loading dose, then 1-2 g qid × 7-10 days

Adult: Ophth gtt TID or more, may decrease frequency as infection improves

P *Child >2 mo:* PO 75 mg/kg or 2 g/m^2 loading dose, then 120-150 mg/kg/day or 4 g/m^2/day in divided doses q6h, not to exceed 6 g/day

Available forms: Tab 500 mg; syr, pediatric susp 500 mg/5 ml; ophth sol 4%

Side effects/adverse reactions

CNS: Headache, insomnia, hallucinations, depression, vertigo, fatigue, anxiety, ***convulsions,*** drug fever, chills, drowsiness
CV: ***Allergic myocarditis***
GI: *Nausea, vomiting, abdominal pain,* stomatitis, ***hepatitis,*** glossitis, pancreatitis, diarrhea, ***enterocolitis,*** anorexia
GU: ***Renal failure, toxic nephrosis,*** increased BUN, creatinine, crystalluria, hematuria, proteinuria
HEMA: ***Leukopenia, thrombocytopenia, agranulocytosis, hemolytic anemia, aplastic anemia***
INTEG: Rash, dermatitis, urticaria, ***Stevens-Johnson syndrome,*** erythema, photosensitivity, alopecia
SYST: ***Anaphylaxis***

Contraindications: Hypersensitivity to sulfonamides and sulfonylureas, thiazide and loop diuretics, salicylates; pregnancy at term

Precautions: Pregnancy **C**, lactation, impaired hepatic

S

function, severe allergy, bronchial asthma

Pharmacokinetics

Absorption	Well absorbed (PO)
Distribution	Widely distributed, crosses placenta
Metabolism	Liver, mostly
Excretion	Breast milk
Half-life	4-7 hr

Pharmacodynamics

	PO	OPHTH
Onset	Unknown	Unknown
Peak	2-4 hr	Unknown

Interactions
Drug/drug:
Individual drugs
Cyclosporin: ↑ nephrotoxicity
Methotrexate: ↑ toxicity
Phenytoin: ↑ folic acid deficiency
Drug classifications
Anticoagulants, oral: ↑ effects of anticoagulant
Hypoglycemics, oral: ↑ effects of hypoglycemics
Thiazide diuretics: ↑ thrombocytopenia

Lab test interferences
False positive: Urinary glucose test

NURSING CONSIDERATIONS
Assessment
- Assess patient for previous sensitivity reaction
- Assess patient for signs and symptoms of infection including characteristics of wounds, sputum, urine, stool, WBC >10,000, temp; obtain baseline information before and during treatment
- Complete C&S testing before beginning drug therapy to identify if correct treatment has been initiated
- Assess for allergic reactions: rash, urticaria, pruritus, chills, fever, joint pain; angioedema may occur a few days after therapy begins. Epinephrine, resuscitation equipment should be on unit for anaphylactic reaction
- Monitor blood studies: CBC, Hct, bilirubin, alk phosphatase monthly if patient is on long-term therapy
- Monitor for bleeding: ecchymosis, bleeding gums, hematuria, stool guaiac daily if on long-term therapy
- Assess for overgrowth of infection: perineal itching, fever, malaise, redness, pain, swelling, drainage, rash, diarrhea, change in cough, sputum

Associated nursing diagnoses
- ✓ Infection, risk for (uses)
- ✓ Diarrhea (adverse reactions)
- ✓ Injury, risk for (adverse reactions)
- ✓ Knowledge deficit (teaching)
- ✓ Noncompliance (teaching)

Implementation
PO route
- Give around the clock to maintain proper blood levels; give with food to increase absorption of drug; do not give within 3 hr of other agents—drug interactions may occur
- Give with 8 oz of water
- Shake liq preparation well before giving; use calibrated device for proper dosing

Patient/family education

- Teach patient to report sore throat, bruising, bleeding, joint pain—may indicate blood dyscrasias (rare)
- Advise patient to contact prescriber if vaginal itching; loose, foul-smelling stools; or furry tongue occur—may indicate superinfection; report itching, rash, pruritus, urticaria
- Instruct patient to take all medication prescribed for the length of time ordered; drug must be taken around the clock to maintain blood levels; medication should not be shared with others

Evaluation

Positive therapeutic outcome

- Absence of signs/symptoms of infection (WBC <10,000, temp WNL, absence of urinary pain, hematuria)
- Reported improvement in symptoms of infection

sulindac

(sul-in'dak)

Apo-Sulin ♣, Clinoril, Novosundac ♣, sulindac

Func. class.: Nonsteroidal antiinflammatory

Chem. class.: Indeneacetic acid derivative

Pregnancy category **C**

Action: Inhibits prostaglandin synthesis by decreasing an enzyme needed for biosynthesis; analgesic, antiinflammatory, antipyretic

➲ Therapeutic Outcome: Decreased pain, inflammation

Uses: Mild to moderate pain, osteoarthritis, rheumatoid, gouty arthritis, ankylosing spondylitis

Dosage and routes

Arthritis

Adult: PO 150 mg bid, may increase to 200 mg bid

Bursitis/acute arthritis

Adult: PO 200 mg bid × 1-2 wk, then reduce dose

Available forms: Tab 150, 200 mg

Side effects/adverse reactions

CNS: Dizziness, drowsiness, fatigue, tremors, confusion, insomnia, anxiety, depression

CV: Tachycardia, peripheral edema, palpitations, dysrhythmias

EENT: Tinnitus, hearing loss, blurred vision

GI: Nausea, anorexia, vomiting, diarrhea, jaundice, ***cholestatic hepatitis,*** constipation, flatulence, cramps, dry mouth, peptic ulcer, ***bleeding, ulceration, perforation***

GU: ***Nephrotoxicity: dysuria, hematuria, oliguria, azotemia***

HEMA: ***Blood dyscrasias***

INTEG: Purpura, rash, pruritus, sweating, photosensitivity

Contraindications: Hypersensitivity, asthma, severe renal disease, severe hepatic disease, active ulcers

S

Precautions: Pregnancy **C**, P lactation, children, bleeding disorders, GI disorders, cardiac disorders, hypersensitivity to other antiinflammatory agents

Pharmacokinetics

Absorption	Well absorbed
Distribution	Not known
Metabolism	Converted to active drug—liver
Excretion	Minimal unchanged kidneys, breast milk
Half-life	7.8 hr; 16.4-hr active metabolite

Pharmacodynamics

	PO
Onset	Unknown
Peak	2 hr
Duration	Unknown

Interactions

Drug/drug:

Individual drugs

Acetaminophen (long-term use): ↑ renal reactions
Alcohol: ↑ adverse reactions
Aspirin: ↓ effectiveness, ↑ adverse reactions
Coumarin: ↑ anticoagulant effects
Digoxin: ↑ toxicity, ↑ levels
Insulin: ↓ insulin effect
Lithium: ↑ toxicity
Methotrexate: ↑ toxicity
Phenytoin: ↑ toxicity
Probenecid: ↑ toxicity
Sulfonylurea: ↑ toxicity

Drug classifications

Anticoagulants: ↑ risk of bleeding
Antihypertensives: ↓ effect of antihypertensives
Antineoplastics: ↑ risk of hematologic toxicity
β-blockers: ↑ antihypertension
Cephalosporins: ↑ risk of bleeding
Diuretics: ↓ effectiveness of diuretics
Glucocorticoids: ↑ adverse reactions
Hypoglycemics: ↓ hypoglycemic effect
Nonsteroidal antiinflammatories: ↑ adverse reactions
Potassium supplements: ↑ adverse reactions
Radiation: ↑ risk of hematologic toxicity
Sulfonamides: ↑ toxicity

Lab test interferences

Increase: Liver function studies, serum potassium, glucose, alk phosphatase

NURSING CONSIDERATIONS

Assessment

- Monitor blood counts during therapy; watch for decreasing platelets; if low, therapy may need to be discontinued, restarted after hematologic recovery; and for blood dyscrasia (thrombocytopenia): bruising, fatigue, bleeding, poor healing

Associated nursing diagnoses

- ✓ Pain (uses)
- ✓ Mobility, impaired physical (uses)
- ✓ Knowledge deficit (teaching)
- ✓ Injury, risk for (adverse reactions)

Implementation

PO route

- Administer with food or milk to decrease gastric symptoms—food slows absorption slightly, does not decrease absorption

Patient/family education

• Advise patient that drug must be continued for prescribed time to be effective; to avoid aspirin, alcoholic beverages
• Caution patient to report bleeding, bruising, fatigue, malaise because blood dyscrasia do occur
• Instruct patient to use caution when driving; drowsiness, dizziness may occur
• Teach patient to take with a full glass of water to enhance absorption; do not crush, break or chew

Evaluation

Positive therapeutic outcome
• Decreased pain
• Decreased inflammation
• Increased mobility

sumatriptan
(soo-ma-trip′tan)
Imitrex
Func. class.: Migraine agent
Chem. class.: 5HT–1-like receptor agonist
Pregnancy category **C**

Action: Binds selectively to the vascular 5-HT-1 receptor subtype and exerts antimigraine effect; causes vasoconstriction in cranial arteries

Therapeutic Outcome: Absence of migraines

Uses: Acute treatment of migraine with or without aura and cluster headache

Dosage and routes

Adult: SC 6 mg or less; may repeat in 1 hr; not to exceed 12 mg/24 hr

Available forms: Inj 6 mg (12 mg/ml); unit of use syringes (0.5 in/ml); self-dosing system, 6-mg single-dose vial (0.5 ml in 2 ml)

Side effects/adverse reactions

CV: *Flushing*
EENT: Throat, mouth, nasal discomfort, vision changes
GI: Abdominal discomfort
INTEG: *Injection site reaction,* sweating
MS: *Weakness, neck stiffness,* myalgia
NEURO: *Tingling, hot sensation, burning, feeling of pressure, tightness, numbness, dizziness, sedation,* headache, anxiety, fatigue
RESP: Chest tightness, pressure

Contraindications: Angina pectoris, history of MI, documented silent ischemia, Prinzmetal's angina, ischemic heart disease, **IV** use, concurrent ergotamine-containing preparations, uncontrolled hypertension, hypersensitivity, basilar or hemiplegic migraine

Precautions: Postmenopausal women, men >40 yr, risk factors for CAD, hypercholesterolemia, obesity, diabetes, impaired hepatic or renal function, pregnancy **C**, lactation, G children, elderly

S

Pharmacokinetics

Absorption	Well absorbed (SC)
Distribution	10%-20% plasma protein binding
Metabolism	Liver (metabolite)
Excretion	Urine, feces
Half-life	2 hr

Pharmacodynamics

	SC
Onset	10-20 min
Peak	10 min-2 hr
Duration	Up to 24 hr (pain relief)

Interactions

Drug/drug:

Individual drugs

Ergotamine: ↑ risk of vasospastic reaction

NURSING CONSIDERATIONS

Assessment

- Assess for tingling, hot sensation, burning, feeling of pressure, numbness, flushing, infection site reaction
- Monitor stress level, activity, reaction, coping mechanisms of patient
- Assess neurologic status: LOC, blurring vision, nausea, vomiting, tingling in extremities preceding headache
- Assess for ingestion of tyramine-containing foods (pickled products, beer, wine, aged cheese), food additives, preservatives, colorings, artificial sweeteners, chocolate, caffeine, which may precipitate these types of headaches

Associated nursing diagnoses

✓ Pain (uses)
✓ Knowledge deficit (teaching)

Implementation

SC route

- Give by SC route only, avoid IM or **IV** administration

Patient/family education

- Teach patient to use the self-dosing system as soon as pain begins, do not use before a migraine is beginning, may repeat dose if migraine returns
- Caution patient not to take more than 2 dose/day or 12 mg/day; allow at least 1 hr between doses
- Caution patient to avoid driving or hazardous activities if dizziness or drowsiness occurs
- Teach patient to report chest tightness, heat, flushing, drowsiness, dizziness, fatigue, or any allergic reactions that occur
- Inform patient to report any side effects to prescriber
- Caution patient to use contraception when taking drug, to notify prescriber if pregnancy is suspected or planned

Evaluation

Positive therapeutic outcome

- Decrease in frequency, severity of headache

tacrine

(tack'rin)

Cognex, Tetrahydroaminoacridine, THA

Func. class.: Reversible cholinersterase

Pregnancy category **C**

Action: Elevates acetylcholine concentrations (cerebral cortex) by slowing degrading of acetylcholine released in cholinergic neutrons; does not alter underlying dementia

Therapeutic Outcome: Improvement in symptoms of dementia in Alzheimer's disease

Uses: Treatment of mild to moderate dementia in Alzheimer's disease

Dosage and routes

Adult: PO 10 mg qid × 6 wk, then 20 mg qid × 6 wk, increase at 6-wk intervals if patient tolerating drug well and if transaminase is within normal limits

Available forms: Cap 10, 20, 30, 40 mg

Side effects/adverse reactions

CNS: ***Dizziness, confusion, insomnia,*** tremor, ***ataxia, somnolence, anxiety, agitation, depression, hallucinations, hostility, abnormal thinking,*** chills, fever

CV: Hypotension or hypertension

GI: ***Nausea, vomiting, anorexia, abdominal pain, constipation,*** dyspepsia, flatulence

GU: ***Frequency, UTI, incontinence***

INTEG: ***Rash,*** flushing

RESP: ***Rhinitis, URI, cough,*** pharyngitis

Contraindications: Hypersensitivity to this drug or acridine derivatives, patients treated with this drug who developed jaundice with a total bilirubin of >3 mg/dl

Precautions: Sick sinus syndrome, history of ulcers, GI bleeding, hepatic disease, bladder obstruction, asthma, pregnancy **C**, lactation, P children

Pharmacokinetics

Absorption	Rapidly absorbed, low
Distribution	55% plasma protein bond
Metabolism	Liver
Excretion	Unknown
Half-life	2-4 hr

Pharmacodynamics

	PO
Onset	Unknown
Peak	Unknown
Duration	Unknown

Interactions

Drug/drug:

Individual drugs

Bethanechol: ↑ effect

Cimetidine: ↑ tacrine level

Succinylcholine: ↑ effect

Theophylline: ↑ toxicity

NURSING CONSIDERATIONS

Assessment

- Monitor B/P for hypotension or hypertension
- Assess mental status: affect, mood, behavioral changes, depression, hallucinations, confusion; conduct suicide assessment
- Assess GI status: nausea, vomiting, anorexia, constipation, abdominal pain; add bulk

T

and increase fluids for constipation
• Assess GU status: urinary frequency, incontinence

Associated nursing diagnoses

✓ Injury, risk for (uses)
✓ Thought processes, altered (uses)
✓ Knowledge deficit (teaching)

Implementation

PO route
• Give dosage adjusted to patient's response no more than q6wk
• Provide assistance with ambulation if needed during beginning therapy; dizziness, ataxia may occur
• Give between meals; if GI symptoms occur, may be given with meals

Patient/family education

• Advise patient to report side effects: twitching, eye spasms; may indicate overdose
• Instruct patient to use drug exactly as prescribed at regular intervals, preferably between meals; may be taken with meals for GI upset
• Advise patient to notify prescriber of nausea, vomiting, diarrhea (dose increased or beginning treatment) or rash, very dark or very light stools, jaundice (delayed onset)
• Caution patient not to increase or abruptly decrease dose; serious consequences may result

Evaluation

Positive therapeutic outcome
• Decrease in confusion, improved mood

Treatment of overdose: Withdraw drug, administer tertiary anticholinergics, provide supportive care

tacrolimus

(tak-roe-li-mus)
Prograf
Func. class.: Immunosuppressant
Chem. clas.: Macrolide
Pregnancy category **C**

Action: Produces immunosuppression by inhibiting lymphocytes (T)

➔ **Therapeutic Outcome:** Prevention of rejection in organ transplant

Uses: Organ transplants—to prevent rejection

Dosage and routes

P ***Adult and child:*** **IV** 0.15 mg/kg/day × 3 days then PO 0.15 mg/kg bid

Available forms: Inj **IV**

Side effects/adverse reactions

CNS: Tremors, headache, insomnia, paresthesia, anxiety, hyperesthesia, numbness, dizziness, fatigue
CV: Hypertension
EENT: Blurred vision, photophobia
GI: Nausea, vomiting, diarrhea, *oral Candida, gum hyperplasia,* ***hepatotoxicity,*** constipation
GU: Urinary tract infections,

albuminuria, hematuria, proteinuria, renal failure
HEMA: Anemia, leukocytosis, thrombocytopenia purpura
INTEG: Rash, flushing, itching, alopecia
META: Hirsutism, hyperglycemia, hyperkalemia, hyperuricemia, hypokalemia, hypomagnesemia
RESP: Pleural effusion, atelectasis, dyspnea

Contraindications: Hypersensitivity

Precautions: Severe renal disease, severe hepatic disease, pregnancy **C**, diabetes mellitus, hyperkalemia, hyperuricemia

Pharmacokinetics

Absorption	Erractically absorbed (PO), completely absorbed (IV)
Distribution	Crosses placenta, 75% protein binding
Metabolism	Liver to metabolite
Excretion	Kidney—minimal, breast milk, bile
Half-life	10 hr

Pharmacodynamics

	PO	IV
Onset	Unknown	Unknown
Peak	1-4 hr	Unknown
Duration	12 hr	12 hr

Interactions

Drug/drug:

Individual drugs
Cyclosporine: ↑ nephrotoxicity, do not use together
Danzoli: ↑ toxicity
Erthromycin: ↑ toxicity
Ibuprofen: ↑ oliguria

NURSING CONSIDERATIONS

Assessment

• Monitor blood studies: Hgb, WBC, platelets during treatment monthly; if leukocytes are <3000/mm^3, or platelets <100,000/mm^3, drug should be discontinued or reduced; decreased hemoglobulin level may indicate bone marrow suppression
• Monitor liver function studies: alk phosphatase, AST (SGOT), ALT (SGPT), amylase, bilirubin, and for hepatotoxicity: dark urine, jaundice, itching, light-colored stools; drug should be discontinued

Associated nursing diagnoses

✓ Infection, risk for (uses)
✓ Knowledge deficit (teaching)

Implementation

PO route
• Give all medications PO if possible; avoid IM inj because bleeding may occur
• Give with meals to reduce GI upset; nausea is common
• Give for several days before transplant surgery; patients should be placed in protective isolation

IV **IV route**
• Give after diluting in 0.9% NaCl or D_5W to a concentration of 0.004 mg/ml to 0.02 mg/ml as a continuous inf

Patient/family education

• Instruct patient to report fever, rash, severe diarrhea, chills, sore throat, fatigue because serious infections may occur; clay-colored stools,

T

cramping may indicate hepatotoxicity
- Caution patient to avoid crowds or persons with known infections to reduce risk of infection

Evaluation

Positive therapeutic outcome
- Absence of graft rejection
- Immunosuppression in autoimmune disorders

tamoxifen

(ta-mox'i-fen)
Nolvadex, Nolvadex-D ✤, Novo-Tamoxifen ✤, Tamofen ✤, Tamone ✤
Func. class.: Antineoplastic
Chem. class.: Antiestrogen hormone
Pregnancy category **D**

Action: Inhibits cell division by binding to cytoplasmic estrogen receptors; resembles normal cell complex but inhibits DNA synthesis and estrogen response of target tissue

Therapeutic Outcome: Prevention of rapidly growing malignant cells

Uses: Advanced breast carcinoma that has not responded to other therapy in estrogen-receptor-positive patients (usually postmenopausal)

Dosage and routes

Adult: PO 10-20 mg bid

Available forms: Tab 10 mg

Side effects/adverse reactions

CNS: Hot flashes, headache, lightheadedness, depression
CV: Chest pain
EENT: Ocular lesions, retinopathy, corneal opacity, blurred vision (high doses)
GI: Nausea, vomiting, altered taste (anorexia)
GU: Vaginal bleeding, pruritus vulvae
HEMA: Thrombocytopenia, leukopenia
INTEG: Rash, alopecia
META: Hypercalcemia

Contraindications: Hypersensitivity, pregnancy **D**

Precautions: Leukopenia, thrombocytopenia, lactation, cataracts

Pharmacokinetics

Absorption	Adequately absorbed (PO)
Distribution	Unknown
Metabolism	Liver—extensively
Excretion	Feces—slowly, small amounts (kidneys)
Half-life	1 wk

Pharmacodynamics

	PO
Onset	Unknown
Peak	4-7 hr
Duration	Unknown

Lab test interferences

Increase: Serum Ca

NURSING CONSIDERATIONS

Assessment

- Monitor CBC, differential, platelet count weekly; withhold drug if WBC is <4000 or plate-

let count is <75,000; notify prescriber of results; monitor calcium levels (hypercalcemia is common)
- Assess for tumor flare: increase in bone, tumor pain during beginning treatment; give analgesics as ordered to decrease pain
- Assess for bleeding: hematuria, guaiac, bruising or petechiae, mucosa or orifices q8h, no rec temp

Associated nursing diagnoses

✓ Injury, risk for (adverse reactions)
✓ Knowledge deficit (teaching)

Implementation

PO route
- Give with food or fluids for GI upset; do not break, crush, or chew enteric products; repeat dose may be needed if vomiting occurs
- Store in light-resistant container at room temp

Patient/family education

- Instruct patient to report any complaints, side effects to health care prescriber; if dose is missed, do not double next dose
- Advise patient that vaginal bleeding, pruritus, hot flashes, can occur, and are reversible after discontinuing treatment
- Instruct patient to report immediately decreased visual acuity, which may be irreversible; stress need for routine eye exams
- Inform patient about who should be told about tamoxifen therapy
- Advise patient to report vaginal bleeding immediately; that tumor flare—increase in size or tumor, increased bone pain—may occur and will subside rapidly; may take analgesics for pain; that premenopausal women must use mechanical birth control method because ovulation may be induced (teratogenic drug)
- Caution patient to use sunscreen and protective clothing to prevent burns because photosensitivity is common
- Teach patient that hair loss may occur during treatment; a wig or hairpiece may make patient feel better; new hair may be different in color, texture
- Inform patient rash or lesions are temporary and may become large during beginning therapy

Evaluation

Positive therapeutic outcome
- Decreased spread of malignant cells in breast cancer

temazepam

(tem-az-a-pam)
Razepam, Restoril, Temazepam
Func. class.: Sedative/hypnotic
Chem. class.: Benzodiazepine
Pregnancy category **X**
Controlled substance schedule **IV** (USA)
schedule **F** (Canada)

T

Action: Produces CNS depression at limbic, thalamic, hypothalamic levels of the CNS; may be mediated by neurotransmitter γ-aminobutyric acid (GABA); results are sedation, hypnosis, skeletal muscle relaxation, anticonvulsant activity, anxiolytic action

➡ Therapeutic Outcome: Decreased insomnia

Uses: Insomnia (short-term)

Dosage and routes

Adult: PO 15-30 mg hs

Available forms: Cap 7.5, 15, 30 mg; tab 15, 30 mg

Side effects/adverse reactions

*CNS: **Lethargy, drowsiness, daytime sedation,*** dizziness, confusion, light headedness, headache, anxiety, irritability

CV: Chest pain, pulse changes

GI: Nausea, vomiting, diarrhea, heartburn, abdominal pain, constipation, anorexia

HEMA: Leukopenia, granulocytopenia (rare)

Contraindications: Hypersensitivity to benzodiazepines, pregnancy **X**, lactation, intermittent porphyria

Precautions: Anemia, hepatic disease, renal disease, suicidal individuals, drug abuse, **G** elderly, **P** psychosis, child <15 yr, acute narrow-angle glaucoma, seizure disorders

Pharmacokinetics

Absorption	Well absorbed (PO)
Distribution	Widely distributed, crosses placenta, crosses blood-brain barrier
Metabolism	Liver
Excretion	Kidneys, breast milk
Half-life	10-20 hr

Pharmacodynamics

	PO
Onset	½ hr
Peak	2-3 hr
Duration	6-8 hr

Interactions

Drug/drug:

Individual drugs

Alcohol: ↑ CNS depression
Cimetidine: ↑ action
Disulfiram: ↑ action
Fluoxetine: ↑ action
Isoniazid: ↑ action
Ketoconazole: ↑ action
Levodopa: ↓ action of levodopa
Metoprolol: ↑ action
Propoxyphene: ↑ action
Propranolol: ↑ action
Rifampin: ↓ action of temazepam
Theophylline: ↓ sedative effects
Valproic acid: ↑ action

Drug classifications

Analgesics, opioid: ↑ CNS depression
Antidepressants: ↑ CNS depression
Antihistamines: ↑ CNS depression
Barbiturates: ↓ effect of temazepam
Contraceptives: ↑ effect

Lab test interferences

Increase: AST (SGOT)/ALT (SGPT), serum bilirubin
False increase: 17-OHCS
Decrease: RAIU

NURSING CONSIDERATIONS

Assessment

- Assess mental status: mood, sensorium, anxiety, affect, sleeping pattern, drowsiness, G dizziness, especially elderly; physical dependency, withdrawal symptoms: anxiety, panic attacks, agitation, convulsions, headache, nausea, vomiting, muscle pain, weakness; suicidal tendencies; for indications of increasing tolerance and abuse
- Monitor B/P (lying, standing), pulse; if systolic B/P drops 20 mm Hg, hold drug, notify prescriber
- Monitor blood studies: CBC during long-term therapy; blood dycrasias have occurred rarely; decreased hematocrit, neutropenia may occur
- Monitor hepatic studies: AST (SGOT), ALT (SGPT), bilirubin, creatinine LDH, alk phosphatase
- Monitor I&O; indicate renal dysfunction

Associated nursing diagnoses

✓ Anxiety (uses)
✓ Depression (uses)
✓ Injury, risk for (adverse reactions)
✓ Knowledge deficit (teaching)

Implementation

PO route

- Give with food or milk for GI symptoms; if patient is unable to swallow medication whole, tab may be crushed and mixed with foods or fluids
- Give sugarless gum, hard candy, frequent sips of water for dry mouth

Patient/family education

- Inform patient that drug may be taken with food, and that fluids and tab may be crushed or swallowed whole
- Advise patient not to use for everyday stress or longer than 3 mo unless directed by prescriber; not to take more than prescribed amount; may be habit forming; not to double doses or skip doses
- Caution patient to avoid OTC preparations unless approved by health care prescriber; alcohol and CNS depressants will increase CNS depression
- Advise patient to avoid driving, activities that require alertness, because drowsiness may occur; to avoid alcohol ingestion or other psychotropic medications; to rise slowly or fainting may occur, especially G in elderly; that drowsiness may worsen at beginning of treatment
- Caution patient not to discontinue medication abruptly after long-term use; withdrawal symptoms include vomiting, cramping, tremors, seizures

T

Evaluation

Positive therapeutic outcome

- Decreased anxiety, restlessness, sleeplessness (short-term treatment only)

Treatment of overdose:

Lavage, VS, supportive care

teniposide

(ten-i-poe-side)

Vumon, VM 26

Func. class.: Antineoplastic

Chem. class.: Semisynthetic podophyllotoxin

Pregnancy category D

Action: Inhibits mitotic activity through metaphase to mitosis; inhibits cells from entering mitosis; depresses DNA, RNA synthesis

Therapeutic Outcome: Prevention of rapid growth of malignant cells

Uses: Childhood acute lymphoblastic leukemia (ALL)

Dosage and routes

***Child* IV** INF: Combo teniposide 165 mg/m^2 and cytarabine 300 mg/m^2 2 ×/wk × 8-9 doses or combo teniposide 250 mg/m^2 and vincristine 1.5 mg/m^2 qwk × 4-8 wk and prednisone 40 mg/m^2 PO × 28 days

Available forms: Inj 10 mg/ml

Side effects/adverse reactions

CNS: Headache, fever
CV: Hypotension
GI: Nausea, vomiting, anorexia, ***hepatotoxicity,*** diarrhea, stomatitis
GU: Nephrotoxicity
HEMA: Thrombocytopenia, leukopenia, neutropenia, myelosuppression, anemia
INTEG: Rash, alopecia, phlebitis
RESP: Bronchospasm
SYST: Anaphylaxis

Contraindications: Hypersensitivity, bone marrow depression, severe hepatic disease, severe renal disease, bacterial infection, pregnancy **D**

Precautions: Renal disease, hepatic disease, lactation, P children, gout, depression

Pharmacokinetics

Absorption	Variably absorbed
Distribution	Rapidly distributed, crosses placenta
Metabolism	Liver—some
Excretion	Kidneys, unchanged 45%, breast milk
Half-life	3 hr initial, 15 hr terminal

Pharmacodynamics

Onset	Unknown
Peak	Unknown
Duration	Unknown

Interactions

Drug/drug:

Individual drugs

Radiation: ↑ toxicity, bone marrow suppression

Drug classifications

Antineoplastics: ↑ toxicity, bone marrow suppression
Live virus vaccines: ↑ adverse reactions

NURSING CONSIDERATIONS

Assessment

• Monitor B/P, (baseline and q15 min) during administration

• Monitor CBC, differential, platelet count weekly; withhold drug if WBC is <4000 or platelet count is <75,000; notify prescriber of results and that recovery will take 3 wk
• Assess for dyspnea, rales, unproductive cough, chest pain, tachypnea
• Monitor renal function studies: BUN, serum uric acid, urine CrCl before, during therapy; I&O ratio; report fall in urine output of 30 ml/hr; for decreased hyperuricemia
• Monitor for cold, fever, sore throat (may indicate beginning infection); notify prescriber if these occur
• Assess for bleeding: hematuria, guaiac, bruising or petechiae, mucosa or orifices q8hr, no rec temp; avoid IM inj; use pressure to venipuncture sites
• Identify nutritional status: an antiemetic may need to be prescribed
• Assess for symptoms indicating severe allergic reactions: rash, pruritus, urticaria, itching, flushing, bronchospasm, hypotension; epinephrine and emergency equipment should be nearby

Associated nursing diagnoses

✓ Injury, risk for (adverse reactions)
✓ Body image disturbance (adverse reactions)
✓ Infection, risk for (adverse reactions)
✓ Knowledge deficit (teaching)

Implementation

IV route

• Give by intermittent inf; sol should be prepared by qualified personnel only under controlled conditions; gloves, gown, and mask should be worn
• Use Luer-Loc tubing to prevent leakage, do not let sol come in contact with skin; if contact occurs, wash well with soap and water
• Give after diluting 100 mg/250 ml or more D_5W or 0.9% NaCl to a concentration of 0.2-0.4 mg/ml, inf over 30-60 min; do not use plastic when preparing this inf
• Use hyaluronidase 150 U/ml to 1 ml NaCl to infiltration area, ice compress for treatment of vesicant activity
• This drug should not be given with or mixed with other drugs

Patient/family education

• Teach patient to avoid use of products containing aspirin or ibuprofen, razors, commercial mouthwash because bleeding may occur; to report symptoms of bleeding (hematuria, tarry stools)
• Instruct patient to report signs of anemia, (fatigue, headache, irritability, faintness, shortness of breath)
• Instruct patient to report any changes in breathing or coughing even several mo after treatment
• Advise patient that contraception will be necessary during treatment; teratogenesis may occur
• Caution patient that hair may be lost during treatment; a wig or hairpiece may make patient feel better; new hair will be different in color, texture

- Advise patient to avoid vaccinations during treatment; serious reactions may occur
- Teach patient to report signs/symptoms of infection; fever, chills, sore throat. Patient should avoid crowds, or persons with known infections

Evaluation

Positive therapeutic outcome
- Decreased spread of malignant, leukemic cells

terazosin
(ter-ay′zoe-sin)
Hytrin
Func. class.: Antihypertensive
Chem. class.: Adrenergic blocker (peripherally acting)
Pregnancy category **C**

Action: Peripheral blood vessels are dilated, peripheral resistance lowered; reduction in blood pressure results from α-adrenergic receptors being blocked

➔ **Therapeutic Outcome:** Decreased B/P in hypertension

Uses: Hypertension, as a single agent or in combination with diuretics or β-blockers, BPH

Dosage and routes

Adult: PO 1 mg hs, may increase doses slowly to desired response; not to exceed 20 mg/day

Available forms: Tab 1, 2, 5 mg

Side effects/adverse reactions

CNS: ***Dizziness, headache, drowsiness,*** anxiety, depression, vertigo, weakness, fatigue
CV: Palpitations, orthostatic hypotension, tachycardia, edema, rebound hypertension
EENT: Blurred vision, epistaxis, tinnitus, dry mouth, red sclera, nasal congestion, sinusitis
GI: ***Nausea,*** vomiting, diarrhea, constipation, abdominal pain
GU: Urinary frequency, incontinence, impotence, priapism
RESP: Dyspnea

Contraindications: Hypersensitivity

Precautions: Pregnancy **C**, [P] children, lactation

Pharmacokinetics

Absorption	Well absorbed
Distribution	Not known
Metabolism	Liver—50%
Excretion	Kidneys unchanged—10%, feces unchanged—20%
Half-life	9-12 hr

Pharmacodynamics

	PO
Onset	15 min
Peak	1 hr
Duration	24 hr

Interactions

Drug/drug:

Individual drugs
Alcohol: ↑ CNS depression
Drug classifications
Antihypertensives: ↑ hypotension
Antiinflamatories, nonsteroidal: ↓ antihypertensive effect
Estrogens: ↓ antihypertensive effect
Nitrates: ↑ hypotensive effects
Sympathomimetics: ↓ antihypertensive effect

Lab test interferences

Increase: VMA excretion, 5-HIAA excretion
Interferences: 17-OHCS, 17-KS

NURSING CONSDERATIONS

Assessment

- Monitor B/P, orthostatic hypotension, syncope; check for edema in feet, legs daily; I&O; monitor for weight daily; notify prescriber of changes
- Assess for allergic reactions: rash, fever, pruritus, urticaria; drug should be discontinued if antihistamines fail to help
- Assess for orthostatic hypotension; tell patient to rise slowly from sitting or lying position

Associated nursing diagnoses

- ✓ Cardiac output, decreased (uses)
- ✓ Injury, risk for (adverse reactions)
- ✓ Knowledge deficit (teaching)
- ✓ Noncompliance (teaching)

Implementation

PO route

- Store in tight container at 86° F (30° C) or less
- May be used in combination with other antihypertensives
- May be given with food to prevent GI symptoms

Patient/family education

- Caution patient not to discontinue drug abruptly; the importance of complying with dosage schedule, even if feeling better; if dose is missed take as soon as remembered; take medication at same time each day
- Teach patient not to use OTC products (cough, cold, allergy) unless directed by prescriber; also to avoid large amounts of caffeine
- Emphasize the need to rise slowly to sitting or standing position to minimize orthostatic hypotension
- Teach patient to notify prescriber of mouth sores, sore throat, fever, swelling of hands or feet, irregular heartbeat, chest pain
- Caution patient to report excessive perspiration, dehydration, vomiting, diarrhea; may lead to fall in B/P
- Caution patient that drug may cause dizziness, fainting, lightheadedness; may occur during 1st few days of therapy; to avoid hazardous activities
- Teach patient how to take B/P, and normal readings for age group; to take B/P q7 days

Evaluation

Positive therapeutic outcome

- Decreased B/P in hypertension

Treatment of overdose: Administer volume expanders or vasopressors; discontinue drug; place patient in supine position

terbinafine

(ter-bin'a-feen)

Lamisil

Func. class.: Topical antifungal

Chem. class.: Synthetic allylamine derivative

Pregnancy category **B**

Action: Interferes with cell membrane permeability in fungi such as *T. rubrum, T. mentagrophytes, T. tonsurans, E. floccosum, M. canis, M. audouinii, M. gypseum, Candida;* broad-spectrum antifungal

➔ **Therapeutic Outcome:** Fungistatic/fungicidal against susceptible organisms: *Tinea pedis, Tinea cruris, Tinea corporis, Tinea versicolor*

Uses: *Tinea cruris, Tinea corporis, Tinea pedis*

Dosage and routes

Massage into affected area, surrounding area qd or bid, continue for 7-14 days, not to exceed 4 wk

Available forms: Cream 1%

Side effects/ adverse reactions

INTEG: Burning, stinging, dryness, itching, local irritation

Contraindications: Hypersensitivity

Precautions: Pregnancy **B**, P lactation, children

Pharmacokinetics

Absorption	Minimally absorbed
Distribution	None
Metabolism	None
Excretion	None
Half-life	Unknown

Pharmacodynamics

Onset	Unknown
Peak	Unknown
Duration	Unknown

Interactions: None

NURSING CONSIDERATIONS

Assessment

- Assess skin for fungal infections: peeling, dryness, itching before and throughout treatment
- Assess for continuing infection: increased size, number of lesions

Associated nursing diagnoses

✓ Skin integrity, impaired (uses)
✓ Infection, risk for (uses)
✓ Knowledge deficit (teaching)

Implementation

Topical route

- Apply to affected area, surrounding area; do not cover with occlusive dressings
- Store below 30° C (86° F)

Patient/family education

- Teach patient proper hygiene: hand-washing technique, nail care, use of con-

comitant topical agents if prescribed
• Advise patient to wear cotton clothing; to use clean towel and dry body well; to avoid contact with mucous membranes; to avoid covering areas unless directed to by prescriber
• Advise patient to report excessive itching, burning
• Instruct patient how to apply; massage cream into affected area and surrounding skin in AM, PM; effects observed within 1 wk, continue 1-2 wk after symptoms decrease; wash hands after application

Evaluation

Positive therapeutic outcome
• Decrease in size, number of lesions

terbutaline

(ter-byoo′te-leen)
Brethaire, Brethine, Bricanyl
Func. class.: Selective β_2-agonist; bronchodilator
Chem. class.: Catecholamine
Pregnancy category **B**

Action: Relaxes bronchial smooth muscle by direct action on β_2-adrenergic receptors through accumulation of cAMP at β-adrenergic receptor sites. Results are bronchodilation, diuresis, and CNS and cardiac stimulation

Therapeutic Outcome: Bronchodilation with ease of breathing

Uses: Bronchospasm

Investigational uses: Premature labor

Dosage and routes

Bronchospasm

P *Adult and child >12 yr:* Inh 2 puffs q1min, then q4-6h; PO 2.5-5 mg q8h; SC 0.25 mg q8h

Premature labor

Adult: **IV** inf: 0.01 mg/min, increased by 0.005 mg q10min, not to exceed 0.025 mg/min; SC 0.25 mg q1h; PO 5 mg q4h × 48 h, then 5 mg q6h as maintenance for above doses

Available forms: Tab 2.5, 5 mg; aerosol 0.2 mg/actuation; inj 1 mg/ml

Side effects/adverse reactions

CNS: Tremors, anxiety, insomnia, headache, dizziness, stimulation
CV: Palpitations, tachycardia, hypertension, dysrhythmias, ***cardiac arrest***
GI: Nausea, vomiting

Contraindications: Hypersensitivity to sympathomimetics, narrow-angle glaucoma, tachydysrhythmias

Precautions: Pregnancy **B**, cardiac disorders, hyperthyroidism, diabetes mellitus, prostatic hypertension, lactation, G elderly, hypertension, glaucoma

T

Pharmacokinetics

Absorption	Well absorbed (SC), partially absorbed (PO)
Distribution	Unknown
Metabolism	Liver—partially
Excretion	Unknown
Half-life	Unknown

Pharmacodynamics

	PO	INH	SC	IV
Onset	½ hr	5-15 min	10-15 min	Rapid
Peak	1-2 hr	1-2 hr	½-1 hr	Unknown
Duration	4-8 hr	4-6 hr	1½-4 hr	Unknown

Interactions

Drug/drug:

Drug classifications

Beta-adrenergic blockers: Block therapeutic effect

Bronchodilators, aerosol: ↑ action of bronchodilator

MAOI: ↑ chance of hypertensive crisis

Sympathominetics: ↑ adrenergic side effects

NURSING CONSIDERATIONS

Assessment

- Monitor respiratory function: vital capacity, forced expiratory volume, ABGs, lung sounds, heart rate, rhythm (baseline)
- Determine that patient has not received theophylline therapy before giving dose; assess client's ability to self-medicate
- Monitor for evidence of allergic reactions; paradoxical bronchospasm; withhold dose; notify prescriber

Associated nursing diagnoses

- ✓ Airway clearance, ineffective (uses)
- ✓ Impaired gas exchange (uses)
- ✓ Knowledge deficit (teaching)
- ✓ Noncompliance (teaching)

Implementation

Aerosol route

- Give after shaking; ask patient to exhale, place mouthpiece in mouth, then inhale slowly; hold breath, remove, exhale slowly; allow at least 1 min between inh
- Store in light-resistant container, do not expose to temp over 86° F (30° C)

PO route

- Give PO with meals to decrease gastric irritation; tab may be crushed and mixed with foods and fluids

SC route

- Do not give by IM route

IV **IV route**

- Give at 5 μg q 10 min until contractions are stopped, use inf pump for correct dose; after ½-1 hr with no contraction decrease dose by 5 μg; switch to PO dose when possible

Syringe compatibility:

Doxapram

Y-site compatibility:

Insulin

Additive incompatibility:

Bleomycin

Additive compatibility:

Aminophylline

Patient/family education

- Advise patient not to use OTC medications; extra stimulation may occur; to use this medication before other medications and allow at least 5 min between each to prevent overstimulation
- Teach patient how to use inhaler; review package insert with patient; to avoid getting aerosol in eyes because blurring may result; to wash inhaler in warm water qd and dry; to avoid smoking, smoke-filled rooms, persons with respiratory infections
- Teach patient that paradoxical bronchospasm may occur and to stop drug immediately and notify health care prescriber; to limit caffeine products such as chocolate, coffee, tea, and colas
- Instruct patient on administration of dose, not to use more than prescribed; serious side effects may occur; if taking PO regularly and dose is missed, take when remembered; space other doses on new time schedule

Evaluation

Positive therapeutic outcome
- Absence of dyspnea, wheezing after 1 hr
- Improved airway exchange
- Improved ABGs

Treatment of overdose:
Administer a β_2-adrenergic blocker

terconazole
(ter-kon′a-zole)
Terazol 3, Terazol 7
Func. class.: Local antiinfective
Chem. class.: Antifungal
Pregnancy category **C**

Action: Interferes with fungal DNA replication; binds sterols in fungal cell membranes, which increases permeability, leaking of nutrients

Therapeutic Outcome: Fungistatic/fungicidal against susceptible organisms: *Candida* only

Uses: Vaginal, vulval, vulvovaginal candidiasis (moniliasis)

Dosage and routes
Adult: Vag 5 g (1 applicator) hs × 7 days

Available forms: Vag cream 0.4%

Side effects/adverse reactions
GU: Vulvovaginal burning, itching, pelvic cramps
INTEG: Rash, urticaria, stinging, burning
MISC: Headache, body pain

Contraindications: Hypersensitivity

Precautions: Children <2 yrs, pregnancy, lactation

T

Pharmacokinetics

Absorption	Minimally absorbed
Distribution	Unknown
Metabolism	Liver—rapidly
Excretion	Feces, kidneys
Half-life	Unknown

Pharmacodynamics

Onset	Unknown
Peak	Unknown
Duration	Unknown

Interactions: None

NURSING CONSIDERATIONS

Assessment

- Assess for allergic reaction: burning, stinging, itching, discharge, soreness

Associated nursing diagnoses

- ✓ Skin integrity, impaired (uses)
- ✓ Infection, risk for (uses)
- ✓ Knowledge deficit (teaching)

Implementation

Topical route

- Administer 1 applicatorful every night high into the vagina
- Store at room temp in dry place

Patient/family education

- Instruct patient in asepsis (hand washing) before, after each application
- Teach patient to apply with applicator only; to avoid use of any other vaginal product unless directed by prescriber; sanitary napkin may prevent soiling of undergarments
- Instruct patient to abstain from sexual intercourse until treatment is completed; reinfection and irritation may occur
- Advise patient to notify prescriber if symptoms persist

Evaluation

Positive therapeutic outcome

- Decreased in itching or white discharge (vaginal)

terfenadine

(ter-fen′i-deen)

Seldane

Func. class.: Antihistamine

Chem. class.: Butyrophenone derivative

Pregnancy category **C**

Action: Acts on blood vessels, GI, respiratory systems by competing with histamine for H_1-receptor site; decreases allergic response by blocking histamine

➔ **Therapeutic Outcome:** Absence of allergy symptoms and rhinitis

Uses: Rhinitis, allergy symptoms

Dosage and routes

P ***Adult and child >12 yr:*** PO 60 mg bid

P ***Child <12 yr:*** PO 15-30 mg bid

Available forms: Tab 60 mg, 120 mg ♣; oral susp 6 mg/ml ♣

Side effects/adverse reactions

CNS: Dizziness, poor coordination
CV: Life-threatening dysrhythmias (rare)
GI: Anorexia, increased liver function tests, dry mouth
GU: Retention
RESP: Increased thick secretions

Contraindications: Hypersensitivity, severe hepatic disease

Precautions: Pregnancy **C**

Pharmacokinetics

Absorption	Completely absorbed
Distribution	Not known
Metabolism	Liver—extensively
Excretion	Feces, biliary
Half-life	Biphasic 3½ hr, 16-23 hr

Pharmacodynamics

	PO
Onset	1-2 hr
Peak	3-6 hr
Duration	6-12 hr

Interactions

Drug/drug:

Individual drugs
Alcohol: ↑ CNS depression
Atropine: ↑ anticholinergic reactions
Azithromycin: ↑ dysrhythmias
Clarithromycin: ↑ dysrhythmias
Disopyramide: ↑ anticholinergic reactions
Erythromycin: ↑ dysrhythmias
Fluconazole: ↑ dysrhythmias
Haloperidol: ↑ anticholinergic reactions
Intraconazole: ↑ dysrhythmias
Ketoconazole: ↑ dysrhythmias
Miconazole: ↑ dysrhythmias
Quinidine: ↑ anticholinergic reactions

Drug classifications
Antidepressants: ↑ anticholinergic reactions
Antihistamines: ↑ anticholinergic reactions
CNS depressants: ↑ CNS depression
MAOI: ↑ anticholinergic effect
Narcotics: ↑ CNS depression
Phenothiazines: ↑ anticholinergic reactions
Sedative/hypnotics: ↑ CNS depression

Lab test interferences

False negative: Skin allergy tests (discontinue antihistamines 3 days prior to testing)

NURSING CONSIDERATIONS

Assessment

- Assess respiratory status: rate, rhythm, increase in bronchial secretions, wheezing, chest tightness; provide fluids to 2 L/day to decrease secretions thickness
- Monitor I&O ratio: be alert for urinary retention, frequency, dysuria, especially G elderly; drug should be discontinued if these occur
- Monitor CBC during long-term therapy; blood dyscrasias may occur but are rare

Associated nursing diagnoses

- ✓ Airway clearance, ineffective (uses)
- ✓ Injury, risk for (adverse reactions)
- ✓ Knowledge deficit (teaching)

T

✓ Noncompliance (teaching—overuse)

Implementation

PO route

- Give on an empty stomach 1 hr ac or 2 hr pc to facilitate absorption
- Store in tight, light-resistant container

Patient/family education

- Teach all aspects of drug uses; to notify prescriber if dizziness occurs; to avoid driving or other hazardous activity if dizziness occurs; to avoid alcohol or other CNS depressants that may potentiate effect
- Advise patient to take 1 hr ac or 2 hr pc to facilitate absorption
- Caution patient not to exceed recommended dose; dysrhythmias may occur
- Advise patient that hard candy, gum, frequent rinsing of mouth may be used for dryness

Evaluation

Positive therapeutic outcome

- Absence of running or congested nose, rashes

Treatment of overdose:

Administer ipecac syrup or lavage, diazepam, vasopressors, barbiturates (short-acting)

testosterone cypionate/testosterone enanthate/ testosterone propionate 🔑

Andro L.A. 200, Delatest, Delatestryl, Durathate-200, Everone 100, Everone 200, Testone LA 100, Testone LA 200, testosterone enanthate, Testrin PA, Andro-Cyp 100, Andro-Cyp 200, Andronate 100, Andronate 200, depAndro 100, depAndro 200, Depotest 100, Depotest 200, Depo-Testosterone, Duratest-100, Duratest-200, testosterone cypionate, Testred Cypionate, Testex, testosterone propionate

Func. class.: Androgenic anabolic steroid

Chem. class.: Halogenated testosterone derivative

Pregnancy category X

Action: Increases weight by building body tissue; increases potassium, phosphorus, chloride, nitrogen levels; increases bone development; responsible for maintenance of secondary sex characteristics (male)

➡ Therapeutic Outcome: Increased hormone levels in eunuchoidism, decreased tumor growth in female breast cancer, onset of male puberty

Uses: Female breast cancer, eunuchoidism, male climacteric, oligospermia, impotence, osteoporosis

Dosage and routes

Oligospermia

Adult: IM 100-200 mg q4-6 wk (cypionate or enanthate)

Breast cancer

Adult: IM 50-100 mg 3 ×/wk (propionate) or 200-400 mg q2-4 wk (cypionate or enanthate)

Male climacteric/ eunuchoidism/eunuchism

Adult: IM 10-25 mg 2-4 ×/wk (propionate)

Available forms: Propionate inj 25, 50, 100 mg/ml; enanthate inj 100, 200 mg/ml; cypionate inj 50, 100, 200 mg/ml

Side effects/adverse reactions

CNS: Dizziness, headache, fatigue, tremors, paresthesias, flushing, sweating, anxiety, lability, insomnia, carpal tunnel syndrome
CV: Increased B/P
EENT: Conjunctional edema, nasal congestion
ENDO: Abnormal GTT
GI: Nausea, vomiting, constipation, weight gain, ***cholestatic jaundice***
GU: Hematuria, amenorrhea, vaginitis, decreased libido, decreased breast size, clitoral hypertrophy, testicular atrophy
INTEG: Rash, acneiform lesions, oily hair and skin, flushing, sweating, acne vulgaris, alopecia, hirsutism
MS: Cramps, spasms

Contraindications: Severe renal disease, severe cardiac disease, severe hepatic disease, hypersensitivity, pregnancy **X**, lactation, genital bleeding (abnormal)

Precautions: Diabetes mellitus, CV disease, MI

Pharmacokinetics

Absorption	Well but slowly absorbed
Distribution	Crosses placenta
Metabolism	Liver
Excretion	Kidneys, breast milk
Half-life	8 days (cypionate) 10-100 min (Base)

Pharmacodynamics

	IM (base)	IM (cypionate)	IM (enanthate)	IM (propionate)
Onset	Unknown	Unknown	Unknown	Unknown
Peak	Unknown	Unknown	Unknown	Unknown
Duration	1-3 days	2-4 wk	2-4 wk	1-3 days

Interactions

Drug/drug:

Individual drugs

ACTH: ↑ edema
Insulin: ↓ effects of insulin
Oxyphenbutazone: ↑ effects of oxyphenbutazone

Drug classifications

Adrenal steroids: ↑ edema
Anticoagulants: ↑ pro-time
Oral antidiabetics: ↑ effects of oral antidiabetics

T

Lab test interferences

Increase: Serum cholesterol, blood glucose, urine glucose
Decrease: Serum Ca, serum K, T_4, T_3, thyroid ^{131}I uptake test, urine 17-OHCS, 17-KS, PBI

NURSING CONSIDERATIONS

Assessment

- Monitor patient's weight daily; notify prescriber if weekly weight gain is >5 lb; assess I&O ratio; be alert for decreasing urinary output, increasing edema
- Monitor B/P q4h
- Assess growth rate in adolescent because growth rate may be uneven (linear/bone growth) if used for extended periods
- Monitor electrolytes: potassium, sodium, chloride, calcium; cholesterol
- Monitor liver function studies: ALT (SGOT), AST (SGPT), bilirubin
- Assess edema, hypertension, cardiac symptoms, jaundice
- Assess mental status: affect, mood, behavioral changes, aggression
- Assess signs of masculinization in female: increased libido, deepening of voice, decreased breast tissue, enlarged clitoris, menstrual irregularities; male: gynecomastia, impotence, testicular atrophy
- Assess hypercalcemia: lethargy, polyuria, polydipsia, nausea, vomiting, constipation; drug may have to be decreased
- Assess hypoglycemia in diabetics because oral antidiabetic action is increased

Associated nursing diagnoses

- ✓ Infection, risk for (adverse reactions)
- ✓ Injury, risk for (adverse reactions)
- ✓ Knowledge deficit (teaching)

Implementation

- Administer diet with increased calories, protein; decreased sodium if edema occurs
- Administer supportive drug if anemia occurs

IM route

- Give titrated dose; use lowest effective dose
- Give IM deep into upper outer quadrant of gluteal muscle; route can be painful

Patient/family education

- Inform patient that drug needs to be combined with complete health plan: diet, rest, exercise
- Caution patient to notify prescriber if therapeutic response decreases; not to discontinue this medication abruptly
- Inform women patients to report menstrual irregularities; about changes in sex characteristics
- Discuss that 1-3 mo course is necessary for response in breast cancer

Evaluation

Positive therapeutic outcome

- Decrease size of tumor in breast cancer
- Increased androgen levels

tetracaine
(tet'ra-caine)
Pontocaine Eye, Pontocaine HCl, tetracaine, Supracaine ✦
Func. class.: Ophthalmic anesthetic/topical anesthetic
Chem. class.: Ester
Pregnancy category C

Action: Decreases ion permeability by stabilizing neuronal membrane

Uses: Cataract extraction, tonometry, gonioscopy, removal of foreign objects, corneal suture removal, glaucoma surgery (Ophth); pruritus, sunburn, toothache, sore throat, cold sores, oral pain, rectal pain and irritation, control of gagging (top)

Dosage and routes
P *Adult and child:* Instill 1-2 gtt before procedure; oint ½-1 in to lower conjunctival fornix
P *Adult and child:* Top apply to affected area 1 oz for adult ¼ oz for child; Sol 2%; aero spray, liq, 0.5% oint, gel, 1% cream (top)

Available forms: Sol 0.5%; oint 0.5%

Side effects/adverse reactions
EENT: *Blurred vision, stinging, burning, lacrimation, photophobia,* conjunctival redness
INTEG: *Contact dermatitis;* rash, burning, stinging, tenderness (top)
SYST: CNS stimulation, CNS and CV depression

Contraindications: Hypersensitivity to PABA, application to large areas

Precautions: Abnormal levels of plasma esterases, allergies, hyperthyroidism, hypertension, cardiac disease, pregnancy **C**; denuded skin (top)

Pharmacokinetics

Absorption	Minimally absorbed
Distribution	Minimally distributed
Metabolism	None
Excretion	Lacrimation (ophth)
Half-life	Short

Pharmacodynamics

	OPH	TOP
Onset	15-30 sec	1 min
Peak	Unknown	Unknown
Duration	15-20 min	½-1 hr

Interactions
Drug classifications
Sulfonamides: ↓ antibacterial action (ophth)

NURSING CONSIDERATIONS
Assessment
- Assess pain: location, duration, characteristics before and after administration
- Assess for infection: redness, drainage, inflammation—this drug should not be used until infection is treated
- Assess for previous hypersensitivity to anesthetics

T

Associated nursing diagnoses

- ☑ Pain (uses)
- ☑ Sensory-perceptual alteration: visual (uses) (ophth)
- ☑ Knowledge deficit (teaching)

Implementation

Ophth route

- Provide protective covering for eye
- Store at room temp in air-tight, light-resistant container; refrigerate

Top route

- Apply to gums as needed for teething pain
- Provide lozenges for temporary sore throat pain
- Store in air-tight, light-resistant container; do not freeze, puncture, or incinerate aerosol container

Patient/family education

- Caution patient to avoid contact with eyes
- Instruct patient not to use for prolonged periods: use for <1 wk; if condition persists, prescriber should be notified
- Advise patient to report change in vision, with blurring or loss of sight, trouble breathing, sweating, flushing
- Caution patient not to touch or rub eye, which may further damage eye
- Inform patient that someone must drive the patient home after the appointment

Evaluation

Positive therapeutic outcome

- Absence of pain

tetracycline

(tet-ra-sye'kleen)

Achromycin, Achromycin V, Alatel, Apo-Tetra ✱, Nor-Tet, Novotetra ✱, Nu-Tetra ✱, Panmycin, Robitet, Sumycin 250, Sumycin 500, Sumycin Syrup, Teline, Teline 500, Tetracap, tetracycline HCl, tetracycline HCl Syrup, Tetracyn, Tetralan 250, Tetralan 500, Tetralan Syrup, Tetralean ✱, Tetram

Func. class.: Broad-spectrum antiinfective

Chem. class.: Tetracycline

Pregnancy category **D**

Action: Inhibits protein synthesis and phosphorylation in microorganisms; bacteriostatic

➡ **Therapeutic Outcome:** Bactericidal action against susceptible organisms; gram-positive pathogens: *Bacillus antracis, Clostridium perfringens, Clostridium tetani, Listeria monocytogenes, Nocardia, Pripionibacterium acnes, Actinomyces isrealii;* gram-negative pathogens *Hemophilus influenzae, Legionella pneumophilia, Yersenia entercolitica, Yersinia pestis, Neisseria gonorrhoeae, Neisseria meningitidis*

Uses: Syphilis, chlamydia trachomatis, gonorrhea, lymphogranuloma venereum, uncommon gram-positive, gram-negative organisms, rickettsial infections

Dosage and routes

Adult: PO 250-500 mg q6h; IM 250 mg/day or 150 mg q12h; **IV** 250-500 mg q8-12h

P *Child >8 yr:* PO 25-50 mg/kg/day in divided doses q6h; IM 15-25 mg/kg/day in divided doses q8-12h; **IV** 10-20 mg/kg/day in divided doses q12h

Gonorrhea

Adult: PO 1.5 g, then 500 mg qid for a total of 9 g over 7 days

Chlamydia trachomatis

Adult: PO 500 mg qid × 7 days

Syphilis

Adult: PO 2-3 g in divided doses × 10-15 days; if syphilis duration >1 yr, must treat 30 days

Brucellosis

Adult: PO 500 mg qid × 3 wk with 1 g streptomycin IM 2 ×/day × 1 wk, and 1 ×/day the second wk

Urethral syndrome in women

Adult: PO 500 mg qid × 7 days

Acne

Adult: 1 g/day in divided doses; maintenance 125-500 mg/day

Available forms: Oral susp 125 mg/5 ml, cap 100, 200, 500 mg; tab 100, 250, 500 mg; powder for inj

Side effects/adverse reactions

CNS: Fever, headache, paresthesia
CV: Pericarditis
EENT: Dysphagia, glossitis, decreased calcification (permanent discoloration) of deciduous teeth, oral candidiasis
GI: Nausea, abdominal pain, *vomiting, diarrhea,* anorexia, enterocolitis, ***hepatotoxicity,*** flatulence, abdominal cramps, epigastric burning, stomatitis
GU: Increased BUN
HEMA: Eosinophilia, neutropenia, thrombocytopenia, leukocytosis, hemolytic anemia
INTEG: Rash, urticaria, photosensitivity, increased pigmentation, ***exfoliative dermatitis,*** pruritus, ***angioedema***

Contraindications: Hypersensitivity to tetracyclines, P children <8 yr, pregnancy **D**, lactation

Precautions: Renal disease, hepatic disease

Pharmacokinetics

Absorption	60%-80% (PO), lower (IM)
Distribution	Widely distributed, some in CSF; crosses placenta
Metabolism	Not metabolized
Excretion	Unchanged—kidneys
Half-life	6-10 hr

Pharmacodynamics

	PO
Onset	1-2 hr
Peak	2-3 hr

T

Interactions

Drug/drug:

Individual drugs

Calcium: Forms chelates, ↓ absorption
Carbamazepine: ↑ effect of carbamazepine
Colestipol: ↓ absorption of tetracycline
Cholestyramine: ↓ absorption of tetracycline
Iron: Forms chelates, ↓ absorption
Magnesium: Forms chelates, ↓ absorption
Phenytoin: ↓ effect of tetracycline
Sucralfate: Prevents absorption of tetracycline

Drug classifications

Anticoagulants, oral: ↑ effect of anticoagulants
Barbiturates: ↓ effect of tetracycline
Contraceptives, oral: ↓ effect of oral contraception

Drug/food:

↓ absorption with dairy products; forms insoluble chelate

Lab test interferences

Increase (false): Urinary catecholamines
False negative: Urine glucose with Clinistix, Tes-Tape

NURSING CONSIDERATIONS

Assessment

- Assess patient for previous sensitivity reaction
- Assess patient for signs and symptoms of infection including characteristics of wounds, sputum, urine, stool, WBC >10,000, temp; obtain baseline information before and during treatment
- Complete C&S testing before beginning drug therapy to identify if correct treatment has been initiated
- Assess for allergic reactions: rash, urticaria, pruritus, chills, fever, joint pain; angioedema may occur a few days after therapy begins—epinephrine, resuscitation equipment should be on unit for anaphylactic reaction
- Identify urine output; if decreasing, notify prescriber (may indicate nephrotoxicity); also, increased BUN, creatinine
- Monitor blood studies: AST (SGOT), ALT (SGPT), CBC, Hct, bilirubin, LDH, alk phosphatase, monthly if patient is on long-term therapy
- Assess bowel pattern qd; if severe diarrhea occurs, drug should be discontinued
- Monitor for bleeding: ecchymosis, bleeding gums, hematuria, stool guaiac daily if on long-term therapy; blood dyscrasias may occur
- Assess for overgrowth of infection: perineal itching, fever, malaise, redness, pain, swelling, drainage, rash, diarrhea, change in cough, sputum

Associated nursing diagnoses

- ✓ Infection, risk for (uses)
- ✓ Diarrhea (adverse reactions)
- ✓ Injury, risk for (adverse reactions)
- ✓ Knowledge deficit (teaching)
- ✓ Noncompliance (teaching)

Implementation

PO route

- Give around the clock to maintain proper blood levels; give with food to increase absorption of drug; do not give within 3 hr of other agents—drug actions may occur
- Give with 8 oz of water
- Shake liq preparation well before giving; use calibrated device for proper dosing

Patient/family education

- Teach patient to report sore throat, bruising, bleeding, joint pain—may indicate blood dyscrasias (rare)
- Advise patient to use a sunscreen when outdoors to decrease photosensitivity reaction
- Advise patient to contact prescriber if vaginal itching; loose, foul-smelling stools; furry tongue occur that may indicate superimposed infection; report itching, rash, pruritus, urticaria
- Instruct patient to take all medication prescribed for the length of time ordered; drug must be taken around the clock to maintain blood levels; do not give medication to others

Evaluation

Positive therapeutic outcome

- Absence of signs/symptoms of infection (WBC <10,000, temp WNL, absence of red, draining wounds)
- Reported improvement in symptoms of infection

tetrahydrozoline

(tet-ra-hye-dro'zoe-leen)

Tyzine HCl, Tyzine Pediatric

Func. class.: Nasal decongestant

Chem. class.: Sympathomimetic amine

Pregnancy category **C**

Action: Produces vasoconstriction (rapid, long-acting) of arterioles, thereby decreasing fluid exudation, mucosal engorgement

Therapeutic Outcome: Absence of nasal congestion

Uses: Nasal congestion, adjunct in otitis media

Dosage and routes

P *Adult and child >6 yr:* Instill 2-4 gtt or sprays q4-6h prn (0.1%)

P *Child 2-6 yr:* Instill 2-3 gtt q4-6h prn (0.05%)

Available forms: Sol 0.05%, 0.1%

Side effects/adverse reactions

CNS: *Anxiety, restlessness, tremors, weakness, insomnia, dizziness,* fever, headache

EENT: *Irritation, burning, sneezing, stinging, dryness, rebound congestion*

GI: Nausea, vomiting, anorexia

INTEG: Contact dermatitis

Contraindications: Hypersensitivity to sympathomimetic amines

P **Precautions:** Child <6 yr, G elderly, diabetes, cardiovascular disease, hypertension, hyperthyroidism, increased ICP, prostatic hypertrophy, pregnancy **C**, glaucoma

Pharmacokinetics

Absorption	Minimally absorbed (usually)
Distribution	None
Metabolism	None
Excretion	None
Half-life	Unknown

Pharmacodynamics

Onset	1 min
Peak	Unknown
Duration	4-6 hr

Interactions

Drug/drug:

Individual drugs

Mecamylamine: ↑ hypotension

Methyldopa: ↑ hypotension

Reserpine: ↑ hypotension

Drug classifications

β-adrenergic blockers: ↑ hypertension

MAOIs: ↑ hypertension

NURSING CONSIDERATIONS

Assessment

- Assess for redness, swelling, pain in nasal passages before and during treatment
- Assess for systemic absorption: hypertension, tachycardia; notify prescriber—systemic absorption occurs at high doses or with prolonged use

Associated nursing diagnoses

- ✓ Airway clearance, ineffective (uses)
- ✓ Knowledge deficit (teaching)
- ✓ Noncompliance (teaching)

Implementation

Nasal route

- Have patient tilt head back, squeeze bulb to create a vacuum and draw correct amount of sol into dropper, insert 2 gtts of sol into nostril, repeat in other nostril
- Store in light-resistant containers; do not expose to high temp or let sol come into contact with aluminum
- Give for <4 consecutive days
- Ensure environmental humidification to decrease nasal congestion, dryness

Patient/family education

- Advise patient that stinging may occur for several applications; drying of mucosa may be decreased by environmental humidification
- Caution patient to notify prescriber if irregular pulse, insomnia, dizziness, or tremors occur
- Teach patient proper administration to avoid systemic absorption
- Advise patient to rinse dropper with very hot water to prevent contamination

Evaluation

Positive therapeutic outcome

- Decreased nasal congestion

theophylline

(thee-off'i-lin)

Accurbron, Aerolate III, Aerolate Jr., Aerolate Slo-Phyllin, Aerolate Sr., Aquaphyllin, Asmalix, Bronkodyl, Constant-T, Elixomin, Elixophyllin, Elixophyllin SR, Lanophyllin, Quibron-T Dividose, Quibron-T/SR Dividose, Respbid, Slo-Bid Gyrocaps, Slo-Phyllin Gyrocaps, Sustaire, Theolair-SR, Theo-24, Theobid Duracaps, Theobid Jr. Duracaps, Theochron, Theoclear-80, Theoclear L.A., Theo-Dur, Theo-Dur Sprinkle, Theolair, Theolair-SR, Theophylline, Theophylline and 5% Dextrose, Theophylline Extended Release, Theophylline Oral, Theophylline S.R., Theo-Sav, Theospan-SR, Theostat 80, Theovent, Theox, T-Phy, Uniphyl

Func. class.: Spasmolytic, bronchodilator

Chem. class.: Xanthine, ethylenediamine

Pregnancy category C

Action: Relaxes smooth muscle of respiratory system by blocking phosphodiesterase, which increases cAMP, which increases bronchodilation, diuresis, circulation, CNS stimulation

Therapeutic Outcome: Ability to breathe without difficulty

Uses: Bronchial asthma, bronchospasm of COPD, chronic bronchitis

Dosage and routes

Bronchospasm, bronchial asthma

Adult: PO 100-200 mg q6h; dosage must be individualized; rec 250-500 mg q9-12h

P *Child:* PO 50-100 mg q6h, not to exceed 12 mg/kg/24 h

COPD, chronic bronchitis

Adult: PO 30-660 q6-8h pc (sodium glycinate)

P *Child >12 yr:* PO 220-330 mg q6-8h pc (sodium glycinate)

P *Child 6-12 yr:* PO 330 mg q6-8h pc (sodium glycinate)

P *Child 3-6 yr:* PO 110-165 mg q6-8h pc (sodium glycinate)

P *Child 1-3 yr:* PO 55-110 mg q6-8h pc (sodium glyinate)

Available forms: Cap 50, 100, 200, 250 mg; tab 100, 125, 200, 225, 250, 300 mg; tab time-release 100, 200, 250, 300, 400, 500 mg; cap time-release 50, 65, 100, 125, 130, 200, 250, 260, 300, 400, 500 mg; elix 80, 11.25 mg/15 mg; sol 80 mg/15 ml; liq 80, 150, 160 mg/15 ml; susp 300 mg/15 ml

Side effects/adverse reactions

CNS: Anxiety, restlessness, insomnia, dizziness, convulsions, headache, lightheadedness, muscle twitching

T

CV: Palpitations, sinus tachycardia, hypotension, other dysrhythmias, fluid retention with tachycardia
GI: Nausea, vomiting, anorexia, diarrhea, bitter taste, dyspepsia, gastric distress
INTEG: Flushing, urticaria
RESP: Increased rate

Contraindications: Hypersensitivity to xanthines, tachydysrhythmias

G **Precautions:** Elderly, CHF, cor pulmonale, hepatic disease, active peptic ulcer disease, diabetes mellitus, hyperthyroidism, hypertension,
P children, pregnancy **C**

Pharmacokinetics

Absorption	Well absorbed (PO), slowly absorbed (ext rel)
Distribution	Crosses placenta, widely distributed
Metabolism	Liver
Excretion	Kidneys, breast milk
Half-life	3-13, increased in liver disease, CHF, elderly

Pharmacodynamics

	PO	PO-ER	IV
Onset	Rapid	Slow	Immediate
Peak	1 hr	4-8 hr	Inf end
Duration	6 hr	12-24 hr	6-8 hr

Interactions

Drug/drug:

Individual drugs
Cimetidine: ↑ action of theophylline
Proprandolol: ↑ action of theophylline
Erythromycin: ↑ action of theophylline
Lithium: ↓ effect of lithium
Drug classifications
Beta blockers: cardiotoxicity

NURSING CONSIDERATIONS

Assessment

- Monitor theophylline blood levels (therapeutic level is 10-20 µg/ml); toxicity may occur with small increase above 20 µg/ml
- Monitor I&O; diuresis
G occurs; dehydration may result
P in elderly or children
- Assess for signs of toxicity: irritability, insomnia, restlessness, tremors, nausea, vomiting
- Monitor respiratory rate, rhythm, depth; auscultate lung fields bilaterally; notify prescriber of abnormalities
- Assess for allergic reactions: rash, urticaria; if these occur, drug should be discontinued

Associated nursing diagnoses

✓ Airway clearance, ineffective (uses)
✓ Knowledge deficit (teaching)

Implementation

PO route
- Give PO pc to decrease GI symptoms; absorption may be affected

Patient/family education

- Advise patient to check OTC medications, current prescription medications for ephedrine, which will increase stimulation, and to avoid alcohol, caffeine
- Caution patient to avoid

hazardous activities; dizziness may occur

- Inform patient that if GI upset occurs, to take drug with 8 oz water; avoid food; absorption may be decreased
- Teach patient not to crush, dissolve, or chew slow-release products
- Teach patient that contents of bead-filled cap may be sprinkled over food for P children's use
- Advise patient to notify prescriber of toxicity: nausea, vomiting, anxiety, insomnia, convulsions
- Advise patient to notify prescriber of change in smoking habit; dosage may have to be changed

Evaluation

Positive therapeutic outcome

- Ability to breathe more easily

thiamine (vitamin B_1)

Betaxin ✤, Betalin S, Biamine, Revitonus, Thiamilate, thiamine HCl, vitamin B

Func. class.: Vitamin B_1

Chem. class.: Water soluble

Pregnancy category **A**

Action: Needed for pyruvate metabolism, carbohydrate metabolism

➔ **Therapeutic Outcome:** Prevention and treatment of thiamine deficiency

Uses: Vitamin B_1 deficiency or polyneuritis, cheilosis adjunct with thiamine beriberi, Wernicke-Korsakoff syndrome, pellagra, metabolic disorders

Dosage and routes

Beriberi

Adult: IM 10-500 mg tid × 2 wk, then 5-10 mg qd × 1 mo

P *Child:* IM 10-50 mg qd × 4-6 wk

Anemia/alcoholism/pregnancy/pellagra

Adult: PO 100 mg qd

P *Child:* PO 10-50 mg qd in divided doses

Beriberi with cardiac failure

P *Adult and child:* **IV** 100-500 mg

Wernicke's encephalopathy

Adult: **IV** 500 mg or less, then 100 mg bid

Available forms: Tab 50, 100, 250, 500 mg; inj 100 mg/ml; enteric-coated tab 20 mg

Side effects/adverse reactions

CNS: Weakness, restlessness

CV: ***Collapse, pulmonary edema,*** hypotension

EENT: Tightness of throat

GI: Hemorrhage, ***nausea, diarrhea***

INTEG: ***Angioneurotic edema,*** cyanosis, sweating, warmth

SYST: ***Anaphylaxis***

Contraindications: Hypersensitivity

Precautions: Pregnancy **A**

Pharmacokinetics

Absorption	Well absorbed (PO, IM) completely absorbed (IV)
Distribution	Widely distributed
Metabolism	Liver
Excretion	Kidneys (unchanged—excess amounts)
Half-life	Unknown

Pharmacodynamics

	PO/IM/IV
Onset	Unknown
Peak	Unknown
Duration	Unknown

Interactions

Drug/drug:

Drug classifications

Neuromuscular blockers: ↑ effect

NURSING CONSIDERATIONS

Assessment

- Monitor thiamine levels throughout treatment
- Assess nutritional status: yeast, beef, liver, whole or enriched grains, legumes

Associated nursing diagnoses

✓ Nutrition: less than body requirements (uses)
✓ Knowledge deficit (teaching)

Implementation

IV **IV route**

- **IV** undiluted given over 5 min or diluted with **IV** sol and given as an inf at a rate of 100 mg or less/5 min or more

Y-site compatibility:

Famotidine

Additive incompatibilities:

Barbiturates; sol with neutral or alkaline pH, such as carbonates, bicarbonates, citrates and acetates; erythromycin, kanamycin, or streptomycin

IM route

- Give by IM inj; rotate sites if pain and inflammation occur; do not mix with alkaline sol; Z-track to minimize pain
- Application of cold may decrease pain
- Store in tight, light-resistant container

Patient/family education

- Teach patient necessary foods to be included in diet: yeast, beef, liver, legumes, whole grains

Evaluation

Positive therapeutic outcome

- Absence of nausea, vomiting, anorexia, insomnia, tachycardia, paresthesias, depression, muscle weakness

thiethylperazine

(thye-eth-il-per′a-zeen)

Norzine, Torecan

Func. class.: Antiemetic

Chem. class.: Phenothiazine, piperazine derivative

Pregnancy category **C**

Action: Acts centrally by blocking chemoreceptor trigger zone, which in turn acts on vomiting center

Therapeutic Outcome: Control of nausea, vomiting

Uses: Nausea, vomiting

Dosage and routes

Adult: PO/IM/rec 10 mg/qd-tid

Available forms: Tab 10 mg; supp 10 mg; inj 5 mg/ml

Side effects/adverse reactions

CNS: Euphoria, depression, restlessness, tremor, extrapyramidal symptoms, ***convulsions,*** drowsiness
CV: Circulatory failure, tachycardia, postural hypotension, ECG changes
GI: Nausea, vomiting, anorexia, dry mouth, diarrhea, constipation, weight loss, metallic taste, cramps
GU: Urinary retention, dark urine
RESP: Respiratory depression

Contraindications: Hypersensitivity to phenothiazines, coma, seizure, encephalopathy, bone marrow depression

Precautions: Children < 2 yr, pregnancy **C**, elderly

Pharmacokinetics

Absorption	Readily absorbed
Distribution	Crosses placenta
Metabolism	Liver
Excretion	Kidneys, breast milk
Half-life	Unknown

Pharmacodynamics

	PO	REC	IM
Onset	45-60 min	45-60 min	Unknown
Peak	Unknown	Unknown	Unknown
Duration	4 hr	Unknown	Unknown

Interactions

Drug/drug:

Drug classifications

Antacids: ↓ absorption
Anticholinergics: ↑ anticholinergic effects
Antidepressants: ↑ CNS depression
Antidiarrheals, adsorbent: ↓ absorption
Antihistamines: ↑ CNS depression
Antihypertensives: ↑ hypotension
Antithyroid agents: ↑ agranulocytosis
Barbiturate anesthetics: ↑ CNS depression
Beta adrenergics: ↑ effects of both drugs
General anesthetics: ↑ CNS depression
MAOI: ↑ CNS depression
Narcotics: ↑ CNS depression
Sedative/hypnotics: ↑ CNS depression

NURSING CONSIDERATIONS

Assessment

- Monitor I&O ratio, palpate bladder if low urinary output occurs, especially in elderly; urinalysis recommended before, during prolonged therapy
- Monitor bilirubin, CBC, liver function studies monthly
- Assess affect, orientation, LOC, reflexes, gait, coordination, sleep pattern disturbances

T

- Monitor B/P with patient in sitting, standing, and lying positions; take pulse and respirations q4h during initial treatment; establish baseline before starting treatment; report drops of 30 mm Hg
- Check for dizziness, faintness, palpitations, tachycardia on rising; severe orthostatic hypotension is common
- Identify for neuroleptic malignant syndrome: hyperpyrexia, muscle rigidity, increased CPK, altered mental status; drug should be discontinued
- Assess for extrapyramidal symptoms including akathisia (inability to sit still, no pattern to movements), tardive dyskinesia (bizarre movements of the jaw, mouth, tongue, extremities), pseudoparkinsonism (tremors, pill rolling, shuffling gait); antiparkinson drug should be prescribed
- Assess for constipation, urinary retention daily; if these occur, increase bulk, water in diet

Associated nursing diagnoses

- ✓ Thought processes, altered (uses)
- ✓ Coping, ineffective individual (uses)
- ✓ Knowledge deficit (teaching)
- ✓ Noncompliance (teaching)

Implementation

IM route

- Give IM inj in large muscle mass; aspirate to avoid **IV** administration; give slowly. Have patient remain supine for 1 hr after administration

Patient/family education

- Teach patient to use good oral hygiene; frequent rinsing of mouth, sugarless gum for dry mouth
- Caution patient to avoid hazardous activities until drug response is determined—dizziness, blurred vision may occur
- Inform patient that orthostatic hypotension occurs often and to rise from sitting or lying position gradually
- Instruct patient to remain lying down after IM inj for at least 30 min
- Advise patient to avoid hot tubs, hot showers, tub baths, since hypotension may occur
- Inform patient that heat stroke may occur in hot weather, and to take extra precautions to stay cool
- Teach patient to avoid OTC preparations (cough, hay fever, cold) unless approved by prescriber because serious drug interactions may occur; avoid use with alcohol, CNS depressants because increased drowsiness may occur
- Inform patient to use a sunscreen and sunglasses to prevent burns
- Teach patient about extrapyramidal symptoms
- Instruct patient to report sore throat, malaise, fever, bleeding, mouth sores; if these occur, CBC should be drawn and drug discontinued

Evaluation

Positive therapeutic outcome

- Absence of nausea, vomiting

thioguanine (6-TG)

(thye-oh-gwah'neen)

thioguanine, Lanvis ✤

Func. class.: Antineoplastic-antimetabolite

Chem. class.: Purine analog

Pregnancy category D

Action: Interferes with synthesis, utilization of purine nucleotides; S phase of cell cycle specific

➔ Therapeutic Outcome: Prevention of rapidly growing malignant cells

Uses: Acute leukemias, chronic granulocytic leukemia, lymphomas, multiple myeloma, solid tumors

Dosage and routes

P *Adult and child:* PO 2 mg/kg/day, then increase slowly to 3 mg/kg/day after 4 wk

Available forms: Tab 40 mg

Side effects/adverse reactions

GI: Nausea, vomiting, anorexia, diarrhea, stomatitis, ***hepatotoxicity***, gastritis, jaundice

GU: ***Renal failure***, hyperuricemia, oliguria

HEMA: ***Thrombocytopenia, leukopenia, myelosuppression, anemia***

INTEG: Rash, dermatitis, dry skin

Contraindications: Prior drug resistance, leukopenia (2500/mm^3), thrombocytopenia (<100,000/mm^3), anemia, pregnancy **D**

Precautions: Liver disease

Pharmacokinetics

Absorption	Variably absorbed, 30%
Distribution	Crosses placenta
Metabolism	Liver—extensively
Excretion	Kidneys
Half-life	11 hr

Pharmacodynamics

	PO
Onset	Unknown
Peak	Unknown
Duration	Unknown

Interactions

Drug/drug:

Individual drugs

Radiation: ↑ toxicity, bone marrow suppression

Drug classifications

Antineoplastics: ↑ toxicity, bone marrow suppression

Lab test interferences

Increase: Uric acid (blood, urine)

NURSING CONSIDERATIONS

Assessment

- Assess buccal cavity q8h for dryness, sores or ulceration, white patches, oral pain, bleeding, dysphagia; obtain prescription for viscous lidocaine (Xylocaine)

T

• Assess symptoms indicating severe allergic reaction: rash, pruritus, urticaria, purpuric skin lesions, itching, flushing
• Monitor CBC, differential, platelet count weekly; withhold drug if WBC count is <4000/mm^3 or platelet count is <100,000/mm^3, notify prescriber of results if WBC <20,000/mm^3, platelets </50,800/mm^3
• Assess for increased uric acid levels, swelling, joint pain (primarily in extremities); patient should be well hydrated to prevent urate deposits
• Monitor renal function studies: BUN, creatinine, serum uric acid, urine CrCl before and during therapy; I&O ratio; report fall in urine output to <30 ml/hr
• Monitor temp q4h (may indicate beginning of infection)
• Monitor liver function tests before and during therapy (bilirubin, AST (SGOT), ALT (SGPT), LDH) as needed or monthly; yellowing of skin, sclera, dark urine, clay-colored stools, itchy skin, abdominal pain, fever, diarrhea
• Assess for bleeding: hematuria, stool guaiac, bruising or petechiae, mucosa or orifices q8h; inflammation of mucosa, breaks in skin
• Identify edema in feet, joint pain, stomach pain, shaking; prescriber should be notified
• Identify inflammation of mucosa, breaks in skin

Associated nursing diagnoses

✓ Injury, risk for (adverse reactions)
✓ Body image disturbance (adverse reactions)
✓ Infection, risk for (adverse reactions)
✓ Knowledge deficit (teaching)

Implementation

• Avoid contact with skin (very irritating), wash completely to remove
• Give fluids **IV** or PO before chemotherapy to hydrate patient
• Give antiemetic 30-60 min before giving drug to prevent vomiting, and prn; antibiotics for prophylaxis of infection
• Give top or syst analgesics for pain
• Provide liq diet: carbonated beverages; gelatin may be added if patient is not nauseated or vomiting
• Provide rinsing of mouth tid-qid with water, club soda; brushing of teeth bid-qid with soft brush or cotton-tipped applicators for stomatitis; use unwaxed dental floss

PO route

• Give 1 hr ac or 2 hr pc to prevent vomiting

Patient/family education

• Inform patient that contraceptive measures are recommended during therapy Caution patient to avoid use of products containing aspirin or ibuprofen, razors, commercial mouthwash, bleeding may occur; to report symptoms of bleeding (hematuria, tarry stools)
• Advise patient to report signs of anemia, (fatigue, headache, irritability, faintness, shortness of breath)

• Caution patient not to have any vaccinations without the advice of the prescriber—serious reactions can occur

Evaluation

Positive therapeutic outcome
• Prevention of rapid division of malignant cells

thiopental

(thye-oh-pen'tal)
Pentothal, thiopental sodium
Func. class.: General anesthetic
Chem. class.: Barbiturate
Pregnancy category **C**
Controlled substance schedule **III**

Action: Acts in reticular-activating system to produce anesthesia, raise seizure threshold

Therapeutic Outcome: Sedation, decreased seizure, decreased intracranial pressure

Uses: Short general anesthesia, narcoanalysis, induction anesthesia before other anesthetics

Investigational uses: Increased intracranial pressure

Dosage and routes

Induction
Adult: **IV** 210-280 mg or 3-5 ml/kg

General anesthetic
Adult: **IV** 50-75 mg given at 20-40 sec intervals

Narcoanalysis
Adult: **IV** 100 mg/min, not to exceed 50 ml/min

Sedation or narcosis
Adult: Rec 12-20 mg/lb

Increased intracranial pressure
Adult: 1.5-3.5 mg/kg

Available forms: Inj 250, 400, 500 mg/g, rectal sus 400 mg/g

Side effects/adverse reactions

CNS: Retrograde amnesia, prolonged somnolence
CV: Tachycardia, hypotension, ***myocardial depression, dysrhythmias***
EENT: Sneezing, coughing
INTEG: Chills, *shivering,* necrosis, pain at inj site
MS: Muscle irritability
RESP: ***Respiratory depression, bronchospasm***

Contraindications: Hypersensitivity, status asthmaticus, hepatic/intermittent porphyrias

Precautions: Severe cardiovascular disease, renal disease, hypotension, liver disease, myxedema, myasthenia gravis, asthma, increased intracranial pressure, pregnancy **C**

Pharmacokinetics

Absorption	Rapidly absorbed (rectal)
Distribution	Rapidly—CNS, redistributed to other organs, crosses placenta
Metabolism	Extensively—liver, small amounts converted to phenobarbital
Half-life	11½ hr; ↑ in obese and pregnant patients (term)

Pharmacodynamics

	IV	RECT
Onset	½-1 sec	8-10 min
Peak	Unknown	Unknown
Duration	10-30 min	Unknown

Interactions

Drug/drug:

Individual drugs

Alcohol: ↑ CNS depression
Ketamine: ↑ Hypotension

Drug classifications

Antidepressants: ↑ CNS depression
Antihistamines: ↑ CNS depression
Diuretics: ↑ Hypotension
Narcotics: ↑ CNS depression
Sedatives/hypnotics: ↑ CNS depression

Lab test interferences

False increase: Sulfobromophthalein

NURSING CONSIDERATIONS

Assessment

- Monitor inj site for redness, pain, swelling
- Assess degree of amnesia in elderly; may be increased [G]
- Assess anterograde amnesia
- Assess vital signs for recovery period in obese patient because half-life may be extended

Associated nursing diagnoses

- ✓ Anxiety (uses)
- ✓ Knowledge deficit (teaching)
- ✓ Noncompliance (teaching)

Implementation

[IV] IV route

- Dilute with D_5W, 0.9% NaCl, or sterile water for inj; do not use colored sol or sol with a precipitate
- Give test dose before administering 25-75 mg, wait 1-2 sec for response
- Give by continual inf after diluting in compatible sol and give slowly

Syringe compatibilities:

Aminophylline, hydrocortisone sodium succinate, neostigmine, pentobarbital, scopolamine, tubocurarine

Syringe incompatibilities:

Benzquinamide, chlorpromazine, dimenhydrinate, diphenhydramine, ephedrine, glycopyrrolate, meperidine, morphine, pentazocine, prochlorperazine, promethazine, propiomazine

Additive compatibilities:

Chloramphenicol, hydrocortisone sodium succinate, pentobarbital, potassium chloride

Additive incompatibilities:

Amikacin, cephapirin, chlorpromazine, codeine, dimenhydrinate, diphenhydramine, hydromorphone, regular insulin, levorphanol, meperidine, methadone, morphine, penicillin G potassium, prochlorperazine, promazine, promethazine, succinylcholine

Solution compatibilities: D_5/0.45% NaCl, D_5W, multiple electrolyte sol, 0.45% NaCl, 0.9% NaCl, 1/6 M sodium lactate

Solution incompatibilities: Dextrose/Ringer's, lactated Ringer's inj combinations, D_{10}/0.9% NaCl, $D_{10}W$, Ringer's, lactated Ringer's inj

Patient/family education

- Caution patient to avoid hazardous activities until drowsiness, weakness subside
- Inform patient that amnesia occurs; events may not be remembered

Evaluation

Positive therapeutic outcome

- Induction of sedation, general anesthesia

Treatment of overdose: Discontinue drug; administer vasopressor agents or anticholinergics, artificial ventilation

thioridazine

(thye-or-rid'a-zeen)

Mellaril, Mellaril Concentrate, Mellaril-5, Novoridazine ✱, thioridazine HCl

Func. class.: Antipsychotic/neuroleptic

Chem. class.: Phenothiazine, piperidine

Pregnancy category C

Action: Depresses cerebral cortex, hypothalamus, limbic system, which control activity, aggression; blocks neurotransmission produced by dopamine at synapse; exhibits strong α-adrenergic, anticholinergic blocking action; mechanism for antipsychotic effects is unclear

➔ **Therapeutic Outcome:** Decreased signs and symptoms of psychosis

Uses: Psychotic disorders, schizophrenia, behavioral problems in children, alcohol withdrawal as adjunct, anxiety, major depressive disorders, organic brain syndrome

Dosage and routes

Psychosis

Adult: PO 25-100 mg tid, max dose 800 mg/day; dose is gradually increased to desired response, then reduced to minimum maintenance

Depression/behavioral problems/organic brain syndrome

Adult: PO 25 tid, range from 10 mg bid-qid to 50 mg tid-qid

P ***Child 2-12 yr:*** PO 0.5-3 mg/kg/day in divided doses

Available forms: Tab 10, 15, 25, 50, 100, 150, 200, 300 mg; conc 30, 100 mg/ml; susp 25, 100 mg/5 ml, syrup 10 mg/15 ml

Side effects/adverse reactions

CNS: Extrapyramidal symptoms (rare): pseudoparkin-

T

sonism, akathisia, dystonia, tardive dyskinesia, ***seizures, headache,*** confusion
CV: Orthostatic hypotension, ***cardiac arrest,*** ECG changes, ***tachycardia***
EENT: Blurred vision, glaucoma, dry eyes
GI: Dry mouth, nausea, vomiting, anorexia, constipation, diarrhea, jaundice, weight gain
GU: Urinary retention, urinary frequency, enuresis, impotence, amenorrhea, gynecomastia
HEMA: Anemia, ***leukopenia, leukocytosis, agranulocytosis***
INTEG: Rash, photosensitivity, dermatitis
RESP: ***Laryngospasm,*** dyspnea, ***respiratory depression***

Contraindications: Hypersensitivity, blood dyscrasias, coma, P child <2 yr, brain damage, bone marrow depression

Precautions: Pregnancy **C**, lactation, seizure disorders, hypertension, hepatic disease, cardiac disease

Pharmacokinetics

Absorption	Variably absorbed (Tab)
Distribution	Widely distributed, high concentrations in CNS, crosses placenta
Metabolism	Liver, extensively, GI mucosa
Excretion	Kidneys, breast milk
Half-life	26-36 hr

Pharmacodynamics

	PO
Onset	Erratic
Peak	2-4 hr
Duration	8-12 hr

Interactions

Drug/drug:

Individual drugs

Alcohol: ↑ effects of both drugs, oversedation
Aluminum hydroxide: ↓ absorption
Bromocriptine: ↓ antiparkinson activity
Disopyramide: ↑ anticholinergic effects
Epinephrine: ↑ toxicity
Guanethidine: ↓ antihypertensive response
Levodopa: ↓ antiparkinson activity
Lithium: ↓ chlorpromazine levels, ↑ extrapyramidal symptoms, masking of lithium toxicity
Magnesium hydroxide: ↓ absorption
Norepinephrine: ↓ vasoresponse, ↑ toxicity
Phenobarbital: ↓ effectiveness, ↑ metabolism

Drug classifications

Antacids: ↓ absorption
Anticholinergics: ↑ anticholinergic effects
Antidepressants: ↑ CNS depression
Antidiarrheals, adsorbent: ↓ absorption
Antihistamines: ↑ CNS depression
Antihypertensives: ↑ hypotension
Antithyroid agents: ↑ agranulocytosis
Barbiturate anesthetics: ↑ CNS depression
Beta adrenergics: ↑ effects of both drugs
General anesthetics: ↑ CNS depression
MAOI: ↑ CNS depression
Narcotics: ↑ CNS depression

Sedative/hypnotics: ↑ CNS depression

Lab test interferences

Increase: Liver function tests, cardiac enzymes, cholesterol, blood glucose, prolactin, bilirubin, PBI, cholinesterase. ^{131}I, alk phosphatase, leukocytes, granulocytes, platelets
Decrease: Hormones (blood and urine)
False positive: Pregnancy tests, PKU, urine bilirubin
False negative: Urinary steroids, 17-OHCS

NURSING CONSIDERATIONS

Assessment

• Assess mental status: orientation, mood, behavior, presence of hallucinations, and type before initial administration and monthly; this drug should significantly reduce psychotic behavior
• Check for swallowing of PO medication; check for hoarding or giving of medication to other patients
• Monitor I&O ratio, palpate bladder if low urinary output G occurs, especially in elderly; urinalysis recommended before, during prolonged therapy
• Monitor bilirubin, CBC, liver function studies monthly
• Assess affect, orientation, LOC, reflexes, gait, coordination, sleep pattern disturbances
• Monitor B/P sitting, standing and lying, take pulse and respirations q4h during initial treatment; establish baseline before starting treatment; report drops of 30 mm Hg; obtain baseline ECG, Q-wave and T-wave changes
• Check for dizziness, faintness, palpitations, tachycardia on rising; severe orthostatic hypotension is common
• Identify for neuroleptic malignant syndrome: hyperpyrexia, muscle rigidity, increased CPK, altered mental status; drug should be discontinued
• Assess for extrapyramidal symptoms including akathisia (inability to sit still, no pattern to movements), tardive dyskinesia (bizarre movements of the jaw, mouth, tongue, extremities), pseudoparkinsonism (ragged, tremors, pill rolling, shuffling gate)—an antiparkinson drug should be prescribed
• Assess for constipation, urinary retention daily; if these occur, increase bulk, water in diet

Associated nursing diagnoses

✓ Thought processes, altered (uses)
✓ Coping, ineffective individual (uses)
✓ Knowledge deficit (teaching)
✓ Noncompliance (teaching)

Implementation

PO route
• Administer drug in liq form mixed in glass of juice or cola if hoarding is suspected; do not mix in caffeine drinks, tannics, pectins
G • Decrease dose in elderly; metabolism is slowed in the elderly
• PO with full glass of water, milk; or give with food to decrease GI upset
• Store in tight, light-resistant container, oral sol in amber bottle

Patient/family education

- Teach patient to use good oral hygiene; frequent rinsing of mouth, sugarless gum for dry mouth
- Advise patient to avoid hazardous activities until drug response is determined; dizziness, blurred vision are common
- Inform patient that orthostatic hypotension occurs often and to rise from sitting or lying position gradually; to avoid hot tubs, hot showers, tub baths because hypotension may occur
- Instruct patient that in hot weather, heat stroke may occur; take extra precautions to stay cool
- Caution patient to avoid abrupt withdrawal of this drug, or extrapyramidal symptoms may result; drug should be withdrawn slowly
- Teach patient to avoid OTC preparations (cough, hay fever, cold) unless approved by prescriber—serious drug interactions may occur; avoid use with alcohol, CNS depressants—increased drowsiness may occur
- Advise patient to use a sunscreen and sunglasses to prevent burns
- Teach patient about extrapyramidal symptoms and necessity for meticulous oral hygiene because oral candidiasis may occur
- Advise patient to take antacids 2 hr before or after this drug
- Instruct patient to report sore throat, malaise, fever, bleeding, mouth sores; if these occur, CBC should be drawn and drug discontinued

Evaluation

Positive therapeutic outcome

- Decrease in emotional excitement, hallucinations, delusions, paranoia
- Reorganization of patterns of thought, speech

Treatment of overdose: Lavage if orally ingested; provide airway; *do not induce vomiting or use epinephrine*

thiotepa

(thye-oh-tep'a)

thiotepa

Func. class.: Antineoplastic

Chem. class.: Alkylating agent

Pregnancy category **D**

Action: Responsible for cross-linking DNA strands leading to cell death; activity is not cell–cycle-specific

Therapeutic Outcome: Prevention of rapidly growing malignant cells

Uses: Hodgkin's disease, lymphomas; breast, ovarian, lung, bladder, cancer; neoplastic effusions

Dosage and routes

Adult: **IV** 50.2 mg/kg × 5 days, then 0.2 mg/kg q1-3 wk

Neoplastic effusions

Adult: Intracavity 10-15 mg

Bladder cancer

Adult: Instill 60 mg/60 ml water for inj instilled in bladder for 2 hr once weekly × 4 wk

Available forms: Inj 15 mg, powder for inj

Side effects/adverse reactions

CNS: Dizziness, headache
GI: Nausea, vomiting, anorexia, stomatitis
GU: Hyperuricemia, ***hematuria, amenorrhea, azoospermia***
HEMA: Thrombocytopenia, leukopenia, pancytopenia
INTEG: Rash, pruritus

Contraindications: Hypersensitivity, pregnancy **D**

Precautions: Radiation therapy, bone marrow suppression, impaired renal or hepatic function

Pharmacokinetics

Absorption	Variably absorbed
Distribution	Unknown
Metabolism	Liver—extensively
Excretion	Kidneys
Half-life	Unknown

Pharmacodynamics

	IV
Onset	Unknown
Peak	Unknown
Duration	Unknown

Interactions

Drug/drug:

Individual drugs

Radiation: ↑ toxicity, bone marrow suppression
Succinylcholine: ↑ apnea

Drug classifications

Antineoplastics: ↑ toxicity bone marrow suppression

NURSING CONSIDERATIONS

Assessment

- Assess buccal cavity q8h for dryness, sores or ulceration, white patches, oral pain, bleeding, dysphagia; obtain prescription for viscous lidocaine (Xylocaine)
- Assess symptoms indicating severe allergic reaction: rash, pruritus, urticaria, itching, flushing
- Monitor CBC, differential, platelet count weekly; withhold drug if WBC count is <4000/mm^3 or platelet count is <100,000/mm^3; notify prescriber of results if WBC <20,000/mm^3, platelets <150,000/mm^3
- Assess for increased uric acid levels, swelling, joint pain (primarily in extremities); patient should be well hydrated to prevent urate deposits
- Monitor renal function studies: BUN, creatinine, serum uric acid, urine CrCl before and during therapy; I&O ratio; report fall in urine output to <30 ml/hr
- Monitor temp q4h (may indicate beginning of infection)
- Monitor liver function tests before and during therapy [bilirubin, AST (SGOT), ALT (SGPT), LDH] as needed or monthly; yellowing of skin, sclera, dark urine, clay-colored stools, itchy skin, abdominal pain, fever, diarrhea
- Assess for bleeding: hematuria, stool guaiac, bruising or petechiae, mucosa or orifices

q8h; inflammation of mucosa, breaks in skin

- Identify dyspnea, rales, unproductive cough, chest pain, tachypnea
- Identify effects of alopecia on body image; discuss feelings about body changes

Associated nursing diagnoses

- ✓ Injury, risk for (adverse reactions)
- ✓ Body image disturbance (adverse reactions)
- ✓ Infection, risk for (adverse reactions)
- ✓ Knowledge deficit (teaching)

Implementation

- Give fluids **IV** or PO before chemotherapy to hydrate patient
- Give antacid before oral agent, give drug after evening meal, before bedtime; antiemetic 30-60 min before giving drug to prevent vomiting, and prn; antibiotics for prophylaxis of infection
- Give top or syst analgesics for pain
- Give liq diet: carbonated beverages; gelatin may be added if patient is not nauseated or vomiting
- Provide rinsing of mouth tid-qid with water, club soda; brushing of teeth bid-qid with soft brush or cotton-tipped applicators for stomatitis; use unwaxed dental floss

IV **IV route**

Direct route

- Give **IV** after diluting 15 mg/1.5 ml of sterile H_2O for inj; give over 1-3 min

Intermittent inf

- May be further diluted in 50-100 ml D_5W, 0.9% NaCl, Ringer's, LR

Syringe compatibilities:

Procaine HCl, (2%), epinephrine 1:1000

Instill route

- Reconstitute solution, then mix 60 mg/30-60 ml sterile water; instill is by Foley catheter; patient's position may be changed every few min; the patient must retain sol for 2 hr to provide for cell death

Intracavity route

- Reconstitute sol and administer by effusion tube as directed

Patient/family education

- Caution patient to avoid use of products containing aspirin or ibuprofen, razors, commercial mouthwash because bleeding may occur; to report symptoms of bleeding (hematuria, tarry stools)
- Advise patient to report signs of anemia, (fatigue, headache, irritability, faintness, shortness of breath)
- Advise patient to report any changes in breathing or coughing even several mo after treatment; to avoid crowds or persons with respiratory or other infections
- Inform patient that hair may be lost during treatment; a wig or hairpiece may make patient feel better; new hair may be different in color, texture
- Caution patient not to have any vaccinations without the advice of the prescriber because serious reactions can occur
- Advise patient that contraception is needed during treat-

ment and for several mo after the completion of therapy

Evaluation

Positive therapeutic outcome
- Prevention of rapid division of malignant cells

thiothixene

(thye-oh-thix'een)

Navane, thiothixene

Func. class.: Antipsychotic/neuroleptic

Chem. class.: Thioxanthene

Pregnancy category C

Action: Depresses cerebral cortex, hypothalamus, limbic system, which control activity, aggression; block neurotransmission produced by dopamine at synapse; exhibits strong α-adrenergic blocking action; mechanism for antipsychotic effects is unclear

Therapeutic Outcome: Decreased signs and symptoms of psychosis

Uses: Psychotic disorders, schizophrenia, acute agitation

Dosage and routes

Adult: PO 2-5 mg bid-qid depending on severity of condition; dose gradually increased to 15-30 mg if needed; IM 4 mg bid-qid; max dose 30 mg qd; administer PO dose as soon as possible

Available forms: Cap 1, 2, 5, 10, 20 mg; conc 5 mg/ml; inj 2 mg/ml; powder for inj 5 mg/ml

Side effects/adverse reactions

CNS: *Extrapyramidal symptoms: pseudoparkinsonism, akathisia, dystonia, tardive dyskinesia,* seizures, *headache*

CV: *Orthostatic hypotension,* hypertension, ***cardiac arrest,*** ECG changes, ***tachycardia***

EENT: Blurred vision, glaucoma

GI: *Dry mouth, nausea, vomiting, anorexia, constipation,* diarrhea, jaundice, weight gain

GU: Urinary retention, urinary frequency, enuresis, impotence, amenorrhea, gynecomastia

HEMA: Anemia, ***leukopenia, leukocytosis, agranulocytosis***

INTEG: *Rash,* photosensitivity, dermatitis

RESP: ***Laryngospasm,*** dyspnea, ***respiratory depression***

Contraindications: Hypersensitivity, blood dyscrasias, child <12 yr, bone marrow depression, circulatory collapse, CNS depression, coma, alcoholism, CV disease, hepatic disease, Reye's syndrome, narrow-angle glaucoma

Precautions: Pregnancy **C**, lactation, seizure disorders, hypertension, hepatic disease

T

Pharmacokinetics

Absorption	Well absorbed (PO, IM)
Distribution	Widely distributed, crosses placenta
Metabolism	Liver
Excretion	Kidneys, breast milk
Half-life	34 hr

Pharmacodynamics

	PO	IM
Onset	Slow	15-30 min
Peak	2-8 hr	1-6 hr
Duration	Up to 12 hr	Up to 12 hr

Interactions

Drug/drug:

Individual drugs

Alcohol: ↑ effects of both drugs, oversedation
Aluminum hydroxide: ↓ absorption
Bromocriptine: ↓ antiparkinson activity
Disopyramide: ↑ anticholinergic effects
Epinephrine: ↑ toxicity
Guanethidine: ↓ antihypertensive response
Levodopa: ↓ antiparkinson activity
Lithium: ↓ chlorpromazine levels, ↑ extrapyramidal symptoms, masking of lithium toxicity
Magnesium hydroxide: ↓ absorption
Norepinephrine: ↓ vasoresponse, ↑ toxicity
Phenobarbital: ↓ effectiveness, ↑ metabolism

Drug classifications

Antacids: ↓ absorption
Anticholinergics: ↑ anticholinergic effects
Antidepressants: ↑ CNS depression
Antidiarrheals, adsorbent: ↓ absorption
Antihistamines: ↑ CNS depression
Antihypertensives: ↑ hypotension
Antithyroid agents: ↑ agranulocytosis
Barbiturate anesthetics: ↑ CNS depression
Beta adrenergics: ↑ effects of both drugs
General anesthetics: ↑ CNS depression
MAOI: ↑ CNS depression
Narcotics: ↑ CNS depression
Sedative/hypnotics: ↑ CNS depression

Lab test interferences

Increase: Liver function tests, cardiac enzymes, cholesterol, blood glucose, prolactin, bilirubin, PBI, cholinesterase. ^{131}I, alk phosphatase, leukocytes, granulocytes, platelets
Decrease: Hormones (blood and urine)
False positive: Pregnancy tests, PKU, urine bilirubin
False negative: Urinary steroids, 17-OHCS

NURSING CONSIDERATIONS

Assessment

- Assess mental status: orientation, mood, behavior, presence of hallucinations, and type before initial administration and monthly; this drug should significantly reduce psychotic behavior
- Check for swallowing of PO medication; check for hoarding or giving of medication to other patients
- Monitor I&O ratio, palpate bladder if low urinary output occurs, especially in elderly; urinalysis recommended before, during prolonged therapy
- Monitor bilirubin, CBC, liver function studies monthly
- Assess affect, orientation, LOC, reflexes, gait, coordination, sleep pattern disturbances
- Monitor B/P sitting, standing and lying, take pulse and respirations q4h during initial

treatment; establish baseline before starting treatment; report drops of 30 mm Hg; obtain baseline ECG, Q-wave and T-wave changes
- Check for dizziness, faintness, palpitations, tachycardia on rising; severe orthostatic hypotension is common
- Identify for neuroleptic malignant syndrome: hyperpyrexia, muscle rigidity, increased CPK, altered mental status; drug should be discontinued
- Assess for extrapyramidal symptoms including akathisia (inability to sit still, no pattern to movements), tardive dyskinesia (bizarre movements of the jaw, mouth, tongue, extremities), pseudoparkinsonism (ragged, tremors, pill rolling, shuffling gait); an antiparkinson drug should be prescribed
- Assess for constipation, urinary retention daily; if these occur, increase bulk, water in diet

Associated nursing diagnoses

- ✓ Thought processes, altered (uses)
- ✓ Coping, ineffective individual (uses)
- ✓ Knowledge deficit (teaching)
- ✓ Noncompliance (teaching)

Implementation

PO route
- Give drug in liq form mixed in glass of juice or cola if hoarding is suspected; do not mix in caffeine drinks, tannics, pectins
- Give decreased dose to elderly because metabolism is G slowed in the elderly
- Give PO with full glass of water, milk; or give with food to decrease GI upset
- Store in tight, light-resistant container; store oral sol in amber bottle

IM route
- Dilute 10 mg vial/2.2 ml sterile water for inj to 5 mg/ml
- Inj in deep muscle mass, do not give SC; do not administer sol with a precipitate

Patient/family education

- Teach patient to use good oral hygiene; frequent rinsing of mouth, sugarless gum for dry mouth
- Advise patient to avoid hazardous activities until drug response is determined; dizziness, blurred vision is common
- Inform patient that orthostatic hypotension occurs often and to rise from sitting or lying position gradually and to remain lying down after IM inj for at least 30 min; tell patient to avoid hot tubs, hot showers, tub baths because hypotension may occur; tell patient that in hot weather, heat stroke may occur, so to take extra precautions to stay cool
- Caution patient to avoid abrupt withdrawal of this drug, or extrapyramidal symptoms may result; drug should be withdrawn slowly
- Teach patient to avoid OTC preparations (cough, hayfever, cold) unless approved by prescriber, because serious drug interactions may occur; avoid use with alcohol, CNS depressants because increased drowsiness may occur
- Caution patient to use a sunscreen and sunglasses to prevent burns

T

• Teach patient about extrapyramidal symptoms and necessity of meticulous oral hygiene because oral candidiasis may occur
• Tell patient to take antacids 2 hr before or after this drug
• Advise patient to report sore throat, malaise, fever, bleeding, mouth sores; if these occur, CBC should be measured and drug discontinued

Evaluation

Positive therapeutic outcome
• Decrease in emotional excitement, hallucinations, delusions, paranoia
• Reorganization of patterns of thought, speech

Treatment of overdose: Lavage if orally ingested; provide airway; *do not induce vomiting or use epinephrine*

thyroid USP (desiccated)

(thye-roid)

Armour Thyroid, Cholaxin ✦, S-P-T, Thyrar, Thyroid Strong, thyroid USP

Func. class.: Thyroid hormone

Chem. class.: Active thyroid hormone in natural state and ratio

Pregnancy category **A**

Action: Increases metabolic rates; controls protein synthesis; increases cardiac output, renal blood blow, O_2 consumption, body temp, blood volume, growth, development at cellular level

➡ **Therapeutic Outcome:** Correction of lack of thyroid hormone

Uses: Hypothyroidism, cretinism, myxedema

Dosage and routes

Hypothyroidism

Adult: PO 65 mg qd, increased by 65 mg q30d until desired response; maintenance dose 65-195 mg qd

G *Geriatric:* PO 7.5-15 mg qd, double dose q6-8w until desired response

Cretinism/juvenile hypothyroidism

P *Child over 1 yr:* PO up to 180 mg qd titrated to response

P *Child 4-12 mo:* PO 30-60 mg qd

P *Child 1-4 mo:* PO 15-30 mg qd; may increase q2w; titrated to response; maintenance dose 30-45 mg qd

Myxedema

Adult: PO 16 mg qd, double dose q2w, maintenance 65-195 mg/day

Available forms: Tab 15, 30, 60, 90, 120 mg; enteric-coated tab 30, 60, 120 mg; sugar-coated tab 30, 60, 120, 180 mg; cap pork 60, 90, 120, 180 mg; tab bovine 30, 60, 120 mg

Side effects/adverse reactions

CNS: Insomnia, tremors, headache, thyroid storm
CV: Tachycardia, palpita-

tions, angina, dysrhythmias, hypertension, ***cardiac arrest***
GI: Nausea, diarrhea, increased or decreased appetite, cramps
MISC: Menstrual irregularities, weight loss, sweating, heat intolerance, fever

Contraindications: Adrenal insufficiency, MI, thyrotoxicosis

G **Precautions:** Elderly, angina pectoris, hypertension, ischemia, cardiac disease, pregnancy **A**, lactation

Pharmacokinetics

Absorption	Well absorbed (PO)
Distribution	Widely distributed, does not cross placenta
Metabolism	Liver, tissues
Excretion	Feces via bile, breast milk
Half-life	T_3—2 days; T_4—1 wk

Pharmacodynamics

	PO
Onset	1 hr
Peak	12-48 hr
Duration	Unknown

Interactions
Drug/drug:
Individual drugs
Cholestyramine: ↓ absorption of thyroid hormone
Colestipol: ↓ absorption of thyroid hormone
Digitalis: ↓ effect of digitalis
Insulin: ↑ requirement for insulin
Phenytoin (IV): ↑ release of thyroid hormone

Drug classifications
Amphetamines: ↑ CNS, cardiac stimulation
Beta-adrenergic blockers: ↓ effect of beta blockers
Decongestants: ↑ CNS, cardiac stimulation
Oral anticoagulants: ↑ requirements for anticoagulants
Vasopressors: ↑ CNS, cardiac stimulation

Lab test interferences
Increase: CPK, LDH, AST (SGOT), PBI, blood glucose
Decrease: TSH, ^{131}I uptake test, uric acid, triglycerides

NURSING CONSIDERATIONS
Assessment

- Identify if the patient is taking anticoagulants, antidiabetic agents; document on chart
- Take B/P, pulse before each dose; monitor I&O ratio and weight every day in same clothing, using same scale, at same time of day
- Monitor height, weight, psychomotor development, and growth rate if given to a P child
- Monitor T_3, T_4, FTIs, which are decreased; radioimmunoassay of TSH, which is increased; radio uptake, which is increased if patient is on too low a dose of medication
- Monitor pro-time—patient may require decreased dosage of anticoagulant; check for bleeding, bruising
- Assess for increased nervousness, excitability, irritability, which may indicate that dose of medication is too high, usually after 1-3 wk of treatment

T

• Assess cardiac status: angina, palpitation, chest pain, change G in vital signs; the elderly patient may have undetected cardiac problems and baseline ECG should be completed before treatment

Associated nursing diagnoses

✓ Knowledge deficit (teaching)
✓ Noncompliance (teaching)

Implementation

PO route

• Give in AM if possible as a single dose to decrease sleeplessness; at same time each day to maintain drug level
• Give only for hormone imbalances; not to be used for obesity, male infertility, menstrual conditions, lethargy; give lowest dose that relieves symptoms; lower dose to the G elderly and in cardiac diseases
• Store in tight, light-resistant container
• Wean patient off medication 4 wk before RAIU test

Patient/family education

• Teach patient that drug is not a cure but controls symptoms and that treatment is long-term
• Instruct patient to report excitability, irritability, anxiety, sweating, heat intolerance, chest pain, palpitations, which indicate overdose
• Advise patient not to switch brands unless approved by prescriber; bioavailability may differ; do not take with food; absorption will be decreased
• Teach patient that drug may be discontinued after giving birth; thyroid panel will be evaluated after 1-2 mo
• Teach patient that hyperthy- P roid child will show almost immediate behavior/ personality change; that hair P loss will occur in child and is temporary
• Caution patient that drug is not to be taken to reduce weight
• Caution patient to avoid OTC preparations containing iodine; read labels; other medications should not be used unless approved by health-care prescriber
• Teach patient to avoid iodine-containing food: iodized salt, soybeans, tofu, turnips, certain kinds of seafood and bread

Evaluation

Positive therapeutic outcome

• Absence of depression
• Weight loss, increased diuresis, pulse, appetite
• Absence of constipation, peripheral edema, cold intolerance, pale, cool dry skin, brittle nails, alopecia, coarse hair, menorrhagia, night blindness, paresthesias, syncope, stupor, coma, rosy cheeks
• Improved levels of T_3, T_4 by laboratory tests
P • Child: Age-appropriate weight, height, and psychomotor development

Treatment of overdose: Withhold dose for up to 1 wk, acute overdose—gastric lavage or induce emesis, then activated charcoal; provide supportive treatment to control symptoms

ticarcillin clavulanate
(tye-kar-sill-in)
Chem. class: Broad-spectrum antibiotic
Func. class.: Extended-spectrum penicillin
Pregnancy category **B**

Action: Interferes with cell wall replication of susceptible organisms; osmotically unstable cell wall swells, bursts from osmotic pressure

➔ **Therapeutic Outcome:** Resolution of infection

Uses: Respiratory, soft tissue, urinary tract infections; bacterial septicemia; effective for gram-positive cocci *(S. aureus, S. faecalis, S. pneumoniae)*, gram-negative cocci *(N. gonorrhoeae)*, gram-positive bacilli *(C. perfringens, C. tetani)*, gram-negative bacilli *(Bacteroides, F. nucleatum, E. coli, P. mirabilis, Salmonella, M. morganii, P. rettgeri, Enterobacter, P. aeruginosa, Serratia, Peptococcus, Peptostreptococcus, Eubacterium)*

Dosage and routes
Adult: **IV** inf 1 vial containing ticarcillin 3 g, clavulanate K 0.1 g q4-6h, infuse over 30 min

P *Child <60 kg:* 200-300 mg ticarcillin/kg/day in divided doses q4-6h

Available forms: Inj IM, **IV** 3 g ticarcillin and 0.1 g clavulanate; **IV** inf 3 g ticarcillin and 0.1 g clavulanate

Side effects/adverse reactions
CNS: Lethargy, hallucinations, anxiety, depression, twitching, ***coma, convulsions***
GI: Nausea, vomiting, diarrhea, increased AST (SGOT), ALT (SGPT), abdominal pain, glossitis, colitis
GU: Oliguria, proteinuria, hematuria, *vaginitis, moniliasis,* ***glomerulonephritis***
HEMA: Anemia, increased bleeding time, ***bone marrow depression, granulocytopenia***
META: Hypokalemia, hypokalemia, alkalosis, hypernatremia

Contraindications: Hypersensitivity to penicillins

Precautions: Hypersensitivity to cephalosporins, pregnancy **B**

Pharmacokinetics

Absorption	Completely absorbed (IV)
Distribution	Widely distributed, crosses blood-brain barrier
Metabolism	Liver
Excretion	Kidneys
Half-life	64-68 min

Pharmacodynamics

	IV
Onset	Unknown
Peak	30-45 min
Duration	4 hr

T

Interactions
Drug/drug:
Individual drugs
Cholestyramine: ↓ absorption of thyroid hormone
Colestipol: ↓ absorption of thyroid hormone
Digitalis: ↓ effect of digitalis

Insulin: ↑ requirement for insulin
Phenytoin (IV): ↑ release of thyroid hormone

Drug classifications

Amphetamines: ↑ CNS, cardiac stimulation
Beta-adrenergic blockers: ↓ effect of beta blockers
Decongestants: ↑ CNS, cardiac stimulation
Oral anticoagulants: ↑ requirements for anticoagulants
Vasopressors: ↑ CNS, cardiac stimulation

Lab test interferences

False positive: Urine glucose, urine protein Coombs' test

NURSING CONSIDERATIONS

Assessment

- Monitor I&O ratio; report hematuria, oliguria because penicillin in high doses is nephrotoxic
- Monitor any patient with compromised renal system because drug is excreted slowly in poor renal system function; toxicity may occur rapidly
- Monitor liver studies: AST (SGOT), ALT (SGPT)
- Monitor studies: WBC, RBC, H&H, bleeding time
- Monitor renal studies: urinalysis, protein, blood
- Obtain C&S test results before initiating drug therapy; drug may be given as soon as culture is taken
- Assess bowel pattern before, during treatment
- Assess skin eruptions after administration of penicillin to 1 wk after discontinuing drug
- Assess respiratory status: rate, character, wheezing, and tightness in chest
- Assess allergies before initiation of treatment, reaction of each medication; highlight allergies on chart, Kardex

Associated nursing diagnoses

✓ Infection, risk for (uses)
✓ Knowledge deficit (teaching)

Implementation

IV **IV route**

- Give **IV** after diluting 3.1 g or less/13 ml of sterile H_2O or NaCl (200 mg/ml), shake; may further dilute in 50-100 ml or more normal saline, D_5W, or LR sol and run over ½ hr
- Give drug after C&S has been completed
- Have adrenalin, suction, tracheostomy set, endotracheal intubation equipment available
- Give adequate fluid intake (2 L) during diarrhea episodes
- Obtain scratch test results to assess allergy after securing order from prescriber—usually done when penicillin is only drug of choice
- Store at room temp, reconstituted sol for 12-24 hr or 3-7 days refrigerated

Patient/family education

- Advise patient that culture may be taken after completed course of medication
- Instruct patient to report sore throat, fever, fatigue (may indicate super infection)
- Advise patient to wear or carry Medic Alert ID if allergic to penicillins

Evaluation

Positive therapeutic outcome
- Absence of fever, purulent drainage, redness, inflammation

Treatment of overdose:
Withdraw drug, maintain airway, administer epinephrine, aminophylline, O_2, **IV** corticosteroids for anaphylaxis

ticlopidine
(tye-cloe'pi-deen)
Ticlid
Func. class.: Platelet aggregation inhibitor
Pregnancy category **B**

Action: Inhibits first and second phases of ADP-induced effects in platelet aggregation

Therapeutic Outcome: Decreased stroke by decreasing platelet aggregation

Uses: Reducing the risk of stroke in high-risk patients

Dosage and routes
Adult: PO 250 mg bid with food

Available forms: Tab 250 mg

Side effects/adverse reactions
GI: Nausea, vomiting, diarrhea, GI discomfort, ***cholestatic jaundice, hepatitis,*** increased cholesterol LDL, VLDL
HEMA: Bleeding (epistaxis, hematuria, conjunctival hemorrhage, GI bleeding), agranulocytosis, neutropenia, thrombocytopenia
INTEG: Rash, pruritus

Contraindications: Hypersensitivity, active liver disease, blood dyscrasias

Precautions: Past liver disease, renal disease, elderly, pregnancy **B**, lactation, children, increased bleeding risk

Pharmacokinetics

Absorption	Well absorbed (PO)
Distribution	Unknown
Metabolism	Liver—extensively
Excretion	Kidneys—unchanged drug
Half-life	Increased with repeat dosing; 4-5 days (multiple doses)

Pharmacodynamics

	PO
Onset	Unknown
Peak	1-3 hr
Duration	Unknown

Interactions
Drug/drug:
Individual drugs
Aspirin: ↑ bleeding tendencies
Cimetidine: ↑ effects of ticlopidine
Digoxin: ↓ plasma levels of ticlopidine
Theophylline: ↑ effects theophylline
Drug classifications
Antacids: ↓ plasma levels of ticlopidine
Anticoagulants: ↑ bleeding tendencies

NURSING CONSIDERATIONS

Assessment

- Monitor liver function studies: AST (SGOT), ALT (SGPT), bilirubin, creatinine if patient is on long-term therapy (4 mo or more)
- Monitor blood studies: CBC, Hct, Hgb, pro-time if patient is on long-term therapy; thrombocytopenia, neutropenia may occur

Associated nursing diagnoses

✓ Injury, risk for (uses)
✓ Knowledge deficit (teaching)

Implementation

PO route

- Give with food to decrease gastric symptoms

Patient/family education

- Advise patient that blood work will be necessary during treatment
- Advise patient to report any unusual bleeding to prescriber
- Instruct patient to take with food or just after eating to minimize GI discomfort
- Caution patient to report side effects such as diarrhea, skin rashes, subcutaneous bleeding, signs of cholestasis (yellow skin and sclera, dark urine, light-colored stools)

Evaluation

Positive therapeutic outcome

- Absence of stroke

timolol

(tye'moe-lole)

Apo-Timol ✦, Blocadren, timolol maleate, Timoptic

Func. class.: Antihypertensive; antiglaucoma

Chem. class.: Nonselective β-blocker

Pregnancy category **C**

Action: Competitively blocks stimulation of β-adrenergic receptor within vascular smooth muscle; produces chronotropic, inotropic activity (decreases rate of SA node discharge, increases recovery time), slows conduction of AV node, decreases heart rate, which decreases O_2 consumption in myocardium; also decreases renin-aldosterone-angiotensin system; at high doses inhibits β-2 receptors in bronchial system

➡ **Therapeutic Outcome:** Decreased B/P, decreased arrhythmias, absence of death from MI, decreased aqueous humor in the eye, absence of migraine headaches

Uses: Mild to moderate hypertension, sinus tachycardia, persistent atrial extrasystoles, tachydysrhythmias, prophylaxis of angina pectoris, reduction of mortality after MI

Investigational uses: Mitral valve prolapse, hypertrophic cardiomyopathy, thyrotoxicosis, tremors, anxiety, pheochromocytoma, tachyarrhythmias, angina pectoris

Dosage and routes

Hypertension

Adult: PO 10 mg bid, or 20 mg qd, may increase by 10 mg q2-3d, not to exceed 60 mg/day

Myocardial infarction

Adult: 10 mg bid beginning 1-4 wk after MI

Glaucoma

Adult: Ophth i gtt qd or bid

P *Child:* Ophth i gtt qd or bid (0.25% sol only)

Migraine headache prevention

Adult: PO 10 mg BID, or 20 mg qd, may increase to 30 mg/day, 20 mg in AM, 10 mg in PM

Available forms: Tab 5, 10, 20 mg; ophth sol 0.25%, 0.5%

Side effects/adverse reactions

CNS: Insomnia, dizziness, hallucinations, anxiety
CV: Hypotension, bradycardia, ***CHF,*** edema, chest pain, bradycardia, claudication
EENT: Visual changes, sore throat, *double vision,* dry burning eyes
GI: Nausea, vomiting, ***ischemic colitis,*** diarrhea, *abdominal pain,* ***mesenteric arterial thrombosis***
GU: Impotence, urinary frequency
HEMA: ***Agranulocytosis, thrombocytopenia, purpura***
INTEG: Rash, alopecia, pruritus, fever
META: Hypoglycemia
MUSC: Joint pain, muscle pain
RESP: ***Bronchospasm,*** dyspnea, cough, rales

Contraindications: Hypersensitivity to β-blockers, cardiogenic shock, heart block (2nd, 3rd degree), sinus bradycardia, CHF, cardiac failure

Precautions: Major surgery, pregnancy **C**, lactation, diabetes mellitus, renal disease, thyroid disease, COPD, well-compensated heart failure, CAD, nonallergic bronchospasm

Pharmacokinetics

Absorption	Well absorbed (PO), ophth (minimal)
Distribution	Not known
Metabolism	Liver—extensively
Excretion	Breast milk
Half-life	3-4 hr

Pharmacodynamics

	PO
Onset	Unknown
Peak	2-4 hr
Duration	12-24 hr

Interactions

Drug/drug:

Individual drugs

Alcohol: ↑ hypotension (large amounts)
Epinephrine: Alpha-adrenergic stimulation
Hydralazine: ↑ hypotension, bradycardia
Indomethacin: ↓ antihypertensive effect

Insulin: ↑ hypoglycemia
Methyldopa: ↑ hypotension, bradycardia
Phenytoin (IV): ↑ myocardial depression
Prazosin: ↑ hypotension, bradycardia
Reserpine: ↑ hypotension, bradycardia
Thyroid: ↓ effectiveness
Verapamil: ↑ myocardial depression

Drug classifications
Antihypertensives: ↑ hypertension
β_2 agonists: ↓ bronchodilation
Cardiac glycosides: ↑ bradycardia
Nitrates: ↑ hypotension
Theophyllines: ↓ bronchodilation

Lab test interferences

False increase: Urinary catecholamines

NURSING CONSIDERATIONS

Assessment

- Monitor B/P during beginning treatment, periodically thereafter; pulse q4h; note rate, rhythm, quality: apical/radial pulse before administration; notify prescriber of any significant changes (pulse <50 bpm)
- Check for baselines in renal, liver function tests before therapy begins
- Assess for edema in feet, legs daily, monitor I&O, daily weight; check for jugular vein distention, rales, bilaterally, dyspnea (CHF)
- Monitor skin turgor, dryness of mucous membranes for hydration status, especially G elderly

Associated nursing diagnoses

✓ Cardiac output, decreased (uses)
✓ Injury, risk for physical (side effects)
✓ Knowledge deficit (teaching)
✓ Noncompliance (teaching)

Implementation

PO route

- Given ac, hs, tab may be crushed or swallowed whole; give with food to prevent GI upset; reduced dosage in renal dysfunction
- Store protected from light, moisture; place in cool environment

Patient/family education

- Teach patient not to discontinue drug abruptly; taper over 2 wk; may cause precipitate angina if stopped abruptly
- Advise patient not to use OTC products containing α-adrenergic stimulants (such as nasal decongestants, cold preparations); to avoid alcohol, smoking and to limit sodium intake as prescribed
- Teach patient how to take pulse and B/P at home—advise patient when to notify prescriber
- Instruct patient to comply with weight control, dietary adjustments, modified exercise program
- Advise patient to carry/wear Medic Alert ID to identify drug being taken, any allergies; tell patient drug controls symptoms but does not cure
- Caution patient to avoid hazardous activities if dizziness, drowsiness is present

• Teach patient to report symptoms of CHF; difficult breathing, especially on exertion or when lying down; night cough; swelling of extremities or bradycardia; dizziness; confusion; depression; fever
• Teach patient to take drug as prescribed, not to double doses, skip doses; take any missed doses as soon as remembered if at least 4 hr until next dose

Evaluation

Positive therapeutic outcome
• Decreased B/P in hypertension (after 1-2 wk)
• Absence of dysrhythmias

Treatment of overdose: Lavage, **IV** atropine for bradycardia, **IV** theophylline for bronchospasm, digitalis, O_2, diuretic for cardiac failure, hemodialysis, **IV** glucose for hyperglycemia, **IV** diazepam (or phenytoin) for seizures

tobramycin

(toe-bra-mye'sin)
Nebcin, tobramycin sulfate, Tobrex
Func. class.: Antiinfective
Chem. class.: Aminoglycoside
Pregnancy category **D**

Action: Interferes with protein synthesis in bacterial cell by binding to ribosomal subunit, causing inaccurate peptide sequence to form in protein chain, causing bacterial death

Therapeutic Outcome: Bactericidal effects for the following organisms: *P. aeruginosa, E. coli, Enterobacter, Providencia, Citrobacter, Staphylococcus, Proteus, Klebsiella, Serratia*

Uses: Severe systemic infections of CNS, respiratory, GI, urinary tract, bone, skin, soft tissues, eye

Dosage and routes

Adult: IM/**IV** 3 mg/kg/day in divided doses q8h; may give up to 5 mg/kg/day in divided doses q6-8h

P *Child:* IM/**IV** 6-7.5 mg/kg/day in 3-4 equal divided doses

P *Neonates <1 wk:* IM up to 4 mg/kg/day in divided doses q12h; **IV** up to 4 mg/kg/day in divided doses q12h diluted in 50-100 mg NS or D_5W; give over 30-60 min

Available forms: Inj 10, 40 mg/ml; powder for inj 1.2 g; inj 20 mg/2 ml, 0.3% ophth

Side effects/adverse reactions

CNS: Confusion, depression, numbness, tremors, ***convulsions,*** muscle twitching, ***neurotoxicity,*** dizziness, vertigo
CV: Hypotension, hypertension, palpitation
EENT: Ototoxicity, deafness, visual disturbances, tinnitus
GI: Nausea, vomiting, anorexia, increased ALT (SGOT), AST (SGPT), bilirubin, hepatomegaly, ***hepatic necrosis,*** splenomegaly

T

GU: Oliguria, hematuria, renal damage, azotemia, renal failure, nephrotoxicity
HEMA: Agranulocytosis, thrombocytopenia, leukopenia, eosinophilia, anemia
INTEG: Rash, burning, urticaria, dermatitis, alopecia

Contraindications: Severe renal disease, hypersensitivity to aminoglycosides

P **Precautions:** Neonates, mild renal disease, pregnancy **D**, myasthenia gravis, lactation, hearing deficits, Parkinson's disease

Pharmacokinetics

Absorption	Well absorbed (IM), completely absorbed (IV)
Distribution	Widely distributed in extracellular fluids
Metabolism	Minimal—liver
Excretion	Mostly unchanged (>90%) kidneys
Half-life	2-3 hr, increased in renal disease

Pharmacodynamics

	IM	IV	OPH
Onset	Rapid	Rapid	Rapid
Peak	1 hr	Inf end	Unknown

Interactions
Drug/drug:
Individual drugs
Amphotericin B: ↑ Ototoxicity, neurotoxicity, nephrotoxicity
Cisplatin: ↑ Ototoxicity, neurotoxicity, nephrotoxicity
Ethacrynic acid: ↑ Ototoxicity, neurotoxicity, nephrotoxicity
Furosemide: ↑ Ototoxicity, neurotoxicity, nephrotoxicity
Mannitol: ↑ Ototoxicity, neurotoxicity, nephrotoxicity
Methoxyflurane: ↑ Ototoxicity, neurotoxicity, nephrotoxicity
Polymyxin: ↑ Ototoxicity, neurotoxicity, nephrotoxicity
Succinylcholine: ↑ Neuromuscular blockade, respiratory depression
Vancomycin: ↑ Ototoxicity, neurotoxicity, nephrotoxicity
Drug classifications
Anesthetics: ↑ Neuromuscular blockade, respiratory depression
Aminoglycosides: ↑ Otoxicity, neurotoxicity, neurotoxicity
Nondepolarizing neuromuscular blockers: ↑ Neuromuscular blockade, respiratory depression

NURSING CONSIDERATIONS
Assessment
- Assess patient for previous sensitivity reaction

Syst route
- Assess patient for signs and symptoms of infection including characteristics of wounds, sputum, urine, stool WBC >10,000, temp; obtain baseline information before and during treatment
- Complete C & S testing before beginning drug therapy to identify if correct treatment has been initiated
- Assess for allergic reactions: rash, urticaria, pruritus, chills, fever, joint pain
- Identify urine output; if decreasing, notify prescriber (may indicate nephrotoxicity); also, obtain BUN, creatinine, urine CrCl (<80 ml/min) values

- Monitor blood studies: AST (SGOT), ALT (SGPT), CBC, Hct, bilirubin, LDH, alk phosphatase, Coombs' test monthly if patient is on long-term therapy
- Monitor electrolytes: potassium, sodium, chloride monthly if patient is on long-term therapy
- Monitor for bleeding: ecchymosis, bleeding gums, hematuria, stool guaiac daily if patient is on long-term therapy
- Assess for overgrowth of infection: perineal itching, fever, malaise, redness, pain, swelling, drainage, rash, diarrhea, change in cough, sputum
- Obtain weight before treatment; calculation of dosage is usually based on ideal body weight, but may be calculated on actual body weight
- Monitor I&O ratio; urinalysis daily for proteinuria, cells, casts; report sudden change in urine output
- Monitor VS during inf, watch for hypotension, change in pulse
- Assess **IV** site for thrombophlebitis including pain, redness, swelling q30 min, change site if needed; apply warm compresses to discontinued site
- Obtain serum peak, drawn at 30-60 min after **IV** inf or 60 min after IM inj, trough level drawn just before next dose; blood level should be 2-4 times bacteriostatic level
- Monitor for deafness by audiometric testing, ringing, roaring in ears, vertigo; assess hearing before, during, after treatment
- Monitor for dehydration: high sp gr, decrease in skin turgor, dry mucous membranes, dark urine
- Monitor for overgrowth of infection including increased temp, malaise, redness, pain, swelling, perineal itching, diarrhea, stomatitis, change in cough, sputum

Associated nursing diagnoses

- ✓ Infection, risk for (uses)
- ✓ Diarrhea (adverse reactions)
- ✓ Injury, risk for (adverse reactions)
- ✓ Knowledge deficit (teaching)
- ✓ Noncompliance (teaching)

Implementation

IM route

- Give deeply in large muscle mass

IV **IV route**

- Give **IV** diluted in 50-100 ml NS $D_{10}W$, D_5/0.9% NaCl, 0.9% NaCl, Ringers, LR, D_5W (adult), infuse over 20-60 min
- Flush after inf with D_5W, 0.9% NaCl

Syringe incompatibilities:

Cefamandole, clindamycin, heparin, sargramositim

Y-site compatibilities:

Acyclovir, amsacrine, amiodarone, ciprofloxacin, cyclophosphamide, enalaprilat, esmolol, fluconazole, fludarabine, foscarnet, furosemide, hydromorphone, insulin (regular), labetalol, magnesium sulfate, meperidine, morphine, perphenazine, tolazoline, zidovudine

T

Additive incompatibilities:
Cefamandole, floxacillin

Additive compatibilities:
Aztreonam, bleomycin, calcium gluconate, cefoxitin, ciprofloxacin, clindamycin, furosemide, metronidazole, ranitidine, verapamil

Patient/family education
Syst route
- Teach patient to report sore throat, bruising, bleeding, joint pain—may indicate blood dyscrasias (rare)
- Advise patient to contact prescriber if vaginal itching, loose, foul-smelling stools, furry tongue occur—may indicate superimposed infection
- Advise patient to notify prescriber of diarrhea with blood or pus, which may indicate pseudomembranous colitis

Evaluation
Positive therapeutic outcome
- Absence of signs/symptoms of infection (WBC <10,000, temp WNL, absence of red, draining wounds)
- Reported improvement in symptoms of infection

Treatment of overdose:
Withdraw drug, hemodialysis, exchange transfusion in the newborn, monitor serum levels of drug, may give ticarcillin or carbenicillin

tocainide
(toe-kay'nide)
Tonocard
Func. class.: Antidysrhythmic (Class IB)
Chem. class.: Lidocaine analog
Pregnancy category **C**

Action: Increases electrical stimulation threshold of ventricle, His-Purkinje system, which stabilizes cardiac membrane and decreases automaticity

➔ **Therapeutic Outcome:** Decreased ventricular dysrhythmia

Uses: PVCs, ventricular tachycardia

Dosage and routes
Adult: PO 600 mg loading dose, then 400 mg q8h

Available forms: Tab 400, 600 mg

Side effects/adverse reactions
CNS: Headache, dizziness, involuntary movement, confusion, psychosis, restlessness, irritability, paresthesias, tremors, ***seizures***
CV: Hypotension, bradycardia, angina, PVCs, ***heart block, cardiovascular collapse, arrest, CHF,*** chest pain, tachycardia
EENT: Tinnitus, blurred vision, hearing loss
GI: Nausea, vomiting, anorexia, diarrhea, hepatitis

HEMA: Blood dyscrasias: leukopenia, agranulocytosis, hypoplastic anemia, thrombocytopenia
INTEG: Rash, urticaria, edema, swelling
RESP: Dyspnea, ***respiratory depression, pulmonary fibrosis***

Contraindications: Hypersensitivity to amides, severe heart block

Precautions: Pregnancy **C**, P lactation, children, renal disease, liver disease, CHF, respiratory depression, myasthenia gravis, blood dyscrasias

Pharmacokinetics

Absorption	Well absorbed (PO)
Distribution	Widely distributed, crossed blood-brain barrier
Metabolism	Liver
Excretion	Kidney (up to 50% unchanged)
Half-life	10-17 hr

Pharmacodynamics

	PO
Onset	1 hr
Peak	½-2 hr
Duration	8-12 hr

Interactions
Drug/drug:
Individual drugs
Cimetidine: ↓ levels of tocainide
Digoxin: ↑ blood levels, ↑ toxicity
Disopyramide: ↑ levels, ↑ toxicity
Flecainide: ↑ levels, ↑ toxicity
Lidocaine: ↑ effect
Mexiletine: ↑ levels, ↑ toxicity
Phenytoin: ↑ blood levels
Procainamide: ↑ levels, ↑ toxicity
Quinidine: ↑ levels, ↑ toxicity
Warfarin: ↑ level, ↑ bleeding
Drug classifications
Beta blockers: ↑ dysrhythmias, arrest
Calcium channel blockers: ↑ dysrhythmias, arrest

Lab test interferences
Increase: CPK

NURSING CONSIDERATIONS
Assessment

- Assess for oxygenation or perfusion deficit: decreased B/P, chest pain, dizziness, loss of consciousness
- Assess respiratory status: auscultate lung fields for bibasilar crackles in patients with advanced CHF
- Assess for urinary retention: check for pain, abdominal absorption, palpate bladder; check males with benign prostatic hypertrophy—anticholinergic reaction may cause retention
- Monitor I&O ratio; electrolytes: (potassium, sodium, chloride); watch for decreasing urinary output, possible retention
- Monitor liver function studies: AST (SGOT), ALT (SGPT), bilirubin, alk phosphatase
- Monitor ECG to determine drug effectiveness; measure PR, QRS, QT intervals; check for PVCs, other dysrhythmias; monitor B/P for hypotension, hypertension; for rebound hypertension after 1-2 hr

T

• Monitor patient for CNS symptoms: confusion, psychosis, numbness, depression, involuntary movements; if these occur, drug should be discontinued
• Assess pulmonary toxicity: dyspnea, fatigue, cough, fever, chest pain; drug should be discontinued if these occur
• Assess cardiac rate, respiration: rate, rhythm, character, chest pain, ventricular tachycardia, supraventricular tachycardia or fibrillation

Associated nursing diagnoses

✓ Cardiac output, decreased (uses)
✓ Impaired gas exchange (adverse reactions)
✓ Knowledge deficit (teaching)

Implementation

PO route

• Give with meals for GI upset occurrences

Patient/family education

• Inform patient or family of reason for use of medication and expected results
• Teach patient method for taking pulse at home and what to report to prescriber
• Advise patient to avoid hazardous activities until drug response is known; dizziness, confusion, sedation may occur
• Advise patient to use a Medic-Alert bracelet or other ID indicating medications taken, condition, and prescriber's name and phone number
• Instruct patient to report bleeding, bruising, respiratory symptoms, chills, fever, sore throat to prescriber

Evaluation

Positive therapeutic outcome

• Decreased dysrhythmias

Treatment of overdose: Defibrillation, vasopressor for hypotension

tolazamide

(tole-az'a-mide)

Tolamide, tolazimide, Tolinase

Func. class.: Antidiabetic, oral

Chem. class.: Sulfonylurea (1st generation)

Pregnancy category **C**

Action: Causes functioning β-cells in pancreas to release insulin, leading to drop in blood glucose levels; may improve binding to insulin receptors or increase the number of insulin receptors with prolonged administration; may also reduce basal hepatic glucose secretion; this drug is not effective if patient lacks functioning β-cells

➡ **Therapeutic Outcome:** Decreased blood glucose levels in diabetes mellitus

Uses: Type II (NIDDM) diabetes mellitus

Dosage and routes

Adult: PO 100 mg/day for FBS <200 mg/dl or 250 mg/

day for FBS >200 mg/dl; dose should be titrated to patient response (1 g or less/day)

Available forms: Tab 100, 250, 500 mg scored

Side effects/adverse reactions

CNS: Headache, weakness, fatigue, lethargy, dizziness, vertigo, tinnitus
ENDO: Hypoglycemia
GI: Nausea, vomiting, diarrhea, constipation, gas, ***hepatotoxicity, jaundice,*** heartburn
HEMA: Leukopenia, thrombocytopenia, agranulocytosis, aplastic anemia, pancytopenia, hemolytic anemia
INTEG: Rash, (rare) allergic reactions, pruritus, urticaria, eczema, photosensitivity, erythema

Contraindications: Hypersensitivity to sulfonylureas, juvenile or brittle diabetes

Precautions: Pregnancy **C**, G elderly, cardiac disease, thyroid disease, severe hypoglycemic reactions, renal disease, hepatic disease

Pharmacokinetics	
Absorption	Well absorbed (PO)
Distribution	Bile
Metabolism	Liver to metabolites
Excretion	Kidneys (unchanged)
Half-life	7 hr

Pharmacodynamics	PO
Onset	1 hr
Peak	4-8 hr
Duration	12-24 hr

Interactions

Drug/drug:

Individual drugs

Chloramphenicol: ↑ hypoglycemia
Cimetidine: ↑ hypoglycemia
Diazoxide: ↓ effect of both drugs
Guanethidine: ↑ hypoglycemia
Insulin: ↑ hypoglycemia
Methyldopa: ↑ hypoglycemia
Phenobarbital: ↓ action of acetohexamide
Phenytoin: ↓ action of acetohexamide
Rifampin: ↓ action of acetohexamide

Drug classifications

Anticoagulants, oral: ↑ hypoglycemia
Calcium channel blockers: ↓ action of acetohexamide
Corticosteroids: ↓ action of acetohexamide
Diuretics, thiazide: ↓ action of acetohexamide
Estrogens: ↓ action of acetohexamide
MAOI: ↑ hypoglycemia
Nonsteroidal antiinflammatories: ↑ hypoglycemia
Oral contraceptives: ↓ action of acetohexamide
Phenothiazines: ↓ action of acetohexamide
Salicylates: ↑ hypoglycemia
Sulfonamides: ↑ hypoglycemia
Sympathomimetics: ↓ action of acetohexamide
Thyroid agents: ↓ action of acetohexamide

NURSING CONSIDERATIONS

Assessment

- Assess for hypoglycemic/

T

hyperglycemic reactions that can occur soon pc; hypoglycemic reactions (sweating, weakness, dizziness, anxiety, tremors, hunger); hyperglycemic reactions

• Monitor CBC (baseline, q3mo) during treatment; check liver function tests periodically AST (SGOT), LDH and renal studies: BUN, creatinine during treatment

Associated nursing diagnoses

✓ Nutrition, altered: more than body requirements (uses)
✓ Nutrition altered: less than body requirements (adverse reactions)
✓ Injury, risk for (adverse reactions)
✓ Knowledge deficit (teaching)
✓ Noncompliance (teaching)

Implementation

• Conversion from other oral hypoglycemic agents or insulin dosage of <40 U/day; change may be made without gradual dosage change

• Patients taking insulin of >40 U/day convert gradually by receiving oral hypoglycemic and 50% of previous insulin dosage for 3-5 days

• Monitor serum or urine glucose and ketones 3 times/day during conversion

PO route

• Give drug 30 min before breakfast; if large dose is required, may be divided into two; give with meals to decrease GI upset and provide best absorption

• Give tab crushed and mixed with meal or fluids for patients with difficulty swallowing

• Store in tight container in cool environment

Patient/family education

• Teach patient to check for symptoms of cholestatic jaundice: dark urine, pruritus, yellow sclera; if these occur, prescriber should be notified

• Teach patient to use capillary blood glucose test or Chemstrip 3 ×/day

• Teach patient symptoms of hypo/hyperglycemia, what to do about each

• Inform patient that drug must be continued on daily basis; explain consequence of discontinuing drug abruptly

• Teach patient to take drug in morning to prevent hypoglycemic reactions at night

• Caution patient to avoid OTC medications unless prescribed by a prescriber

• Teach patient that diabetes is lifelong illness; that this drug is not a cure

• Instruct patient that all food included in diet plan must be eaten to prevent hypoglycemia

• Advise patient to carry Medic Alert ID for emergency purposes, and to carry a glucagon emergency kit

Evaluation

Positive therapeutic outcome

• Decrease in polyuria, polydipsia, polyphagia, clear sensorium, absence of dizziness, stable gait

Treatment of overdose:

Glucose 25 g **IV**, via dextrose 50% sol, 50 cc, or 1 mg glucagon

tolazoline
(toe-laz'a-leen)
Priscoline
Func. class.: Peripheral vasodilator
Chem. class.: Imidazoline derivative
Pregnancy category **C**

Action: Peripheral vasodilation occurs by direct relaxation on vascular smooth muscle; also has weak α- and β-adrenergic properties

Therapeutic Outcome: Decreased pulmonary hypertension

Uses: Persistent pulmonary hypertension of newborn; also hypoxic pulmonary hypertension

Dosage and routes
P *Newborn:* **IV** 1-2 mg/kg via scalp vein; **IV** inf 1-2 mg/kg/hr

Available forms: Inj 25 mg/ml

Side effects/adverse reactions
CV: Orthostatic hypotension, ***tachycardia,*** dysrhythmias, hypertension, ***cardiovascular collapse***
GI: Nausea, vomiting, diarrhea, peptic ulcer, ***GI hemorrhage, hepatitis***
GU: Edema, oliguria, hematuria
HEMA: Thrombocytopenia, leukopenia
INTEG: Flushing, tingling, rash, chills, sweating, increased pilomotor activity
RESP: Pulmonary hemorrhage

Contraindications: Hypersensitivity, CVA, CAD

Precautions: Pregnancy **C**, active peptic ulcer, lactation, mitral stenosis

Pharmacokinetics	
Absorption	Complete (IV)
Distribution	Unknown
Metabolism	Liver
Excretion	Kidneys
Half-life	3-10 hr

Pharmacodynamics	IV
Onset	½ hr
Peak	½-1 hr
Duration	3-4 hr

Interactions
Drug/drug:
Alcohol: ↑ effects
Epinephrine: ↓ B/P, rebound hypertension
Drug classifications
Beta blockers: ↑ effects
Antihypertensives: ↑ effects

NURSING CONSIDERATIONS
Assessment
- Monitor ABGs, electrolytes, P VS in newborn
- Monitor B/P, pulse during treatment until stable; take B/P with patient in lying and standing position; orthostatic hypotension is common
- Monitor hepatic tests: AST (SGOT), ALT (SGPT), bilirubin; liver enzymes may increase

T

• Monitor blood studies: CBC, platelets; watch for thrombocytopenia, agranulocytosis
• Monitor hepatic involvement: nausea, vomiting, jaundice; drug should be discontinued if this occurs
• Monitor for bleeding from GI tract: coffee grounds vomitus, increased pulse, pain in upper gastric area
• Assess affected areas for changes in temp, color

Associated nursing diagnoses

✓ Tissue, perfusion, altered (uses)
✓ Knowledge deficit (teaching)

Implementation

IV route

• Give **IV** undiluted; give 10 mg or less over 1 min; in scalp vein may be diluted in D_5, D_5NS, LR, NS, ½NS, Ringer's sol; run over 1 hr
• Give ordered analgesic if headache develops
• Give intraarterially to patient in supine position
• Give to patient who is sitting or lying down during treatment
• Store at room temp, protect from light

Patient/family education

• Advise patient to report jaundice, dark urine, joint pain, fatigue, malaise, bruising, easy bleeding, which may indicate blood dyscrasias
• Instruct patient that it is necessary to quit smoking to prevent excessive vasoconstriction if prescribed for PVD
• Caution to avoid hazardous activities until stabilized on medication; dizziness may occur

Evaluation

Positive therapeutic outcome

• Decrease in pulmonary hypertension or pulse volume, increased temperature in extremities, ability to walk without pain

Treatment of overdose: Administer **IV** fluids, position patient's head in low position

tolbutamide

(tole-byoo'ta-mide)

Mobenol ♣, **Novobutamide** ♣, **Orinase, tolbutamide, Tolbutone** ♣

Func. class.: Antidiabetic

Chem. class.: Sulfonylurea (1st generation)

Pregnancy category C

Action: Causes functioning β-cells in pancreas to release insulin, leading to drop in blood glucose levels; may improve binding to insulin receptors or increase the number of insulin receptors with prolonged administration; may also reduce basal hepatic secretion; not effective if patient lacks functioning β-cells

Therapeutic Outcome: Decreased blood glucose levels in diabetes mellitus

Uses: Type II (NIDDM) diabetes mellitus

Dosage and routes

Adult: PO 1-2 g/day in divided doses, titrated to patient response, **IV** 1 g (Fajan's test)

Available forms: Tab 250, 500 mg scored, 1 g inj

Side effects/adverse reactions

CNS: Headache, weakness, paresthesia, tinnitus, dizziness, vertigo
ENDO: Hypoglycemia
GI: Nausea, fullness, heartburn, ***hepatotoxicity, cholestatic jaundice,*** taste alteration, diarrhea
HEMA: Leukopenia, thrombocytopenia, agranulocytosis, aplastic anemia, increased AST (SGOT), ALT (SGPT), alk phosphatase
INTEG: Rash, allergic reactions, pruritus, urticaria, eczema, photosensitivity, erythema
MS: Joint pains

Contraindications: Hypersensitivity to sulfonylureas, juvenile or brittle diabetes

Precautions: Pregnancy **C**, G elderly, cardiac disease, thyroid disease, severe hypoglycemic reactions, renal disease, hepatic disease

Pharmacokinetics

Absorption	Well absorbed (PO)
Distribution	Bile
Metabolism	Liver to metabolites
Excretion	Kidneys (unchanged)
Half-life	4-7 hr

Pharmacodynamics

	PO
Onset	1 hr
Peak	3-5 hr
Duration	6-12 hr

Interactions

Drug/drug:

Individual drugs

Chloramphenicol: ↑ hypoglycemia
Cimetidine: ↑ hypoglycemia
Diazoxide: ↓ effect of both drugs
Guanethidine: ↑ hypoglycemia
Insulin: ↑ hypoglycemia
Methyldopa: ↑ hypoglycemia
Phenobarbital: ↓ action of acetohexamide
Phenytoin: ↓ action of acetohexamide
Rifampin: ↓ action of acetohexamide

Drug classifications

Anticoagulants, oral: ↑ hypoglycemia
Calcium channel blockers: ↓ action of acetohexamide
Corticosteroids: ↓ action of acetohexamide
Diuretics, thiazide: ↓ action of acetohexamide
Estrogens: ↓ action of acetohexamide
MAOI: ↑ hypoglycemia
Nonsteroidal antiinflammatories: ↑ hypoglycemia
Oral contraceptives: ↓ action of acetohexamide
Phenothiazines: ↓ action of acetohexamide
Salicylates: ↑ hypoglycemia
Sulfonamides: ↑ hypoglycemia
Sympathomimetics: ↓ action of acetohexamide

Thyroid agents: ↓ action of acetohexamide

NURSING CONSIDERATIONS

Assessment

- Assess for hypoglycemic/hyperglycemic reactions that can occur soon pc; hypoglycemic reactions (sweating, weakness, dizziness, anxiety, tremors, hunger); hyperglycemic reactions
- Monitor CBC (baseline, q3mo) during treatment; check liver function tests periodically AST (SGOT), LDH and renal studies: BUN, creatinine during treatment

Associated nursing diagnoses

- ✓ Nutrition, altered: more than body requirements (uses)
- ✓ Nutrition altered: less than body requirements (adverse reactions)
- ✓ Injury, risk for (adverse reactions)
- ✓ Knowledge deficit (teaching)
- ✓ Noncompliance (teaching)

Implementation

- Conversion from other oral hypoglycemic agents or insulin dosage of <40 U/day; change may be made without gradual dosage change.
- Patients taking >40 U/day of insulin convert gradually by receiving oral hypoglycemic and 50% of previous insulin dosage for 3-5 days.
- Monitor serum or urine glucose and ketones 3 times/day during conversion.

PO route

- Give drug 30 min before breakfast—if large dose is required, may be divided into two; give with meals to decrease GI upset and provide best absorption
- Give tab crushed and mixed with meal or fluids for patients with difficulty swallowing
- Store in tight container in cool environment

Patient/family education

- Teach patient to check for symptoms of cholestatic jaundice: dark urine, pruritus, yellow sclera; if these occur, prescriber should be notified
- Teach patient to use capillary blood glucose test or Chemstrip 3 ×/day
- Teach patient symptoms of hypo/hyperglycemia, what to do about each
- Instruct patient that drug must be continued on daily basis; explain consequence of discontinuing drug abruptly
- Teach patient to take drug in AM to prevent hypoglycemic reactions at night
- Caution patient to avoid OTC medications unless prescribed by a prescriber
- Teach patient that diabetes is lifelong illness; that this drug is not a cure
- Instruct patient that all food included in diet plan must be eaten to prevent hypoglycemia
- Advise patient to carry Medic-Alert ID and a glucagon emergency kit for emergency purposes

Evaluation

Positive therapeutic outcome

- Decrease in polyuria, polydipsia, polyphagia, clear sensorium, absence of dizziness, stable gait

Treatment of overdose: Glucose 25 g **IV**, via dextrose 50% sol, 50 cc or 1 mg glucagon

tolmetin

(tole'met-in)

Tolectin DS, Tolectin 200, Tolectin 600, tolmetin sodium

Func. class.: Nonsteroidal antiinflammatory

Chem. class.: Pyrrole acetic acid derivative

Pregnancy category B

Action: Inhibits prostaglandin synthesis by decreasing an enzyme needed for biosynthesis; analgesic, antiinflammatory, antipyretic

Therapeutic Outcome: Decreased pain, inflammatory

Uses: Mild to moderate pain, osteoarthritis, rheumatoid arthritis

Dosage and routes

Adult: PO 400 mg tid-qid, not to exceed 2 g/day

Child >2 yr: PO 15-30 mg/kg/day in 3 or 4 divided doses

Available forms: Cap 400 mg; tab 200, 600 mg

Side effects/adverse reactions

CNS: Dizziness, drowsiness, fatigue, tremors, confusion, insomnia, anxiety, depression

CV: Tachycardia, peripheral edema, palpitations, dysrhythmias, hypertension

EENT: Tinnitus, hearing loss, blurred vision

GI: Nausea, anorexia, vomiting, diarrhea, jaundice, ***cholestatic hepatitis,*** constipation, flatulence, cramps, dry mouth, peptic ulcer, ulceration, bleeding, perforation

GU: ***Nephrotoxicity: dysuria, hematuria, oliguria, azotemia, pseudoproteinuria***

HEMA: ***Blood dyscrasias***

INTEG: Purpura, rash, pruritus, sweating

Contraindications: Hypersensitivity, asthma, severe renal disease, severe hepatic disease, ulcer disease

Precautions: Pregnancy **B**, lactation, children, bleeding disorders, GI disorders, cardiac disorders, hypersensitivity to other antiinflammatory agents, peptic ulcer disease

Pharmacokinetics

Absorption	Well absorbed
Distribution	Not known
Metabolism	Extensively
Excretion	Unchanged kidneys—20%
Half-life	3-3½ hr

Pharmacodynamics

	PO
Onset	Unknown
Peak	2 hr
Duration	Unknown

Interactions

Drug/drug:

Individual drugs

Acetaminophen (long-term use): ↑ renal reactions

Alcohol: ↑ adverse reactions

Aspirin: ↓ effectiveness, ↑ adverse reactions
Coumarin: ↑ anticoagulant effects
Digoxin: ↑ toxicity, ↑ levels
Insulin: ↓ insulin effect
Lithium: ↑ toxicity
Methotrexate: ↑ toxicity
Phenytoin: ↑ toxicity
Probenecid: ↑ toxicity
Sulfonylurea: ↑ toxicity

Drug classifications

Anticoagulants: ↑ risk of bleeding
Antihypertensives: ↓ effect of antihypertensives
Antineoplastics: ↑ risk of hematologic toxicity
β-blockers: ↑ antihypertension
Cephalosporins: ↑ risk of bleeding
Glucocorticoids: ↑ adverse reactions
Hypoglycemics: ↓ hypoglycemic effect
Diuretics: ↓ effectiveness of diuretics
Nonsteroidal antiinflammatories: ↑ adverse reactions
Potassium supplements: ↑ adverse reactions
Radiation: ↑ risk of hematologic toxicity
Sulfonamides: ↑ toxicity

Lab test interferences

Increase: Serum potassium, liver function studies, BUN
False positive: Urine protein

NURSING CONSIDERATIONS

Assessment

• Monitor blood counts during therapy; watch for decreasing platelets; if low, therapy may need to be discontinued, restarted after hematologic recovery; and for blood dyscrasia (thrombocytopenia): bruising, fatigue, bleeding, poor healing

Associated nursing diagnoses

✓ Pain (uses)
✓ Mobility, impaired physical (uses)
✓ Injury, risk for (adverse reactions)
✓ Knowledge deficit (teaching)

Implementation

PO route

• Administer with food or milk to decrease gastric symptoms—food will slow absorption slightly, but will not decrease absorption

Patient/family education

• Inform patient that drug must be continued for prescribed time to be effective; to avoid aspirin, alcoholic beverages
• Caution patient to report bleeding, bruising, fatigue, malaise because blood dyscrasias do occur
• Instruct patient to use caution when driving; drowsiness, dizziness may occur
• Teach patient to take with a full glass of water to enhance absorption; do not crush, break or chew

Evaluation

Positive therapeutic outcome

• Decreased pain
• Decreased inflammation
• Increased mobility

tolnaftate
(tole-naf'tate)
Absorbine Antifungal, Absorbine Jock Itch, Absorbine Jr. Antifungal, Aftate For Athlete's Foot, Aftate For Jock Itch, Desenex Spray, Genaspor, NP-27, Quinsana Plus, Tinactin, Ting, tolnaftate, Zeasorb-AF

Func. class.: Local anti-infective
Chem. class.: Antifungal

Pregnancy category C

Action: Interferes with fungal cell membrane, which increases permeability, leaking of cell nutrients

Therapeutic Outcome: Fungistatic/fungicidal against susceptible organisms: *Tinea pedis, Tinea cruris, Tinea corporis, Tinea versicolor*

Uses: *Tinea pedis, Tinea cruris, Tinea corporis, Tinea capitis, Tinea unguium, Tinea versicolor*

Dosage and routes
Adult and child: Top apply to affected area bid for 2-6 wk, rub in

Available forms: Cream, powder, aerosol powder, aerosol liq, gel, pump spray liq 1%

Side effects/adverse reactions
INTEG: Rash, urticaria, stinging

Contraindications: Hypersensitivity, nail infections

Precautions: Pregnancy **C**, lactation

Pharmacokinetics

Absorption	Minimally absorbed
Distribution	Unknown
Metabolism	Liver
Excretion	Feces, kidneys
Half-life	Unknown

Pharmacodynamics

Onset	Unknown
Peak	Unknown
Duration	Unknown

Interactions: None

NURSING CONSIDERATIONS
Assessment
- Assess skin for fungal infections: peeling, dryness, itching before and throughout treatment
- Monitor for allergic reaction: burning, stinging, swelling, redness, dermatitis, rash; drug should be discontinued

Associated nursing diagnoses
- ✓ Skin integrity, impaired (uses)
- ✓ Infection, risk for (uses)
- ✓ Knowledge deficit (teaching)

Implementation
Top route
- Apply enough medication to cover lesions completely
- Apply after cleansing with soap, water before each application; dry well

• Store at room temp in dry place

Patient/family education

• Instruct patient to wear gloves while applying medication so as to prevent further infection; not to cover with occlusive dressings
• Teach patient that long-term therapy may be needed to clear infection (2 wk-6 mo depending on organism); compliance is needed even after feeling better
• Teach patient proper hygiene: hand-washing technique, nail care, use of concomitant top agents if prescribed
• Advise patient to avoid use of OTC creams, ointments, lotions unless directed
• Instruct patient to use asepsis (hand washing) before, after each application; to change socks and shoes once a day during treatment of tinea pedis
• Advise patient to inform health care prescriber if infection persists or returns; if blisters, burning, oozing, swelling occur
• Inform patient to avoid alcohol, since nausea, vomiting, hypertension may occur
• Caution patient to use sunscreen or avoid direct sunlight to prevent photosensitivity
• Instruct patient to notify health care prescriber of sore throat, fever, skin rash, which may indicate overgrowth of organisms

Evaluation

Positive therapeutic outcome
• Decrease in size, number of lesions
• Decrease in itching or white patches around vulva

trace elements (chromium, copper, iodide, manganese, selenium, zinc)

Concentrated Multiple Trace Elements, ConTE-PAK-4, M.T.E.-4 Concentrated, M.T.E.-5, M.T.E.-5 Concentrated, M.T.E.-6, M.T.E.-6 Concentrated, M.T.E.-7, MulTE-PAK-4, MulTE-PAK-5, Multiple Trace Element, Multiple Trace Element Neonatal, Multiple Trace Element Pediatric, Neotrace 4, Ped TE-PAK-4, Pedtrice-4, P.T.E.-4, P.T.E.-5

Func. class.: Mineral supplement
Chem. class.:

Pregnancy category C

Action: Needed for adequate absorption and synthesis of amino acids

Therapeutic Outcome: Replacement for mineral deficiencies

Uses: Prevention of trace element deficiency, a component of TPN

Dosage and routes

Usual dosage may be given in TPN sol

Adult: **IV** 10-15 μg qd

P *Child:* **IV** 0.14-0.20 µg/kg/day

Copper
Adult: **IV** 0.5-1.5 mg/day
P *Child:* **IV** .05-0.2 mg/kg/day

Iodine
Adult: **IV** 1 µg/kg/day

Manganese
Adult: **IV** 1-3 mg/day

Selenium
Adult: 40-120 µg/day
P *Child:* 3 µg/kg/day

Zinc
Adult: **IV** 2-4 mg/day
P *Child:* **IV** 0.05 mg/kg/day

Available forms: Many forms available—see particular elements

Side effects/adverse reactions

ZINC: Vomiting, oliguria, hypothermia, vision changes, tachycardia, jaundice, coma
SELENIUM: Alopecia, depression, vomiting, GI cramping, nervousness, garlic smell
MANGANESE: Incoordination, headache, irritability, lability, slurred speech, impotence
IODINE: Headache, edema of eyelids, acne, metallic taste, sore mouth, running nose
COPPER: Personality changes, diarrhea, weakness, photophobia, muscle weakness
CHROMIUM: Seizures, coma, nausea, vomiting, ulcers, renal/hepatic toxicity

Precautions: Liver, biliary disease, pregnancy **C**, lactation, severe vomiting or diarrhea

Pharmacokinetics

Absorption	Completely absorbed (IV)
Distribution	Widely distributed
Metabolism	Unknown
Excretion	Depends on element
Half-life	Unknown

Pharmacodynamics

	IV
Onset	Unknown
Peak	Unknown
Duration	Unknown

Interactions: None

NURSING CONSIDERATIONS

Assessment

- Assess trace element levels; notify prescriber if low copper 0.07-0.15 mg/ml, zinc 0.05-0.15 mg/100 ml, manganese 4-20 µg/100 ml, selenium 0.1-0.19 µg/ml
- Assess trace element deficiency if patient is receiving TPN for extended period
- Obtain calorie count to identify nutritional definitions
- Assess for toxicity to individual element (see side effects/adverse reactions)

Associated nursing diagnoses

✓ Nutrition: less than body requirements (uses)
✓ Knowledge deficit (teaching)

Implementation

IV **IV route**
- Give by **IV** inf, often mixed with TPN sol

T

- Discard unused portions
- Give by continuous inf diluted in 1 L or more **IV** sol; give at prescribed rate

Patient/family education

- Explain reason for and expected results of medication

Evaluation

Positive therapeutic outcome

- Absence of element deficiency

tranylcypromine

(tran-ill-sip′roe-meen)

Parnate

Func. class: Antidepressant—MAOI

Chem. class: Nonhydrazine

Pregnancy category **C**

Action: Increases concentrations of endogenous epinephrine, norepinephrine, serotonin, dopamine in storage sites in CNS by inhibition of MAO; increased concentration reduces depression

Therapeutic Outcome: Decreased symptoms of depression after 2-3 wk

Uses: Depression, when uncontrolled by other means

Dosages and routes

Adult: PO 10 mg bid; may increase to 30 mg/day after 2 wk

Available forms: Tab 10 mg

Side effects/adverse reactions

CNS: *Dizziness, drowsiness,* confusion, headache, anxiety, tremors, stimulation, weakness, hyperreflexia, mania, insomnia, fatigue, weight gain

CV: *Orthostatic hypotension, hypertension, dysrhythmias,* ***hypertensive crisis***

EENT: Blurred vision

ENDO: SIADH-like syndrome

GI: Constipation, dry mouth, nausea, vomiting, *anorexia,* diarrhea, weight gain

GU: Change in libido, frequency

HEMA: Anemia

INTEG: Rash, flushing, increased perspiration

Contraindications: Hypersensitivity to MAOIs, elderly, hypertension, CHF, severe hepatic disease, pheochromocytoma, severe renal disease, severe cardiac disease

Precautions: Suicidal patients, convulsive disorders, severe depression, schizophrenia, hyperactivity, diabetes mellitus, pregnancy **C**

Pharmacokinetics

Absorption	Well absorbed
Distribution	Crosses placenta
Metabolism	Liver, extensively
Excretion	Kidneys, breast milk
Half-life	Unknown

Pharmacodynamics

	PO
Onset	Unknown
Peak	Unknown
Duration	Unknown

Interactions

Drug/drug:

Individual drugs
Alcohol: ↑ CNS depression
Fluoxetine: ↑ serious reactions
Guanethidine: ↓ hypertensive crisis
Paroxetine: ↑ serious reactions
Drug classifications
Analgesics (opioid): ↑ CNS depression
Antidepressants, tricyclic: ↑ hypertensive crisis
Antihypertensives: ↑ hypotension

Drug/food:

Tyramine: ↑ hypertensive crisis

NURSING CONSIDERATIONS

Assessment

- Monitor B/P (lying, standing), pulse q4h; if systolic B/P drops 20 mm hg hold drug, notify prescriber; take vital signs q4h in patients with cardiovascular disease
- Monitor hepatic studies: AST (SGOT), ALT (SGPT), bilirubin
- Check weight qwk; appetite may increase with drug
- Assess mental status: mood, sensorium, affect, suicidal tendencies; increase in psychiatric symptoms: depression, panic
- Monitor urinary retention, constipation; constipation is P more likely to occur in chil- G dren or elderly
- Assess for withdrawal symptoms: headache, nausea, vomiting, muscle pain, weakness; do not usually occur unless drug was discontinued abruptly
- Identify alcohol consumption; if alcohol is consumed, hold dose until morning

Associated nursing diagnoses

✓ Coping, ineffective individual (uses)
✓ Injury, risk for (side effects)
✓ Knowledge deficit (teaching)
✓ Noncompliance (teaching)

Implementation

PO route

- Give with food or milk for GI symptoms; crush if patient is unable to swallow medication whole
- Store at room temp; do not freeze

Patient/family education

- Advise patient that therapeutic effects may take 2-3 wk
- Teach patient to use caution in driving or other activities requiring alertness because of drowsiness, dizziness, blurred vision; to avoid rising quickly from sitting to standing, espe- G cially elderly
- Caution patient to avoid alcohol ingestion, other CNS depressants
- Advise patient not to discontinue medication quickly after long-term use: may cause nausea, headache, malaise
- Advise patient to increase fluids, bulk in diet if constipation, urinary retention occur, G especially elderly
- Teach patient to take gum, hard sugarless candy, or frequent sips of water for dry mouth
- Teach patient to avoid high-tyramine foods; cheese (aged), sour cream, beer, wine, pickled products, liver, raisins, bananas,

T

figs, avocados, meat tenderizers, chocolate, yogurt; increased caffeine
- Teach patient to report headache, palpitation, neck stiffness
- Instruct patient to carry Medic-Alert Bracelet or ID with medications taken, condition treated, and prescriber's name and phone number

Evaluation

Positive therapeutic outcome
- Decrease in depression
- Absence of suicidal thoughts

Treatment of overdose: Lavage, activated charcoal, monitor electrolytes, vital signs, diazepam **IV**, $NaHCO_3$

trazodone

(tray'zoe-done)

Desyrel, Desyrel Dividose, trazodone HCl

Func. class.: Antidepressant, miscellaneous

Chem. class.: Triazolopyridine

Pregnancy category C

Action: Selectively inhibits serotonin uptake by brain, potentiates behavioral changes

➡ **Therapeutic Outcome:** Decreased symptoms of depression after 2-3 wk

Uses: Depression

Investigational uses: Chronic pain syndromes

Dosage and routes:

Adult: PO 150 mg/day in divided doses; may increase by 50 mg/day q3-4d, not to exceed 600 mg/day

Available forms: Tab 50, 100, 150, 300 mg

Side effects/adverse reactions

CNS: Dizziness, drowsiness, confusion, headache, anxiety, tremors, stimulation, weakness, insomnia, nightmares, G EPS (elderly), increase in psychiatric symptoms

CV: Orthostatic hypotension, ECG changes, tachycardia, ***hypertension,*** palpitations

EENT: Blurred vision, tinnitus, mydriasis

GI: Diarrhea, dry mouth, nausea, vomiting, ***paralytic ileus,*** increased appetite, cramps, epigastric distress, jaundice, ***hepatitis,*** stomatitis

GU: Retention, ***acute renal failure, priapism***

HEMA: ***Agranulocytosis, thrombocytopenia, eosinophilia, leukopenia***

INTEG: Rash, urticaria, sweating, pruritus, photosensitivity

Contraindications: Hypersensitivity to tricyclic antidepressants, recovery phase of MI, convulsive disorders, prostatic hypertrophy

Precautions: Suicidal patients, severe depression, increased intraocular pressure, narrow-angle glaucoma, urinary retention, cardiac disease, hepatic disease, hyperthyroidism, electroshock therapy, elective surgery, pregnancy **C**

Pharmacokinetics

Absorption	Well absorbed
Distribution	Widely distributed
Metabolism	Liver, extensively
Excretion	Kidneys—unchanged minimally
Half-life	4½-7½ hr

Pharmacodynamics

	PO
Onset	Unknown
Peak	Unknown
Duration	Unknown

Interactions

Drug/drug:

Individual drugs

Alcohol: ↑ CNS depression
Cimetidine: ↑ levels, ↑ toxicity
Clonidine: Severe hypotension, avoid use
Disulfiram: Organic brain syndrome
Fluoxetine: ↑ levels, ↑ toxicity
Guanethidine: ↓ effects

Drug classifications

Analgesics:↑ CNS depression
Anticholinergics: ↑ side effects
Antihistamines: ↑ CNS depression
Antihypertensives: may block antihypertensive effect
Barbiturates: ↑ effects
Benzodiazepines: ↑ effects
CNS depressants: ↑ effects
MAOI: hypertensive crisis, convulsions
Oral contraceptives: ↑ effects, toxicity
Phenothiazines: ↑ toxicity
Sedative/hypnotics: ↑ CNS depression
Sympathomimetics, indirect-acting: ↓ effects

Drug/smoking:

↑ metabolism, ↓ effects

Lab test interferences

Increase: Serum bilirubin, blood glucose, alk phosphatase
Decrease: VMA, 5-HIAA, blood glucose
False increase: Urinary catecholamines

NURSING CONSIDERATIONS

Assessment

- Monitor B/P (lying, standing), pulse q4h; if systolic B/P drops 20 mm hg hold drug, notify prescriber; take vital signs q4h in patients with cardiovascular disease
- Monitor blood studies: CBC, leukocytes, differential, cardiac enzymes if patient is receiving long-term therapy
- Monitor hepatic studies: AST (SGOT), ALT (SGPT), bilirubin
- Check weight qwk; appetite may increase with drug
- Assess ECG for flattening of T wave, bundle branch block, AV block, dysrhythmias in cardiac patients
- Assess for EPS primarily in G elderly; rigidity, dystonia, akathisia
- Assess mental status: mood, sensorium, affect, suicidal tendencies; increase in psychiatric symptoms: depression, panic
- Monitor urinary retention, constipation; constipation is P more likely to occur in children G or elderly
- Assess for withdrawal symptoms: headache, nausea, vomiting, muscle pain,

T

weakness; do not usually occur unless drug was discontinued abruptly
- Identify alcohol consumption; if alcohol is consumed, hold dose until AM

Associated nursing diagnoses

✓ Coping, ineffective individual (uses)
✓ Injury, risk for (adverse reactions)
✓ Knowledge deficit (teaching)
✓ Noncompliance (teaching)

Implementation

PO route
- Give with food or milk for GI symptoms; crush if patient is unable to swallow medication whole
- Give dosage hs if oversedation occurs during day; may take entire dose hs; G elderly may not tolerate once/day dosing
- Store at room temp; do not freeze

Patient/family education

- Teach patient that therapeutic effects may take 2-3 wk
- Teach patient to use caution in driving or other activities requiring alertness because of drowsiness, dizziness, blurred vision; to avoid rising quickly from sitting to standing, G especially elderly
- Caution patient to avoid alcohol ingestion, other CNS depressants
- Teach patient not to discontinue medication quickly after long-term use: may cause nausea, headache, malaise
- Advise patient to wear sunscreen or large hat because photosensitivity occurs
- Teach patient to increase fluids, bulk in diet if constipation, urinary retention occur, G especially elderly
- Advise patient to take gum, hard sugarles candy, or frequent sips of water for dry mouth

Evaluation

Positive therapeutic outcome
- Decrease in depression
- Absence of suicidal thoughts

Treatment of overdose: ECG monitoring, induce emesis, lavage, activated charcoal, administer anticonvulsant

tretinoin (vitamin A acid, retinoic acid)

(tret'i-noyn)

Retin-A, Stievaa ✤

Func. class.: Vitamin A acid/acne product
Chem. class.: Tretinoin derivative

Pregnancy category **C**

Action: Decreases cohesiveness of follicular epithelium, decreases microcomedone formation

Uses: Acne vulgaris (grades 1-3)

Investigational uses: Skin cancer

Dosage and routes

P *Adult and child:* Top cleanse area, apply hs; cover lightly

Available forms: Top cream 0.05%, 0.01%; top gel 0.025%, 0.01%; top liq 0.05%

Side effects/adverse reactions

INTEG: Rash, stinging, warmth, redness, erythema, blistering, crusting, peeling, contact dermatitis, hypopigmentation, hyperpigmentation

Contraindications: Hypersensitivity

Precautions: Pregnancy **C**, lactation, eczema, sunburn

Pharmacokinetics

Absorption	Small amounts
Distribution	Unknown
Metabolism	Unknown
Excretion	Kidneys
Half-life	Unknown

Pharmacodynamics

	TOP
Onset	Unknown
Peak	Unknown
Duration	Unknown

Interactions

Drug/drug:

Individual drugs

Benzyl peroxide: ↑ peeling
Resorcinol: ↑ peeling
Salicylic acid: ↑ peeling
Sulfur: ↑ peeling

Drug classifications

Abrasive soaps: ↑ peeling
Alcohol astringents: ↑ peeling

NURSING CONSIDERATIONS

Assessment

- Assess part of body involved, including time involved, what helps or aggravates condition, cysts, dryness, itching. Lesions may become worse at beginning of treatment

Associated nursing diagnoses

- ✓ Skin integrity, impaired (uses)
- ✓ Body image disturbances (uses)
- ✓ Knowledge deficit (teaching)

Implementation

Top route

- Apply once daily before hs; cover area lightly using gauze
- Store at room temp
- Wash hands after application

Liq

- Apply with gloves or cotton; apply only to affected areas

Patient/family education

- Instruct patient to avoid application on normal skin, and to avoid getting cream in eyes, nose, other mucous membranes
- Advise patient to avoid sunlight, sunlamps or to use protective clothing or sunscreen to prevent burns
- Advise patient that treatment may cause warmth, stinging; dryness; peeling will occur
- Inform patient that cosmetics may be used over drug; not to use shaving lotions
- Inform patient that rash may occur during first 1-3 wk of therapy
- Caution patient that drug does not cure condition; only relieves symptoms; that therapeutic results may be seen in

T

2-3 wk but may not be optimal until after 6 wk

Evaluation

Positive therapeutic outcome

- Decrease in size and number of lesions

triamcinolone

(trye-am-sin'oh-lone)

Aristocort, Atolone, Kenacort, Azmacort, Cenocort A-40, Kenaject-40, Kenalog, Kenalog-10, Kenalog-40, Tac-3, Tac-40, Triam-A, triamcinolone acetonide, Triamonide 40, Amcort, Aristocort Forte, Aristocort Intralesional, Articulose L.A., Cenocort Forte, triamcinolone, Triam Forte, Triamolone 40, Trilone, Trisoject, Aristospan Intra-Articular, Aristospan Intralesional, Tri-Kort, Trilog

Func. class.: Corticosteroid; antiinflammatory

Chem. class.: Glucocorticoid, intermediate-acting

Pregnancy category **C**

Action: Decreases inflammation by suppression of migration of polymorphonuclear leukocytes, fibroblasts, reversal to increase capillary permeability and lysosomal stabilization

➔ **Therapeutic Outcome:** Decreased inflammation, normal immune response

Uses: Severe inflammation, immunosuppression, neoplasms, asthma (steroid dependent), collagen, respiratory, dermatologic disorders

Dosage and routes

Adult: PO 4-12 mg/day in divided doses qd-qid; IM 40 mg qwk (acetonide, or diacetate), 5-48 mg into neoplasms (diacetate, acetonide), 2-40 mg into joint or soft tissue (diacetate, acetonide), 0.5 mg/sq in of affected intralesional skin (hexacetonide), 2-20 mg into joint or soft tissue (hexacetonide)

P *Child:* PO 117 μg/kg/day as a single dose or divided doses

Asthma

Adult: Inh 2 tid-qid, not to exceed 16 Inh/day

P *Child 6-12 yr:* Inh 1-2 tid-qid, not to exceed 12 inh/day

Available forms: Tab 1, 2, 4, 8, 16 mg; syr 2 mg/5 ml, 4.85 mg/5 ml; inj 25, 40 mg/ml diacetate; inj 3, 10, 40 mg/ml acetonide; inj 5, 20 mg/ml hexacetonide; inh 100 μg/spray; intranasal 55 μg/spray

Side effects/adverse reactions

CNS: Depression, flushing, sweating, headache, mood changes

*CV: Hypertension, **circulatory collapse, thrombophlebitis, embolism,*** tachycardia, edema

EENT: Fungal infections, increased intraocular pressure, blurred vision

GI: Diarrhea, nausea, abdominal distention, ***GI hemorrhage, increased appetite, pancreatitis***
HEMA: ***Thrombocytopenia***
INTEG: Acne, poor wound healing, ecchymosis, petechiae
MS: Fractures, osteoporosis, weakness

Contraindications: Psychosis, hypersensitivity, idiopathic thrombocytopenia, acute glomerulonephritis, amebiasis, fungal infections, nonasthmatic bronchial disease, child <2 yr, AIDS, TB

Precautions: Pregnancy **C**, diabetes mellitus, glaucoma, osteoporosis, seizure disorders, ulcerative colitis, CHF, myasthenia gravis, renal disease, esophagitis, peptic ulcer

Interactions

Drug/drug:

Individual drugs

Amphotericin B: ↑ hypokalemia
Azlocillin: ↑ hypokalemia
Insulin: ↑ need for insulin
Mezlocillin: ↑ hypokalemia
Phenytoin: ↓ action, ↑ metabolism
Piperacillin: ↑ hypokalemia
Rifampin: ↓ action, ↑ metabolism
Ticarcillin: ↑ hypokalemia

Drug classifications

Barbiturates: ↓ action, ↑ metabolism
Diuretics: ↑ hypokalemia
Hypoglycemia agents: ↑ need for hypoglycemic agents

Lab test interferences

Increase: Cholesterol, sodium, blood glucose, uric acid, calcium, urine glucose
Decrease: Calcium, potassium, T_4, T_3, thyroid ^{131}I uptake test, urine 17-OHCS, 17-KS, PBI
False negative: Skin allergy tests

Pharmacokinetics

Absorption	Well absorbed (PO, IM)
Distribution	Crosses placenta, widely distributed
Metabolism	Liver—extensively
Excretion	Kidney, breast milk
Half-life	2-5 hr, adrenal suppression 3-4 days

NURSING CONSIDERATIONS

Assessment

- Monitor potassium, blood sugar, urine glucose while on long-term therapy; hypokalemia and hyperglycemia
- Monitor weight daily; notify prescriber of weekly gain >5 lb; I&O ratio; be alert for decreasing urinary output and increasing edema
- Monitor B/P q4h, pulse; notify prescriber if chest pain occurs
- Monitor plasma cortisol levels during long-term therapy (normal level; 138-635

Pharmacodynamics

	PO	IM	TOP	INH	INTRANASAL
Onset	Unknown	Unknown	Min to hr	1-2 wk	Unknown
Peak	1-2 hr	1-2 hr	Hr to days	Unknown	2-3 wk
Duration	3 days	Unknown	Hr to days	Unknown	Unknown

nmol/L SI units when drawn at 8 AM); adrenal function periodically for HPA axis suppression
• Assess for infection: increase temp, WBC even after withdrawal of medication; drug masks infection symptoms
• Potassium depletion: paresthesias, fatigue, nausea, vomiting, depression, polyuria, dysrhythmias, weakness
• Assess mental status: affect, mood, behavioral changes, aggression
• Assess nasal passages during long-term treatment for changes in mucus (nasal)
• Monitor temp; if fever develops, drug should be discontinued
• Assess for systemic absorption: increased temp, inflammation, irritation (top)

Associated nursing diagnoses

✓ Infection, risk for (adverse reactions)
✓ Knowledge deficit (teaching)
✓ Noncompliance (noncompliance)

Implementation

IM route
• Give IM inj deeply in large mass, rotate sites, avoid deltoid, use 21-gauge needle
• Give in one dose in AM to prevent adrenal suppression; avoid SC administration—may damage tissue

PO route
• Give with food or milk to decrease GI symptoms

Inh route
• Give inh with water to decrease possibility of fungal infections; titrated dose, use lowest effective dose
• Give after cleaning aerosol top daily with warm water, dry thoroughly
• Store in cool environment; do not puncture or incinerate container

Top route
• Apply only to affected areas; do not get in eyes
• Apply medication, then cover with occlusive dressing (only if prescribed), seal to normal skin, change q12h; systemic absorption may occur
• Apply only to dermatoses; do not use on weeping, denuded, or infected areas
• Cleanse skin before applying drug
• Use treatment for a few days after area has cleared
• Store at room temp

Nasal route
• Have patient clear nasal passages before administration; use decongestant if needed; shake inhaler, invert, tilt head backward, insert nozzle into nostril, away from septum; hold other nostril closed and depress activator, inhale through nose, exhale through mouth

Patient/family education

• Advise patient that ID as steroid user should be carried
• Instruct patient to notify patient if therapeutic response decreases; dosage adjustment may be needed; not to discontinue abruptly; adrenal crisis can result
• Caution patient to avoid OTC products: salicylates, alcohol in cough products, cold preparations unless directed by prescriber

• Advise patient on all aspects of drug usage including cushingoid symptoms
• Teach patient symptoms of adrenal insufficiency: nausea, anorexia, fatigue, dizziness, dyspnea, weakness, joint pain
• Teach patient that long-term therapy may be needed to clear infection (1-2 mo depending on type of infection)

Nasal route

• Instruct patient to clear nasal passages if sneezing attack occurs, repeat dose
• Advise patient to continue using product even if mild nasal bleeding occurs; is usually transient
• Teach patient method of instill after providing written instruction from manufacturer

Inh route

• Teach patient proper administration technique; to wash inhaler with warm water and dry after each use
• Teach patient all aspects of drug usage including cushingoid symptoms

Top route

• Instruct patient to avoid sunlight on affected area; burns may occur

Evaluation

Positive therapeutic outcome

• Decrease in runny nose (nasal)
• Decreased dyspnea, wheezing, dry rales on auscultation (inh)
• Ease of respirations, decreased inflammation
• Absence of severe itching, patches on skin, flaking (top)

triamterene

(try-am'ter-een)

Dyrenium

Func. class.: Potassium-sparing diuretic

Chem. class.: Pteridine derivative

Pregnancy category **C**

Action: Acts primarily on distal tubule to inhibit reabsorption of sodium, chloride; increase potassium retention and conserve hydrogen ions

Therapeutic Outcome: Diuretic and antihypertensive effect while retaining potassium

Uses: Edema, hypertension, diuretic-induced hypokalemia

Dosage and routes

Adult: PO 100 mg bid pc, not to exceed 300 mg/day

Available forms: Cap 50, 100 mg

Side effects/adverse reactions

CNS: Weakness, headache, dizziness
ELECT: Hyperkalemia, hyponatremia, hypochloremia
GI: Nausea, diarrhea, vomiting, dry mouth, jaundice, liver disease
GU: ***Azotemia, interstitial nephritis,*** increased BUN, creatinine, renal stones, bluish discoloration of urine
HEMA: ***Thrombocytopenia, megaloblastic anemia,*** low folic acid levels

T

INTEG: Photosensitivity, rash

Contraindications: Hypersensitivity, anuria, severe renal disease, hyperkalemia

Precautions: Dehydration, hepatic disease, lactation, CHF, renal disease, cirrhosis, pregnancy **C,** lactation

Pharmacokinetics

	PO
Absorption	GI tract; well absorbed
Distribution	Crosses placenta
Metabolism	Liver
Excretion	Renal; breast milk
Half-life	3 hr

Pharmacodynamics

	PO
Onset	2 hr
Peak	6-8 hr
Duration	12-16 hr

Interactions

Drug/drug:

Individual drugs

Indomethacin: ↑ nephrotoxicity

Lithium: ↑ action, toxicity

Drug classifications

ACE inhibitors: ↑ hyperkalemia

Antihypertensives: ↑ action

Diuretics, potassium-sparing: ↑ hyperkalemia

Nonsteroidal antiinflammatories: ↓ nephrotoxicity

Potassium products: ↑ hyperkalemia

Salt substitutes: ↑ hyperkalemia

Drug/food:

Potassium foods: ↑ hyperkalemia

Lab test interferences

Interfere: Quinidine serum levels LDH

NURSING CONSIDERATIONS

Assessment

- Monitor manifestations of hyperkalemia: *RENAL:* acidic urine, reduced urine osmolality, nocturia, polyuria, polydipsia *CARDIAC:* hypotension, broad T wave, U wave, ectopy, tachycardia, weak pulse *NEURO:* muscle weakness, altered LOC, drowsiness, apathy, lethargy, confusion, depression, anorexia, nausea, cramps, constipation, distension, paralytic ileus, hypoventilation, respiratory muscle weakness
- Monitor for manifestations of hyponatremia: *CV:* ↑ B/P, cold, clammy skin, hypo- or hypervolemia; *GI:* anorexia, nausea, vomiting, diarrhea, abdominal cramps; *NEURO:* lethargy, increased ICP, confusion, headache, seizures, coma, fatigue, tremors, hyperreflexia
- Monitor for manifestations of hyperchloremia: *NEURO:* weakness, lethargy, coma; *RESP:* deep rapid breathing
- Assess fluid volume status: I&O ratios and record, weight, distended red veins, crackles in lung, color, quality and sp gr of urine, skin turgor, adequacy of pulses, moist mucous membranes, bilateral lung sounds, peripheral pitting edema. Dehydration symptoms of de-

creasing output, thirst, hypotension, dry mouth and mucous membranes should be reported.

- Monitor electrolytes: potassium, sodium, calcium, magnesium; also include BUN, ABGs, uric acid, CBC, blood sugar

Associated nursing diagnoses

- ✓ Urinary elmination, altered (adverse reactions)
- ✓ Fluid volume deficit (adverse reactions)
- ✓ Fluid volume excess (uses)
- ✓ Knowledge deficit (teaching)

Implementation

- Give in AM to avoid interference with sleep

PO route

- With food, if nausea occurs

Patient/family education

General

- Teach patient to take medication early in the day to prevent nocturia
- Instruct the patient to take with food or milk if GI symptoms of nausea and anorexia occur
- Teach patient to maintain a record of weight on a weekly basis and notify prescriber of weight loss of 5 lb
- Caution the patient that this drug causes an increase in potassium levels, that foods high in potassium should be avoided; refer to dietician for assistance planning
- Caution the patient not to exercise in hot weather, and stand for prolonged periods of time because orthostatic hypotension will be enhanced
- Advise patient to wear protective clothing and sunscreen in the sun to prevent photosensitivty
- Teach patient not to use alcohol, or any over-the-counter medications without prescriber's approval because serious drug reactions may occur
- Emphasize the need to contact prescriber immediately if muscle cramps, weakness, nausea, dizziness, or numbness occur
- Teach patient to take own B/P and pulse and record
- Advise patient that dizziness and confusion may occur; avoid driving or other hazardous activities if alertness is decreased
- Teach patient to continue taking medication even if feeling better; this drug controls symptoms but does not cure the condition
- Advise the patient with hypertension to continue other medical treatment (exercise, weight loss, relaxation techniques, cessation of smoking)

Evaluation

Positive therapeutic outcome

- Prevention of hypokalemia (diuretic use)
- Decreased edema
- Decreased B/P
- Increased diuresis

Treatment of overdose:

Lavage if taken orally; monitor electrolytes; administer sodium bicarbonate for K^2 6.5 mEq/L; monitor hydration, CV, renal status

triazolam

(trye-az'oh-lam)

Apo-Triazo ♣, Halcion, Novotriolam ♣, Nu-Triazol ♣

Func. class.: Sedative-hypnotic

Chem. class.: Benzodiazepine

Pregnancy category **X**

Controlled substance schedule **IV** (USA), schedule **F** (Canada)

Action: Produces CNS depression at limbic, thalamic, hypothalamic levels of CNS; may be mediated by neurotransmitter; γ-aminobutyric acid (GABA); results are sedation, hypnosis, skeletal muscle relaxation, anticonvulsant activity, anxiolytic action

➔ **Therapeutic Outcome:** Decreased anxiety, insomnia

Uses: Insomnia (short-term)

Dosage and routes

Adult: PO 0.125-0.5 mg hs

G *Elderly:* PO 0.125-0.25 mg hs

Available forms: Tab 0.125, 0.25, 0.5 mg

Side effects/adverse reactions

CNS: Headache, lethargy, drowsiness, daytime sedation, dizziness, confusion, lightheadedness, anxiety, irritability, amnesia, poor coordination

CV: Chest pain, pulse changes

GI: Nausea, vomiting, diarrhea, heartburn, abdominal pain, constipation

HEMA: Leukopenia, granulocytopenia (rare)

Contraindications: Hypersensitivity to benzodiazepines, pregnancy **X**, lactation, intermittent porphyria

Precautions: Anemia, hepatic disease, renal disease, suicidal G individuals, drug abuse, elderly, P psychosis, child <15 yr, acute narrow-angle glaucoma, seizure disorders

Pharmacokinetics

Absorption	Well absorbed (PO)
Distribution	Widely distributed, crosses placenta, crosses blood-brain barrier
Metabolism	Liver
Excretion	Kidneys, breast milk
Half-life	2-3 hr

Pharmacodynamics

	PO
Onset	½ hr
Peak	Unknown
Duration	6-8 hr

Interactions

Drug/drug:

Individual drugs

Alcohol: ↑ CNS depression
Cimetidine: ↑ action
Disulfiram: ↑ action
Fluoxetine: ↑ action
Isoniazid: ↑ action
Ketoconazole: ↑ action
Levodopa: ↓ action of levodopa
Metoprolol: ↑ action
Propoxyphene: ↑ action
Propranolol: ↑ action

Rifampin: ↓ action of triazolam
Theophylline: ↓ sedative effects
Valproic acid: ↑ action
Drug classifications
Analgesics, opioid: ↑ CNS depression
Antidepressants: ↑ CNS depression
Antihistamines: ↑ CNS depression
Barbiturates: ↓ effect of triazolam
Contraceptives: ↑ effect

Lab test interferences

Increase: AST (SGOT)/ALT (SGPT), serum bilirubin
False increase: 17-OHCS
Decrease: RAIU

NURSING CONSIDERATIONS

Assessment

- Assess patient's mental status: mood, sensorium, anxiety, affect, sleeping pattern, drowsiness, dizziness, especially G elderly; physical dependency, withdrawal symptoms: anxiety, panic attacks, agitation, convulsions, headache, nausea, vomiting, muscle pain, weakness; suicidal tendencies; for indications of increasing tolerance and abuse
- Monitor patient's B/P (lying, standing), pulse; if systolic B/P drops 20 mm Hg, hold drug, notify prescriber
- Monitor blood studies: CBC during long-term therapy; blood dycrasias have occurred rarely; decreased hematocrit, neutropenia may occur
- Monitor hepatic studies: AST (SGOT), ALT (SGPT), bilirubin, creatinine LDH, alk phosphatase
- Monitor I&O; indicate renal dysfunction

Associated nursing diagnoses

✓ Anxiety (uses)
✓ Depression (uses)
✓ Injury, risk for (adverse reactions)
✓ Knowledge deficit (teaching)

Implementation

PO route

- Give with food or milk for GI symptoms; if patient is unable to swallow medication whole, tab may be crushed and mixed with foods or fluids
- Give sugarless gum, hard candy, frequent sips of water for dry mouth

Patient/family education

- Advise patient that drug may be taken with food, or fluids and tab may be crushed or swallowed whole
- Caution patient not to use for everyday stress or longer than 3 mo unless directed by prescriber; not to take more than prescribed amount; may be habit forming; not to double doses or skip doses
- Instruct patient to avoid OTC preparations unless approved by health care prescriber; alcohol and CNS depressants will increase CNS depression
- Caution patient to avoid driving, activities that require alertness because drowsiness may occur; to avoid alcohol ingestion or other psychotropic medications; to rise slowly or fainting may occur, especially

T

G elderly; that drowsiness may worsen at beginning of treatment

• Advise patient not to discontinue medication abruptly after long-term use; withdrawal symptoms include vomiting, cramping, tremors, seizures

Evaluation

Positive therapeutic outcome

• Decreased anxiety, restlessness, sleeplessness (short-term treatment only)

Treatment of overdose: Lavage, VS, supportive care

trifluoperazine

(trye-floo-oh-per'a-zeen)

Novoflurazine ✦, Solazine ✦, Stelazine, Suprazine, Terfluzine, trifluoperazine HCl, Triflurin

Func. class.: Antipsychotic/neuroleptic

Chem. class.: Phenothiazine, piperazine

Pregnancy category C

Action: Depresses cerebral cortex, hypothalamus, limbic system, which control activity, aggression; blocks neurotransmission produced by dopamine at synapse; exhibits strong α-adrenergic, anticholinergic blocking action; mechanism for antipsychotic effects is unclear

➡ **Therapeutic Outcome:** Decreased signs and symptoms of psychosis

Uses: Psychotic disorders, nonpsychotic anxiety, schizophrenia

Dosage and routes

Adult: PO 2-5 mg bid, usual range 15-20 mg/day, may require 40 mg/day or more; IM 1-2 mg q4-6h

P *Child >6 yr:* PO 1 mg qd or bid; IM *not recommended for children,* but 1 mg may be given qd or bid

Nonpsychotic anxiety

Adult: PO 1-2 mg bid, not to exceed 5 mg/day; do not give longer than 12 wk

Available forms: Tab 1, 2, 5, 10, 20 mg; conc 10 mg/ml; inj 2 mg/ml

Side effects/adverse reactions

CNS: Extrapyramidal symptoms: pseudoparkinsonism, akathisia, dystonia, tardive dyskinesia, ***seizures,*** *headache,* ***neuroleptic malignant syndrome***

CV: Orthostatic hypotension, hypertension, ***cardiac arrest,*** ECG changes, ***tachycardia***

EENT: Blurred vision, glaucoma, dry eyes

GI: Dry mouth, nausea, vomiting, anorexia, constipation, diarrhea, jaundice, weight gain

GU: Urinary retention, urinary frequency, enuresis, impotence, amenorrhea, gynecomastia

HEMA: Anemia, ***leukopenia, leukocytosis, agranulocytosis***

INTEG: Rash, photosensitivity, dermatitis

RESP: Laryngospasm, dyspnea, ***respiratory depression***

Contraindications: Hypersensitivity, cardiovascular disease, coma, blood dyscrasias, severe hepatic disease, child <6 yr, glaucoma

Precautions: Breast cancer, seizure disorders, pregnancy **C,** lactation, diabetes mellitus, respiratory conditions, prostatic hypertrophy

Pharmacokinetics

Absorption	Variably absorbed (tab), well absorbed (IM)
Distribution	Widely distributed, high concentrations in CNS, crosses placenta
Metabolism	Liver—extensively
Excretion	Kidneys, breast milk
Half-life	Unknown

Pharmacodynamics

	PO	IM
Onset	Rapid	Immediate
Peak	2-3 hr	1 hr
Duration	12 hr	12 hr

Interactions

Drug/drug:

Individual drugs

Alcohol: ↑ effects of both drugs, oversedation
Aluminum hydroxide: ↓ absorption
Bromocriptine: ↓ antiparkinson activity
Disopyramide: ↑ anticholinergic effects
Epinephrine: ↑ toxicity
Guanethidine: ↓ antihypertensive response
Levodopa: ↓ antiparkinson activity
Lithium: ↓ chlorpromazine levels, ↑ extrapyramidal symptoms, masking of lithium toxicity
Magnesium hydroxide: ↓ absorption
Norepinephrine: ↓ vasoresponse, ↑ toxicity
Phenobarbital: ↓ effectiveness, ↑ metabolism

Drug classifications

Antacids: ↓ absorption
Anticholinergics: ↑ anticholinergic effects
Antidepressants: ↑ CNS depression
Antidiarrheals, adsorbent: ↓ absorption
Antihistamines: ↑ CNS depression
Antihypertensives: ↑ hypotension
Antithyroid agents: ↑ agranulocytosis
Barbiturate anesthetics: ↑ CNS depression
Beta adrenergics: ↑ effects of both drugs
General anesthetics: ↑ CNS depression
MAO inhibitors: ↑ CNS depression
Narcotics: ↑ CNS depression
Sedative/hypnotics: ↑ CNS depression

Lab test interferences

Increase: Liver function tests, cardiac enzymes, cholesterol, blood glucose, prolactin, bilirubin, PBI, cholinesterase. I, alk phosphatase, leukocytes, granulocytes, platelets
Decrease: Hormones (blood and urine)
False positive: Pregnancy tests, PKU, urine bilirubin
False negative: Urinary steroids, 17-OHCS

T

NURSING CONSIDERATIONS

Assessment

- Assess mental status: orientation, mood, behavior, presence of hallucinations, and type before initial administration and monthly; drug should significantly reduce psychotic behavior
- Check for swallowing of PO medication; check for hoarding or giving of medication to other patients
- Monitor I&O ratio, palpate bladder if low urinary output **G** occurs, especially in elderly; urinalysis recommended before, during prolonged therapy
- Monitor bilirubin, CBC, liver function studies monthly
- Assess affect, orientation, LOC, reflexes, gait, coordination, sleep pattern disturbances
- Monitor B/P sitting, standing and lying, take pulse and respirations q4h during initial treatment; establish baseline before starting treatment; report drops of 30 mm Hg; obtain baseline ECG, Q-wave and T-wave changes
- Check for dizziness, faintness, palpitations, tachycardia on rising; severe orthostatic hypotension is common
- Identify for neuroleptic malignant syndrome: hyperpyrexia, muscle rigidity, increased CPK, altered mental status; drug should be discontinued
- Assess for extrapyramidal symptoms including akathisia (inability to sit still, no pattern to movements), tardive dyskinesia (bizarre movements of the jaw, mouth, tongue, extremities), pseudoparkinsonism (ragged, tremors, pill rolling, shuffling gait); an antiparkinson drug should be prescribed
- Assess for constipation, urinary retention daily; if these occur, increase bulk, water in diet

Associated nursing diagnoses

✓ Thought processes, altered (uses)
✓ Coping, ineffective individual (uses)
✓ Knowledge deficit (teaching)
✓ Noncompliance (teaching)

Implementation

PO route

- Drug in liq form mixed in glass of juice or cola if hoarding is suspected; do not mix in caffeine drinks, tannics, pectins
- **G** Decreased dose in elderly; metabolism is slowed in the elderly
- PO with full glass of water, milk; or give with food to decrease GI upset
- Storage in tight, light-resistant container, oral sol in amber bottle

IM route

- Inj in deep muscle mass, do not give SC; do not administer sol with a precipitate

Patient/family education

- Teach patient to use good oral hygiene; frequent rinsing of mouth, sugarless gum for dry mouth
- Caution patient to avoid hazardous activities until drug response is determined; dizziness, blurred vision is common
- Inform patient that orthostatic hypotension occurs often and to rise from sitting or lying position gradually and to re-

main lying down after IM inj for at least 30 min
• Caution patient to avoid tubs, hot showers, tub baths because hypotension may occur
• Instruct patient that heat stroke may occur in hot weather, so to take extra precautions to stay cool
• Advise patient to avoid abrupt withdrawal of this drug, or extrapyramidal symptoms may result; drug should be withdrawn slowly
• Teach patient to avoid OTC preparations (cough, hay fever, cold) unless approved by prescriber because serious drug interactions may occur; avoid use with alcohol, CNS depressants because increased drowsiness may occur
• Advise patient to use a sunscreen and sunglasses to prevent burns
• Teach patient about extrapyramidal symptoms and necessity of meticulous oral hygiene because oral candidiasis may occur
• Advise patient to take antacids 2 hr before or after this drug
• Instruct patient to report sore throat, malaise, fever, bleeding, mouth sores; if these occur, CBC should be drawn and drug discontinued

Evaluation

Positive therapeutic outcome
• Decrease in emotional excitement, hallucinations, delusions, paranoia
• Reorganization of patterns of thought, speech

Treatment of overdose: Lavage if orally ingested; provide airway; *do not induce vomiting or use epinephrine*

trihexyphenidyl

(trye-hex-ee-fen'i-dill)

Artane, Artane Sequels, Novohexidyl ✦, Trihexy-2, Trihexy-5, trihexyphenidyl HCl, Trihexane

Func. class.: Cholinergic blocker; antiparkinson

Chem. class.: Synthetic tertiary amine

Pregnancy category **C**

Action: Blocks central muscarinic receptors, which decreases involuntary movements, sweating, salivation

➔ Therapeutic Outcome: Decreased involuntary movements

Uses: Parkinson symptoms, drug-induced extrapyramidal symptoms

Dosage and routes

Parkinson symptoms

Adult: PO 1 mg, increased by 2 mg q3-5d to a total of 6-10 mg/day

Drug-induced extrapyramidal symptoms

Adult: PO 1 mg/day; usual dose 5-15 mg/day

Available forms: Tab 2, 5 mg; cap sus-rel 5 mg; elix 2 mg/5 ml

Side effects/adverse reactions

CNS: Confusion, anxiety, restlessness, irritability, delu-

T

sions, hallucinations, headache, sedation, depression, incoherence, dizziness, flushing, weakness
CV: Palpitations, tachycardia, postural hypotension
EENT: Blurred vision, photophobia, dilated pupils, difficulty swallowing, dry eyes, increased intraocular tension, angle-closure glaucoma
GI: Dryness of mouth, constipation, nausea, vomiting, abdominal distress, ***paralytic ileus***
GU: Urinary hesitancy, urinary retention, dysuria
INTEG: Urticaria, rash
MISC: Suppression of lactation, nasal congestion, decreased sweating, increased temp, hyperthermia, heat stroke, numbness of fingers
MS: Weakness, cramping

Contraindications: Hypersensitivity, narrow-angle glaucoma, myasthenia gravis, GI/GU obstruction, tachycardia, myocardial ischemia, unstable CV disease, prostatic hypertrophy

Precautions: Pregnancy **C**, G elderly, lactation, tachycardia, abdominal obstruction, infection, P children, gastric ulcer

Pharmacokinetics

Absorption	Well absorbed
Distribution	Unknown
Metabolism	Unknown
Excretion	Unknown
Half-life	Unknown

Pharmacodynamics

	PO	PO-ER
Onset	1 hr	Unknown
Peak	2-3 hr	Unknown
Duration	6-12 hr	Up to 24 hr

Interactions

Drug/drug:

Individual drugs
Alcohol: ↑ CNS depression
Disopyramide: ↑ anticholinergic effects
Quinidine: ↑ anticholinergic effects
Drug classifications
Analgesics: ↑ CNS depression
Antacids: ↓ absorption
Antidepressants, tricyclic: ↑ anticholinergic effects
Antihistamines: ↑ anticholinergic effects
Phenothiazines: ↑ anticholinergic effects
Sedatives/hypnotics: ↑ CNS depression

NURSING CONSIDERATIONS

Assessment

- Monitor I&O ratio; retention commonly causes decreased urinary output, distention, frequency, incontinence
- Assess for Parkinsonism, extrapyramidal symptoms: shuffling gait, muscle rigidity, involuntary movements, pill rolling, muscle spasms, drooling before and during treatment
- Monitor for urinary hesitancy, retention; palpate bladder if retention occurs
- Monitor for constipation, cramping, pain in abdomen, abdominal distention; increase fluids, bulk, exercise if this occurs

• Assess for tolerance over long-term therapy; dose may have to be increased or changed
• Assess for mental status: affect, mood, CNS depression, worsening of mental symptoms during early therapy

Associated nursing diagnoses

✓ Physical mobility, impaired (uses)
✓ Knowledge deficit (teaching)

Implementation

PO route
• Give with or pc to prevent GI upset; may give with fluids other than water; offer hard candy, frequent drinks, gum to relieve dry mouth
• Give at hs to avoid daytime drowsiness in patient with parkinsonism
• Store at room temp

Patient/family education

• Teach patient to use caution in hot weather; drug may increase susceptibility to stroke because perspiration is decreased; patient should remain indoors
• Teach patient not to discontinue this drug abruptly; to taper off over 1 wk to prevent withdrawal symptoms (insomnia, involuntary movements, anxiety, tachycardias)
• Caution patient to avoid driving or other hazardous activities; drowsiness, dizziness may occur
• Advise patient to avoid OTC medications: cough, cold preparations with alcohol, antihistamines unless directed by prescriber; increased CNS depression may occur
• Instruct patient to rise from sitting or recumbent position slowly to minimize orthostatic hypotension
• Advise patient to use gum, hard candy, frequent sips of water to decrease dry mouth; if dry mouth continues, saliva substitutes may be prescribed
• Instruct patient that doses should not be doubled, but missed dose may be taken up to 2 hr before next dose

Evaluation

Positive therapeutic outcome
• Absence of involuntary movements (pill-rolling, tremors, muscle spasms)

trimethaphan

(trye-meth′a-fan)
Arfonad
Func. class.: Antihypertensive
Chem. class.: Ganglionic blocker
Pregnancy category **D**

Action: Occupies receptor site, prevents acetylcholine from attaching to postsynaptic nerve endings in sympathetic ganglia

T

➔ **Therapeutic Outcome:** Decreased B/P

Uses: Hypertensive emergencies; production of controlled hypotension during surgery; acute aortic dissection

Dosage and routes

Hypertension, severe

Adult: **IV**—dilute 500 mg in 500 ml of 5% dextrose inj, run at 3-4 mg/min, adjust to maintain B/P at desired rate; range 0.3-6 mg/min

P *Child:* **IV** 50-150 μg/kg/min, adjust to maintain B/P at desired rate

Controlled hypotension during surgery

Adult: **IV** 3-4 mg/min, then 300 μg-6mg/min

Aortic dissection

Adult: **IV** 1-4 mg/min, then increased to maintain B/P

Available forms: Inj **IV** 50 mg/ml

Side effects/adverse reactions

CNS: Headache, agitation, weakness, restlessness
CV: Orthostatic hypotension, angina, tachycardia, edema
EENT: Blurred vision, diplopia, pupillary dilation
GI: Nausea, vomiting, anorexia, dry mouth, diarrhea, constipation, ileus
GU: Urinary retention
INTEG: Rash, urticaria, pruritus
RESP: Respiratory arrest

Contraindications: Uncorrected respiratory insufficiency, hypersensitivity, pregnancy **D**, hypovolemic shock, glaucoma, uncorrected anemia

G **Precautions:** Elderly, debilitated, allergy-prone individuals; cardiac disease, degenerative CNS disease, hepatic disease, renal disease, diabetes mellitus, Addison's disease, P children

Pharmacokinetics

Absorption	Completely absorbed (IV)
Distribution	Crosses placenta
Metabolism	Small amount metabolized—liver
Excretion	Kidneys, unchanged
Half-life	Unknown

Pharmacodynamics

	IV
Onset	Rapid
Peak	Unknown
Duration	15 min

Interactions

Drug/drug:

Individual drugs

Procainamide: ↑ hypotension
Succinylcholine: ↑ neuromuscular blockade
Tubocurarine: ↑ neuromuscular blockade

Drug classifications

Anesthetics: ↑ hypotension
Antihypertensives: ↑ hypotension
Diuretics: ↑ hypotension
Nitrates: ↑ hypotension

NURSING CONSIDERATIONS

Assessment

- Monitor B/P during beginning treatment, periodically thereafter; pulse q4h; note rate, rhythm, quality; apical/radial pulse before administration; notify prescriber of any significant changes (pulse <50 bpm)
- Check for baselines in renal, liver function tests before therapy begins

• Assess for edema in feet, legs daily; monitor I&O, daily weight; check for jugular vein distention, rales bilaterally, dyspnea (CHF)
• Monitor skin turgor, dryness of mucous membranes for hydration status, especially G elderly

Associated nursing diagnoses

✓ Cardiac output, decreased (uses)
✓ Injury, risk for (adverse effects)
✓ Knowledge deficit (teaching)
✓ Noncompliance (teaching)

Implementation

IV **IV route**
• Give by continuous inf after diluting 500 mg (10 ml)/500 ml 0.9% NaCl, D_5W, Ringer's to 1 mg/ml; give at prescribed rate using an **IV** pump; titrate to patient's response
• Use only freshly prepared sol; elevate patient's head to control B/P; ensure that artificial ventilation equipment is available

Y-site compatibilities:

Heparin, hydrocortisone, potassium chloride, vitamin B with C

Additive incompatibilities:

Alkaline solutions, bromides, gallamine, thiopental, tubocurarine

Patient/family education

• Explain to patient reason for medication and expected result
• Caution patient to remain recumbent during treatment to prevent orthostatic hypotension

Evaluation

Positive therapeutic outcome
• Decreased B/P, primarily systolic B/P

Treatment of overdose:

Administer vasopressors, phenylephrine, mephentermine

trimethobenzamide

(trye-meth-oh-ben'za-mide)
Arrestin, Benzacot, Brogan, Stemetic, T-Gen, Tebamide, Ticon, Tigan, Tijet-20, Tribun, Trimazide, trimethobenzamide, trimethobenzamide HCl
Func. class.: Antiemetic, anticholinergic
Chem. class.: Ethanolamine derivative
Pregnancy category **C**

Action: Acts centrally by blocking chemoreceptor trigger zone, which in turn acts on vomiting center

➔ **Therapeutic Outcome:** Absence of nausea and vomiting

Uses: Nausea, vomiting, prevention of postoperative vomiting

Dosage and routes

Postoperative vomiting
Adult: IM/rec 200 mg before or during surgery; may repeat 3 hr after

T

Discontinuing anesthesia

P ***Child 13-40 kg:*** PO/rec 100-200 mg tid-qid

P ***Child <13 kg:*** PO/rec 100 mg tid-qid

Nausea/vomiting

Adult: PO 250 mg tid-qid; IM/rec 200 mg tid-qid

Available forms: Cap 100, 250, mg; supp 100, 200 mg; inj 100 mg/ml

Side effects/adverse reactions

CNS: Drowsiness, restlessness, headache, dizziness, insomnia, confusion, nervousness, tingling, *vertigo,* extrapyramidal symptoms
CV: Hypertension, hypotension, palpitations
EENT: Dry mouth, blurred vision, diplopia, nasal congestion, photosensitivity
GI: Nausea, anorexia, diarrhea, vomiting, constipation
INTEG: Rash, urticaria, fever, chills, flushing

Contraindications: Hypersensitivity to narcotics, shock, P children (parenterally)

P **Precautions:** Children, cardiac G dysrhythmias, elderly, asthma, pregnancy **C**, prostatic hypertrophy, bladder-neck obstruction, narrow-angle glaucoma, stenosing peptic ulcer, pyloroduodenal obstruction

Pharmacokinetics

Absorption	Unknown
Distribution	Unknown
Metabolism	Liver, extensively
Excretion	Kidneys
Half-life	Unknown

Pharmacodynamics

	PO	IM	REC
Onset	20-40 min	15 min	10-40 min
Peak	Unknown	Unknown	Unknown
Duration	3-4 hr	2-3 hr	3-4 hr

Interactions

Drug/drug:

Individual drugs

Alcohol: ↑ CNS depression

Drug classifications

Analgesics: ↑ CNS effect
Antidepressants: ↑ CNS effect
Antihistamines: ↑ CNS effect
CNS depressants: ↑ CNS effect
Sedative/hypnotics: ↑ CNS effect

NURSING CONSIDERATIONS

Assessment

- Monitor VS, B/P; check patients with cardiac disease more often
- Assess for signs of toxicity of other drugs or masking of symptoms of disease: brain tumor, intestinal obstructions
- Observe for drowsiness, dizziness
- Assess for nausea, vomiting before and after treatment

Associated nursing diagnoses

✓ Knowledge deficit (teaching)

Implementation

IM route

- Administer IM inj in large muscle mass; aspirate to avoid **IV** administration

PO route
- Cap may be swallowed whole or opened and mixed with food or fluids

Patient/family education

- Teach patient to use good oral hygiene; frequent rinsing of mouth, sugarless gum for dry mouth
- Caution patient to avoid hazardous activities until drug response is determined, drowsiness may occur
- Inform patient that orthostatic hypotension occurs often and to rise from sitting or lying position gradually and to remain lying down after IM inj for at least 30 min
- Advise patient to avoid hot tubs, hot showers, tub baths because hypotension may occur
- Inform patient that in hot weather, heat stroke may occur; take extra precautions to stay cool
- Teach patient to avoid OTC preparations (cough, hayfever, cold) unless approved by prescriber because serious drug interactions may occur; avoid use with alcohol, CNS depressants because increased drowsiness may occur
- Teach patient about extrapyramidal symptoms
- Instruct patient to report sore throat, malaise, fever, bleeding, mouth sores; if these occur, CBC should be drawn and drug discontinued

Evaluation

Positive therapeutic outcome
- Decreased nausea, vomiting

triprolidine

(trye-proe'li-deen)
Actidil, Alleract, Myidil, triprolidine HCl
Func. class.: Antihistamine
Chem. class.: Alkylamine, H_1-receptor antagonist
Pregnancy category C

Action: Acts on blood vessels, GI, respiratory systems by competing with histamine for H_1-receptor site; decreases allergic response by blocking histamine

Therapeutic Outcome: Absence of allergy symptoms and rhinitis

Uses: Rhinitis, allergy symptoms

Dosage and routes

Adult: PO 2.5 mg tid-qid
P ***Child >6 yr:*** PO 1.25 mg tid-qid
P ***Child 4-6 yr:*** PO 0.9 mg tid-qid
P ***Child 2-4 yr:*** PO 0.6 mg tid-qid
P ***Child 4 mo-2 yr:*** PO 0.3 mg tid-qid

Available forms: Tab 2.5 mg; syr 1.25 mg/5 ml

Side effects/adverse reactions

CNS: Dizziness, drowsiness, poor coordination, fatigue, anxiety, euphoria, confusion, paresthesia, neuritis
CV: Hypotension, palpitations, tachycardia

T

EENT: Blurred vision, dilated pupils, tinnitus, nasal stuffiness, dry nose, throat, mouth
GI: *Constipation,* dry mouth, nausea, vomiting, anorexia, diarrhea
GU: *Retention,* dysuria, frequency
HEMA: Thrombocytopenia, agranulocytosis, hemolytic anemia
INTEG: Rash, urticaria, photosensitivity
RESP: Increased thick secretions, wheezing, chest tightness

Contraindications: Hypersensitivity to H_1-receptor antagonist, acute asthma attack, lower respiratory tract disease

Precautions: Increased IOP, renal disease, cardiac disease, hypertension, bronchial asthma, seizure disorder, stenosed peptic ulcers, hyperthyroidism, prostatic hypertrophy, bladder neck obstruction, pregnancy **C**

Pharmacokinetics

Absorption	Well absorbed
Distribution	Widely distributed, crosses blood-brain barrier
Metabolism	Liver—extensively
Excretion	Kidneys
Half-life	5 hr

Pharmacodynamics

	PO
Onset	15-60 min
Peak	1-2 hr
Duration	6-8 hr

Interactions

Drug/drug:

Individual drugs
Alcohol: ↑ CNS depression
Atropine: ↑ anticholinergic reactions
Disopyramide: ↑ anticholinergic reactions
Haloperidol: ↑ anticholinergic reactions
Quinidine: ↑ anticholinergic reactions

Drug classifications
Antidepressants: ↑ anticholinergic reactions
Antihistamines: ↑ anticholinergic reactions
CNS depressants: ↑ CNS depression
MAO inhibitors: ↑ anticholinergic effect
Narcotics: ↑ CNS depression
Phenothiazines: ↑ anticholinergic reactions
Sedative/hypnotics: ↑ CNS depression

Lab test interferences

False negative: Skin allergy tests (discontinue antihistamines 3 days before testing)

NURSING CONSIDERATIONS

Assessment

- Assess respiratory status: rate, rhythm, increase in bronchial secretions, wheezing, chest tightness; provide fluids to 2 L/day to decrease thickness of secretions
- Monitor I&O ratio: be alert for urinary retention, frequency, dysuria, especially in **G** elderly; drug should be discontinued if these occur
- Monitor CBC during long-term therapy; blood dyscrasias may occur but are rare

Associated nursing diagnoses

- ✓ Airway clearance, ineffective (uses)
- ✓ Injury, risk for (adverse reactions)
- ✓ Knowledge deficit (teaching)
- ✓ Noncompliance (teaching—overuse)

Implementation

PO route

- Give on an empty stomach, 1 hr ac or 2 hr pc after meals to facilitate absorption
- Store in tight, light-resistant container

Patient/family education

- Teach patient all aspects of drug uses; to notify prescriber if confusion, sedation, hypotension occur; to avoid driving or other hazardous activity if drowsiness occurs; to avoid alcohol or other CNS depressants that may potentiate effect
- Advise patient to take medication 1 hr ac or 2 hr pc to facilitate absorption
- Caution patient not to exceed recommended dose because dysrhythmias may occur
- Inform patient that hard candy, gum, frequent rinsing of mouth may be used for dryness

Evaluation

Positive therapeutic outcome

- Absence of running or congested nose, rashes

Treatment of overdose:

Administer ipecac syrup or lavage, diazepam, vasopressors, barbiturates (short-acting)

tubocurarine 🔑

(too-boh-cure-a-reen)

Tubarine ✱, Tubocuraine

Func. class.: Neuromuscular blocker

Chem. class.: Synthetic curariform

Pregnancy category **C**

Action: Inhibits transmission of nerve impulses by binding with cholinergic receptor sites, antagonizing action of acetylcholine; no analgesic response

➡ Therapeutic Outcome: Skeletal muscle paralysis during anesthesia

Uses: Facilitation of endotracheal intubation, skeletal muscle relaxation during mechanical ventilation, surgery, or general anesthesia

Dosage and routes

Adult: **IV** Bol 0.4-0.5 mg/kg, then 0.08-0.10 mg/kg 20-45 min after 1st dose if needed for prolonged procedures

Available forms: Inj 3 mg/ml, (20 U/ml)

Side effects/adverse reactions

CV: Bradycardia, tachycardia, increased, decreased B/P
EENT: Increased secretions
INTEG: Rash, flushing, pruritus, urticaria
RESP: ***Prolonged apnea, bronchospasm, cyanosis, respiratory depression***

T

Contraindications: Hypersensitivity

Precautions: Pregnancy **C**, cardiac disease, lactation, P children <2 yr, electrolyte imbalances, dehydration, neuromuscular disease, respiratory disease

Pharmacokinetics

Absorption	Complete bioavailability (IV)
Distribution	Extensive, crosses placenta
Metabolism	Liver, small amount
Excretion	Kidneys—unchanged (30%-75%), bile (11%)
Half-life	2 hr

Pharmacodynamics

	IV	IM
Onset	1 min	15-30 min
Peak	5 min	Unknown
Duration	½-1½ hr	Unknown

Interactions

Drug/drug:

Individual drugs

Clindamycin: ↑ paralysis, length and intensity
Colistin: ↑ paralysis, length and intensity
Lidocaine: ↑ paralysis, length and intensity
Lithium: ↑ paralysis, length and intensity
Magnesium: ↑ paralysis, length and intensity
Polymyxin B: ↑ paralysis, length and intensity
Procainamide: ↑ paralysis, length and intensity
Quinidine: ↑ paralysis, length and intensity
Succinylcholine: ↑ paralysis, length and intensity

Drug classifications

Aminoglycosides: ↑ paralysis, length and intensity
Beta blockers: ↑ paralysis, length and intensity
Diuretics, potassium-losing: ↑ paralysis, length and intensity
General anesthesia: ↑ paralysis, length and intensity

NURSING CONSIDERATIONS

Assessment

- Monitor for electrolyte imbalances (potassium, magnesium), before drug is used; electrolyte imbalances may lead to increased action of this drug
- Monitor vital signs (B/P, pulse, respirations, airway) until fully recovered; rate, depth, pattern of respirations, strength of hand grip; patient should be intubated before use
- Monitor recovery: decreased paralysis of face, diaphragm, leg, arm, rest of body; residual weakness and respiratory problems may occur during recovery period
- Monitor allergic reactions: rash, fever, respiratory distress, pruritus; drug should be discontinued

Associated nursing diagnoses

✓ Breathing pattern, ineffective (uses)
✓ Communication, impaired verbal (adverse reactions)
✓ Fear (adverse reactions)
✓ Knowledge deficit (teaching)

Implementation

IV **IV route**

- Using peripheral nerve stimulator by anesthesiologist to determine neuromuscular

blockade; deep tendon reflexes should be monitored during extended periods
• Give **IV** undiluted by direct **IV** over 1-1½ min, (only by qualified person, usually an anesthesiologist)

Additive incompatibilities:
Barbiturates, sodium bicarbonate, trimethophan

Syringe compatibilities:
Pentobarbital, thiopental

Solution compatibilities:
D_5, $D_{10}W$, 0.9% NaCl, 0.45% NaCl, Ringer's, LR, dextrose/Ringer's or dextrose/LR combinations

Patient/family education

• Provide reassurance if communication is difficult during recovery from neuromuscular blockade
• Provide explanation to patients regarding all procedures or treatments; patient will remain conscious if anesthesia is not given also

Evaluation

Positive therapeutic outcome
• Paralysis of jaw, eyelid, head, neck, rest of body as evaluated by peripheral nerve stimulator

Treatment of overdose:

Edrophonium or neostigmine, atropine, monitor VS; patient may require mechanical ventilation

undecylenic acid (topical)

(un-de'sye-len-ik)
Caldesene, Cruex, Decylenes, Desenex, Desenex Maximum Strength, Protectol
Func. class.: Local antiinfective
Chem. class.: Antifungal, antibacterial
Pregnancy category **C**

Action: Interferes with fungal cell membrane permeability

Therapeutic Outcome: Absence of itching and white patches of the skin

Uses: Tinea cruris, tinea pedis, diaper rash, minor skin iritations

Dosage and routes

Adult and child: Top apply to affected areas bid

Available forms: Powder 10, 15, 19%, oint 22%, cream 8, 20%, foam 10%, soap 97.5 g/bar

Side effects/adverse reactions

INTEG: Rash, urticaria, stinging, burning

Contraindications: Hypersensitivity

Precautions: Pregnancy **C**, lactation; impaired circulation; diabetes mellitus; broken, pustular skin; puncture wounds

U

Pharmacokinetics

Absorption	Minimally absorbed
Distribution	Unknown
Metabolism	Liver
Excretion	Feces, kidneys
Half-life	2-3 days

Pharmacodynamics

Onset	Unknown
Peak	Unknown
Duration	Unknown

Interactions: None

NURSING CONSIDERATIONS

Assessment

- Assess skin for fungal infections: peeling, dryness, itching before and throughout treatment
- Monitor for allergic reaction: burning, stinging, swelling, redness, dermatitis, rash; drug should be discontinued

Associated nursing diagnoses

- ✓ Skin integrity, impaired (uses)
- ✓ Infection, risk for (uses)
- ✓ Knowledge deficit (teaching)

Implementation

Top route

- Apply enough medication to cover lesions completely
- Apply after cleansing area with soap, water before each application; dry well
- Store medication at room temp in dry place

Patient/family education

- Instruct patient to apply with glove to prevent further infection; not to cover with occlusive dressings
- Teach patient that long-term therapy may be needed to clear infection (2 wk-6 mo depending on organism); compliance is needed even after feeling better
- Teach patient proper hygiene: hand-washing technique, nail care, use of concomitant top agents if prescribed
- Caution patient to avoid use of OTC creams, ointments, lotions unless directed by prescriber
- Instruct patient to use medical asepsis (hand washing) before, after each application; to change socks and shoes once a day during treatment of tinea pedis
- Advise patient to report to health care prescriber if infection perisits or recurs; if blisters, burning, oozing, swelling
- Caution patient to avoid alcohol because nausea, vomiting, hypertension may occur
- Caution patient to use sunscreen or avoid direct sunlight to prevent photosensitivity
- Advise patient to notify health care prescriber of sore throat, fever, skin rash, which may indicate overgrowth of organisms

Evaluation

Positive therapeutic outcome

- Decrease in size, number of lesions
- Decrease in itching or white patches around vulva

urokinase

(yoor-oh-kin'ase)

Abbokinase, Abbokinase Open-Cath

Func. class.: Thrombolytic enzyme

Chem. class.: β-hemolytic streptococcus filtrate (purified)

Pregnancy category B

Action: Promotes thrombolysis by directly converting plasminogen to plasmin

Therapeutic Outcome: Lysis of emboli, or thrombosis in various parts of the body

Uses: Venous thrombosis, pulmonary embolism, arterial thrombosis, arterial embolism, arteriovenous cannula occlusion, lysis of coronary artery thrombi after MI

Dosage and routes

Lysis of pulmonary emboli

Adult: **IV** 4400 IU/kg/hr × 12-24 hr, not to exceed 200 ml; then **IV** heparin, then anticoagulants

Coronary artery thrombosis

Adult: Instill 6000 IU/min into occluded artery for 1-2 hr after giving **IV** bol of heparin 2500-10,000 U

May also give as **IV** inf of 2-3 million U over 45-90 min

Venous catheter occlusion

Adult: Instill 5000 IU into line, wait 5 min, then aspirate; repeat aspiration attempts q5min × ½ hr; if occlusion has not been removed, then cap line and wait ½-1 hr, then aspirate; may need 2nd dose if still occluded

Available forms: Inj

Side effects/adverse reactions

CNS: Headache, fever,
CV: Hypertension, dysrhythmias
EENT: Periorbital edema
GI: Nausea
HEMA: Decreased Hct, ***bleeding***
INTEG: Rash, urticaria, phlebitis at **IV** inf site, itching, flushing
MS: Low back pain
RESP: Altered respirations, SOB, ***bronchospasm***
SYST: GI, GU, intracranial, retroperitoneal bleeding; surface bleeding; ***anaphylaxis***

Contraindications: Hypersensitivity, active bleeding, intraspinal surgery, neoplasms of CNS, ulcerative colitis/enteritis, severe hypertension, renal disease, hepatic disease, hypocoagulation, COPD, subacute bacterial endocarditis, rheumatic valvular disease, cerebral embolism/thrombosis/hemorrhage, intraarterial diagnostic procedure or surgery (10 days), recent major surgery

Precautions: Arterial emboli from left side of heart, pregnancy **B**

U

Pharmacokinetics

Absorption	Completely (IV)
Distribution	Unknown
Metabolism	Liver
Excretion	Kidneys
Half-life	10-20 min

Pharmacodynamics

	IV
Onset	Rapid
Peak	Rapid
Duration	12 hr

Interactions

Drug/drug:

Individual drugs

Aspirin: ↑ bleeding
Dipyridamole: ↑ bleeding
Heparin: ↑ bleeding
Plicamycin: ↑ bleeding
Valproic acid: ↑ bleeding

Drug classifications

Cephalosporins: ↑ bleeding
Anticoagulants, oral: ↑ bleeding
Nonsteroidal antiinflammatories: ↑ bleeding

Lab test interferences

Increase: PT, APTT, TT

NURSING CONSIDERATIONS

Assessment

• Monitor VS, B/P, pulse, respirations (including peripheral), neurologic signs, temp at least q4hr; temp >104° F (40° C) indicates internal bleeding; monitor rhythm closely; ventricular dysrhythmias may occur with hyperfusion; monitor heart, breath sounds, neuro status, peripheral pulses

• Assess for bleeding during first hr of treatment: hematuria, hematemesis, bleeding from mucous membranes, epistaxis, ecchymosis; guaiac all body fluids, stools; blood studies (Hct, platelets, PTT, PT, TT, APTT) before starting therapy; PT or APTT must be less than 2 × control before starting therapy TT or PT q3-4h during treatment

• Assess allergy: fever, rash, itching, chills; mild reaction may be treated with antihistamines; report to health care prescriber

• Monitor ECG on monitor, watch for segment changes, changes in rhythm; sinus bradycardia, ventricular tachycardia, accelerated idioventricular rhythm may occur because of reperfusion

Associated nursing diagnoses

✓ Tissue perfusion, altered (uses)
✓ Injury, high risk for (adverse reactions)
✓ Impaired gas exchange (uses)

Implementation

IV **IV route**

Int IV

• Give **IV** loading dose over 30 min to avoid hypotension

• **IV** after dilution with 4-5 g/250 ml NS, D_5W, LR, give over 1 hr; may give by continuous inf after loading dose(s) of 1 g/hr diluted in 50-100 ml of compatible sol; use inf pump; do not give by direct **IV**

• Give heparin therapy after thrombolytic therapy is discontinued, TT, ACT, or APTT less than 2 × control (about 3-4 hr)

• Avoid invasive procedures, inj, rec temp

• Apply pressure for 30 sec to minor bleeding sites; 30 min to sites of atrial puncture, followed by pressure dressing; inform prescriber if this does not attain hemostasis; apply pressure dressing
• Store powder at room temp or refrigerate; protect from excessive light

Additive incompatibilities:
Do not mix with other medications

Patient/family education
• Teach patient reason for medication, signs and symptoms of bleeding, allergic reactions, when to notify health care prescriber

Evaluation
Positive therapeutic outcome
• Lysis of thrombi or emboli

vancomycin
(van-koe-mye'sin)
Vancocin, vancomycin HCL
Func. clas.: Anti-infective, misc.
Chem. class.: Tricyclic glycopeptide
Pregnancy category **C**

Action: Inhibits bacterial cell wall synthesis

➔ **Therapeutic Outcome:** Bactericidal for the following organisms: Staphylococci, Streptococci, Pneumoniae, Corynebacterium, Clostridium

Uses: Resistant staphylococcal infections, pseudomembranous colitis, staphylococcal enterocolitis, group A beta-hemolytic streptococci, endocarditis prophylaxis for dental procedures

Dosage and routes
Serious staphylococcal infections
Adult: **IV** 500 mg (7.5 mg/kg) q6h or 1 g (15 mg/kg) q12h max 4 g/day
P *Child:* **IV** 40 mg/kg/day divided q6-12h
P *Neonates:* **IV** 15 mg/kg initially followed by 10 mg/kg q8-12 h

Pseudomembranous/staphylococcal enterocolitis
Adult: PO 500 mg 2 g/day in 3-4 divided doses for 7-10 days
P *Child:* PO 40 mg/kg/day divided q6h, not to exceed 2 g/day
P *Neonates:* PO 10 mg/kg/day in divided doses

Endocarditis prophylaxis
Adult: **IV** 1 g over 1 hr, 1 hr before dental procedure
P *Child:* 20 mg/kg over 1 hr, 1 hr before procedure

Available forms: Pulvules 125, 250 mg; powder for oral sol 1, 10 g; powder for inj **IV** 500 mg, 1-g, 5-g, 10-g, vials

Side effects/adverse reactions
CV: Cardiac arrest, vascular collapse

V

EENT: Ototoxicity, permanent deafness, tinnitus
GI: Nausea
GU: Nephrotoxicity, increased BUN, creatinine, albumin, fatal uremia
HEMA: Leukopenia, eosinophilia, neutropenia
INTEG: Chills, fever, rash, thrombophlebitis at inj site, urticaria, pruritus, necrosis (Redman's syndrome)
RESP: Wheezing, dyspnea
SYST: Anaphylaxis

Contraindications: Hypersensitivity, decreased hearing

Precautions: Renal disease, G pregnancy **C**, lactation, elderly, P neonates

Pharmacokinetics

Absorption	Poorly absorbed (PO), completely absorbed (IV)
Distribution	Widely distributed, crosses placenta
Metabolism	Liver
Excretion	PO—feces, IV—kidneys
Half-life	4-8 hr

Pharmacodynamics

	IV
Onset	Immediate
Peak	Inf end

Interactions

Drug/drug:

Individual drugs
Amphotericin B: ↑ toxicity
Bacitracin: ↑ toxicity
Cisplatin: ↑ toxicity
Polymyxin B: ↑ toxicity
Drug classifications
Cephalosporins: ↑ toxicity

NURSING CONSIDERATIONS

Assessment

- Monitor I&O ratio; report hematuria, oliguria because nephrotoxicity may occur
- Monitor any patient with compromised renal system; drug is excreted slowly in poor renal system function; toxicity may occur rapidly
- Monitor blood studies: WBC
- Obtain C&S before drug therapy; drug may be given as soon as culture is taken
- Assess auditory function during, after treatment; hearing loss, ringing, roaring in ears; drug should be discontinued
- Monitor B/P during administration; sudden drop may indicate Redman's syndrome
- Assess for signs of infection
- Assess respiratory status: rate, character, wheezing, tightness in chest
- Identify allergies before treatment, reaction of each medication; place allergies on chart in bright letters; notify all people giving drugs

Associated nursing diagnoses

✓ Infection, risk for (uses)
✓ Knowledge deficit (teaching)

Implementation

IV **IV route**

- Give after reconstitution with 10 ml sterile water for inj (500 mg/10 ml); further dilution is needed for **IV**, 500 mg/100 ml NS, D_5W given as int inf over 1 hr
- Give antihistamine if Redman's syndrome occurs: decreased B/P, flushing of neck, face

• Give dose based on serum concentration
• Store at room temp for up to 2 wk after reconstitution
• Have adrenalin, suction, tracheostomy set, endotracheal intubation equipment on unit; anaphylaxis may occur
• Provide adequate intake of fuids (2 L) to prevent nephrotoxicity

Patient/family education

• Teach patient aspects of drug therapy: need to complete entire course of medication to ensure organism death (7-10 days); culture may be taken after completed course of medication
• Advise patient to report sore throat, fever, fatigue; could indicate superinfection
• Instruct patient that drug must be taken in equal intervals around clock to maintain blood levels

Evaluation

Positive therapeutic outcome
• Absence of fever, sore throat

vasopressin

(vay-soe-press'in)
Pitressin Synthetic, Pressyn
Func. class.: Pituitary hormone
Chem. class.: Lysine vasopressin
Pregnancy category **C**

Action: Promotes reabsorption of water by action on renal tubular epithelium; causes vasoconstriction on muscles in the GI system

Therapeutic Outcome: Increased osmolality, decreased urine output in diabetes insipidus

Uses: Diabetes insipidus (nonnephrogenic/nonpsychogenic), abdominal distention postoperatively, bleeding esophageal varices

Dosage and routes

Diabetes insipidus

Adult: IM/SC 5-10 units bid-qid prn; IM/SC 2.5-5 units q2-3 days (Pitressin Tannate) for chronic therapy

P *Child:* IM/SC 2.5-10 units bid-qid prn; IM/SC 1.25-2.5 units q2-3 days (Pitressin Tannate) for chronic therapy

Abdominal distention

Adult: IM 5 units, then q3-4h, increasing to 10 units if needed (aqueous)

Available forms: Inj 20, 5 U/ml (tannate), spray, cotton pledgets

Side effects/adverse reactions

CNS: Drowsiness, headache, lethargy, flushing
CV: Increased B/P
EENT: Nasal irritation, congestion, rhinitis
GI: Nausea, heartburn, cramps
GU: Vulval pain, uterine cramping
MISC: Tremor, sweating, vertigo, urticaria, bronchial constriction

Contraindications: Hypersensitivity, chronic nephritis

Precautions: CAD, pregnancy **C**

Pharmacokinetics

Absorption	Erratically absorbed (IM)
Distribution	Widely distributed extracellular fluid
Metabolism	Liver—rapidly
Excretion	Kidneys, unchanged
Half-life	10-20 min

Pharmacodynamics

	IM	NASAL
Onset	Unknown	1 hr
Peak	Unknown	Unknown
Duration	3-8 hr	3-8 hr

Interactions

Drug/drug:

Individual drugs

Alcohol: ↓ response
Carbamazepine: ↑ response
Chlorpropamide: ↑ response
Clofibrate: ↑ response
Demeclocycline: ↓ response
Epinephrine (large doses): ↓ response
Heparin: ↓ response
Lithium: ↓ response

Drug classifications

Ganglionic blockers: ↑ vasopressor response

NURSING CONSIDERATIONS

Assessment

- Monitor nasal mucosa for irritation if given by intranasal spray
- Assess intranasal use: nausea, congestion, cramps, headache; usually decreased with decreased dose
- Monitor pulse, B/P when giving drug **IV** or SC
- Monitor I&O ratio, weight daily; check for edema in extremities; if water retention is severe, diuretic may be prescribed; check for water intoxication: lethargy, behavioral changes, disorientation, neuromuscular excitability

Associated nursing diagnoses

- ✓ Fluid volume excess (side effects)
- ✓ Fluid volume deficit (uses)
- ✓ Knowledge deficit (teaching)

Implementation

IM route

- May be given IM/SC for diagnosis of diabetes insipidus
- Give patient 16 oz water at administration to prevent nausea, vomiting, cramping

Patient/family education

- Teach patient technique for nasal instillation: to insert tube into nasal cavity to instill drug
- Caution patient to avoid OTC products for cough, hay fever products because these preparations may contain epinephrine, decrease drug response; do not use with alcohol
- Advise patient to wear Medic Alert ID specifying therapy, disease process (diabetes insipidus)

Evaluation

Positive therapeutic outcome

- Absence of severe thirst
- Decreased urine output, osmolality

vecuronium bromide
(ve-kure-oh'nee-yum)
Norcuron
Func. class.: Neuromuscular blocker
Chem. class.: Synthetic curariform
Pregnancy category C

Action: Inhibits transmission of nerve impulses by binding with cholinergic receptor sites, antagonizing action of acetylcholine; no analgesic response

Therapeutic Outcome: Skeletal muscle paralysis during anesthesia

Uses: Facilitation of endotracheal intubation; skeletal muscle relaxation during mechanical ventilation, surgery, or general anesthesia

Dosage and routes

***Adult and child >9 yr:* IV** bol 0.08-0.10 mg/kg, then 0.010-0.015 mg/kg for prolonged procedures

Available forms: 10 mg/5 ml vial

Side effects/adverse reactions

CNS: Skeletal muscle weakness or paralysis (rarely)
RESP: ***Prolonged apnea, possible respiratory paralysis***

Contraindications: Hypersensitivity

Precautions: Pregnancy **C**, cardiac disease, lactation, children <2 yr, electrolyte imbalances, dehydration, neuromuscular disease, respiratory disease

Pharmacokinetics

Absorption	Completely absorbed (IV)
Distribution	Rapid—to extracellular fluids
Metabolism	Liver (20%)
Excretion	Kidneys—unchanged (35%)
Half-life	1½ hr, increased in liver disease

Pharmacodynamics

	IV
Onset	1 min
Peak	5 min
Duration	15-25 min

Interactions

Drug/drug:

Individual drugs

Clindamycin: ↑ paralysis, length and intensity
Colistin: ↑ paralysis, length and intensity
Lidocaine: ↑ paralysis, length and intensity
Lithium: ↑ paralysis, length and intensity
Magnesium: ↑ paralysis, length and intensity
Polymyxin B: ↑ paralysis, length and intensity
Procainamide: ↑ paralysis, length and intensity
Quinidine: ↑ paralysis, length and intensity
Succinylcholine: ↑ paralysis, length and intensity

Drug classifications

Aminoglycosides: ↑ paralysis, length and intensity
Beta blockers: ↑ paralysis, length and intensity

V

Diuretics, potassium-losing: ↑ paralysis, length and intensity
General anesthesia: ↑ paralysis, length and intensity

NURSING CONSIDERATIONS

Assessment

- Monitor for electrolyte imbalances (potassium, magnesium), before drug is used; electrolyte imbalances may lead to increased action of this drug
- Monitor patient's vital signs (B/P, pulse, respirations, airway) until fully recovered; rate, depth, pattern of respirations, strength of hand grip; patient should be intubated before use
- Monitor patient's recovery: decreased paralysis of face, diaphragm, leg, arm, rest of body; residual weakness and respiratory problems may occur during recovery period
- Monitor allergic reactions: rash, fever, respiratory distress, pruritus; drug should be discontinued

Associated nursing diagnoses

✓ Breathing pattern, ineffective (uses)
✓ Communication, impaired verbal (adverse reactions)
✓ Fear (adverse reactions)
✓ Knowledge deficit (teaching)

Implementation

IV **IV route**

- Using peripheral nerve stimulator by anesthesiologist to determine neuromuscular blockade; deep tendon reflexes should be monitored during extended periods
- Give by direct **IV** after reconstituting with bacteriostatic water, over 5 min, D_5W, 0.9% NaCl or LR
- Give by direct **IV** after reconstituting dose in 5-10 ml; give by titrating to patient response
- Give by continuous inf after diluting to 10-20 mg/100 ml and by titrating to patient response (only by qualified person, usually an anesthesiologist); do not administer IM
- Store in light-resistant area

Y-site compatibilities:
Aminophylline, cefazolin, cefuroxime, cimetidine, cotrimoxazole, dobutamine, dopamine, epinephrine, esmolol, fentanyl, gentamicin, heparin, hydrocortisone sodium succinate, isoproterenol, lorazepam, midazolam, morphine, nitroglycerin, ranitidine, sodium nitroprusside, vancomycin

Y-site incompatibility:
Barbiturates

Syringe incompatibility:
Barbiturates

Patient/family education

- Provide reassurance if communication is difficult during recovery from neuromuscular blockade
- Provide explanation to patients regarding all procedures or treatments; patient will remain conscious if anesthesia is not given also

Evaluation

Positive therapeutic outcome

- Paralysis of jaw, eyelid, head,

neck, rest of body as evaluated by peripheral nerve stimulator

Treatment of overdose: Edrophonium or neostigmine, atropine, monitor VS; may require mechanical ventilation

venlafaxine

(ven-laa-fax'een)

Effexor

Func. class.: Second-generation antidepressant

Chem. class.:

Pregnancy category C

Action: Potent inhibitor of neuronal serotinin and norepinephrine uptake, weak inhibitor of dopamine; no muscarinic, histaminergic, or α-adrenergic receptors in vitro

Therapeutic Outcome: Relief of depression

Uses: Depression

Dosage and routes

Adult: PO 75 mg/day in 2 or 3 divided doses; taken with food, may be increased to 150 mg/day; if needed may be further increased to 225 mg/day; increments of 75 mg/day should be made at intervals of no less than 4 days; some hospitalized patients may require up to 375 mg/day in 3 divided doses

Available forms: Tab scored 25, 37.5, 50, 75, 100 mg

Side effects/adverse reactions

CNS: *Emotional lability, vertigo,* apathy, ataxia, CNS stimulation, euphoria, hallucinations, hostility, increased libido, hypertonia, hypotonia, psychosis

CV: *Migraine,* angina pectoris, extrasystoles, hypotension, syncope, thrombophlebitis

EENT: *Abnormal vision, ear pain,* cataract, conjunctivitis, corneal lesions, dry eyes, otitis media, photophobia

GI: *Dysphagia, eructation,* colitis, gastritis, gingivitis, rectal hemorrhage, stomatitis, stomach and mouth ulceration

GU: *Anorgasmia, dysuria, hematuria, metrorrhagia, vaginitis, impaired urination,* albuminaria, amenorrhea, kidney calculus, cystitis, nocturia, breast and bladder pain, polyuria, uterine hemorrhage, vaginal hemorrhage, moniliasis

INTEG: Ecchymosis, acne, alopecia, brittle nails, dry skin, photosensitivity

META: *Peripheral edema, weight gain,* diabetes mellitus, edema, glycosuria, hyperlipemia, hypokalemia

MS: Arthritis, bone pain, bursitis, myasthenia tenosynovitis

RESP: *Bronchitis, dyspnea,* asthma, chest congestion, epistaxis, hyperventilation, laryngitis

SYST: *Accidental injury, malaise, neck pain,* enlarged abdomen, cyst, facial edema, hangover effect, hernia

Contraindications: Hypersensitivity

Precautions: Mania, pregnancy **C**, lactation, children, elderly

Pharmacokinetics

Absorption	Well absorbed
Distribution	Widely distributed, 27% protein binding
Metabolism	Liver—extensively
Excretion	Kidneys, 87%
Half-life	5-7 hr, 11-13 hr

Pharmacodynamics

	PO
Onset	Unknown
Peak	Unknown
Duration	Unknown

Interactions

Drug/drug:

Drug classifications

MAOI: Hypertensive crisis, convulsions

Lab test interferences

Increase: Serum bilirubin, blood glucose, alk phosphatase
Decrease: VMA, 5-HIAA
False increase: Urinary catecholamines

NURSING CONSIDERATIONS

Assessment

- Monitor B/P (lying, standing), pulse q4h; if systolic B/P drops 20 mm hg hold drug, notify prescriber; take vital signs q4h in patients with cardiovascular disease
- Monitor blood studies: CBC, leukocytes, differential, cardiac enzymes if patient is receiving long-term therapy
- Monitor hepatic studies: AST (SGOT), ALT (SGPT), bilirubin
- Check weight qwk; appetite may increase with drug
- Assess mental status: mood, sensorium, affect, suicidal tendencies; increase in psychiatric symptoms: depression, panic
- Monitor urinary retention, constipation; constipation is more likely to occur in children or elderly
- Assess for withdrawal symptoms: headache, nausea, vomiting, muscle pain, weakness; do not usually occur unless drug was discontinued abruptly
- Identify alcohol consumption; if alcohol is consumed, hold dose

Associated nursing diagnoses

- ✓ Coping, ineffective individual (uses)
- ✓ Injury, risk for physical (side effects)
- ✓ Knowledge deficit (teaching)
- ✓ Noncompliance (teaching)

Implementation

PO route

- Give with food or milk for GI symptoms
- Crush if patient is unable to swallow medication whole
- Store at room temp; do not freeze

Patient/family education

- Teach patient that therapeutic effects may take 2-3 wk
- Teach patient to use caution in driving or other activities requiring alertness because of

drowsiness, dizziness, blurred vision; to avoid rising quickly from sitting to standing, especially elderly

G

- Teach patient to avoid alcohol ingestion, other CNS depressants

Evaluation

Positive therapeutic outcome

- Decreased depression
- Absence of suicidal thoughts

Treatment of overdose: ECG monitoring, induce emesis, lavage, activated charcoal, administer anticonvulsant

verapamil

(ver-ap'a-mil)

Calan, Calan SR, Isoptin, Isoptin SR, verapamil HCl, Verelan

Func. class.: Calcium-channel blocker; antihypertensive; antianginal

Chem. class.: Phenylalkylamine

Pregnancy category **C**

Action: Inhibits calcium ion influx across cell membrane during cardiac depolarization; produces relaxation of coronary vascular smooth muscle; peripheral vascular smooth muscle; dilates coronary vascular arteries; increases myocardial oxygen delivery in patients with vasospastic angina

Therapeutic Outcome: Decreased angina pectoris, dysrhythmias, B/P

Uses: Chronic stable angina pectoris, vasospastic angina, dysrhythmias, hypertension

Investigational uses: Prevention of migraine headaches, ventricular outflow obstruction in hypertrophic cardiomyopathy

Dosage and routes

Adult: PO 80 mg tid or qid, increase qwk; **IV** bol 5-10 mg >2 min, repeat if necessary in 30 min

P *Child 0-1 yr:* **IV** bol 0.1-0.2 mg/kg >2 min with ECG monitoring, repeat if necessary in 30 min

P *Child 1-15 yr:* **IV** bol 0.1-0.3 mg/kg over >2 min, repeat in 30 min, not to exceed 10 mg in a single dose

Available forms: Tab 40, 80, 120 mg; sus-rel tab, 120, 180, 240 mg; inj 2.5 mg/ml; sus-rel cap 120, 180, 240 mg

Side effects/adverse reactions

CNS: Headache, drowsiness, dizziness, anxiety, depression, weakness, insomnia, confusion, light-headedness

CV: Edema, ***CHF,*** bradycardia, hypotension, palpitations, AV block

GI: Nausea, diarrhea, gastric upset, constipation, increased liver function studies

GU: Nocturia, polyuria

Contraindications: Sick sinus syndrome, 2nd- or 3rd-degree heart block, hypotension less than 90 mm Hg systolic, cardiogenic shock, severe CHF

Precautions: CHF, hypotension, hepatic injury, pregnancy P C, lactation, children, renal disease, concomitant β-blocker therapy

Pharmacokinetics

Absorption	Well absorbed (PO)
Distribution	Not known
Metabolism	Liver—extensively
Excretion	Kidneys
Half-life	Biphasic 4 min, 3-7 hr

Pharmacodynamics

	PO	PO-ER	IV
Onset	1-2 hr	Unknown	1-5 min
Peak	½-1½ hr	5-7 hr	3-5 min
Duration	3-7 hr	24 hr	2 hr

Interactions

Drug/drug:

Individual drugs
Alcohol: ↑ hypotension
Carbamazepine: ↑ toxicity
Digoxin: ↑ digoxin levels, ↑ bradycardia, CHF
Phenobarbital: ↓ effectiveness
Phenytoin: ↓ effectiveness
Propranolol: ↑ toxicity

Drug classifications
Antihypertensives: ↑ hypotension
Beta-adrenergic blockers: ↑ bradycardia, CHF
Nitrates: ↑ nitrates

NURSING CONSIDERATIONS

Assessment

- Assess fluid volume status: I&O ratio and record; weight; distended red veins; crackles in lung; color; quality, and specific gravity of urine; skin turgor; adequacy of pulses; moist mucous membranes; bilateral lung sounds; peripheral pitting edema—dehydration symptoms of decreasing output, thirst, hypotension, dry mouth, and mucous membranes should be reported
- Monitor B/P and pulse, pulmonary capillary wedge pressure (PCWP), central venous pressure, index, often during inf; if B/P drops 30 mm Hg, stop inf and call prescriber
- Monitor ALT (SGPT), AST (SGOT), bilirubin daily; if these are elevated, hepatotoxicity is suspected
- Monitor if platelets are <150,000/mm^3—if so, drug is usually discontinued and another drug started
- Assess for extravasation: change site q48h
- Monitor cardiac status: B/P, pulse, respiration, ECG

Associated nursing diagnoses

✓ Cardiac output, decreased (uses)
✓ Knowledge deficit (teaching)

Implementation

PO route

- Give once a day, with food for GI symptoms

IV **IV route**

- Give by direct **IV** undiluted (Y-site, three-way stopcock) over at least 2 min; to prevent serious hypotension, patient should be recumbent for 1 hr or more

Syringe compatibilities:
Amrinone, heparin, milrinone

Y-*site incompatibilities:*

Albumin, ampicillin, mezlocillin, nafcillin, oxacillin, sodium bicarbonate

Y-*site compatibilities:*

Amrinone, azlocillin, carbenicillin, dobutamine, dopamine, famotidine, hydralazine, meperidine, methicillin, milrinone, penicillin G potassium, piperacillin, ticarcillin

Patient/family education

- Caution patient to avoid hazardous activities until stabilized on drug, dizziness is no longer a problem
- Instruct patient to limit caffeine consumption; to avoid alcohol and OTC drugs unless directed by prescriber
- Advise patient to comply with medical regimen: diet, exercise, stress reduction, drug therapy; to notify prescriber of irregular heart beat, shortness of breath, swelling of feet and hands, pronounced dizziness, constipation, nausea, hypotension
- Teach patient to use as directed even if feeling better; may be taken with other cardiovascular drugs (nitrates, beta blockers)

Evaluation

Positive therapeutic outcome

- Decreased anginal pain
- Decreased dysrhythmias
- Decreased B/P

Treatment of overdose:

Defibrillation, atropine for AV block, vasopressor for hypotension

vinblastine (VLB)

(vin-blast'een)

Alkaban-AQ, Velban, Velbe ✤, Velsar, vinblastine sulfate

Func. class.: Antineoplastic

Chem. class.: Vinca rosea alkaloid

Pregnancy category **D**

Action: Inhibits mitotic activity, arrests cell cycle at metaphase; inhibits RNA synthesis, blocks cellular use of glutamic acid needed for purine synthesis; a vesicant

Therapeutic Outcome: Prevention of rapid growth of malignant cells, immunosuppressive

Uses: Breast, testicular cancer; lymphomas; neuroblastoma; Hodgkin's, non-Hodgkin's lymphomas; mycosis fungoides; histiocytosis; Kaposi's sarcoma

Dosage and routes

Adult: **IV** 0.1 mg/kg or 3.7 mg/m^2 q wk or q2 wk, not to exceed 0.5 mg/kg or 18.5 mg/m^2 q wk

P *Child:* 2.5 mg/m^2 then dose of 3.75, 5.0, 6.25 and 7.5 at 7-day intervals

Available forms: Inj powder 10 mg for 10 ml **IV** inj

Side effects/adverse reactions

CNS: Paresthesias, peripheral neuropathy, depression, headache, ***convulsions***

V

CV: Tachycardia, orthostatic hypotension
GI: Nausea, vomiting, ileus, ***anorexia, stomatitis,*** constipation, abdominal pain, GI and rectal bleeding, ***hepatotoxicity,*** pharyngitis
GU: Urinary retention, ***renal failure***
HEMA: ***Thrombocytopenia, leukopenia, myelosuppression***
INTEG: Rash, alopecia, photosensitivity
META: SIADH
RESP: ***Fibrosis, pulmonary infiltrate***

Contraindications: Hypersensitivity, P infants, pregnancy **D**

Precautions: Renal disease, hepatic disease

Pharmacokinetics

Absorption	Complete bioavailability (IV)
Distribution	Crosses blood-brain barrier slightly
Metabolism	Liver—active antineoplastic
Excretion	Biliary, kidneys
Half-life	Triphasic—35 min, 53 min, 19 hr

Pharmacodynamics

	IV
Onset	Unknown
Peak	Unknown
Duration	Unknown

Interactions

Drug/drug:

Individual drugs

Live virus vaccines: ↑ adverse reactions
Mitomycin: Bronchospasm
Radiation: ↑ toxicity, bone marrow suppression

Drug classifications

Antineoplastics: ↑ toxicity, bone marrow suppression

NURSING CONSIDERATIONS

Assessment

- Monitor B/P, (baseline and q15 min) during administration
- Monitor CBC, differential, platelet count weekly; withhold drug if WBC is <4000 or platelet count is <75,000; notify prescriber of results, recovery will take 3 wk
- Assess for dyspnea, rales, unproductive cough, chest pain, tachypnea
- Monitor renal function studies: BUN, serum uric acid, urine CrCl before, during therapy; I&O ratio; report fall in urine output of 30 ml/hr; for decreased hyperuricemia
- Monitor for cold, fever, sore throat (may indicate beginning infection); notify health care prescriber if these occur
- Assess for bleeding: hematuria, guaiac, bruising or petechiae, mucosa or orifices q8h, no rectal temp; avoid IM inj; use pressure to venipuncture sites
- Identify nutritional status: an antiemetic may need to be prescribed
- Assess for symptoms indicating severe allergic reactions: rash, pruritus, urticaria, itching, flushing, bronchospasm, hypotension; epinephrine and crash cart should be nearby

Associated nursing diagnoses

✓ Injury, risk for (adverse reactions)

✓ Body image disturbance (adverse reactions)
✓ Infection, risk for (adverse reactions)
✓ Knowledge deficit (teaching)

Implementation

IV route

- Give by intermittent inf
- Sol should be prepared by qualified personnel only under controlled conditions
- Use Luer-Loc tubing to prevent leakage; do not let sol come in contact with skin; if contact occurs, wash well with soap and water
- Administer **IV** after diluting 10 mg/10 ml NaCl; give through Y-tube or 3-way stopcock or directly over 1 min
- Hyaluronidase 150 U/ml in 1 ml NaCl, warm compress for extravasation for vesicant activity treatment

Syringe compatibilities:

Bleomycin, cisplatin, cyclophosphamide, droperidol, fluorouracil, leucovorin, methotrexate, metoclopramide, mitomycin, ondansetron, vincristine

Y-site compatibilities:

Bleomycin, cisplatin, cyclophosphamide, doxorubicin, droperidol, fluorouracil, heparin, leucovorin, methotrexate, metoclopramide, mitomycin, ondansetron, sargramostim vincristine

Y-site incompatibility:

Furosemide

Patient/family education

- Teach patient to avoid use of products containing aspirin or ibuprofen, razors, commercial mouthwash because bleeding may occur; to report symptoms of bleeding (hematuria, tarry stools)
- Instruct patient to report signs of anemia, (fatigue, headache, irritability, faintness, shortness of breath)
- Caution patient to report any changes in breathing or coughing even several mo after treatment
- Advise patient that contraception will be necessary during treatment; teratogenesis may occur
- Inform patient that hair may be lost during treatment; a wig or hairpiece may make patient feel better; new hair will be different in color, texture
- Advise patient to avoid vaccinations during treatment; serious reactions may occur
- Teach patient to report signs/symptoms of infection: fever, chills, sore throat; patient should avoid crowds and persons with known infections

Evaluation

Positive therapeutic outcome

- Decreased spread of malignant cells

vincristine (VCR)

(vin-kris'teen)

Oncovin, Vincasar PFS, vincristine sulfate

Func. class.: Antineoplastic

Chem. class.: Vinca alkaloid

Pregnancy category **D**

Action: Inhibits mitotic activity, arrests cell cycle at metaphase; inhibits RNA synthesis, blocks cellular use of glutamic acid needed for purine synthesis; a vesicant

Therapeutic Outcome: Prevention of rapid growth of malignant cells, immunosuppression

Uses: Breast, lung cancer; lymphomas; neuroblastomas; Hodgkin's disease; acute lymphoblastic and other leukemias; rhabdomyosarcoma, Wilms' tumor; osteogenic and other sarcomas

Dosage and routes

Adult: **IV** 1-2 mg/m^2/wk, not to exceed 2 mg

P *Child:* **IV** 1.5-2 mg/m^2/wk, not to exceed 2 mg

Available forms: Inj 1 mg/ml

Side effects/adverse reactions

CNS: Decreased reflexes, numbness, weakness, motor difficulties, CNS depression, cranial nerve paralysis, ***seizures***

CV: Orthostatic hypotension

GI: Nausea, vomiting, anorexia, stomatitis, constipation, ***paralytic ileus, abdominal pain, hepatotoxicity***

HEMA: Thrombocytopenia, leukopenia, myelosuppression, anemia

INTEG: Alopecia

Contraindications: Hypersensitivity, P infants, pregnancy **D**

Precautions: Renal disease, hepatic disease, hypertension, neuromuscular disease

Pharmacokinetics

Absorption	Complete bioavailability
Distribution	Rapidly, widely distributed; blood-brain barrier
Metabolism	Liver
Excretion	Biliary, in feces, crosses placenta
Half-life	Triphasic 0.85 min, 7.4 min, 1.64 min

Pharmacodynamics

	IV
Onset	Unknown
Peak	Unknown
Duration	1 wk

Interactions

Drug/drug:

Individual drugs

L-asparaginase: ↓ metabolism of vincristine

Mitomycin: ↑ bronchospasm

Radiation: ↑ toxicity, bone marrow suppression

Drug classifications

Antineoplastics: ↑ toxicity, bone marrow suppression

Live virus vaccines: ↓ antibody response

NURSING CONSIDERATIONS

Assessment

- Monitor CBC, differential, platelet count weekly; withhold drug if WBC is <4000 or platelet count is <75,000; notify prescriber of results; platelets may increase or decrease
- Assess neurologic status: paresthesia, weakness, cranial nerve palsies, orthostatic hypotension, lethargy, agitation,

psychosis; notify health care prescriber

- Monitor renal function studies: BUN, serum uric acid, urine CrCl before, during therapy; I&O ratio; report fall in urine output of 30 ml/hr; for decreased hyperuricemia, hyponatremia, and increased fluid retention (SIADH)
- Monitor for cold, fever, sore throat (may indicate beginning infection)
- Identify for increased uric acid levels, joint pain in extremities; increase fluid intake to 2-3 L/day unless contraindicated

Associated nursing diagnoses

✓ Injury, risk for (adverse reactions)
✓ Body image disturbance (adverse reactions)
✓ Infection, risk for (adverse reactions)
✓ Knowledge deficit (teaching)

Implementation

IV route

- Administer **IV** after diluting with diluent provided or 1 mg/10 ml of sterile H_2O or NaCl; give through Y-tube or 3-way stopcock or directly over 1 min
- Hyaluronidase 150 U/ml in 1 ml NaCl; apply warm compress for extravasation

Syringe compatibilities:

Bleomycin, cisplatin, cyclophosphamide, droperidol, fluorouracil, leucovorin, methotrexate, metoclopramide, mitomycin, ondansetron, vincristine

Syringe incompatibility:

Furosemide

Y-*site compatibilities:*

Bleomycin, cisplatin, cyclophosphamide, droperidol, fluorouracil, leucovorin, methotrexate, metoclopramide, mitomycin, ondansetron, sargramostim, vincristine

Y-*site incompatibility:*

Furosemide

Patient/family education

- Teach patient to avoid use of products containing aspirin or ibuprofen, razors, commercial mouthwash because bleeding may occur; to report symptoms of bleeding (hematuria, tarry stools)
- Instruct patient to report signs of anemia, (fatigue, headache, irritability, faintness, shortness of breath)
- Caution patient to report any changes in breathing or coughing, even several mo after treatment
- Advise patient that contraception will be necessary during treatment; teratogenesis may occur
- Inform patient that hair may be lost during treatment; a wig or hairpiece may make patient feel better; new hair will be different in color, texture
- Advise patient to avoid vaccinations during treatment; serious reactions may occur
- Teach patient to report signs/symptoms of infection: fever, chills, sore throat; patient should avoid crowds, or persons with known infections

Evaluation

Positive therapeutic outcome

- Decreased spread of malignancies

vinorelbine

(vi-nor′el-bine)

Navelbine

Func. class.: Antineoplastic

Chem. class.: Semisynthetic Vinca alkaloid

Pregnancy category **D**

Action: Inhibits mitotic activity, arrests cell cycle at metaphase; inhibits RNA synthesis, blocks cellular use of glutamic acid needed for purine synthesis; a vesicant

➡ **Therapeutic Outcome:** Decreased spread of malignancy

Uses: Breast cancer; unresectable, advanced non–small-cell lung cancer (NSCLC) stage IV; may be used alone or in combination with cisplatin for stage III or IV NSCLC

Dosage and routes

Adult: **IV** 30 mg/m^2 qwk

Breast cancer

Adult: **IV** 30 mg/m^2 qwk

Available forms: Inj **IV**, powder 10 mg for 10 ml **IV** inj

Side effects/adverse reactions

CNS: Paresthesias, peripheral neuropathy, depression, headache, ***convulsions,*** weakness, jaw pain

GI: Nausea, vomiting, ileus, *anorexia, stomatitis,* constipation, abdominal pain, GI, diarrhea, ***hepatotoxicity***

HEMA: Neutropenia, anemia, thrombocytopenia

INTEG: Rash, alopecia, photosensitivity

META: SIADH

MS: Myalgia

Contraindications: Hypersensitivity, P infants, pregnancy **D**

Precautions: Renal disease, hepatic disease

Pharmacokinetics	
Absorption	Poor bioavailability (<50%)
Distribution	Unknown
Metabolism	Liver—to metabolite
Excretion	Bile
Half-life	43 hr

Pharmacodynamics	IV
Onset	Unknown
Peak	1-2 hr
Duration	Unknown

Interactions

Drug/drug:

Individual drugs

Fluorouracil: ↑ toxicity a possibility

NURSING CONSIDERATIONS

Assessment

- Monitor B/P, (baseline and q15 min) during administration

• Monitor CBC, differential, platelet count weekly; withhold drug if WBC is <4000 or platelet count is <75,000; notify prescriber of results, recovery will take 3 wk
• Assess for dyspnea, rales, unproductive cough, chest pain, tachypnea
• Monitor renal function studies: BUN, serum uric acid, urine CrCl before, during therapy, I&O ratio; report fall in urine output of 30 ml/hr; for decreased hyperuricemia
• Monitor for cold, fever, sore throat (may indicate beginning infection); notify health care prescriber if these occur
• Assess for bleeding: hematuria, guaiac, bruising or petechiae, mucosa or orifices q8h: no rectal temp; avoid IM inj; use pressure to venipuncture sites
• Identify nutritional status: an antiemetic may need to be prescribed
• Assess for symptoms indicating severe allergic reactions: rash, pruritus, urticaria, itching, flushing, bronchospasm, hypotension; epinephrine and crash cart should be nearby

Associated nursing diagnoses

✓ Injury, risk for (adverse reactions)
✓ Body image disturbance (adverse reactions)
✓ Infection, risk for (adverse reactions)
✓ Knowledge deficit (teaching)

Implementation

IV **IV route**
• Hyaluronidase 150 U/ml in 1 ml NaCl, warm compress for extravasation for vesicant activity treatment
• Antacid before oral agent; give drug after evening meal before bedtime
• Antiemetic 30-60 min before giving drug and prn to prevent vomiting

Cont inf
• Give 40 mg/m^2 q 3 wk after **IV** Bol of 8 mg/m^2; may be given in combination with doxorubicin, fluorouracil, cisplatin

Patient/family education

• Teach patient to use liq diet: cola, Jell-O; dry toast or crackers may be added if patient is not nauseated or vomiting
• Advise patient to rinse mouth 3-4 × day with water and brush teeth 2-3 × day with soft brush or cotton-tipped applicators for stomatitis; use unwaxed dental floss
• Inform patient that a nutritious diet with iron, vitamin supplements is necessary

Evaluation

Positive therapeutic outcome
• Decreased spread of malignant cells

vitamin A

Aquasol A, Del-Vi-A, Vitamin A
Func. class.: Vitamin, fat-soluble
Chem. class.: Retinol
Pregnancy category **A**

V

Action: Needed for normal bone and tooth development, visual dark adaptation, skin disease, mucosa tissue repair, assists in production of adrenal steroids, cholesterol, RNA

Therapeutic Outcome: Prevention, absence of vitamin A deficiency

Uses: Vitamin A deficiency

Dosage and routes

P ***Adult and child >8 yr:*** PO 100,000-500,000 IU qd 3 days, then 50,000 qd × 2 wk; dose based on severity of deficiency; maintenance 10,000-20,000 IU for 2 mo

P ***Child 1-8 yr:*** IM 5,000-15,000 IU qd × 10 days

P ***Infants <1 yr:*** IM 5,000-15,000 IU × 10 days

Maintenance

P ***Child 4-8 yr:*** IM 15,000 IU qd × 2 mo

P ***Child <4 yr:*** IM 10,000 IU qd × 2 mo

Available forms: Cap 10,000, 25,000, 50,000 IU; drops 5000 IU; inj 50,000 IU/ml; tab 10,000, 25,000, 50,000 IU

Side effects/adverse reactions

CNS: Headache, increased intracranial pressure, intracranial hypertension, lethargy, malaise
EENT: Gingivitis, papilledema, exophthalmos, inflammation of tongue and lips
GI: Nausea, vomiting, anorexia, abdominal pain, ***jaundice***
INTEG: Drying of skin, pruritus, increased pigmentation, night sweats, alopecia
MS: Arthraglia, retarded growth, hard areas on bone
META: Hypomenorrhea, hypercalcemia

Contraindications: Hypersensitivity to Vit A, malabsorption syndrome (PO)

Precautions: Lactation, impaired renal function, pregnancy **A**

Pharmacokinetics

Absorption	Rapidly absorbed
Distribution	Stored in liver, kidneys, lungs
Metabolism	Liver
Excretion	Breast milk
Half-life	Unknown

Pharmacodynamics

	PO/IM
Onset	Unknown
Peak	Unknown
Duration	Unknown

Interactions

Drug/drug:

Individual drugs

Cholestyramine: ↓ absorption of Vitamin A
Colestipol: ↓ absorption of Vitamin A
Mineral oil: ↓ absorption of Vitamin A

Drug classifications

Corticosteroids: ↑ levels of Vitamin A
Oral contraceptives: ↑ level of Vitamin A

Lab test interferences

False increase: Bilirubin, serum cholesterol

NURSING CONSIDERATIONS

Assessment

- Assess nutritional status: increase intake of yellow and dark green vegetables, yellow/orange fruits, vitamin A-fortified foods, liver, egg yolks
- Assess vitamin A deficiency: decreased growth; night blindness; dry, brittle nails; hair loss; urinary stones; increased infection; hyperkeratosis of skin; drying of cornea
- Identify vitamin A deficiency by plasma vitamin A, carotene level
- Assess for chronic vitamin A toxicity: increased calcium, BUN, glucose, cholesterol, triglyceride level

Associated nursing diagnoses

✓ Nutrition: less than body requirements (uses)
✓ Knowledge deficit (teaching)

Implementation

PO route

- With food (PO) for better absorption; do not give **IV** because anaphylaxis may occur
- Store in tight, light-resistant container

Patient/family education

- Instruct patient that if dose is missed, it should be omitted
- Inform patient that ophth exams may be required periodically throughout therapy
- Instruct patient not to use mineral oil while taking this drug because absorption will be decreased
- Advise patient to notify a prescriber of nausea, vomiting, lip cracking, loss of hair, headache
- Caution patient not to take more than the prescribed amount

Evaluation

Positive therapeutic outcome

- Increase in growth rate, weight
- Absence of dry skin and mucous membranes, night blindness

Treatment of overdose: Discontinue drug

(vitamin B_{12}) cyanocobalamin/ (vitamin B_{12}a) hydroxocobalamin

(sye-an-oh-koe-bal′a-min)

Acti-B_{12} ✱, Alphamine, Anacobin ✱, Bedoz ✱, B_{12}, Resin, Cobex, Crystamine, Crysti-12, Cyanoject, Cyomin, Hydrobexan, Hydro Cobex, Rubesol-1000, Rubion ✱, Rubramin PC, Vitamin B_{12}

Func. class.: Vitamin B_{12}, water-soluble vitamin

Chem. class.:

Pregnancy category A

Action: Needed for adequate nerve functioning, protein and carbohydrate metabolism, normal growth, RBC development and cell reproduction

➔ **Therapeutic Outcome:** Prevention, correction of vitamin B_{12} deficiency

Uses: Vitamin B_{12} deficiency; pernicious anemia; Vitamin B_{12} malabsorption syndrome; Schilling test; increased requirements with pregnancy, thyrotoxicosis, hemolytic anemia, hemorrhage, renal and hepatic disease

Dosage and routes

Adult: PO 25 μg qd × 5-10 days, maintenance 100-200 mg IM qmo; IM/SC 30-100 μg qd × 5-10 days, maintenance 100-200 μg IM qmo

P *Child:* PO 1 μg qd × 5-10 days, maintenance 60 μg IM qmo or more; IM/SC 1-30 μg qd × 5-10 days, maintenance 60 μg IM qmo or more

Pernicious anemia/ malabsorption syndrome

Adult: IM 100-1000 μg qd × 2 wk, then 100-1000 μg IM qmo

P *Child:* IM 100-500 μg over 2 wk or more given in 100-500 μg doses, then 60 μg IM/SC monthly

Schilling test

P *Adult and child:* IM 1000 μg in one dose

Available forms: Tab 25, 50, 100, 250, 500, 1000 μg; inj 100, 120, 1000 μg/ml

Side efects/adverse reactions

CNS: Flushing, optic nerve atrophy

CV: CHF, peripheral vascular thrombosis, *pulmonary edema*

GI: Diarrhea

INTEG: Itching, rash, pain at site

META: Hypokalemia

SYST: Anaphylactic shock

Contraindications: Hypersensitivity, optic nerve atrophy

Precautions: Pregnancy **A,** P lactation, children, cardiac disease, uremia, iron deficiency, folic acid deficiency

Pharmacokinetics

Absorption	Well absorbed (IM, SC)
Distribution	Crosses placenta
Metabolism	Stored in liver, kidney, stomach
Excretion	50%-90% (urine), breast milk
Half-life	Unknown

Pharmacodynamics

	PO/IM/SC
Onset	Unknown
Peak	Unknown
Duration	Unknown

Interactions

Drug/drug:

Individual drugs

Alcohol: ↓ absorption

Aminosalicylic acid: ↓ absorption

Chloramphenicol: ↓ absorption

Cimetidine: ↓ absorption

Colchicine: ↓ absorption

Drug classifications

Aminoglycosides: ↓ absorption

Anticonvulsants: ↓ absorption

Potassium products: ↓ absorption

Lab test interferences

False positive: Intrinsic factor

NURSING CONSIDERATIONS

Assessment

- Assess for deficiency: anorexia, dyspepsia or exertion, palpitations, paresthesias, psychosis, visual disturbances, pallor, red inflamed tongue, neuropathy, edema of legs
- Monitor potassium levels during beginning treatment in patients with megaloblastic anemia
- Monitor CBC for increase in reticulocyte count during 1st wk of therapy, then increase in RBC and hemoglobin; folic acid levels, vitamin B_{12} levels
- Assess nutritional status: egg yolks, fish, organ meats, dairy products, clams, oysters, which are good sources for Vit B_{12}
- Monitor for pulmonary edema or worsening of CHF in cardiac patients

Associated nursing diagnoses

- ✓ Nutrition; less than body requirements (uses)
- ✓ Knowledge deficit (teaching)
- ✓ Noncompliance (teaching) (overuse)

Implementation

PO route

- Give with fruit juice to disguise taste; administer immediately after mixing
- Give with meals if possible for better absorption

IM route

- Give by IM inj for pernicious anemia for life unless contraindicated

IV **IV route**

- May be mixed with TPN sol, but **IV** route is not recommended

Y-site compatibilities: Heparin, hydrocortisone sodium succinate, potassium chloride

Solution compatibilities: Dextrose/Ringer's or lactated Ringer's combinations, dextrose/saline combinations, D_5W, $D_{10}W$, 0.45% NaCl, Ringer's or lactated Ringer's sol, ascorbic acid

Patient/family education

- Instruct patient that treatment must continue for life if diagnosed as having pernicious anemia
- Advise patient to eat well-balanced diet from the food pyramid and comply with dietary recommendation
- Caution patient not to exceed the RDA of vitamin B_{12} because adverse reactions may occur

Evaluation

Positive therapeutic outcome

- Decreased anorexia, dyspnea on exertion, palpitations, paresthesias, psychosis, visual disturbances, edema of legs
- Prevention or correction of vitamin B_{12} deficiency

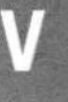

Treatment of overdose: Discontinue drug

vitamin D (cholecalciferol, vitamin D_3) ergocalciferol, (vitamin D_2)
Calciferol, Drisdol, Radiostol ♣, Radiostol Forte ♣, Delta-D, Vitamin D, Vitamin D_3
Func. class.: Vitamin D
Chem. class: Fat soluble
Pregnancy category: **A** (**D** if >RDA)

Action: Needed for regulation of calcium, phosphate levels; normal bone development; parathyroid activity; neuromuscular functioning

➔ **Therapeutic Outcome:** Prevention of rickets, osteomalacia, normal calcium/phosphate levels

Uses: Vitamin D deficiency, rickets, renal osteodystrophy, hypoparathyroidism, hypophosphatemia, psoriasis, rheumatoid arthritis

Dosage and routes

Deficiency

Adult: PO/IM 12,000 IU qd, then increased to 500,000 IU/day

P ***Child:*** PO/IM 1500/5000 IU qd × 2-4 wk, may repeat after 2 wk or 600,000 IU as single dose

Hypoparathyroidism

P ***Adult and child:*** PO/IM 200,000 IU given with 4 g calcium tab

Available forms: Tab 400, 1000, 50,000 IU; cap 25,000, 50,000; oral sol 8000 IU/ml; inj 500,000 IU/ml, 500,000 IU/5 ml

Side effects/adverse reactions

CNS: Fatigue, weakness, drowsiness, ***convulsions,*** headache, psychosis
CV: Hypertension, dysrhythmias
GI: Nausea, vomiting, anorexia, cramps, diarrhea, constipation, metallic taste, dry mouth, decreased libido
GU: Polyuria, nocturia, ***hematuria, albuminuria, renal failure***
INTEG: Pruritus, photophobia
MS: Decreased bone growth, early joint pain, early muscle pain

Contraindications: Hypersensitivity, hypercalcemia, renal dysfunction, hyperphosphatemia

Precautions: Cardiovascular disease, renal calculi, pregnancy **A**

Pharmacokinetics

Absorption	Well absorbed
Distribution	Stored in liver
Metabolism	Liver, sun
Excretion	Bile, kidney
Half-life	12-22 hr

Pharmacodynamics

	PO	IM
Onset	Unknown	Unknown
Peak	4 hr	Unknown
Duration	15-20 days	Unknown

Interactions

Drug/drug:

Individual drugs

Cholestyramine: ↓ absorption of vitamin D
Colestipol: ↓ absorption of vitamin D
Mineral oil: ↓ absorption of vitamin D

Drug classifications

Corticosteroids: ↓ effects
Cardiac glycosides: ↑ dysrhythmias
Diuretics, thiazide: ↑ hypercalcuria

Lab test interferences

False increase: Cholesterol

NURSING CONSIDERATIONS

Assessment

• Monitor BUN, urinary calcium, AST (SGOT), ALT (SGPT), cholesterol, creatinine, uric acid, chloride, magnesium, electrolytes, urine pH, phosphate—may increase; calcium should be kept at 9-10 mg/dl; vitamin D 50-135 IU/dl, phosphate 70 mg/dl; ALK phosphatase—may be decreased
• Monitor for increased blood level—toxic reactions may occur rapidly
• Assess for dry mouth, metallic taste, polyuria, bone pain, muscle weakness, headache, fatigue, tinnitus, change in LOC, irregular pulse, dysrhythmias, increased respirations, anorexia, nausea, vomiting, cramps, diarrhea, constipation—may indicate hypercalcemia
• Assess renal status: decreased urinary output (oliguria, anuria), edema in extremities, weight gain 5 lb, periorbital edema
• Assess nutritional status, diet for sources of vitamin D (milk, cod, halibut, salmon, sardines, egg yolk) calcium (dairy products, dark green vegetables), phosphates (dairy products)

Associated nursing diagnoses

✓ Nutrition, less than body requirements (uses)
✓ Knowledge deficit (teaching)

Implementation

PO route

• PO may be increased q4wk depending on blood level
• Store in airtight, light-resistant container at room temp

IM route

• Give deeply in large muscle mass, administer slowly, aspirate to avoid **IV** administration, rotate inj site

Patient/family education

• Advise patient to omit dose if missed; to avoid vitamin supplements unless directed by prescriber
• Inform patient of necessary foods to be included in diet
• Advise patient to keep appointments for evaluation because therapeutic and toxic levels are narrow
• Instruct patient to report weakness, lethargy, headache, anorexia, loss of weight; to report nausea, vomiting, abdominal cramps, diarrhea, constipation, excessive thirst, polyuria, muscle and bone pain

• Caution patient to decrease intake of antacids and laxatives containing magnesium

Evaluation

Positive therapeutic outcome
• Calcium levels 9-10 ml/dl
• Decreasing symptoms of bone disease

vitamin E

Amino-Opti-E, Aquasol E, Daltose ✤, E-Complex-600, E-Ferol, E-Vitamin Succinate, E-200 I.U. Softgels, Gordo-Vite E, Tocopherol, vitamin E, Vita-Plus E Softgells, Vitec

Func. class.: Vitamin E
Chem. class.: Fat soluble

Pregnancy category **A**

Action: Needed for digestion and metabolism of polyunsaturated fats, decreases platelet aggregation, decreases blood clot formation, promotes normal growth and development of muscle tissue, prostaglandin synthesis

➡ **Therapeutic Outcome:** Prevention and treatment of vitamin E deficiency

Uses: Vitamin E deficiency, impaired fat absorption, hemolytic anemia in premature neonates, prevention of retrolental fibroplasia, sickle cell anemia, supplement in malabsorption syndrome

Dosage and routes

Deficiency

Adult: PO 60-75 IU qd, not to exceed 300 IU/day

P *Child:* PO 1 mg/0.6 g of dietary fat

Prevention of deficiency

Adult: PO 30 u/day

Top

P *Adult and child:* Top apply to affected areas as needed

Available forms: Cap 100, 200, 400, 500, 600, 800 ✤, 1000 IU; tab 100, 200, 400 IU; drops 50 mg/ml; chew tab 400 U; ointment, cream, lotion, oil

Side effects/adverse reactions

CNS: Headache, fatigue
CV: Increased risk thrombophlebitis
EENT: Blurred vision
GI: Nausea, cramps, diarrhea
GU: Gonadal dysfunction
INTEG: Sterile abscess, contact dermatitis
META: Altered metabolism of hormones, thyroid, pituitary, adrenal, altered immunity
MS: Weakness

Contraindications: None significant

Precautions: Pregnancy **A**

Pharmacokinetics

Absorption	20%-80% (PO)
Distribution	Widely distributed, stored in fat
Metabolism	Liver
Excretion	Bile
Half-life	Unknown

Pharmacodynamics

	PO
Onset	Unknown
Peak	Unknown
Duration	Unknown

Interactions

Drug/drug:

Individual drugs

Cholestyramine: ↓ absorption
Colestipol: ↓ absorption
Mineral oil: ↓ absorption
Sucralfate: ↓ absorption

Drug classification

Oral anticoagulants: ↑ action of anticoagulants

NURSING CONSIDERATIONS

Assessment

- Monitor vitamin E levels during treatment
- Assess nutritional status: intake of wheat germ, dark green leafy vegetables, nuts, eggs, liver, vegetable oils, dairy products, cereals
- Assess for vitamin E deficiency (usually in neonates): irritability, restlessness, hemolytic anemia

Associated nursing diagnoses

✓ Nutrition: less than body requirements (uses)
✓ Knowledge deficit (teaching)

Implementation

PO route

- PO: administer with or pc
- Chewable tab: chew well
- Sol: may be dropped in mouth or mixed with food
- Store in tight, light-resistant container

Top route

- Apply top to moisturize dry skin

Patient/family education

- Inform patient necessary foods to be included in diet high in vitamin E
- Instruct patient to omit if dose missed
- Instruct patient to avoid vitamin supplements unless directed by prescriber because overdose may occur

Evaluation

Positive therapeutic outcome

- Absence of hemolytic anemia
- Adequate Vitamin E levels
- Improvement in skin lesions
- Decrease in edema

warfarin

(war'far-in)

Coumadin, Sofarin, warfarin sodium, Warfilone Sodium ✱

Func. class.: Anticoagulant
Chem. class:

Pregnancy category **D**

Action: Interferes with blood clotting by indirect means; depresses hepatic synthesis of Vitamin K-dependent coagulation factors (II, VII, IX, X)

➡ **Therapeutic Outcome:** Prevention of clotting

Uses: Pulmonary emboli, deep vein thrombosis, MI, atrial dysrhythmias, postcardiac valve replacement

Dosage and routes

Adult: PO 10-15 mg/day × 3 days, then titrated to prothrombin time qd

Available forms: Tab 1 mg, 2, 2.5, 5, 7.5, 10 mg; inj 50 mg/2 ml

Side effects/adverse reactions

CNS: Fever
GI: Diarrhea, nausea, vomiting, anorexia, stomatitis, cramps, ***hepatitis***
GU: Hematuria
HEMA: Hemorrhage, agranulocytosis, leukopenia, eosinophilia
INTEG: Rash, dermatitis, urticaria, alopecia, pruritus

Contraindications: Hypersensitivity, hemophilia, leukemia with bleeding, peptic ulcer disease, thrombocytopenic purpura, hepatic disease (severe), severe hypertension, subacute bacterial endocarditis, acute nephritis, blood dyscrasias, pregnancy **D**, eclampsia, preeclampsia, lactation

Precautions: Alcoholism, G elderly

Pharmacokinetics

Absorption	Well absorbed (PO), completely absorbed
Distribution	Crosses placenta, 99% plasma protein binding
Metabolism	Liver
Excretion	Kidney, feces (active, inactive metabolites)
Half-life	½-2½ days

Pharmacodynamics

	PO
Onset	12-24 hr
Peak	½-3 days
Duration	3-5 days

Lab test interferences

Increase: T_3 uptake
Decrease: Uric acid

NURSING CONSIDERATIONS

Assessment

- Monitor blood studies (Hct, occult blood in stools) q3mo; partial prothrombin time, which should be 1½-2 × control, PTT; often done qd, APTT, ACT; platelet count q2-3 days; thrombocytopenia may occur
- Monitor B/P, watch for increasing signs of hypertension
- Assess for bleeding: bleeding gums, petechiae, ecchymosis, black tarry stools, hematuria, epistaxis; decreased B/P may indicate bleeding and possible hemorrhage
- Assess for fever, skin rash, urticaria
- Assess for needed dosage change q1-2 wk

Associated nursing diagnoses

- ✓ Injury, risk for (uses, adverse reactions)
- ✓ Tissue perfusion, altered (uses)
- ✓ Knowledge deficit (teaching)

Implementation

PO route

- Warfarin is usually given with **IV** heparin for 3 or more days, warfarin blood level may take several days

IV **IV route**

- Protect from light, **IV** form is in short supply

Patient/family education

- Caution patient to avoid OTC preparations unless directed by prescriber—may cause serious drug interactions
- Advise patient that drug may be withheld during active bleeding (menstruation), depending on condition
- Advise patient to use soft-bristle toothbrush to avoid bleeding gums, avoid contact sports, use electric razor, avoid IM inj
- Instruct patient to carry a Medic-Alert ID identifying drug taken
- Advise patient to report any signs of bleeding: gums, under skin, urine, stools
- Teach patient to read food labels—limited intake of vitamin K foods is necessary to maintain consistent prothrombin levels

Evaluation

Positive therapeutic outcome

- Decrease of deep vein thrombosis
- Prothrombin time (1.3-2.0 × control)

xylometazoline

(xye-loe-met-az'oh-leen)

Otrivin, Otrivin Pediatric Nasal Drops, xylometazoline HCl

Func. class.: Nasal decongestant

Chem. class.: Sympathomimetic amine

Pregnancy category C

Action: Dilates arterioles of nasal membrane, which decreases congestion

Therapeutic Outcome: Absence of nasal congestion

Uses: Nasal congestion; adjunct in otitis media

Dosage and routes

Adult and child >12 yr: Instill 2-3 gtt or 2 sprays q8-10h (0.1%)

P ***Child <12 yr:*** Instill 2-3 gtt or 1% spray q8-10h (0.05%)

Available forms: Sol 0.05%, 0.1%

Side effects/adverse reactions

EENT: Irritation, burning, sneezing, stinging, dryness, rebound congestion

INTEG: Contact dermatitis

Contraindications: Hypersensitivity to sympathomimetic amines

Precautions: Pregnancy **C**, glaucoma

Pharmacokinetics	
Absorption	Unknown
Distribution	Unknown
Metabolism	Unknown
Excretion	Unknown
Half-life	Unknown

Pharmacodynamics	
Onset	5-10 min
Peak	Unknown
Duration	5-6 hr

X

NURSING CONSIDERATIONS

Assessment

- Assess for redness, swelling, pain in nasal passages before and during treatment
- Assess for systemic absorption: hypertension, tachycardia; notify prescriber; systemic absorption occurs at high doses or prolonged use

Associated nursing diagnoses)

✓ Airway clearance, ineffective (uses)
✓ Knowledge deficit (teaching)
✓ Noncompliance (teaching)

Implementation

Nasal route

- Have patient tilt head back, squeeze bulb to create a vacuum and draw correct amount of sol into dropper, insert 2 gtt of sol into nostril, repeat in other nostril
- Store in light-resistant container; do not expose to high temp or let sol come into contact with aluminum
- Give for <4 consecutive days
- Ensure environmental humidification to decrease nasal congestion, dryness

Patient/family education

- Advise patient that stinging may occur for several applications; drying of mucosa may be decreased by environmental humidification
- Caution patient to notify prescriber if irregular pulse, insomnia, dizziness, or tremors occur
- Teach patient proper administration to avoid systemic absorption
- Advise patient to rinse dropper with very hot water to prevent contamination

Evaluation

Positive therapeutic outcome

- Decreased nasal congestion

zalcitabine

(zal-sit'a-bin)
HIVID, ddC, Dideoxycitidine
Func. class.: Antiviral
Chem. class.: Synthetic pyrimidine nucleoside analog of 2′-deoxycytidine
Pregnancy category **C**

Action: Inhibits HIV replication by the conversion of this drug by cellular enzymes to an active antiviral metabolite

➡ **Therapeutic Outcome:** Improved symptoms of HIV infection

Uses: Advanced HIV infections in adults and children >13 yrs who have ben unable to use zidovudine or who have not responded to treatment

Dosage and routes

Adult: PO combined with zidovudine in advanced HIV infection: 0.75 mg administered concomitantly with 200 mg zidovudine q8h; dosage reduction not necessary for patients weighing >30 kg; in presence of peripheral neuropathy initiate dose at 0.375 mg q8h of zalcitabine

Available forms: Tab 0.375 and 0.75 mg

Side effects/adverse reactions

CNS: Headache, peripheral neuropathy, seizures, confusion, anxiety, hypertonia, abnormal thinking, asthenia, insomnia, CNS depression, pain, dizziness, chills, fever
CV: Hypertension, vasodilation, dysrhythmia, snycope, palpitation, tachycardia
EENT: Ear pain, otitis, photophobia, visual impairment
GI: Pancreatitis, diarrhea, nausea, vomiting, abdominal pain, constipation, stomatitis, dysplasia, liver abnormalities, oral ulcers, flatulence, taste perversion, dry mouth, oral thrush, melena, increased ALT (SGOT), AST (SGPT), alk phosphatase, amylase, increased bilirubin
GU: Uric acid, ***toxic nephropathy,*** polyuria
HEMA: ***Leukopenia, granulocytopenia, thrombocytopenia,*** anemia
INTEG: Rash, pruritus, alopecia, sweating, acne
MS: Myalgia, arthritis, myopathy, muscular atrophy
RESP: Cough, pneumonia, dyspnea, asthma, hypoventilation

Contraindications: Hypersensitivity

Precautions: Renal, hepatic disease, pregnancy **C,** lactation, P children (<13 yr), patients with peripheral neuropathy

Pharmacokinetics

Absorption	Minimally absorbed (PO)
Distribution	Unknown
Metabolism	Liver
Excretion	Unknown
Half-life	1.62 hr, increased in renal disease

Pharmacodynamics

	PO
Onset	Unknown
Peak	1½-2½
Duration	Unknown

Interactions

Drug/drug:

Individual drugs

Amphotericin B: ↑ neurotoxicity, nephrotoxicity
Interferon: ↑ neurotoxicity, nephrotoxicity
Methotretate: ↑ neurotoxicity, nephrotoxicity
Probenecid: ↑ neurotoxicity, nephrotoxicity

Drug classifications

Aminoglycosides: ↑ neurotoxicity, nephrotoxicity

NURSING CONSIDERATIONS

Assessment

- Assess for peripheral neuropathy: tingling or pain in hands and feet, distal numbness; if these occur during therapy, drug may be decreased or discontinued
- Assess for pancreatitis: abdominal pain, nausea, vomiting, elevated liver enzymes; drug should be discontinued because condition can be fatal
- P Assess children by dilated retinal examination q6mo to rule out retinal depigmentation
- Monitor CBC, differential,

platelet count qmo; withhold drug if WBC is <4000 or platelet count is <75,000; notify prescriber of results
• Monitor renal function studies; BUN, serum uric acid, urine CrCl before, during therapy; these may be elevated throughout treatment
• Monitor temp q4h, may indicate beginning infection
• Monitor liver function tests before, during therapy (bilirubin, AST (SGOT), ALT (SGPT), amylase, alk phosphatase as needed or qmo

Associated nursing diagnoses

✓ Infection, risk for (uses)
✓ Injury, risk for (adverse reactions)
✓ Knowledge deficit (teaching)

Implementation

PO route
• Give on empty stomach, q8h around the clock

Patient/family education

• Advise patient to take on empty stomach; not to take dapsone at same time as ddC; to use exactly as prescribed
• Instruct patient to report signs of infection: increased temp, sore throat, flu symptoms; to avoid crowds and those with known infections
• Caution patient to report signs of anemia; fatigue, headache, faintness, shortness of breath, irritability
• Advise patient to report bleeding; avoid use of razors or commercial mouthwash
• Inform patient that hair may be lost during therapy (rare); a wig or hairpiece may make patient feel better
• Caution patient to avoid OTC products or other medications without approval of prescriber
• Caution patient not to have any sexual contact without use of a condom, that needles should not be shared, that blood from infected individual should not come in contact with another's mucus membranes

Evaluation

Positive therapeutic outcome
• Absence of infection; symptoms of HIV

zidovudine

(zye-doe'vue-deen)
Apo-Zidovudine ♣, Azidothymidine, AZT, Novo-AZT ♣, Retrovir
Func. class.: Antiviral
Chem. class.: Thymidine analog
Pregnancy category **C**

Action: Inhibits replication of HIV by incorporating into cellular DNA by viral reverse transcriptase, thereby terminating the cellular DNA chain

Uses: Symptomatic HIV infections (AIDS, ARC), confirmed *P. carinii* pneumonia, or absolute CD4 lymphocytes <200/mm^3

Dosage and routes

Adult: PO 200 mg q4h; may

have to stop treatment if severe bone marrow depression occurs, and restart after bone marrow recovery; **IV** 1-2 mg/kg q4h initiate PO as soon as possible

Available forms: Cap 100 mg; Inj 200 mg/20 ml; oral syr 50 mg/5 ml

Side effects/adverse reactions

CNS: Fever, headache, malaise, diaphoresis, dizziness, *insomnia,* paresthesia, somnolence, chills, tremor, twitching, anxiety, confusion, depression, lability, vertigo, loss of mental acuity
EENT: Taste change, hearing loss, photophobia
GI: *Nausea,* vomiting, diarrhea, anorexia, cramps, *dyspepsia,* constipation, dysphagia, *flatulence,* rec bleeding, mouth ulcer
GU: Dysuria, polyuria, frequency, hesitancy
HEMA:* *Granulocytopenia, anemia
INTEG: Rash, acne, pruritus, urticaria
MS: Myalgia, arthralgia, muscle spasm
RESP: Dyspnea

Contraindications: Hypersensitivity

Precautions: Granulocyte count <1000/mm^3 or Hgb <9.5 g/dl, pregnancy **C**, lactation, P children, severe renal disease, severe hepatic function

Pharmacokinetics

Absorption	Well absorbed (PO), completely absorbed (IV)
Distribution	Widely distributed—crosses placenta, CSF
Metabolism	Liver—mostly
Excretion	Kidneys
Half-life	1 hr

Pharmacodynamics

	PO	IV
Onset	Unknown	Rapid
Peak	½-1½ hr	Inf end
Duration	Unknown	Unknown

Interactions

Drug/drug:

Individual drugs

Amphotericin B: ↑ neurotoxicity, nephrotoxicity
Interferon: ↑ neurotoxicity, nephrotoxicity
Methotretate: ↑ neurotoxicity, nephrotoxicity
Probenecid: ↑ neurotoxicity, nephrotoxicity

Drug classifications

Aminoglycosides: ↑ neurotoxicity, nephrotoxicity

NURSING CONSIDERATIONS

Assessment

- Assess for peripheral neuropathy: tingling or pain in hands and feet, distal numbness; if these occur, drug may be decreased or discontinued
- Assess for pancreatitis: abdominal pain, nausea, vomiting, elevated liver enzymes; drug should be discontinued because condition can be fatal
- P Assess children by dilated retinal examination q6mo to rule out retinal depigmentation

• Monitor CBC, differential, platelet count qmo; withhold drug if WBC is <4000 or platelet count is <75,000; notify prescriber of results
• Monitor renal function studies; BUN, serum uric acid, urine CrCl before, during therapy; these may be elevated throughout treatment
• Monitor temp q4h, may indicate beginning infection
• Monitor liver function tests before, during therapy (bilirubin, AST (SGOT), ALT (SGPT)) amylase, alkaline phosphatase prn or qmo

Associated nursing diagnoses

✓ Infection, risk for (uses)
✓ Injury, risk for physical injury (adverse reactions)
✓ Knowledge deficit (teaching)

Implementation

PO route
• Give on empty stomach, q4h around the clock

IV **IV route**
• Give by intermittent inf after diluting with D_5W. Give over 1 hr (<4 mg/ml), do not give by direct **IV**

Y-site compatibilities:

Acyclovir, amikacin, amphotericin B, aztreonam, ceftazidine, ceftriaxone, cimetidine, clindamycin, dexamethasone, dobutamine, dopamine, erythromycin lactobionate, fluconazole, fludarabine, gentamicin, heparin, imipenem/cilastatin, lorazepam, metoclopramide, morphine, nafcillin, ondansetron, oxacillin, pentamidine, phenylephrine, piperacillin, potassium chloride, ranitidine, sargramostim, tobramycin, trimethoprim-sulfamethoxazole, vancomycin

Additive incompatibilities:

Blood products or protein solutions

Patient/family education

• Caution patient to take on empty stomach; not to take dapsone at same time as ddl; to use exactly as prescribed
• Advise patient to report signs of infection: increased temp, sore throat, flu symptoms; to avoid crowds and those with known infections
• Instruct patient to report signs of anemia: fatigue, headache, faintness, shortness of breath, irritability
• Advise patient to report bleeding; avoid use of razors or commercial mouthwash
• Inform patient that hair may be lost during therapy (rare); a wig or hairpiece may make patient feel better
• Caution patient to avoid OTC products or other medications without approval of prescriber
• Caution patient not to have any sexual contact without use of a condom, needles should not be shared, blood from infected individual should not come in contact with another's mucus membranes

Evaluation

Positive therapeutic outcome
• Decreased infection; symptoms of HIV

zinc sulfate

Orazinc, PMS Egozine ♣, Verazinc, Zinca-Pak, Zincate, Zinc 15, Zinc-220, zinc sulfate

Func. class.: Trace element; nutritional supplement

Pregnancy category A

Action: Needed for adequate healing, bone and joint development, taste and smell (23% zinc)

➔ Therapeutic Outcome: Replacement of zinc

Uses: Prevention of zinc deficiency, adjunct to Vitamin A therapy

Investigational uses: Wound healing

Dosage and routes

Dietary supplement

Adult: PO 25-50 mg/day

***Nutritional supplement* (IV)**

Adult: 2.5-4 mg/day, may increase by 2 mg/day if needed

P *Child to 5 yr:* **IV** 100 μg/kg/day

P *Infants: <1500 gm to 3 kg;* **IV** 300 μg/kg/day

Available forms: Tab 66, 110 mg; cap 220 mg; inj 1 mg, 5 mg/ml

Side effects/adverse reactions

GI: Nausea, vomiting, cramps, heartburn, ulcer formation

OVERDOSE: Diarrhea, rash, dehydration, restlessness

Precautions: Pregnancy **A**

Pharmacokinetics

Absorption	Poorly absorbed (PO), completely absorbed (IV)
Distribution	Widely distributed
Metabolism	Liver
Excretion	90%—feces, 10%—kidneys
Half-life	Unknown

Pharmacodynamics

	PO/IV
Onset	Unknown
Peak	Unknown
Duration	Unknown

Interactions

Drug/drug:

Individual drugs

Tetracycline: ↓ absorption of tetracycline

NURSING CONSIDERATIONS

Assessment

- Monitor zinc levels during treatment

Associated nursing diagnoses

✓ Nutrition: less than body requirements (uses)

✓ Knowledge deficit (teaching)

Implementation

PO route

- Give with meals to decrease gastric upset; restrict dairy products, caffeine, which decrease absorption

IV route

- Part of total parenteral nutrition (TPN)

Patient/family education

- Inform patient that element must be taken for 2 mo to be effective
- Advise patient to report immediately nausea, diarrhea, rash, severe vomiting, restlessness, abdominal pain, tarry stools

Evaluation

Positive therapeutic outcome

- Absence of zinc deficiency
- Improved wound healing

zolpidem

(zole-pi′dem)

Ambien

Func. class.: Sedative-hypnotic

Chem. class.: Nonbenzodiazepine of imidazopyridine class

Pregnancy category B

Action: Produces CNS depression at limbic, thalamic, hypothalamic levels of CNS; may be mediated by neurotransmitter aminobutyric acid (GABA); results are sedation, hypnosis, skeletal muscle relaxation, anticonvulsant activity, anxiolytic action

Therapeutic Outcome: Ability to sleep, sedation

Uses: Insomnia, short-term treatment

Dosage and routes

Adult: PO 10 mg hs × 7-10 days only; total dose should not exceed 10 mg

Available forms: Tab 5 mg, 10 mg

Side effects/adverse reactions

CNS: *Headache, lethargy, drowsiness, daytime sedation, dizziness, confusion, lightheadedness, anxiety, irritability, amnesia, poor coordination*

CV: *Chest pain, palpitation*

GI: *Nausea, vomiting, diarrhea, heartburn, abdominal pain, constipation*

Contraindications: Hypersensitivity to benzodiazepines

Precautions: Anemia, hepatic disease, renal disease, suicidal individuals, drug abuse, elderly, psychosis, child <18 yr, seizure disorders, pregnancy **B**, lactation

Pharmacokinetics

Absorption	Rapidly absorbed (PO)
Distribution	Unknown
Metabolism	Liver—inactive metabolite
Excretion	Kidneys, breast milk
Half-life	2½ hr, increased in elderly

Pharmacodynamics

	PO
Onset	Unknown
Peak	Unknown
Duration	Unknown

Interactions

Drug/drug:

Individual drugs

Alcohol: ↑ CNS depression
Fluoxetine: ↑ action
Propoxyphene: ↑ action

Drug classifications

Analgesics, opioid: ↑ CNS depression
Antidepressants: ↑ CNS depression
Antihistamines: ↑ CNS depression
Sedative/hypnotics: ↑ CNS depression

Drug/food:

↓ absorption

Lab test interferences

Increase: ALT (SGPT), AST (SGOT), serum bilirubin
Decrease: RAI uptake
False increase: Urinary 17-OHCS

NURSING CONSIDERATIONS

Assessment

- Assess mental status: mood, sensorium, anxiety, affect, sleeping pattern, drowsiness, G dizziness, especially elderly; physical dependency, withdrawal symptoms: anxiety, panic attacks, agitation, convulsions, headache, nausea, vomiting, muscle pain, weakness; suicidal tendencies; for indications of increasing tolerance and abuse
- Monitor B/P (lying, standing), pulse; if systolic B/P drops 20 mm Hg, hold drug, notify prescriber
- Monitor blood studies: CBC during long-term therapy; blood dycrasias have occurred rarely; decreased hematocrit, neutropenia may occur
- Monitor hepatic studies: AST (SGOT), ALT (SGPT), bilirubin, creatinine LDH, alk phosphatase
- Monitor I&O for renal dysfunction

Associated nursing diagnoses

✓ Anxiety (uses)
✓ Depression (uses)
✓ Injury, risk for (adverse reactions)
✓ Knowledge deficit (teaching)

Implementation

PO route

- Give ½-1 hr before hs for sleeplessness; give several hr before patient is to arise (to avoid hangover)
- Store in tight container in cool environment

Patient/family education

- Instruct patient that drug may be taken with food, or fluids and tab may be crushed or swallowed whole
- Caution patient not to use for everyday stress or longer than 3 mo unless directed by prescriber; not to take more than prescribed amount; may be habit forming; not to double or skip doses
- Caution patient to avoid OTC preparations unless approved by health care prescriber; alcohol and CNS depressants will increase CNS depression
- Advise patient to avoid driving, activities that require alertness, because drowsiness may occur; to avoid alcohol ingestion or other psychotropic

medications; to rise slowly or fainting may occur, especially elderly; that drowsiness may worsen at beginning of treatment

• Instruct patient not to discontinue medication abruptly after long-term use; withdrawal symptoms include vomiting, cramping, tremors, seizures

Evaluation

Positive therapeutic outcome

• Ability to sleep at night

• Decreased amount of early morning awakening if taking drug for insomnia

Treatment of overdose:

Lavage, VS, supportive care

SECTION III

DRUG CATEGORIES

ALPHA-ADRENERGIC BLOCKERS

Action: Binds to α-adrenergic receptors, causing dilatation of peripheral blood vessels; lowers peripheral resistance, resulting in decreased blood pressure.
Uses: Used for pheochromocytoma, prevention of tissue necrosis, and sloughing associated with extravasation of IV vasopressors.
Side effects/adverse reactions: The most common side effects are hypotension, tachycardia, nasal stuffiness, nausea, vomiting, and diarrhea.
Contraindications: Hypersensitive reactions may occur, and allergies should be identified before these products are given. Patients with myocardial infarction, coronary insufficiency, angina, or other evidence of coronary artery disease should not use these products.
Pharmacokinetics: Onset, peak, and duration vary among products.
Interactions: Vasoconstrictive and hypertensive effects of epinephrine are antagonized by α-adrenergic blockers.

NURSING CONSIDERATIONS

Assessment

- Monitor electrolytes: potassium, sodium chloride, carbon dioxide
- Monitor weight daily, I&O
- Monitor B/P with patient lying, standing before starting treatment, q4h thereafter
- Assess for nausea, vomiting, diarrhea
- Assess for skin turgor, dryness of mucous membranes for hydration status

Associated nursing diagnoses

✓ Altered tissue perfusion (uses)
✓ Risk for injury (adverse reactions)
✓ Sleep pattern disturbance (adverse reactions)

Implementation

PO Route

- Start with low dose, gradually increasing to prevent side effects
- Give with food or milk for GI symptoms

Evaluation

- Therapeutic response: decreased B/P, increased peripheral pulses

Patient/family education

- Caution patient to avoid alcoholic beverages
- Advise patient to report dizziness, palpitations, fainting

- Instruct patient to change position slowly or fainting may occur
- Teach patient to take drug exactly as prescribed; to avoid all OTC products (cough, cold, allergy) unless directed by prescriber

Generic Names

phenoxybenzamine (p. 1095) phentolamine (p. 1097)

ANESTHETICS—GENERAL/LOCAL

Action: Anesthetics (general) act on the CNS to produce tranquilization and sleep before invasive procedures. Anesthetics (local) inhibit conduction of nerve impulses from sensory nerves.

Uses: General anesthetics are used to premedicate for surgery, and for induction and maintenance in general anesthesia. For local anesthetics, refer to individual product listing for indications.

Side effects/adverse reactions: The most common side effects are dystonia, akathisia, flexion of arms, fine tremors, drowsiness, restlessness, and hypotension. Also common are chills, respiratory depression, and laryngospasm.

Contraindications: Persons with CVA, increased intracranial pressure, severe hypertension, cardiac decompensation should not use these products, since severe adverse reactions can occur.

G **Precautions:** Anesthetics (general) should be used with caution in the elderly, cardiovascular disease (hypotension, bradydysrhythmias), renal
P disease, liver disease, Parkinson's disease, children <2 yr. The precaution for anesthetics (local) is pregnancy.

Pharmacokinetics: Onset, peak, and duration vary widely among products. Most products are metabolized in the liver and excreted in urine.

Interactions: MAOIs, tricyclics, phenothiazines may cause severe hypotension or hypertension when used with local anesthetics. CNS depressants will potentiate general and local anesthetics.

NURSING CONSIDERATIONS

Assessment

- Monitor VS q10 min during IB administration, q30 min after IM dose

Associated nursing diagnoses

General

✓ Risk for injury (adverse reactions)

✓ Knowledge deficit (teaching)

Local

✓ Pain (uses)

✓ Knowledge deficit (teaching)

Implementation

- Give anticholinergic preoperatively to decrease secretions
- Administer only with crash cart, resuscitative equipment nearby
- Provide quiet environment for recovery to decrease psychotic symptoms

Evaluation

- Therapeutic response: maintenance of anesthesia, decreased pain

---

Generic Names

General anesthetics:
droperidol (p. 511)
fentanyl citrate (p. 581)
  fentanyl citrate/droperidol
ketamine (p. 777)
methohexital (p. 884)
tetracaine (p. 1309)

Local anesthetics:
🔑 lidocaine HCl (p. 805)
midazolam (p. 925)
propofol (p. 1174)
thiopental (p. 1323)

ANTACIDS

Action: Antacids are basic compounds that neutralize gastric acidity and decrease the rate of gastric emptying. Products are divided into those containing aluminum, magnesium, calcium, or a combination of these.

Uses: Hyperacidity is decreased by antacids in conditions such as peptic ulcer disease, reflux esophagitis, gastritis, or hiatal hernia.

Side effects/adverse reactions: The most common side effect caused by aluminum-containing antacids is constipation, which may lead to fecal impaction and bowel obstruction. Diarrhea occurs often when magnesium products are given. Alkalosis may occur when systemic products are used. Constipation occurs more frequently than laxation with calcium carbonate. The release of CO_2 from carbonate-containing antacids causes belching, abdominal distention, and flatulence. Sodium bicarbonate may act as a systemic antacid and produce systemic electrolyte disturbances and alkalosis. Calcium carbonate and sodium bicarbonate may cause rebound hyperacidity and milk-alkali syndrome. Alkaluria may occur when products are used on a long-term basis, particularly in persons with abnormal renal function.

Contraindications: Sensitivity to aluminum or magnesium products may cause hypersensitive reactions. Aluminum products should not be used by persons sensitive to aluminum; magnesium products should not be used by persons sensitive to magnesium. Check for sensitivity before administering.

Precautions: Magnesium products should be given cautiously to patients with renal insufficiency and during pregnancy and lactation. Sodium content of antacids may be significant; use with caution for patients with hypertension, CHF, or those on a low-sodium diet.

Pharmacokinetics: Duration is 20-40 min. If ingested 1 hr pc, acidity is reduced for at least 3 hr.

Interactions: Drugs whose effects may be increased by some antacids: quinidine, amphetamines, pseudoephedrine, levodopa, valproic acid, dicumarol. Drugs whose effects may be decreased by some antacids: cimetadine, corticosteroids, ranitidine, iron salts, phenothiazines, phenytoin, digoxin, tetracyclines, ketoconazole, salicylates, isoniazid.

NURSING CONSIDERATIONS

Assessment

- Assess for aggravating and alleviating factors of epigastric pain or hyperacidity; identify the location, duration, and characteristics of epigastric pain
- Assess GI symptoms, including constipation, diarrhea, abdominal pain; if severe abdominal pain with fever occurs, these drugs should not be given
- Assess renal symptoms, including increasing urinary pH, electrolytes

Associated nursing diagnoses

- ✓ Pain (uses)
- ✓ Constipation (adverse reactions)
- ✓ Diarrhea (adverse reactions)

Implementation

- Give all products with an 8-oz glass of water to ensure absorption in the stomach
- Give another antacid if constipation occurs with aluminum products

Evaluation

- Therapeutic response: absence of epigastric pain, decreased acidity

Patient/family education

- Advise patient not to take other drugs within 1-2 hr of antacid administration, since antacids may impair absorption of other drugs

Generic Names

aluminimum hydroxide (p. 93)
bismuth subsalicylate (p. 210)
calcium carbonate (p. 245)
magaldrate (p. 837)
magnesium oxide (p. 839)
sodium bicarbonate (p. 1245)

ANTIANGINALS

Action: The antianginals are divided into the nitrates, calcium channel blockers, and β-adrenergic blockers. The nitrates dilate coronary arteries, causing decreased preload, and dilate systemic arteries, causing decreased afterload. Calcium channel blockers dilate coronary arteries, decrease SA/AV node conduction. β-Adrenergic blockers decrease heart rate so that myocardial O_2 use is decreased. Dipyridamole selectively dilates coronary arteries to increase coronary blood flow.

Uses: Antianginals are used in chronic stable angina pectoris, unstable angina, vasospastic angina. Some (i.e., calcium channel blockers and β-blockers) may be used as dysrhythmias and in hypertension.

Side effects/adverse reactions: The most common side effects are postural hypotension, headache, flushing, dizziness, nausea, edema, and drowsiness. Also common are rash, dysrhythmias, and fatigue.

Contraindications: Persons with known hypersensitivity, increased intracranial pressure, or cerebral hemorrhage should not use some of these products.

Precautions: Antianginals should be used with caution in postural P hypotension, pregnancy, lactation, children, renal disease, and hepatic injury.

Pharmacokinetics: Onset, peak, and duration vary widely among coronary products. Most products are metabolized in the liver and excreted in urine.

Interactions: Please check individual monographs, since interactions vary widely among products.

NURSING CONSIDERATIONS

Assessment

- Orthostatic B/P, pulse

- Assess for pain: duration, time started, activity being performed, character
- Assess for tolerance if taken over long period
- Assess for headache, lightheadedness, decreased B/P; may indicate a need for decreased dosage

Associated nursing diagnoses

- ✓ Altered tissue perfusion: cardiopulmonary (uses)
- ✓ Pain (uses)
- ✓ Risk for injury (uses)
- ✓ Knowledge deficit (teaching)
- ✓ Decreased cardiac output (adverse reactions)

Implementation

- Store protected from light, moisture; place in cool environment

Evaluation

- Therapeutic response: decreased, prevention of anginal pain

Patient/family education

- Instruct patient to keep tabs in original container
- Instruct patient not to use OTC products unless directed by prescriber
- Advise patient to report bradycardia, dizziness, confusion, depression, fever
- Teach patient to take pulse at home; advise when to notify prescriber
- Advise patient to avoid alcohol, smoking, sodium intake
- Advise patient to comply with weight control, dietary adjustments, modified exercise program
- Teach patient to carry Medic Alert ID to identify drug being taken, allergies
- Caution to make position changes slowly to prevent fainting

Generic Names

Nitrates:

amyl nitrite (p. 146)
isosorbide (p. 766)
🔑 nitroglycerin (p. 998)

β-adrenergic blockers:

atenolol (p. 162)
dipyridamole (p. 484)
metoprolol (p. 912)

Calcium channel blockers:

amlodipine (p. 119)
bepridil (p. 197)
diltiazem (p. 470)
nadolol (p. 960)
nicardipine (p. 989)
nifedipine (p. 994)
🔑 propranolol (p. 1178)
🔑 verapamil (p. 1399)

ANTICHOLINERGICS

Action: Anticholinergics inhibit the muscarinic actions of acetylcholine at receptor sites in the autonomic nervous system; anticholinergics are also known as antimuscarinic drugs.

Uses: Anticholinergics are used for a variety of conditions: gastrointestinal anticholinergics are used to decrease motility (smooth muscle tone) in the GI, biliary, and urinary tracts and for their ability to decrease gastric secretions (propantheline, glycopyrrolate); decreasing involuntary movements in parkinsonism (benztropine, trihexyphenidyl); bradydysrhythmias (atropine); nausea and vomiting (scopolamine); and as cycloplegic mydriatics (atropine, hematropine, scopalamine, cyclopentolate, tropicamide).

Side effects/adverse reactions: The most common side effects are dry mouth, constipation, urinary retention, urinary hesitancy, headache, and dizziness. Also common is paralytic ileus.

Contraindications: Persons with narrow angle glaucoma, myasthenia gravis, or GI/GU obstruction should not use some of these products.

Precautions: Anticholinergics should be used with caution in patients G who are elderly, pregnant, or lactating or in those with prostatic hypertrophy, CHF, or hypertension; use with caution in presence of high environmental temp.

Pharmacokinetics: Onset, peak, and duration vary widely among products. Most products are metabolized in the liver and excreted in urine.

Interactions: Increased anticholinergic effects may occur when used with MAOIs and tricyclic antidepressants and amantadine. Anticholinergics may cause a decreased effect of phenothiazines and levodopa.

NURSING CONSIDERATIONS

Assessment

- Assess I&O ratio; retention commonly causes decreased urinary output
- Assess for urinary hesitancy, retention; palpate bladder if retention occurs
- Assess for constipation; increase fluids, bulk, exercise if this occurs
- Identify tolerance over long-term therapy; dosage may need to be increased or changed
- Assess mental status: affect, mood, CNS depression, worsening of mental symptoms during early therapy

Associated nursing diagnoses

✓ Decreased cardiac output (uses)

✓ Constipation (adverse reactions)
✓ Knowledge deficit (teaching)

Implementation

IV IM/IV Routes

- Give parenteral dose with patient recumbent to prevent postural hypotension
- Give parenteral dose slowly; keep in bed for at least 1 hr after dose; monitor VS
- Give after checking dose carefully; even slight overdose could lead to toxicity

PO Route

- Give with or after meals to prevent GI upset; may give with fluids other than water
- Store at room temp
- Give hard candy, frequent drinks, sugarless gum to relieve dry mouth

Evaluation

- Therapeutic response: decreased secretions, absence of nausea and vomiting

Patient/family education

- Caution patient to avoid driving and other hazardous activities; drowsiness may occur
- Advise patient to avoid OTC medication: cough, cold preparations with alcohol, antihistamines unless directed by prescriber

---

Generic Names

🔑 atropine (p. 169)
🔑 benztropine (p. 194)
biperiden (p. 206)
glycopyrrolate (p. 653)
propantheline (p. 1172)
scopolamine (p. 1230)
trihexyphenidyl (p. 1377)

ANTICOAGULANTS

Action: Anticoagulants interfere with blood clotting by preventing clot formation.

Uses: Anticoagulants are used for deep vein thrombosis, pulmonary emboli, myocardial infarction, open heart surgery, disseminated intravascular clotting syndrome, atrial fibrillation with embolization, and in transfusion and dialysis.

Side effects/adverse reactions: The most serious adverse reactions are hemorrhage, agranulocytosis, leukopenia, eosinophilia, and thrombocytopenia, depending on the specific product. The most common side effects are diarrhea, rash, and fever.

Contraindications: Persons with hemophilia, leukemia with bleeding, peptic ulcer disease, thrombocytopenic purpura, blood dyscrasias, acute nephritis, and subacute bacterial endocarditis should not use these products.

G **Precautions:** Anticoagulants should be used with caution in alcoholism, elderly, and pregnancy.

Pharmacokinetics: Onset, peak, and duration vary widely among products. Most products are metabolized in the liver and excreted in urine.

Interactions: Salicylates, steroids, and nonsteroidal antiinflammatories will potentiate the action of anticoagulants. Anticoagulants may cause serious effects; please check individual monographs.

NURSING CONSIDERATIONS

Assessment

- Monitor blood studies (Hct, platelets, occult blood in stools) q3 mo
- Monitor partial prothrombin time, which should be 1½-2 × control, PPT; often qd, APTT, ACT
- Monitor B/P; watch for increasing signs of hypertension
- Monitor for bleeding gums, petechiae, ecchymosis, black tarry stools, hematuria
- Monitor for fever, skin rash, urticaria
- Monitor for needed dosage change q1-2wk

Associated nursing diagnoses

✓ Altered tissue perfusion (uses)
✓ Risk for injury (side effects)
✓ Knowledge deficit (teaching)

Implementation

SC Route

- Give at same time each day to maintain steady blood levels
- Do not massage area or aspirate when giving SC inj; give in abdomen between pelvic bones; rotate sites; do not pull back on plunger, leave in for 10 sec; apply gentle pressure for 1 min

- Do not change needles
- Avoid all IM inj that may cause bleeding
- Store in tight container (PO dose)

Evaluation

- Therapeutic response: decrease of deep vein thrombosis

Patient/family education

- Advise patient to avoid OTC preparations that may cause serious drug interactions unless directed by prescriber
- Inform patient that drug may be held during active bleeding (menstruation), depending on condition
- Caution patient to use soft-bristle toothbrush to avoid bleeding gums; avoid contact sports; use electric razor
- Instruct patient to carry a Medic-Alert ID identifying drug taken
- Instruct patient to report any signs of bleeding: gums, under skin, urine, stools

---

Generic Names

enoxaparin (p. 525)
🗝 heparin (p. 681)
🗝 warfarin (p. 1415)

ANTICONVULSANTS

Action: Anticonvulsants are divided into the barbiturates (p. 1466), benzodiazepines (p. 1468), hydantoins, succinimides, and miscellaneous products. Barbiturates and benzodiazepines are discussed in separate sections. Hydantoins act by inhibiting the spread of seizure activity in the motor cortex. Succinimides act by inhibiting spike and wave formation; they also decrease amplitude, frequency, duration, and spread of discharge in seizures.

Uses: Hydantoins are used in generalized tonic-clonic seizures, status epilepticus, and psychomotor seizures. Succinimides are used for absence of (petit mal) seizures. Barbiturates are used in generalized tonic-clonic and cortical focal seizures.

Side effects/adverse reactions: Bone marrow depression is the most life-threatening adverse reaction associated with hydantoins or succinimides. The most common side effects are GI symptoms. Other common side effects for hydantoins are gingival hyperplasia and CNS effects such as nystagmus, ataxia, slurred speech, and confusion.

Contraindications: Hypersensitive reactions may occur, and allergies should be identified before these products are given.

Precautions: Persons with renal or hepatic disease should be watched closely.
Pharmacokinetics: Onset, peak, and duration vary widely among products. Most products are metabolized in the liver and excreted in urine, bile, and feces.
Interactions: Decreased effects of estrogens, oral contraceptives (hydantoins).

NURSING CONSIDERATIONS

Assessment

- Monitor renal function studies, including BUN, creatinine, serum uric acid, urine creatinine clearance before and during therapy
- Monitor blood studies: RBC, Hct, Hgb, reticulocyte counts weekly for 4 wk then monthly
- Monitor hepatic studies: AST (SGOT), ALT (SGPT), bilirubin, creatinine
- Assess mental status, including mood, sensorium, affect, behavioral changes; if mental status changes, notify prescriber
- Assess for eye problems, including need for ophth examinations before, during, and after treatment (slit lamp, fundoscopy, tonometry)
- Assess for allergic reaction, including red raised rash; if this occurs, drug should be discontinued
- Assess for blood dyscrasias, including fever, sore throat, bruising, rash, jaundice
- Monitor toxicity, including bone marrow depression, nausea, vomiting, ataxia, diplopia, cardiovascular collapse, Stevens-Johnson syndrome

Associated nursing diagnoses

✓ Risk for injury (uses)
✓ Noncompliance (teaching)
✓ Sleep pattern disturbance (adverse reactions)

Implementation

PO Route

- Give with food, milk to decrease GI symptoms
- Good oral hygiene is important for patients taking hydantoins

Evaluation

- Therapeutic response, including decreased seizure activity; document on patient's chart

Patient/family education

- Advise patient to carry ID card or Medic Alert bracelet stating drugs taken, condition, prescriber's name, phone number
- Advise patient to avoid driving, other activities that require alertness

---

Generic Names

Hydantoins:
phenytoin (p. 1102)

Succinimides:
ethosuximide (p. 556)

Miscellaneous:
acetazolamide (p. 56)
carbamazepine (p. 252)
clonazepam (p. 380)
diazepam (p. 444)
felbamate (p. 574)
magnesium sulfate (p. 839)

Barbiturates:
amobarbital (p. 121)
phenobarbital (p. 1090)
primidone (p. 1149)
thiopental (p. 1323)

ANTIDEPRESSANTS

Action: Antidepressants are divided into the tricyclics, MAOIs, and miscellaneous antidepressants. The tricyclics work by blocking reuptake of norepinephrine and serotonin into nerve endings and increasing action of norepinephrine and serotonin in nerve cells. MAOIs act by increasing concentrations of endogenous epinephrine, norepinephrine, serotonin, dopamine in storage sites in CNS by inhibition of MAO; increased concentration reduces depression.

Uses: Antidepressants are used for depression and in some cases P enuresis in children.

Side effects/adverse reactions: The most serious adverse reactions are paralytic ileus, acute renal failure, hypertension, and hypertensive crisis, depending on the specific product. Common side effects are dizziness, drowsiness, diarrhea, dry mouth, urinary retention, and orthostatic hypotension.

Contraindications: The contraindications for antidepressants are convulsive disorders, prostatic hypertrophy, severe renal, hepatic, cardiac disease depending on the type of medication.

Precautions: Antidepressants should be used cautiously in suicidal patients, severe depression, schizophrenia, hyperactivity, diabetes mel-G litus, pregnancy, and the elderly.

Pharmacokinetics: Onset, peak, and duration vary widely among products. Most products are metabolized in the liver and excreted in urine.

Interactions: Please check individual monographs, since interactions vary widely among products.

NURSING CONSIDERATIONS

Assessment

- Monitor B/P (lying, standing), pulse q4h; if systolic B/P drops 20 mm Hg, hold drug, notify prescriber; take VS q4h in patients with cardiovascular disease
- Monitor blood studies: CBC, leukocytes, differential, cardiac enzymes if patient is receiving long-term therapy
- Monitor hepatic studies: AST (SGOT), ALT (SGPT), bilirubin, creatinine
- Monitor weight weekly; appetite may increase with drug
- G Monitor for EPS primarily in elderly: rigidity, dystonia, akathisia
- Assess mental status: mood, sensorium, affect, suicidal tendencies, increase in psychiatric symptoms (depression, panic)
- P G Check for urinary retention, constipation; constipation is more likely to occur in children, elderly
- Assess for withdrawal symptoms: headache, nausea, vomiting, muscle pain, weakness; do not usually occur unless drug was discontinued abruptly
- Identify alcohol consumption; if alcohol is consumed, hold dose until AM

Associated nursing diagnoses

✓ Ineffective individual coping (uses)
✓ Risk for injury (uses/adverse reactions)
✓ Knowledge deficit (teaching)

Implementation

PO Route

- Give increased fluids, bulk in diet if constipation, urinary retention occur
- Give with food or milk for GI symptoms
- Give gum, hard candy, or frequent sips of water for dry mouth
- Store in tight container at room temp; do not refreeze
- Provide assistance with ambulation during beginning therapy, since drowsiness/dizziness occurs

Evaluation

- Therapeutic response: decreased depression

Patient/family education

- Teach patient that therapeutic effects may take 2-3 wk
- Advise patient to use caution in driving or other activities requiring alertness because of drowsiness, dizziness, blurred vision
- Caution patient to avoid alcohol ingestion, other CNS depressants
- Instruct patient not to discontinue medication quickly after long-term use; may cause nausea, headache, malaise
- Instruct patient to wear sunscreen or large hat, since photosensitivity may occur

---

Generic Names

Tricyclics:
amitriptyline (p. 116)
amoxapine (p. 124)
clomipramine (p. 377)
doxepin (p. 503)
imipramine (p. 722)
nortriptyline (p. 1005)

Miscellaneous:
bupropion (p. 231)
fluoxetine (p. 613)
maprotiline (p. 845)
paroxetine (p. 1047)
sertraline (p. 1240)
trazodone (p. 1362)
venlafaxine (p. 1397)

MAOIs:
phenelzine (p. 1087)
tranylcypromine (p. 1360)

ANTIDIABETICS

Action: Antidiabetics are divided into the insulins that decrease blood sugar, phosphate, and potassium and increase blood pyruvate and lactate; and oral antidiabetics that cause functioning β-cells in the pancreas to release insulin, improves the effect of endogenous and exogenous insulin.

Uses: Insulins are used for ketoacidosis and diabetes mellitus types I (IDDM) and II (NIDDM); oral antidiabetics are used for stable adult-onset diabetes mellitus type II (NIDDM).

Side effects/adverse reactions: The most common side effect of insulin and oral antidiabetics is hypoglycemia. Other adverse reactions for oral antidiabetics include blood dyscrasias, hepatotoxicity, and, rarely, cholestatic jaundice. Adverse reactions for insulin products include allergic responses and, more rarely, anaphylaxis.

Contraindications: Hypersensitive reactions may occur, and allergies should be identified before these products are given. Oral antidiabetics should not be used in juvenile or brittle diabetes, diabetic ketoacidosis, severe renal disease, or severe hepatic disease.

G **Precautions:** Oral antidiabetics should be used with caution in the elderly, in cardiac disease, pregnancy, lactation, and in the presence of alcohol.

Pharmacokinetics: Onset, peak, and duration vary widely among products. Oral antidiabetics are metabolized in the liver, with metabolites excreted in urine, bile, and feces.

Interactions: Interactions vary widely among products. Check individual monograph for specific information.

NURSING CONSIDERATIONS

Assessment

- Monitor blood, urine glucose levels during treatment to determine diabetes control (oral products)
- Monitor fasting blood glucose, 2 hr PP (60-100 mg/dl normal fasting level) (70-130 mg/dl—normal 2-hr level)
- Assess for hypoglycemic reaction that can occur during peak time

Associated nursing diagnoses

✓ Altered nutrition: more than body requirements (uses)

Implementation

SC Route

- Give insulin after warming to room temp by rotating in palms to prevent lipodystrophy from injecting cold insulin
- Give human insulin to those allergic to beef or pork
- Rotate inj sites when giving insulin; use abdomen, upper back, thighs, upper arm, buttocks; keep a record of sites

PO Route

- Give oral antidiabetic 30 min ac

Evaluation

- Therapeutic response, including decrease in polyuria, polydipsia, polyphagia, clear sensorium, absence of dizziness, stable gait

Patient/family education

- Advise patient to avoid alcohol and salicylates except on advice of prescriber
- Teach patient symptoms of ketoacidosis: nausea, thirst, polyuria, dry mouth, decreased B/P, dry, flushed skin, acetone breath, drowsiness, Kussmaul respirations

- Teach patient symptoms of hypoglycemia: headache, tremors, fatigue, weakness; and that candy or sugar should be carried to treat hypoglycemia
- Advise patient to test urine for glucose/ketones tid if this drug is replacing insulin
- Advise patient to continue weight control, dietary restrictions, exercise, hygiene

---

Generic Names

Oral antidiabetics:
acetohexamide (p. 60)
chlorpropamide (p. 342)
🔑 insulin, isophane suspension (p. 732)
🔑 insulin, regular (p. 737)
🔑 insulin, regular concentrated (p. 740)
insulin, zinc suspension (extended) (p. 745)
insulin, zinc suspension (Lente) (p. 742)
insulin, zinc suspension (prompt) (p. 747)
tolazamide (p. 1348)
tolbutamide (p. 1352)

ANTIDIARRHEALS

Action: Antidiarrheals work by various actions including direct action on intestinal muscles to decrease GI peristalsis; or by inhibiting prostaglandin synthesis responsible for GI hypermotility; acting on mucosal receptors responsible for peristalsis; or decreasing water content of stools.

Uses: Antidiarrheals are used for diarrhea of undetermined causes.

Side effects/adverse reactions: The most serious adverse reactions of some products are paralytic ileus, toxic megacolon, and angioneurotic edema. The most common side effects are constipation, nausea, dry mouth, and abdominal pain.

Contraindications: Persons with severe ulcerative colitis, pseudomembranous colitis with some products.

G P **Precautions:** Antidiarrheal should be used with caution in the elderly, pregnancy, lactation, children, dehydration.

Pharmacokinetics: Onset, peak, and duration vary widely among products. Most products are metabolized in the liver and excreted in urine.

Interactions: Please check individual monographs, since interactions vary widely among products.

NURSING CONSIDERATIONS

Assessment

- Monitor electrolytes (potassium, sodium, chloride) if on long-term therapy
- Monitor bowel pattern before; for rebound constipation after termination of medication
- Assess response after 48 hr; if no response, drug should be discontinued
- P Identify dehydration in children

Associated nursing diagnoses

✓ Diarrhea (uses)
✓ Constipation (adverse reactions)
✓ Fluid volume deficit (adverse reactions)
✓ Knowledge deficit (teaching)

Implementation

PO Route

- Give for 48 hr only

Evaluation

- Therapeutic response: decreased diarrhea

Patient/family education

- Advise patient to avoid OTC products
- Caution patient not to exceed recommended dose

Generic Names

bismuth subsalicylate (p. 210)
diphenoxylate (p. 482)
kaolin/pectin (p. 776)
loperamide (p. 824)

ANTIDYSRHYTHMICS

Action: Antidysrhythmics are divided into four classes and miscellaneous antidysrhythmics:

- Class I increases the action potential duration and the effective refractory period and reduces disparity in the refractory period between a normal and infarcted myocardium; further subclasses include Ia, Ib, Ic

- Class II decreases the rate of SA node discharge, increases recovery time, slows conduction through the AV node, and decreases heart rate, which decreases O_2 consumption in the myocardium
- Class III increases the action potential duration and the effective refractory period
- Class IV inhibits calcium ion influx across the cell membrane during cardiac depolarization; decreases SA node discharge, decreases conduction velocity through the AV node
- Miscellaneous antidysrhythmics include those such as adenosine, which slows conduction through the AV node, and digoxin, which decreases conduction velocity and prolongs the effective refractory period in the AV node

Uses: These products are used for PVCs, tachycardia, hypertension, atrial fibrillation, angina pectoris.

Side effects/adverse reactions: Side effects and adverse reactions vary widely among products.

Contraindications: Contraindications vary widely among products.

Precautions: Precautions vary widely among products.

Pharmacokinetics: Onset, peak, and duration vary widely among products.

Interactions: Interactions vary widely among products; check individual monograph for specific information.

NURSING CONSIDERATIONS

Assessment

- Monitor ECG continuously to determine drug effectiveness, PVCs, or other dysrhythmias
- Assess for dehydration or hypovolemia
- Monitor B/P continuously for hypotension, hypertension
- Monitor I&O ratio
- Monitor serum potassium
- Assess for edema in feet and legs daily

Associated nursing diagnoses

✓ Altered tissue perfusion: cardiopulmonary (uses)
✓ Decreased cardiac output (uses)
✓ Diarrhea (adverse reactions)
✓ Impaired gas exchange (adverse reactions)

Evaluation

- Therapeutic response, including decrease in B/P in hypertension, decreased B/P, edema moist rales in CHF

Patient/family education

- Advise patient to comply with dosage schedule, even if patient is feeling better
- Instruct patient to report bradycardia, dizziness, confusion, depression, fever

---

Generic Names

ANTIFUNGALS (SYSTEMIC)

Action: Antifungals act by increasing cell membrane permeability in susceptible organisms by binding sterols and decreasing potassium, sodium, and nutrients in the cell.

Uses: Antifungals are used for infections of histoplasmosis, blastomycosis, coccidioidomycosis, cryptococcosis, aspergillosis, phycomycosis, candidiasis, sporotrichosis causing severe meningitis, septicemia, and skin infections.

Side effects/adverse reactions: The most serious adverse reactions include renal tubular acidosis, permanent renal impairment, anuria, oliguria, hemorrhagic gastroenteritis, acute liver failure, and blood dyscrasias. Some common side effects include hypokalemia, nausea, vomiting, anorexia, headache, fever, and chills.

Contraindications: Persons with severe bone depression or hypersensitivity should not use these products.

Precautions: Antifungals should be used with caution in renal disease, pregnancy, and hepatic disease.

Pharmacokinetics: Onset, peak, and duration vary widely among products. Most products are metabolized in the liver and excreted in urine.

Interactions: Please check individual monographs, since interactions vary widely among products.

NURSING CONSIDERATIONS

Assessment

- Monitor VS q15-30 min during first inf; note changes in pulse, B/P
- Monitor I&O ratio; watch for decreasing urinary output, change in sp gr; discontinue drug to prevent permanent damage to renal tubules
- Monitor blood studies; CBC, potassium, sodium, calcium, magnesium q2 wk
- Monitor weight weekly; if weight increases over 2 lb/wk, edema is present; renal damage should be considered
- Assess for renal toxicity: increasing BUN, is >40 mg/dl or if serum creatinine >3 mg/dl; drug may be discontinued or dosage reduced
- Assess for hepatotoxicity: increasing AST (SGOT), ALT (SGPT), alkaline phosphatase, bilirubin
- Assess for allergic reaction: dermatitis, rash; drug should be discontinued; antihistamines (mild reaction) or epinephrine (severe reaction) administered
- Assess for hypokalemia: anorexia, drowsiness, weakness, decreased reflexes, dizziness, increased urinary output, increased thirst, paresthesias
- Assess for ototoxicity: tinnitus (ringing, roaring in ears), vertigo, loss of hearing (rare)

Associated nursing diagnoses

✓ Risk for infection (uses)

✓ Risk for injury (adverse reactions)

✓ Knowledge deficit (teaching)

Implementation

IV IV route

- Give by IV using in-line filter (mean pore diameter >1 μm) using distal veins; check for extravasation, necrosis q8h
- Give drug only after C&S confirms organism, drug needed to treat condition; make sure drug is used in life-threatening infections

- Provide protection from light during inf; cover with foil
- Give symptomatic treatment as ordered for adverse reactions: aspirin, antihistamines, antiemetics, antispasmodics
- Store protected from moisture and light; diluted sol is stable for 24 hr

Evaluation

- Therapeutic response: decreased fever, malaise, rash, negative C&S for infecting organism

Patient/family education

- Teach patient that long-term therapy may be needed to clear infection (2 wk-3 mo depending on type of infection)

Generic Names

amphotericin B (p. 134)
fluconazole (p. 597)
flucytosine (p. 599)
griseofulvin (p. 660)
itraconazole (p. 771)
ketoconazole (p. 779)
miconazole (p. 922)
nystatin (p. 1007)

ANTIHISTAMINES

Action: Antihistamines compete with histamines for H_1 receptor sites. They antagonize in varying degrees most of the pharmacologic effects of histamines.

Uses: Products are used to control the symptoms of allergies, rhinitis, and pruritus.

Side effects/adverse reactions: Most products cause drowsiness; however, two of the newer products, astemizole and terfenadine, products little, if any, drowsiness. Other common side effects are headache and thickening of bronchial secretions. Serious blood dyscrasias may occur, but are rare. Urinary retention, GI effects occur with many of these products.

Contraindications: Hypersensitivity to H_1-receptor antagonists occurs rarely. Patients with acute asthma and lower respiratory tract disease should not use these products, since thick secretions may result. Other contraindications include narrow angle glaucoma, bladder neck obstruction, stenosing peptic ulcer, symptomatic prostatic hypertrophy, newborn, lactation.

Precautions: These products must be used cautiously in conjunction with intraocular pressure, since they increase intraocular pressure. Caution should also be used in patients with renal and cardiac disease, G hypertension, and seizure disorders, pregnancy, lactation and in the elderly.

Pharmacokinetics: Onset varies from 20-60 min, with duration lasting 4-12 hr. In general, pharmacokinetics vary widely among products.

Interactions: Barbiturates, narcotics, hypnotics, tricyclic antidepressants, and alcohol can increase CNS depression when taken with antihistamines.

NURSING CONSIDERATIONS

Assessment

- Check I&O ratio; be alert for urinary retention, frequency, dysuria; drug should be discontinued if these occur
- Assess for blood dyscrasias: thrombocytopenia, agranulocytosis (rare)
- Assess for respiratory status, including rate rhythm, increase in bronchial secretions, wheezing, chest tightness
- Assess for cardiac status, including palpitations, increased pulse, hypotension
- Assess CBC during long-term therapy, since hemolytic anemia, although rare, may occur
- Administer with food or milk to decrease GI symptoms; absorption may be decreased slightly
- Administer whole (sustained-release tab)
- Provide hard candy, gum, frequent rinsing of mouth for dryness

Associated nursing diagnoses

✓ Ineffective airway clearance (uses)

Evaluation

- Therapeutic response: absence of allergy symptoms, itching

Patient/family education

- Advise patient to notify prescriber if confusion, sedation, hypotension occur
- Caution patient to avoid driving and other hazardous activity if drowsiness occurs
- Instruct patient to avoid concurrent use of alcohol and other CNS depressants
- Inform patient to discontinue a few days before skin testing

Generic Names

astemizole (p. 160)
azatadine (p. 178)
brompheniramine (p. 223)
chlorpheniramine (p. 336)
clemastine (p. 366)
cyproheptadine (p. 414)
diphenhydramine (p. 479)
loratidine (p. 827)
promethazine (p. 1169)
terfenadine (p. 1304)
triprolidine (p. 1383)

ANTIHYPERTENSIVES

Action: Antihypertensives are divided into angiotensin converting enzyme (ACE) inhibitors, β-adrenergic blockers, calcium channel blockers, centrally acting adrenergics, diuretics, peripherally acting antiadrenergics, and vasodilators. β-Blockers, calcium channel blockers, and diuretics are discussed in separate sections. ACE inhibitors selectively suppress renin-angiotensin I to angiotensin II; dilatation of arterial and venous vessels occurs. Centrally acting adrenergics act by inhibiting the sympathetic vasomotor center in the CNS, which reduces impulses in the sympathetic nervous system; blood pressure, pulse rate, and cardiac output decrease. Peripherally acting antiadrenergics inhibit sympathetic vasoconstriction by inhibiting release of norepinephrine and/or depleting norepinephrine stores in adrenergic nerve endings. Vasodilators act on arteriolar smooth muscle by producing direct relaxation or vasodilatation; a reduction in blood pressure, with concomitant increases in heart rate and cardiac output, occurs.

Uses: Used for hypertension and for heart failure not responsive to conventional therapy. Some products are used in hypertensive crisis, angina, and for some cardiac dysrhythmias.

Side effects/adverse reactions: The most common side effects are marked hypotension, bradycardia, tachycardia, headache, nausea, and vomiting. Side effects and adverse reactions may vary widely between classes and specific products.

Contraindications: Hypersensitive reactions may occur, and allergies should be identified before these products are given. Antihypertensives should not be used in patients with heart block or in children.

Precautions: Antihypertensives should be used with caution in the elderly, in dialysis patients, and in the presence of hypovolemia, leukemia, and electrolyte imbalances.

Pharmacokinetics: Onset, peak, and duration vary widely among products. Most products are metabolized in the liver, with metabolites excreted in urine, bile, and feces.

Interactions: Interactions vary widely among products; check individual monograph for specific information.

NURSING CONSIDERATIONS

Assessment

- Monitor blood studies: neutrophil; decreased platelets occur with many of the products
- Monitor renal studies: protein, BUN, creatinine; watch for increased levels, which may indicate nephrotic syndrome; obtain baselines in renal and liver function studies before beginning treatment
- Assess for edema in feet and legs daily
- Identify allergic reaction, including rash, fever, pruritus, urticaria: drug should be discontinued if antihistamines fail to help
- Identify symptoms of CHF: edema, dyspnea, wet rales, B/P
- Assess for renal symptoms: polyuria, oliguria, frequency

Associated nursing diagnoses

✓ Altered tissue perfusion (uses)
✓ Decreased cardiac output (uses)
✓ Diarrhea (adverse reactions)
✓ Impaired gas exchange (adverse reactions)

Implementation

- Place patient in supine or Trendelenburg position for severe hypotension

Evaluation

- Therapeutic response: decrease in B/P in hypotension; decreased B/P, edema, moist rales in CHF

Patient/family education

- Instruct patient to comply with dosage schedule, even if feeling better
- Advise patient to rise slowly to sitting or standing position to minimize orthostatic hypotension

---

Generic Names

ACE inhibitors: benazepril (p. 189)

enalapril (p. 522)
fosinopril (p. 631)
quinapril (p. 1198)
ramipril (p. 1203)

Centrally acting adrenergics:
clonidine (p. 382)
guanabenz (p. 663)
guanfacine (p. 670)
methyldopa (p. 892)

Peripherally acting antiadrenergics:
guanadrel (p. 665)
guanethidine (p. 668)
prazosin (p. 1142)
reserpine (p. 1208)
terazosin (p. 1298)

Vasodilators:
diazoxide (p. 447)
hydralazine (p. 687)
minoxidil (p. 934)
nitroprusside (p. 1001)

Antidrenergic:
combined α-/β-blocker—labetalol (p. 785)

ANTIINFECTIVES

Action: Antiinfectives are divided into several groups, which include but are not limited to penicillins, cephalosporins, aminoglycosides, sulfonamides, tetracyclines, monobactam, erythromycins, and quinolones. These drugs inhibit the growth and replication of susceptible bacterial organisms.

Uses: Used for infections of susceptible organisms. These products are effective against bacterial, rickettsial, and spirochete infections.

Side effects/adverse reactions: The most common side effects are nausea, vomiting, and diarrhea. Adverse reactions include bone marrow depression and anaphylaxis.

Contraindications: Hypersensitive reactions may occur, and allergies should be identified before these products are given. Cross-sensitivity can occur between products of different classes (penicillins or cephalosporins). Often persons allergic to penicillins are also allergic to cephalosporins.

Precautions: Antiinfectives should be used with caution in persons with renal and liver disease.

Pharmacokinetics: Onset, peak, and duration vary widely among products. Most products are metabolized in the liver, and metabolites are excreted in urine, bile, and feces.

Interactions: Interactions vary widely among products; check individual monograph for specific information.

NURSING CONSIDERATIONS

Assessment

- Assess for nephrotoxicity, including increased BUN, creatinine
- Monitor blood studies: AST (SGOT), ALT (SGPT), CBC, Hct, bilirubin; test monthly if patient is on long-term therapy
- Monitor bowel pattern qd; if severe diarrhea occurs, drug should be discontinued
- Monitor urine output; if decreasing, notify prescriber; may indicate nephrotoxicity
- Assess for allergic reaction, including rash, fever, pruritus, urticaria; drug should be discontinued
- Assess for bleeding: ecchymosis, bleeding gums, hematuria, stool guaiac daily
- Assess for overgrowth of infection: perineal itching, fever, malaise, redness, pain, swelling, drainage, rash, diarrhea, change in cough, sputum

Associated nursing diagnoses

✓ Risk for infection (uses)
✓ Diarrhea (adverse reactions)

Implementation

- Give for 10-14 days to ensure organism death, prevention of superinfection
- Give after C&S completed; drug may be taken as soon as culture is obtained

Evaluation

- Therapeutic response: absence of fever, fatigue, malaise, draining wounds

Patient/family education

- Teach patient to comply with dosage schedule, even if feeling better
- Advise patient to report sore throat, bruising, bleeding, joint pain; may indicate blood dyscrasias (rare)

Generic Names

Aminoglycosides:
amikacin (p. 99)
azithromycin (p. 181)
clarithromycin (p. 364)
gentamicin (p. 645)
kanamycin (p. 773)
neomycin (p. 979)
netilmicin (p. 983)

streptomycin (p. 1264)
tobramycin (p. 1343)

Cephalosporins:
cefaclor (p. 268)
cefadroxil (p. 271)
cefamandole (p. 273)
cefazolin (p. 276)
cefixime (p. 279)
cefmetazole (p. 281)
cefonicid (p. 283)
cefoperazone (p. 286)
🔑 cephalexin (p. 310)
cephalothin (p. 312)
cephapirin (p. 315)
cephradine (p. 318)

Penicillins:
amoxicillin/clavulanate (p. 127)
ampicillin/sulbactam (p. 138)
cloxacillin (p. 389)
dicloxacillin (p. 453)
imipenem/cilastatin (p. 719)
methicillin (p. 877)
mezlocillin (p. 920)
nafcillin (p. 963)
oxacillin (p. 1018)
penicillin G benzathine (p. 1054)
penicillin G potassium (p. 1057)
penicillin G procaine (p. 1060)
🔑 penicillin G sodium (p. 1063)
penicillin V (p. 1066)
piperacillin (p. 1115)
ticarcillin/clavulanate (p. 1337)

Sulfonamides:
sulfasalazine (p. 1279)
sulfisoxazole (p. 1283)

Tetracyclines:
doxycycline (p. 508)
minocycline (p. 931)
tetracycline (p. 1310)

ANTINEOPLASTICS

Action: Antineoplastics are divided into alkylating agents, antimetabolites, antibiotic agents, hormonal agents, and miscellaneous agents. Alkylating agents act by cross-linking strands of DNA. Antimetabolites act by inhibiting DNA synthesis. Antibiotic agents act by inhibiting RNA synthesis and by delaying or inhibiting mitosis. Hormones alter the effect of androgens, luteinizing hormone, follicle-stimulating hormone, or estrogen by changing the hormonal environment.

Uses: Uses vary widely among products and classes of drugs. They are used to treat leukemia, Hodgkin's disease, lymphomas, and other tumors throughout the body.

Side effects/adverse reactions: Most products cause thrombocytopenia, leukopenia, and anemia, and, if these reactions occur, the drug may need to be stopped until the problem is corrected. Other side effects include nausea, vomiting, glossitis, and hair loss. Some products also cause hepatotoxicity, nephrotoxicity, and cardiotoxicity.

Contraindications: Hypersensitive reactions may occur, and allergies should be identified before these products are given. Also, persons with severe liver and kidney disease should not use these products unless the benefits outweigh the risks.

Precautions: Persons with bleeding, severe bone marrow depression, or renal or hepatic disease should be watched closely.

Pharmacokinetics: Onset, peak, and duration vary widely among products. Most products cross the placenta and are excreted in breast milk and in urine.

Interactions: Toxicity may occur when used with other antineoplastics or radiation.

NURSING CONSIDERATIONS

Assessment

- Monitor CBC, differential, platelet count weekly; withhold drug if WBC is <4000 or platelet count is <75,000; notify prescriber of results
- Monitor renal function studies, including BUN, creatinine, serum uric acid, and urine creatinine clearance before and during therapy
- Monitor I&O ratio; report fall in urine output of 30 ml/hr
- Monitor temp q4h (may indicate beginning infection)
- Monitor liver function tests before and during therapy (bilirubin, AST [SGOT], ALT [SGPT], LDH) prn or monthly
- Assess for bleeding, including hematuria, guaiac, brusing or petechiae, mucosa, or orifices q8h; obtain prescription for viscous lidocaine (Xylocaine)
- Identify yellowing of skin, sclera, dark urine, clay-colored stools, itchy skin, abdominal pain, fever, diarrhea
- Assess for edema in feet, joint pain, stomach pain, shaking
- Assess for inflammation of mucosa, breaks in skin

Associated nursing diagnoses

✓ Risk for infection (adverse reactions)
✓ Altered nutrition: less than body requirements (adverse reactions)
✓ Altered oral mucous membrane (adverse reactions)

Implementation

- Check IB site for irritation; phlebitis
- Have epinephrine available for hypersensitivity reaction
- Give antibiotics for prophylaxis of infection
- Provide strict medical asepsis, protective isolation if WBC levels are low

- Provide comprehensive oral hygiene, using careful technique and soft-bristle brush

Evaluation

- Therapeutic response: decreased tumor size

Patient/family education

- Advise patient to report signs of infection, including increased temp, sore throat, malaise
- Instruct patient to report signs of anemia, including fatigue, headache, faintness, shortness of breath, irritability
- Instruct patient to report bleeding and to avoid use of razors and commercial mouthwash

---

Generic Names

Alkylating agents:
busulfan (p. 235)
carboplatin (p. 257)
carmustine (p. 262)
chlorambucil (p. 323)
cisplatin (p. 361)
cyclophosphamide (p. 409)
dacarbazine (p. 419)
lomustine (p. 822)
mechlorethamine (p. 849)
melphalan (p. 857)
streptozocin (p. 1267)
thiotepa (p. 1328)

Antimetabolites:
cytarabine (p. 416)
doxorubicin (p. 505)
etoposide (p. 562)
fludarabine (p. 601)
fluorouracil (p. 611)
mercaptopurine (p. 866)
thioguanine (6-TG) (p. 1321)

Antibiotic agents:
bleomycin (p. 216)
dactinomycin (p. 421)
daunorubicin (p. 428)
methotrexate (p. 886)
mitomycin (p. 937)
mitoxantrone (p. 942)
plicamycin (p. 1126)

Hormonal agents:
aminoglutethimide (p. 108)
estramustine (p. 550)
flutamide (p. 624)
goserelin acetate (p. 658)
leuprolide (p. 793)
megestrol (p. 856)
mitotane (p. 940)
tamoxifen (p. 1292)

Miscellaneous agents:
altretamine (p. 90)
asparaginase (p. 155)
interferon alfa-2A, interferon alfa-2B (p. 750)
pentostatin (p. 1076)
procarbazine (p. 1157)
vinblastine (p. 1401)
vincristine (p. 1403)

ANTIPARKINSONIAN AGENTS

Action: Antiparkinsonian agents are divided into cholinergics and dopamine agonists. Cholinergics work by the blocking or competing at central acetylcholine receptors; dopamine agonists work by decarboxylation to dopamine or by activation of dopamine receptors; monoamine oxidase type B inhibitors increase dopamine activity by inhibiting MAO type B activity.

Uses: These agents are used alone or in combination for patients with Parkinson's disease.

Side effects/adverse reactions: Side effects and adverse reactions vary widely among products. The most common side effects include involuntary movements, headache, numbness, insomnia, nightmares, nausea, vomiting, dry mouth, and orthostatic hypotension.

Contraindications: Persons with hypersensitivity, narrow angle glaucoma, and undiagnosed skin lesions should not use these products.

Precautions: Antiparkinsonian agents should be used with caution in P pregnancy, lactation, children, renal, cardiac, hepatic disease, and affective disorder.

Pharmacokinetics: Onset, peak, and duration vary widely among products. Most products are metabolized in the liver and excreted in urine.

Interactions: Please check individual monographs, since interactions vary widely among products.

NURSING CONSIDERATIONS

Assessment

- Monitor B/P, respiration
- Mental status: affect, behavioral changes, depression, complete suicide assessment

Associated nursing diagnoses

✓ Risk for injury (uses)
✓ Risk for impaired mobility (uses)
✓ Knowledge deficit (teaching)

Implementation

- Give drug up until NPO before surgery
- Adjust dosage depending on patient response
- Give with meals; limit protein taken with drug
- Give only after MAOIs have been discontinued for 2 wk

- Assist with ambulation, during beginning therapy if needed
- Test for diabetes mellitus and acromegaly if on long-term therapy

Evaluation

- Therapeutic response: decrease in akathisia, improvement in mood

Patient/family education

- Advise patient to change positions slowly to prevent orthostatic hypotension
- Instruct patient to report side effects: twitching, eye spasm; indicate overdose
- Advise patient to use drug exactly as prescribed; if drug is discontinued abruptly, parkinsonian crisis may occur

Generic Names

amantadine (p. 95)
benztropine (p. 194)
biperiden (p. 206)
bromocriptine (p. 220)
carbidopa/levodopa (p. 254)
levodopa (p. 798)
selegiline (p. 1236)
trihexyphenidyl (p. 1377)

ANTIPSYCHOTICS

Action: Antipsychotics/neuroleptics are divided into several subgroups: phenothiazines, thioxanthenes, butyrophenones, dibenzoxazepines, dibenzodiazepines, and indolones and other heterocyclic compounds. Although chemically different, these subgroups share many pharmacologic and clinical properties. All antipsychotics work to block postsynaptic dopamine receptors in the brain that are responsible for psychotic behavior, including hallucinations, delusions, and paranoia.

Uses: Antipsychotic behavior is decreased in conditions such as schizophrenia, paranoia, and mania. These agents are also effective for severe anxiety, intractable hiccups, nausea, vomiting, behavioral problems in children, and before surgery for relaxation.

Side effects/adverse reactions: The most common side effects include extrapyramidal symptoms such as pseudoparkinsonism, akathisia, dystonia, and tardive dyskinesia, which may be controlled by use of antiparkinsonian agents. Serious adverse reactions such as hypotension, agranulocytosis, cardiac arrest, and laryngospasm have occurred. Other common side effects include dry mouth and photosensitivity.

Contraindications: Persons with liver damage, severe hypertension or coronary disease, cerebral arteriosclerosis, blood dyscrasias, bone marrow depression, parkinsonism, severe depression, or narrow angle glaucoma, children <12 yr, or persons withdrawing from alcohol or barbiturates should not use antipsychotics until these conditions are corrected.

Precautions: Caution must be used when antipsychotics are given to the elderly, since metabolism is slowed and adverse reactions can occur rapidly. Hepatic and renal disease may cause poor metabolism and excretion of the drug. Seizure threshold is decreased with these products; increases in the dose of anticonvulsants may be required. Persons with diabetes mellitus, prostatic hypertrophy, chronic respiratory disease, and peptic ulcer disease should be monitored closely.

Pharmacokinetics: Onset, peak, and duration vary widely with different products and routes. Products are metabolized by the liver, are excreted in urine as metabolites, are highly bound to plasma proteins, cross the placenta, and enter breast milk. Half-life can be extended over 3 days.

Interactions: Because other CNS depressants can cause oversedation, these combinations should be used carefully. Anticholinergics may decrease the therapeutic actions of phenothiazines and also cause increased anticholinergic effects.

NURSING CONSIDERATIONS

Assessment

- Monitor bilirubin, CBC, liver function studies monthly, since these drugs are metabolized in the liver and excreted in urine
- Monitor I&O ratio: palpate bladder if low urinary output occurs, since urinary retention occurs with many of these products
- Assess affect, orientation, LOC, reflexes, gait, coordination, sleep pattern disturbances
- Assess dizziness, faintness, palpitations, tachycardia on rising
- Check B/P with patient lying and standing; wide fluctuations between lying and standing B/P may require dosage or product change, since orthostatic hypotension is occurring
- Assess for EPS, including akathisia, tardive dyskinesia, pseudoparkinsonism

Associated nursing diagnoses

- ✓ Altered thought processes (uses)
- ✓ Sensory-perceptual alterations(uses)

Implementation

- Give antiparkinsonian agent if EPS occur

- Administer liq concentrates mixed in glass of juice or cola, since taste is unpleasant; avoid contact with skin when preparing liq concentrate or parenteral medications
- Supervise ambulation until stabilized on medication; do not involve in strenuous exercise program, since fainting is possible; patient should not stand still for long periods
- Increase fluids to prevent constipation
- Give sips of water, candy, gum for dry mouth

Evaluation

- Therapeutic response: decrease in excitement, hallucinations, delusions, paranoia, reorganization of thought patterns, speech

Patient/family education

- Advise patient to rise from sitting or lying position gradually, since fainting may occur
- Instruct patient to remain lying down for at least 30 min after IM inj
- Caution patient to avoid hot tubs, hot showers, or tub baths, since hypotension may occur
- Advise patient to wear a sunscreen or protective clothing to prevent burns
- Advise patient to take extra precautions during hot weather to stay cool; heat stroke can occur
- Caution patient to avoid driving and other activities requiring alertness until response to medication is known
- Inform patient that drowsiness or impaired mental/motor activity is evident the first 2 wk, but tends to decrease over time

---

Generic Names

Phenothiazines:

chlorpromazine (p. 338)
fluphenazine (p. 616)
mesoridazine (p. 870)
perphenazine (p. 1082)
prochlorperazine (p. 1159)
promazine (p. 1165)
thioridazine (p. 1325)
thiothixene (p. 1331)
trifluoperazine (p. 1374)

Butyrophenone:

haloperidol (p. 675)

Miscellaneous:

loxapine (p. 834)
molindone (p. 946)
risperidone (p. 1220)

ANTITUBERCULARS

Action: Antituberculars act by inhibiting RNA or DNA, or interfering with lipid and protein synthesis, thereby decreasing tubercle bacilli replication.
Uses: Antituberculars are used for pulmonary tuberculosis.
Side effects/adverse reactions: They vary widely among products. Most products can cause nausea, vomiting, anorexia, and rash. Serious adverse reactions include renal failure, nephrotoxicity, ototoxicity, and hepatic necrosis.
Contraindications: Persons with severe renal disease or hypersensitivity should not use these products.
Precautions: Antituberculars should be used with caution in pregnancy, lactation, and hepatic disease.
Pharmacokinetics: Onset, peak, and duration vary widely among products. Most products are metabolized in the liver and excreted in urine.
Interactions: Please check individual monographs, since interactions vary widely among products.

NURSING CONSIDERATIONS

Assessment

- Assess for signs of anemia: Hct, Hgb, fatigue
- Monitor liver studies weekly: ALT (SGPT), AST (SGOT), bilirubin
- Monitor renal status before treatment and monthly thereafter: BUN, creatinine, output, sp gr, urinalysis
- Monitor hepatic status: decreased appetite, jaundice, dark urine, fatigue

Associated nursing diagnoses

✓ Risk for infection (uses)
✓ Risk for injury (adverse reactions)
✓ Knowledge deficit (teaching)
✓ Noncompliance (teaching)

Implementation

- Give some of these agents on empty stomach, 1 hr ac (only for isoniazid and rifampin) or 2 hr pc
- Give antiemetic if vomiting occurs
- Give after C&S is completed; monthly to detect resistance

Evaluation

- Therapeutic response: decreased symptoms of TB, culture negative

Patient/family education

- Teach patient that compliance with dosage schedule, duration is necessary
- Teach patient that scheduled appointments must be kept; relapse may occur
- Advise patient to avoid alcohol while taking drug
- Advise patient to report flulike symptoms: excessive fatigue, anorexia, vomiting, sore throat; unusual bleeding, yellowish discoloration of skin/eyes

---

Generic Names

ethambutol (p. 555)
isoniazid (p. 761)
pyrazinamide (p. 1189)
rifabutin (p. 1214)
rifampin (p. 1216)
streptomycin (p. 1264)

ANTITUSSIVES/EXPECTORANTS

Action: Antitussives suppress the cough reflex by direct action on the cough center in the medulla. Expectorants act by liquefying and reducing the viscosity of thick, tenacious secretions.

Uses: Antitussives/expectorants are used to treat cough occurring in pneumonia, bronchitis, TB, cystic fibrosis, and emphysema; as an adjunct in atelectasis (expectorants); and for nonproductive cough (antitussives).

Side effects/adverse reactions: The most common side effects are drowsiness, dizziness, and nausea.

Contraindications: Some products are contraindicated in hypothyroidism, iodine sensitivity, pregnancy, and lactation.

G **Precautions:** Some products should be used cautiously in asthma, elderly, and debilitated patients.

Pharmacokinetics: Onset, peak, and duration vary widely among products. Some products are metabolized in the liver and excreted in urine.

Interactions: Please check individual monographs, since interactions vary widely among products.

NURSING CONSIDERATIONS

Assessment

- Assess cough: type, frequency, character including sputum

Associated nursing diagnoses:

✓ Ineffective breathing pattern (uses)
✓ Ineffective airway clearance (uses)
✓ Knowledge deficit (teaching)

Implementation

- G Give decreased dosage to elderly patients; their metabolism may be slowed
- Increase fluids to liquefy secretions
- Humidify patient's room

Evaluation

- Therapeutic response: absence of cough

Patient/family education

- Advise patient to avoid driving and other hazardous activities until stabilized on this medication
- Caution patient to avoid smoking, smoke-filled rooms, perfumes, dust, environmental pollutants, cleaners that increase cough

---

Generic Names

acetylcysteine (p. 63)
codeine (p. 394)
dextromethorphan (p. 439)
diphenhydramine (p. 479)
guaifenesin (p. 662)
hydrocodone (p. 692)
potassium iodide (p. 1133)

ANTIVIRALS

Action: Antivirals act by interfering with DNA synthesis that is needed for viral replication.

Uses: Antivirals are used for mucocutaneous herpes simplex virus, herpes genitalis (HSV_1, HSV_2), advanced HIV infections, herpes simplex virus encephalitis, varicella-zoster encephalomyelitis.

Side effects/adverse reactions: Serious adverse reactions are fatal metabolic encephalopathy, blood dyscrasias, and acute renal failure. Common side effects are nausea, vomiting, anorexia, diarrhea, headache, vaginitis, and moniliasis.

Contraindications: Persons with hypersensitivity and immunosuppressed individuals with herpes zoster should not use these products.

Precautions: Antivirals should be used with caution in renal disease, liver disease, lactation, pregnancy, and dehydration.
Pharmacokinetics: Onset, peak, and duration vary widely among products. Most products are metabolized in the liver and excreted in urine.
Interactions: Please check individual monographs, since interactions vary widely among products.

NURSING CONSIDERATIONS

Assessment

- Assess for signs of infection, anemia
- Monitor I&O ratio; report hematuria, oliguria, fatigue, weakness; may indicate nephrotoxicity; check for protein in urine during treatment
- Monitor any patient with compromised renal system, since drug is excreted slowly in poor renal system function; toxicity may occur rapidly
- Check liver studies: AST (SGOT), ALT (SGPT)
- Check blood studies: WBC, RBC, Hct, Hgb, bleeding time; blood dyscrasias may occur; drug should be discontinued
- Check renal studies: urinalysis, protein, BUN, creatinine, Cr Cl
- Obtain C&S before drug therapy; drug may be taken as soon as culture is obtained; repeat C&S after treatment
- Assess bowel pattern before, during treatment; if severe abdominal pain with bleeding occurs, drug should be discontinued
- Identify skin eruptions: rash, urticaria, itching
- Assess for allergies before treatment, reaction of each medication; place allergies on chart, Kardex in bright red letters

Associated nursing diagnoses

✓ Risk for infection (uses)
✓ Risk for injury (adverse reactions)
✓ Knowledge deficit (teaching)

Implementation

- Give increased fluids to 3 L/day to decrease crystalluria when given IB
- Store at room temp for up to 12 hr after reconstitution
- Give adequate intake of fluids (2000 ml) to prevent deposit in kidneys

Evaluation

- Therapeutic response: absence of or control of infection

Patient/family education

- Inform patient that drug does not cure infection, just controls symptoms
- Instruct patient to report sore throat, fever, fatigue; could indicate superinfection
- Advise patient that drug must be taken in equal intervals around the clock to maintain blood levels for duration of therapy
- Advise patient to notify prescriber of side effects of bruising, bleeding, fatigue, malaise; may indicate blood dyscrasias

---

Generic Names

🔑 acyclovir (p. 68)
amantadine (p. 95)
didanosine (p. 455)
foscarnet (p. 628)
ganciclovir (p. 641)
idoxuridine (p. 716)
rimantadine (p. 1218)
zalcitabine (p. 1418)
🔑 zidovudine (p. 1420)

BARBITURATES

Action: Barbiturates act by decreasing impulse transmission to the cerebral cortex.

Uses: All forms of epilepsy can be controlled, since the seizure threshold is increased. **P** Uses also include febrile seizures in children, sedation, insomnia, hyperbilirubinemia, chronic cholestasis with some of these products. Ultra-short acting barbiturates are used as anesthetics.

Side effects/adverse reactions: The most common side effects are drowsiness and nausea. Serious adverse reactions such as Stevens-Johnson syndrome and blood dyscrasias may occur with high doses and long-term treatment.

Contraindications: Hypersensitivity may occur, and allergies should be identified before administering. Barbiturates are identified as pregnancy category (D) and should not be used in pregnancy. Other contraindications include porphyria and marked impairment of liver function.

Precautions: Caution must be used when these products are given to **G** the elderly or debilitated; usually smaller doses are needed, since metabolism is slowed. Persons with renal and hepatic disease may show **P** delayed excretion. Barbiturates may produce excitability in children.

Pharmacokinetics: Onset of action can be slow, up to 1 hr, with a peak of 8 hr and a duration of 3-10 hr. These drugs are metabolized by the liver, excreted by the kidneys, cross the placenta, and enter breast milk. **Interactions:** Increased CNS depressant effect may occur with alcohol, MAOIs, sedatives, or narcotics. These products should be used together cautiously. Oral anticoagulants, corticosteroids, griseofulvin, quinidine, oral contraceptives, and theophylline may show a decreased effect when used with barbiturates.

NURSING CONSIDERATIONS

Assessment

- Monitor hepatic and renal studies: AST (SGOT), ALT (SGPT), bilirubin, creatinine, LDH, alkaline phosphatase, BUN if patient is on long-term therapy, since these products are metabolized and excreted by the liver and kidney
- Monitor blood studies: CBC, hematocrit, hemoglobin, and prothrombin time if patient is on long-term therapy, since these products increase the possibility of bleeding and blood dyscrasias
- Identify barbiturate toxicity: hypotension, pulmonary constriction, cold, clammy skin, cyanosis of lips, insomnia, nausea, vomiting, hallucinations, delirium, weakness

Associated nursing diagnoses

✓ Sleep pattern disturbance (uses)
✓ Risk for injury (adverse reactions)

Evaluation

- Therapeutic response: appropriate sedation or seizure control

Patient/family education

- Inform patient that physical dependency may result when used for extended periods (45-90 days, depending on dosage)
- Advise patient to avoid driving and activities that require alertness, since drowsiness and dizziness may occur
- Caution patient to abstain from alcohol and other psychotropic medications unless prescribed by prescriber
- Instruct patient not to discontinue medication abruptly after long-term use; withdrawal symptoms will occur

---

Generic Names

amobarbital (p. 121)
pentobarbital (p. 1073)
phenobarbital (p. 1090)
secobarbital (p. 1233)
thiopental (p. 1323)

BENZODIAZEPINES

Action: Benzodiazepines potentiate the effects of GABA, including any other inhibitory transmitters in the CNS, resulting in decreased anxiety.

Uses: Anxiety is relieved in conditions such as phobic disorders. Benzodiazepines are also used for acute alcohol withdrawal to relieve the possibility of delirium tremens, and some products are used before surgery for relaxation.

Side effects/adverse reactions: The most common side effects are dizziness, drowsiness, blurred vision, and orthostatic hypotension. Most adverse effects are mediated through the CNS. There is a risk for physical dependence and abuse.

Contraindications: Hypersensitivity, acute narrow angle glaucoma, P children <6 months, liver disease (clonazepam), lactation (diazepam).

Precautions: Caution must be used when these products are given to G the elderly or debilitated; usually smaller dosages are needed, since metabolism is slowed. Persons with renal and hepatic disease may show delayed excretion. Clonazepam may increase incidence of seizures.

Pharmacokinetics: Onset of action is ½-1 hr, with a peak of 1-2 hr and a duration of 4-6 hr. These drugs are metabolized by the liver, excreted by the kidneys, cross the placenta, and enter breast milk.

Interactions: Increased CNS depressant effect may occur with other CNS depressants. These products should be used together cautiously. Alcohol should not be used; fatal reactions can occur. The serum concentration and toxicity of digoxin may be increased.

NURSING CONSIDERATIONS

Assessment

- Monitor B/P (with patient lying, standing), pulse; if systolic B/P drops 20 mm Hg, hold drug, notify prescriber; orthostatic hypotension is severe
- Monitor hepatic and renal studies: AST (SGOT), ALT (SGPT), bilirubin, creatinine, LDH, alkaline phosphatase
- Assess for physical dependency, withdrawal symptoms, including headache, nausea, vomiting, muscle pain, weakness after long-term use

Associated nursing diagnoses

✓ Anxiety (uses)

✓ Risk for injury (adverse reactions)

Implementation

- Give with food or milk for GI symptoms; may give crushed if patient is unable to swallow medication whole

Evaluation

- Therapeutic response: relaxation or decreased anxiety

Patient/family education

- Teach patient that drug should not be used for everyday stress or long term; not to take more than prescribed amount, since drug is habit forming
- Caution patient to avoid driving and activities that require alertness, since drowsiness and dizziness occur
- Caution patient to abstain from alcohol and other psychotropic medications unless prescribed by prescriber
- Advise patient not to discontinue medication abruptly after long-term use; withdrawal symptoms will occur

---

Generic Names

alprazolam (p. 84)
chlordiazepoxide (p. 328)
clonazepam (p. 380)
diazepam (p. 444)
flurazepam (p. 620)
halazepam (p. 672)
lorazepam (p. 828)
midazolam (p. 925)
oxazepam (p. 1023)
prazepam (p. 1140)
quazepam (p. 1196)
temazepam (p. 1293)
triazolam (p. 1372)

β-ADRENERGIC BLOCKERS

Action: β-Blockers are divided into selective and nonselective blockers. Nonselective blockers produce a fall in blood pressure without reflex tachycardia or reduction in heart rate through a mixture of β-blocking effects; elevated plasma renins are reduced. Selective β-blockers competitively block stimulation of β_1-receptors in cardiac smooth muscle; these drugs produce chronotropic and inotropic effects.

Uses: β-Blockers are used for hypertension, ventricular dysrhythmias, and prophylaxis of angina pectoris.

Side effects/adverse reactions: The most common side effects are orthostatic hypotension, bradycardia, diarrhea, nausea, vomiting. Serious adverse reactions include blood dyscrasias, bronchospasm, and CHF.

Contraindications: Hypersensitive reactions may occur, and allergies should be identified before these products are given. β-Adrenergic blockers should not be used in heart block, CHF, or cardiogenic shock.

G **Precautions:** β-Blockers should be used with caution in the elderly or in renal and thyroid disease, COPD, CAD, diabetes mellitus, pregnancy, or asthma.

Pharmacokinetics: Onset, peak, and duration vary widely among products. Most products are metabolized in the liver, with metabolites excreted in urine, bile, and feces.

Interactions: Interactions vary widely among products; check individual monograph for specific information.

NURSING CONSIDERATIONS

Assessment

- Monitor renal studies, including protein, BUN, creatinine; watch for increased levels that may indicate nephrotic syndrome; obtain baselines in renal and liver function studies before beginning treatment
- Monitor I&O, weight daily
- Monitor B/P during beginning treatment and periodically thereafter, pulse q4h; note rate, rhythm, quality
- Monitor apical/radial pulse before administration; notify prescriber of significant changes
- Check for edema in feet and legs daily

Associated nursing diagnoses

✓ Altered tissue perfusion (uses)
✓ Decreased cardiac output (uses)
✓ Diarrhea (adverse reactions)
✓ Impaired gas exchange (adverse reactions)

Implementation

- Give PO ac, hs; tab may be crushed or swallowed whole
- Give reduced dosage in renal dysfunction

Evaluation

- Therapeutic response: decrease in B/P in hypertension; decreased B/P, edema, moist rales in CHF

Patient/family education

- Instruct patient to comply with dosage schedule, even if feeling better
- Caution patient to rise slowly to sitting or standing position to minimize orthostatic hypotension

- Advise patient to report bradycardia, dizziness, confusion, depression, fever
- Teach patient to take pulse at home; advise when to notify prescriber
- Instruct patient to comply with weight control, dietary adjustment, modified exercise program
- Advise patient to wear support hose to minimize effects of orthostatic hypotension
- Advise patient not to discontinue drug abruptly; taper over 2 wk; may precipitate angina

---

Generic Names

Selective β_1-receptor blockers:
acebutolol (p. 51)
atenolol (p. 162)
esmolol (p. 543)
metoprolol (p. 912)

Nonselective β_1 and β_2-blockers:
carteolol (p. 264)
nadolol (p. 960)
pindolol (p. 1111)
propranolol (p. 1178)
timolol (p. 1340)

Combined α_1, β_1, and β_2-receptor blocker:
labetalol (p. 785)

BRONCHODILATORS

Action: Bronchodilators are divided into anticholinergics, α/β-adrenergics agonists, β-adrenergic agonists, and phosphodiesterase inhibitors. Anticholinergics act by inhibiting interaction of acetylcholine at receptor sites on bronchial smooth muscle; α/β-adrenergic agonists by relaxing bronchial smooth muscle and increasing diameter of nasal passages; β-adrenergic agonists by action on β_2-receptors, which relaxes bronchial smooth muscle; phosphodiesterase inhibitors by blocking phosphodiesterase and increasing cAMP, which mediates smooth muscle relaxation in the respiratory system.

Uses: Bronchodilators are used for bronchial asthma, bronchospasm associated with bronchitis, emphysema, other obstructive pulmonary diseases, and Cheyne-Stokes respirations, as well as prevention of exercise-induced asthma.

Side effects/adverse reactions: The most common side effects are tremors, anxiety, nausea, vomiting, and irritation in the throat. The most serious adverse reactions include bronchospasm and dyspnea.

Contraindications: Persons with hypersensitivity, narrow angle glaucoma, tachydysrhythmias, and severe cardiac disease should not use some of these products.
Precautions: Bronchodilators should be used with caution in lactation, pregnancy, hyperthyroidism, hypertension, prostatic hypertrophy, and seizure disorders.
Pharmacokinetics: Onset, peak, and duration vary widely among products. Most products are metabolized in the liver and excreted in urine.
Interactions: Please check individual monographs, since interactions vary widely among products.

NURSING CONSIDERATIONS

Assessment

- Monitor respiratory function: vital capacity, FEV, ABGs, lung sounds, heart rate and rhythm

Associated nursing diagnoses

✓ Ineffective airway clearance (uses)
✓ Activity intolerance (uses)
✓ Risk for injury (adverse reactions)
✓ Knowledge deficit (teaching)

Implementation

- Give after shaking; exhale, place mouthpiece in mouth, inhale slowly, hold breath, remove, exhale slowly
- Give gum, sips of water for dry mouth
- Give PO with meals to decrease gastric irritation
- Store in light-resistant container; do not expose to temp over 86° F

Evaluation

- Therapeutic response: absence of dyspnea, wheezing

Patient/family education

- Advise patient not to use OTC medications; extra stimulation may occur
- Teach patient use of inhaler; review package insert with patient; to wash inhaler in warm water qd and dry
- Advise patient to avoid getting aerosol in eyes
- Caution patient to avoid smoking, smoke-filled rooms, persons with respiratory tract infections

Generic Names

CALCIUM CHANNEL BLOCKERS

Action: These products inhibit calcium ion influx across the cell membrane in cardiac and vascular smooth muscle. This action produces relaxation of coronary vascular smooth muscle, dilates coronary arteries, slows SA/AV node conduction, and dilates peripheral arteries.
Uses: These products are used for chronic stable angina pectoris, vasospastic angina, dysrhythmias, hypertension, and unstable angina.
Side effects/adverse reactions: The most common side effects are dysrhythmias and edema. Also common are headache, fatigue, drowsiness, and flushing.
Contraindications: Persons with 2nd- or 3rd-degree heart block, sick sinus syndrome, hypotension of <90 mm Hg systolic, Wolff-Parkinson-White syndrome, or cardiogenic shock should not use these products, since worsening of those conditions may occur.
Precautions: CHF may worsen, since edema may be increased. Hypotension may worsen, since B/P is decreased. Patients with renal and liver disease should use these products cautiously, since they are metabolized in the liver and excreted by the kidneys.
Pharmacokinetics: Onset, peak, and duration vary widely with route of administration. Drugs are metabolized by the liver and excreted in the urine primarily as metabolites.
Interactions: Increased levels of digoxin and theophylline may occur when used with these products. Increased effects of β-blockers and antihypertensives may occur with calcium channel blockers.

NURSING CONSIDERATIONS

Assessment

- Monitor cardiac system, including B/P, pulse, respirations, ECG intervals (PR, QRS, QT)

Associated nursing diagnoses

✓ Altered tissue perfusion: cardiopulmonary (uses)
✓ Decreased cardiac output (adverse reactions)

Implementation

- Give PO ac and hs

Evaluation

- Therapeutic response: decreased anginal pain, decreased B/P, dysrhythmias

Patient/family education

- Teach patient how to take pulse before taking drug; patient should record or graph pulses to identify changes
- Advise patient to avoid hazardous activities until stabilized on this drug, since dizziness occurs frequently
- Inform patient of need for compliance to all areas of medical regimen, including diet, exercise, stress reduction, drug therapy

---

Generic Names

amlodipine (p. 119)
bepridil (p. 197)
diltiazem (p. 470)
felodipine (p. 576)
isradipine (p. 769)
nicardipine (p. 989)
nifedipine (p. 994)
🔑 verapamil (p. 1399)

CARDIAC GLYCOSIDES

Action: Products act by inhibiting sodium and potassium ATPase and then making more calcium available to activate contracted proteins. Cardiac contractility and cardiac output are increased.

Uses: These products are used for CHF, atrial fibrillation, atrial flutter, atrial tachycardia, and rapid digitalization in these disorders.

Side effects/adverse reactions: The most common side effects are cardiac disturbances, headache, hypotension, GI symptoms. Also common are blurred vision and yellow-green halos.

Contraindications: Hypersensitive reactions may occur, and allergies should be identified before these products are given. Also, persons with ventricular tachycardia, ventricular fibrillation, and carotid sinus syndrome should not use these products.

Precautions: Persons with acute MI and those who have or may develop serum potassium, calcium, or magnesium imbalances should use these products cautiously. Also, persons with AV block, severe respiratory disease, hypothyroidism, renal and liver disease, and the G elderly should exercise caution when these drugs are prescribed.

Pharmacokinetics: Onset, peak, and duration vary widely with the route of administration. Digitoxin is inactivated by the liver, and inactive metabolites are excreted in urine. Digoxin is excreted in urine mainly as the parent drug and metabolites.

Interactions: Toxicity may occur when used with diuretics, succinylcholine, quinidine, and thioamines. Increased blood levels may occur with propantheline bromide, spironolactone, quinidine, verapamil, aminoglycosides (PO), amiodarone, anticholinergics, and quinine. Diuretics may increase toxicity.

NURSING CONSIDERATIONS

Assessment

- Montior cardiac system, including B/P, pulse, respirations, and increased urine output
- Monitor apical pulse for 1 min before giving drug; if pulse <60, take again in 1 hr; if <60 notify prescriber
- Monitor electrolytes, including potassium, sodium, chloride, calcium, magnesium; renal function studies, including BUN and creatinine; and blood studies, including AST (SGOT), ALT (SGPT), bilirubin
- Monitor I&O ratio, daily weights
- Monitor therapeutic drug levels

Associated nursing diagnoses

✓ Altered tissue perfusion: cardiopulmonary (uses)
✓ Decreased cardiac output (adverse reactions)

Implementation

- Give potassium supplements if ordered for potassium levels <3

Evaluation

- Therapeutic response: decreased weight, edema, pulse, respiration, and increased urine output

Patient/family education

- Teach patient how to take pulse before taking drug; patient should record or graph pulse to identify changes
- Advise patient to avoid hazardous activities until stabilized on this drug, since dizziness occurs frequently
- Inform patient of need for compliance to all areas of medical regimen, including diet, exercise, stress reduction, drug therapy

Generic Names

digitoxin (p. 461) — Key digoxin (p. 463)

CHOLINERGICS

Action: Cholinergics act by preventing destruction of acetylcholine, which increases concentration at sites where acetylcholine is released; this exaggerates the effects of acetylcholine and facilitates transmission of impulses across myoneural junction. Cholinergics may also act by stimulating receptors for acetylcholine.

Uses: Cholinergics are used for myasthenia gravis, as antagonists of nondepolarizing neuromuscular blockade, postoperative bladder distention and urinary distention, postoperative ileus.

Side effects/adverse reactions: The most serious adverse reactions are respiratory depression, bronchospasm, constriction, laryngospasm, respiratory arrest, convulsions, and paralysis. The most common side effects are nausea, diarrhea, and vomiting.

Contraindications: Persons with obstruction of the intestine or renal system should not use these products.

Precautions: Caution should be used in patients with bradycardia, hypotension, seizure disorders, bronchial asthma, coronary occlusion, P hyperthyroidism, and in lactation and children.

Pharmacokinetics: Onset, peak, and duration vary widely among products. Most products are metabolized in the liver and excreted in urine.

Interactions: Please check individual monographs since interactions vary widely among products.

NURSING CONSIDERATIONS

Assessment

- Monitor VS, respiration q8h
- Monitor I&O ratio; check for urinary retention of incontinence
- Assess for bradycardia, hypotension, bronchospasm, headache, dizziness, convulsions, respiratory depression; drug should be discontinued if toxicity occurs

Associated nursing diagnoses

- ✓ Altered urinary elimination (uses)
- ✓ Ineffective breathing pattern (uses)
- ✓ Knowledge deficit (teaching)
- ✓ Noncompliance (teaching)

Implementation

- Give only with atropine sulfate available for cholinergic crisis
- Give only after all other cholinergics have been discontinued
- Give increased dosages if tolerance occurs
- Give larger doses after exercise or fatigue
- Give on empty stomach for better absorption
- Store at room temp

Evaluation

- Therapeutic response: increased muscle strength, hand grasp, improved muscle gait, absence of labored breathing (if severe)

Patient/family education

- Inform patient that drug is not a cure; it only relieves symptoms (myasthenia gravis)
- Advise patient to wear Medic Alert ID specifying myasthenia gravis, drugs taken

---

Generic Names

bethanechol (p. 204)
edrophonium (p. 520)
neostigmine (p. 981)
physostigmine (p. 1105)
pyridostigmine (p. 1190)

CHOLINERGIC BLOCKERS

Action: Cholinergic blockers inhibit or block acetylcholine at receptor sites in the autonomic nervous system.

Uses: Many products are used to decrease secretions before surgery, to reverse neuromuscular blockade, and to decrease motility of GI, biliary, urinary tracts. Other products are used for parkinsonian symptoms, including dystonia associated with neuroleptic drugs.

Side effects/adverse reactions: The most common side effects are dryness of the mouth and constipation, which can be prevented by frequent rinsing of the mouth and increasing water and bulk in the diet.

Contraindications: Hypersensitivity can occur, and allergies should be identified before administering these products. Persons with GI and GU obstruction should not use these products, since constipation and urinary retention may occur. They are also contraindicated in angle closure glaucoma and myasthenia gravis.

Precautions: Caution must be used when these products are given to G the elderly, since metabolism is slowed. Also, persons with tachycardia or prostatic hypertrophy should use these products with caution.

Pharmacokinetics: Onset, peak, and duration vary with route.
Interactions: Increase in anticholinergic effect occurs when used with narcotics, barbiturates, antihistamines, MAOIs, phenothiazines, amantadine.

NURSING CONSIDERATIONS

Assessment

- Assess I&O ratio; be alert for urinary retention, frequency, dysuria; drug should be discontinued if these occur
- Assess urinary hesitancy, retention; palpate bladder if retention occurs
- Assess constipation; increase fluids, bulk, exercise
- Assess for tolerance over long-term therapy; dosage may need to be changed
- Assess mental status: affect, mood, CNS depression, worsening of mental symptoms during early therapy

Associated nursing diagnoses

✓ Impaired physical mobility (uses)
✓ Pain (uses)

Implementation

- Give with food or milk to decrease GI symptoms
- Give parenteral dose with patient recumbent to prevent postural hypotension; give dose slowly, monitoring VS
- Give hard candy, gum, frequent rinsing of mouth for dryness

Evaluation

- Therapeutic response: absence of cramps, absence of EPS

Patient/family education

- Caution patient to avoid driving and other hazardous activity if drowsiness occurs
- Advise patient to avoid concurrent use of cough, cold preparations with alcohol, antihistamines unless directed by prescriber
- Caution patient to use with caution in hot weather, since medication may increase susceptibility to heat stroke

---

Generic Names

🔑 atropine (p. 169)
🔑 benztropine (p. 194)
biperiden (p. 206)
glycopyrrolate (p. 653)
scopolamine (p. 1230)
trihexyphenidyl (p. 1377)

CORTICOSTEROIDS

Action: Corticosteroids are divided into glucocorticoids and mineralocorticoids. Glucocorticoids decrease inflammation by the suppression of migration of polymorphonuclear leukocytes, fibroblasts, increased capillary permeability, and lysosomal stabilization. They also have varied metabolic effects and modify the body's immune responses to many different stimuli. Mineralocorticoids act by increasing resorption of sodium by increasing hydrogen and potassium excretion in the distal tubule.

Uses: Glucocorticoids are used to decrease inflammation and for immunosuppression. In addition, some products may be given for allergy, adrenal insufficiency, or cerebral edema. Mineralocorticoids are given for adrenal insufficiency or adrenogenital syndrome.

Side effects/adverse reactions: The most common side effects include change in behavior, including insomnia and euphoria; GI irritation, including peptic ulcer; metabolic reactions; including hypokalemia, hyperglycemia, and carbohydrate intolerance; and sodium and fluid retention. Most adverse reactions are dose dependent.

Contraindications: Hypersensitivity may occur and should be identified before administering. Since these products mask infection, they should not be used in systemic fungal infections or amebiasis. Mothers taking pharmacologic doses of corticosteroids should not nurse.

Precautions: Caution must be used when these products are prescribed for diabetic patients, since hyperglycemia may occur. Also, patients with glaucoma, seizure disorders, peptic ulcer, impaired renal function, CHF, hypertension, ulcerative colitis, or myasthenia gravis should be monitored closely if corticosteroids are given. Use with caution in children and the elderly and during pregnancy.

Pharmacokinetics: For oral preparations the onset of action occurs between 1-2 hr, and duration can be up to 2 days, with a half-life of 2-4 days. Pharmacokinetics vary widely among products. These products cross the placenta and appear in breast milk.

Interactions: Decreased corticosteroid effect may occur with barbiturates, rifampin, phenytoin; corticosteroid dosage may need to be increased. There is a possibility of GI bleeding when used with salicylates, indomethacin. Steroids may reduce salicylate levels. When using with digitalis glycosides, potassium-depleting diuretics, and amphotericin, serum potassium levels should be monitored.

NURSING CONSIDERATIONS

Assessment

- Monitor potassium, blood sugar, urine glucose while on long-term therapy; hypokalemia and hyperglycemia are common
- Monitor weight daily; notify prescriber if weekly gain of >5 lb, since these products alter fluid and electrolyte balance
- Assess for potassium depletion, including paresthesias, fatigue, nausea, vomiting, depression, polyuria, dysrhythmias, weakness
- Assess for mental status, including affect, mood, behavioral changes, aggression; if severe personality changes occur, including depression, drug may need to be tapered and then discontinued
- Monitor I&O ratio; be alert for decreasing urinary output and increasing edema
- Monitor plasma cortisol levels during long-term therapy (normal level is 138-635 nmol/L when drawn at 8 AM)
- Assess for infection, including increased temp, WBC, even after withdrawal of medication; drug masks symptoms of infection
- Assess for adrenal insufficiency: nausea, anorexia, fatigue, dizziness, dyspnea, weakness, joint pain

Associated nursing diagnoses

✓ Risk for infection (adverse reactions)
✓ Body image disturbance (adverse reactions)
✓ Risk for violence: self-directed (suicide) (adverse reactions)

Implementation

- Give with food or milk to decrease GI symptoms

Evaluation

- Therapeutic response: decreased inflammation

Patient/family education

- Advise patient that ID as steroid user should be carried
- Advise patient not to discontinue this medication abruptly or adrenal crisis can result
- Teach patient all aspects of drug use, including cushingoid symptoms
- Instruct patient that single daily or alternate-day doses should be taken in the morning before 9 AM (for replacement therapy)
- Instruct patient to take with meals or a snack

Generic Names

Glucocorticoids:
beclomethasone (p. 188)
betamethasone (p. 201)
cortisone (p. 404)
flunisolide (p. 606)
hydrocortisone (p. 695)
methylprednisolone (p. 899)
prednisolone (p. 1144)
prednisone (p. 1146)
triamcinolone (p. 1367)

Mineralocorticoid:
fludrocortisone (p. 603)

DIURETICS

Action: Diuretics are divided into subgroups: thiazides and thiazide-like diuretics, loop diuretics, carbonic anhydrase inhibitors, osmotic diuretics, and potassium-sparing diuretics. Each one of these subgroups differs in its mechanism of action. Thiazides and thiazide-like diuretics increase excretion of water and sodium by inhibiting resorption in the early distal tubule. Loop diuretics inhibit resorption of sodium and chloride in the thick ascending limb of the loop of Henle. Carbonic anhydrase inhibitors increase sodium excretion by decreasing sodium-hydrogen ion exchange throughout the renal tubule. Carbonic anhydrase inhibitors also decrease secretion of aqueous humor in the eye and thus decrease intraocular pressure. Osmotic diuretics increase the osmotic pressure of glomerular filtrate, thus decreasing net absorption of sodium. The potassium-sparing diuretics interfere with sodium resorption at the distal tubule, thus decreasing potassium excretion.

Uses: Blood pressure is reduced in hypertension; edema is reduced in CHF; intraocular pressure is decreased in glaucoma.

Side effects/adverse reactions: Hypokalemia, hyperuricemia, and hyperglycemia occur most frequently with thiazide diuretics. Aplastic anemia, blood dyscrasias, volume depletion, and dehydration may occur when thiazide-like diuretics, loop diuretics, or carbonic anhydrase inhibitors are given. Side effects and adverse reactions vary widely for the miscellaneous products.

Contraindications: Persons with electrolyte imbalances (sodium, chloride, potassium), dehydration, or anuria should not be given these products until the problem is corrected.

G **Precautions:** Caution must be used when diuretics are given to the elderly, since electrolyte disturbances and dehydration can occur rapidly. Hepatic and renal disorders may cause poor metabolism and excretion of the drug.

Pharmacokinetics: Onset, peak, and duration vary widely among the different subgroups of these drugs.

Interactions: Cholestyramine and colestipol decrease the absorption of thiazide diuretics. Concurrent use of thiazides with diazoxide may increase hyperuricemia, hyperglycemia, and antihypertensive effects of thiazides. Ototoxicity may occur when loop diuretics are used with aminoglycosides. Thiazide and loop diuretics may increase therapeutic and toxic effects of lithium.

NURSING CONSIDERATIONS

Assessment

- Monitor weight, I&O daily to determine fluid loss; check skin turgor for dehydration
- Monitor electrolytes: potassium, sodium, chloride: include BUN, blood sugar, CBC, serum creatinine, blood pH, ABGs, uric acid, calcium; electrolyte imbalances may occur quickly
- Monitor B/P with patient lying, standing; postural hypotension may occur, since fluid loss occurs from intravascular spaces first
- Assess for signs of metabolic alkalosis, including drowsiness and restlessness
- Assess for signs of hypokalemia with some products, including postural hypotension, malaise, fatigue, tachycardia, leg cramps, weakness

Associated nursing diagnoses

✓ Fluid volume excess (uses)
✓ Decreased cardiac output (adverse reactions)

Implementation

- Give in AM to avoid interference with sleep if using drug as a diuretic
- Give potassium replacement if potassium is less than 3

Evaluation

- Therapeutic reponse: improvement in edema of feet, legs, sacral area daily if medication is being used in CHF; improvement in B/P if medication is being used as a diuretic; improvement in intraocular pressure if medication is being used to decrease aqueous humor in the eye

Patient/family education

- Teach patient to take drug early in the day (diuretic) to prevent nocturia

---

Generic Names

Thiazides:
hydrochlorothiazide (p. 689)

Thiazide-like:
chlorthalidone (p. 345)
indapamide (p. 727)
metolazone (p. 909)

Loop:
bumetanide (p. 225)
furosemide (p. 633)

Carbonic anhydrase inhibitors:
acetazolamide (p. 56)

Potassium-sparing:
amiloride (p. 102)
spironolactone (p. 1257)
triamterene (p. 1369)

Osmotic:
mannitol (p. 842)

HISTAMINE H_2 ANTAGONISTS

Action: Histamine H_2 antagonists act by inhibiting histamine at H_2 receptor site in parietal cells, which inhibits gastric acid secretion.
Uses: Histamine H_2 antagonists are used for short-term treatment of duodenal and gastric ulcers and maintenance therapy for duodenal ulcer; and for gastroesophageal reflux disease.
Side effects/adverse reactions: The most serious adverse reactions are agranulocytosis, thrombocytopenia, neutropenia, aplastic anemia, exfoliative dermatitis. The most common side effects are confusion (not with rantidine), headache and diarrhea.
Contraindications: Persons with hypersensitivity should not use these products.
P **Precautions:** Caution should be used in pregnancy, lactation, children <16 yr, organic brain syndrome, hepatic disease, renal disease.
Pharmacokinetics: Onset, peak, and duration vary widely among products. Most products are metabolized in the liver and excreted in urine.
Interactions: Antacids interfere with absorption of histamine H_2 antagonists. Check individual monographs for other interactions.

NURSING CONSIDERATIONS

Assessment

- Monitor gastric pH (>5 should be maintained)
- Monitor I&O ratio, BUN, creatinine

Associated nursing diagnoses

✓ Pain (uses)
✓ Risk for injury (bleeding)
✓ Knowledge deficit (teaching)

Implementation

- Give with meals for prolonged drug effect
- Give antacids 1 hr before or 1 hr after cimetidine
- Give **IV** slowly; bradycardia may occur; give over 30 min
- Store of diluted sol at room temp for up to 48 hr

Evaluation

- Therapeutic response: decreaed pain in abdomen

Patient/family education

- Advice patient that gynecomastia, impotence may occur, but is reversible
- Caution patient to avoid driving and other hazardous activities until patient is stabilized on this medication
- Caution patient to avoid black pepper, caffeine, alcohol, harsh spices, extremes in temp of food
- Caution patient to avoid OTC preparations: aspirin, cough, cold preparations
- Inform patient that drug must be continued for prescribed time to be effective
- Advise patient to report bruising, fatigue, malaise; blood dyscrasias may occur

---

Generic Names

cimetidine (p. 354)
famotidine (p. 570)
ranitidine (p. 1206)

IMMUNOSUPPRESSANTS

Action: Immunosuppressants produce immunosuppression by inhibiting T lymphocytes.

Uses: Most products are used for organ transplants to prevent rejection.

Side effects/adverse reactions: The most serious adverse reactions are albuminuria, hematuria, proteinuria, renal failure, and hepatotoxicity. The most common side effects are oral *Candida* infection, gum hyperplasia, tremors, and headache. The most serious adverse reactions for azathioprine are hematologic (leukopenia and thrombocytopenia) and GI (nausea and vomiting). There is a risk of secondary infection.
Contraindications: Products are contraindicated in hypersensitivity.
Precautions: Caution should be used in severe renal disease, severe hepatic disease, and pregnancy.
Pharmacokinetics: Onset, peak, and duration vary widely among products. Most products are metabolized in the liver and excreted in urine.
Interactions: Please check individual monographs, since interactions vary widely among products.

NURSING CONSIDERATIONS

Assessment

- Monitor renal studies: BUN, creatinine at least monthly during treatment, 3 mo after treatment
- Monitor liver function studies: alkaline phosphatase, AST (SGOT), ALT (SGPT), bilirubin
- Monitor drug blood levels during treatment
- Assess for hepatotoxicity: dark urine, jaundice, itching, light-colored stools; drug should be discontinued

Associated nursing diagnoses

✓ Risk for infection (adverse reactions)
✓ Risk for injury (uses)
✓ Knowledge deficit (teaching)

Implementation

- Give for several days before transplant surgery
- Give with meals for GI upset or place drug in chocolate milk
- Give with oral antifungal for *Candida* infections

Evaluation

- Therapeutic response: absence of rejection

Patient/family education

- Advise patient to report fever, chills, sore throat, fatigue, since serious infections may occur
- Caution patient to use contraceptive measures during treatment and for 12 wk after ending therapy

Generic Names

azathioprine (p. 178)
cyclophosphamide (p. 409)
cyclosporine (p. 413)
methotrexate (p. 886)
muromonab-CD3 (p. 957)

LAXATIVES

Action: Laxatives are divided into bulk products, lubricants, osmotics, saline laxative stimulants, and stool softeners. Bulks work by absorbing water and expanding to increase moisture content and bulk in the stool. Lubricants increase water retention in the stool, causing reabsorption of water in the bowel. Stimulants act by increasing peristalsis by direct effect on the intestine. Saline draws water into the intestinal lumen. Osmotics increase distention and promote peristalsis. Stool softeners reduce surface tension of liq in the bowel.

Uses: Laxatives are used as a preparation for bowel, rectal examination, constipation, or as stool softeners.

Side effects/adverse reactions: The most common side effects are nausea, abdominal cramps, and diarrhea.

Contraindications: Persons with GI obstruction, perforation, gastric retention, toxic colitis, megacolon, abdominal pain, nausea, vomiting, and fecal impaction should not use these products.

Precautions: Caution should be used in rectal bleeding, large hemorrhoids, and anal excoriation.

Pharmacokinetics: Onset, peak, and duration vary among products.

Interactions: Please check individual monographs, since interactions vary widely among products.

NURSING CONSIDERATIONS

Assessment

- Monitor blood, urine electrolytes if drug is used often by patient
- Monitor I&O ratio: to identify fluid loss
- Give cause of constipation; identify whether fluids, bulk, or exercise is missing from lifestyle
- Assess for cramping, rectal bleeding, nausea, vomiting; if these symptoms occur, drug should be discontinued

Associated nursing diagnoses

- ✓ Constipation (uses)
- ✓ Diarrhea (adverse reactions)
- ✓ Knowledge deficit (teaching)

Implementation

- Give alone only with water for better absorption; do not take within 1 hr of antacids, milk, or cimetidine

Evaluation

- Therapeutic response: decrease in constipation

Patient/family education

- Teach patient to swallow tab whole; do not chew
- Caution patient not to use laxatives for long-term therapy; bowel tone will be lost; that normal bowel movements do not always occur daily
- Caution patient not to use in presence of abdominal pain, nausea, vomiting
- Advise patient to notify prescriber of abdominal pain, nausea, vomiting
- Advise patient to notify prescriber if constipation is unrelieved or if symptoms of electrolyte imbalance occur: muscle cramps, pain, weakness, dizziness

---

Generic Names

Bulk laxative:
psyllium (p. 1187)

Osmotic agents:
glycerin (p. 651)
lactulose (p. 788)

Saline:
magnesium salts (p. 840)
sodium phosphate/biphosphate (p. 1249)

Stimulants:
bisacodyl (p. 208)
cascara (p. 267)
phenolphthalein (p. 1093)
senna (p. 1238)

Stool softeners:
docusate (p. 492)

OPIOID ANALGESICS

Action: These agents depress pain impulse transmission at the spinal cord level by interacting with opioid receptors. Products are divided into opiates and nonopiates.

Uses: Most products are used to control moderate to severe pain and are used before and after surgery.

Side effects/adverse reactions: GI symptoms, including nausea, vomiting, anorexia, constipation, and cramps are the most common side effects. Other common side effects include lightheadedness, dizziness, sedation. Serious adverse reactions such as respiratory depression, respiratory arrest, circulatory depression, and increased intracranial pressure may result, but are less common and usually dose dependent.

Contraindications: Hypersensitive reactions occur frequently. Check for sensitivity before administering. These drugs should not be used if narcotic addiction is suspected, and they are also contraindicated in acute bronchial asthma and upper airway obstruction.

Precautions: Caution must be used when these products are given to persons with an addictive personality, since the possibility of addiction is so great. Also, persons with increased intracranial pressure may experience an even greater increase in intracranial pressure. Persons with severe heart disease, hepatic or renal disease, respiratory conditions, and seizure disorders should be monitored closely for worsening condition.

Pharmacokinetics: Onset of action is immediate by **IV** route and rapid by IM and PO routes. Peak occurs from 1-2 hr, depending on route, with a duration of 2-8 hr. These agents cross the placenta and appear in breast milk.

Interactions: Barbiturates, other narcotics, hypnotics, antipsychotics, or alcohol can increase CNS depression when taken with narcotics.

NURSING CONSIDERATIONS

Assessment

- Monitor I&O ratio; be alert for urinary retention, frequency, dysuria; drug should be discontinued if these occur
- Assess for respiratory dysfunction, including respiratory depression, rate, rhythm, character; notify prescriber if respirations are <12/min
- Assess for CNS changes: dizziness, drowsiness, hallucinations, euphoria, LOC, pupil reaction
- Assess for allergic reactions: rash, urticaria
- Assess for need for pain medication, use pain scoring

Associated nursing diagnoses

✓ Pain (uses)
✓ Impaired gas exchange (adverse reactions)

Implementation

- Give with antiemetic if nausea or vomiting occurs

- Give when pain is beginning to return; determine dosage interval by patient response
- Provide assistance with ambulation; patient should not be ambulating during drug peak

Evaluation

- Therapeutic response: decrease in pain

Patient/family education

- Advise patient to report any symptoms of CNS changes, allergic reactions, or shortness of breath
- Caution patient that physical dependency may result when used for extended periods
- Teach patient that withdrawal symptoms may occur, including nausea, vomiting, cramps, fever, faintness, anorexia
- Advise patient to avoid alcohol and other CNS depressants

Generic Names

NEUROMUSCULAR BLOCKING AGENTS

Action: Neuromuscular blocking agents are divided into depolarizing and nondepolarizing blockers. They act by inhibiting transmission of nerve impulses by binding with cholinergic receptor sites.

Uses: Neuromuscular blocking agents are used to facilitate endotracheal intubation and skeletal muscle relaxation during mechanical ventilation, surgery, or general anesthesia.

Side effects/adverse reactions: The most serious adverse reactions are prolonged apnea, bronchospasm, cyanosis, respiratory depression, and malignant hyperthermia. The most common side effects are bradycardia and decreased motility.

Contraindications: Persons that are hypersensitive should not be given this product.

Precautions: Caution should be used in pregnancy, thyroid disease,

P collagen disease, cardiac disease, lactation, children <2 yr, electrolyte imbalances, dehydration, neuromuscular disease (myasthenia gravis), and respiratory disease.

Pharmacokinetics: Onset, peak, and duration vary widely among products. Most products are metabolized in the liver and excreted in urine.

Interactions: Aminoglycosides potentiate neuromuscular blockade. See individual monographs.

NURSING CONSIDERATIONS

Assessment

- Monitor for electrolyte imbalances (potassium, magnesium); may lead to increased action of this drug
- Monitor VS (B/P, pulse, respirations, airway) q15 min until fully recovered; rate, depth, pattern of respirations, strength of hand grip
- Monitor I&O ratio; check for urinary retention, frequency, hesitancy
- Assess for recovery: decreased paralysis of face, diaphragm, leg, arm, rest of body
- Assess for allergic reactions: rash, fever, respiratory distress, pruritus; drug should be discontinued

Associated nursing diagnoses

✓ Ineffective breathing pattern (uses)
✓ Risk for injury (adverse reactions)
✓ Knowledge deficit (teaching)

Implementation

- Administer using nerve stimulator by anesthesiologist to determine neuromuscular blockade
- Administer anticholinesterase to reverse neuromuscular blockade
- Administer **IV** undiluted over 1-2 min (only by qualified person, usually an anesthesiologist)
- Store in light-resistant, cool area
- Reassure if communication is difficult during recovery from neuromuscular blockade

Evaluation

- Therapeutic response: paralysis of jaw, eyelid, head, neck, rest of body

Generic Names

NONSTEROIDAL ANTIINFLAMMATORIES

Action: Nonsteroidals decrease prostaglandin synthesis by inhibiting an enzyme needed for biosynthesis.

Uses: Nonsteroidal antiinflammatories are used to treat mild to moderate pain, osteoarthritis, rheumatoid arthritis, and dysmenorrhea.

Side effects/adverse reactions: The most serious adverse reactions are nephrotoxicity (dysuria, hematuria, oliguria, azotemia), blood dyscrasias, and cholestatic hepatitis. The most common side effects are nausea, abdominal pain, anorexia, dizziness, and drowsiness.

Contraindications: Persons with hypersensitivity, asthma, severe renal disease, and severe hepatic disease should not use these products.

P **Precautions:** Caution should be used in pregnancy, lactation, children, bleeding disorders, GI disorders, cardiac disorders, hypersensitivity to other antiinflammatory agents, and the elderly. G

Pharmacokinetics: Onset, peak, and duration vary widely among products. Most products are metabolized in the liver and excreted in urine.

Interactions: Please check individual monographs, since interactions vary widely among products.

NURSING CONSIDERATIONS

Assessment

- Monitor renal, liver, blood studies: BUN, creatinine, AST (SGOT), ALT (SGPT), Hgb, before treatment, periodically thereafter
- Monitor audiometric, ophth examination before, during, and after treatment.
- Check for eye, ear problems: blurred vision, tinnitus, may indicate toxicity

Associated nursing diagnoses

✓ Chronic pain (uses)
✓ Impaired physical mobility (uses)

✓Knowledge deficit (teaching)
✓Noncompliance (teaching)

Implementation

- Give with food to decrease GI symptoms; however, best to take on empty stomach to facilitate absorption
- Store at room temp

Evaluation

- Therapeutic response: decreased pain, stiffness in joints, decreased swelling in joints, ability to move more easily

Patient/family education

- Advise patient to report blurred vision, ringing, roaring in ears; may indicate toxicity
- Caution patient to avoid driving, other hazardous activities if G dizziness, drowsiness occurs, especially elderly
- Advise patient to report change in urine pattern, increased weight, edema, increased pain in joints, fever, blood in urine; indicate nephrotoxicity
- Inform patient that therapeutic effects may take up to 1 mo

---

Generic Names

diclofenac (p. 450)
etodolic acid (p. 560)
fenoprofen (p. 579)
flurbiprofen (p. 623)
ibuprofen (p. 711)
indomethacin (p. 730)
ketoprofen (p. 781)
ketorolac (p. 783)
meclofenamate (p. 852)
nabumetone (p. 958)
naproxen (p. 972)
piroxicam (p. 1123)
sulindac (p. 1285)
tolmetin (p. 1355)

SALICYLATES

Action: Salicylates have analgesic, antipyretic, and antiinflammatory effects. The antiinflammatory and analgesic activities may be mediated through the inhibition of prostaglandin synthesis. Antipyretic action results from inhibition of the hypothalamic heat-regulating center.
Uses: The primary uses of salicylates are relief of mild to moderate pain and fever and in inflammatory conditions such as arthritis, thromboembolic disorders, and rheumatic fever.
Side effects/adverse reactions: The most common side effects are

GI symptoms and rash. Serious blood dyscrasias and hepatotoxicity may result when used for long periods at high doses. Tinnitus or impaired hearing may indicate that blood salicylate levels are reaching or exceeding the upper limit of the therapeutic range.

Contraindications: Hypersensitivity to salicylates is common. Check for sensitivity before administering. Persons with bleeding disorders, GI bleeding, and vitamin K deficiency should not use these products, P since salicylates increase prothrombin time. Children should not use these products, since salicylates have been associated with Reye's syndrome.

Precautions: Caution is needed when salicylates are given to patients with anemia, hepatic or renal disease, or Hodgkin's disease. Caution should also be exercised in pregnancy and lactation.

Pharmacokinetics: Onset of action occurs in 15-30 min, with a peak of 1-2 hr and a duration up to 6 hr. These drugs are metabolized by the liver and excreted by the kidneys.

Interactions: Increased effects of anticoagulants, insulin, methotrexate, heparin, valproic acid, and oral sulfonylureas may occur when used with salicylates. Aspirin may decrease serum concentrations of nonsteroidal antiinflammatory agents.

NURSING CONSIDERATIONS

Assessment

- Monitor hepatic and renal studies: AST (SGOT), ALT (SGPT), bilirubin, creatinine, LDH, alkaline phosphatase, BUN if patient is on long-term therapy, since these products are metabolized and excreted by the liver and kidney
- Monitor blood studies: CBC, Hct, Hgb, and prothrombin time if patient is on long-term therapy, since these products increase the possibility of bleeding and blood dyscrasias
- Assess for hepatotoxicity: dark urine, clay-colored stools, yellowing skin and sclera, itching, abdominal pain, fever, diarrhea, which may occur with long-term use
- Assess for ototoxicity: tinnitus, ringing, roaring in ears; audiometric testing is needed before and after long-term therapy

Associated nursing diagnoses

✓ Pain (uses)
✓ Impaired physical mobility (uses)
✓ Activity intolerance (uses)
✓ Sensory-perceptual alteration: auditory (adverse reactions)
✓ Thermoregulation (uses)

Implementation

- Give with food or milk to decrease gastric irritation; give 30 min ac or 1 hr pc with a full glass of water

Evaluation

- Therapeutic response: decreased pain, fever

Patient/family education

- Advise patient that blood sugar levels should be monitored closely, if patient is diabetic
- Caution patient not to exceed recommended dosage; acute poisoning may result
- Inform patient that therapeutic response takes 2 wk in arthritis
- Caution patient to avoid use of alcohol, since GI bleeding may result
- Advise patient to notify prescriber if ringing in the ears or persistent GI pain occurs
- Advise patient to take with full glass of water to reduce risk of lodging in esophagus

---

Generic Names

aspirin (p. 157)
choline salicylate (p. 350)
magnesium salicylate (p. 840)
salsalate (p. 1225)

THROMBOLYTICS

Action: Thrombolytics activate conversion of plasminogen to plasmin (fibrinolysin): plasmin is able to break down clots (fibrin).

Uses: Thrombolytics are used to treat deep vein thrombosis, pulmonary embolism, arterial thrombosis, arterial embolism, arteriovenous cannula occlusion, lysis of coronary artery thrombi after MI, acute evolving transmural MI.

Side effects/adverse reactions: Serious adverse reactions include GI, GU, intracranial, and retroperitoneal bleeding, and anaphylaxis. The most common side effects are decreased Hct, urticaria, headache, and nausea.

Contraindications: Persons with hypersensitivity, active bleeding, intraspinal surgery, neoplasms of the CNS, ulcerative colitis/enteritis, severe hypertension, renal disease, hepatic disease, hypocoagulation, COPD, subacute bacterial endocarditis, rheumatic valvular disease, cerebral embolism/thrombosis/hemorrhage, intraarterial diagnostic procedure or surgery (10 days), and recent major surgery should not use these products.

Precautions: Caution should be used in arterial emboli from left side of heart and pregnancy.

Pharmacokinetics: Onset, peak, and duration vary widely among products. Most products are metabolized in the liver and excreted in urine.

Interactions: Please check individual monographs, since interactions vary widely among products.

NURSING CONSIDERATIONS

Assessment

- Monitor VS, B/P, pulse, respirations, neurologic signs, temp at least q4h, temp is an indicator of internal bleeding, cardiac rhythm following intracoronary administration; systolic pressure increase of >25 mm Hg should be reported to prescriber
- Assess for neurologic changes that may indicate intracranial bleeding
- Assess retroperitoneal bleeding: back pain, leg weakness, diminished pulses
- Assess for allergy: fever, rash, itching, chill; mild reaction may be treated with antihistamines
- Assess for bleeding during 1st hr of treatment: hematuria, hematemesis, bleeding from mucous membranes, epistaxis, ecchymosis
- Monitor blood studies (Hct, platelets, PTT, PT, TT, APTT) before starting therapy; PT or APTT must be less than 2 times control before starting therapy TT or PT q3-4h during treatment

Associated nursing diagnoses

✓ Risk for injury (uses)

Implementation

- Administer as soon as thrombi identified; not useful for thrombi over 1 wk old
- Administer cryoprecipitate or fresh, frozen plasma if bleeding occurs
- Administer loading dose at beginning of therapy; may require increased loading doses
- Give heparin after fibrinogen level is over 100 mg/dl; heparin inf to increase PTT to 1.5-2 times baseline for 3-7 days
- About 10% of patients have high streptococcal antibody titers requiring increased loading doses

- Give **IV** therapy using 0.8-μm filter
- Store reconstituted sol in refrigerator; discard after 24 hr
- Provide bed rest during entire course of treatment
- Avoid venous or arterial puncture, injection, rec temp
- Provide treatment of fever with acetaminophen or aspirin
- Apply pressure for 30 sec to minor bleeding sites; inform prescriber if this does not attain hemostasis; apply pressure dressing

Evaluation

- Therapeutic response: resolution of thrombosis, embolism

Generic Names

alteplase (p. 88)
anistreplase (p. 148)
streptokinase (p. 1261)
urokinase (p. 1389)

THYROID HORMONES

Action: Increase metabolic rates, resulting in increased cardiac output, O_2 consumption, body temp, blood volume, growth, development at cellular level, respiratory rate, enzyme system activity

Uses: Products are used for thyroid replacement.

Side effects/adverse reactions: The most common side effects include insomnia, tremors, tachycardia, palpitations, angina, dysrhythmias, weight loss, and changes in appetite. Serious adverse reactions include thyroid storm.

Contraindications: Persons with adrenal insufficiency, myocardial infarction, or thyrotoxicosis should not use these products.

G **Precautions:** The elderly and patients with angina pectoris, hypertension, ischemia, cardiac disease, or diabetes mellitus or insipidus should be watched closely when using these products. Caution should be used in pregnancy **A** and lactation.

Pharmacokinetics: Pharmacokinetics vary widely among products; check specific monographs.

Interactions

- Impaired absorption of thyroid products may occur when administered with cholestyramine (separate by 4-5 hr)
- Increased effects of anticoagulants, sympathomimetics, tricyclic antidepressants, catecholamines may occur
- Decreased effects of digitalis, glycosides, insulin, hypoglycemics may occur
- Decreased effects of thyroid products may occur with estrogens

NURSING CONSIDERATIONS

Assessment

- Monitor B/P, pulse before each dose
- Monitor I&O ratio
- Monitor weight qd in same clothing, using same scale, at same time of day
- P • Monitor height, growth rate if given to a child
- Monitor T_3, T_4, which are decreased; radioimmunoassay of TSH, which is increased; ratio uptake, which is decreased if patient is on too low a dosage of medication
- Assess for increased nervousness, excitability, irritability; may indicate too high doses of medication usually after 1-3 wk of treatment
- Assess for cardiac status: angina, palpitation, chest pain, change in VS

Associated nursing diagnoses

✓ Knowledge deficit (teaching)
✓ Noncompliance (teaching)
✓ Body image disturbance (adverse reactions)

Implementation

- Give at same time each day to maintain drug level
- Give only for hormone imbalances; not to be used for obesity, male infertility, menstrual conditions, lethargy
- Remove medication 4 wk before RAIU test

Evaluation

- Therapeutic response: absence of depression; increased weight loss, diuresis, pulse, appetite; absence of constipation, peripheral edema, cold intolerance, pale, cool, dry skin, brittle nails, alopecia, coarse hair, menorrhagia, night blindness, paresthesias, syncope, stupor, coma, rosy cheeks

Patient/family education:

- P • Advise patient that hair loss will occur in child and is temporary
- Advise patient to report excitability, irritability, anxiety; indicates overdose
- Caution patient not to switch brands unless directed by prescriber
- P • Caution patient that hypothyroid child will show almost immediate behavior/personality change
- Advise patient that treatment drug is not to be taken to reduce weight

- Advise patient to avoid OTC preparations with iodine; read labels; to avoid iodine-containing food, iodinized salt, soybeans, tofu, turnips, some seafood, some bread

---

Generic Names

levothyroxine (T_4) (p. 802)
liothyronine (T_3) (p. 810)
liotrix (p. 812)
thyroid USP (p. 1334)

VASODILATORS

Action: Vasodilators act in various ways. Please check individual monograph for specific action.

Uses: Vasodilators are used to treat intermittent claudication, arteriosclerosis obliterans, vasospasm and muscular ischemia, ischemic cerebral vascular disease, hypertension, and angina.

Side effects/adverse reactions: The most common side effects are headache, nausea, hypotension or hypertension, and ECG changes.

Contraindications: Some drugs are contraindicated in acute MI, paroxysmal tachycardia, and thyrotoxicosis.

Precautions: Caution should be used in uncompensated heart disease or peptic ulcer disease.

Pharmacokinetics: Onset, peak, and duration vary widely among products. Most products are metabolized in the liver and excreted in urine.

Interactions: Please check individual monographs, since interactions vary widely among products.

NURSING CONSIDERATIONS

Assessment

- Bleeding time in individuals with bleeding disorders
- Assess cardiac status: B/P, pulse, rate, rhythm, character; watch for increasing pulse

Associated nursing diagnoses

✓ Decreased cardiac output (uses)
✓ Altered tissue perfusion: cardiovascular/pulmonary (uses)
✓ Knowledge deficit (teaching)

Implementation

- Give with meals to reduce GI symptoms

- Store in tight container at room temp

Evaluation

- Therapeutic response: ability to walk without pain, increased temp in extremities, increased pulse volume

Patient/family education

- Inform patient that medication is not cure, may need to be taken continuously
- Advise patient that it is necessary to quit smoking to prevent excessive vasoconstriction
- Advise patient that improvement may be sudden, but usually occurs gradually over several wk
- Instruct patient to report headache, weakness, increased pulse, since drug may need to be decreased or discontinued
- Instruct patient to avoid hazardous activities until stabilized on medication; dizziness may occur

---

Generic Names

amyl nitrite (p. 146)
dipyridamole (p. 484)
hydralazine (p. 687)
minoxidil (p. 934)
papaverine (p. 1045)
tolazoline (p. 1351)

VITAMINS

Action: Action varies widely among products and classes; check specific monographs.

Uses: Vitamins are used to correct and prevent vitamin deficiencies.

Side effects/adverse reactions: There is an absence of side effects or adverse reactions with the water-soluble vitamins (C, B). However, fat-soluble vitamins (A, D, E, K) may accumulate in the body and cause adverse reactions (refer to specific monographs).

Contraindications: Hypersensitive reactions may occur, and allergies should be identified before these products are given.

Pharmacokinetics: Onset, peak, and duration vary widely among products; check individual monograph for specific information.

NURSING CONSIDERATIONS

Associated nursing diagnoses

✓ Altered nutrition, less than body requirements (uses)

Implementation

- Give PO with food for better absorption
- Store in tight, light-resistant container

Evaluation

- Therapeutic response: absence of vitamin deficiency

Patient/family education

- Advise patient not to take more than prescribed amount

Generic Names

Fat-soluble:
phytonadione (p. 1107)
vitamin A (p. 1407)
vitamin D (p. 1412)
vitamin E (p. 1414)

Water-soluble:
ascorbic acid (C) (p. 152)
pyridoxine (B_6) (p. 1192)
riboflavin (B_2) (p. 1213)
thiamine (B_1) (p. 1317)

Miscellaneous:
multivitamins (p. 954)

Appendix A

Infusion Rate Tables

Aminocaproic Acid (*Amicar*)

Suggested Mixing Instructions			
Dilutions	Concentrations	Usual Dose	Suggested Titration
5000 mg/500 ml 5000 mg/250 ml	10 mg/ml 20 mg/ml	*Initial:* 4-5 g during first hr *Maintenance:* 1-1.25 g/hr for 6-8 hr *Maximal:* 30 g in 24 hr	*Give priming dose over first hr *Follow by continuous inf of 1-1.25 g/hr for 6-8 hr or until hemorrhage is controlled

TABLE A-1 Aminocaproic Acid Infusion Rates in Milliliters per Hour

	Concentration	
Dose gm/hr	10 mg/ml	20 mg/ml
0.5	50	25
1	100	50
1.25	125	63
1.5	150	75
2	200	100
3	300	150
4	400	200
5	500	250

From Keen J, et al: *Mosby's critical care and emergency drug reference,* St. Louis, 1994, Mosby–Year Book, Inc.

Aminophylline, Theophylline Ethylenediamine

Suggested Mixing Instructions			
Dilutions	Concentrations	Usual Dose	Suggested Titration
250 mg/250 ml 500 mg/250 ml 1000 mg/250 ml	1 mg/ml 2 mg/ml 4 mg/ml	*Initial:* 0.5-1 mg/kg/hr *Maintenance:* 0.1-0.8 mg/kg/hr *Maximal:* 3 mg/kg/hr	LD over 20 min, start at 0.5 mg/kg/hr and titrate up until desired response, drug level, or signs/symptoms of toxicity

TABLE A-2 Aminophylline Infusion Rates in Milliliters per Hour (Concentration: 1 mg/ml)*

Loading Dose (5.6 mg/kg)	Patient Weight in Kg (lbs)										
	50 (110)	55 (121)	60 (132)	65 (143)	70 (154)	75 (165)	80 (176)	90 (198)	100 (220)	110 (242)	120 (264)
	280 mg	308 mg	336 mg	364 mg	392 mg	420 mg	448 mg	504 mg	560 mg	616 mg	672 mg
Dose in mg/kg/hr											
0.1	5	6	6	7	7	8	8	9	10	11	12
0.2	10	11	12	13	14	15	16	18	20	22	24
0.3	15	17	18	20	21	23	24	27	30	33	36
0.4	20	22	24	26	28	30	32	36	40	44	48
0.5	25	28	30	33	35	38	40	45	50	55	60
0.6	30	33	36	39	42	45	48	54	60	66	72
0.7	35	39	42	46	49	53	56	63	70	77	84
0.8	40	44	48	52	56	60	64	72	80	88	96
0.9	45	50	54	59	63	68	72	81	90	99	108
1.0	50	55	60	65	70	75	80	90	100	110	120
2.0	100	110	120	130	140	150	160	180	200	220	240
3.0	150	165	180	195	210	225	240	270	300	330	360

*When infusion rates fall on the right side of the thick line, a more concentrated drip is indicated.

TABLE A-3 Aminophylline Infusion Rates in Milliliters per Hour (Concentration: 2 mg/ml)

Loading Dose (5.6 mg/kg)	Patient Weight in Kg (lbs)										
	50 (110)	55 (121)	60 (132)	65 (143)	70 (154)	75 (165)	80 (176)	90 (198)	100 (220)	110 (242)	120 (264)
	280 mg	308 mg	336 mg	364 mg	392 mg	420 mg	448 mg	504 mg	560 mg	616 mg	672 mg
	Dose in mg/kg/hr										
0.1	3	3	3	3	4	4	4	5	5	6	6
0.2	5	6	6	7	7	8	8	9	10	11	12
0.3	8	8	9	10	11	11	12	14	15	17	18
0.4	10	11	12	13	14	15	16	18	20	22	24
0.5	13	14	15	16	18	19	20	23	25	28	30
0.6	15	17	18	20	21	23	24	27	30	33	36
0.7	18	19	21	23	25	26	28	32	35	39	42
0.8	20	22	24	26	28	30	32	36	40	44	48
0.9	23	25	27	29	32	34	36	41	45	50	54
1.0	25	28	30	33	35	38	40	45	50	55	60
2.0	50	55	60	65	70	75	80	90	100	110	120
3.0	75	84	90	99	105	114	120	135	150	165	180

TABLE A-4 Aminophylline Infusion Rates in Milliliters per Hour (Concentration: 4 mg/ml)

Loading Dose (5.6 mg/kg)	Patient Weight in Kg (lbs)										
	50 (110)	55 (121)	60 (132)	65 (143)	70 (154)	75 (165)	80 (176)	90 (198)	100 (220)	110 (242)	120 (264)
	280 mg	308 mg	336 mg	364 mg	392 mg	420 mg	448 mg	504 mg	560 mg	616 mg	672 mg
Dose in mg/kg/hr											
0.1	1	1	2	2	2	2	2	2	3	3	3
0.2	3	3	3	3	4	4	4	5	5	6	6
0.3	4	4	5	5	5	6	6	7	8	8	9
0.4	5	6	6	6	7	8	8	9	10	11	12
0.5	6	7	8	8	9	9	10	11	13	14	15
0.6	8	8	9	10	11	11	12	14	15	17	18
0.7	9	10	11	11	12	13	14	16	18	19	21
0.8	10	11	12	13	14	15	16	18	20	22	24
0.9	11	12	14	15	16	17	18	20	23	25	27
1.0	13	14	15	16	18	19	20	23	25	28	30
2.0	25	28	30	33	35	37	40	45	50	55	60
3.0	38	41	45	49	53	56	60	68	75	83	90

Amrinone (*Inocor*)

Suggested Mixing Instructions			
Dilutions	Concentrations	Usual Dose	Suggested Titration
250 mg/250 ml 500 mg/250 ml 1000 mg/250 ml	1000 µg/ml 2000 µg/ml 4000 µg/ml	*Initial:* 2.5-5 µg/kg/min *Maintenance:* 5-10 µg/kg/min *Maximal:* 20 µg/kg/min	5 µg/kg/min q10 min: to optimize CO

TABLE A-5 Amrinone Infusion Rates in Milliliters per Hour (Concentration: 1000 μg/ml)

Loading Dose 0.75 mg/kg over 2-3 min	Patient Weight in Kg (lbs)										
	50 (110)	55 (121)	60 (132)	65 (143)	70 (154)	75 (165)	80 (176)	90 (198)	100 (220)	110 (242)	120 (264)
	38 mg	41 mg	45 mg	49 mg	53 mg	56 mg	60 mg	68 mg	75 mg	83 mg	90 mg
Dose in μg/kg/min											
5	15	17	18	20	21	23	24	27	30	33	36
6	18	20	22	23	25	27	29	32	36	40	43
7	21	23	25	27	29	32	34	38	42	46	50
8	24	26	29	31	34	36	38	43	48	53	58
9	27	30	32	35	38	41	43	49	54	59	65
10	30	33	36	39	42	45	48	54	60	66	72
11	33	36	40	43	46	50	53	59	66	73	79
12	36	40	43	47	50	54	58	65	72	79	86
13	39	43	47	51	55	59	62	70	78	86	94
14	42	46	50	55	59	63	67	76	84	92	101
15	45	50	54	59	63	68	72	81	90	99	108
20	60	66	72	78	84	90	96	108	120	132	144

TABLE A-6 Amrinone Infusion Rates in Milliliters per Hour (Concentration: 2000 μg/ml)

Loading Dose 0.75 mg/kg over 2-3 min	Patient Weight in Kg (lbs)										
	50 (110)	55 (121)	60 (132)	65 (143)	70 (154)	75 (165)	80 (176)	90 (198)	100 (220)	110 (242)	120 (264)
	38 mg	41 mg	45 mg	49 mg	53 mg	56 mg	60 mg	68 mg	75 mg	83 mg	90 mg
Dose in μg/kg/min											
5	8	8	9	10	11	11	12	14	15	17	18
6	9	10	11	12	13	14	14	16	18	20	22
7	11	12	13	14	15	16	17	19	21	23	25
8	12	13	14	16	17	18	19	22	24	26	29
9	14	15	16	18	19	20	22	24	27	30	32
10	15	17	18	20	21	23	24	27	30	33	36
11	17	18	20	21	23	25	26	30	33	36	40
12	18	20	22	23	25	27	29	32	36	40	43
13	20	21	23	25	27	29	31	35	39	43	47
14	21	23	25	27	29	32	34	38	42	46	50
15	23	25	27	29	32	34	36	41	45	50	54
20	30	33	36	39	42	45	48	54	60	66	72

TABLE A-7 Amrinone Infusion Rates in Milliliters per Hour (Concentration: 4000 μg/ml)

Loading Dose 0.75 mg/kg over 2-3 min	Patient Weight in Kg (lbs)										
	50 (110)	55 (121)	60 (132)	65 (143)	70 (154)	75 (165)	80 (176)	90 (198)	100 (220)	110 (242)	120 (264)
	38 mg	41 mg	45 mg	49 mg	53 mg	56 mg	60 mg	68 mg	75 mg	83 mg	90 mg
Dose in μg/kg/min											
5	4	4	5	5	5	6	6	7	8	8	9
6	5	5	5	6	6	7	7	8	9	10	11
7	5	6	6	7	7	8	8	9	11	12	13
8	6	7	7	8	8	9	10	11	12	13	14
9	7	7	8	9	9	10	11	12	14	15	16
10	8	8	9	10	11	11	12	14	15	17	18
11	8	9	10	11	12	12	13	15	17	18	20
12	9	10	11	12	13	14	14	16	18	20	22
13	10	11	12	13	14	15	16	18	20	21	23
14	11	12	13	14	15	16	17	19	21	23	25
15	11	12	14	15	16	17	18	20	23	25	27
20	15	17	18	20	21	23	24	27	30	33	36

Lidocaine HCl (*Xylocaine*), Procainamide HCl (*Pronestyl*), Bretylium (*Bretylol*)

Suggested Mixing Instructions			
Dilutions	Concentrations	Usual Dose	Suggested Titration
500 mg/500 ml 500 mg/250 ml 1000 mg/250 ml 2000 mg/250 ml	1 mg/ml 2 mg/ml 4 mg/ml 8 mg/ml	*Initial:* 1-2 mg/min *Maintenance:* 1-4 mg/min	Start at 1-2 mg/min and titrate for dysrhythmia control

TABLE A-8 Lidocaine/Pronestyl/Bretylium Infusion Rates in Milliliters per Hour

Dose mg/min	Concentrations			
	1 mg/ml	2 mg/ml	4 mg/ml	8 mg/ml
1	60	30	15	8
2	120	60	30	15
3	180	90	45	23
4	240	120	60	30

Dobutamine HCl (*Dobutrex*)

Suggested Mixing Instructions			
Dilutions	Concentrations	Usual Dose	Suggested Titration
250 mg/250 ml 500 mg/250 ml 1000 mg/250 ml	1000 μg/ml 2000 μg/ml 4000 μg/ml	*Initial:* 2.5 μg/kg/min *Maintenance:* 2.5-10 μg/kg/min *Maximal:* 40 μg/kg/min	2.5 μg/kg/min q10 min: to optimize CO

TABLE A-9 Dobutamine Infusion Rates in Milliliters per Hour (Concentration: 1000 μg/ml)*

Dose μg/kg/min	Patient Weight in Kg (lbs)										
	50 (110)	55 (121)	60 (132)	65 (143)	70 (154)	75 (165)	80 (176)	90 (198)	100 (220)	110 (242)	120 (264)
2.5	8	8	9	10	11	11	12	14	15	17	18
5	15	17	18	20	21	23	24	27	30	33	36
7.5	23	25	27	29	32	34	36	41	45	50	54
10	30	33	36	39	42	45	48	54	60	66	72
12.5	38	41	45	49	53	56	60	68	75	83	90
15	45	50	54	59	63	68	72	81	90	99	108
17.5	53	58	63	68	74	79	84	95	105	116	126
20	60	66	72	78	84	90	96	108	120	132	144
22.5	68	74	81	88	96	101	108	122	135	149	162
25	75	83	90	98	105	113	120	135	150	165	180
27.5	83	91	99	108	116	124	132	149	165	182	198
30	91	99	108	118	127	135	144	163	180	199	216
32.5	99	107	117	128	138	146	156	177	195	216	234

*When infusion rates fall on the right side of the thick line, a more concentrated drip is indicated.

TABLE A-10 Dobutamine Infusion Rates in Milliliters per Hour (Concentration: 2000 µg/ml)

Dose µg/kg/min	Patient Weight in Kg (lbs)										
	50 (110)	55 (121)	60 (132)	65 (143)	70 (154)	75 (165)	80 (176)	90 (198)	100 (220)	110 (242)	120 (264)
2.5	4	4	5	5	5	6	6	7	8	8	9
5	8	8	9	10	11	11	12	14	15	17	18
7.5	11	12	14	15	16	17	18	20	23	25	27
10	15	17	18	20	21	23	24	27	30	33	36
12.5	19	21	23	24	26	28	30	34	38	41	45
15	23	25	27	29	32	34	36	41	45	50	54
17.5	26	29	32	34	37	39	42	47	53	58	63
20	30	33	36	39	42	45	48	54	60	66	72
22.5	34	37	41	44	47	51	54	61	68	74	81
25	38	41	45	49	53	56	60	68	75	83	90
27.5	41	45	50	54	58	62	66	74	83	91	99
30	45	50	54	59	63	68	72	81	90	99	108
32.5	49	54	59	63	68	73	78	88	98	107	117

TABLE A-11 Dobutamine Infusion Rates in Milliliters per Hour (Concentration: 4000 μg/ml)

Dose μg/kg/min	Patient Weight in Kg (lbs)										
	50 (110)	55 (121)	60 (132)	65 (143)	70 (154)	75 (165)	80 (176)	90 (198)	100 (220)	110 (242)	120 (264)
2.5	2	2	2	2	3	3	3	3	4	4	5
5	4	4	5	5	5	6	6	7	8	8	9
7.5	6	6	7	7	8	8	9	10	11	12	14
10	8	8	9	10	11	11	12	14	15	17	18
12.5	9	10	11	12	13	14	15	17	19	21	23
15	11	12	14	15	16	17	18	20	23	25	27
17.5	13	14	16	17	18	20	21	24	26	29	32
20	15	17	18	20	21	23	24	27	30	33	36
22.5	17	19	20	22	24	25	27	30	34	37	41
25	19	21	23	24	26	28	30	34	38	41	45
27.5	21	23	25	27	29	31	33	37	41	45	50
30	23	25	27	29	32	34	36	41	45	50	54
32.5	24	27	29	32	34	36	39	44	49	54	59

Dobutamine HCl (*Dobutrex*)

Pediatric Chart			
Suggested Mixing Instructions		Usual Dose	Suggested Titration
Dilutions	Concentrations		
250 mg/500 ml	500 μg/ml	*Initial:* 2.5 μg/kg/min *Maintenance:* 2.5-10 μg/kg/min *Maximal:* 40 μg/kg/min	2.5 μg/kg/min q10 min: to optimize CO

TABLE A-12 Dobutamine Infusion Rates in Milliliters per Hour (Concentration: 500 μg/ml)

Dose μg/kg/min	Patient Weight in Kg (lbs)										
	4 (9)	6 (13)	8 (18)	10 (22)	12 (26)	14 (31)	16 (35)	18 (40)	20 (44)	25 (55)	30 (66)
2	1	1	2	2	3	3	4	4	5	6	7
3	1	2	3	4	4	5	6	6	7	9	11
4	2	3	4	5	6	7	8	9	10	12	14
5	2	4	5	6	7	8	10	11	12	15	18
6	3	4	6	7	9	10	12	13	14	18	22
7	3	5	7	8	8	12	13	15	17	21	25
8	4	6	8	10	12	13	15	17	19	24	29
9	4	6	9	11	13	15	17	19	22	27	32
10	5	7	10	12	14	17	19	22	24	30	36

Dopamine (*Dopastat, Intropin*)

Suggested Mixing Instructions		Usual Dose	Suggested Titration
Dilutions	Concentrations		
200 mg/250 ml 400 mg/250 ml 800 mg/250 ml	800 μg/ml 1600 μg/ml 3200 μg/ml	*Low Dose:* 0.5-2 μg/kg/min (dopaminergic effects) *Intermediate Dose:* 2-10 μg/kg/min (β-1 adrenergic effects) *High Dose:* >10 μg/kg/min (alpha-adrenergic effects)	Increase by 1-4 μg/kg/min q10-30 min until desired response maximum dose: 40 μg/kg/min

TABLE A-13 Dopamine Infusion Rates in Milliliters per Hour (Concentration: 800 μg/ml)*

Dose μg/kg/min	Patient Weight in Kg (lbs)										
	50 (110)	55 (121)	60 (132)	65 (143)	70 (154)	75 (165)	80 (176)	90 (198)	100 (220)	110 (242)	120 (264)
2	8	8	9	10	11	11	12	14	15	17	18
5	19	21	23	24	26	28	30	34	38	41	45
12.5	47	52	56	61	66	70	75	84	94	103	113
15	56	62	68	73	79	84	90	101	113	124	135
17.5	66	70	79	85	92	98	105	118	131	144	158
20	75	83	90	98	105	113	120	135	150	165	180
25	94	103	113	122	131	141	150	169	188	206	225
30	112	124	135	146	158	169	180	203	225	248	270
40	150	165	180	195	210	225	240	270	300	330	360
50	188	206	225	244	263	281	300	338	375	413	450

*When infusion rates fall on the right side of the thick line, a more concentrated drip is indicated.

TABLE A-14 Dopamine Infusion Rates in Milliliters per Hour (Concentration: 1600 μg/ml)*

Dose μg/kg/min	Patient Weight in Kg (lbs)										
	50 (110)	55 (121)	60 (132)	65 (143)	70 (154)	75 (165)	80 (176)	90 (198)	100 (220)	110 (242)	120 (264)
2	4	4	5	5	5	6	6	7	8	8	9
5	9	10	11	12	13	14	15	18	19	21	23
12.5	23	26	28	30	33	35	38	42	47	52	56
15	28	31	34	37	39	42	45	51	56	62	68
17.5	33	36	39	43	46	49	53	59	66	72	79
20	38	41	45	49	53	56	60	68	75	83	90
25	47	52	56	61	66	70	75	85	94	103	113
30	56	62	68	73	79	84	90	101	113	124	135
40	75	83	90	98	105	113	120	135	150	165	180
50	94	103	113	122	131	140	150	169	188	206	225

*When infusion rates fall to the right side of the thick line, a more concentrated infusion rate is indicated.

TABLE A-15 Dopamine Infusion Rates in Milliliters per Hour (Concentration: 3200 µg/ml)

Dose µg/kg/min	Patient Weight in Kg (lbs)										
	50 (110)	55 (121)	60 (132)	65 (143)	70 (154)	75 (165)	80 (176)	90 (198)	100 (220)	110 (242)	120 (264)
2	2	2	2	2	3	3	3	3	4	4	5
5	5	5	6	6	7	7	8	8	9	10	11
12.5	12	13	14	15	16	18	19	21	23	26	28
15	14	15	17	18	20	21	23	25	28	31	34
17.5	16	18	20	21	23	25	26	30	33	36	39
20	19	21	23	24	26	28	30	34	38	41	45
25	23	26	28	30	33	35	38	42	47	52	56
30	28	31	34	37	39	42	45	51	56	62	68
40	38	41	45	49	53	56	60	68	75	83	90
50	47	52	56	61	66	70	75	84	94	103	113

Dopamine (*Dopastat, Intropin*)

Pediatric Chart			
Suggested Mixing Instructions		Usual Dose	Suggested Titration
Dilution	Concentration		
40 mg/100 ml	400 μg/ml	*Low Dose:* 0.5-2 μg/kg/min (dopaminergic effects) *Intermediate Dose:* 2-10 μg/kg/min (β-1 adrenergic effects) *High Dose:* >10 μg/kg/min (alpha-adrenergic effects)	Increase by 1-4 μg/kg/min q10-30 min until desired response maximum dose: 40 μg/kg/min

TABLE A-16 Dopamine Infusion Rates in Milliliters per Hour (Concentration: 400 μg/ml)

Dose μg/kg/min	Patient Weight in Kg (lbs)									
	4 (9)	6 (13)	8 (18)	10 (22)	12 (26)	14 (31)	16 (35)	18 (40)	20 (44)	25 (55)	30 (66)
2	1	2	2	3	4	4	5	5	6	8	9
3	2	3	4	5	5	6	7	8	9	11	14
4	2	4	5	6	7	8	10	11	12	15	18
5	3	5	6	8	9	11	12	14	15	19	23
6	4	5	7	9	11	13	14	16	18	23	27
7	4	6	8	11	13	15	17	19	21	26	32
8	5	7	10	12	14	17	19	22	24	30	36
9	5	8	11	14	16	19	22	24	27	34	41
10	6	9	12	15	18	21	24	27	30	38	45
12	7	11	14	18	22	25	29	32	36	45	54
14	8	13	17	21	25	29	34	38	42	53	63
16	10	14	19	24	29	34	38	43	48	60	72
18	11	16	22	27	32	38	43	49	54	68	81
20	12	18	24	30	36	42	48	54	60	75	90

Esmolol (*Brevibloc*)

Suggested Mixing Instructions		Usual Dose	Suggested Titration
Dilutions	Concentrations		
2500 mg/250 ml 5000 mg/250 ml	10 mg/ml 20 mg/ml	*Initial:* 50 μg/kg/min *Maintenance:* 50-200 μg/kg/min *Maximal:* <300 μg/kg/min	(LD) over 1 min, 50 μg/kg if no response, repeat LD and increase infusion rate in increments of 50 μg/kg/min until desired response

TABLE A-17 Esmolol Infusion Rates in Milliliters per Hour (Concentration: 10 μg/ml)

Loading Dose (500 μg/kg)	Patient Weight in Kg (lbs)										
	50 (110)	55 (121)	60 (132)	65 (143)	70 (154)	75 (165)	80 (176)	90 (198)	100 (220)	110 (242)	120 (264)
	25 mg	28 mg	30 mg	33 mg	35 mg	38 mg	40 mg	45 mg	50 mg	55 mg	60 mg
Dose in mcg/kg/min											
2.5	8	8	9	10	11	11	12	14	15	17	18
5	15	17	18	20	21	23	24	27	30	33	36
7.5	23	25	27	30	32	34	36	41	45	50	54
10	30	33	36	39	42	45	48	54	60	66	72
12.5	38	41	45	49	53	56	60	68	75	83	90
15	45	50	54	59	63	68	72	81	90	99	108
17.5	53	58	63	68	74	79	84	95	105	116	126
20	60	66	72	78	84	90	96	108	120	132	144

TABLE A-18 Esmolol Infusion Rates in Milliliters per Hour (Concentration: 20 μg/ml)

Loading Dose (500 μg/kg)	Patient Weight in Kg (lbs)										
	50 (110)	55 (121)	60 (132)	65 (143)	70 (154)	75 (165)	80 (176)	90 (198)	100 (220)	110 (242)	120 (264)
	25 mg	28 mg	30 mg	33 mg	35 mg	38 mg	40 mg	45 mg	50 mg	55 mg	60 mg
Dose in mcg/kg/min											
2.5	4	4	5	5	5	6	6	7	8	8	9
5	8	8	9	10	11	11	12	14	15	17	18
7.5	11	12	14	15	16	17	18	20	23	25	27
10	15	17	18	20	21	23	24	27	30	33	36
12.5	19	21	23	24	26	28	30	34	38	41	45
15	23	25	27	29	32	34	36	41	45	50	54
17.5	26	29	32	34	37	39	42	47	53	58	63
20	30	33	36	39	42	45	48	54	60	66	72

Epinephrine (*Adrenalin*)

Suggested Mixing Instructions			
Dilutions	Concentrations	Usual Dose	Suggested Titration
1 mg/250 ml 3 mg/250 ml 8 mg/250 ml	4 µg/ml 12 µg/ml 32 µg/ml	*Low:* 1-4 µg/min *Moderate:* 4-12 µg/min *Maximal:* <40 µg/min	Titrate by 1 µg/min increments q5 min until desired response is achieved

TABLE A-19 Epinephrine Infusion Rates in Milliliters per Hour*

Dose µg/min	Concentration		
	4 µg/ml	12 µg/ml	32 µg/ml
1	15	5	2
2	30	10	4
3	45	15	6
4	60	20	8
5	75	25	9
6	90	30	11
7	105	35	13
8	120	40	15
9	135	45	17
10	150	50	19
15		75	29
20		125	38
25		150	47
30			56
35			66
40			75

*When infusion rates fall below the thick line, a more concentrated drip is indicated.

Heparin Sodium

Suggested Mixing Instructions			
Dilutions	Concentrations	Usual Dose	Suggested Titration
10,000 U/500 ml 20,000 U/500 ml 25,000 U/250 ml	20 U/ml 40 U/ml 100 U/ml	*Initial:* loading dose of 5000 U *Maintenance:* 20-40,000 U/24 hr or (800-1600 U/hr)	Rate adjusted according to desired response as measured by clotting tests

TABLE A-20 Heparin Infusion Rates in Milliliters per Hour

Dose U/hr	Concentration		
	20 U/ml	40 U/ml	100 U/ml
500	25	13	5
750	38	19	8
1000	50	25	10
1250	63	31	13
1500	75	38	15
1750	88	44	18
2000	100	50	20

Isoproterenol (*Isuprel*)

Suggested Mixing Instructions		Usual Dose	Suggested Titration
Dilutions	Concentrations		
1 mg/250 ml 2 mg/250 ml 4 mg/250 ml	4 µg/ml 8 µg/ml 16 µg/ml	*Initial:* 0.5 µg/min *Maintenance:* use lowest effective dose *Maximal:* <10 µg/min	Titrate by 0.5-2 µg/min at q5-15 min intervals desired response is achieved

TABLE A-21 Isoproterenol Infusion Rates in Milliliters per Hour

Dose µg/min	Concentration		
	4 µg/ml	8 µg/ml	16 µg/ml
0.5	8	4	2
1	15	8	4
2	30	15	8
4	60	30	15
6	90	45	23
8	120	60	30
10	150	75	38

Nitroglycerin (*Tridil*)

Suggested Mixing Instructions			
Dilutions	Concentrations	Usual Dose	Suggested Titration
25 mg/250 ml 50 mg/250 ml 100 mg/250 ml	100 μg/ml 200 μg/ml 400 μg/ml	*Initial:* 5-10 μg/min *Maintenance:* use lowest effective dose *Maximal:* <200 μg/min	Titrate by 5-10 μg/min increments q5-10 min until angina subsides

TABLE A-22 Nitroglycerine Infusion Rates in Milliliters per Hour

Dose µg/min	Concentration		
	100 µg/ml	200 µg/ml	400 µg/ml
5	3	—	—
10	6	3	2
20	12	6	3
30	18	9	5
40	24	12	6
50	30	15	8
60	36	18	9
70	42	21	10
80	48	24	12
90	54	27	14
100	60	30	15
150	90	45	23
200	120	60	30
250	150	75	38
350	210	105	53

Nitroprusside Sodium (*Nipride, Nitropress*)

Suggested Mixing Instructions			
Dilutions	Concentrations	Usual Dose	Suggested Titration
50 mg/250 ml 100 mg/250 ml 200 mg/250 ml	200 μg/ml 400 μg/ml 800 μg/ml	*Initial:* 0.3 μg/kg/min *Maintenance:* 3-5 μg/kg/min *Maximal:* 10 μg/kg/min	Titrate inf by small increments: q2-3 min according to BP

TABLE A-23 Nitroprusside Infusion Rates in Milliliters per Hour (Concentration: 200 μg/ml)*

Dose	Patient Weight in Kg (lbs)										
μg/kg/min	50 (110)	55 (121)	60 (132)	65 (143)	70 (154)	75 (165)	80 (176)	90 (198)	100 (220)	110 (242)	120 (264)
0.3	5	5	5	6	6	7	7	8	9	10	11
0.5	8	8	9	10	11	11	12	14	15	17	18
1	15	17	18	20	21	23	24	27	30	33	36
2	30	33	36	39	42	45	48	54	60	66	72
3	45	50	54	59	63	68	72	81	90	99	108
4	60	66	72	78	84	90	96	108	120	132	144
5	75	83	90	98	105	113	120	135	150	165	180
6	90	99	108	117	126	135	144	162	180	198	216
7	105	116	126	137	147	158	168	189	210	231	252
8	120	132	144	156	168	180	192	216	240	264	288
9	135	149	162	176	189	203	216	243	270	297	324
10	150	165	180	195	210	225	240	270	300	330	360

*When infusion rates fall on right side of the thick line, a more concentrated drip is indicated.

TABLE A-24 Nitroprusside Sodium Infusion Rates in Milliliters per Hour (Concentration: 400 μg/ml)*

Dose	Patient Weight in Kg (lbs)										
μg/kg/min	50 (110)	55 (121)	60 (132)	65 (143)	70 (154)	75 (165)	80 (176)	90 (198)	100 (220)	110 (242)	120 (264)
0.3	2	2	3	3	3	3	4	4	5	5	5
0.5	4	4	5	5	5	6	6	7	8	8	9
1	8	8	9	10	11	11	12	14	15	17	18
2	15	17	18	20	21	23	24	27	30	33	36
3	23	25	27	30	32	34	36	41	45	50	54
4	30	33	36	39	42	45	48	54	60	66	72
5	38	41	45	49	53	56	60	68	75	83	90
6	45	50	54	59	63	68	72	81	90	99	108
7	53	58	63	68	74	79	84	95	105	116	126
8	60	66	72	78	84	90	96	108	120	132	144
9	68	74	81	88	95	101	108	122	135	149	162
10	75	83	90	98	105	113	120	135	150	165	180

*When infusion rates fall on right side of the thick line, a more concentrated drip is indicated.

TABLE A-25 Nitroprusside Sodium Infusion Rates in Milliliters per Hour (Concentration: 800 µg/ml)

Dose µg/kg/min	Patient Weight in Kg (lbs)										
	50 (110)	55 (121)	60 (132)	65 (143)	70 (154)	75 (165)	80 (176)	90 (198)	100 (220)	110 (242)	120 (264)
0.3	1	1	1	1	2	2	2	2	2	3	3
0.5	2	2	2	2	3	3	3	3	4	4	5
1	4	4	5	5	5	6	6	7	8	8	9
2	8	8	9	10	11	11	12	14	15	17	18
3	11	12	14	15	16	17	18	20	23	25	27
4	15	17	18	20	21	23	24	27	30	33	36
5	19	21	23	24	26	28	30	34	38	41	45
6	23	25	27	29	32	34	36	41	45	50	54
7	26	29	32	34	37	39	42	47	53	58	63
8	30	33	36	39	42	45	48	54	60	66	72
9	34	37	41	44	47	51	54	61	68	74	81
10	38	41	45	49	53	56	60	68	75	83	90

Nitroprusside Sodium (*Nipride Nitropress*)

Pediatric Chart

Suggested Mixing Instructions		Usual Dose	Suggested Titration
Dilution	Concentration		
50 mg/250 ml	200 μg/ml	*Initial:* 0.3 μg/kg/min *Maintenance:* 3-5 μg/kg/min *Maximal:* 10 μg/kg/min	Titrate inf by small increments: q2-3 min according to BP

TABLE A-26 Nitroprusside Sodium Infusion Rates in Milliliters per Hour (Concentration: 200 μg/ml)

Dose μg/kg/min	Patient Weight in Kg (lbs)										
	4 (9)	6 (13)	8 (18)	10 (22)	12 (26)	14 (31)	16 (35)	18 (40)	20 (44)	25 (55)	30 (66)
0.5	1	1	1	2	2	2	2	3	3	4	5
1	1	2	2	3	4	4	5	5	6	8	9
1.5	2	3	3	5	6	6	7	8	9	12	14
2	2	4	5	6	7	8	10	11	12	15	18
2.5	3	5	6	8	9	11	12	14	15	19	23
3	4	5	7	9	11	13	14	16	18	23	27
4	5	7	10	12	14	17	19	22	24	30	36
5	6	9	12	15	18	21	24	27	30	38	45
6	7	11	14	18	22	25	29	32	36	45	54
7	8	13	17	21	25	29	34	38	42	53	63
8	10	14	19	24	29	32	38	43	48	60	72
9	11	16	22	27	32	38	43	49	54	68	81
10	12	18	24	30	36	42	48	54	60	75	90

Norepinephrine (*Levophed*)

Suggested Mixing Instructions		Usual Dose	Suggested Titration
Dilutions	Concentrations		
2 mg/500 ml 4 mg/500 ml 8 mg/500 ml 8 mg/250 ml	4 µg/ml 8 µg/ml 16 µg/ml 32 µg/ml	*Initial:* 8-12 µg/min *Maintenance:* 2-4 µg/min *Maximum:* 40 µg/min	Adjust q2 min as necessary to maintain desired systolic or mean BP

TABLE A-27 Norepinephrine Infusion Rates in Milliliters per Hour

Dose µg/min	Concentration			
	4 µg/ml	8 µg/ml	16 µg/ml	32 µg/ml
4	60	30	15	8
8	120	60	30	15
10	150	75	38	19
12	180	90	45	23
14	210	105	53	26
16	240	120	60	30
18	270	135	68	34
20	300	150	75	38
25	375	188	94	47
30	450	225	113	56
35	525	263	131	66
40	600	300	150	75

Phenylephrine (*Neo-Synephrine*)

Suggested Mixing Instructions		Usual Dose	Suggested Titration
Dilutions	Concentrations		
10 mg/500 ml 10 mg/250 ml 50 mg/500 ml	20 μg/ml 40 μg/ml 100 μg/ml	*Initial:* 100-180 μg/min *Maintenance:* 40-60 μg/min	Titrate to systolic or mean BP, adjust q10-15 min to maintain low normal systolic BP

TABLE A-28 Phenylephrine Infusion Rates in Milliliters per Hour

Dose μg/min	Concentration		
	20 μg/ml	40 μg/ml	100 μg/ml
20	60	30	12
40	120	60	24
60	180	90	36
80	240	120	48
100	300	150	60
120	360	180	72
140	420	210	84
160	480	240	96
180	540	270	108
200	600	300	120

Propofol (*Diprivan*)

Pre-Mixed Solutions			
Dilutions	Concentration	Usual Dose	Suggested Titration
200 mg/20 ml ampule 500 mg/50 ml vial 1,000 mg/100 ml vial	10 mg/ml	*Initial:* 5 µg/kg/min *Maintenance:* 5-50 µg/kg/min *Maximum:* 150 µg/kg/min	Start at 5 µg/kg/min, increase by increments of 5 µg/kg/min q5-10 min until desired level of sedation

TABLE A-29 Diprivan Infusion Rates in Milliliters per Hour (Concentration: 10 μg/ml)

Dose μg/kg/min	Patient Weight in Kg (lbs)										
	50 (110)	55 (121)	60 (132)	65 (143)	70 (154)	75 (165)	80 (176)	90 (198)	100 (220)	110 (242)	120 (264)
5	2	2	2	2	2	2	2	3	3	3	4
10	3	3	4	4	4	5	5	5	6	7	7
15	5	5	5	6	6	7	7	8	9	10	11
20	6	7	7	8	8	9	10	11	12	13	14
25	8	8	9	10	11	11	12	14	15	17	18
30	9	10	11	12	13	14	14	16	18	20	22
35	11	12	13	14	15	16	17	19	21	23	25
40	12	13	14	16	17	18	19	22	24	26	29
45	14	15	16	18	19	20	22	24	27	30	32
50	15	17	18	20	21	23	24	27	30	33	36
60	18	20	22	23	25	27	29	32	36	40	43
70	21	23	25	27	29	32	34	38	42	46	50
80	24	26	29	31	34	36	38	43	48	53	58
90	27	30	32	35	38	41	43	49	54	59	65
100	30	33	36	39	42	45	48	54	60	66	72

Propranolol HCl (*Inderal*)

Suggested Mixing Instructions		Usual Dose	Suggested Titration
Dilutions	Concentrations		
15 mg/500 ml 15 mg/250 ml	30 μg/ml 60 μg/ml	*Initial:* 2 mg/hr *Maintenance:* 2-3 mg/hr	Most patients well controlled on 2-3 mg/hr, if needed can give intermittent bol doses of 1 mg

TABLE A-30 Propranolol Infusion Rates in Milliliters per Hour

Dose mg/hr	Concentration	
	30 μg/ml	60 μg/ml
1	33	17
2	67	33
3	100	50
4	133	67

Vasopressin (*Pitressin*)

Mixing Instructions		Usual Dose	Suggested Titration
Dilutions	Concentrations		
100 U/100 ml 200 U/250 ml	1 U/ml 0.8 U/ml	*Initial:* 0.2 U/min *Maintenance:* increase qh by 0.2 U/min until hemorrhage controlled	Start at 0.2 U/min; Increase in increments of 0.2 U/min q each hr until hemorrhage controlled Maximum dose 1-2 U/min

TABLE A-31 Vasopressin Infusion Rates in Milliliters per Hour

Dose		Concentration	
U/min	U/hr	1 U/ml	0.8 U/ml
0.2	12	12	15
0.4	24	24	30
0.6	36	36	45
0.8	48	48	60
1	60	60	75
1.2	72	72	90
1.4	84	84	105
1.6	96	96	120
1.8	108	108	135
2	120	120	150

Appendix B

Drugs Not to Crush

The following is a partial list of drugs that should not be crushed. Whenever possible it is suggested that if a liquid dosage form of the medication is available, it should be used instead of a crushed tablet. Coated tablets generally should not be crushed because the coating was applied for a specific reason, such as (1) to prevent stomach irritation (e.g., Dulcolax Tablet); (2) to prevent destruction by stomach acids (e.g., Ananase) (3) to produce a prolonged or extended effect (e.g., Dimetapp) or (4) to avoid an unwanted reaction (e.g., chloral hydrate in capsule has a very bitter taste, and Povan tablet will stain the mouth red; Kaon tablets may produce a burning effect on sensitive mucosa).

Afrinol Repetabs
Allerest Capsule
Aminodur Duratab
Artane Sequel
ASA Enseals
Azulfadine Entab
Betaphen-VK
Compazine Spansule
Diamox Sequel
Donnatol Extentab
Drixoral tablet
Ecotrin tablet
E-Mycin tablet
Entozyme tablet
Feosol tablet
Feosol Spansule
Ferro Grad-500 Tab
Isordil Sublingual
Kaon tablet
Nitroglycerin tab
Nitrospan capsule
Ornade Spansule
Quinaglute Duratab
Quinidex Extentab
Slow K tablet
Sudafed SA Capsule
Theo-Dur tablet
Teldrin Capsule
Trental

From McKenry and Salerno: Mosby's pharmacology in nursing, ed 19, St. Louis, 1995, Mosby–Year Book, Inc.

Appendix C

Routine Pediatric and Adult Immunizations

TABLE C-1 Active Immunization of Normal Infants and Children: Recommended Schedule

Age	Vaccines*	Special comments
2 mo	DPT, OPV, H Flu, Hep B	DPT/OPV may be given earlier if endemic to the area.
4 mo	DPT, OPV, H Flu, Hep B	
6 mo	DPT, OPV, H Flu, Hep B	Third dose of OPV may be omitted in low-risk areas.
12 mo	H Flu	
15 mo	MMR	If OPV omitted at 6 mo, it should be administered now.
18 mo	DPT, OPV, Hep B	Hep B is only administered if all previous 3 doses were not given.
4-6 yr	DPT, OPV, MMR	The measles vaccine may be administered alone.
14-16 yr	DT	Diphtheria and tetanus should be given and then repeated every 10 yr.

*Vaccines: *DPT:* diphtheria-pertussis-tetanus; *OPV:* oral polio vaccine; *MMR:* measles-mumps-rubella; *H Flu: Haemophilus* influenza; *Hep B:* hepatitis B.

From McKenry and Salerno: Mosby's pharmacology in nursing, ed 19, St. Louis, 1995, Mosby–Year Book, Inc.

TABLE C-2 Adult Immunization Recommendations (Ages 18 and Older)

Immunizing agent	Indication(s)/dosage schedule
For all adults routinely	
Tetanus toxoid	Management of wounds. IM booster dose every 10 yr.
Diphtheria toxoid	As a preventative or to help in management of contacts with persons with diphtheria. IM dose every 10 yr.
For selected persons	
Influenza vaccine	Elderly persons or persons with chronic disease states. Adults living in high-risk situations: nursing home residents, medical personnel, or healthy persons 65 yr and older. Annually.
Pneumococcal vaccine	High-risk persons, such as those with underlying health problems and healthy elderly persons 65 yr and older. Repeat 6 yr after first dose.
For adolescents and young persons	
Measles vaccine	For persons born after 1956 who have not had measles or have not previously received a live virus vaccine. SC schedule, 2 doses.
Rubella vaccine	For hospital workers, adolescents and adult females up to age 45 who are not immunized and have no laboratory evidence of immunity. SC once.
Hepatitis B vaccine	For persons at high risk of hepatitis exposure, such as health care personnel, hemodialysis patients, drug abusers, those exposed to a family member with hepatitis, and travelers. Three doses are the usual dosage schedule.

From McKenry and Salerno: Mosby's pharmacology in nursing, ed 19, St. Louis, 1995, Mosby–Year Book, Inc.

Appendix D

Combination Products

Aceta with Codeine, Empracet with Codeine No. 3, Tylenol with Codeine No. 3: acetaminophen 300 mg with codeine phosphate 30 mg
Alazide, Altexide: spironolactone 25 mg with hydrochlorothiazide 25 mg
Aldactazide 25/25: spironolactone 25 mg with hydrochlorothiazide 25 mg
Aldactazide 50/50: spironolactone 50 mg with hydrochlorothiazide 50 mg
Aldoclor-15: methyldopa 250 mg with chlorothiazide 15 mg
Aldoclor-150: methyldopa 250 mg with chlorothiazide 150 mg
Aldoclor-250: methyldopa 250 mg with chlorothiazide 250
Aldoril-15: methyldopa 250 mg with hydrochlorothiazide 15 mg
Aldoril-25: methyldopa 250 mg with hydrochlorothiazide 25 mg
Aldoril D30: methyldopa 500 mg with hydrochlorothiazide 30 mg
Aldoril D50: methyldopa 500 mg with hydrochlorothiazide 50 mg
Amaphen with Codeine No 3: acetaminophen 325 mg with butalbital 50 mg, caffeine 40 mg, codeine phosphate 30 mg
Ambenyl: diphenhydramine HCl 12.5 mg/5 ml with codeine phosphate 10 mg/5 ml
Anexsia: hydrocodone bitartrate 7.5 mg with acetaminophen 325 mg
Anexsia with Codeine, Empirin with Codeine 30 mg No. 3: codeine 30 mg with acetaminophen 325 mg
Anguen No. 1: pentaerythritol tetranitrate 20 mg, phenobarbital 15 mg
Anodynos-DHC, DIA-Gesic: acetaminophen 150 mg with aspirin 230 mg, caffeine 30 mg, hydrocodone bitartrate 5 mg
Antrocol: atropine sulfate 0.195 mg with phenobarbital 16 mg
Antrocol Elixir: atropine sulfate 0.039 mg/ml with phenobarbital 3 mg/ml
Apresazide 25/25: hydralazine HCl 25 mg with hydrochlorothiazide 25 mg
Apresazide 50/50: hydralazine HCl 50 mg with hydrochlorothiazide 50 mg
Apresazide 100/50: hydralazine HCl 100 mg with hydrochlorothiazide 50 mg
Apresodex, Apresoline-Esidrix: hydralazine HCl 25 mg with hydrochlorothiazide 15 mg
Aralen Phosphate with Primaquine Phosphate: chloroquine phosphate 300 mg (of chloroquine) with primaquine phosphate 45 mg (of primaquine)
Arcotrate No. 3: pentaerythri-

tol tetranitrate 20 mg, phenobarbital 8 mg

A.S.A. and Codeine Compound No. 3 Pulvules: codeine 30 mg with aspirin 380 mg, caffeine 30 mg

Ascriptin with Codeine No. 2: aspirin 325 mg with codeine phosphate 15 mg, buffers

Ascriptin with Codeine No. 3: aspirin 325 mg with codeine phosphate 30 mg, buffers

Atropine, Demerol Injection: meperidine HCl 50 mg/ml with atropine sulfate 0.4 mg/ml

Atropine, Demerol Injection: meperidine HCl 75 mg/ml with atropine sulfate 0.4 mg/ml

Augmentin, Clavulin: amoxicillin 250 mg with clavulanate potassium 125 mg; amoxicillin 500 mg with clavulanate potassium 125 mg; amoxicillin 125 mg with potassium clavulanate 31.5 mg/5 ml; amoxicillin 250 with potassium clavulanate 31.5 mg/5 ml

Axotal: aspirin 650 mg with butalbital 50 mg

Azo Gantanol, Azo Sulfamethoxazole, UroGantanol: sulfamethoxazole 500 mg with phenazopyridine HCl 100 mg

Azo-Gantrisin, Azo-Suldiazo, Azo-Sulfamethoxazole: sulfisoxazole 500 mg with phenazopyridine HCl 50 mg

B-A-C: aspirin 650 mg with butalbital 50 mg, caffeine 40 mg, buffers

B-A-C No. 3: aspirin 325 mg with butalbital 50 mg, caffeine 40 mg, codeine phosphate 30 mg, buffers

Bancap: acetaminophen 325 mg with butalbital 50 mg

Bancap HC, Dolacet, Hydrocet, Zydone: hydrocodone bitartrate 5 mg with acetaminophen 500 mg

Barbidonna: belladonna alkaloids, atropine sulfate 0.025 mg, hyoscyamine sulfate 0.1286 mg, phenobarbital 16 mg, scopolamine hydrobromide 0.0074 mg

Barbidonna Elixir: belladonna alkaloids, atropine sulfate 0.034 mg/5 ml, hyoscyamine sulfate 0.0174 mg/5 ml, phenobarbital 21.6 mg/ml, scopolamine hydrobromide 0.01 mg/5 ml

Barbidonna No. 2: belladonna alkaloids, atropine sulfate 0.025 mg, hyoscyamine sulfate 0.1286 mg, phenobarbital 32 mg, scopolamine hydrobromide 0.0074 mg

BC Powder: aspirin 650 mg with caffeine 32 mg, salicylamide 195 mg

Belap, Pheno-Bella: belladonna extract 10.8 mg (0.135 mg of alkaloids of belladonna leaf) with phenobarbital 16.2 mg

Belladenal-S: levorotatory belladonna alkaloids malates 0.25 mg (of levorotatory belladonna alkaloids) with phenobarbital 50 mg

Bellalphen, Donnatal, Hyosophen: belladonna alkaloids atropine sulfate 0.0194 mg, hyoscyamine sulfate 0.1037 mg, phenobarbital 16.2 mg, scopolamine hydrobromide 0.0065 mg

Bellergal-S: ergotamine tartrate 0.6 mg with levorotatory belladonna alkaloids malates 0.2 mg (of lavorotatory belladonna alkaloids 40 mg)

Benadryl: diphenhydramine HCl 25 mg with pseudoephedrine HCl 60 mg

Benylin: diphenhydramine HCl 12.5 mg/5 ml with pseudoephedrine HCl 30 mg/5 ml

Benylin DM: dextromethorphan hydrobromide 5 mg/5 ml with guaifenesin 100 mg/5 ml
Bexophene, Darvon Compound 65, Dolene Compound-65, Doxaphene Compound, Propoxyphene-AC, Propoxyphene Compound-65: propoxyphene HCl 65 mg with aspirin 389 mg, caffeine 32.4 mg
Bicillin C-R: 150,000 units (of penicillin G) per ml with penicillin G benzathine 150,000 units (of penicillin G) per ml
Bicillin C-R: penicillin G procaine 300,000 units (of penicillin G) per ml with penicillin G benzathine 300,000 units (of penicillin G) per ml
Bicillin C-R 900/300: penicillin G procaine 150,000 units (of penicillin G) per ml with penicillin G benzathine 450,000 units (of penicillin G) per ml
Biphetamine 12½: dextroamphetamine 6.25 mg, amphetamine 6.25 mg
Biphetamine 20: dextroamphetamine 10 mg, amphetamine 10 mg
Bitrate: pentaerythritol tetranitrate 15 mg, phenobarbital 20 mg
Blanex: chlorzoxazone 250 mg, acetaminophen 300 mg
Bromo-seltzer: acetaminophen 325 mg/capful measure with citric acid 2.224 g/capful measure, sodium bicarbonate 2.871 g/capful measure
Butibel: belladonna extract 15 mg (0.187 mg of alkaloids of belladonna leaf) with butabarbital sodium 15 mg
Butibel Elixir: belladonna extract 15 mg (0.187 mg of alkaloids of belladonna leaf) with butabarbital sodium 15 mg
Cafergot: ergotamine tartrate 1 mg with caffeine 100 mg
Cafergot suppositories: ergotamine tartrate 2 mg, caffeine 100 mg
Caladryl: diphenhydramine HCl 1% with calamine 8%, camphor 0.1%
Calcidrine: codeine 8.4 mg/5 ml with calcium iodide anhydrous 152 mg/5 ml
CAM-AP-ES: hydrochlorothiazide 15 mg, hydralazine 25 mg, reserpine 0.1 mg
Cantri, Vagilia: sulfisoxazole 10% with allantoin 2%, aminacrine HCl 0.2%
Capital and Codeine: codeine 30 mg with acetaminophen 325 mg
Capital with Codeine: acetaminophen 120 mg/5 ml with codeine 12 mg/5 ml
Capozide 25/15: captopril 25 mg with hydrochlorothiazide 15 mg
Capozide 25/25: captopril 25 mg with hydrochlorothiazide 25 mg
Capozide 50/15: captopril 50 mg with hydrothiazide 15 mg
Capozide 50/25: captopril 50 mg with hydrochlorothiazide 25 mg
Carisoprodol Compound, Soprodol Compound, Soma Compound, Soprodol Compound: risoprodol 200 mg with aspirin 325 mg
Clindex, Clinoxide, Clipoxide, Librax, Lidox, Lidoxide: clidinium bromide 2.5 mg with chlordiazepoxide HCl 5 mg
Chardonna-2: belladonna extract 15 mg (0.187 mg of alkaloids of belladonna leaf) with phenobarbital 15 mg

Cherapas, Ser-A-Gen, Ser-Ap-Es, Serathide, Serpazide, Tri-Hydroserpine, Unipres: reserpine 0.1 mg with hydralazine HCl 25 mg, hydrochlorothiazide 15 mg
Children's Hold 4 Hour: dextromethorphan hydrobromide 3.75 mg with phenylpropanolamine HCl 6.25 mg
Chlorofon-F, Chlorzone Forte, Paracet Forte, Parafon Forte, Zoxaphen: chlorzoxazone 250 mg with acetaminophen 300 mg
Chloroserp-250, Chloroserpine-250, Diupres-250: reserpine 0.125 mg with chlorothiazide 250 mg
Chloroserp-500, Chloroserpine-500, Diupres-500: reserpine 0.125 mg with chlorothiazide 500 mg
Clindex, Clinoxide, Clipoxide, Librax, Lidox: chlordiazepoxide HCl 5 mg with clidinium bromide 2.5 mg
Co-Gesic, Damacet-P, Duradyne, Hy-Phen, Norcet, Vicodin: hydrocodone bitartrate 5 mg with acetaminophen 500 mg
Codalan No. 1: acetaminophen 500 mg with caffeine 30 mg, codeine phosphate 8 mg
Codalan No. 2: acetaminophen 500 mg with caffeine 30 mg, codeine phosphate 15 mg
Codalan No. 3: acetaminophen 500 mg with caffeine 30 mg, codeine phosphate 30 mg
Codoxy, Percodan, Roxiprin: oxycodone HCl 4.5 mg, oxycodone terephthalate 0.38 mg with aspirin 325 mg
Combipres 0.1 mg: clonidine HCl 0.1 mg with chlorthalidone 15 mg
Combipres 0.2 mg: clonidine HCl 0.2 mg with chlorthalidone 15 mg
Comtrex: dextromethorphan hydrobromide 10 mg with acetaminophen 325 mg, chlorpheniramine maleate 2 mg, phenylpropanolamine hydrochloride 12.5 mg
Comtrex: dextromethorphan hydrobromide 3.3 mg/5 ml with acetaminophen 108.3 mg/5 ml, chlorpheniramine maleate 0.67 mg/5 ml, phenylpropanolamine HCl 4.2 mg/5 ml
Conar: dextromethorphan hydrobromide 15 mg with acetaminophen 300 mg, guaifenesin 100 mg, phenylephrine HCl 10 mg
Conar Expectorant: dextromethorphan hydrobromide 15 mg/5 ml with guaifenesin 100 mg/5 ml, phenylephrine HCl 10 mg/5 ml
Conar Syrup: dextromethorphan hydrobromide 15 mg/5 ml with phenylephrine HCl 10 mg/5 ml
Congespirin: phenylpropanolamine HCl 6.25 mg/5 ml with acetaminophen 130 mg/5 ml
Congespirin, Aspirin-Free: acetaminophen 81 mg with phenylephrine HCl 81 mg
Contac Jr.: dextromethorphan hydrobromide 5 mg/5 ml with acetaminophen 160 mg/5 ml, pseudoephedrine HCl 15 mg/5 ml
Contac Severe Cold Formula, Nyquil Nighttime Cold Medicine, Nytime Cold Medicine, Quiet Nite: dextromethorphan hydrobromide 5 mg/5 ml with acetaminophen 167 mg/5 ml, doxylamine succinate 1.25 mg/5

ml, pseudoephedrine HCl 10 mg/5 ml

Copavin Pulvules: codeine sulfate 15 mg with papaverine HCl 15 mg

Corzide 40/5: bendroflumethiazide 5 mg with nadolol 40 mg

Corzide 80/5: bendroflumethiazide 5 mg with nadolol 80 mg

CoTylenol: dextromethorphan hydrobromide 5 mg/5 ml with acetaminophen 108.3 mg/5 ml, chlorpheniramine maleate 0.67 mg/5 ml, pseudoephedrine HCl 10 mg/5 ml

CoTylenol Cold Medication Tablets: dextromethorphan hydrobromide 15 mg with acetaminophen 325 mg, chlorpheniramine maleate 2 mg, pseudoephedrine HCl 30 mg

Cremacoat 3: dextromethorphan hydrobromide 6.7 mg/5 ml with guaifenesin 66.7 mg/5 ml, phenylpropanolamine HCl 12.5 mg/5 ml

Cremacoat 4: dextromethorphan hydrobromide 6.7 mg/5 ml with doxylamine succinate 2.5 mg/5 ml, phenylpropanolamine HCl 12.5 mg/5 ml

Cyclomydril Ophthalmic: cyclopentolate HCl 0.2%, phenylephrine HCl 1%

Cystex: methenamine 165 mg, salicylamide 65 mg, sodium salicylate 97 mg, benzoic acid 32 mg

Damason-P: hydrocodone bitartrate 5 mg with aspirin 224 mg, caffeine 32 mg

Darvocet-N 50, Propoxyphene Napsylate with Acetaminophen Tablets: acetaminophen 325 mg with propoxyphene napsylate 50 mg

Darvocet-N 100, Doxapap-N, Propacet-100: propoxyphene napsylate 100 mg with acetaminophen 650 mg

Darvon Compound Pulvules: aspirin 389 mg with caffeine 32.4 mg propoxyphene HCl 32 mg

Darvon Compound-65 Pulvules, Dolene Compound-65, SK-65-Compound: aspirin 389 mg with caffeine 32.4 mg, propoxyphene HCl 65 mg

Darvon with A.S.A. Pulvules: aspirin 325 mg with propoxyphene HCl 65 mg

Darvon-N and A.S.A.: aspirin 325 mg with propoxyphene napsylate 100 mg

Decadron with Xylocaine: dexamethasone PO_4 4 mg, lidocaine HCl 10 mg/ml

Deconamine: pseudoephedrine HCl 60 mg with chlorpheniramine maleate 4 mg

Demerol APAP: acetaminophen 300 mg with meperidine HCl 50 mg

Demi-Regroton: chlorthalidone 25 mg with reserpine 0.125 mg

Deprol: meprobamate 400 mg with benactyzine HCl 1 mg

Dihydrocodeine Compound Modified, Synalgos: aspirin 356.4 mg with caffeine 30 mg and dihydrocodeine bitartrate 16 mg

Dilantin with Phenobarbital: phenytoin sodium 100 mg, phenobarbital 32 mg

Dilantin with Phenobarbital: phenobarbital 16 mg, phenytoin sodium 100 mg

Dimetane-DX Cough Syrup: dextromethorphan hydrobromide 10 mg/5 ml with brompheniramine maleate 2 mg/5 ml, pseudoephedrine HCl 30 mg/5 ml

Dimycor: pentaerythritol tetranitrate 10 mg, phenobarbital 15 mg

Diupres-250: chlorothiazide 250 mg, reserpine 0.125 mg

Diupres-500: chlorothiazide 50 mg, reserpine 0.125 mg

Diurese, Matatensin No. 4, Trichlormethiazide with Reserpine Tablets, Trichlortensin: trichlormethiazide 4 mg with reserpine 0.1 mg

Diutensen: methyclothiazide 2.5 mg with cryptenamine tannates 2 mg (of cryptenamine)

Diutensen: reserpine 0.1 mg with methyclothiazide 2.5 mg

Diutensin-R: methyclothiazide 25 mg with reserpine 0.1 mg

Dolene AP-65: acetaminophen 650 mg with propoxyphene HCl 65 mg

Donnagel-PG: powdered opium 24 mg, Kaolin 6 g, pectin 142.8 mg, hyoscyamine SO_4 0.1037 mg, atropine SO_4 0.0194 mg, scopolamine hydrobromide 0.0065 mg, alcohol 5%/30 ml susp

Donnagel Suspension: Kaolin 6 g, pectin 142.8 mg, hyoscyamine SO_4 0.1037 mg, atropine SO_4 0.0194 mg, scopolamine hydrobromide 0.0065 mg, alcohol 3.8%/30 ml susp

Donnatal: belladonna alkaloids atropine sulfate 0.0194 mg, hyoscyamine sulfate 0.1037 mg, phenobarbital 32.4 mg, scopolamine hydrobromide 0.0065 mg

Donnatal Elixir, Hyosophen Elixir: belladonna alkaloids atropine sulfate 0.0194 mg/5 ml, hyoscyamine sulfate 0.1037 mg/5 ml, phenobarbital 16.2 mg/5 ml, scopolamine hydrobromide 0.0065/5 ml

Donnatal Extentabs: belladonna alkaloids atropine sulfate 0.0582 mg, hyoscyamine sulfate 0.3111 mg, phenobarbital 48.6 mg, scopolamine hydrobromide 0.0195 mg

Donnatal, Hyosophen: belladonna alkaloids atropine sulfate 0.0194 mg, hyoscyamine sulfate 0.1037 mg, phenobarbital 16.2 mg, scopolamine hydrobromide 0.0065 mg

Dorcol Children's Cough Syrup: dextromethorphan hydrobromide 5 mg/5 ml with guaifenesin 50 mg/5 ml, pseudoephedrine HCl 15 mg/5 ml

DUO-Medihaler: isoproterenol HCl 160 μg/metered spray with phenylephrine bitartrate 240 μg/metered spray

Dyazide: hydrochlorothiazide 25 mg with triamterene 50 mg

E-Pilo: epinephrine bitartrate 1%, pilocarpine HCl 1%, 2%, 3%, 4%, 6%

Empirin with Codeine 15 mg No. 2: codeine 15 mg with aspirin 325 mg

Empirin with Codeine 60 mg No. 4: aspirin 325 mg with codeine phosphate 60 mg

Empracet with Codeine Phosphate 60 mg No. 4, Tylenol with Codeine No. 4: acetaminophen 300 mg with codeine phosphate 60 mg

Endecon, Phenapap No. 2: phenylpropanolamine HCl 25 mg with acetaminophen 325 mg

Enduronyl-Forte, Eserdine Forte, Methyclothiazide and Deserpidine Tablets 5 mg/0.5

mg, Methy-Deserpidine Forte, Methy-Deserpidine Strong: methyclothiazide 5 mg with deserpidine 0.5 mg
Enduronyl, Eserdine, Methychlothiazide, Deserpidine Tablets 5 mg/0.25 mg: deserpidine 0.25 mg with methychlothiazide 5 mg
Entex: guaifenesin 200 mg with phenylephrine HCl 5 mg with phenylpropanolamine HCl 45 mg
Entex LA: guaifenesin 400 mg with phenylpropanolamine HCl 75 mg
Epromate, Equagesic, Equazine-M, Hepto-M, Mepro Compound, Meprogesic, Micranin: meprobamate 200 mg with aspirin 325 mg
Equagesic, Equazine-M, Mepro-Analgesic, Mepor Compound, Micrainin: aspirin 325 mg with meprobamate 200 mg
Ergocaff: ergotamine tartrate 1 mg, caffeine 100 mg
Esgic, Fioricet: acetaminophen 325 mg with butalbital 50 mg, caffeine 40 mg
Esimil: guanethidine monosulfate 10 mg (equivalent to guanethidine sulfate 8.4 mg) with hydrochlorothiazide 25 mg
Estratest: esterified estrogens 1.25 mg, methyltestosterone 2.5 mg
Estratest HS: esterified estrogens 0.625 mg, methyltestosterone 1.25 mg
Etrafon 2-10: perphenazine 2 mg, amitriptyline HCl 10 mg
Etrafon: perphenazine 2 mg, amitriptyline HCl 10 mg
Etrafon-A: perphenazine 4 mg, amitriptyline HCl 10 mg
Etrafon-Forte: perphenazine 4 mg, amitriptyline HCl 25 mg
Euthroid-½: levothyroxine sodium 30 μg, liothyronine sodium 7.5 μg
Euthroid-1: levothyroxine sodium 60 μg, liothyronine sodium 15 μg
Euthroid-2: levothyroxine sodium 120 μg, liothyronine sodium 30 μg
Euthroid-3: levothyroxine sodium 180 μg, liothyronine sodium 45 μg
Eutron Filmtab: pargyline HCl 25 mg with methyclothiazide 5 mg
Excedrin: acetaminophen 194 mg with aspirin 227 mg, caffeine 33 mg, buffers
Excedrin: aspirin 250 mg with acetaminophen 250 mg, caffeine 65 mg
Excedrin P.M.: acetaminophen 500 mg with diphenhydramine citrate 38 mg
Exna-R Tablets: benzthiazide 50 mg, reserpine 0.125 mg
Femguard, Sulfa-Gyn, Sultrin, Sulfa, Trysul: miscellaneous sulfonamide-sulfonamide sulfabenzamide 3.7.%, sulfacetamide 2.85%, sulfiazole 3.42%, and urea 0.64%
Fermalox: ferrous SO_4 200 mg, magnesium hydroxide, dried aluminum hydroxide gel 200 mg
Ferocyl: iron (fumarate) 50 mg, docusate sodium 100 mg
Fero-Sequels: iron (fumarate) 50 mg, docusate sodium 100 mg
Fiorinal: aspirin 325 mg with butalbital 50 mg, caffeine 40 mg
Fiorinal with Codeine No. 1: aspirin 325 mg with butalbital 50 mg, caffeine 40 mg, codeine phosphate 7.5 mg
Fiorinal with Codeine No. 2: aspirin 325 mg with butalbital 50 mg, caffeine 40 mg, and codeine phosphate 15 mg

Fiorinal with Codeine No. 3: aspirin 325 mg with butalbital 50 mg, caffeine 40 mg, codeine phosphate 30 mg
Gemnisyn: acetaminophen 325 mg with aspirin 325 mg
Hexalol: methenamine 40.8 mg, phenyl salicylate 18.1 mg, atropine SO_4 0.03, hyoscyamine 0.03 mg, benzoic acid 4.5 mg, methylene blue 5.4 mg
Hybephen: belladonna alkaloids atropine sulfate 0.0233 mg, hyoscyamine sulfate 0.1277 mg, phenobarbital 15 mg, scopolamine hydrobromide 0.0094 mg
Hydergine: dihydroergocorine mesylate 0.167 mg
Hydrogesic: hydrocodone bitartrate 7.5 mg with acetaminophen 650 mg
Hydromox R: quinethazone 50 mg with reserpine 0.125 mg
Hydropres-25, Hydro-Reserpine-25, Hydroserp, Hydroserpine No. 1, Hydrosine 25 mg, Mallopress: reserpine 0.125 mg with hydrochlorothiazide 25 mg
Hydropres-50, Hydro-Reserpine-50, Hydroserp, Hydroserpine No. 2, Hydrosine 50 mg, Hydrotensin, Hydroserpalan: reserpine 0.125 mg with hydrochlorothiazide 50 mg
Inderide 40/25, Propranolol HCl, Hydrochlorothiazide Tablets 40/25: propranolol HCl 40 mg with hydrochlorothiazide 25 mg
Inderide 80/25, Propranolol HCl, Hydrochlorothiazide Tablets 80/25: propranolol HCl 80 mg with hydrochlorothiazide 25 mg
Inderide LA 80/50: propranolol HCl 80 mg with hydrochlorothiazide 50 mg
INH: isoniazid 1 tablet, isoniazid 300 mg
Iophen DM, Tussi-Organidin DM: Dextromethorphan hydrobromide 10 mg/5 ml with iodinated glycerol 30 mg/5 ml
Isoptop-ES: pilocarpine HCl 2%, physostigmine salicylate 0.25%
Kinesed: belladonna alkaloids atropine sulfate 0.02 mg, hyoscyamine sulfate 0.12 mg, phenobarbital 16 mg, scopolamine hydrobromide 0.007 mg
Levsin with Phenobarbital Tablets, Anaspaz: hyoscyamine sulfate 0.125 mg with phenobarbital
Levsinex with Phenobarbital Elixir: hyoscyamine sulfate 0.125 mg/5 ml with phenobarbital 15 mg/5 ml
Levsinex with Phenobarbital Time-caps: hyoscyamine sulfate 0.375 mg with phenobarbital 45 mg
Levsin-PB: hyoscyamine sulfate 0.125 mg/ml with phenobarbital 15 mg/ml
Librax: chlordiazepoxide HCl 5 mg, clidinium bromide 2.5 mg
Limbitrol 5-12.5: chlordiazepoxide 5 mg, amitriptyline HCl 12.5 mg
Limbitrol 10-25: chlordiazepoxide 10 mg, amitriptyline HCl 25 mg
Lobac: chlorzoxazone 250 mg, acetaminophen 300 mg
Lopressor HCT 50/25: metoprolol tartrate 50 mg with hydrochlorothiazide 25 mg
Lopressor HCT 100/25: metoprolol tartrate 100 mg with hydrochlorothiazide 25 mg

M-KYA, Q-VEL: quinine SO_4 64.8 mg, vit. E. 400 U, lecithin
Maxzide: hydrochlorothiazide 50 mg with triamterene 75 mg
Mediqueall: dextromethorphan hydrobromide 15 mg with pseudoephedrine HCl 30 mg
Menrium 5-2: chlordiazepoxide 5 mg with esterified estrogens 0.2 mg
Menrium 5-4 chlordiazepoxide 5 mg with esterified estrogens 0.4 mg
Menrium 10-4: chlordiazepoxide 10 mg with esterified estrogens 0.4 mg
Mepergan: meperidine HCl 25 mg/ml with promethazine HCl 25 mg/ml
Mepergan Fortis: meperidine HCl 50 mg with promethazine HCl 25 mg
Metatensin No. 2: reserpine 0.1 mg with trichlormethiazide 2 mg
Midol Caplets: aspirin 454 mg with caffeine 32.4 mg, cinnamedrine HCl 14.9 mg
Midol PMS Caplets: acetaminophen 500 mg with pamabrom 25 mg, pyrilamine maleate 15 mg
Migral: ergotamine tartrate 1 mg, caffeine 50 mg, cyclizine HCl 25 mg
Milprem-200, PMB 200: meprobamate 200 mg with conjugated estrogens 0.45 mg
Milprem-400, PMB 400: meprobamate 400 mg with conjugated estrogens 0.45 mg
Minizide 1: prazosin HCl 1 mg (of prazosin) with polythiazide 0.5 mg
Minizide 2: prazosin HCl 2 mg (of prazosin) with polythiazide 0.5 mg
Minizide 5: prazosin HCl 5 mg (of prazosin) with polythiazide 0.5 mg
Mixtard injection: 100 mg/ml isophane purified pork insulin susp, purified pork insulin inj
Moduretic: amiloride HCl 5 mg, hydrochlorothiazide 50 mg
Morphine, Atropine Sulfate Injection: morphine sulfate 16 mg/ml with atropine sulfate 0.4 mg/ml
Murocoll-2: scopolamine hydrobromide 0.3%, phenylephrine hydrochloride 10%
Mus-Lax: chlorzoxazone 250 mg, acetaminophen 300 mg
Myapap with Codeine, Tylenol with Codeine: acetaminophen 120 mg/5 ml with codeine phosphate 12 mg/5 ml
Mysteclin F: amphotericin B 25 mg/5 ml with tetracycline equivalent to tetracycline HCl 25 mg/5 ml
Mysteclin-F: amphotericin B 50 mg with tetracycline equivalent to tetracycline HCl 250 mg
Mysteclin-F: tetracycline equivalent to 125 mg tetracycline HCl per 5 ml with amphotericin B 25 mg/5 ml
Mysteclin-F: tetracycline equivalent to 350 mg tetracycline HCl with amphotericin B 50 mg/5 ml
Mysteclin-F Syrup: tetracycline equivalent to 125 mg tetracycline HCl per 5 ml with amphotericin B 25 mg/5 ml
Naldecon-DX Adult: dextromethorphan hydrobromide 15 mg/5 ml with guaifenesin 200 mg/5 ml, phenylpropanolamine HCl 18 mg/5 ml
Naldecon-DX Children's Syrup: dextromethorphan hydrobromide 7.5 mg/5 ml with guaifenesin 100 mg/5 ml, phe-

nylpropanolamine HCl 9 mg/5 ml

Naldegisic: acetaminophen 325 mg with pseudoephedrine HCl 15 mg

Naquival: trichlormethiazide 4 mg, reserpine 0.1 mg

Naturetin with K 2.5, mg: bendroflumethiazide 2.5, potassium chloride 500 mg

Naturetin with K 5 mg: bendroflumethiazide 5 mg with potassium chloride 500 mg

Neosporin G.U. Irrigant: polymyxin B sulfate 200,000 units (of polymyxin B)

Nitrotym-Plus: nitroglycerin 2.5 mg, butabarbital 48 mg

Norgesic: orphenadrine citrate 25 mg, aspirin 385 mg, caffeine 30 mg

Norgesic Forte: orphenadrine citrate 50 mg, aspirin 770 mg, caffeine 60 mg

Normozide 100/25: labetalol hydrochloride 100 mg, hydrochlorothiazide 25 mg

Normozide 200/25: labetalol hydrochloride 200 mg, hydrochlorothiazide 25 mg

Normozide 300/25: labetalol hydrochloride 300 mg, hydrochlorothiazide 25 mg

Novahistine Cough and Cold Formula: dextromethorphan hydrobromide 10 mg/5 ml with chlorpheniramine maleate 2 mg/5 ml, pseudoephedrine HCl 30 mg/5 ml

Opium and Belladonna: powdered opium 60 mg with belladonna extract 15 mg (equivalent to belladonna alkaloids 0.2 mg)

Oreticyl 25: deserpidine 0.125 mg with hydrochlorothiazide 25 mg

Oreticyl 50: deserpidine 0.125 mg with hydrochlorothiazide 50 mg

Oreticyl Forte: deserpidine 0.25 mg with hydrochlorothiazide 50 mg

Ornex: phenylpropanolamine HCl 12.5 mg with acetaminophen 325 mg

Orthoxicol Cough Syrup: dextromethorphan hydrobromide 10 mg/5 ml with methoxyphenamine HCl 17 mg/5 ml

Oxymycin, Terramycin Intramuscular Solution: oxytetracycline 50 mg/ml with lidocaine 2%

Pamprin: acetaminophen 325 mg with pamabrom 25 mg, pyrilamine maleate 12.5 mg

Pamprin Maximum Cramp Relief: acetaminophen 500 mg with pamabrom 25 mg, pyrilamine maleate 15 mg

Paracet Forte: chlorzoxazone 250 mg, acetaminophen 300 mg

Parepectolin: opium 15 mg, kaolin 5.85 g, pectin 162 mg, alcohol 0.69%/30 ml susp

Pathibamate-200: meprobamate 200 mg with tridihexethyl chloride 25 mg

Pathibamate-400: meprobamate 400 mg with tridihexethyl chloride 25 mg

Pediazole: erythromycin ethylsuccinate 200 mg (of erythromycin) per 5 ml with sulfisoxazole acetyl 600 mg (of sulfisoxazole) per 5 ml

Penntuss: codeine polistirex equivalent to codeine 10 mg/5 ml with chlorpheniramine polistirex equivalent to chlorpheniramine maleate 4 mg/5 ml

Perbuzem: pentaerythritol tetranitrate 10 mg, butabarbital 15 mg

Percodan-Demi: aspirin 325 mg with oxycodone HCl 2.25 mg, oxycodone terephthalate 0.19 mg
Percogesic: acetaminophen 325 mg with phenyltoloxamine citrate 30 mg
Peri-Colace: docusate sodium 100 mg with cusanthranol 30 mg
Persistin: salsalate 487.5 mg with aspirin 162.5 mg
Phenaphen with Codeine No. 2: acetaminophen 325 mg with codeine phosphate 15 mg
Phenaphen with Codeine No. 2, Proval No. 3: codeine 30 mg with acetaminophen 325 mg
Phenaphen with Codeine No. 3, Proval No. 2: acetaminophen 325 mg with codeine phosphate 30 mg
Phenaphen with Codeine No. 4: acetaminophen 325 mg with codeine phosphate 60 mg
Phenaphen-650 with Codeine: acetaminophen 650 mg with codeine phosphate 30 mg
Phenergan: promethazine HCl 6.25 mg/5 ml with phenylephrine HCl 5 mg/5 ml
Phenergan-D: promethazine HCl 6.25 mg with pseudoephedrine HCl 60 mg
Phenergan VC Syrup, Promethazine HCl VC: promethazine HCl 6.25 mg/5 ml with phenylephrine HCl 5 mg/5 ml
Phenergan with Dextromethorphan: dextromethorphan hydrobromide 15 mg/5 ml with promethazine HCl 6.35 mg/5 ml
Phrenilin: acetaminophen 325 mg with butalbital 50 mg
Phrenilin Forte: acetaminophen 650 mg, butalbital 50 mg
Phrenilin with Codeine No. 3: acetaminophen 325 mg, butalbital 50 mg, codeine phosphate 30 mg
Polycillin-PRB: ampicillin trihydrate 3.5 g with probenecid 1 g
Polyflex: chlorzoxazone 250 mg, acetaminophen 300 mg
Propoxyphene HCl/65, Wygesic: acetaminophen 650 mg, propoxyphene HCl 65 mg
Principen with Probenecid: ampicillin trihydrate 3.5 g with probenecid 1 g
Prunicodeine: terpin hydrate 29 mg/5 ml, codeine sulfate 10 mg/5 ml
Rautrax: rauwolfia 50 mg, flumethiazide 400 mg, potassium chloride 400 mg
Rautrax-N: bendroflumethiazide 4 mg, rauwolfia serpentina 50 mg, potassium chloride 400 mg
Rauzide: bendroflumethiazide 4 mg, rauwolfia serpentina 50 mg
Regroton: reserpine 0.25 mg, chlorthalidone 50 mg
Renese-R: reserpine 0.25 mg, polythiazide 2 mg
Rifamate: isoniazid 150 mg with rifampin 300 mg
Rimactane: isoniazid 2 capsules, rifampin 300 mg
Rimactane: rifampin 1 tablet, isoniazid 300 mg
Rimactane: rifampin 2 capsules, rifampin 300 mg
Robaxisal, Robomol/ASA: methocarbamol 400 mg, aspirin 325 mg
Robitussin-DM: dextromethorphan hydrobromide 15 mg/5 ml, guaifenesin 100 mg/5 ml
Roxicet: oxycodone HCl 5

mg/5 ml, acetaminophen 325 mg/5 ml
S-A-C: salicylamide 230 mg, acetaminophen 150 mg, caffeine 30 mg
Salimeth Forte: salicylamide 600 mg, acetaminophen 250 mg
S.B.P.: secobarbital sodium 50 mg, butabarbital sodium 30 mg, phenobarbital 15 mg
Ser-a-Gen: hydrochlorothiazide 15 mg, hydralazine hydrochloride 25 mg, reserprine 0.1 mg
Serpasil-Apresoline HCl No. 1: hydralazine HCl 25 mg, reserpine 0.1 mg
Serpasil-Apresoline HCl No. 2: hydralazine HCl 25 mg, reserpine 0.2 mg
Serpasil-Esidrix No. 1: reserpine 0.1 mg, hydrochlorothiazide 25 mg
Serpasil-Esidrix No. 2: reserpine 0.1 mg, hydrochlorothiazide 50 mg
Simron: iron (gluconate) 10 mg, polysorbate 20, 400 mg
Sine-Aid: acetaminophen 325 mg, pseudoephedrine HCl 30 mg
Sine-Aid Extra Strength Caplets, Tylenol Sinus Maximum Strength Caplets: acetaminophen 500 mg, pseudoephedrine HCl 30 mg
Sine-Off Extra Strength, Sinutab: acetaminophen 500 mg, pseudoephedrine HCl 30 mg
Sinubid: acetaminophen 600 mg, phenylpropanolamine HCl 100 mg, phenyltoloxamine citrate 66 mg
Sinutab Maximum Nighttime: acetaminophen 167 mg/5 ml, diphenhydramine HCl 8.3 mg/5 ml, pseudoephedrine HCl 10 mg/5 ml
Sinutab II Maximum, Tylenol Maximum Strength Sinus: acetaminophen 500 mg, pseudoephedrine HCl 30 mg
SK-APAP with Codeine, Tylenol with Codeine No. 2: codeine 5 mg with acetaminophen 300 mg
Skelez: chlorzoxazone 250 mg, acetaminophen 300 mg
Soma Compound: carisoprodol 200 mg, aspirin 325 mg
Soma Compound with Codeine: codeine 16 mg, aspirin 325 mg, carisoprodol 200 mg
Spec-T: Phenylpropanolamine 10.5 mg with Benzocaine 10 mg, Phenylephrine HCl 5 mg
Spec-T Sore Throat Cough Suppressant: dextromethorphan hydrobromide 10 mg with benzocaine 10 mg
Spironazide: spironolactone 25 mg, hydrochlorothiazide 25 mg
Spirozide: spironolactone 25 mg, hydrochlorothiazide 25 mg
Sudafed Cough Syrup: dextromethorphan hydrobromide 5 mg/5 ml with guaifenesin 100 mg/5 ml, pseudoephedrine HCl 15 mg/5 ml
Sultrin: miscellaneous sulfonamide-sulfonamide sulfabenzamide 184 mg, sulfacetamide 143.75 mg, sulfathiazole 172.5 mg, urea 31.83 mg
Talacen: pentazocine HCl 25 mg (of pentazocine) with acetaminophen 650 mg
Talwin Compound Caplets: aspirin 325 mg with pentazocine HCl 12.5 mg (of pentazocine)
Tenoretic 50: atenolol 50 mg with chlorthalidone 25 mg
Tenoretic 100: atenolol 100 mg with chlorthalidone 25 mg
Terpin Hydrate and Codeine: terpin hydrate 85 mg/5 ml with

dextromethorphan hydrobromide 10 mg/5 ml (with alcohol 39%-44%)
Terramycin Intramuscular Solution: oxytetracycline 125 mg/ml with lidocaine 2%
T-Gesic: hydrocodone bitartrate 5 mg with acetaminophen 325 mg, butalbital 30 mg, caffeine 40 mg
Thiacide: methenamine mandelate 500 mg, potassium acid phosphate 250 mg
Thyrolar-¼: levothyroxine sodium 12.5 mg, liothyronine sodium 3.1 μg
Thyrolar-½: levothyroxine sodium 25 μg, liothyronine sodium 6.25 μg
Thyrolar-1: levothyroxine sodium 50 μg, liothyronine sodium 12.5 μg
Thyrolar-2: levothyroxine sodium 100 μg, liothyronine sodium 25 μg
Thyrolar-3: levothyroxine sodium 150 μg, liothyronine sodium 37.5 μg
Timentin Inj: ticarcillin disodium 3 g with clavulanate potassium 100 mg
Timolide 10/25: timolol maleate 10 mg with hydrochlorothiazide 25 mg
TracTabs 2X: methenamine 120 mg, methylene blue 6 mg, phenyl salicylate 30 mg, atropine 0.06, hyoscyamine SO_4 0.03 mg, benzoic acid 7.5 mg
Trendar: acetaminophen 325 mg with pamabrom 25 mg
Triaminic-DM Cough Formula: dextromethorphan hydrobromide 10 mg/5 ml with phenylpropanolamine HCl 12.5 mg/5 ml
Triaminicol: dextromethorphan hydrobromide 10 mg/5 ml with chlorpheniramine maleate 2 mg/5 ml, phenylpropanolamine HCl 12.5 mg/5 ml
Triavil 2-10, Triavil 4-10, Triavil 2-25, Triavil 4-25 (see Etrafon—same products) Triavil 4-50: perphenazine 4 mg, amitriptyline HCl 50 mg
Tri-Barb Capsules: phenobarbital 32 mg, butabarbital sodium 32 mg, secobarbital sodium 32 mg
Trigesic: aspirin 230 mg with acetaminophen 125 mg, caffeine 30 mg
Triple Sulfa: sulfadiazine 167 mg, sulfamerazine 167 mg, sulfamethazine 167 mg
Tuinal 200 mg Pulvules: secobarbital sodium 100 mg with amobarbital sodium 100 mg
Tylenol with Codeine No. 1: acetaminophen 300 mg with codeine phosphate 7.5 mg
Tylenol with Codeine No. 2: acetaminophen 300 mg with codeine phosphate 15 mg
Tylenol with Codeine No. 3: acetaminophen 300 mg with codeine phosphate 30 mg
Tylenol with Codeine No. 4: acetaminophen 300 mg with codeine phosphate 60 mg
Tylox: acetaminophen 500 mg with oxycodone HCl 5 mg
Unasyn Inj: ampicillin sodium 1 g with sulbactam sodium 500 mg; ampicillin sodium 2 g with sulbactam sodium 1 g
Unipres: hydrochlorothiazide 15 mg, reserpine 0.1 mg, hydralazine hydrochloride 25 mg
Urisedamine: methenamine mandelate 500 mg, hyoscyamine 0.15 mg
Urobiotic-250: oxytetracycline HCl 250 mg (of oxytetracycline) with phenazopyridine HCl 50

mg, sulfamethizole 250 mg
Uroquid-Acid No. 2: methenamine mandelate 500 mg, sodium acid phosphate 500 mg
Vanquish Caplets: aspirin 227 mg with acetaminophen 194 mg, caffeine 30 mg, buffers
Vaseretic: enalapril maleate 10 mg with hydrochlorothiazide 25 mg
Vicks Childrens Cough Syrup: dextromethorphan hydrobromide 3.5 mg/5 ml with guaifenesin 25 mg/5 ml
Vicks Cough Silencers: dextromethorphan hydrobromide 2.5 mg with benzocaine 1 mg
Vicks Daycare: dextromethorphan hydrobromide 10 mg with acetaminophen 325 mg, guaifenesin 100 mg, pseudoephedrine HCl 30 mg
Vicks Daycare: dextromethorphan hydrobromide 3.3 mg/5 ml with acetaminophen 108.3 mg/5 ml, guaifenesin 33.3 mg/5 ml, pseudoephedrine HCl 10 mg/5 ml
Vicks Formula 44 Cough Control Discs: dextromethorphan hydrobromide 5 mg with benzocaine 1.25 mg
Vicks Formula 44 Cough Mixture: dextromethorphan hydrobromide 15 mg/5 ml with doxylamine succinate 3.75 mg/5 ml
Vicks Formula 44D: dextromethorphan hydrobromide 10 mg/5 ml with guaifenesin 6.7 mg/5 ml, pseudoephedrine HCl 20 mg/5 ml
Vicks Formula 44M: dextromethorphan hydrobromide 7.4 mg/5 ml with acetaminophen 125 mg/5 ml, guaifenesin 50 mg/5 ml, pseudoephedrine HCl 15 mg/5 ml
Wigraine: ergotamine tartrate 1 mg, caffeine 100 mg, levorotatory belladonna alkaloids 0.1 mg, phenacetin 130 mg
Wigraine Suppositories: ergotamine tartrate 2 mg, caffeine 100 mg, tartaric acid 21.5 mg
Wyanoids: belladonna extract 15 mg (0.19 mg of alkaloids of belladonna leaf) with ephedrine 3 mg
Zoxaphen: chlorzoxazone 250 mg, acetaminophen 300 mg
Ziradyl: diphenhydramine HCl 2% with zinc oxide 2%

Appendix E

Controlled Substance Chart

DRUGS	UNITED STATES	CANADA
Heroin, LSD, peyote, marijuana, mescaline	Schedule I	Schedule H
Opium (morphine), meperidine, amphetamines, cocaine, short-acting barbiturates (secobarbital)	Schedule II	Schedule G
Glutethimide, paregoric, phendimetrazine	Schedule III	Schedule F
Chloral hydrate, chlordiazepoxide, diazepam, mazindol, meprobamate, phenobarbital (Canada-G)	Schedule IV	Schedule F
Antidiarrheals with opium (Canada-G), antitussives	Schedule V	Schedule F

Appendix F

FDA Pregnancy Categories

- **A** No risk demonstrated to the fetus in any trimester
- **B** No adverse effects in animals, no human studies available
- **C** Only given after risks to the fetus are considered; animal studies have shown adverse reactions, no human studies available
- **D** Definite fetal risks, may be given in spite of risks if needed in life-threatening conditions
- **X** Absolute fetal abnormalities; not to be used anytime during pregnancy

Appendix G

Nomogram for Calculation of Body Surface Area

Place a straight edge from the patient's height in the left column to his weight in the right column. The point of intersection on the body surface area column indicates the body surface area (BSA). Reproduced from Behrman RE, and Vaughn VC (editors): Nelson's textbook of pediatrics, ed 12, Philadelphia, 1983. WB Saunders.

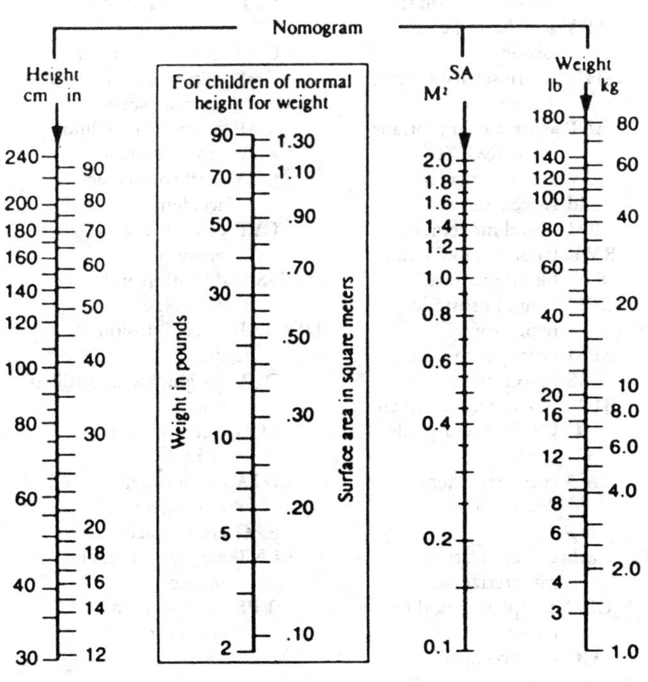

Appendix H

Commonly Used Abbreviations

abd abdomen
ABG arterial blood gas
ac before meals
ACE angiotensin-converting enzyme
ADA American Diabetes Association
ADH antidiuretic hormone
ALT alanine aminotransferase
ANA antinuclear antibody
AP anteroposterior
APTT activated partial thromboplastin time
ASA acetylsalicylic acid, aspirin
ASHD arteriosclerotic heart disease
AST aspartate aminotransferase (SGOT)
AV atrioventricular
bid twice a day
BM bowel movement
BMR basal metabolic rate
B/P blood pressure
BPH benign prostatic hypertrophy
BPM beats per minute
BS blood sugar
BUN blood urea nitrogen
C Celsius (centigrade)
Ca cancer
CAD coronary artery disease
cap capsule
Cath catheterization or catheterize
CBC complete blood cell count
CC chief complaint
cc cubic centimeter
CHF congestive heart failure
cm centimeter
CNS central nervous system
CO_2 carbon dioxide
CONT continuous
COPD chronic obstructive pulmonary disease
CPAP continuous positive airway pressue
CPK creatinine phosphokinase
CPR cardiopulmonary resuscitation
CrCl creatinine clearance
C&S culture and sensitivity
C sect cesarean section
CSF cerebrospinal fluid
CV cardiovascular
CVA cerebrovascular accident
CVP central venous pressure
D&C dilatation and curettage
DIR INF direct infusion
dr dram
D_5W 5% glucose in distilled water
ECG electrocardiogram (EKG)
EDTA ethylenediamine tetraacetic acid
EEG electroencephalogram
EENT ear, eye, nose, and throat
EPS extrapyramidal symptom

ESR erythrocyte sedimentation rate
EXT REL extended release
EXTRA STREN SUSP extra strength suspension
FBS fasting blood sugar
FHT fetal heart tones
FSH follicle-stimulating hormone
g gram
GABA γ-aminobutyric acid
GI gastrointestinal
gr grain
GTT glucose tolerance test
gtt drops
GU genitourinary
H_2 histamine$_2$
HCG human chorionic gonadotropin
Hct hematocrit
HDCV human diploid cell rabies vaccine
Hgb hemoglobin
H & H hematocrit and hemoglobin
5-HIAA 5-hydroxyindoleacetic acid
HIV human immunodeficiency virus (AIDS)
H_2O water
HOB head of bed
HR heart rate
hr hour
hs at bedtime
IgG immunoglobulin G
IM intramuscular
INF infusion
INH inhalation
inj injection
I&O intake and output
IPPB intermittent positive-pressure breathing
ITP idiopathic thrombocytopenic purpura
IUD intrauterine device
IV intravenous
IVP intravenous pyelogram
K potassium
kg kilogram
L liter
lb pound
LDH lactic dehydrogenase
LE lupus erythematosus
LH luteinizing hormone
LLQ left lower quadrant
LMP last menstrual period
LOC level of consciousness
LR lactated Ringer's solution
LUQ left upper quadrant
M meter
m minim
m^2 square meter
MAOI monoamine oxidase inhibitor
mEq milliequivalent
mg milligram
μg microgram
MI myocardial infarction
min minute
ml milliliter
mm millimeter
mo month
Na sodium
neg negative
NPO nothing by mouth (Lat. *nulla per os*)
NS normal saline
O_2 oxygen
OBS organic brain syndrome
OD right eye
OR operating room
os left eye
OTC over-the-counter
OU each eye
oz ounce
p̄ after
P56 plasma-lyte 56

$PaCO_2$ arterial carbon dioxide tension (pressure)
PaO_2 arterial oxygen tension (pressure)
PAT paroxysmal atrial tachycardia
PBI protein-bound iodine
PCWP pulmonary capillary wedge pressure
PEEP positive end-expiratory pressure
PERRLA pupils equal, round, react to light and accommodation
pH hydrogen ion concentration
PO by mouth
postop postoperative
PP postprandial
preop preoperative
prn as required
PT prothrombin time
PTT partial thromboplastin time
PVC premature ventricular contraction
q every
qAM every morning
qd every day
qh every hour
q2h every 2 hours
q3h every 3 hours
q4h every 4 hours
q6h every 6 hours
q12h every 12 hours
qid four times daily
qod every other day
qPM every night
qs sufficient quantity
qt quart
R right
RAIU radioactive iodine uptake
RBC red blood count or cell
RLQ right lower quadrant
ROM range of motion
RUQ right upper quadrant
SC subcutaneous
SIMV synchronous intermittent mandatory ventilation
SL sublingual
SLE systemic lupus erythematosus
SOB shortness of breath
sol solution
ss one half
suppos suppository
sus rel sustained release
Syr syrup
T&A tonsillectomy and adenoidectomy
tab tablet
tbsp tablespoon
temp temperature
tid three times daily
tinc tincture
TPN total parenteral nutrition
top topical
TRANS transdermal
TSH thyroid-stimulating hormone
tsp teaspoon
TT thrombin time
U unit
UA urinalysis
UTI urinary tract infection
UV ultraviolet
vag vaginal
VMA vanillylmandelic acid
vol volume
VS vital sign
WBC white blood cell count
wk week
wt weight
yr year
$>$ greater than
$<$ less than
$=$ equal
$^\circ$ degree
% percent
γ gamma
β beta

Appendix I

Bibliography

American Society of Health-System Pharmacists: American hospital formulary service drug information '95, Bethesda, Md, 1995, The Society.
Clark J, Queener S, and Karb V: Pharmacologic basis of nursing practice, ed 4, St. Louis, 1993, Mosby–Year Book, Inc.
Drug information for the health care professional (USP DI), ed 15, United States Pharmaceutical Convention, Rockville, Md, 1995.
Gahart B: Intravenous medications, ed 10, St. Louis, 1994, Mosby–Year Book, Inc.
Goodman A and others: Goodman and Gilman's the pharmacological basis of therapeutics, ed 8, New York, 1990, Pergamon Press.
McKenry LM and Salerno E: Mosby's pharmacology in nursing, ed 19, St. Louis, 1995, Mosby–Year Book, Inc.
Tissel L: Handbook on injectable drugs, ed 8, Bethesda, Md, 1994, American Society of Hospital Pharmacists, Inc.

Appendix J

IV Drug/Solution Compatibility Chart

			D_5					
	D_5	D_{10}	½S	S	NS	R	LR	OTHER
Acetazolamide	C	C	C	C	C	C	C	
Acyclovir	C							
$Alpha_1$-proteinase inhibitor								Sterile water for inj
Alprostadil	C	C			C			
Alteplase								Sterile water for inj
Amdinocillin	C	C	C	C	C	C	C	D_5 in R
Amikacin	C				C			
Aminocaproic acid			C	C	C	C		D in distilled water
Ammonium Cl					C			May add KCl to solution
Amphotericin B	C							
Ampicillin	C				C			
Amrinone lactate					C			0.45% saline
Antithrombin III	C				C			Sterile water for inj
Ascorbic acid	C				C	C	C	Sodium lactate
Azlocillin	C		C		C			
Atenolol	C				C			0.45% saline
Aztreonam	C	C			C	C	C	Normosol-R
Bretylium tosylate	C				C			
Cefamandole	C				C			
Cefazolin	C				C			
Cefotetan	C				C			
Cefoxitin	C	C			C	C	C	Aminosol
Ceftrazidime	C		C	C	C	C	C	M/G Sodium lactate
Ceftriaxone	C				C			
Cefuroxime	C		C	C		C		M/G Sodium lactate
Cephalothin	C				C	C	C	M/G Sodium lactate

This chart is not inclusive and is based on manufacturers' recommendations.

Key

C = Compatible
C_5 = Dextrose 5%
D_{10} = Dextrose 10%
D_5½S = Dextrose 5% in saline 0.45%
D_5S = Dextrose 5% in saline 0.9%
NS = Sodium chloride 0.9% (normal saline)
R = Ringer's solution
LR = Lactated Ringer's solution

	D_5	D_{10}	D_5 ½S	D_5 S	NS	R	LR	OTHER
Cephapirin	C				C			
Ciprofloxacin	C				C			
Cyclosporine	C				C			Use only glass containers
Dobutamine					C			Sodium lactate
Dopamine	C		C	C	C		C	M/G Sodium lactate
Doxycycline	C				C			Invert sugar 10%
Edetate Na	C	C						Isotonic saline
Ganciclovir	C				C	C	C	
Gentamicin	C				C			Normosol-R
Heparin Na	C	C			C	C		
Ifosfamide	C				C		C	Sterile water for inj
Isoproterenol	C			C	C	C		Invert sugar 5% & 10%
Kanamycin	C				C			
Metaraminol	C			C	C	C	C	Normosol-R
Methicillin	C			C				
Metoclopramide	C			C		C	C	
Mezlocillin	C	C	C	C	C	C	C	Fructose 5%
Moxalactam	C	C	C	C	C	C	C	M/G Sodium lactate
Netilmicin	C	C		C	C	C	C	Normosol-R
Norepinephrine	C	C		C			C	
Nitroglycerin	C	C			C			
Piperacillin	C			C	C		C	
Ritodrine	C							
Ticarcillin	C				C		C	
Tobramycin	C				C			
Vidarabine	C	C			C			

Disorders Index

P

R

S

Index

Entries can be identified as follows: generic name, Trade Name, DRUG CATEGORY, *Combination Product.*

Entries can be identified as follows: generic name, Trade Name, DRUG CATEGORY, *Combination Product.*

Entries can be identified as follows: generic name, Trade Name, DRUG CATEGORY, *Combination Product.*

Entries can be identified as follows: generic name, Trade Name, DRUG CATEGORY, *Combination Product.*

Entries can be identified as follows: generic name, Trade Name, DRUG CATEGORY, *Combination Product*.

Entries can be identified as follows: generic name, Trade Name, DRUG CATEGORY, *Combination Product.*

Entries can be identified as follows: generic name, Trade Name, DRUG CATEGORY, *Combination Product.*

Entries can be identified as follows: generic name, Trade Name, DRUG CATEGORY, *Combination Product.*

F

Entries can be identified as follows: generic name, Trade Name, DRUG CATEGORY, *Combination Product.*

G

Entries can be identified as follows: generic name, Trade Name, DRUG CATEGORY, *Combination Product.*

H

Entries can be identified as follows: generic name, Trade Name, DRUG CATEGORY, *Combination Product.*

Entries can be identified as follows: generic name, Trade Name, DRUG CATEGORY, *Combination Product*.

Entries can be identified as follows: generic name, Trade Name, DRUG CATEGORY, *Combination Product.*

Entries can be identified as follows: generic name, Trade Name, DRUG CATEGORY, *Combination Product.*

Entries can be identified as follows: generic name, Trade Name, DRUG CATEGORY, *Combination Product.*

Entries can be identified as follows: generic name, Trade Name, DRUG CATEGORY, *Combination Product.*

Entries can be identified as follows: generic name, Trade Name, DRUG CATEGORY, *Combination Product.*

Entries can be identified as follows: generic name, Trade Name, DRUG CATEGORY, *Combination Product.*

O

P

Entries can be identified as follows: generic name, Trade Name, DRUG CATEGORY, *Combination Product.*

Entries can be identified as follows: generic name, Trade Name, DRUG CATEGORY, *Combination Product.*

Entries can be identified as follows: generic name, Trade Name, DRUG CATEGORY, *Combination Product.*

Entries can be identified as follows: generic name, Trade Name, DRUG CATEGORY, *Combination Product*.

Entries can be identified as follows: generic name, Trade Name, DRUG CATEGORY, *Combination Product.*

Entries can be identified as follows: generic name, Trade Name, DRUG CATEGORY, *Combination Product.*

U

Entries can be identified as follows: generic name, Trade Name, DRUG CATEGORY, *Combination Product.*

Entries can be identified as follows: generic name, Trade Name, DRUG CATEGORY, *Combination Product.*

Entries can be identified as follows: generic name, Trade Name, DRUG CATEGORY, *Combination Product.*

COLOR PLATES

PHOTO ATLAS OF DRUG ADMINISTRATION

A

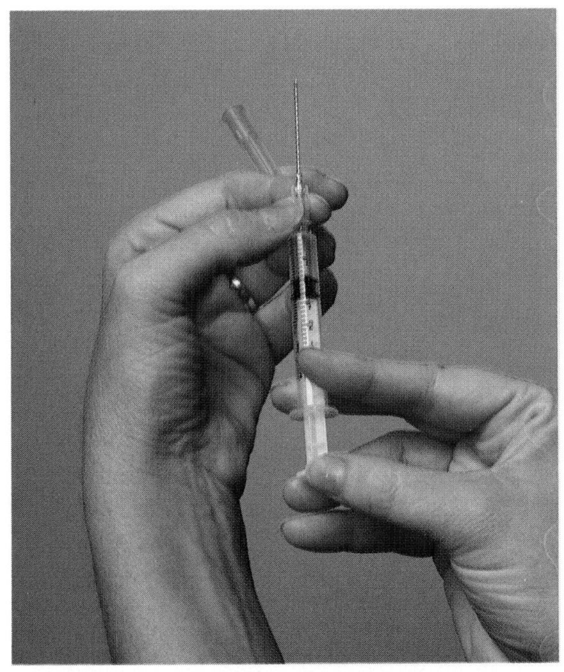

Figure 1 Preparing an injection from a vial. **A,** Take syringe and remove needle cap. Pull back on plunger to draw amount of air into syringe equivalent to volume of medication to be aspirated from vial. *Continued.*

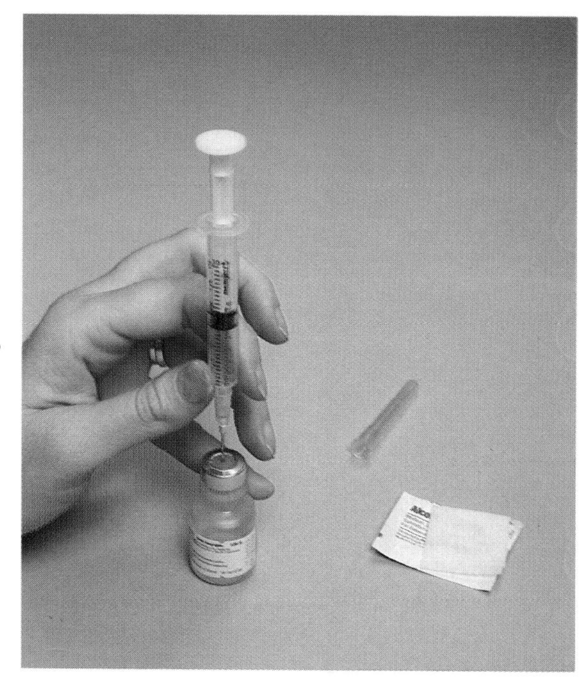

Figure 1, cont'd **B,** Insert tip of needle, with bevel pointing up, through center of rubber seal. Apply pressure of tip of needle during insertion.

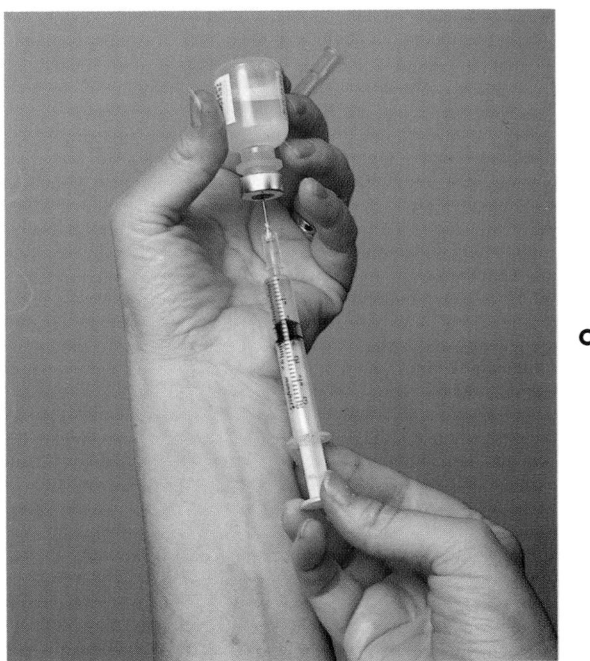

C

Figure 1, cont'd C, Allow air pressure to fill syringe gradually with medication. Pull back slightly on plunger if necessary.

Continued.

D

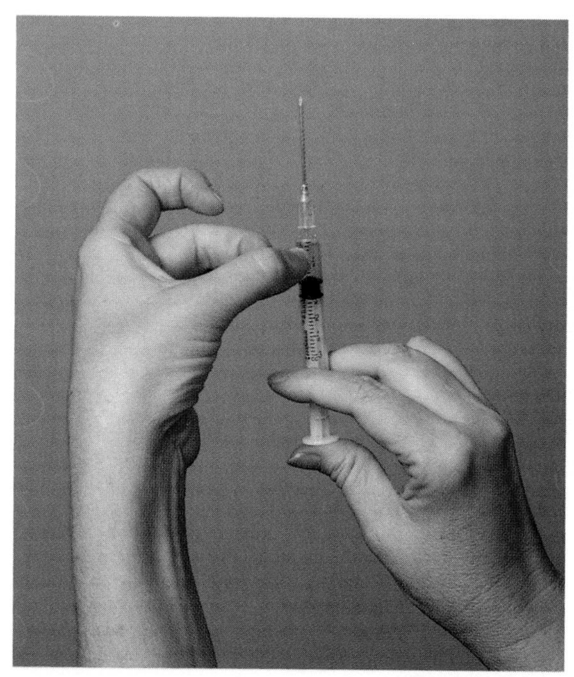

Figure 1, cont'd **D,** Remove remaining air from syringe by holding it and needle upright. Tap barrel to dislodge air bubbles. Draw back slightly on plunger and then push plunger upward to eject air.

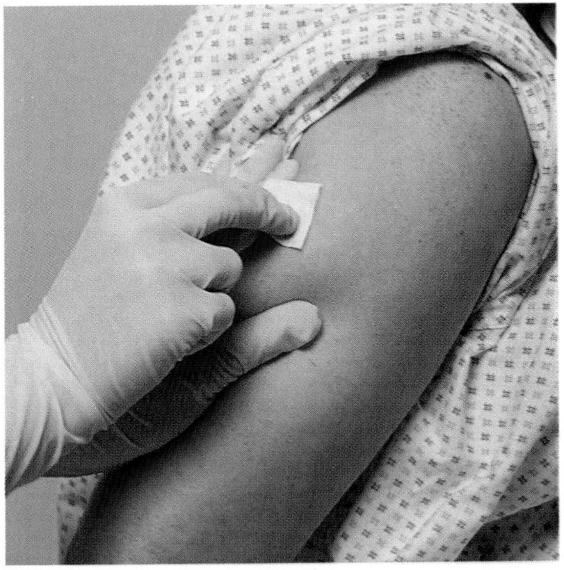

Figure 2 Administering an injection. Cleanse site with antiseptic swab. Apply swab at center of site and rotate outward in circular direction for about 5 cm (2 inches).

A

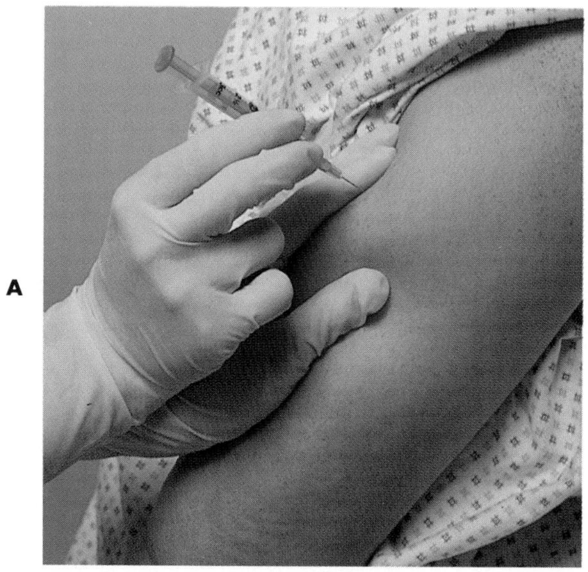

Figure 3 **A,** Hold syringe correctly between thumb and forefinger of dominant hand.

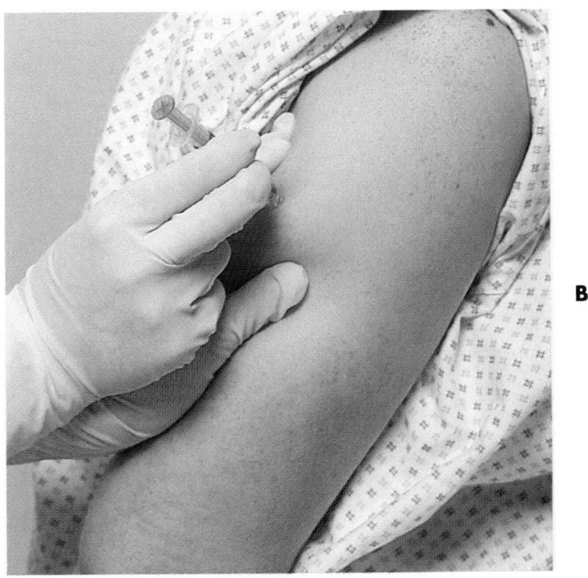

B

Figure 3, cont'd B, Position nondominant hand at proper anatomical landmarks and spread skin tightly. Inject needle quickly at a 90° angle (IM).

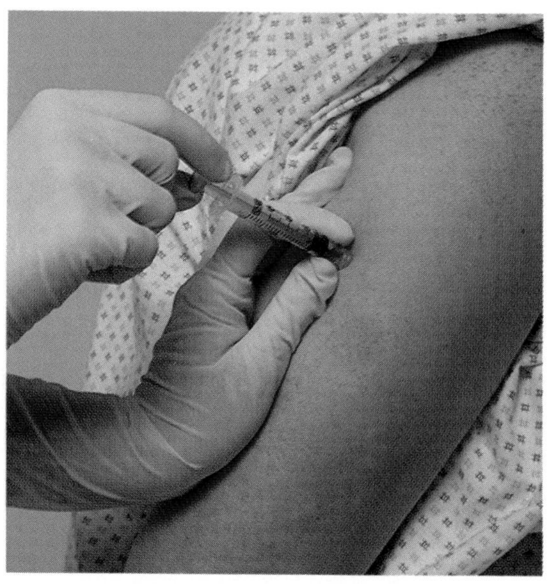

Figure 4 Move dominant hand to end of plunger. Avoid moving syringe while pulling back on plunger (IM).

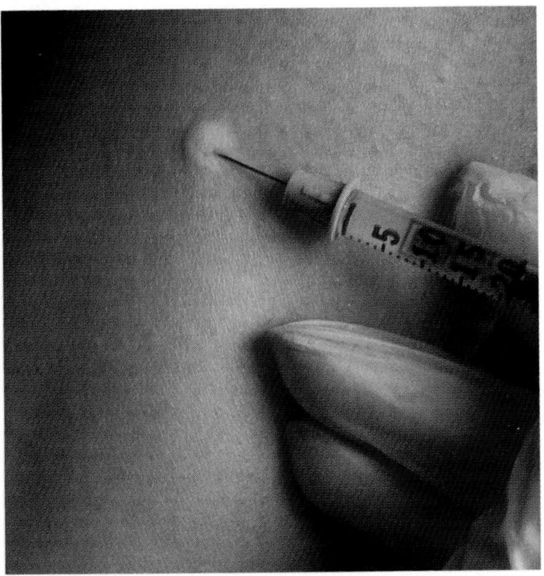

Figure 5 During intradermal injection, note formation of small bleb on the skin's surface.

A

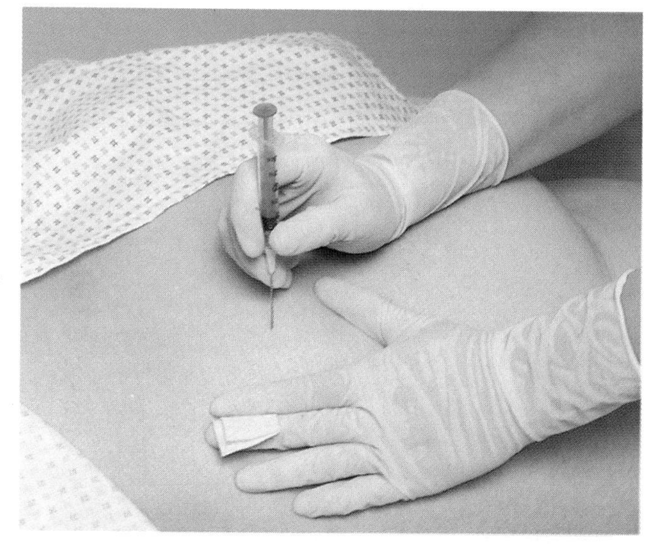

B

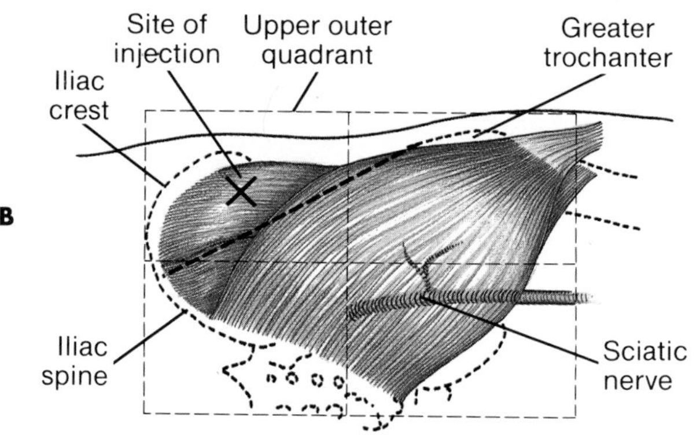

Figure 6 **A,** Site of IM injection into the left dorsogluteal muscle. **B,** Imaginary diagonal line extending from the posterior iliac spine to the greater trochanter is the landmark for selecting the dorsogluteal injection site.

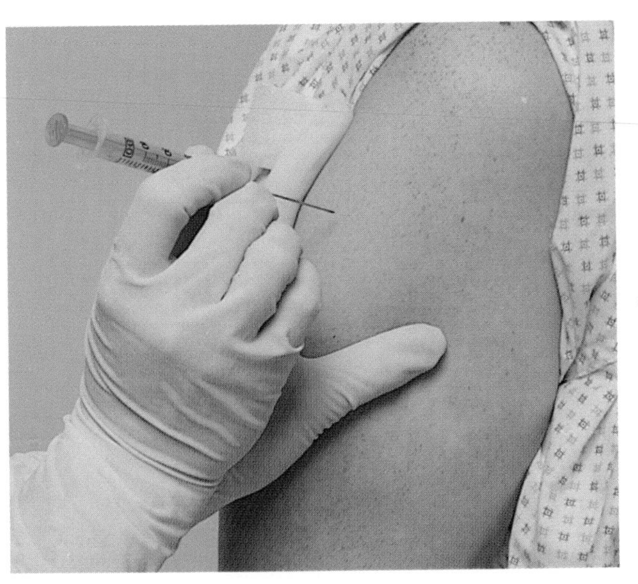

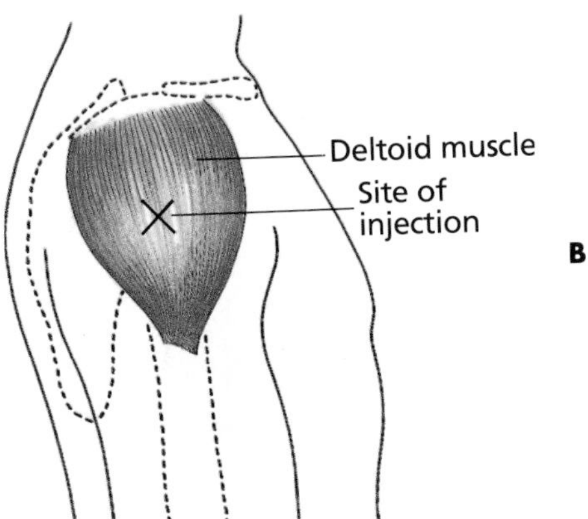

Figure 7 **A,** Site of IM injection into the deltoid muscle. **B,** Site of deltoid muscle injection below acromion process.

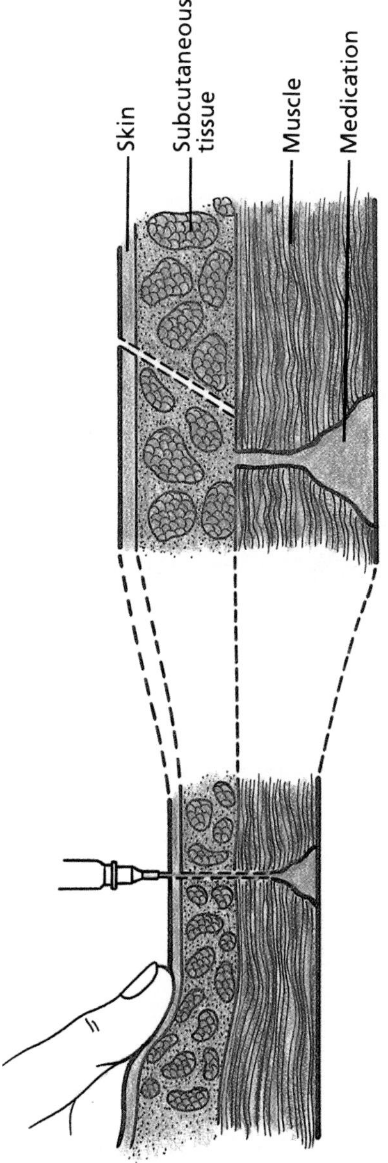

Figure 8 The Z-track method of injection prevents the deposit of medication through sensitive tissues.

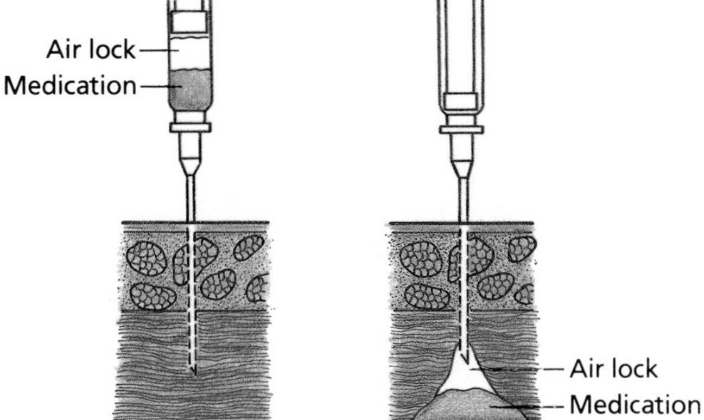

Figure 9 Administering IM injection by the air-lock technique prevents tracking of medication through SQ tissues.

A

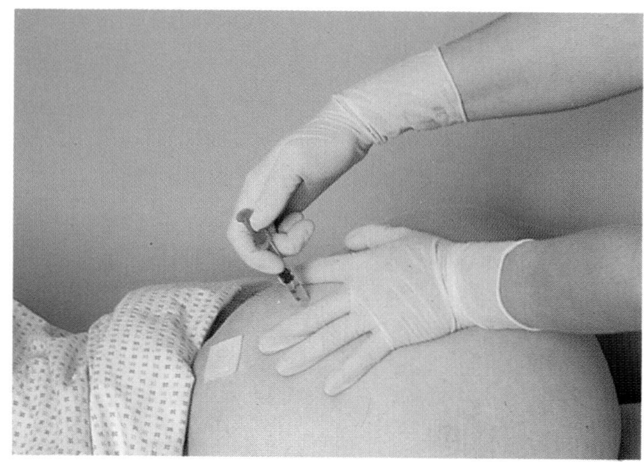

B

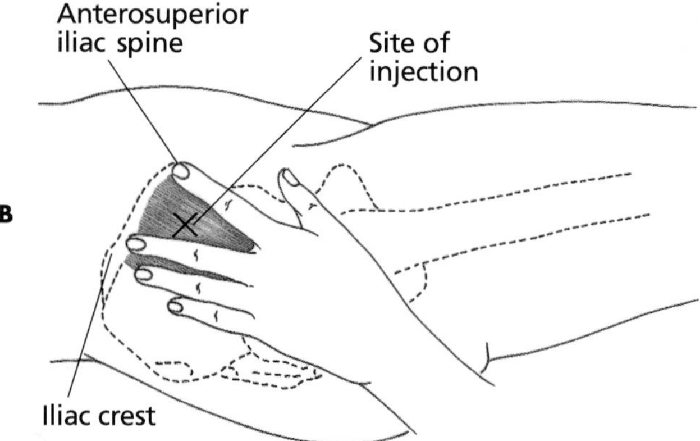

Figure 10 **A,** Injection site into ventrogluteal muscle avoids major nerves and blood vessels. **B,** Anatomical view of ventrogluteal muscle injection site.

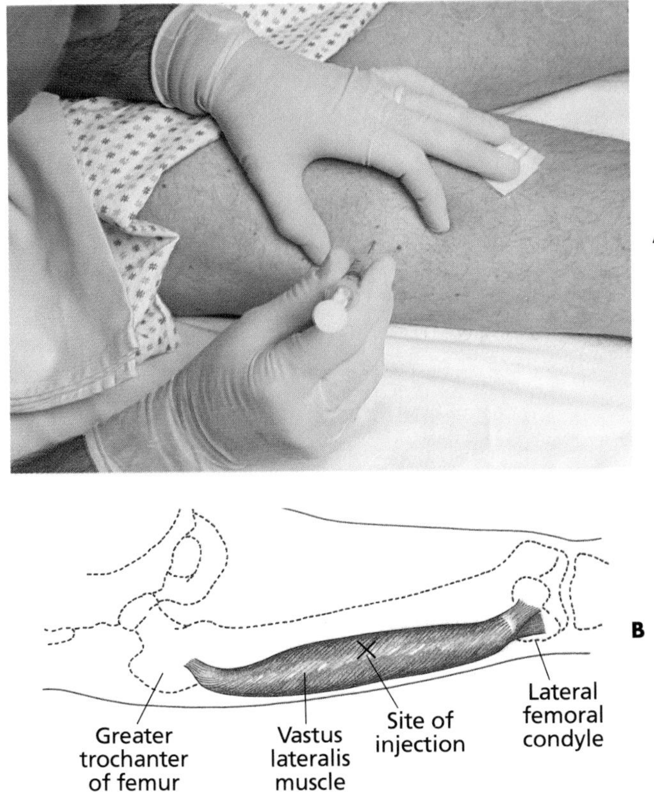

Figure 11 **A,** Injection site into the vastus lateralis muscle. **B,** Anatomical view of the site for IM injection into the vastus lateralis muscle.

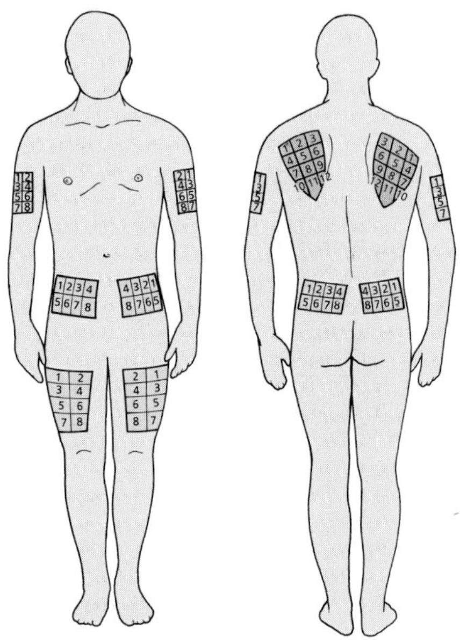

Figure 12 Common sites for SQ injections. Note how sites might be rotated.

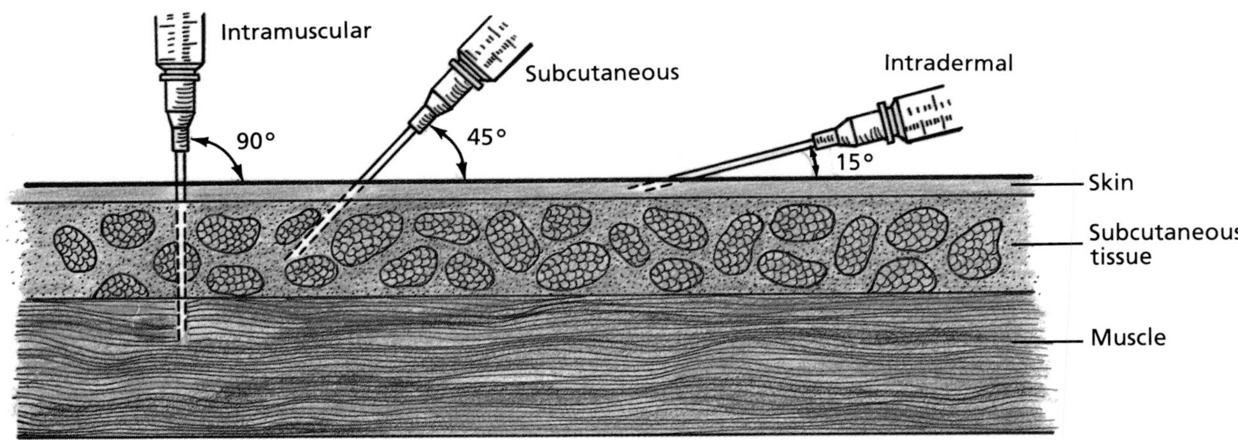

Figure 13 Comparison of the angles of insertion for IM (90°), SQ (45°), and intradermal (15°) injections.

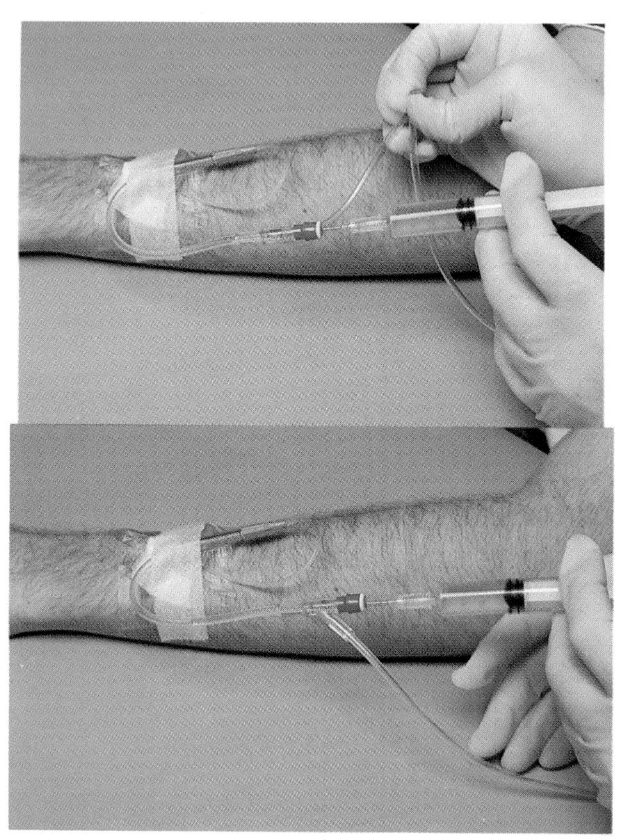
A
B

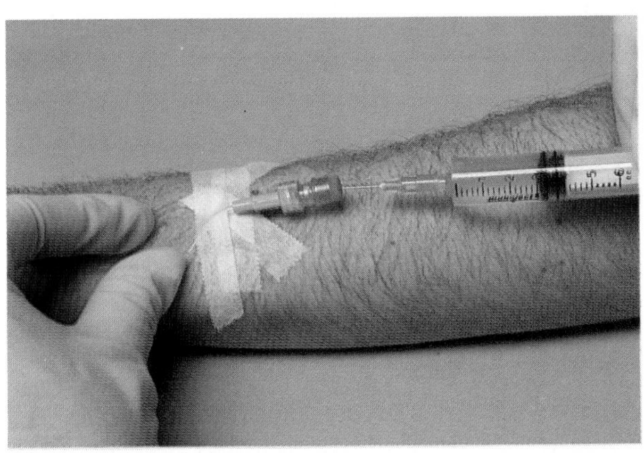

C

Figure 14 **A,** Occlude IV line by pinching tubing just above injection port. **B,** Inject medication slowly after aspirating with no blood return. **C,** Administering medications by IV push. Insert needle of syringe containing prepared drug through center of diaphragm.

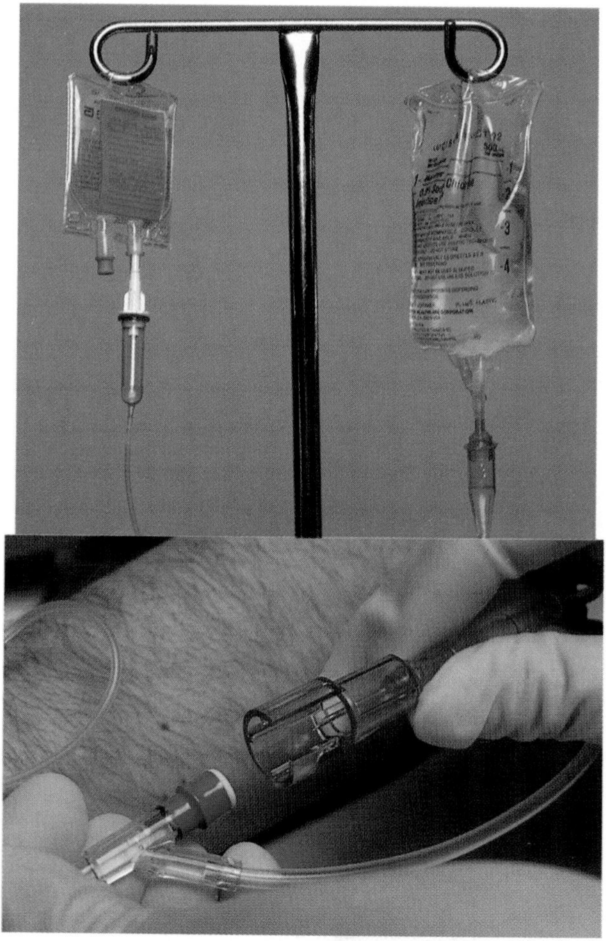

B

Figure 15 Administering IV medication by piggyback or volume administration sets. **A,** Hang medication bag at or above level of main fluid bag. A hook may be used to lower main line. **B,** Connect covered sterile needle of piggyback to injection port of main line.

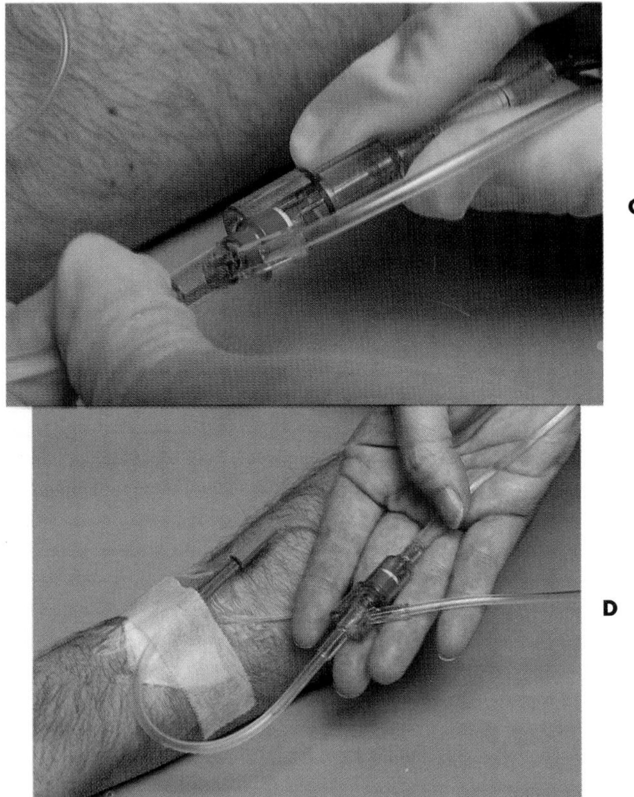

Figure 15, cont'd **C,** Connect covered sterile needle to end of infusion tubing after removing cover. **D,** Use needle-lock device to secure needle of secondary piggyback through injection port of main line.

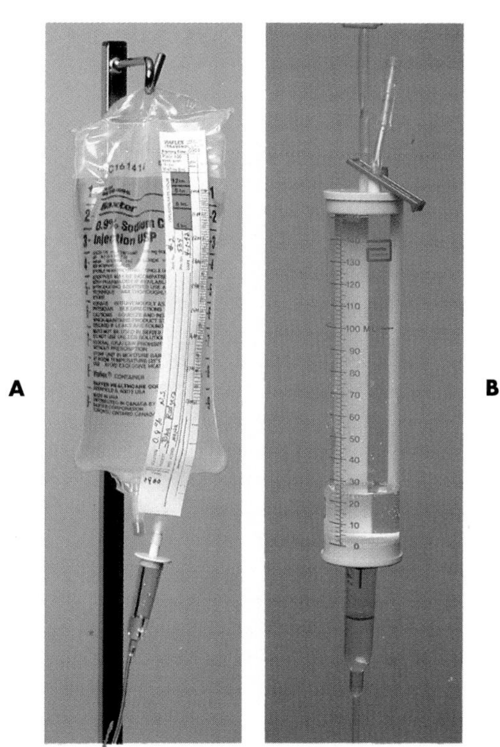

Figure 16 **A,** Regulate IV infusion and check IV periodically. **B,** Fill Volutrol with desired amount of fluid (50 to 100 ml) by opening clamp between Volutrol and main IV bag.

A

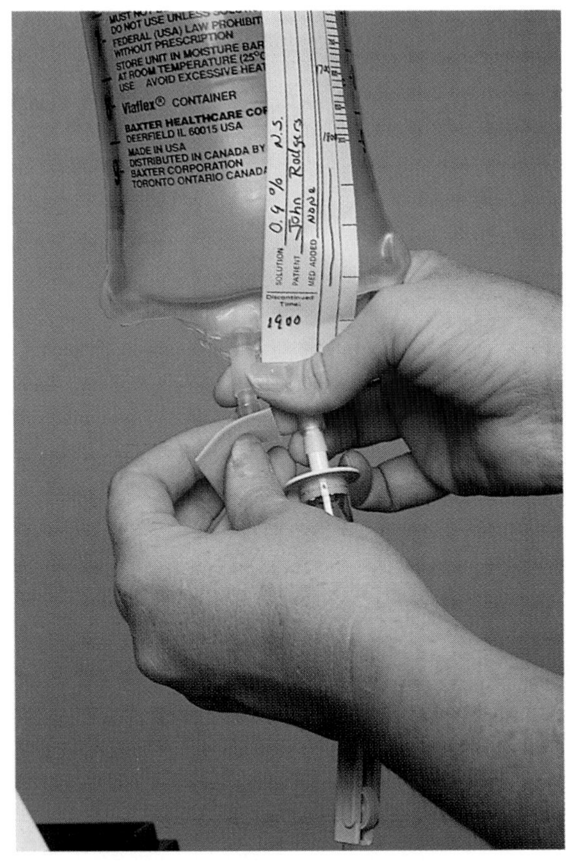

Figure 17 **A,** Wipe medication port with alcohol or antiseptic swab before adding medication to existing container.

Continued.

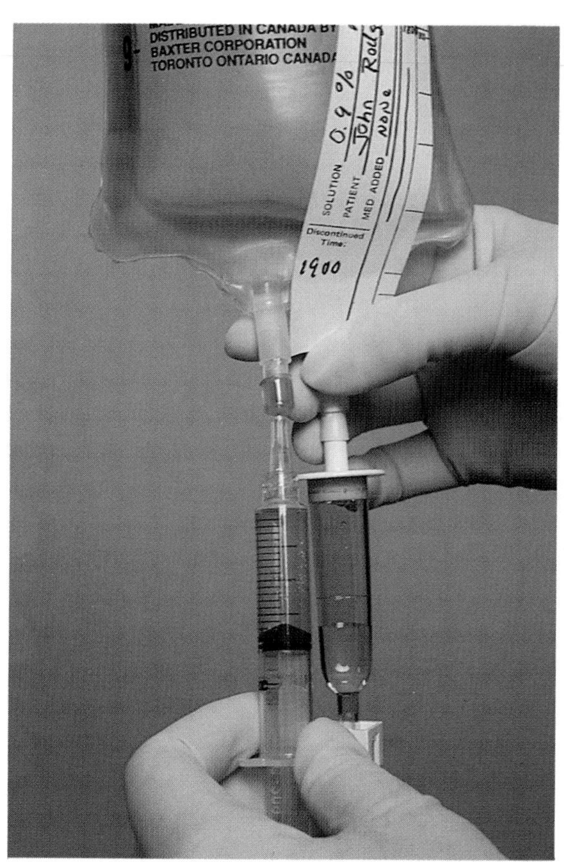

Figure 17, cont'd **B,** Adding medication to IV fluid containers. Remove needle cap from syringe through center of injection port or site and then inject medication.

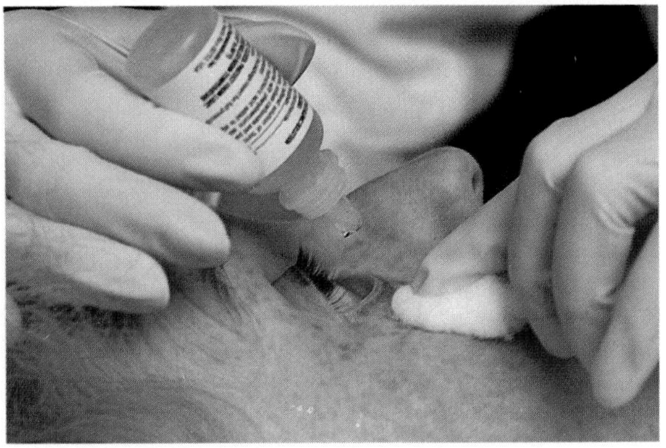

Figure 18 Instilling eye drops. Rest dominant hand on client's forehead; hold eye dropper ½ to ¾ inch above conjunctive sac; drop prescribed medication in conjunctival sac.

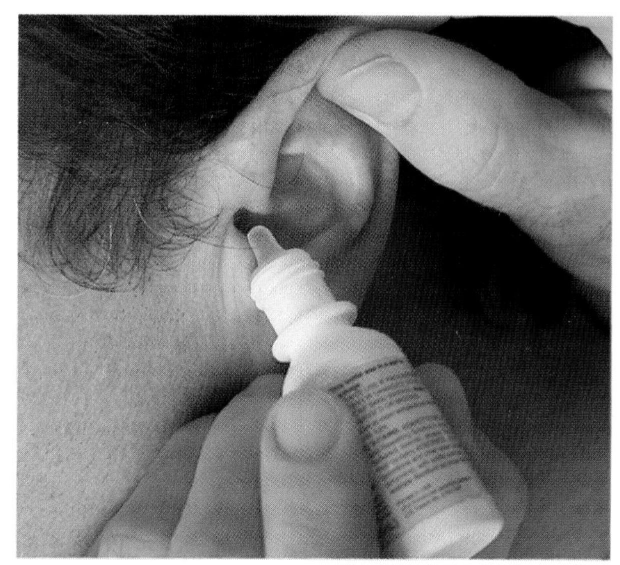

Figure 19 Instilling ear drops. **A,** Straighten ear canal by pulling auricle upward and outward (adult), or down and back (child).

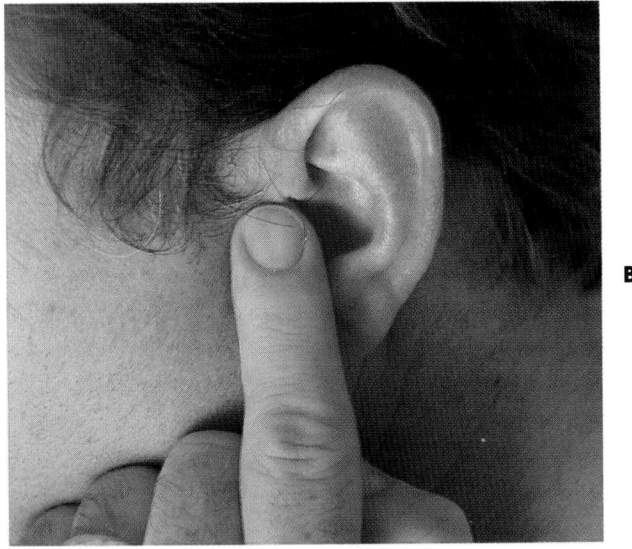

Figure 19, cont'd **B,** Client should remain side-lying for 2 to 3 minutes. Apply gentle pressure to tragus of ear.

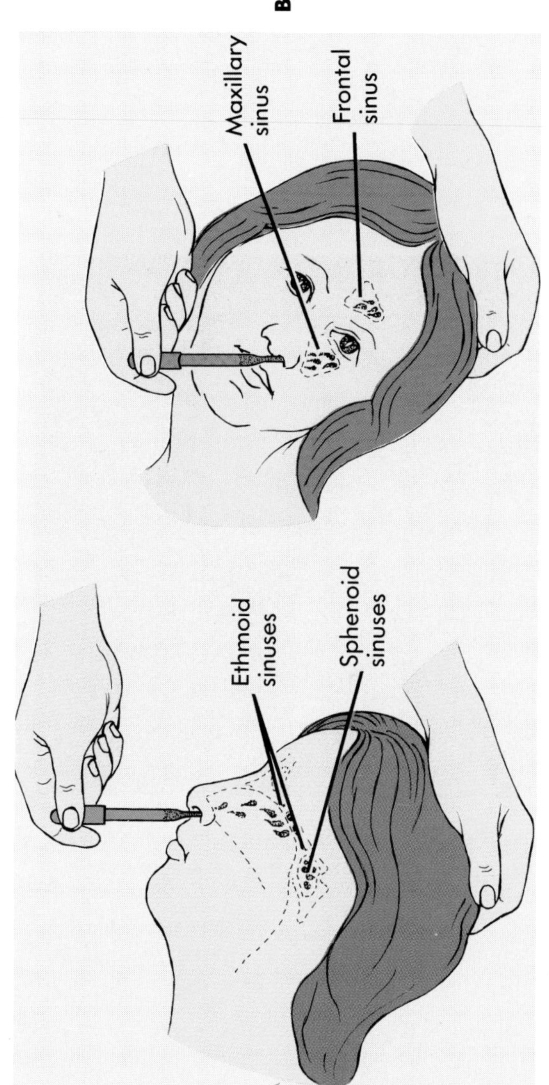

Figure 20 Instilling nose drops. **A,** Hold dropper ½ inch above nares and instill prescribed number of drops toward midline of ethmoid bone. **B,** Turn head to side to be treated and tilt back over edge of bed or pillow.

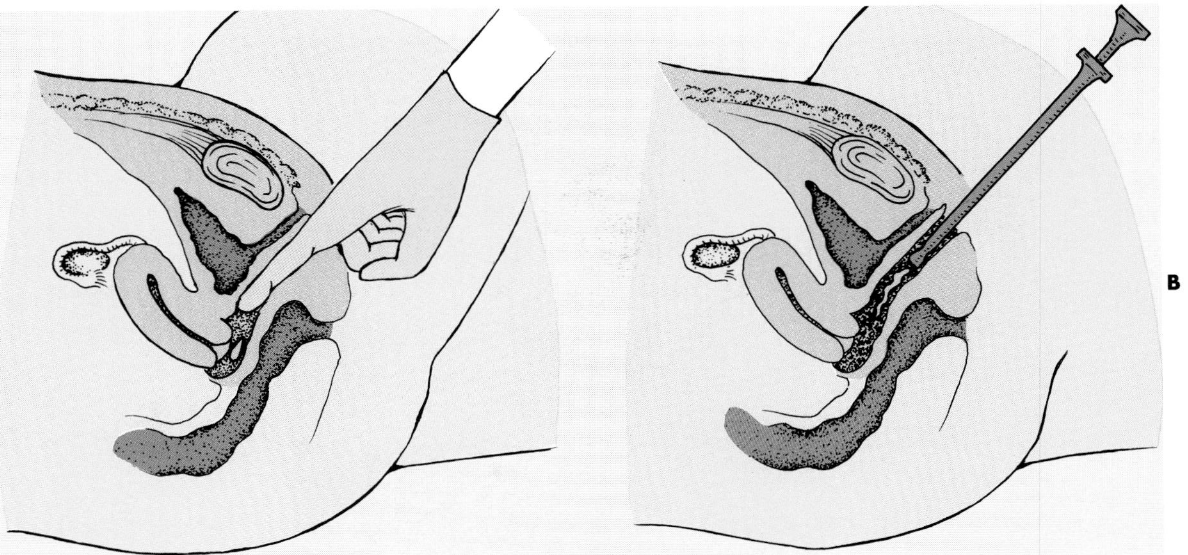

Figure 21. Suppository insertion. **A,** With gloved hand, insert suppository. **B,** With nondominant gloved hand, insert applicator 2 to 3 inches; push plunger to deposit medication.

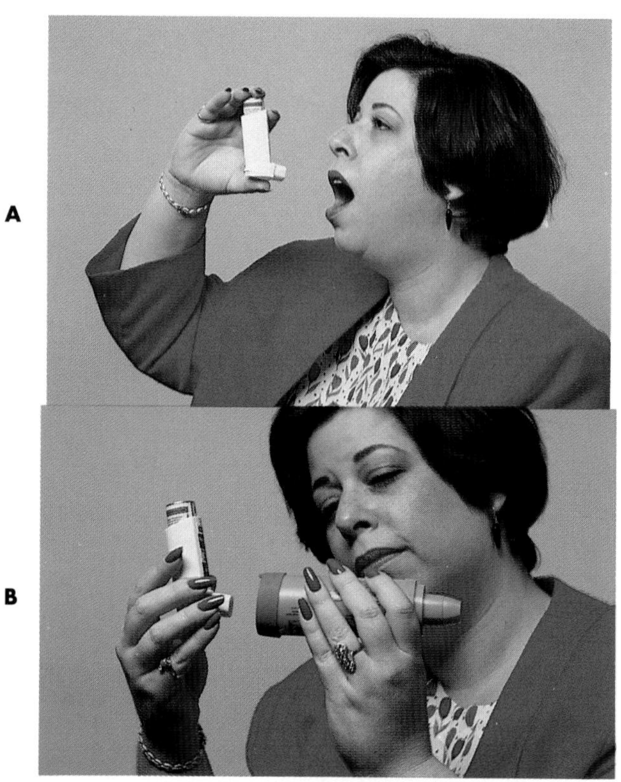

Figure 22 Inhaler use. **A,** Tilt head back and breathe out. **B,** Attach spacer to mouthpiece of inhaler. **C,** Place mouthpiece of inhaler or spacer in mouth. **D,** Press down on inhaler to release one pass of medication while inhaling slowly.

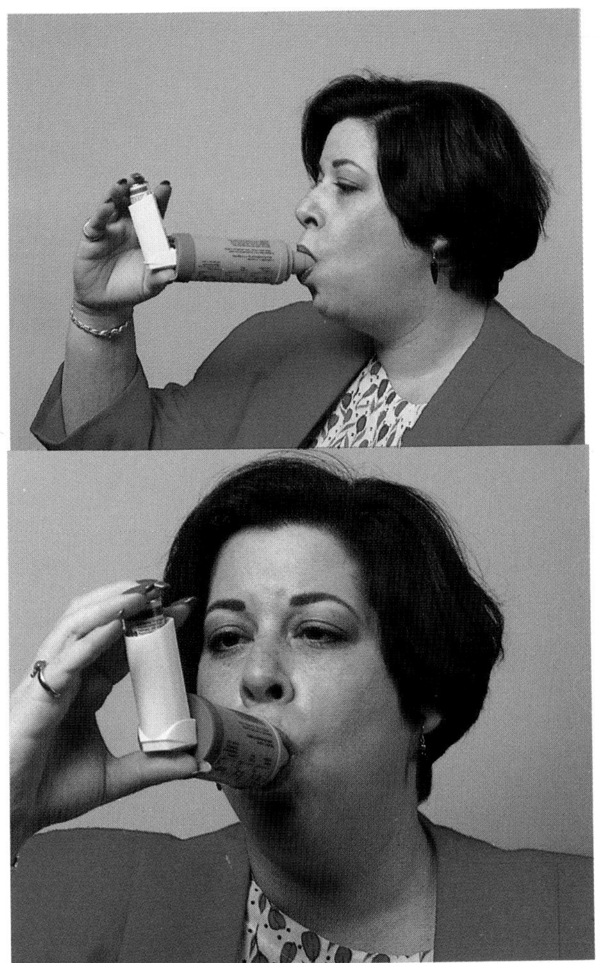

C

D